Handbook of Experimental Pharmacology

Continuation of Handbuch der experimentellen Pharmakologie

Vol. 69

Pharmacology of the Eye

Contributors

G. J. Chader · J. Cunha-Vaz · P. H. Fischer · R. W. Flower
B. R. Friedland · I. Gery · M. O. Hall · M.-H. Heinemann
L. M. Jampol · T. R. Jones · P. L. Kaufman · J. C. Le Douarec
I. H. Leopold · V. J. Lotti · T. H. Maren · K. Masuda
D. M. Maurice · S. Mishima · R. B. Nussenblatt · M. Pandolfi
A. Patz · J. R. Polansky · A. M. Potts · W. H. Prusoff · T. W. Reid
J. R. Robinson · M. Rosenberg · M. L. Sears · D. Seigel · H. Shichi
J. Stjernschantz · C. A. Stone · R. N. Weinreb · T. Wiedman

Editor

M. L. Sears

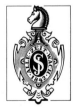

Springer-Verlag Berlin Heidelberg New York Tokyo 1984

Professor Dr. MARVIN L. SEARS
Department of Ophthalmology and Visual Science
School of Medicine
Yale University
333 Cedar Street
New Haven, CT 06510/USA

With 147 Figures

ISBN 3-540-12578-7 Springer-Verlag Berlin Heidelberg New York Tokyo
ISBN 0-387-12578-7 Springer-Verlag New York Heidelberg Berlin Tokyo

© by Springer-Verlag Berlin Heidelberg 1984
Printed in Germany

The use of registered names, trademarks, etc. in this publication does not imply, even in the absence of a specific statement, that such names are exempt from the relevant protective laws and regulations and therefore free for general use.

Product liability: The publisher can give no guarantee for information about drug dosage and application thereof contained in this book. In every individual case the respective user must check its accuracy by consulting other pharmaceutical literature.

Typesetting, printing and bookbinding: Brühlsche Universitätsdruckerei, Giessen
2122/3130-543210

Preface

Roots of the theory and practice of ocular pharmacology may be traced to the ancient Mesopotamian code of Hammurabi and then to several papyri reflecting the clinical interests of the Egyptians. The evolution of its art and science was irregularly paced until the nineteenth century when Kohler, in 1884, proved the anesthetic effect of cocaine on the cornea, and when Fraser, Laquer, Schmiedeberg, Meyer, and others studied the pharmacology of the autonomic nervous system by way of observations of the pupil. Advances in the past few decades have been nothing short of explosive. How can the student, physician, or basic research scientist stay in touch with these electrifying studies? To help with the answer to this question, the authors set as their goal the development of increased understanding so that the student, research scientist, and ophthalmologist can cope with the latest discoveries. The authors want to narrow what appears to be an ever-increasing gap between basic science and ophthalmology. The basic aspects of pharmacology have been presented in light of the natural physiology. In this regard, while distinctions among endogenous mechanisms, drug effects, and the pathogenesis of disease are to be separately recognized, appreciation must be given to the concept that both the desirable and unwanted manifestations or functions caused by either disease or drugs must very often represent a *quantitative* change in normal metabolic pathways. "The most likely way, therefore, to get any insight into the nature of those parts of creation, which come within our observations, must in all reason, be to number, weigh and measure," as Stephen Hales (1677–1761) wrote (*Vegetable Staticks*. Watson, New York 1969). The authors have, wherever possible, in this first effort at a text in ocular pharmacology, attempted to guide themselves by a quantitative approach.

The current text includes reports of articles up to the end of 1982. The authors have not considered treatment of the topic of therapeutics per se. In particular, the drug device and drug delivery areas have not been discussed. Numerous recent references deal with these subjects anyway. This book is not intended to cover clinical ocular pharmacology, but rather to provide a sound foundation on which the use of drugs in ocular therapy can be based. The authors will have considered their goal accomplished if an improved understanding has been provided for the reader and increased pleasure has been given to those particularly interested in pharmacology as applied to the eye.

New Haven   MARVIN L. SEARS

List of Contributors

G. J. CHADER, Laboratory of Vision Research, National Eye Institute, National Institutes of Health, Bldg. 6, Rm. 222, Bethesda, MD 20205/USA

J. CUNHA-VAZ, Department of Ophthalmology, University of Coimbra, Coimbra, Portugal

P. H. FISCHER, Department of Oncology, University of Wisconsin, School of Medicine, Madison, WI 53792/USA

R. W. FLOWER, Applied Physics Laboratory, Johns Hopkins Road, Laurel, MD 20810/USA

B. R. FRIEDLAND, Department of Pharmacology and Therapeutics, University of Florida, College of Medicine, Gainesville, FL 32610/USA

I. GERY, Laboratory of Vision Research, National Eye Institute, National Institutes of Health, Bldg. 6, Rm. 232, Bethesda, MD 20205/USA

M. O. HALL, Jules Stein Eye Institute, UCLA Medical Center, Los Angeles, CA 90024/USA

M.-H. HEINEMANN, Memorial Sloan-Kettering Cancer Center, 1275 York Avenue, New York, NY 10021/USA

L. M. JAMPOL, Sickle Cell Eye Clinic, University of Illinois, Department of Ophthalmology, Medical Center, Hospital Eye and Ear Infirmary, 1855 W. Taylor Street, Chicago, IL 60612/USA

T. R. JONES, Department of Ophthalmology and Visual Science, Yale University, School of Medicine, 333 Cedar Street, New Haven, CT 06510/USA

P. L. KAUFMAN, Department of Ophthalmology, University of Wisconsin, Hospital Clinics, 600 Highland Avenue, Madison, WI 53792/USA

J. C. LEDOUAREC, Searle Research and Development, Sophia Antipolis, B.P. 23, F-06562 Valbonne Cedex

I. H. LEOPOLD, Department of Ophthalmology, University of California, College of Medicine, Irvine, CA 92717/USA

V. J. LOTTI, Merck Sharp and Dohme Research Laboratories, West Point, PA 19486/USA

T. H. MAREN, Department of Pharmacology and Therapeutics, University of Florida, College of Medicine, The J. Hillis Miller Health Center, Gainesville, FL 32610/USA

K. MASUDA, Department of Ophthalmology, School of Medicine, University of Tokyo, 113 Hongo, 7-3-1 Bunkyo-ku, Tokyo, Japan

D. M. MAURICE, Division of Ophthalmology, Department of Surgery, Stanford University, School of Medicine, Stanford, CA 94305/USA

S. MISHIMA, Department of Ophthalmology, School of Medicine, University of Tokyo, 113 Hongo, 7-3-1 Bunkyo-ku, Tokyo, Japan

R. B. NUSSENBLATT, Laboratory of Vision Research, National Eye Institute, National Institutes of Health, Bldg. 6, Room 232, Bethesda, MD 20205/USA

M. PANDOLFI, Department of Ophthalmology, University of Lund, Malmö General Hospital, S-21401 Malmö; King Faisal University, Department of Ophthalmology, Khobar Teaching Hospital, P.O. Box 2208, Al-Khobar, Saudi Arabia

A. PATZ, Retinal Vascular Center, Wilmer Ophthalmological Institute, Johns Hopkins Hospital, 601 North Broadway, Baltimore, MD 21205/USA

J. R. POLANSKY, Department of Ophthalmology, School of Medicine, University of California, Parnassus Avenue, San Francisco, CA 94143/USA

A. M. POTTS, Department of Ophthalmology, School of Medicine, University of Louisville, Kentucky Lions Eye Institute, 301 E. Muhammad Ali Blvd., Louisville, KY 40202/USA

W. H. PRUSOFF, Department of Pharmacology, Yale University, School of Medicine, 333 Cedar Street, New Haven, CT 06510/USA

T. W. REID, Department of Ophthalmology and Visual Science, Yale University, School of Medicine, 333 Cedar Street, New Haven, CT 06510/USA

J. R. ROBINSON, School of Pharmacy, University of Wisconsin, 425 N. Charter Street, Madison, WI 53706/USA

M. ROSENBERG, Department of Ophthalmology, University of Illinois, Medical Center, Hospital Eye and Ear Infirmary, 1855 W. Taylor Street, Chicago, IL 60612/USA

M. L. SEARS, Department of Ophthalmology and Visual Science, School of Medicine, Yale University, 333 Cedar Street, New Haven, CT 06510/USA

D. SEIGEL, Clinical Trials Section, Office of Biometry and Epidemiology, National Eye Institute, National Institutes of Health, Bldg. 31, Room 6A.16, Bethesda, MD 20205/USA

H. SHICHI, Institute of Biological Sciences, Oakland University, Rochester, MI 48063/USA

J. STJERNSCHANTZ, Department of Ophthalmology, School of Medicine, Yale University, 333 Cedar Street, New Haven, CT 06510/USA

C. A. STONE, Merck Sharp and Dohme Research Laboratories, West Point, PA 19486/USA

R. N. WEINREB, Department of Ophthalmology, Glaucoma Service, University of Texas Health Sciences Center at Dallas, 5323 Harry Hines Blvd., Dallas, TX 75235/USA

T. WIEDMAN, School of Pharmacy, University of Wisconsin, 425 N. Charter Street, Madison, WI 53706/USA

Contents

CHAPTER 1

The History of Ophthalmic Therapeutics
M.-H. HEINEMANN. With 7 Figures 1

References 16

CHAPTER 2

Ocular Pharmacokinetics
D. M. MAURICE and S. MISHIMA. With 20 Figures

Abbreviations 19
A. Introduction 20
    I. Objectives 20
    II. Compartments and Barriers 22
    III. Routes of Administration and Penetration 22
        1. Topical Administration 23
        2. Local Injection 24
        3. Systemic Administration 25
    IV. Animal Models and Human Experimentation 25
        1. Animal Models 25
        2. Human Experiments 26
B. Topical Administration 26
    I. Factors Involved in Intraocular Penetration 26
        1. The Tears and Contact with Ocular Surface 26
        2. Corneal Penetration 31
        3. Conjunctiva and Sclera 36
        4. Intraocular Structures 37
        5. Metabolism of Drugs During Intraocular Penetration 39
    II. Compartmental Analysis 41
        1. Compartmentation 41
        2. Two-Compartment Model 43
        3. Tear Patterns 49
        4. Other Compartments 52
        5. Kinetics of Ocular Responses to Drugs 53
        6. Parameter Determination 59
    III. Conclusions and Recommendations 66

C. Local Injections 67
    I. Subconjunctival 67
        1. Regurgitation 67
        2. Depot Dynamics 68
        3. Aqueous Humor Concentration 68
        4. Entry Pathways 70
        5. Vitreous Penetration 71
        6. Retrobulbar Injection 71
    II. Intravitreal Injection 72
        1. Diffusion in Vitreous 72
        2. Loss from the Vitreous Chamber 72
        3. Drug Kinetics 75
        4. Application to Humans 77
D. Systemic Administration 77
    I. Intraocular Drug Penetration 77
        1. Structures Related to Entry from Blood 78
        2. The Blood–Vitreous Barrier 79
        3. Chemical Factors in Drug Penetration 80
        4. Drug Distribution in the Eye 82
    II. Compartmental Analysis 84
        1. Formulation of Aqueous Humor Dynamics 84
        2. One-Compartment Approximation 86
        3. Changes in Aqueous Concentration 88
        4. Kinetics of Intracameral Penetration 89
        5. Penetration into the Vitreous 91
        6. Penetration into the Cornea and Lens 93
    III. Conclusions and Recommendations 95
E. Kinetics in Ocular Disease 96
    I. Inflammation and its Models 96
    II. Effects on Ocular Parameters 97
        1. Permeability 97
        2. Active Transport 98
        3. Vasomotor Effects 99
    III. Effects on Drug Kinetics 99
        1. Topical Application 99
        2. Systemic Penetration 100
        3. Periocular Injection 101
        4. Intravitreal Injection 101
F. Conclusion 101
References 102

CHAPTER 3

Biotransformation and Drug Metabolism. H. SHICHI. With 25 Figures

A. Introduction 117
B. Hepatic Drug-Metabolizing Systems 118

Contents

    I. Microsomal Electron Transport Systems (Phase I Enzymes) . . . 118
       1. Cytochrome P-450 119
       2. NADPH · Cytochrome P-450 Reductase 120
       3. Cytochrome b_5 and NADH · Cytochrome b_5 Reductase 121
   II. Reactions Catalyzed by the Cytochrome P-450 System 121
       1. Oxidative Reactions 121
       2. Reductive Reactions 126
  III. Conjugation Reactions (Phase II Reactions) 127
       1. Glucuronidation 128
       2. Sulfation 129
       3. Acetylation 130
       4. Conjugation with Amino Acids 131
       5. Methylation 132
       6. Conjugation with Glutathione 133
   IV. Induction of Drug-Metabolizing Enzymes 135
C. Ocular Drug Metabolism 138
    I. Aryl Hydrocarbon Hydroxylase Induction in the Eye 138
   II. Tissue Distribution of Drug-Metabolizing Enzymes in the Eye . . 139
  III. Drug Toxicity – An Experimental Approach 141
D. Concluding Remarks 142
References 143

CHAPTER 4

Cholinergics

P. L. KAUFMAN, T. WIEDMAN, and J. R. ROBINSON. With 11 Figures

A. Chemistry Related to Biological Activity 149
    I. Cholinergic Neurotransmission 149
   II. Direct-Acting Agonists 150
       1. Muscarinic Agents 150
       2. Nicotinic Agents 153
  III. Indirect-Acting Agonists: Anticholinesterases 154
       1. Carbamates 154
       2. Organophosphorous Compounds 156
B. Ocular Anatomy/Physiology Relevant to Cholinergic Mechanisms:
   Acute Effects of Cholinergic Drugs 156
    I. Lacrimation 156
   II. Cornea 157
  III. Lens 158
  IV. Pupillary Movement and Accommodation 159
   V. Aqueous Humor Formation, Removal, and Composition;
      Blood–Aqueous Barrier 161
       1. Basic Anatomy and Physiology 161
       2. Acute Effects of Cholinergic Drugs 163

  VI. Retina 168
  VII. Oculorotary and Respiratory Skeletal Muscles 169
C. Longer-Term Effects of Cholinergic Drugs or Altered Cholinergic
  Neurotransmission 170
    I. Cholinergic Sensitivity in Ocular Smooth Muscles 170
      1. Physiologically and Pharmacologically Induced Alterations . . 170
      2. Disease-Induced Alterations 174
      3. Surgically Induced Alterations 175
    II. Cholinergic Toxicity 175
      1. Lens (Cataractogenesis) 175
      2. Iris/Ciliary Muscle/Trabecular Meshwork 178
References 180

CHAPTER 5a

Autonomic Nervous System: Adrenergic Agonists
M. L. SEARS. With 21 Figures

A. Introduction 193
B. Cellular Sites and Mechanism of Adrenergic Action 193
C. Modulation and Interaction of Receptor Types 195
D. Sensitivity 196
E. Stereoisomerism 197
F. Storage, Release, and Degradation 198
    I. Monoamine Oxidase 198
    II. Catechol-O-methyltransferase 199
G. Pharmacokinetics 200
    I. Penetration 200
    II. Distribution and Accumulation 200
    III. Duration 200
    IV. Action of Drugs on Intraocular Pressure 201
H. Tissue Functions 201
    I. Lacrimal Gland 201
    II. Cornea and Lens 202
    III. Iris 203
 J. Blood Flow 205
K. Intraocular Pressure 207
L. Other Interactions 228
    I. Guanyl Cyclase 228
    II. Steroids and Adrenergics 229
    III. Adrenergics and Prostaglandins 229
    IV. Adrenergics and Ocular Pigment 230
M. Retina 231
References 233

CHAPTER 5b

Autonomic Nervous System: Adrenergic Antagonists
V.J. Lotti, J.C. LeDouarec, and C.A. Stone

A. Introduction 249
B. Beta-Adrenergic Antagonists 249
   I. Animal Pharmacology 249
     1. Intraocular Pressure 249
     2. Aqueous Humor Dynamics 257
     3. Interactions with Beta-Adrenergic Receptors in the Eye 258
     4. Mechanisms of Action on Intraocular Pressure 262
     5. Ocular Penetration and Distribution 264
     6. Other Ocular Pharmacology 265
   II. Clinical Pharmacology 267
     1. Intraocular Pressure 267
     2. Aqueous Humor Dynamics 268
     3. Beta-Adrenergic Receptor Blockade in the Eye 268
     4. Mechanisms of Action 269
     5. Ocular Penetration 269
C. Alpha-Adrenergic Antagonists 270
   I. Animal Pharmacology 270
     1. Selective Alpha-Adrenergic Antagonists 270
     2. Alpha- and Beta-Adrenergic Antagonists (Labetalol) 271
   II. Clinical Pharmacology 272
References 272

CHAPTER 6

Carbonic Anhydrase: Pharmacology of Inhibitors and Treatment of Glaucoma
B.R. Friedland and T.H. Maren. With 10 Figures

A. History 279
B. Pharmacology of the Clinically Used Carbonic Anhydrase Inhibitors . 281
C. Physiology of Ocular Carbonic Anhydrase Inhibition 288
   I. Aqueous Humor Dynamics 288
   II. Aqueous Flow 289
   III. Relation to Pressure 289
   IV. Chemical Mechanisms of Flow 290
   V. Relation to Systemic Effects 293
   VI. Pharmacology of the Inhibitors Related to Ocular Effect and
     Enzyme Inhibition 293
D. Clinical Uses of Carbonic Anhydrase Inhibitors 297
   I. Glaucoma 297
   II. Miscellaneous Uses and Effects 298
E. Urolithiasis with Carbonic Anhydrase Inhibitors 299
F. Other Toxic Effects 300
G. Summary 303
References 303

CHAPTER 7

Autacoids and Neuropeptides. J. STJERNSCHANTZ. With 5 Figures

A. Introduction 311
B. Prostaglandins, Prostacyclin, Thromboxane, and Lipoxygenase Products 312
    I. General Background 312
    II. Occurrence and Biosynthesis in the Eye 314
    III. Elimination 315
    IV. Effects in the Eye 316
        1. Blood Flow 316
        2. Blood–Aqueous Barrier and Formation of Aqueous Humor . 317
        3. Intraocular Pressure 321
        4. Outflow of Aqueous Humor 322
        5. Iridial and Ciliary Smooth Muscles 322
        6. Miscellaneous Effects 323
    V. Interaction with the Autonomic and Sensory Nervous Systems
       in the Eye 323
    VI. Pathophysiological Considerations 325
        1. Immediate Response to Injury of the Eye 325
        2. Inflammation of the Eye 327
        3. Other Disorders in the Eye Possibly Involving Prostaglandins . 328
C. Histamine 329
    I. General Background 329
    II. Occurrence and Effects in the Eye 330
    III. Pathophysiological Considerations 331
D. 5-Hydroxytryptamine 332
    I. General Background 332
    II. Occurrence and Effects in the Eye 332
E. Plasma Kinins 334
    I. General Background 334
    II. Effects in the Eye 334
F. The Renin–Angiotensin System 336
    I. General Background 336
    II. Occurrence in the Eye 337
G. Substance P 337
    I. General Background 337
    II. Distribution in the Eye 338
    III. Effects in the Eye 339
        1. Retina 339
        2. Iridial Smooth Muscles 339
        3. Ocular Circulation and Blood–Aqueous Barrier 340
        4. Intraocular Pressure 341
        5. Formation and Outflow of Aqueous Humor 341
H. Enkephalins 342
    I. General Background 342
    II. Occurrence and Effects in the Eye 342
 J. Neurotensin 342

K. Hypothalamic Peptides Regulating the Adenohypophysis 343
    I. Somatostatin 343
    II. Thyrotropin-Releasing Hormone 343
    III. Luteinizing-Hormone-Releasing Hormone 344
L. Peptide Hormones Secreted by the Neurohypophysis 344
    I. General Background 344
    II. Effects of Antidiuretic Hormone in the Eye 344
    III. Effects of Oxytocin in the Eye 346
M. Melanocyte-Stimulating Hormones 346
    I. Effects in the Eye 346
N. Vasoactive Intestinal Polypeptide 347
    I. General Background 347
    II. Localization and Effects in the Eye 347
O. Glucagon 348
P. Gastrin/Cholecystokinin 348
Q. Summary 349
References 350

CHAPTER 8

Vitamin A. G.J. CHADER. With 6 Figures

A. Introduction 367
B. Retinoid Structure 368
C. Retinoid Properties 369
D. Retinoid Identification 370
    I. Spectral Methods 371
    II. Fluorescence Methods 372
    III. Colorimetric Methods 372
    IV. High-Pressure Liquid Chromatography 373
E. Retinoid Metabolism 373
F. Retinoid Uptake 375
G. Retinoid Action 376
    I. The Visual Process 376
    II. Glycoprotein Biosynthesis 379
    III. Hormone-like Action 379
References 380

CHAPTER 9

Anti-Infective Agents. I. H. LEOPOLD

A. Introduction 385
B. Accurate Diagnosis and Drug Choice 385
    I. Mechanisms of Action 385
    II. Penetration and Absorption 390
        1. Protein and Tissue Binding 390
        2. The Blood – Aqueous Barrier 390

  3. Physicochemical Influences 391
  4. Aqueous and Uveoscleral Outflow 391
 III. Limiting Factors 391
  1. Age 391
  2. Renal Disease 392
  3. Liver Disease 392
  4. Enzymes 392
  5. Pregnancy 392
  6. Ocular Damage and Disease 392
 IV. Routes of Administration 393
  1. Topically Applied Antibiotic Drops 398
  2. Continuous Corneal Lavage with Antibiotic Solutions . . . 399
  3. Subconjunctival Injections of Antibiotics 401
  V. Use of Antibiotics in Combination 402
  1. Prevention of Emergence of Drug-Resistant Mutants . . . 402
  2. Treatment of Mixed Infections 402
  3. Initial Treatment of Vision-Threatening Infections 402
  4. Antibiotic Synergism and Antagonism 403
 VI. Adverse Drug Interactions 406
C. Postoperative Intraocular Infections (Endophthalmitis) 409
  I. Incidence 412
 II. Results of Therapy 413
 III. Contributory Factors 413
  1. Sources of Infection in the Surgical Environment 413
  2. Ophthalmic Operative Area 413
  3. Influence of Host Tissue 414
  4. Organisms Responsible for Intraocular Infection 414
 IV. Antibiotic Prophylaxis 415
  V. Use of Steroids 416
 VI. Vitrectomy 416
D. Antibiotics 417
  I. Penicillin Derivatives 417
  1. Ampicillin 418
  2. Amoxicillin 418
  3. Carbenicillin 418
  4. Ticarcillin 419
 II. Probenecid 420
 III. Cephalosporins 420
 IV. Aminoglycosides 423
  1. Streptomycin and Dihydrostreptomycin 423
  2. Gentamicin 424
  3. Tobramycin 424
  4. Neomycin 425
  5. Kanamycin 426
  6. Amikacin 426
  7. Spectinomycin 427
  8. Others 427

V. Erythromycin 427
VI. Lincomycin 428
VII. Clindamycin 429
VIII. Oleandomycin 429
IX. Carbomycin 429
X. Spiramycin 430
XI. Novobiocin 430
XII. Ristocetin 430
XIII. Vancomycin 430
XIV. Bacitracin 431
XV. Polymyxin B 431
XVI. Soframycin 432
XVII. Colistin 432
XVIII. Sulfonamides 433
XIX. Trimethoprim-Sulfamethoxazole 434
XX. Chloramphenicol 434
    1. Penetration and Absorption 435
    2. Toxicity and Side Effects 435
XXI. Tetracyclines 437
    1. Penetration and Absorption 437
    2. Fluorescence 438
    3. Toxicity and Side Effects 439
XXII. Pyrimethamine 439
    1. Value 440
    2. Toxicity 440
    3. Penetration and Dosage 441
XXIII. Drugs Used in the Treatment of Fungal Infections 441
    1. Griseofulvin, Nystatin, and Amphotericin B 441
    2. 5-Fluorocytosine 443
    3. Imidazoles 443
XXIV. Diethylcarbamazine in the Treatment of Onchocerciasis 444
References 446

CHAPTER 10a

Anti-Inflammatory Agents: Steroids as Anti-Inflammatory Agents
J.R. POLANSKY and R.N. WEINREB. With 18 Figures

A. Introduction 459
B. Historical Development 459
    I. Cortisone 459
    II. Use of Steroids in Ophthalmology 461
C. Steroid Therapy 466
    I. Activity of Steroid Compounds 466
        1. Potency 466
        2. Absorption and Distribution 470
        3. Metabolism 473

II. Routes of Administration 475
    1. Topical 475
    2. Periocular 480
    3. Systemic 482
    4. Intravitreal 484
III. Therapeutic Approaches 485
    1. Specific Clinical Problems and Controversies 485
    2. Current Assessment 490
IV. Complications 490
    1. Glaucoma 491
    2. Cataract 500
    3. Other Ocular Effects 502
    4. Systemic Complications 503
D. Cellular and Molecular Mechanisms 505
    I. The Immune System 505
        1. Leukocyte Kinetics and Function 506
        2. Vascular and Inflammatory Effects 512
        3. Ocular Immune Mechanisms 514
    II. The Glucocorticoid Receptor 514
        1. The Target Cell 515
        2. Cellular Sensitivity and Modulation of Steroid Responses . . . 517
        3. Permissive Effects and Hormonal Interactions 520
        4. Glucocorticoid Receptors in Ocular Tissues 521
        5. Implications 523
References 524

CHAPTER 10b

Anti-Inflammatory Agents: Nonsteroidal Anti-Inflammatory Drugs
K. MASUDA. With 4 Figures

A. Introduction 539
B. Mechanism of Action of Nonsteroidal Anti-Inflammatory Drugs . . . 539
C. Salicylates 542
D. Indomethacin 543
E. Pyrazolon Derivatives 545
F. Propionic Acid Derivatives 546
G. Anthranilic Acid Derivatives 548
References 548

CHAPTER 11

Chemotherapy of Ocular Viral Infections and Tumors
P. H. FISCHER and W. H. PRUSOFF. With 6 Figures

A. Introduction 553
B. Clinically Available Antiviral Agents 554
    I. 5-Iodo-2′-deoxyuridine (Idoxuridine) 554

1. Synthesis 554
2. Antiviral Activity 555
3. Effects on Normal Cells 555
4. Mechanism of Action 556
II. 9-β-D-Arabinofuranosyladenine (Adenine, Arabinoside, Vidarabine) 557
1. Synthesis 557
2. Antiviral Activity 558
3. Effects on Normal Cells 558
4. Mechanism of Action 559
III. 5-Trifluoromethyl-2'-deoxyuridine (Trifluorothymidine, Viroptic,
Trifluridine) 559
1. Synthesis 559
2. Antiviral Activity 559
3. Effects on Normal Cells 560
4. Mechanism of Action 560
C. Newer Agents Under Development 561
I. 9-(2-Hydroxyethoxymethyl)guanine (Acyclovir, Acycloguanosine) . 561
1. Synthesis 561
2. Antiviral Activity 561
3. Effects on Normal Cells 563
4. Mechanism of Action 563
II. 5-Ethyl-2'-deoxyuridine (Aedurid) 564
1. Synthesis 564
2. Antiviral Activity 564
3. Effects on Normal Cells 565
4. Mechanism of Action 565
III. E-5-(2-Bromovinyl)-2'-deoxyuridine 565
IV. 1-(2-Deoxy-2-fluoro-β-D-arabinosyl)-5-iodo-cytosine 566
V. 5-Iodo-5'-amino-2',5'-dideoxyuridine 566
1. Synthesis 566
2. Antiviral Activity 567
3. Effects on Normal Cells 567
4. Mechanism of Action 567
VI. Phosphonoacetate and Phosphonoformate (Foscarnet) 568
1. Synthesis 568
2. Antiviral Activity 569
3. Effects on Normal Cells 569
4. Mechanism of Action 570
References 570

CHAPTER 12

Immunosuppressive Drugs
I. GERY and R. B. NUSSENBLATT. With 8 Figures

A. Introduction 585
B. Alkylating Agents 587

I. Chemical Structure and Metabolism 588
II. Mode of Action 589
III. Effects on the Immune System 589
C. Antimetabolic Drugs 590
I. Purine Analogs 590
1. Mode of Action 591
2. Effects on the Immune System 591
II. Pyrimidine Analogs 592
1. Mode of Action 593
2. Effects on the Immune System 593
III. Folic Acid Analogs 593
1. Mode of Action 593
2. Effects on the Immune System 594
D. Cyclosporin A 594
I. Mode of Action 595
II. Effects on the Immune System 596
E. Antilymphocyte Sera 597
I. Preparations 597
II. Mode of Action 597
III. Effects on the Immune System 598
IV. Adverse Side Effects 598
F. Ionizing Irradiation 599
G. Immunosuppressive Agents of Potential Future Use 599
H. Immunosuppressive Agents in Ocular Conditions 599
I. Cyclophosphamide 600
II. Chlorambucil 600
III. Azathioprine 600
IV. Methotrexate 601
V. Cyclosporin A 601
VI. Antilymphocyte Sera 601
VII. Adverse Side Effects 601
References 602

CHAPTER 13

Anticoagulants, Fibrinolytics, and Hemostatics
M. PANDOLFI. With 3 Figures

A. Introduction: The Hemostatic Mechanism 611
B. Anticoagulants 614
I. Direct Anticoagulants (Heparin) 614
II. Indirect Anticoagulants 615
III. Contraindications: Precautions in Ophthalmology 616
C. Fibrinolytics 617
I. Commonly Used Fibrinolytic Agents 617
1. Streptokinase 617
2. Urokinase 617
3. Plasmin 618

    II. Therapeutic Thrombolysis: Effect on Hemostasis 618
   III. Fibrinolytics in Ophthalmology 619
       1. Occlusion of the Central Retinal Vein 619
       2. Hemorrhages in the Anterior Chamber and Vitreous Body . 620
D. Hemostatics 621
    I. Specific 622
       1. Substitution Therapy 622
       2. Antifibrinolytics 623
   II. Nonspecific 625
References 625

CHAPTER 14

Oxygen. R. W. FLOWER, M. O. HALL, and A. PATZ

A. Introduction 627
B. Oxygen and the Adult Eye 627
C. Oxygen and the Immature Eye 630
    I. Retrolental Fibroplasia 630
   II. Monitoring Oxygen Administration in the Nursery 632
D. Oxygen Interaction with Other Drugs 633
    I. Anti-Inflammatory Agents 633
   II. Antioxidants in Retrolental Fibroplasia 633
       1. α-Tocopherol 633
       2. Superoxide Dismutase 634
       3. Other Antioxidants 636
E. Conclusions 636
References 636

CHAPTER 15

The Alipathic Alcohols. A. M. POTTS

A. General 639
B. Ocular Effects of Single Doses of Ethanol in Nonhabituated Individuals 640
    I. Muscle Balance 640
   II. Extraocular Muscles in Action 640
  III. Nystagmus 642
  IV. Intraocular Muscles 643
       1. The Iris 643
       2. Accommodation 643
   V. Electrophysiological Measurements 643
  VI. Miscellaneous Measurements of Visual Function 645
 VII. Intraocular Pressure 646
C. The Special Case of Disulfiram (Antabuse) 646
D. Chronic Alcoholism and the Eye 646
E. Methanol 647
References 649

CHAPTER 16

Photosensitizing Substances. A. M. Potts. With 1 Figure

A. Direct Action of Ultraviolet Light on Skin 655
  I. Mechanism of Ultraviolet Action 655
  II. Direct Action of Light on the Eye 656
B. Photosensitization 657
  I. Mechanism 658
  II. Ocular Effects 659
C. Photosensitizing Substances 660
  I. Exogenous Photosensitizers 660
  II. Endogenous Photosensitizers 662
D. Conclusions 665
References 665

CHAPTER 17

Trace Elements in the Eye. T. R. Jones and T. W. Reid. With 1 Figure

A. Introduction 667
B. Iron 670
C. Zinc 672
D. Copper 674
E. Selenium 676
F. Vanadium 678
G. Chromium 679
H. Conclusion 680
References 681

CHAPTER 18

Clinical Trials. D. Seigel

A. A Strategy of Research 687
B. Planning the Trial 688
  I. Defining the Research Goals 688
  II. Sample Size 689
  III. The Ethical Basis 689
C. Conducting the Trial 690
  I. Bias 690
  II. Data Monitoring 691
  III. Follow-up 691
D. Analysis of the Results 692
  I. Adherence 692
  II. Eyes Come in Twos 693
  III. Variable Duration of Follow-up 694
  IV. Tests of Significance and Data Analysis 695
E. A Greater Awareness 696
References 697

CHAPTER 19a

Diagnostic Agents in Ophthalmology: Sodium Fluorescein and Other Dyes
L. M. JAMPOL and J. CUNHA-VAZ. With 1 Figure

A. Sodium Fluorescein. 699
    I. Introduction 699
    II. Defects of the Corneal and Conjunctival Epithelia 700
    III. Use for Applanation Tonometry 701
    IV. Fitting of Contact Lenses 701
    V. Assessment of the Lacrimal System 702
    VI. The Seidel Test – Documentation of Appearance of Aqueous
        Humor in the Cul-de-Sac 703
    VII. Measurement of the Rate of Aqueous Humor Formation. . . . 704
    VIII. Measurement of Arm – Retina Circulation Times and Retinal
        Transit Times 704
    IX. Fundus and Iris Fluorescein Angiography 705
    X. Assessment of the Blood – Ocular Barriers 707
        1. Aqueous Fluorophotometry 708
        2. Vitreous Fluorophotometry 708
        3. Histopathology 709
B. Rose Bengal. 710
C. Indocyanine Green 710
D. Other Dyes for Retinal and Choroidal Angiography 711
E. Other Dyes for Vital Staining of the Conjunctiva and Cornea 711
References 712

CHAPTER 19b

Diagnostic Agents in Ophthalmology: Drugs and the Pupil
M. ROSENBERG and L. M. JAMPOL

A. Introduction 715
B. The Sympathetic Nervous System 715
    I. Epinephrine 716
    II. Cocaine. 717
    III. Hydroxyamphetamine 717
C. The Parasympathetic Nervous System 718
D. Distinction Between Pharmacologic Blockade and Oculomotor Nerve
    Palsy 719
E. Diagnosis of Accommodative Esotropia 720
References 720

Subject Index 721

CHAPTER 1

The History of Ophthalmic Therapeutics

M.-H. Heinemann

The complex course which characterizes the development of medical thought is, above all, a manifestation of the individual and collective diversity of human beings and the diseases which afflict them. The history of ocular therapeutics is no exception. The use of medical therapeutics in the treatment of eye diseases is as old as medicine itself, and its history is an interesting one, documented well into antiquity and generously supplied with engaging personalities and dramatic events. In its study one quickly uncovers an innate charm due largely to the spiritual kinship between the modern physician and his professional forebears. The more this kinship is reinforced, the more solid will be the foundations of modern medical thought and the more productive its continued development.

In general terms, the history of ocular therapeutics is characterized by a laborious evolutionary process in which mysticism slowly gave way to empiricism and rationalism. To reach its present position – on a solid basis of objective reasoning and sound experimentation – ocular therapeusis has progressed inexorably but by a circuitous path, periods of relative social and intellectual enlightenment having alternated with periods of cultural and scientific retrenchment. Ophthalmology was more deeply rooted in mysticism than other medical specialties, largely because of the immeasurable importance of the eye as the preeminent sense organ. As perceived by primitive man, sight was the most precious gift, blindness the most horrific affliction. The absence of any fundamental understanding of the structure and function of the eye, knowledge which would only truly begin to manifest itself in the Renaissance after the decline of Dogma and Scholasticism, served to reinforce the supernatural aura surrounding the eye, and thus hindered a rational approach to the treatment of disease. This gradually changed as the social and cultural attitudes influencing ophthalmology as a science and clinical specialty came to be generated by a quest for knowledge rather than by awe and fear.

In searching for a starting point for an overview of the history of ocular pharmacology, one is inevitably drawn to the Old and Middle Kingdoms of ancient Egypt. Egyptian medical culture, which spanned several millennia, was itself strongly influenced by Nubian and Central African cultures to the south and Sumerian and Oriental influences to the east, and there are certainly references to ocular therapeusis that predate Egyptian records, most notably in the Mesopotamian Code of Hammurabi (ca. 1,950 B.C.) (GHALIOUNGUI 1963). But in Egypt the fusion of anatomic study and applied therapeutics was carefully incorporated into a highly organized social system. Although deeply rooted in mysticism, pharaonic medicine at its peak developed to a point where a certain degree of empiricism could coexist with the rites and incantations which formed the cornerstone of

Egyptian culture. As a result, priests became medical specialists, temples were centers of clinical medicine, and the materia medica grew ever more expansive.

Ocular disease was of particular interest to the Egyptians, largely because of the ravages of trachoma and other external diseases. Oculists were, therefore, particularly valuable to society and held a special place among the ever-expanding group of medical specialists. They were the wards of the god Thoth, the ibis-headed deity of wisdom and knowledge, who had magically restored the sight of Horus, a healing god who had been blinded by Seth, the god of plague. Our ties to Egyptian mythology are not too remote, as a symbolic representation of the eye of Horus adorns most prescriptions and is the unquestioned symbol of medical therapeutics. The Egyptians believed that the eye and visual process were manifestations of divine ominipotence, and the priests of the cults of Douaou and Horus became powerful and famous as a result of their expertise in the treatment of eye disease (HELBLING 1980). Most of our knowledge of Egyptian medicine is derived from the nine principal medical papyri, of which the Ebers Papyrus (ca. 1,550 B.C.), acquired in Thebes in 1862, and the Edwin Smith Papyrus (ca. 1,600 B.C.), obtained in 1872, are the best known. The Edwin Smith Papyrus clearly demonstrates that the prevailing medical practice was clinical in its orientation and based upon bedside observation and a rudimentary understanding of anatomy and physiology. The Egyptians, however, did not fully capitalize on their anatomic interests, as most eyes of the deceased were placed, undissected, in canopic jars.

The Ebers Papyrus, an amalgam of medical sources compiled during the reign of Amenophis I, is the longest and most expansive papyrus, and contains a richly detailed materia medica. Nine pages of the papyrus are devoted to ocular diseases and their treatment. External diseases, particularly the stigmata of trachoma, such as cicatricial entropion, trichiasis, and corneal leukomata, appear to have been particularly nettlesome (BRYAN 1931). Included are drugs with undeniable pharmacologic activity, such as copper salts, calcium carbonate, sulfur, hyoscyamus, and recinus reeds. Copper carbonate was used cosmetically around the eyes and legend has it that was Imhotep (2,800 B.C.), who was the greatest of Egyptian physicians and was eventually deified, was the first to discover the beneficial properties of malachite in the treatment of trachoma. His wife had been stricken with the disease and he sought divine intervention, which came in the form of a vision directing him to prepare a poultice of animal excrement on the copper plate his wife used for her makeup. The poultice reacted with the malachite and Imhotep's wife was cured by the treatment. Other medications cited in the Ebers Papyrus were used in rituals of transfer to cure blindness; the application of porcine vitreous humor was thought to be effective in this way. Other agents were used for their noxious effect, presumably to ward off evil spirits, as in the case of the use of fish bile to reverse corneal leukomata. In all, the Ebers Papyrus contains well over 100 prescriptions for the treatment of ophthalmic disease, including some that to the modern physician may seem uncannily prescient, such as the treatment of nyctalopia by applications of bovine liver (GHALIOUNGUI 1963). Medications were often to be administered intraocularly as well as topically, and practitioners were instructed how to fashion hollow reeds or, more dramatically, vulture feathers into needles for this purpose.

In the final analysis, the absence of sound scientific thinking meant that the use of medicinal plants and chemicals by the Egyptians was based more often on legend and ritual than upon observation and experimentation; however, this did not in any way diminish the profound effect of these works on later influential writers such as Dioscorides (40–90 A.D.) and Georg Bartisch (1535–1606). Furthermore, central to the primitive materia medica was the belief that therapeutic substances were identified by a signature or external characteristic which signified their medical properties, as in the use of applications of goose grease in the treatment of xanthelasma.

It is important to note that the extant medical papyri were essentially compilations of practical remedies written for the benefit of practitioners, and did not belong to the official texts, such as the *Hermetic Books of Thoth*, which contained the closely guarded knowledge that formed the basis for medical and religous teaching. Partly as a result of the increasing centralization of knowledge, the spirit of rationality that characterizes the most valuable parts of the medical papyri was lost as medical practice and teaching became more strictly ritualized.

The heirs to the Egyptian medical tradition were the physicians of preclassical Greece. The degree to which the Greeks were influenced is evident in the writings of Aristotle, especially in the *Politics*, and in the works of the historian Herodotus, who studied the Egyptian medical system in depth. The cultural diversity of the Greek people, as well as the geographic constraints of their homeland, prompted the Greeks to establish networks of communication with the world around them, particularly Egypt, Mesopotamia, and Phoenicia. As a result, Greece began to benefit from the rich cultural diversity that flowed to its shores. The medicine of preclassical, Homeric Greece (ca. 1,000 B.C.) was the domain of cults worshiping the healing god Aesculapius. As with the Egyptians, the focal point of medical activity was the temple, which in addition to being a religous center also served as hospital and medical school. Medicine in this salubrious atmosphere was, however, little advanced from that which had preceded it. Patients who congregated at Epidaurus and other temples often had to depend upon therapeutic dreams and votive offerings for their cures. The turning point occurred on the island of Cos with the birth of Hippocrates in 460 B.C. Hippocrates was to become the guiding influence of medicine, displacing the myriad gods and spirits from their positions of importance. The environment of Athens during its Golden Age was a catalyst for the expression of new ideas, and art, natural science, and philosophy combined as never before. As a result, despite the encumbrance of the Pythagorean concept of the fundamental humors, Ionian medicine was able to develop in such a way that the prevailing medical knowledge could be synthesized into a scientific system and, more importantly, the physician could use his reason and clinical skills to best advantage. The technical standards established during the Ionian school were the direct result of the transition of medical thought from the constraints of ritual to the freedom of philosophic self-expression. The physician-priest had become the physician-philosopher, and had become part of a system in which medical knowledge could not only be accumulated but also passed on effectively. Science was recognized for what it was, an implicit quest for truth, and medicine became a science truly based upon clinical observation.

From a practical standpoint, however, ophthalmic therapeutics would remain mired so long as the basic pathophysiological processes of the eye remained unknown. The hippocratic system of therapeutics was based upon the premise of assisting *physis*, the body's innate ability to heal itself. In this way treatment was individualized, and as a result, careful clinical observation was encouraged. Disease was thought to be the result of imbalances in the fundamental humors, and just as these imbalances were thought to be highly variable, so was the patient's response. The morbid state of humoral imbalance manifested itself as fever or inflammation, the state of *pepsis*. Recovery depended either upon the removal of the offending humors by surgical means – venesection or the like – or by excretion (MAGNUS 1901). The *Corpus Hippocraticum*, compiled in Alexandria by the Pharaon Ptolemy Sloter (323–285 B.C.), contains hundreds of therapeutic remedies for the most part based upon the existing Egyptian materia medica. The treatment of trachoma, for example, depended upon conjunctival abrasion using milesian wool, the process of *ophthalmoxipis*, followed by topical administration of copper salts. The *Corpus Hippocraticum* is full of richly detailed clinical information on the treatment of photophobia, excessive lacrimation, strabismus, nystagmus, and a wide variety of external diseases.

The hippocratic teachings flourished in the benevolent environment of Alexandria during the third century B.C., and were widely disseminated by Sloter. Important scientific discoveries were made by Herophilus of Chalcedon (ca. 300 B.C.), whose public dissections included demonstrations of the retina, vitreous, and ciliary body, and by Erasistratus (310–250 B.C.), who studied the innervation and circulation of the central nervous system. Alexandria continued to be an important center of medical knowledge long after Rome established preeminence, and the Alexandrian pharmacist Heracleides of Tarentum (ca. 150 A.D.) was one of the earliest medical botanists.

The effects of the rapid expansion of the Roman Empire upon medical therapeutic practice were far reaching and long-lasting. Greek and Alexandrian medical thought was quickly incorporated into the Roman medical system, the influence of which followed the great military advances of the Empire's legions. The most important writers of this period were Celsus (25 B.C.–50 A.D.), Galen (138–201 A.D.), Pliny (23–79 A.D.), and Dioscorides (40–90 A.D.).

From a therapeutic standpoint, the most influential figure to emerge was the Greek physician and medical botanist Pedacius Dioscorides. His five-volume materia medica, *De Universa Medicina*, was the definitive pharmacopoeia of antiquity, and was widely used during the Renaissance, as is evidenced by the many editions that were printed in the fifteenth and sixteenth centuries (NIELSEN 1974). The ophthalmic medications presented by Dioscorides and his contemporaries were largely in the form of collyria, cake-like ointment sticks in which drugs and mineral substances were incorporated into a base of gum resins which had to be triturated with rainwater, vinegar, or other liquids of presumed therapeutic efficacy before use. The medications could be prepared ahead of time, stored, and easily transported. Stamped collyria embellished with the seals of military physicians and engraved with information on pharmaceutical content and use have been unearthed in areas once occupied by Roman forces throughout northern Europe, and are of great medical as well as archeological interest (NIELSEN 1974). Collyria as popularized by the Romans became the most common means of dispensing ocular medications in the eighteenth century. An example is a collyrium prescription for the treatment of purulent ophthalmia in the *Nouveau Traité des Maladies des Yeux* by Charles de Saint Yves, published in 1767. The prescription requires one ounce of *tuttie preparé* (zinc oxide), two scruples of *heametite preparé* (ferric oxide), 12 grains of *meilleur aloes preparé* (best aloes), *four grains of ground pearls*, and a sufficent quantity of *graisse de vipère* (snake gall) (St. Yves 1767). This prescription is little different from those that Dioscorides published for treatment of *lippitudo*, or ophthalmia, which included instructions for the preparation of artificial hematite from heated lodestone, Indian aloes, *lapis calaminaris* (zinc silicate), and fish gall (Wellman 1906). Dioscorides' greatest contributions were the classification of therapeutics according to the clinical presentation of the diseases they were meant to cure, and his advocacy of the use of *Lacryma papaveris* (opium) as a soporific and painkiller.

His materia medica included a broad classification of plants with therapeutic properties, including species of mimosa plants, frequently used by the Egyptians; extract of aloes, touted to be a cure for a wide variety of ocular diseases; chelidonium latex, used as a base for many collyria; and frankincense. Myrrh, also popular with Egyptian oculists, was a common ingredient of collyria, especially for the treatment of leukomata and blepharitis. *Opabalsamum* (balsam extract) was thought to have magical powers and to be able to restore sight, as was the mythical plant *opopanaceum*.

The materia medica also included many mineral substances, mostly natural ores and salts which also had their origins in the alchemical laboratories in Egypt. The Egyptian advances in metallurgy, especially with respect to their skill in handling copper, quickly found application in the treatment of trachoma and other diseases. *Aerugo* (copper acetate) was frequently used by the Romans, as were copper carbonate, malachite, and azurite. Alum was used as an astringent. Useful byproducts of copper smelting included *cadmia* (zinc silicate), extensively used in the treatment of conjunctivitis. Other mineral substances with therapeutic effectiveness were *cinnabar* (mercury sulfide) and *stibium* (antimony). Frequently mentioned but of much more dubious therapeutic value are animal substances such as *castoreum* (extract of the scent glands and testicles of beavers), *crocodilonium stercus* (crocodile excrement), *cornu cervi* (extract of stag antlers), and many varieties of animal gall (Nielsen 1974). Fish gall as an eye medication was used extensively in the seventeenth century, in large measure due to the fact that in the Lutheran Bible approved by the Synod of Dordrecht there is a passage in the Apocrypha, in the Book of Tobit, describing the healing of blindness by using fish gall to dissolve leukomata. One wonders if readers of the King James version of the Bible were equally enthusiastic about this form of therapy. Although the vast majority of the medications presented in these ancient pharmacopoeias at best did their patient no harm, there were some effective medications, such as those containing copper and zinc, alum, opium, and the anti-infective substance galbanum gum, which preceded the introduction of resorcinol by Unna in 1886 by nearly two millennia (Unna 1886).

Caius Plinius Secundus, Pliny the Elder (23–79 A.D.), a contemporary of Dioscorides, wrote the encyclopedic *Historia Mundi* and *Historia Naturalis*, which contain a vast materia medica. Although not a physician himself, he shared a native-born Roman's mistrust of physicians, and strove through his work to upgrade the quality of medicine. He encouraged physicians to prepare their own collyria, lest they and their patients be the victims of unscrupulous practitioners capitalizing on their own pharmacopoeias. Like the volumes of Dioscorides, Pliny's work had a broad readership centuries later, the first printed editions appearing in Vienna in 1469. Of more contemporary interest is the observation by Neuberger as cited by Castiglioni that Karl Himly (1771–1837), upon reading Pliny's descriptions of the use of anagallis extract prior to cataract surgery, was inspired in 1800 to study the cycloplegic effects of belladonna (CASTIGLIONI 1941).

The teachings of Aurelius Celsus (25 B. C.–50 A. D.) in *De Re Medicinae* include some of the most important ophthalmologic writings of antiquity. His descriptions of the structure and function of the lens and the treatment of cataract were important milestones (SNYDER 1967). He encouraged the use of mandrake root in the treatment of painful ophthalmias, and also took clinical advantage of the mydriatic effect of hyoscyamine. However, the cynosure of Roman medicine was Claudius Galen (138–201 A. D.) of Pergamon, whose voluminous body of work was to become the unquestioned standard of medical science. *De Usu Partium Corporis Humani, Methodus Medendi*, and *De Morborum Causis* were widely circulated and used religiously until the time of Vesalius. Book IV of *De Compositione Medicamentorum Secundum Locus* contains hundreds of prescriptions for the preparation of collyria. As it had earlier with the Egyptians, medical thought began to stagnate under the Romans; authoritarian galenic dogma was to prevail throughout the Dark Ages, and it was left to a small group of savants, primarily Byzantine and Arabian masters, to preserve the medical knowledge that had come before. Aetius of Amida (502–575) wrote extensively on diseases of the eye and compiled a large materia medica preserved in the classic work the *Tetrabiblion* (HIRSCHBERG 1899). The most important of the Arabian physicians was Rhazes (860–896), who made Baghdad the foremost medical center of his time. He meticulously compiled the elaborate pharmacopoeia *Liber Medicinalis ad Almansorem*, the *Liber Continens*, and the *Liber ad Pestilencia*, which is of interest for the discussion of ocular smallpox and its treatment. Another influential work was the *Tadkirat*, the bible of Arabian oculists written by Ali ibn Isa (940–1010). In its are described some 130 diseases of the eye and their treatments, remedies still in use in many parts of the Arabic-speaking world.

Almost coincidentally with the decline of the Arabian civilizations, Europe slowly began to rise from the abyss of illiteracy and ignorance. The founding of the School of Salerno in the eleventh century heralded the return of intellectual freedom in medicine. Important works dating from this period include the *Regimen Sanitatis Salernitalum* and the formulary *Antidotarium Nicolai Salernitani*. One of the most important figures in Salerna was Benvenutus GRASSUS (ca. 1150), whose *De Oculis Eorumque Egritudinibus et Curis*, first printed in 1474, is the earliest printed work on eye disease. Grassus was fundamentally galenic in his approach to disease and blamed most ocular problems, including cataract, on the ingress of foreign humors into the eye. The rigid dogmatism of the Church, which had readily accepted the monotheistic teachings of Galen, finally began to erode in the fifteenth century when the religious and scientific reformations first manifested them-

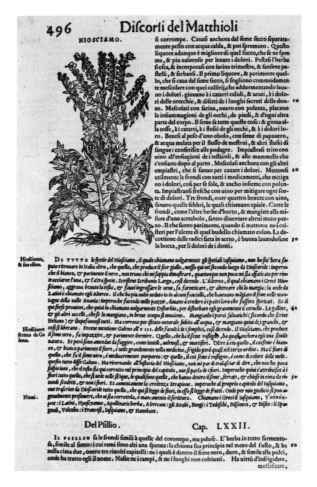

Fig. 1. Page from Mattioli's *Commentary on Dioscorides* featuring an etching of *Hyoscyamus niger* accompanied by a descriptive text on its medical properties. (Yale University School of Medicine Library)

selves. Just as the centralized power of the Church was being undermined by the new forces of trade, scientific thought and medicine were to be revolutionized by the teachings of Copernicus (1473–1543) and Paracelsus (1493–1541). *De Gradibus*, by Paracelsus, a compilation of chemical therapeutics based upon iatrochemical theories, was anticlerical in its orientation and effectively refuted the fundamental galenic doctrines. Such heretical thinking was not immediately accepted, but with the publication of *De Humani Corporis Fabrica* by Andreas Vesalius (1514–1564) in 1543, a new era in medicine unquestionably began. The intellectually liberating climate that was evolving was to produce an unprecedented harvest of scientific knowledge from men such as Francis Bacon, Reneé Descartes, Johannes Kepler, and Constantijn Huygens.

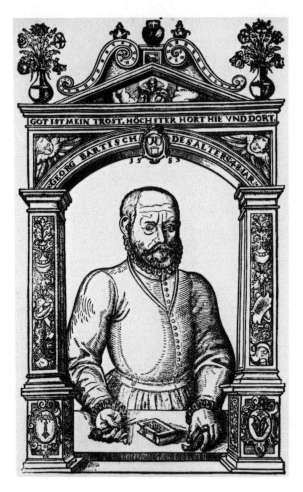

Fig. 2. Frontispiece of the *Augendienst* of Georg Bartisch with the author depicted with couching needle. (Yale University School of Medicine Library)

Just as anatomy and physics flourished during the sixteenth century, so did pharmacology. The iatrochemical, almost alchemic theories of Paracelsus encouraged the investigation of the therapeutic usefulness of metals, while the importation of exotic plant life into Italy stimulated medical botanists. The Renaissance physician-botanists, such as Mattioli (1501–1577), whose *Commentary on Dioscorides* (Fig. 1) was the preeminent pharmacopoeia of its time (Mattioli 1576), and Valerius Cordus (1515–1544), author of the *Dispensatorium*, sought a rational system of therapeutics. After the publication of the *Nuovo Receptario Composito* in Florence in 1498, the first pharmacopoeia printed, the dissemination of more scientifically prepared materia medica continued unabated. Important ophthalmologic works to appear were the *Ophthalmodouleia, das ist, Augendienst* (Fig. 2) of Georg Bartisch (1583); the *Traité des Maladies de l'Oeil* by Jacques Guil-

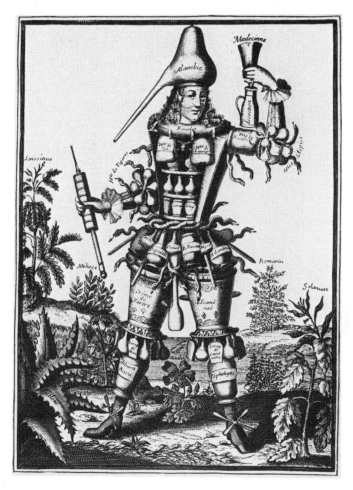

Fig. 3. An eighteenth-century caricature of an apothecary dressed in the materia medica of his time. (HOLLANDER 1921)

lemeau (1550–1612), a student of Ambrose Paré (published in 1585); and *A Briefe Treatise Touching the Preservation of the Eie* by Walter Bayley (1529–1592) (published in 1586). Bartisch's beautifully illustrated work was the first medical book on eye disease written in the modern vernacular, and its materia medica draws extensively on the *Tadkirat*, Galen, Dioscorides, and Celsus (HERFORT 1962).

The revolutionary advances in anatomy, physiology, and chemistry during the seventeenth century were to have a profound effect on ophthalmic therapeutics. Lazare Rivière (1589–1655), a chemist and physician of Montpellier, wrote extensively on the clinical approach to cataract and was enmeshed in the controversy regarding the beneficial effects of antimony which raged throughout Europe. The introduction of cinchona bark in 1632 by Jesuit priests under Cardinal de Luga from Peru revolutionized pharmacology more than any other single event. Drugs

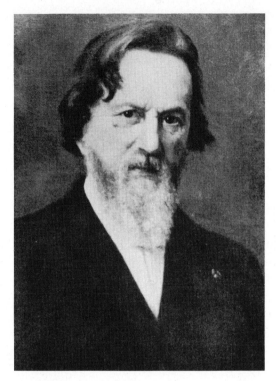

Fig. 4. Frans Cornelis Donders (1818–1889)

were now sought for their specific properties rather than for their galenic purgative effect.

Antoine Maitre-Jan (1650–1730) observed in 1682 the anterior dislocation of the lens during couching, and his subsequent postmortem dissection of a woman whose cataract had been couched demonstrated conclusively that it was an opacification of the lens which resulted in cataract (MAITRE-JAN 1707). The *Traité de la Cataracte et du Glaucome* by Michel Brisseau (1676–1743) contained concise pathologic and anatomic descriptions of normal and diseased eyes, and confirmed the veracity of Maitre-Jan's observations (BRISSEAU 1707). In 1707 Charles de Saint Yves (1667–1736) removed fragments of a lens that had prolapsed into the anterior chamber and became the first to report cataract extraction (SAINT YVES 1722). The institutionalization of ophthalmology was soon to follow with the establishment of a lectureship in ophthalmology in Vienna by Empress Maria Theresa. The appointment of Joseph Barth as the first professor of ophthalmology in Europe fully brought the specialty into the mainstream of the other cultural and scientific influences of the Age of Enlightenment (Fig. 3). A strong ophthalmologic tradition had been established when Barth was succeeded by J. A. Schmidt (1759–1809) and by George Joseph Beer (1763–1821), who later trained Carl Friedrich von Graefe, the father of Albrecht von Graefe. Scientific perceptions generated in this new intellectual climate quickly spread. In the United Kingdom publication of James

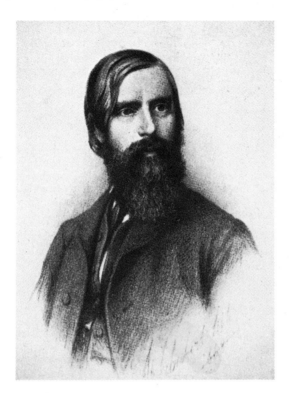

Fig. 5. Albrecht von Graefe (1828–1870)

Wardrop's (1782–1869) *Essays on the Morbid Anatomy of the Human Eye*, a classification of ocular disease based on pathophysiology and anatomy (1808), and of William Mackenzie's (1791–1868) *Practical Treatise on Diseases of the Eye* (1830) were events that had profound effects upon the understanding of the processes of disease and treatment. The latter treatise underscored the hardness of the globe as an essential feature of glaucoma.

Belladonna drugs were introduced into ophthalmic practice by Franz Resinger (1787–1855), who used them during examination (REISINGER 1825), and by Schmidt, who reported the use of hyoscyamine in the treatment of iritis in 1801. Karl Himly, who together with Schmidt founded the first ophthalmologic journal, *Ophthalmologische Bibliothek*, used atropine for mydriasis before cataract surgery, and his observations of the lens through a dilated pupil enabled him to classify cataract properly for the first time. Later in the century, Frans Donders (1818–1889) (Fig. 4) and Albrecht von Graefe (1828–1870) (Fig. 5) directed their prodigious talents to the study of the actions and uses of belladonna drugs (DONDERS 1864; VON GRAEFE 1854). Their lively correspondence on these matters carried on between Utrecht and Berlin is of considerable interest.

Donders and von Graefe corresponded on a broad spectrum of ophthalmic subject matter, ranging from early experiences with the ophthalmoscope to discussions of medical history. Many illustrious colleagues appear in the letters –

Heinrich Muller (1820–1864), professor at Würzburg; Richard Liebreich (1830–1917), associate of Virchow; von Helmholtz; and Theodor Leber (1840–1917), who at the time was von Graefe's assistant. A number of interesting letters are illustrative of the achievements in ophthalmic pharmacology. For example, in a letter written in June 1853 (WEVE and TEN DOESSCHATE 1935), von Graefe discusses with Donders his paper on the action of belladonna which was to appear in the Dutch literature:

> I fully share your recent views on the activity of belladonna. The substance penetrates the cornea and has a direct effect on the iris – in rabbits, the more one reduces the membrane by removing individual bits of cornea, the quicker it works. If one injects the aqueous humor from an eye treated with atropine into the anterior chamber, the pupil dilates. I have carried out experiments on 20 of my patients to discover how the spectrum is seen after operation for cataract; in 16 cases it was clearly established that these patients see a wide band of color beyond violet, which in some is almost as wide as our violet.

In a letter dated 4 July 1862 (WEVE and TEN DOESSCHATE 1935), von Graefe asks Donders' opinion of Fraser's recently published report on the action of the Calabar bean – physostigmine:

> What do you think of the Calabar bean? I have set up quite a few experiments involving it, and have been amazed at the results. I am particularly struck by the fact that glaucomatous pupils (even in the case of a half-atropic iris) manifest a proportion of the effect. This is really of use where iridectomy is concerned. It works quite independently on the lens, as I have proved in the case of a man without any iris. The accommodation phenomenon lasts one hour, the myosis a few days; the former consists of an increase in the refractive state (on average of one-eighth) and a shortening of the near point after recovery from the myosis-dependent impairment (by approximately 1/30). It passes into the anterior chamber and acts directly on the nerves of the iris; as with atropine, the effect is completely lacking in birds, or at least quite different. The experiments following administration of atropine drops are very interesting.

Topical eserine was introduced for the treatment of glaucoma by Ludwig Laqueur (1876). Laqueur (1839–1909) (Fig. 6), who himself suffered from the disease and had undergone peripheral iridectomies performed by Johann Horner, wrote eloquently of his experiences (1909). The history of the discovery of physostigmine and its later introduction into medical practice is an interesting one. The story begins in Old Calabar, the erstwhile slave-trading headquarters of West Africa located in the Cross River basin near the Bight of Biafra. The area was plagued by disease, corruption, and the internecine power struggles of the violently divided indigenous population. A member of the British military presence established to enforce the ban on slavery, a young medical officer named William Daniell, witnessed the use of Calabar beans during the Efik trials by ordeal, and reported his findings. These reports stimulated the interest of Robert Christison, the venerable internist and pharmacologist at the University of Edinburgh. He began to experiment with some samples he had been given by a missionary, and even went so far as to ingest extracts of the beans himself, an exercise which provided the material for articulate descriptions of the parasympathomimetic effects of the drugs. It was left to Christison's assistant, Thomas Fraser, to isolate the active ingredient, which he named eserine. Fraser's own experiments documented the miotic effects on the pupil (1863), and it was not long before another Edinburgh physician, Douglas Argyll Robertson, became interested in the drug and suggested its use in the treatment of iris prolapse and iritis (1863).

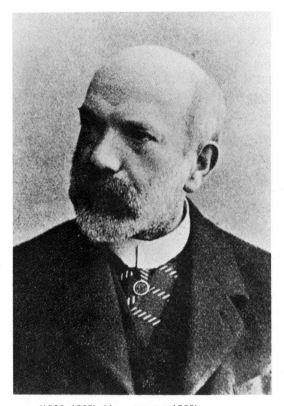

Fig. 6. Ludwig Laqueur (1839–1909). (Anonymous 1909)

Fraser (1841–1920) was 21 at the time of the publication of this thesis on the therapeutic uses of the Calabar bean, for which he was awarded the Gold Medal by the University of Edinburgh. Born in Calcutta and educated in Scotland, Fraser went on to a brilliant career at Edinburgh, where he assumed the Chair of Pharmacology upon Christison's retirement. He contributed significantly to the university's vaunted medical reputation in the late nineteenth century. He was one of the first to apply knowledge of chemical structures to pharmacologic action, especially in the study of quaternary ammonium bases. Codeine, morphine, strychnine, and a host of other substances fell under his scrutiny. He was much interested in the antagonistic action of physostigmine and atropine, although he never realized the potential value of these drugs in ophthalmic practice. Here Fraser (1863) describes the effects of physostigmine applied topically to his own left eye:

A small drop of syrupy extract was placed on the point of a thin probe, and applied to the conjunctiva over the left eyeball. A copious discharge of tears immediately occurred.

In five minutes, the left pupil was a little contracted, and very evidently so in eight minutes, the left being one half the size of the right. In ten minutes, the pupil was one sixteenth of an inch in diameter. Vision with this was imperfect, the visual distance being lessened, but the iris was mobile. A slightly painful sensation was now experienced in the supraorbital region of the left side, and a sensation of heat in the left eyeball. In thirty minutes, no change had occurred in the right pupil; the left was a mere speck. Vision with the left eye was almost lost; there was a little redness, and tenderness on exposure to light. In one hour and a half, all disagreeable sensations had gone, the dimness of vision was less marked, but extreme contraction of the pupil continued. In four hours, the dimness of vision disappeared; but the contraction of the left pupil continued unchanged for twenty-four hours.

During the nineteenth century great advances were also being made in the field of ocular bacteriology. The treatment and prophylaxis of ophthalmia neonatorum was to be one of the great triumphs of nineteenth-century ocular therapeusis. As early as 1795, James Ware (1756–1812) had published the first clinical descriptions of neonatal gonorrheal ophthalmitis, and in 1807 Benjamin Gibson reported the communicability of the disorder and identified vaginal secretions as the source of the infections. Although silver nitrate had been used for centuries, most notably by Angelus Sala in the sixteenth century, it was not until 1835 that Étienne Julliard first reported its use and efficacy in the treatment of gonococcal ophthalmia. Nearly 50 years were to pass after this important report was published before Karl Credé (1819–1892), Professor of Obstetrics at Leipzig, was to advocate the prophylactic instillation of 2% silver nitrate into the eyes of neonates (CREDÉ 1884). Credé's contribution to ophthalmology coincided with a new awareness of infectious disease and the value of preventive medicine. This was the era of Louis Pasteur (1822–1895), whose work on virulent disease and preventive inoculation received the attention it deserved, and of Robert Koch (1843–1910), who discovered the tubercle bacillus and was engaged in the perfection of steam sterilization.

The importance of asepsis and the role of microorganisms in the development of wound infections was stressed by Alfred Carl Graefe (1830–1899), who in 1884 routinely began to use corrosive sublimate as a disinfectant for cataract surgery (GRAEFE 1889), applying Lord Lister's principles to ophthalmology. Preoperative conjunctival sterilization was later popularized by K. K. Lundsgard (1867–1931).

In the 1880s ophthalmic surgery was to be revolutionized in yet another way. One of the most outstanding contributions to the field of ocular therapeutics and surgery was the introduction of cocaine as a topical anesthetic agent by Karl Koller (1857–1944) (Fig. 7) in 1884. In the mid-nineteenth century the introduction of general anesthetic agents such as ether and nitrous oxide by W. T. G. Morton (1819–1868), Humphrey Davy (1788–1829), and others had a tremendous impact on general surgery but found little application in eye surgery, although Henry Willard Williams (1821–1895), the advocate of the corneal suture, used ether anesthesia routinely at the Boston City Hospital in the 1860s. Although cocaine had been isolated by Albert Niemann in 1858, it was not until 1879 that Vasili Anrep described its anesthetic properties when applied to the skin. Koller studied in Vienna under von Arlt and later in Utrecht under Snellen and Donders. He apparently collaborated with Sigmund Freud while both were working at the Allgemeines Krankenhaus in Vienna, where Freud studied the physiological effects of cocaine in the hope that it might be used in the treatment of morphine addiction. Within months of the publication of Koller's report cocaine was being used in a wide variety of ophthalmic procedures, and later that year Hermann Knapp (1832–1911) reported performing a retrobulbar injection of cocaine prior to an enucleation procedure.

By the end of the nineteenth century the dramatic advances in basic science, pathology, experimental physiology, and bacteriology ensured that clinical ophthalmology would be based upon sound concepts which would carry it into a new age

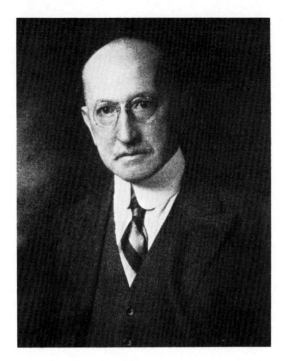

Fig. 7. Carl Koller (1857–1944). (Bloom 1944)

of technological and scientific achievements. The many contributions made by von Graefe, Donders, and Helmholtz and their skill as teachers were largely responsible for bringing ophthalmology into the modern era. But this was also the era of Mooren (1828–1899), who studied sympathetic ophthalmia; of La Grange (1852–1928), who invented fistulizing procedures for glaucoma; of Parinaud (1844–1905), who described tuberculous conjunctivitis; of Morax (1866–1934), who studied trachoma and diplobacillary conjunctivitis; of Otto Haab (1860–1931), whose classic works on external and fundus disease greatly advanced medical ophthalmology; of Ernst Fuchs (1851–1930); and of Julius Hirschberg (1843–1925).

Studies of muscarinic drugs and histamine by Schmeideberg (1838–1921), founder of the *Archiv für experimentelle Pathologie und Pharmakologie*, as well as the studies of sympathomimetic drugs by his student Hans Meyer (1853–1939), pioneered the investigative pharmacology of the autonomic nervous system and its effectors. Thomas Fraser, in addition to his work on physostigmine, made many other contributions correlating chemical structure with function. J. J. Abel (1865–1935) was the first to isolate epinephrine from the adrenal gland and made early contributions to the study of hormones and autonomic effectors. The pioneering work by Koch and by Pasteur and his student Ernst Roux (1852–1933), who introduced serologic antisyphilitic therapy, laid the groundwork for Paul Ehrlich's (1854–1915) truly revolutionary techniques of chemotherapy. Ehrlich's perseverance in searching for the effective arsenical substances in the treatment of syphilis set standards of methodology which would have a great impact upon the search for more effective pharmacologic agents.

Despite these and more recent advances that have been made in the field of ocular therapeutics, it is clear that each new fragment of knowledge generates unanswered questions. Looking at scientific progress from this perspective, we must take heed of the fact that we are, after all, not so far removed from our professional forebears as to have lost our appreciation for the aura surrounding the eye and the diseases that affect it, or our ability to marvel at the secrets of this astounding organ system.

References

Anonymous (1909) Ludwig Laqueur (1839–1909). Klin Monatsbl Augenheilkd 47:537 (obituary)

Argyll Robertson D (1863) The Calabar bean as a new agent in ophthalmic practice. Edin Med J 8:815–820

Bartisch G (1583) Ophthalmodouleia, das ist, Augendienst. Stöckel, Dresden

Bayley W (1586) A briefe treatise touching the preservation of the eie sight. Waldegrave, London

Bloom S (1944) Carl Koller. Arch Ophthalmol 31:344 (obituary)

Brisseau M (1707) Traité de la catarcte et du glaucoma. d'Houry, Paris

Bryan CP (1931) The papyrus Ebers. Appleton, New York

Castiglioni A (1941) A history of medicine. Knopf, New York

Cordus V (1546) Pharmacorum omnium, quae quidem in usus sunt, conficiendorum ratio, vulgo vocant dispensatorium pharmacopolarum. Petreium, Norimbergae

Credé KSF (1884) Die Verhütung der Augenentzündung der Neugeborenen. Hirschwald, Berlin

Donders FC (1864) On the anomalies of accommodation and refraction of the eye. Translated from the author's manuscript by WD Moore. New Sydenham Society, London

Fraser TR (1863) On the characters, actions and therapeutic uses of the bean of Calabar. Edin Med J 9:36–56

Ghalioungui P (1963) Magic and medical science in ancient Egypt. Hodder and Stoughton, London

Graefe AC (1889) Fortgesetzter Bericht über die mittelst antiseptischer Wundbehandlung erzielten Erfolge der Staaroperationen. Arch Ophthalmol 35:248–264

Grassus B (1474) De oculis eorumque egritudinibus et curis. Severinus de Ferrara, Ferrara

Guillemeau J (1585) Traité des maladies de l'oeil. Massé, Paris

Heibling M (1980) Der altägyptische Augenkranke, sein Arzt und seine Götter. Juris, Zürich

Herfort K (1962) Antike und arabische Elemente in den Rezepten von Georg Bartischs Augendienst. Albrecht von Graefes, Arch Klin Exp Ophthalmol 164:303–320

Hirschberg J (1899) Geschichte der Augenheilkunde, Erstes Buch: Geschichte der Augenheilkunde im Altertum. Veit, Leipzig

Hollander E (1921) Die Karikatur und Satire in der Medizin. Emke, Stuttgart

Julliard EF (1835) De l'emploi de l'excision et de la cautérisation a l'aide du nitrate d'argent fondu dans l'opthalmie blennorrhagique. Thèse 26, Paris

Koller C (1884) Vorläufige Mittheilung über locale Anästhesierung am Auge. Klin Monatsbl Augenheilkd 22:60–63

Laqueur L (1876) Ueber eine neue therapeutische Verwendung des Physostigmin. Zbl Med Wiss 14:421–422

Laqueur L (1909) Geschichte meiner Glaukomerkrankung. Klin Monatsbl Augenheilkd 47:639–646

Mackenzie W (1830) A practical treatise on diseases of the eye. Longman, London

Magnus M (1901) Die Augenheilkunde der Alten. Kern, Breslau

Maître-Jan A (1707) Traité des maladies de l'oeil. Le Febure, Troyes

Mattioli PA (1576) Commentary on Dioscorides. Venice

Nielsen H (1974) Ancient ophthalmologic agents. Odense University Press, Odense

Reisinger F (1825) Ophthalmologische Versuche bey Thieren mit dem Hyoscyamin und Atropin. Med Chir Ztg 1:237–253

Saint Yves C de (1722) Nouveau traité des maladies des yeux. Le Mercier, Paris

Schmidt JA (1801) Ueber Nachstaar und Iritis nach Staaroperationem. Abhandl Med Chir Josephs-Acad Wien 2:209–292

Snyder C (1967) Our ophthalmic heritage. Little, Brown, Boston

Unna PG (1886) Ichthyol und Resorcin als Repräsentanten der Gruppe reduzierter Heilmittel. Voss, Hamburg

Von Graefe FWEA (1854) Notiz über die Behandlung der Mydriasis. Albrecht von Graefes Arch Ophthalmol 2:202–257

Wardrop J (1808) Essays on the morbid anatomy of the human eye. G Ramsay, Edinburgh

Wellman M (1906) Dioscorides, De materia medica. Weidmann, Berolini

Weve HJM, ten Doesschate G (1935) Die Briefe Albrecht von Graefe's an F.C. Donders (1852–1870). Enke, Stuttgart, pp 15

CHAPTER 2

Ocular Pharmacokinetics

D. M. MAURICE and S. MISHIMA

Abbreviations. Nearly 100 symbols are used in the mathematical development of kinetic theory in this chapter. The majority of them appear only transiently and are defined where they are used, so that no purpose would be served by listing them here. Most of those that are used more generally are illustrated in Fig. 4 and are listed below, but a few others are neither in the figure nor in accordance with standard convention: owing to other uses for the more common symbols, the thickness of a tissue layer and its area are referred to as q and Q; readers may remember them from the German *quer* and *Quadrat*. In place of the abbreviation AUC for area under the curve, the symbol U is used, and specifically U_d for the area under the tear concentration curve.

The most common symbols used for the ocular compartments are shown in Fig. 1, and the entire set is listed here for convenience: d, tears; c, cornea; a, anterior aqueous humor; h, posterior aqueous humor; v, vitreous body; l, crystalline lens; p, blood plasma; r, undefined reservoir; b, applied drop; s, tissue fluid of corneal stroma; z, ciliary body secretion.

For the labeling of compartments, transfer coefficients, and permeability coefficients, a slightly modified version of the system of DUKE-ELDER and MAURICE (1957) has been adopted. The concentration in and volume of a compartment x are called C_x and V_x, and the mass of drug it contains, m_x. The transfer coefficient between compartments x and y referred to the volume of y is denoted k_{xy}, and referred to the volume of x is denoted k_{yx}; in the original system they were called $k_{y \cdot xy}$ and $k_{x \cdot xy}$.

Established usage provides an exception to the rule for some commonly used transfer coefficients. Thus, k_c is the transfer coefficient between cornea and aqueous humor, referred to the volume of the cornea; k_o, loss coefficient out of the anterior chamber to the blood; k_i, entry coefficient from plasma to anterior chamber; α, loss coefficient from the tears. A and B are the apparent elimination and absorption coefficients of the aqueous humor in the open two-compartment model comprising the anterior chamber and cornea.

r_{ca} denotes the ratio of the drug concentration in the cornea (mass per total volume of tissue) to that in the aqueous humor at steady state. g_{ca} is the corresponding ratio while the two concentrations are declining in parallel as the drug is eliminated from the eye. r_{ap} is the ratio of the drug concentration in the aqueous humor to its free concentration in the plasma. When the total concentration in the plasma is considered, the symbol r'_{ap} is employed.

A. Introduction

I. Objectives

The tissues of the eye are protected from noxious substances in the environment or bloodstream by a variety of mechanisms: notably a tear secretion continuously flushing its surface, an impermeable surface epithelium, and a transport system actively clearing the retina of agents potentially able to disturb the visual process. From the point of view of medical therapy, it is unfortunate that these mechanisms sometimes make it difficult to assure an effective concentration of a drug at the intended site. The difficulties can be compounded by the structure of the globe itself, where many of its internal structures are isolated at a distance from the blood and from the outside surface of the eye. A major problem, then, in ocular therapeutics is how to circumvent these structural obstacles and protective mechanisms and bring about the desired biological response, e.g., changes in pupil diameter or in counts of viable bacteria in the vitreous body, without creating high concentrations of the drug elsewhere in the eye or body which could have unpleasant or dangerous effects.

Ocular pharmacokinetics is the systematic study of the changes of concentration in the tissues of the eye when a drug is administered in different dosage forms, by different routes, and according to various schedules. Ultimately, it should be possible to predict these changes knowing only a limited number of the chemical and physical properties of the drug. In order to achieve these objectives it is necessary to analyze the penetration of a drug to its site of action in terms of the barriers offered to its passage by the separate tissues comprising the eye. This analysis is assisted by the wealth of information available from physiological studies, which has allowed these barriers to be identified and the obstruction they offer to a number of substances to be measured, and has clarified the nature of the circulation in the intraocular and lacrimal fluids.

Investigations of drug penetration into the eye have unfortunately not been concerned with a kinetic analysis of the process but have been restricted to finding out whether therapeutic concentrations can be achieved and maintained by means of a particular schedule of administration. This information is valuable, but does not allow a comparison between one drug and another in terms of the barrier offered by any cell layer that restricts entry. Frequently, it is not even possible to predict the effect on the concentrations within the eye of changing the schedule of administration. Furthermore, most experiments have been carried out in the rabbit, and it is not certain how far they apply to humans.

It is the main purpose of this chapter to develop a kinetic analysis for each method of clinical administration. The published literature has been examined to extract as much information as possible characterizing the passage of drugs across the tissues. While sifting this information, it became evident what improvements in the design of drug penetration experiments are desirable if the data they provide are to have a more general significance.

The methods of compartmental analysis used correspond in most respects to those of systemic pharmacokinetics. However, the study of intraocular dynamics grew up independently of that field, and the distinctive properties of the eye lend themselves to special emphasis on limited relationships between neighboring media

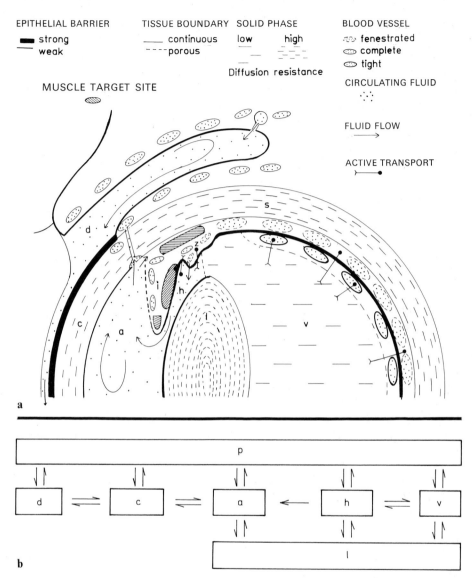

Fig. 1. a Synopsis of the tissues and fluids that make up the eye, showing the barriers and diffusion resistances and the transport and flow systems that regulate drug movement. **b** Compartmental system used to model ocular pharmacokinetics. *p*, plasma; *d*, tear fluid; *c*, cornea; *a*, anterior chamber; *h*, posterior chamber; *l*, lens; *i*, iris; *z*, ciliary body; *s*, sclera; *v*, vitreous body.

such as the aqueous humor and the vitreous humor or cornea. In this respect ocular kinetics has the unusual advantage that a number of noninvasive techniques are available to monitor changes in concentration of agents in individual eyes so that human and animal data can be directly related. Some of these methods make use of the biological responses of the eye to active agents, and this subject will be dealt with in a later section. Another technique, of wider application, is the use of fluorescent substances as tracers, which allows concentration determinations to be made in all the transparent media of the living eye. Most use has been made of fluorescein, a nontoxic compound without pharmacologic activity, unbound by the tissues, and measurable at very low concentrations. It appears that many lipophobic drugs obey kinetics similar to those of fluorescein in the eye.

II. Compartments and Barriers

Our present knowledge of the structural constraints that control the movement of substances within the eye is summarized in Fig. 1 a. Solid media, where diffusion limits the rate of movement, are denoted by dashed areas, the concentration of the dashes corresponding to the obstruction – thus substances diffuse easily through the vitreous but only slowly in the lens. A cellular barrier between these media is shown by a thick line, the thickness corresponding to its resistance. The absolute value of these barriers is dependent on the lipid solubility of the solute, but probably their relative importance stays the same for any particular drug (see Table 3; Sect. B.II.6.a).

Blood vessels of three types are shown: the very permeable, fenestrated choriocapillaris, the capillaries with tight junctions in the retina, and the capillaries with leaky junctions elsewhere. Some active transport systems that could be of importance in affecting drug dynamics are indicated, and the direction of flow of the secreted fluids is shown by arrows.

The more important compartments that make up the kinetic system of the eye and their interrelationships are illustrated schematically in Fig. 1 b. As can be seen, they essentially form a chain of five elements, each one of which carries out exchanges with the plasma. The three intraocular compartments are also linked to the lens, but these exchanges are relatively limited because of the high resistance to diffusion in that tissue.

In principle, the entire system could be modeled on a computer, and the concentration changes in any chamber following the introduction of a drug at any other point could be calculated, allowance being made for the absence of mixing in several of the compartments. At present there are not sufficient data to allow such a system to be assembled for any drug of clinical importance. Furthermore, establishing values for the barriers is more readily carried out by analyzing the concentration changes in a limited number of neighboring compartments, and this is more relevant to the therapeutic situation.

III. Routes of Administration and Penetration

This section briefly describes various methods of administering drugs to the eye and identifies the pathway by which they penetrate the media. In practice, the great majority of prescriptions are for drops or oral forms that may conveniently be self-administered.

1. Topical Administration

Introducing the drug directly into the conjunctival sac so that it mixes with the tear fluid and bathes the entire corneal and conjunctival surfaces is adequate for the treatment of most external conditions of the eye and those of the anterior segment. Generally, a watery drop of about 50 µl is allowed to fall on the eye from a dropper. The drop is sometimes made viscous in an attempt to increase the contact time of the drug with the eye; to prolong contact further, ointments are instilled into the conjunctival sac.

There are two main pathways of entry from the conjunctival sac into the anterior segment: across the cornea and across the conjunctiva. Direct entry from the tears into the anterior chamber occurs across the cornea, and the major barrier to penetration is the epithelium, except in the case of very lipophilic compounds, to which the cell layers offer virtually no resistance; the stroma is then the barrier. There is a loss of drug to the limbal circulation, but this is not of major importance, as will be shown later.

By blocking access of the drug to either the corneal or the conjunctival surface, several workers have confirmed that the latter route of entry to the anterior chamber is of lesser importance. In one series of experiments (DOANE et al. 1978), where the conjunctival sac of a rabbit was filled with radiolabeled hydrocortisone solution, 70 times less drug entered the aqueous humor when the solution was denied contact with the cornea. Similar results were found with pilocarpine.

That portion of the material which crosses the conjunctiva and is not lost to the blood in passage can then diffuse into the sclera. In the limbal zone it has the possibility of entering the anterior chamber directly or diffusing sideways into the corneal stroma. Slightly more posteriorly it may have direct access to the base of the ciliary body and iris. A sectional dilation of the pupil after the localized application of epinephrine to the conjunctiva bears witness to the existence of this route in the human eye (BIENFANG 1973). Over most of the globe, however, any substance that crossed the conjunctiva and sclera would come into contact with the heavily vascularized choroid, and the greater part of it would be washed into the general circulation. The return of drug to the eye through the general circulation after its absorption into the blood can be tested by measurements in the contralateral eye, and can be of significance in rabbits but is unlikely to be of importance in humans.

Once in the anterior chamber, the drug circulates in the aqueous humor and has access to the anterior surface of the iris and the portion of the lens exposed by the pupil. The margin of the pupil forms a valve on the lens, and convective flow back into the posterior chamber does not occur in normal eyes. This has been disputed by SHERMAN et al. (1978), who found a movement of fluorescein from the anterior to the posterior chamber in cannulated monkey eyes. However, both in rabbits (CUNHA-VAZ and MAURICE 1969; HOLM and KRAKAU 1966) and humans (HOLM 1968; NAGATAKI 1975) a relatively unstained fluid is seen to flow through the pupil into the brightly fluorescent anterior chamber after the systemic or topical administration of fluorescein. In humans, but perhaps not rabbits (COLE and MONRO 1976), aqueous humor flows through the base of the iris to the suprachoroidal space, and this could bring a drug into contact with the base of the ciliary body.

Effective drug concentrations need to be maintained in the eye for extended periods of time – even permanently – yet the effect of a drop is transitory, lasting only a few hours. Attempts have been made to prolong the action of topical applications by introducing devices which gradually release the drug into the tear fluid over a period of time. The devices range from simple expedients, such as a contact lens soaked in a solution of the active material, to an insert engineered to release the drug at a constant rate over a considerable period of time.

Iontophoresis is the enhancement of the penetration of a charged solute across the corneal or conjunctival epithelium by establishing an electrical gradient of the appropriate polarity across it. The pathways are essentially those followed in topical instillation, although it is possible to restrict the area of penetration to that of the electrode.

2. Local Injection

One certain way of circumventing the eye's natural barriers to drug penetration and of establishing a definite concentration within it is to introduce the drug directly into the globe. Injection directly into the anterior chamber has no definite advantages except during the course of other intraocular surgical intervention because drugs can be made to reach useful concentrations in the anterior segment by other methods. It is sometimes not possible to achieve an adequate penetration into the vitreous chamber, however, except by intravitreal injections. Injected material will diffuse through the entire vitreous body from a depot and will come directly in contact with the whole area of retinal surface. Furthermore, it can be carried into the anterior chamber by the flow of aqueous humor and will permeate the cornea and all the anterior structures. Fear of causing harm to the eye has limited this treatment to the most acutely threatening diseases, in practice to endophthalmitis.

In subconjunctival injections, 0.5–1 ml fluid is injected, which dissects through the tissues raising a large bleb that spreads backward and sideways around the corneal periphery. Further spreading and absorption of the fluid causes the bleb to flatten, but it takes several hours to disappear totally. The injection of large volumes in the rabbit raises a bleb which can cover part of the corneal surface, and regurgitation out of the needle hole is a common occurrence in this species (Wine et al. 1964). Injection beneath Tenon's capsule is treated as a distinct maneuver by some authors, and Swan et al. (1956) found that a 50 µl injection of epinephrine brought on a more rapid onset of mydriasis in this location. However, larger volumes of fluid are likely to spread and escape from beneath the capsule, so that most of the drug will be subconjunctival regardless of where it was orignally injected. Furthermore, it is unlikely that a thin layer of connective tissue like the capsule could offer more than a transient obstacle to diffusion.

From a position beneath the conjunctiva, a drug could follow the pathways previously described for transconjunctival penetration: directly into the anterior chamber, directly to the ciliary body, or through the root of the iris or across the sclera into the vitreous. Where there is regurgitation (through the needle hole) into the conjunctival sac in the rabbit, entry across the cornea can occur. Similarly, where prolapse of the bleb over the cornea occurs, over a large area in the rabbit but perhaps in a limited zone around the limbus in man, serial penetration across the conjunctival and corneal epithelia may take place. Entry pathways from the subconjunctival site will be considered in more detail in Sect. C.II.4.

Injection of drugs deep into the orbit is sometimes practiced in an attempt to give them access to the posterior intraocular structures or the vessels and nerves leading to the globe. Retrobulbar injections of fluorescein solution have been made into the orbits of human eyes that were about to be enucleated (MIYAKE and OHT-SUKI (1981). In histological sections the sclera and choroidal stroma were found to be stained, as well as tissue spaces in the ciliary muscle and the stroma of the ciliary processes. Observations of the fundus in vivo showed that some dye penetrated into the vitreous body, but the amount was not quantified.

3. Systemic Administration

Systemic dosage, whether by ingestion or parenteral injection, is an effective method of bringing a drug to all parts of the eye through the bloodstream. It can directly enter the stroma of the iris and can pass into the newly formed aqueous humor from the ciliary processes. The cornea is exposed to the drug both from the limbal capillaries and the aqueous humor. The conjunctival and deeper vessels bring the drug to the outside of the globe. The retina and vitreous body may obtain therapeutic levels from either the choroidal or retinal circulation and from the posterior chamber to a lesser extent. In very many cases this is prevented by structural barriers in the retinal capillaries and in the pigmented epithelia of the retina and ciliary body, as well as by active transport mechanisms removing the drug from the eye.

The systemic route suffers from the disadvantage that all the organs of the body are subjected to the action of the drug, when only a very small volume of tissue in the eye needs the treatment.

IV. Animal Models and Human Experimentation

1. Animal Models

The ultimate purpose of pharmacokinetic studies is to benefit patients, and the findings of such studies need to be related to the human eye. Little advance can be made without following concentration changes of drugs in the inner structures of the eye, so that generally these studies cannot be carried out on people, and alternatives need to be found. Enucleated eyes are unsuitable because an intact circulation is essential in many investigations, and the integrity of the delicate corneal epithelium must be assured in others. Reliance has to be placed on experiments on living animals, therefore. Although monkeys have occasionally been used because of their greater similarity to man, the most frequently used animal model is the rabbit. It is necessary, then, to consider how closely its ocular physiology resembles that of the human.

First of all, the pattern of blinking in the two species is very different – the rabbit blinks only four or five times in an hour – and the tear drainage systems show notable dissimilarities. Fortunately, because of the accessibility of this system in humans it is not necessary to rely heavily on the animal model. The permeability of the cell layers of the cornea seems to be significantly lower in humans (see Table 3). The aqueous humor dynamics are similar in the two species, however (see

Tables 1–3, Sects. B.I.5.b, B.II.6.a, and D.I.4.a), although the presence of the uveoscleral outflow system in humans may be important (see Sect. B.I.4.a) when the deeper penetration of drugs is considered. In the posterior sector, the anatomic arrangement of the retinal layer in the rabbit is unusual; its vessels are restricted to a horizontal streak and lie upon a thick layer of myelinated nerves instead of being intraretinal. The exchange dynamics between blood and vitreous have been little investigated in man, and so it is not possible to state whether it is similar in the rabbit, but at least there is no evidence of a profound difference.

2. Human Experiments

When an animal model is fully understood, it becomes necessary to carry out experiments on the human eye in order to find out to what extent the model can be used to predict its behavior. Some of these experiments can be of a noninvasive type, using as a measure of the local concentration either inert tracers such as fluorescein or autonomic agents which give rise to readily monitored physiological responses. On occasion, however, one must establish the kinetics of an antibiotic or of an anti-inflammatory agent, and then it is necessary to collect a tissue or fluid sample from a patient's eye. Since this collection involves an extra intraocular procedure not intended for the patient's benefit, its ethical justification may be questioned. It is important that the purpose of the experiment be clearly defined and that care be taken in its design to extract as much significant information from it as is possible. Investigators should consider in advance exactly what point is to be established and whether further measurements taken at the time of the experiment would allow wider conclusions to be drawn, and they should terminate a series when its purpose is achieved. (The writers believe that similar criteria should be applied to experiments carried out on animals.) Concentration measurements in both the tissues and fluids of the eye may be possible after enucleation for melanoma, and a few globes may provide as much information as many samples of aqueous humor alone extracted from patients operated on for cataract. This procedure may be easier to justify.

B. Topical Administration

I. Factors Involved in Intraocular Penetration

1. The Tears and Contact with Ocular Surface

Topical application is by far the most common route of delivery of a drug to the eye, but it leaves much to be desired as a means of establishing a predictable level within the tissues. How much drug penetrates the eye is dependent upon the extent to which the drop is diluted by the tear fluid present in the conjunctival sac and how rapidly it is washed out by the tear flow. It is these factors that demonstrate the greatest variability among individual humans and may result in large differences between human and the rabbit, the principal species used in the study of drug penetration. The characteristics of the tear distribution and flow therefore deserve particular attention.

a) Tears

The tear film is a watery layer which covers the corneal surface with a uniform layer about 8 μm thick (MISHIMA 1965; EHLERS 1965a) and also coats the conjunctiva, filling in and bridging the folds in the tissue. Its total volume averages 8 μl in adult human eyes (MISHIMA et al. 1966) and about the same in the rabbit (CHRAI et al. 1973).

Apart from a somewhat raised potassium level, the composition of the freshly secreted tear fluid is similar to that of plasma dialysate (IWATA 1973). The fluid collected from the conjunctival sac contains a proportion of proteins derived from the blood or from the secretory glands of the conjunctiva (ELLISON et al. 1981). They may bind drugs, for example pilocarpine (MIKKELSON et al. 1973), and appreciably reduce their effective concentration in the tear fluid.

The tear film is stabilized by mucin produced by the goblet cells of the conjunctiva, and it is covered by a very thin lipid film of meibomian gland secretion, which restricts the evaporation of water. Most of the watery secretion is produced by the lacrimal glands, from which it is conducted to the globe by numerous ducts in the upper tarsal plate in man, but by a single duct close to the lateral canthus in the rabbit (GOLDSTEIN et al. 1967).

If fluorescein is instilled into the conjunctival sac, its concentration in the precorneal tear film can be followed for up to an hour by means of a slit-lamp fluorophotometer. The dye is washed out of the sac by the constant secretion and drainage of the tears and is also absorbed across the conjunctiva. Under quiet conditions it undergoes an exponential fall in concentration, the half-life of the exponential drop varying from 2 to 20 min in normal subjects (MISHIMA et al. 1966), which corresponds to an average tear secretion rate of the order of 1 μl/min and a loss coefficient of about 6 h^{-1}. This tenfold range of washout times, affecting as it does all substances dissolved in the tear film, must be a major cause of variability in patients' responses to topically applied drugs. The average turnover rate of tears slows with age (FURUKAWA and POLSE 1978).

More irregular kinetics are observed immediately after instillation, while the dye is still mixing throughout the conjunctival sac, and at any time a faster turnover rate may result from ocular irritation, yawning, or emotional responses which lead to an increase in watery tear flow. The tearing that occurs from painful stimuli can wash substances out of the conjunctival sac within a minute (MAURICE 1971). On the other hand, tear flow is heavily suppressed during general anesthesia (KRUPIN et al. 1977) in humans and is lowered by local anesthesia in rabbits (PATTON and ROBINSON 1975). According to MURAI (1976), the turnover rate drops by about one-half when the eyes are closed.

Framing the palpebral aperture are the marginal tear strips, capillary columns of fluid which fill the angle between the lid margins and the cornea and conjunctiva and cover the punctae in the human eye. Freshly secreted tears run down the inner surface of the upper lid into the superior tear strip and flow around the eye, emptying through the punctae into the nose. Between the marginal tear strips and the precorneal tear film, and most probably extending also over the scleral regions, there is a line where a thinning of the watery layer occurs (McDONALD and BRUBAKER 1971). This line, which moves with the lids, forms a barrier to diffusion, as can be shown by injecting fluorescein through a fine cannula directly into the tear strip, where it remains without spreading onto the corneal surface if the lids do not move.

When the eye is open and the lids are still, the lacrimal fluid is divided into three separate compartments: a stagnant layer covering the exposed cornea and conjunctiva; a layer moistening the conjunctiva under the lids, mostly stagnant but in humans providing a passage for tears in the upper fornix; and the marginal tear strips along which the tear flow occurs (MAURICE 1973, 1980). Mixing between the three compartments occurs during a blink, and a substance dissolved in the precorneal film is redistributed at this time. In the absence of blinking, the precorneal film is not replaced, and its exchanges with the underlying tissue continue in isolation. This may contribute to a difference in the penetration of a drug between the rabbit and the human because of their very different rates of blinking.

In the rabbit, PATTON and ROBINSON (1975) estimated the average flow rate of tears to be 0.66 µl min^{-1}, and LONGWELL et al. (1976), who directly cannulated the drainage duct, found a value of 0.78 µl min^{-1}. Since the total volume of lacrimal fluid is 7.5 µl, this flow rate should lead to a loss constant of 6 h^{-1} for substances dissolved in the tears, and a figure of 5 h^{-1} for technetium loss was determined experimentally by CHRAI et al. (1973). The turnover rates in rabbits and humans are on average very much the same, therefore. Considerably larger values are found in the stimulated eye (SIEG and ROBINSON 1977) or on deviations from physiological pH (CONRAD et al. 1978), but the flow returns to baseline after topical anesthesia (PATTON and ROBINSON 1975). The position of the animal's head, when it is under anesthesia, has a noticeable effect on drainage (SIEG and ROBINSON 1974).

b) Contact with Ocular Surface

The quantity of drug crossing into the cornea or conjunctiva is determined by the area under the curve that relates its concentration in the tear film to the time; this area is the precise definition of what is commonly known as contact time. Under natural conditions the area is largely a function of the total volume of tear fluid moistening the area and of the rate at which fresh fluid is secreted and drained. In clinical practice, the time a drug dwells in the tears can be modified by a variety of techniques, which may be as simple as increasing the viscosity of an eye drop or may employ highly engineered devices. Although contact time can be modified in this way, it is difficult to control absolutely because of the variation in tear flow rates of different patients.

The sequence of events that follows the topical instillation of a single watery drop is not simple, nor is it fully understood. The size of a drop is nominally 50 µl, but such a volume cannot be retained between the eyelids, and a large fraction of it will run onto the cheek according to the position of the head and the force of the blink reflex in response to instillation. The excess volume of 10–20 µl that remains on the eye is rapidly removed by the drainage system, which pumps out about 2 µl on each blink. During these blinks the drug dissolved in the instilled fluid is mixed to some extent with the tear fluid in the conjunctival fornices; it becomes diluted in the process, so that the concentration arrived at in the tear film when the excess fluid has drained off averages about one-third that of the original drop (SUGAYA and NAGATAKI 1978), but this value is quite variable. During and

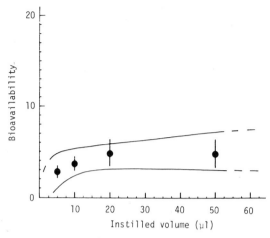

Fig. 2. The bioavailability of pilocarpine after instillation of various volumes of 0.5% solution into the eyes of five subjects. The bioavailability was determined from the pupil response, which was well below its maximum. (SUGAYA and NAGATAKI 1978)

after this initial mixing (CHRAI et al. 1973), the drug concentration is constantly reduced by the normal secretion and drainage of tears and by absorption across the conjunctival surface, and it undergoes a continual decline in a more or less exponential manner, as seen with fluorescein. In the case of certain drugs, some authors (RIDLEY 1958; SIDIKARO and JONES 1981) have noted a slowing up of the rate of loss after the concentration has dropped to a low level. This slowed loss may occur because drug initially dissolved in the conjunctival epithelium is returned to the tear film.

Some drugs cause unpleasant side effects elsewhere in the body after absorption across the mucous membranes of the eye and nose, and it is beneficial to reduce the amount instilled. From the preceding paragraph, it can be concluded that above a certain volume the size of the drop is unimportant, since the excess spills harmlessly but wastefully onto the skin, where most will be wiped away. Below this there is a range where the efficacy falls as the drop volume rises because the excess fluid is drained off and absorbed from the nasolacrimal passages without having had appreciable contact with the cornea. Both in the rabbit (PATTON 1977) and human (SUGAYA and NAGATAKI 1978) eye it has been found that increasing the size of a pilocarpine drop above about 20 µl does not lead to a greater penetration, and that a 5 µl drop exhibits about one-half the maximum efficacy (Fig. 2).

Various mechanical maneuvers have been proposed to delay the drainage of an instilled drop out of the eye so that the intraocular concentration can be increased, or prolonged at an effective level. Obstructing the tear outflow pathway or pulling out the lower lid for a period of time have been advocated in order to increase the penetration. Since the concentration of a drug in the tear film only falls 10% in a minute, on average, these manipulations would have to be continued for several minutes to create a worthwhile effect if they acted only to delay the washout, and it is more probable that their action is to increase the initial saturation of the film. Since this could only increase penetration of a drug two or three times, the simpler alternative of repeating the instillation once or twice at 10-min intervals should be considered, unless systemic toxicity is a danger.

A distinction needs to be made between techniques intended to cause a raised concentration of drug in the eye at the time of instillation – pulsed delivery – and those designed to extend the time for which an effective concentration remains in the eye – sustained delivery. It is evident that increasing the peak concentration by a pulsed delivery system will inevitably lead to an extension of the time any lesser concentration is present. Although this may be valuable therapeutically, it does not constitute true sustained delivery, and for many drugs the therapeutic index is not wide enough for it to be employed. Moreover, it is a poor way to prolong drug levels, since for each doubling of the aqueous humor level, the extension in time will only be about 1 h in most cases. It will be demonstrated later (Sect. B.II.3.c) that, unless a maneuver slows the rate of loss of drug from the tears very considerably, the effect on the time course of the drug in the anterior segment is not significantly affected and the device may be considered a pulsed delivery system.

A sustained delivery device with an exponential decline in the rate of drug release would have to be replaced within one or two half-lives in order not to cause excessive concentration swings within the eye. Even if it were replaced after one half-life, only 50% of the material in the device would be wasted at the expense of a 2:1 swing in concentration. These figures seem acceptable if compared to the performance of single drops.

The limiting form of sustained delivery is continuous delivery, in which a constant concentration of drugs is maintained in the tear film. These systems have been reviewed by SHELL (1982), and two types have been produced. In the first, a solution of drug is constantly run into the conjunctival sac by means of a tube connected to a reservoir and pump. The second is the Ocusert, a solid device which is inserted in the conjunctival sac. The device contains an inner wafer saturated with the drug, and this is sandwiched between two membranes, whose porosity is designed to allow the drug to leach out slowly. In this way a precise and constant delivery of pilocarpine to the tear film over a period of a week may be assured.

The addition of a polymer to increase the viscosity of a drop has been shown to augment the action of drugs both in humans and rabbits. Studies with fluorescein show that the increase in penetration that can be achieved is limited to 50%–100%, and that this maximum rise can be achieved with solutions which are only slightly viscous (ADLER et al. 1971; PATTON and ROBINSON 1975). Most probably this is a result of greater initial saturation of the tear film, not a slower rate of washout (ADLER et al. 1971; SUGAYA and NAGATAKI 1978).

Ointments, either simple, where the drug is dissolved or suspended in an oil or grease, or compound, where it is incorporated in a biphasic dispersion of water in oil or oil in water, are also used in order to increase drug penetration. They are undoubtedly able to effect a manifold increase in the action of a drug and also to prolong it, especially if the eyelids are held closed after instillation. They probably create a reservoir of drug, particularly if it is fat-soluble, which is only slowly blinked away. The mechanics and the kinetics of the process are likely to differ considerably between man and rabbit. A thorough discussion of the behavior of multiphase preparations in the eye has been given by SIEG and ROBINSON (1975, 1977). They experimented in the rabbit, and some question must remain about how far their conclusions can be applied to humans. In the case of fluorometholone crystals, profiles of the aqueous humor drug concentration were similar whether the crystals were suspended in water or in ointment, as long as the drug was in excess. The tear film was probably saturated by microcrystals of the undissolved drug. This conclusion would also apply to results with chloramphenicol (HONEGGER 1961), which penetrated to the same extent whether given as a crystalline suspension in grease or dissolved in grease by means of an emulsifier. SIEG and ROBINSON (1977) also studied pilocarpine as a water-in-oil emulsion, in which the drug is dissolved in the aqueous phase. Penetration of the cornea was the same whether its epithelium was intact or abraded, and it was concluded that availability of the drug was limited by the area of free surface between the ointment and the tear film. A similar effect occurs with a suspension of dexamethasone acetate (LEIBOWITZ et al. 1978). This hypothesis should be investigated in humans with test substances which are less lipid-soluble and less pharmacologically active.

2. Corneal Penetration

a) Barriers

The cornea may be treated as a three-layered structure consisting of a sheet of connective tissue, the stroma, covered on both surfaces with cellular layers. On the external surface is the multilayered epithelium, and on the inside is the endothelium, a single sheet of cells. The outer, squamous, cells of the epithelium are joined by tight junctions that create an extremely resistant barrier to the passage of lipophobic solutes such as fluorescein. When the tear film or the stroma is intensely stained with this dye, the epithelial cells show no fluorescence on examination with the slit lamp, so that it probably penetrates to the anterior chamber by way of the paracellular spaces (KAISER and MAURICE 1964). That the permeabilities to positive and negative ions are similar suggests the same conclusion (KLYCE 1975). There is a negative potential of about 30 mV on the surface of the rabbit cornea, developed as a result of ion transport. This would have only a minor effect on the penetration of ionized materials from the tear film, and it is not present on the human eye.

When a solute is lipid-soluble, its rate of penetration across the epithelium increases. Most drugs used in ophthalmology are in this class, undoubtedly as a result of a process similar to natural selection; if they were not lipophilic they would not have penetrated the cornea sufficiently to exhibit any therapeutic activity.

The permeability of the corneal endothelium of the rabbit has been studied in greater detail than that of the epithelium, and its value has been determined for a number of small ions and lipophobic solutes. The permeabilities found, both in vivo and in vitro, agree in falling on a monotonic curve (MAURICE, to be published a), where the value depends almost entirely on the molecular weight of the solute and is independent of its charge. Drugs which exhibit lipid solubility may be expected to pass across the cell layer more rapidly, as they do the epithelium, and some metabolites, notably glucose, cross at an accelerated rate by a process of facilitated transfer (HALE and MAURICE 1969). The endothelium is a low-resistance barrier, and for small ions its permeability is about 200 times greater than that of the epithelium; this disproportion increases for larger solutes. The behavior of the endothelial layer suggests that hydrophilic materials permeate principally by way of the paracellular spaces, and this hypothesis is reinforced by the finding that the action of cold increases its resistance to the diffusion of small ions in proportion to the increase in the viscosity of water (MAURICE 1969).

The stroma of the cornea has a tendency to swell, which results in aqueous humor being sucked into the tissue across the endothelial layer. This fluid is pumped out by an active mechanism resident in the endothelial cells. However, solutes diffuse across the cell layer so freely that their passage in either direction is not appreciably affected by the active or passive flux of water.

The corneal stroma is made up of several hundred lamellae composed of collagen fibrils embedded in a ground substance largely consisting of glycosaminoglycan chains which bear numerous negative charges along their length. This is a comparatively open structure which allows diffusion of all solutes below a certain molecular size; this cut-off point corresponds to a molecular weight of 500,000 in the normal stroma, but for larger molecules there may be diffusion when the stroma is edematous. The rate of diffusion is about two and a half times slower than in free solution for the smallest solutes, and about ten times slower for a protein of the size of albumin.

b) Compartments

The human cornea is on average 0.52 ± 0.04 (SD) mm thick in the center but more toward its edges; it is 11 mm in diameter, and it weighs about 70 mg. In the rabbit the thickness is uniform over the surface, and it increases with age, ranging from 0.35 mm to 0.45 mm. Its weight is of the order of 80 mg, and the ratio of this to that of the aqueous humor is 0.29 (MAURICE 1955).

The stroma occupies about 90% of the corneal thickness and is the principal reservoir for hydrophilic drugs dissolved in the tissue. Virtually all the water in this tissue is available as a solvent for molecules of small size (MAURICE 1970). There is evidence that some solutes bind to the tissue, probably as a result of its negative charge, and this shows up for small ions as a relative surplus of Na. Fluorescein, although it bears an overall negative charge, has also been shown to bind to the stroma. In vivo experiments indicate that its equilibrium concentration ratio between tissue and aqueous humor is of the order of 1.7 both in human (JONES and MAURICE 1966; SAWA et al. 1981) and rabbit eyes (OTA et al. 1974). However, the binding is loose in this case and does not introduce any notable nonlinearities into the kinetics. It can be considered as reducing the effective concentration of dye in the stroma, or as giving rise to an increase in the apparent volume of the tissue.

The epithelial water is probably not accessible to lipid-insoluble drugs, but when they are lipid-soluble, as in the case of pilocarpine (SIEG and ROBINSON 1976), they can enter the cell layer, which becomes an alternative reservoir. The high concentration of such drugs suggests they are not restricted to the lipid membranes but are also dissolved in the cytosol; their distribution and dynamics have been little investigated, however. The endothelium, only 3 μm thick, can be ignored as a reservoir for solutes. The stroma is populated by numerous keratocytes, which have a total volume about one-half that of the epithelium, and these might also be expected to act as a reservoir for lipophilic drugs. No experiments have been done to test this possibility, however, and no data have been published that suggest that it is important.

c) Drug Chemistry

It is well established that as the lipid solubility of solutes increases the more easily they penetrate cell membranes. The same is true for penetration across cellular layers, and the effect is more marked in those epithelia which show a very high resistance to the passage of lipophobic substances.

SWAN and WHITE (1942) showed that naphthylamine readily penetrates across the epithelium and, in fact, the resistance of the cell layer appeared to be negligible, since the amount of amine entering the stroma was not affected after scraping it off. The substitution of further ionized groups, particularly sulfonic acid, reduced the lipid solubility of the molecule, and successively lowered the epithelial permeability. A substituted phenyl ring traversed the epithelium 100 times more slowly than the corresponding substituted naphthalene compound, showing that molecular size was not a decisive factor in determining the rate at which such compounds penetrate cell membranes. The relative permeability of the cornea to a series of carbonic anhydrase inhibitors showed a strong correlation with lipid solubility (see Fig. 3).

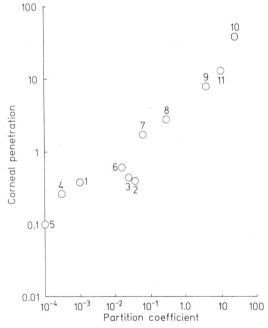

Fig. 3. Relation of penetration of a drug across the cornea to its chloroform/pH 7.2 buffer partition coefficient for a series of carbonic anhydrase inhibitors: *1*, acetazolamide; *2*, 2-isopentenylamino-1,3,4-thiadiazole-5-sulfonamide; *3*, 2-benzoylamino-1,3,4-thiadiazole-5-sulfonamide; *4*, bromacetazolamide; *5*, benzolamide; *6*, 5-imino-4-methyl-Δ-1,3,4-thiadiazole-2-sulfonamide; *7*, methazolamide; *8*, trifluormethazolamide; *9*, trichlormethazolamide; *10*, ethoxzolamide; *11*, chlorzolamide (CL-13 580). (MAREN et al. 1983)

Substances that pass completely freely across the cell layers will still encounter a barrier in the cornea corresponding to the diffusional resistance of the stroma. As will be discussed later (Sect. B.II.2.d), for those which have a molecular weight comparable to that of fluorescein (330), the limiting permeability of the cornea is of the order of 0.1 cm h^{-1}.

Several biological effects of a solute, including its cell membrane permeability, undergo a rise and then a fall as its partition coefficient between an organic solvent and water increases; this relationship approximates to being parabolic (HANSCH and CLAYTON 1973; FLYNN and YALKOWSKY 1972). Correspondingly, an increase in permeability of the cornea followed by a drop has been reported in the case of N-alkyl p-aminobenzoate esters (MOSHER and MIKKELSON 1979), steroids (SCHOENWALD and WARD 1978), and substituted anilines (KISHIDA and OTORI 1980) as the partition coefficient of the congener increases. All these substances penetrate the cornea readily, and the maximum permeability values in each group correspond to that of the stroma alone, showing that the epithelium becomes a negligible barrier. Although the studies showed penetration was linear with time, in no case was it determined that it was linear with applied concentration, so that the results should be interpreted with caution. Since this is likely to be an important area of investigation in ocular pharmacokinetics, it may be noted that, apart from linearity, it is also desirable to check with an inert tracer that the epithelium is undamaged either by the agent being studied at the concentration employed or by other experimental procedures.

Many drugs are weak acids or bases whose degree of ionization and hence their lipid solubility is considerably affected by pH. Changes in the pH of the conjunctival sac are not fully neutralized for about 30 min (LONGWELL et al. 1976), so that the reaction of the instilled eye drop can have a prolonged influence on the ionization of the drug in the tear film. SWAN and WHITE (1942) showed that the penetration of procaine increases more than tenfold on changing its reaction from pH 7 to 9.5, and that this range corresponds to the conversion of the fully ionized base to its undissociated form. Similar results were obtained by COGAN and HIRSCH (1944) for various weak bases and alkaloids, and they have been confirmed by several workers, e.g., BOBERG-ANS et al. (1959) and CONRAD et al. (1978). However, other factors, such as drug stability and irritation to the eye, are generally considered more important than corneal permeability in adjusting the reaction of eye drops (HIND and GOYAN 1947; RIEGELMAN and VAUGHAN 1958).

It is often stated that a drug must be in an associated form to penetrate the epithelium and must dissociate into an ionized form to diffuse across the stroma. This statement requires interpretation; once in solution in the stromal tissue fluid, diffusion will occur whether the molecule bears a charge or not. However, movement from the cell layer into the aqueous phase will certainly be assisted if the drug can assume a hydrophilic form.

d) Concentration

α) *Linearity.* The amount of drug crossing the cornea is generally assumed to be proportional to the concentration in the tear film, but there is very little evidence bearing on this point. In the case of the Na ion, this proportionality was found to be true on the concentration being changed over a range of 50–1,500 mEq/l (MAURICE 1955). The penetration of tritiated pilocarpine has been reported to be linear over the range $10^{-6} - 10^{-1}$ M (CHRAI and ROBINSON 1974).

On the other hand, the curve relating the flux of procaine to concentration is very nonlinear; saturation is seen at a concentration of about 50 mM, and signs of nonlinearity are shown at one-tenth of that (SWAN and WHITE 1942). It is evident that the passage of a procaine molecule is blocked by the presence of high concentrations of others, and it is probable that the solubility of the drug in the cell membranes is limited and that saturation is restricting the permeability.

Experimental data for other drugs are confused by the absence of osmotic control (see below), but it may be expected that lipophobic solutes will exhibit linear behavior, while it can be suspected that lipophilic solutes may show some degree of nonlinearity.

β) *Osmotic Effects.* A further aspect of the drug concentration in an eye drop is the effect on its osmotic pressure. Because the tear film is very thin, it rapidly comes into osmotic equilibrium with the blood. If it is assumed that, after the introduction of a hyperosmotic drop, the excess fluid osmotically pulled across the conjunctiva is immediately drained away, so that the tear film does not thicken, the time constant of approach to equilibrium can be calculated to be $2 \sigma L_p C_d / q_d$, where L_p is the hydraulic conductivity of the conjunctiva, σ the reflection coefficient, C_d the concentration of ions in normal tear fluid, and q_d the tear film thickness. The values of σL_p for the corneal epithelium and endothelium are not very different (MISHIMA and HEDBYS 1967), and accepting an intermediate value for the conjunctival epithelium and taking the known value of 8 μm for q_d, a time constant of about 10 s is calculated. By labeling hypertonic drops with fluorescein, a complete dilution to isotonicity was found within 15 s by MAURICE (1971), and by collecting tears and measuring their tonicity, HOLLY and LAMBERTS (1981) arrived at a half-life of about 20 s for the approach to equilibrium.

Accordingly, if the concentration of a drug is increased so as to make its solution hypertonic, a very rapid dilution results when a drop is instilled, and the penetration is not raised above that of an isotonic solution. Hypotonic drops, on the other hand, should lose water to the conjunctiva until their tonicity is raised to that of the blood, and this may lead to a higher concentration in the tear film than would be anticipated. The changes in fluorescence of the tear film after a dilute fluorescein drop was instilled corresponded to this hypothesis (MAURICE 1971).

Most subjects feel some irritation from an eye drop which is twice as concentrated as a 0.9% saline solution (TROLLE-LASSEN 1958). On the other hand, a single drop which is ten times more concentrated than normal saline, even though it stings the eye, does not stimulate a tear flow and so cause drug to be flushed out of the eye (MAURICE 1971).

e) Iontophoresis

It is hardly necessary to point out that for iontophoresis to be effective the drug must be in an ionized form and the polarity of the electrode must be such as to drive the ions into the tissue. The current will be shared among any ions that are present, so that the presence of any ionized material other than the drug lowers its effectiveness. In any case, most of the current will be carried by a small ion of the opposite charge, Na or Cl, emerging from the tissue.

This technique would be most valuable for drugs such as gentamicin, which are not lipid-soluble and penetrate the epithelium with great difficulty. In the case of a large ion, the passage of a current of 1 mA/cm^2 has been theoretically calculated to lead to an increase in the penetration of about 600 times over that which occurs by diffusion alone in the absence of the current (MAURICE, to be published b). Ratios of this order of magnitude have been reported for iodide (TRICHTEL and TRICHTEL 1959), fluorescein, and gentamicin (MAURICE, to be published b). For most drugs lower numbers are found, e.g., 40 times for penicillin (VON SALLMANN 1947), suggesting that they can penetrate by routes not accessible to ions.

3. Conjunctiva and Sclera

a) Conjunctiva

The conjunctiva is a membrane of connective tissue covered by a multilayered epithelium continuous with that of the cornea. Its total area is 16 cm^2 in the human eye (EHLERS 1965 b). In addition to epithelial cells it contains goblet cells, which secrete the tear film mucin, and some islands of accessory lacrimal glands. It is moderately vascularized and in its palpebral area overlies vascularized tissue. Its permeability has not been well studied but appears to be greater than that of the corneal epithelium (MAURICE 1973), so that an appreciable loss of drugs from the tear fluid could take place across it. LEE and ROBINSON (1979) calculated that the loss of pilocarpine by absorption was similar to the loss by tear drainage in the rabbit, and this proportion would be similar for salicylate in humans, according to the results of Schirmer (MAURICE 1973).

The conjunctival epithelium, like that of the cornea, can form a reservoir for lipid-soluble drugs (SENDELBECK et al. 1975; HAMARD et al. 1975), and may be expected to return them to the tear film once the level in it has dropped as a result of drainage. The nictitating membrane in rabbits absorbs a quantity of drug that is significant compared to that in the conjunctiva (LEE and ROBINSON 1979; HAMARD et al. 1975).

Topically applied drugs making contact with the eye outside the corneal limbus encounter two obstacles: the first is the barrier to diffusion offered by the conjunctival epithelium, and the second is the loss to the blood before the drug has the opportunity to continue its penetration into the deeper tissue. The drug that enters the bloodstream is joined by that which later crosses the mucous membranes of the nasal lacrimal duct or mouth or passes across the stomach epithelium, and behaves as if it were injected systemically.

b) Sclera

The sclera is a layer of connective tissue varying in thickness from 1 mm at the posterior pole to 0.3 mm under the insertion of the muscles in the human eye. It is perforated by numerous holes which carry the veins and arteries to the uvea and retina, but is itself very poorly vascularized. BILL (1965) found that serum albumin or red dextran (molecular weight 40,000) injected suprachoroidally in the living rabbit will penetrate into the tissue. In vitro experiments on the anterior beef sclera showed that most solutes, including large-molecular-weight proteins but excluding some anionic dyes, diffused across the tissue but rather more slowly than in the corneal stroma. The drugs penicillin and hydrocortisone moved across at approximately the same rate, and their diffusion constant in the tissue was of the order of 2×10^{-3} cm^2 h^{-1}, about 12 times slower than in free solution, while the restriction on the movement of pilocarpine was somewhat less (MAURICE and POLGAR 1977).

4. Intraocular Structures

a) Anterior and Posterior Chambers

The aqueous humor is contained in two cavities of unequal volume, the anterior and posterior chambers. The anterior chamber volume in man decreases with age as a result of the continued growth of the lens, and falls from about 0.25 ml in youth to 0.1 ml in old age; a representative value of 0.2 ml will be adopted in this chapter. The anterior chambers of young laboratory rabbits have a volume of about 0.25 ml, and they increase to about 0.3 ml with maturity; their posterior chamber volume is 0.055 ml.

Fresh aqueous humor is continuously secreted by the ciliary processes into the posterior chamber and flows in bulk into the anterior chamber through the pupil. It then drains out of the eye through either the conventional or the unconventional channels. By the conventional route the fluid passes into the veins through a porous system situated in the angle between the iris and the cornea. The unconventional route consists of tissue spaces in the iris root and loose connective tissue between the ciliary muscles and the suprachoroid, from where the aqueous humor flows through the sclera to the extraocular connective tissue (BILL 1971). The aqueous flow through the unconventional route was estimated to be 4%–14% of the total in the human eye (BILL and PHILLIPS 1971), but in the rabbit and cat it is almost negligible (BILL 1971).

The rate of aqueous outflow through the conventional route is proportional to the difference between the pressure in the anterior chamber and that in the veins (GOLDMANN 1951). With a steady intraocular pressure, the rate of aqueous formation is equal to the rate of aqueous drainage through the two main outflow routes.

b) Iris

The iris, a mobile diaphragm separating the anterior and posterior chambers, is formed of a connective tissue stroma covered by two layers of epithelium on the posterior surface. The stroma is built up of collagen fibers arranged in a cross-network to allow for extensive movement (ROHEN 1961), and is densely populated with melanocytes and fibroblasts. The tissue is porous, and macromolecules dissolved in it freely communicate with the aqueous humor across its anterior surface (GREGERSEN 1958; SMELSER and ISHIKAWA 1962). Thus the iris stroma may be regarded as a part of the anterior chamber compartment from the point of view of pharmacokinetics. However, the iris pigments absorb various drugs, modifying their distribution in the eye and their kinetics; this has been reviewed by Mishima (1981).

Hogan et al. (1971) and Raviola (1977) have reviewed the ultrastructural basis of the anterior segment barriers. The endothelial cells of the iris capillaries have no fenestrae and are connected by discontinuous macula occludens. Electron-dense markers injected intravenously are held within the vessel lumen, but solutes of small molecular weight can probably escape between the cells (Cunha-Vaz et al. 1966; Bellhorn 1980). The rate at which the transfer occurs depends on species and age (Szalay et al. 1975) as well as the molecular size of the solute. Dyes are used for these observations, and their passage could be missed because of dilution in the stromal fluid and aqueous humor. The diffusion of fluorescein into the anterior chamber from the iris surface has been observed in vivo (Maurice 1967a) when the thermal circulation of the aqueous humor is suppressed. The reverse movement, into the vessels from the anterior chamber, has been directly noted by freeze-drying the eye (Sherman et al. 1978). Since the aqueous freely communicates with the porous iris stroma, drugs entering the anterior chamber have ready access to the iris vessels and can be lost by passage into the blood.

The sphincter pupillae muscles run circularly around the pupil near the pupillary border, and the dilator muscles, which are modified cells of the inner layer of the iris epithelium, run radially in the most posterior layer of the stroma. The former muscles are supplied mainly by cholinergic nerves and the latter mainly by adrenergic nerves with predominantly α-receptors. Abundant varicose adrenergic nerve fibers are present in the iris and take up exogenously administered catecholamines (Kramer and Potts 1969; Bhattacherjee 1971), modifying the pharmacokinetics of these drugs.

c) Ciliary Body

The ciliary body is divided into two parts: in front, the pars plicata, consisting of about 70 ciliary processes which project into the posterior chamber, and behind, the relatively flat pars plana, which borders on the anterior vitreous body. The outer part of the ciliary body is composed largely of the ciliary muscles, whose bundles of fibers are separated by loose connective tissue. The inner surface is lined by an epithelium formed by two layers of cells, the outer pigmented and the inner nonpigmented, and the latter is believed to be the main site of aqueous humor secretion. Its cells are interconnected on their apical side by a zonula occludens, which forms a tight barrier (Raviola and Raviola 1978).

The ciliary processes are filled with a connective tissue stroma which has a rich vascular supply. In the rabbit, the capillaries have a total surface area of about 7.7 cm^2, comparable to that of the ciliary processes themselves (Baurmann 1930). The blood flow is very high, about 2 ml min^{-1} g^{-1} tissue in the monkey (Alm et al. 1973). The capillary endothelium is characterized by abundant fenestrae and the junctional complexes are discontinuous (Hirsch et al. 1978). Various electron-dense markers injected intravenously appear quickly in the stroma of the ciliary processes, as well as in the spaces between the pigmented cells and those between the pigmented and nonpigmented cells. The further movement of these substances is stopped at the zonulae occludentes connecting the nonpigmented epithelial cells. Due to the leaky nature of the capillaries, the ciliary process stroma has a high protein content, about 70% of that in the serum, and its turnover rate is high (BILL 1968).

Intravenously injected tracers move from the ciliary processes through the iris root into the anterior chamber (VEGGE et al. 1976). Determination of the protein fractions in the anterior chamber aqueous (DERNOUCHAMPS and HERMANS 1975) lead to an estimate of the pore radius of the blood–aqueous barrier of about 10 nm; this probably corresponds to the permeability of the capillaries of the ciliary processes. The capillaries in the ciliary muscle have thick walls, and their endothelial cells have no fenestrae and do not allow passage of electron-dense markers (RAVIOLA 1977).

d) Lens

The lens is an epithelial tissue in which the mass of the cells are elongated into fibers which lie parallel to each other in the cortex, forming layers which are wrapped around a central nucleus consisting of hard condensed cellular material. The fibers are closely packed, with narrow intercellular spaces which interdigitate in places. They are connected by gap junctions which are mostly in a low resistance state (GOODENOUGH 1979). The anterior surface is lined with cuboidal epithelium whose cells are attached to each other with a zonula occludens. The tissue is enclosed by the capsule, an elastic layer permeable to macromolecules, analogous to the basement membrane of the epithelium.

Most tissues in the eye are thin and bathed on either side by constantly renewed fluids, so that drug absorbed from these fluids will be returned to them with little delay. The lens, on the other hand, is a solid mass of cells, so that solutes that penetrate it from the vitreous body or aqueous humor are not washed out readily but slowly diffuse through the whole mass. The movement of the ionic procion dyes through the lens cortex has been observed on the microscopic scale by RAE (1974). Dye in the extracellular space will diffuse through this space without entering fibers. When it is injected into a fiber, it will move into neighboring fibers, presumably through the specialized junctions in the cell membranes. The diffusion of fluorescein in mass has been followed, and the rate of penetration across the epithelial surface as well as that of diffusion in the lens cortex has been established (KAISER and MAURICE 1964). The dye spreads laterally in the cortex more rapidly than it penetrates, and it forms a colored shell beneath the surface of the tissue. The behavior of rhodamine B, a lipid-soluble dye, has also been directly observed (COUSINS et al., to be published), and it appears to be similar to that of fluorescein. Some of the dye that enters the lens diffuses out again and can be calculated to be the major source of solutes in the anterior chamber 2 days after topical application. Because substances can spread around the lens parallel to its surfaces, the tissue could act as an exchange pathway between the vitreous body and the anterior chamber.

5. Metabolism of Drugs During Intraocular Penetration

Some drugs are broken down by the tissues during intraocular penetration, and not only the original compounds but also the metabolites appear in the anterior chamber. This process generally results in a loss of activity of the drug, but attempts have been made to exploit it in the case of prodrugs, where the breakdown product is designed to have superior qualities to the parent compound.

It is difficult to provide a theoretical treatment of how the intraocular kinetics are affected by this metabolic activity. A slow breakdown of the drug might be taken account of by an additional negative exponential term but, in general, accurate information as to where and how fast it is taking place would be necessary (Rowland and Tozer 1980).

a) Breakdown of Drugs

Pilocarpine is inactivated by the tissues of the anterior segment of the eye (Schonberg and Ellis 1969), and although part of this may be due to reversible binding of the drug to the tissues (Newsome and Stern 1974), enzymatic hydrolysis is appreciable (Ellis et al. 1972). Sendelbeck et al. (1975) found, after instillation of pilocarpine in the rabbit eye, that about 40% of the material in the cornea and 75% of that in the anterior chamber were metabolites of pilocarpine, mainly pilocarpic acid. The rate constant of pilocarpine metabolism in the albino rabbit eye was estimated to be about 10^{-2} h^{-1} (Makoid and Robinson 1979), which is much less than its ocular transfer coefficients, so that this metabolism is of minor significance in its kinetics. A considerably higher pilocarpine metabolism, of the order of 1 h^{-1} (Lee et al. 1980), is found in the cornea of the pigmented rabbit, which will contribute to the relative ineffectiveness of this drug in the pigmented compared to the albino animal.

Atropine esterase, inherited through an incompletely dominant trait (Ambache 1955), is present in the serum of a large proportion of rabbits, and lesser activities are found in the iris, ciliary body, and cornea (Miichi et al., to be published). The mydriatic response to atropine is significantly less in a rabbit with positive atropine esterase than one without the enzyme, indicating that this enzyme may have a significant effect on the ocular pharmacokinetics of the drug.

Catechol O-methyltransferase and monoamine oxidase activities are found in the iris-ciliary body of the rabbit eye (Waltmann and Sears 1964; Shanthaveerappa and Bourne 1964), and probably also in the cornea (Anderson et al. 1980). One to two hours after instillation of epinephrine its major metabolites are found in the anterior chamber (Anderson et al. 1980), but its inactivation occurs mainly by absorptive uptake to the adrenergic nerves abundantly present in the iris and ciliary body (Kramer et al. 1972; Bhattacherjee 1970).

Some antiviral drugs are particularly subject to metabolic breakdown, probably in the corneal epithelium. After instillation of 5-iodo-2′-deoxyuridine (IDU) into the rabbit eye, 2′-deoxyuridine and iodouracil appear in the anterior chamber, but this does not occur without the presence of the corneal epithelium (O'Brien and Edelhauser 1977). Similarly, adenine arabinoside is almost completely converted to hypoxanthine arabinoside (Pavan-Langston et al. 1973) in the presence of the corneal epithelium (O'Brien and Edelhauser 1977). On the other hand, trifluorothymidine penetrates the anterior chamber of the intact rabbit eye without significant alteration (O'Brien and Edelhauser 1977).

Several steroids are also subject to metabolism, and their metabolites can be recovered from the anterior chamber. While tetrahydrotriamcinolone penetrates the human eye virtually unaltered, triamcinolone is broken down to give two unidentified metabolites (SUGAR et al. 1972). Prednisolone acetate, dexamethasone, corticosterone, and fluorometholone are also metabolized. After topical application of cortisone acetate in the rabbit eye, cortisone and hydrocortisone are recovered from the anterior chamber (HAMASHIGE and POTTS 1955).

Fluorescein is not the inactive tracer it was once thought to be, and in the bloodstream it is quickly converted to the much less fluorescent glucuronide (CHEN et al. 1980). There is at present no evidence that the enzymes responsible are active in the tissues of the eye.

b) Prodrugs

A compound which is not necessarily potent itself but is metabolized in the tissue and releases an active product is called a "prodrug." An early example of such a material was penethamate, an ester of penicillin which is hydrolyzed in vivo. This was found, in rabbits, to penetrate the vitreous body readily from the blood, whereas penicillin does not (BLEEKER and MAAS 1958).

Dipivalyl epinephrine is hydrolyzed rapidly in the cornea, mainly in the epithelium, with a rate constant of about 0.26 min^{-1}, and its metabolite, epinephrine, is released into the anterior chamber (ANDERSON et al. 1980). By virtue of a high lipid solubility, dipivalyl epinephrine penetrates the cornea readily, and the permeability of the rabbit epithelium to this substance is about ten times greater than that of epinephrine in the rabbit (WEI et al. 1978) and 17 times greater in humans (MANDELL et al. 1978; MISHIMA 1981). In consequence, effects comparable to those of standard drops of epinephrine can be produced by much more dilute solutions of the prodrug. After breakdown of the prodrug in the eye, the released epinephrine appears to follow its own kinetics.

II. Compartmental Analysis

1. Compartmentation

Compartment theory has been widely used in pharmacokinetic analysis, but often lacks practical value when applied to more than the simplest systems. This has led some workers, such as SMOLEN (1973, 1978), to abandon it in favor of engineering control theory, a powerful technique which does not require models to be constructed but equally does not allow the specific mechanisms controlling drug transfer between the tissues to be identified. One problem associated with compartmental analysis is the need for curve stripping or equivalent forms of data fitting, which, if incautiously applied, can result in large errors in assessing exchanges between compartments or in misidentifying the compartments themselves (see Fig. 6).

On the other hand, when the compartments can be clearly identified and their apparent volumes and their transfer coefficients checked by in vivo or in vitro experiments, a valid model of the biological system can be constructed which is valuable for predicting how drug kinetics will alter if these parameters are changed. Experimental disagreement with the predictions of the model can be useful, furthermore, in stimulating investigation into the presence of previously unidentified compartments or of deviations from linear kinetics.

The eye has the advantage that its major compartments are visible in the living condition, so that by using fluorescent tracers the concentration and distribution

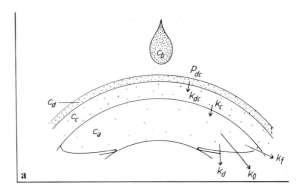

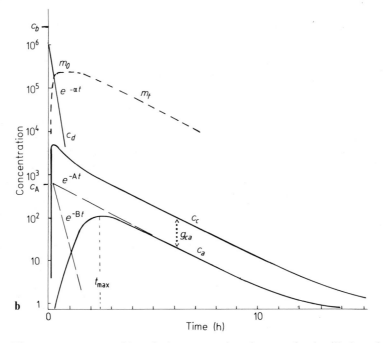

Fig. 4. a The compartments and **b** typical concentration changes after instillation of a drug into the eye. The drop, concentration C_b, is immediately diluted on instillation. The concentration in the tear film, C_d, then undergoes an exponential decline with a rate constant α. Drug transfer to the cornea, giving rise to a tissue concentration, C_c, is controlled by the permeability of the epithelium, P_{dc}, and described by a transfer coefficient, k_{dc}; it is complete in 10–20 min. The drug then crosses the endothelium to build up a concentration in the aqueous, C_a, and the exchange is described by a transfer coefficient, k_c. The aqueous concentration rises to a maximum at time t_{max}, and its profile is described by the apparent elimination and absorption coefficients, A and B. The corresponding exponential components intersect at a concentration C_A. For a period of time, the corneal and aqueous concentrations decline exponentially in parallel, their ratio being g_{ca}. Return of drug from reservoirs in the lens or elsewhere slows up the rate of fall when the aqueous concentration reaches a low value. k_d, coefficient of diffusional exchange; k_o, coefficient of loss; k_f, coefficient of outflow.

The *ordinate* is labeled in arbitrary units of concentration, and the total mass of drug in the eye, m_t, is shown on an unrelated arbitrary scale; m_o, mass of initial depot in the eye

of the dye within them may be continuously recorded without ambiguity. The compartmental models derived in this way can be applied with some confidence to that of drugs in the eye in general.

The principal compartments involved in the topical application of a drug are illustrated in Fig. 4, which also shows approximately how the concentrations will change within them. It can be noted that over appreciable periods of time the concentration in a compartment such as the tear film or cornea may run a simple exponential course. In some instances (see Sect. B.II.2), defining this exponential may provide sufficient information as to the kinetics of a drug. Generally, however, the kinetics in the anterior segment are controlled by two components, the cornea and aqueous humor, and to describe them adequately a two-compartment model is necessary.

2. Two-Compartment Model

a) Definition

In order to analyze the exchanges occurring within the eye after the topical administration of a drug, the complex system illustrated in Fig. 1 b is simplified to its more important components, shown in Fig. 5. This represents a two-compartment open system of conventional pharmacokinetics. The assumptions required to make it valid are that: (i) loss of drug to the tears from the cornea is negligible; (ii) entry into the aqueous humor from the tears other than through the cornea is negligible; (iii) exchanges between the cornea and blood at the limbus are unimportant; and (iv) exchanges of the aqueous humor with the posterior reservoir are negligible. The validity of assumptions (iii) and (iv) will be discussed later in this section; (ii) has already been considered; the truth of (i) follows from the low permeability of the epithelium to most substances.

The kinetics within the compartments are controlled by three coefficients shown in Fig. 5. In this, k_o is the transfer coefficient from the aqueous humor to the blood, which is defined by:

$$\frac{dC_a}{dt} = k_o(C_p r_{ap} - C_a), \tag{1}$$

where C_a and C_p are the concentrations in the aqueous humor and blood plasma and r_{ap} is the value of the ratio C_a/C_p at steady state.

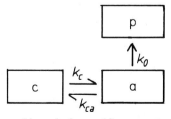

Fig. 5. The cornea (c), aqueous (a), and plasma (p) compartments, abstracted from Fig. 1b, that are used in the kinetic treatment of topical drug application. k_c and k_{ca} are transfer coefficients between the cornea and aqueous humor, and k_o is the loss coefficient from the aqueous to the plasma, which maintains zero concentration

The transfer coefficient k_c describes the exchange of a drug between the cornea and the aqueous humor and is referred to the volume of the cornea. It is defined by:

$$\frac{dC_c}{dt} = k_c(C_a r_{ca} - C_c), \tag{2}$$

where C_c, the corneal concentration, will be defined as the mass of drug in the entire cornea divided by the total volume of the tissue, V_c.

The transfer coefficient k_{ca} is also for exchange between the cornea and aqueous humor but is referred to the volume of the aqueous humor. It is related to k_c (an abbreviation of k_{ac}) by:

$$\frac{k_{ca}}{k_c} = \frac{V_c}{V_a} r_{ca}, \tag{3}$$

where V_a is the volume of the anterior chamber. The equilibrium ratio r_{ca} is the value of the ratio C_c/C_a when dC_c/dt is zero; if the drug is in simple solution in the stromal tissue fluid, the ratio will have a value of about 0.75; if it accumulates in the cornea, for example by reversible binding to the stroma or by solution in cell membranes, the ratio will be much larger than unity. The expression $r_{ca}V_c$ can be termed the apparent volume of the cornea. Since V_c and V_a are determined, only two of the parameters k_{ca}, k_c, and r_{ca} are independent; in the remainder of this chapter, k_c and r_{ca} will generally be used in formulating equations.

The time scale of most exchanges in the eye is of the order of hours, and the units of h^{-1} will be used for the transfer coefficients, since this brings their values conveniently into the range of whole numbers.

b) Concentration Changes

If a depot of drug is created in the cornea at zero time, and the concentration in the anterior chamber is initially zero, the simple model of Fig. 5 predicts (Jones and Maurice 1966) that the aqueous humor concentration will obey the equation:

$$C_a = C_A(e^{-At} - e^{-Bt}), \tag{4}$$

where C_A is a constant which depends on the initial loading of the cornea.

The corresponding equation for the cornea is:

$$C_c = \frac{C_A}{k_{ca}}\left\{(B - k_c)e^{-At} - (A - k_c)e^{-Bt}\right\} \tag{5}$$

and for the total mass of drug in the eye:

$$m_t = \frac{V_a C_A}{k_c}(Be^{-At} - Ae^{-Bt}). \tag{6}$$

If m_o is the mass of the initial depot in the eye:

$$m_o = \frac{V_c C_A}{k_c}(B - A) \tag{7}$$

and from Eq. (4):

$$C_a = \frac{m_o k_c}{V_a(B - A)}(e^{-At} - e^{-Bt}) \tag{8}$$

A and B, the apparent elimination and absorption coefficients (Fig. 4), are defined by:

$$A + B = k_c + k_{ca} + k_o \tag{9}$$

$$AB = k_c k_o. \tag{10}$$

The concentration of fluorescein in the human anterior chamber was shown to follow the double exponential form of Eq. (4) very closely after its introduction into the cornea by iontophoresis (Fig. 6), and the mass to obey Eq. (6) (JONES and MAURICE 1966). In reality, there is a delay in the rise in concentration of fluorescein in the anterior chamber as a result of the time taken for it to diffuse across the cornea. This may be accounted for by writing Eq. (4) in the form

$$C_a = C_A \left\{ e^{-A(t - t_0)} - e^{-B(t - t_0)} \right\}, \tag{11}$$

where t_o is the time lag. Equations (5) and (6) will be altered correspondingly.

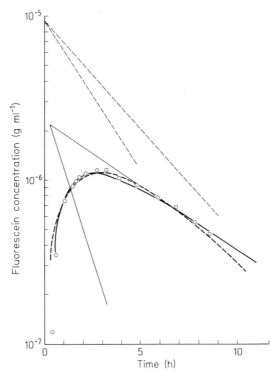

Fig. 6. The *points* represent measurements of fluorescein concentration in the anterior chamber of a human subject (RK from JONES and MAURICE 1966) after iontophoresis of fluorescein into the cornea at zero time. The *continuous curve through the points* was fitted in that paper according to the equation $C_a = C_A (e^{-At} - e^{-Bt})$, with elimination and absorption coefficients A and B of 0.18 h^{-1} and 0.84 h^{-1}, corresponding to the *two continuous straight lines* in the figure. The dangers of curve fitting over short periods of time are illustrated by an arbitrary pair of alternative values of A and B, 0.30 h^{-1} and 0.42 h^{-1}, which are indicated by the *dashed lines* and *curve*. This curve fits the points as well as the continuous line, and confirmation of the latter's validity came from measurements extended over 24 h

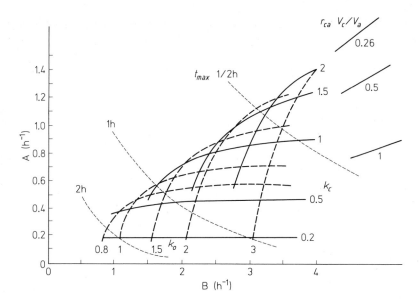

Fig. 7. The families of curves of k_o (loss coefficient from the aqueous to the plasma) *(dashed lines)* and k_c (transfer coefficient between the cornea and aqueous humor) *(continuous lines)* corresponding to experimental values of elimination and absorption coefficients A and B. The curves were calculated from Eqs. (7) and (8) using a value of $r_{ca} V_c/V_a$ applicable to the human eye. The time at which the concentration in the aqueous humor reaches its maximum, t_{max}, is also plotted from the equations; $t_{max} = ln (A/B)/(A-B)$. It will be noted that in general there are two pairs of values of k_c and k_o corresponding to each combination of A and B. Since k_o has a minimum value equal to k_f (coefficient of outflow; about 0.7 h^{-1}), there is a unique solution below the corresponding curve. The slope of the envelope to the curves is given by: $1 + 2r_{ca} V_c/V_a - 2 \{(r_{ca} V_c/V_a)^2 + r_{ca} V_c/V_a\}^{1/2}$. The value of 0.75 was assigned to r_{ca} on the assumption that the drug is in simple solution in the stromal tissue fluid. This value will increase if the drug is bound in the tissue or dissolved in the epithelium, and the slope will diminish, as shown

Because of the quadratic nature of the relationship expressed by Eqs. (3), (9), and (10), there are generally two alternative pairs of values of k_c and k_o corresponding to each pair of A and B (Fig. 7). There is also a limiting ratio of A to B that cannot be exceeded. The solution of the equations depends on the ratio r_{ca}, and the effect of increasing its value is indicated in Fig. 7. It is important to determine this value if there is any question whether the drug is not simply dissolved in the stromal water, and this will require measurements to be taken when an equilibrium has been set up between the cornea and aqueous humor, for example in experiments in which the drug is given systemically or the isolated cornea is perfused with the drug in solution.

In principle, values of both A and B can be obtained if the C_a curve is well defined. As is seen from Fig. 6, even when very smooth data points are available, it is necessary to continue the measurements for many hours before the coefficients can be established without ambiguity. Moreover, when the data points cannot be obtained noninvasively from a single subject but are assembled from separate samples of aqueous humor, their scatter is such that a very large number of experiments are needed to establish the coefficients, particularly B, to an acceptable accuracy. These experiments need to be carried out both at the early times, when C_a is rising, and later, when it is falling.

c) Cornea–Aqueous Transfer Relationship

Because B is always larger than A, Eqs. (5) and (6) predict that at a long time after the delivery of the drug both the aqueous and corneal concentrations should decline in a simple exponential manner with a rate coefficient of A. The logarithms of the two concentrations should plot as parallel straight lines as shown in Fig. 4. This behavior is observed in the case of fluorescein, and the parallel decline can be followed for almost two log cycles of concentration before the curves become nonlinear as a result of the return of the drug to the anterior chamber from the lens or iris (KAISER and MAURICE 1964). Many drugs follow the same pattern, although the nonlinearity may appear earlier.

A method of deriving k_o and k_c has been described (MAURICE 1980), where B is not necessary for the calculations but is replaced by g_{ca}, the ratio of C_c/C_a which holds during the parallel linear decline (Fig. 4). A mass balance for the anterior chamber can be described: $V_a dC_a/dt = - dm_c/dt - k_o C_a V_a$, where m_c is the mass of drug in the cornea.

Hence: $dC_a/C_a dt = - (m_c/C_a V_a)(dm_c/m_c dt) - k_o$.

During the period of parallel linear decline:

$$A = - \frac{dC_a}{C_a dt} = - \frac{dm_c}{m_c dt} = \frac{k_o}{1 + m_c/C_a V_a}.$$

Thus, remembering that $g_{ca} = C_c/C_a$:

$$k_o = A(1 + g_{ca} V_c/V_a). \qquad (12)$$

Thus the value of k_o can be derived from the slope A and the ratio g_{ca} without the ambiguity of an alternative solution; moreover, it is not necessary to know the value of r_{ca}. Figure 8 plots k_o as a function of A and g_{ca}.

Further, by dividing Eq. (2) by C_c we obtain:

$$\frac{dC_c}{C_c dt} = k_c \left(\frac{C_a}{C_c} r_{ca} - 1 \right) \cdot = A$$

Thus, when the concentrations in the aqueous and cornea are declining in parallel:

$$k_c = \frac{A}{1 - r_{ca}/g_{ca}}. \qquad (13)$$

Figure 8 also displays how k_c varies with A and g_{ca}, on the assumption that r_{ca} is 0.75, corresponding to simple solution of the drug in the stromal tissue fluid. It will be seen that when g_{ca} is large compared to r_{ca} its exact value will be unimportant, and k_c will approximate to A.

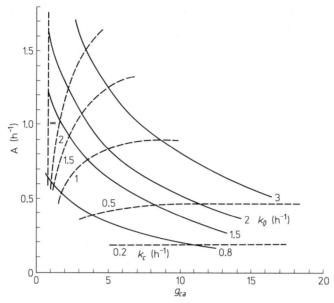

Fig. 8. Curves relating k_o (loss coefficient from aqueous to plasma) (*continuous lines*) and k_c (transfer coefficient between cornea and aqueous) (*dashed lines*) to A (elimination coefficient) and g_{ca} (ratio between corneal and aqueous concentrations), according to Eqs. (12) and (13). The calculations are made for the rabbit eye $V_c/V_a = 0.28$ on the assumption that $r_{ca} = 0.75$

It may be noted also that the restriction that the aqueous and corneal curves be parallel is not essential to the derivation of Eq. (13), so that the value of g_{ca} and the slope of $\ln C_c$ at any instant in time are sufficient to establish k_c. Equation (13) is analogous to Eq. (44) used in systemic drug dynamics.

d) Stroma-Controlled Exchange

As the lipid solubility of a drug increases, the barrier offered by the cellular layers drops. Ultimately, their resistance can become negligible compared to that of the stroma, and the rate of diffusion of the drug in this tissue will then be the controlling factor in determining corneal exchanges. Some transfer relationships are readily calculated under these conditions. Since the rate of diffusion of substances in the stroma seems to be primarily determined by their molecular size, it will be assumed for purposes of illustration that drugs have a diffusion constant D_s similar to that determined for fluorescein, 1×10^{-6} cm²/s (MAURICE 1960).

It is readily seen that the permeability of the cornea becomes $P_c = D_s/q_s$, where q_s is the stromal thickness. For the rabbit, where q_s is about 0.36 mm, P_c will be close to 0.1 cm h^{-1}.

The transfer coefficient between the cornea and aqueous humor will be a complicated function, but when approaching steady state it will be approximated by (CRANK 1975): $k_c = \pi^2 D_s/4q_s$, which has a value 7 h^{-1} for the rabbit. This will provide an upper limit for the rate at which a drug can leave the eye if the transfer out of the anterior chamber to the blood is instantaneous.

Finally, the lag time for diffusion across the stroma, obtained by extrapolating back to the time axis the curve showing the initial rise in aqueous humor concentration, will be approximated by the formula (CRANK 1975) $t_o = q_s/6D_s$, which for the human cornea leads to a value of 0.011 h. This is similar to the minimum values found for the time lag of pupil responses after the instillation of mydriatics (see Sect. B.II.5.c).

3. Tear Patterns

Although a drug can be introduced into the cornea in a matter of seconds, for example, by iontophoresis, more usually it penetrates from the tear fluid over a more extended period of time. As discussed earlier (Sect. B.I.1.b), the drug can be made to persist longer in the eye if its loss from the tears is delayed by means of a device. This situation requires a modification to Eqs. (4) and (5). Only two tear concentration profiles need to be considered. One is continuous delivery, where the concentration is constant, and the other is first-order kinetics, where the concentration drops off exponentially with time.

a) Zero Order

If a constant tear film concentration, $\bar{C}_d$, is maintained over a prolonged period, a steady state will by created in the tissues of the eye. According to the two-compartment model with a low epithelial permeability, P_{dc}, the steady-state aqueous humor concentration, $\bar{C}_a$, is given by:

$$\bar{C}_a = \frac{\bar{C}_d Q_c P_{dc}}{V_a k_o},\tag{14}$$

where Q_c is the corneal surface area. The rise to the steady-state value follows the equation

$$C_a = \bar{C}_a \left(1 + \frac{B}{A-B} e^{-At} - \frac{A}{A-B} e^{-Bt}\right).\tag{15}$$

The steady-state corneal concentration is given by:

$$\bar{C}_c = \bar{C}_a \frac{k_{ca} + k_o}{k_{ca}},\tag{16}$$

where k_{ca} is the aqueous-cornea transfer coefficient referred to the aqueous volume.

b) Area Under Curve

The contact time between the drug instilled in a drop and the corneal surface can be expressed as the area, U_d, under the curve relating tear film concentration to time, so that

$$U_d = \int_0^\infty C_d dt.$$

If fresh tears are formed at a constant flow rate, f_d, and they are well mixed with the tear volume, V_d, resident in the conjunctival sac, then α, the turnover rate of solutes in the conjunctival area, will be given by:

$$\alpha = \frac{f_d}{V_d}.$$

(17)

If a concentration C_o is originally established in the tear film, U_d is given by:

$$U_d = \int_0^\infty C_o e^{-\alpha t} dt$$

$$= \frac{C_o}{\alpha}.$$

(18)

If a small quantity of drug, dm_d, is released by a device into the conjunctival sac, it will give rise to concentration dm_d/V_d. The value of U_d resulting from this increment of drug is therefore given by $dU_d = dm_d/\alpha V_d$, so that

$$U_d = \frac{m_d}{f_d}.$$

(19)

Thus the area under the curve is not dependent on how the drug is scheduled to leave the device but only on the total amount released, m_d; this is known as Dost's principle (Gladtke and von Hattingberg 1979). As long as m_d does not change, U_d should not be affected if the equivalent tear volume, V_d, is artificially increased, as when a soft contact lens is inserted in the eye. However, such an increase will cause a fall in α, as shown by Eq. (17).

Hull et al. (1974 b) found that instilling a drop of prednisolone phosphate into a rabbit eye carrying a soft lens gave rise to the same concentration inside the eye after 4 h as that found in a normal eye, in accordance with the expectation above. On the contrary, Asseff et al. (1973) found that about three times more pilocarpine entered the eye from a soft contact lens than from the same amount of drug applied as a 5 μl drop of 8% solution. One reason why the drop was less effective may be that the excess volume of fluid was blinked away before the drug had a chance to mix into the tear film.

c) Pulsed and Sustained Delivery

An exponential decline in tear film concentration is soon established after a drop is instilled into the eye or a simple insert is used to deliver the drug. As pointed out in the previous section, the U_d for a given mass of drug should not be affected by the use of a delivery device, but by delaying its release the concentration profile in the ocular tissues can be altered. A device will generally deliver a greater quantity of drug to the eye than a drop, but if the release time is short compared to the elimination coefficient, A, it will not affect the intraocular kinetics. This is defined as pulse delivery.

The effect on the aqueous humor concentration profile of changing the loss coefficient from the tears, α, while keeping the initial tear film concentration constant is shown in Fig. 9. In the domain of pulse delivery, there is a linear relationship between C_a and $1/\alpha$. As the release time is prolonged, a point is reached where the concentration profile within the eye is extended. Ultimately, when α is smaller than A, it will take control of how the concentration within the eye falls off with

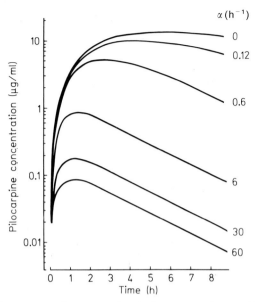

Fig. 9. Calculated time course of concentration in the aqueous humor (C_a) of the human eye after instilling 1 drop of pilocarpine solution. The effect of altering the loss coefficient from the tears, α, is demonstrated. The value of A is 0.34 h^{-1}, and an effect on the shape of the curve is noticeable at $\alpha = 0.6$ h^{-1} and the shift to sustained delivery is complete at $\alpha = 0.12$ h^{-1}. The inverse relationship between α and C_a at large values of α may also be noted. The curves, from MISHIMA (1981), were derived by computer but may also be calculated from Eq. (20)

time. This corresponds to sustained delivery. It is seen in Fig. 9 that for pilocarpine, whose value of A is about 0.3 h^{-1}, sustained delivery starts for a value of α between 0.6 and 0.12 h^{-1}.

Generalized equations for this and other situations have been provided by MAKOID and ROBINSON (1979) but require computer solutions. The concentration curve of the aqueous humor can be calculated explicitly in the following manner. The concentration in the anterior chamber at time t, if a small quantity of drug, dm_c, has been introduced into the cornea at time t', is given by:

$$dC_a = \frac{dm_c k_c}{V_a(B-A)} (e^{-A(t-t')} - e^{-B(t-t')})$$

from Eq. (8). The value of dm_c is given by $dm_c = k_{dc} V_c C_o e^{-\alpha t'} dt'$, where C_o is the initial tear film concentration at time zero and k_{dc} is the transfer coefficient across the epithelium. By integration from time zero to t, the concentration in the aqueous humor follows the relation:

$$C_a = \frac{C_o k_{dc} k_c V_c}{(B-A) V_a} \left(\frac{e^{-\alpha t} - e^{-At}}{A - \alpha} - \frac{e^{-\alpha t} - e^{-Bt}}{B - \alpha} \right). \tag{20}$$

Where α is zero, Eq. (20) becomes identical with Eq. (15).

4. Other Compartments

The validity of some of the assumptions made in setting up the two-compartment model will now be examined. We will be concerned with estimating the exchanges with compartments that were previously ignored.

a) Limbal Exchange

As a first approximation, the loss of material from the cornea to the blood around its circumference may be treated as equivalent to the drop in concentration of an infinite cylinder when its curved surface is kept at zero concentration (Crank 1975). After a short period of time the drop will be monoexponential, and for the cornea

$$C_c = K \exp\left(-\frac{D_p \beta_1^2}{P^2} t\right),$$

where K is a constant and $\beta_1 = 2.4$, D_p is the diffusion coefficient of the material in the plane of the cornea and P is the radius of the circle where the concentration is zero, about 1 mm beyond the anatomic limbus (Allansmith et al. 1979). Thus the loss coefficient across the limbus will be:

$$\frac{dC_c}{C_c dt} = -5.7 \frac{D_p}{P^2}. \tag{21}$$

In the rabbit P is about 7 mm, and therefore in the case of fluorescein, whose diffusion rate in the stroma is is 1×10^{-6} cm^2 s^{-1}, the loss coefficient across the limbus will be about 4×10^{-2} h^{-1} compared to the total apparent elimination coefficient A, which is 0.2 h^{-1} for this dye. One-fifth of the loss should be across the limbus, therefore, but the figure will be several times smaller for most drugs because they exchange more rapidly across the endothelium than fluorescein (see Sect. B.II.6.a; Table 3). The error in ignoring the loss to the blood generally will be less than the errors of measurements of concentration, and it is ignored in the remainder of this chapter.

If it is desired to make the correction, it is readily shown that Eq. (12) is to be replaced by:

$$k_o = A(1 + m g_{ca} V_c / V_a) \tag{22}$$

and Eq. (13) by:

$$k_c = \frac{mA}{1 - r_{ca}/g_{ca}}, \tag{23}$$

where m is the fraction of the total loss from the cornea that goes by way of the anterior chamber.

b) Posterior Reservoir

Not all the drug that is lost from the aqueous humor passes directly into the blood by drainage or absorption into the capillaries of the iris. The anterior cortex of the lens and a variety of cells in the iris can take up the drug. A small, slow passage through the lens cortex into the vitreous body can also occur, as well as a direct penetration into it through the iris and the posterior chamber, which could be significant for lipid-soluble drugs, according to the results of Maren et al. (1983).

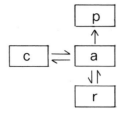

Fig. 10. Compartmental model used to account for the changes in pilocarpine concentration in the anterior chamber after the instillation of a drop. p, plasma; c, cornea; a, anterior chamber; r, reservoir. (MAKOID and ROBINSON 1979)

Some part of the material that is absorbed can be returned to the anterior chamber when the aqueous humor concentration declines to a low value. This leads to a nonlinearity at the tail end of the aqueous and corneal monoexponential curves (Fig. 4).

These effects could be expected to be greater for drugs which are lipid-soluble and can penetrate better into the posterior cellular structures. This appears to be the case, for fluorescein shows no nonlinearities until the aqueous concentration has dropped to 1/100 of its peak (KAISER and MAURICE 1964; JONES and MAURICE 1966), whereas pilocarpine deviates from a straight line within one-tenth (MAKOID and ROBINSON 1979). These workers found that the experimental points could be adequately accounted for by adding a single closed compartment to the two-chamber model (Fig. 10).

5. Kinetics of Ocular Responses to Drugs

a) Biological Responses

The extent of the reversible pharmacologic response of an organ may often be an instantaneous function of the drug concentration in its biophase, so that the time course of this response would reflect that of the change in drug concentration in the tissue. On this basis, the pharmacokinetics of a given drug may be analyzed from the response it provokes, provided that the relationship between the response and the concentration of the drug in the biophase is known. However, this relationship is difficult to derive for most pharmacologic responses of the body, since drug concentrations are usually determined in the serum, and the concentration in the biophase of the organ remains unknown.

As an exception, the responses of the intraocular smooth muscles – miosis, mydriasis, and accommodation – are particularly suited for pharmacokinetic analysis because: (i) an exact dose–response relationship can be obtained using isolated muscle specimens; (ii) methods of exact measurement of the in vivo response are available; (iii) the in vitro and in vivo dose–response relationship can be readily compared; and (iv) the penetration kinetics of instilled drugs have been studied in detail in both the rabbit and human eye, and can be compared with the kinetics of responses.

Although all the above advantages do not apply, limited pharmacokinetic analyses have also been performed for the responses to drugs of the intraocular pres-

sure and of corneal sensation. There are a number of other quantifiable variables
in the eye which can be measured in vivo and which are affected by drugs, e.g.,
aqueous humor flow rate, blink rate, and the electroretinogram, for which an analysis has not been attempted. The acute response to injury which can be characterized by changes in intraocular pressure and the permeability of the blood–ocular
barrier and the more chronic models of uveitis characterized by cellular responses
are of particular interest because of the importance of anti-inflammatory agents in
ocular therapeutics.

A complication in the use of the biological responses as an index of biophase
concentration, as well as in the use of autonomic agents as chemical tracers, is that
the parameters determined may themselves be affected by the administration of the
drug. Thus the instillation of pilocarpine will change the tear flow rate, the rate of
aqueous secretion, and the volume of the anterior chamber. The values of k_o measured by the use of this substance are likely to be different from those found with
inert tracers; moreover, they may change during the course of the experiment.

b) Dose–Response Relationship in the Pupil

LEVY (1964) administered an anticholinergic agent to mice and attempted to calculate the elimination rate of the drug constant from the decline of the mydriatic response on the basis of a simple dose–response relationship. Studies have been carried out (SCHOENWALD and SMOLEN 1971; SMOLEN 1971) on the pupil response of
the rabbit using a non-linear dose–response relationship obtained by the intravenous administration of a drug. They developed a function to convert the pupil response into parameters which describe the drug concentration in the biophase of
the sphincter muscle. A computer program was designed to estimate the drug's bioavailability from the pharmacologic data. However, the same data can readily be
converted to yield a linear dose–response relationship for the pupil by calculating
a response coefficient according to the principle of WAGNER (1968). This method
allows the intraocular kinetics of topically administered miotic and mydriatic
drugs to be established explicitly, and has yielded pharmacokinetic coefficients for
the human eye (YOSHIDA and MISHIMA 1975; MISHIMA 1981).

The dose–response relationship of the isolated iris sphincter muscle of the human eye to carbachol and pilocarpine follows a typical sigmoid curve; the maximal
response to both drugs is similar, which suggests that pilocarpine should be considered a full agonist. From this maximal response, R_{max}, and the response, R, to
a submaximal concentration of the drug, C, a response coefficient $R_l = R/(R_{max} - R)$
can be calculated. The experimental data are found to follow the equation:

$$R_l = \varrho C \tag{24}$$

where ϱ is a proportionality constant (OHARA 1977). This linear relationship is
found to be valid for numerous in vitro responses in a variety of species (MISHIMA
1981). Both the isolated iris strip preparation of the sphincter and the whole-mount
iris preparation have been used, and carbachol, pilocarpine, acetylcholine, atropine, epinephrine, and isoproterenol have been tested. It can be concluded, therefore, that Eq. (24) is a valid description of the dose–response relationship of the
sphincter and dilator muscles of the iris.

To define the response coefficient in vivo, measurements of pupil diameter are
used, and it is necessary to know the limits of movement of the tissue. In the human

eye the smallest pupil diameter that can be attained by miotic drugs has been estimated to be 1 mm, and the largest diameter after mydriatic drugs to be 8.5 mm (LOEWENFELD and NEWSOME 1971; YOSHIDA and MISHIMA 1975). Denoting the diameter before the drug as D_o mm and after the drug as D mm, the response (R) and the maximum response (R_{max}) are defined as follows: $R=(D_o-D)$, $R_{max}=(D_o-1)$ for the miotic response; and $R=(D-D_o)$, $R_{max}=(8.5-D_o)$ for the mydriatic response.

The linearized response, R_l, is then written:

$$R_l=\frac{D_o-D}{D-1} \tag{25}$$

for the miotic response, or:

$$R_l=\frac{D-D_o}{8.5-D} \tag{26}$$

for the mydriatic response.

The pupil diameter has been measured at intervals after instilling various concentrations of pilocarpine or tropicamide into the eyes of normal volunteers. The linearized response, R_l, was calculated for the peak response and was plotted on a log–log scale against the corresponding concentration of the instilled drug; the relationship was found to be linear with a slope of unity. Accordingly:

$$R_l=\varrho' C_b. \tag{27}$$

Assuming that the drug transfer from tears to aqueous follows first-order kinetics, a comparison of Eqs. (24) and (27) leads to the conclusion that R_l calculated from the pupil diameter is proportional to the drug concentration in the biophase of the iris muscles (MISHIMA 1981).

The in vivo mydriatic response to epinephrine differs from that to tropicamide in not following the linear relationship of Eq. (27) in either the rabbit or human eye. Since Eq. (24) applies to the response of the isolated iris preparation to this drug, it seems that the biophase concentration in vivo is not linearly related to the concentration applied. This might result from the absorption of epinephrine by the varicose adrenergic nerves of the iris.

c) Kinetics of Pupil Responses

The linearized response, R_l, may be calculated from the pupil diameter and plotted against time after instillation, as in Fig. 11. Its value increases in proportion to the applied drug concentration, and the curves for different concentrations are congruent, which confirms that R_l is proportional to the biophase drug concentration. The R_l-time curves for pilocarpine and for tropicamide are similar and can be fitted by Eq. (11) in the form:

$$R_l=R_L\{e^{-A(t-t_0)}-e^{-B(t-t_0)}\}, \tag{28}$$

where R_L is the value of R_l at the interception of the A and B components of the curve and t_o is the time lag between the instillation and the first response.

A similar analysis was made for results published in the literature (MISHIMA 1981), and the apparent elimination and absorption rate constants, A and B, are

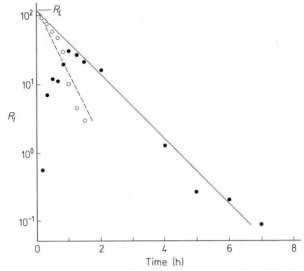

Fig. 11. Time course of the linearized pupil response, R_l, to tropicamide after instillation of a 0.5% solution in a normal subject. *Filled circles* show values of R_l; *open circles* show the derivation of absorption rate constant B. R_L is intercept A and B components according to Eq. (28). (Yoshida and Mishima 1975)

Table 1. Pharmacokinetic coefficients of pupil and cycloplegic responses in human eyes. (Mishima 1981)[a]

Drug	A(h)$^{-1}$	B(h)$^{-1}$	t_o(h)	t_{max}(h)	k_c(h)$^{-1}$	k_o(h^{-1})
			PUPIL			
Pilocarpine						
Blue eyes	0.46				0.5–0.6	1–2
		1.2–2.4	0.14	1–1.6	(0.8–1.8)	(0.6–0.7)
Brown eyes	0.36					
Tropicamide	0.7	1.5–4	0.13	0.6–1	0.8	1.5–4
					(1–4)	(1)
Homatropine						
Blue eyes	0.31				0.3	1.9–2.4
		2.1–2.5	0.25	1.3		
Brown eyes	0.19					
Scopolamine	0.025					
Atropine	0.017					
Phenylephrine	0.63	2.1	0.3	1.2	0.8	1.7
					(1.4)	(0.95)
			ACCOMMODATION			
Tropicamide	1.5	3.2	0.1	0.6	–	–
Cyclopentolate	0.44	2.3	0.15	1.1	0.5	2.1
					(1.6)	(0.65)
Homatropine	0.35	1.3	0.2	1.6	0.4	1.1
Scopolamine	0.022	2.9	0.1	1.8	0.022	2.9
Atropine	0.012	1.5	0.1	3.4	0.012	1.5

[a] The values of k_c and k_o are derived from A and B by means of Fig. 7. Where two alternative sets of values are admissible, the less probable pair is placed in parentheses

listed in Table 1 for various drugs. It is of interest that the apparent elimination rate constants of pilocarpine and homatropine are faster in blue eyes than in dark eyes. This can be attributed to binding of these drugs to the pigment of the anterior uvea, which then releases the drug slowly (MISHIMA 1981). A and B can be converted to k_c and k_o by means of Fig. 7, and these values are presented in Table 1. Two pairs of coefficients can be derived from the figure; in some cases one value of k_o is below k_f, and the corresponding pair can be rejected. Where both pairs are admissible, that which agrees with the values found for other drugs (Table 2) is preferred and the other is set in brackets in Table 1.

Numerous reports cited by MISHIMA (1981) agree that a greater ocular pigmentation reduces the effect of many miotic and mydriatic drugs as well as the drop in intraocular pressure caused by pilocarpine or epinephrine, and suggest that this is a result of the drug binding to uveal pigment with a consequent drop in its concentration in the biophase. Antibiotics such as clindamycin (TABBARA and O'CONNOR 1975) may also be bound by the pigment, which would lead to a reduction of their activity after they had penetrated into the eye; it is possible, on the other hand, that their slow release from binding could result in a prolongation of their action.

d) Cycloplegic Response

After the instillation of cycloplegic drugs, the amplitude of accommodation is reduced. In this case, the maximum response will be the state of zero amplitude of accommodation and the response coefficient is given by

$$R_l = \frac{\Delta_o - \Delta}{\Delta}, \tag{29}$$

where Δ_o and Δ are the amplitudes of accommodation before and after the action of the drug. The linearized response, R_l, was calculated from the peak cycloplegic responses after the instillation of various concentrations of tropicamide (YOSHIDA 1976), and it was found that Eq. (27) applies. This was confirmed (MISHIMA 1981) from the published results of SMITH (1974).

On this basis, the kinetics of the cycloplegic responses to various drugs were analyzed, and the pharmacokinetic coefficients that were extracted are listed in Table 1. The elimination rate constants are slightly less than those found for the mydriatic responses for the same drugs, but they are in the same range. The lag time and the peak time of cycloplegia are also similar to those found for the mydriatic responses, indicating that the time required for the drug to reach the ciliary muscles and the iris sphincter muscles is similar. The rapid access of the drug to the ciliary muscles may be accounted for either by uveoscleral aqueous flow, which would carry the drug to the site from the anterior chamber, or to its direct passage from the tear film across the sclera. The thickness and properties of the sclera and cornea are sufficiently alike to make it difficult to distinguish between the two routes (MAURICE and POLGAR 1977; Sect. B.II.2.d).

e) Pharmacokinetics of Surface Anesthetics in the Cornea

Using a Cochet-Bonnet esthesiometer, MATSUMOTO et al. (1981) measured the corneal sensitivity threshold at 1 min intervals after instilling different concentrations of lidocaine and benoxinate into the eyes of normal volunteers. The maximum anesthetic effect was reached very rapidly, within 2–3 min with lidocaine and 1–2 min with benoxinate. The duration of the effect was defined as the interval between the time of instillation and that at which the corneal sensitivity threshold returned to its predrug level. These durations were plotted against the logarithm of the concentration and resulted in a linear relationship. Such a relationship is found in a one-compartment model, and the data may be analyzed according to the equation of Levy (1971):

$$\log C - \log C_{\min} = t_d k_e / 2.3, \tag{30}$$

where C and $C_{\min}$ are the concentration of a drug and the least effective concentration of the drug respectively, t_d is the duration of the effect, and k_e is the elimination rate constant of the drug from the corneal epithelium. This constant was about $5\,h^{-1}$ for lidocaine and $6\,h^{-1}$ for benoxinate. From the published data of Polse et al. (1978), the elimination rate constant is calculated to be $5\,h^{-1}$ for proparacaine. The same analysis can be performed on published data for animal corneas (Gerlough 1931; Susina et al. 1962; Smolen and Siegel 1968) and gives similar rate constants. These values of k_e are the same as those found for α, the normal loss rate from the tears, and this suggests that the receptors for the anesthetic might be in equilibrium with the tear fluid.

f) Intraocular Pressure Response

After the instillation of a hypotensive agent, the intraocular pressure generally falls to its lowest value in 2–3 h and then slowly returns to the original level. The pressure response is the final result of complex interactions in the target tissue, and a linearized response coefficient cannot readily be derived. An analysis according to the two-compartment model is therefore not immediately feasible, and the one-compartment approximation of Levy has been applied to the elimination phase of

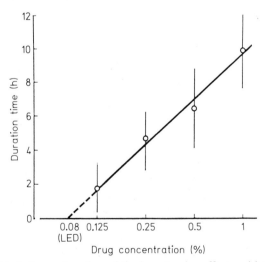

Fig. 12. Relationship between duration of the hypotensive effect and befunolol concentration after its topical instillation in eight normal subjects. *Vertical bars*, SD of determinations; *LED*, least-effect concentration. Duration of effect defined as time from peak effect to return to baseline value of intraocular pressure. (Mishima 1981)

the kinetics. The duration of the hypotensive effect is defined as the interval between the time of the peak effect and that at which the pressure returned to the original level. This is plotted against the logarithm of concentrations of befunolol, a β-adrenergic antagonist, in Fig. 12. A linear relationship is evident, and the results may be analyzed on the basis of Eq. (30).

The slope of the regression line in Fig. 12 may be called the rate of effect disappearance, instead of the elimination rate constant. Its intercept with the concentration axis gives the least effective concentration of the drug. Knowledge of the rate of effect disappearance and the least effective concentration is useful in determining the therapeutic concentration of a drug and the optimal frequency of its application (MISHIMA 1981; TAKASE et al. 1978).

6. Parameter Determination

a) Endothelial Transfer Coefficient

In principle, if the rise and fall of the aqueous humor concentration of a drug is measured after its topical administration, it should be possible to evaluate the coefficients A and B and derive k_c as shown in Fig. 7. In fact, examination of about 300 papers reporting such experiments revealed only three or four sets of data that were

Table 2. Pharmacokinetic parameters for drug exchange between aqueous and cornea derived from A and g_{ca} according to Fig. 8[a]

Drug	A (h^{-1})	g_{ca}	$k_c(h^{-1})$	$k_o(h^{-1})$
Gentamicin	$0.2^b (0.15)^c$		~ 0.2	
Penicillin	$0.7^{d,e}$	9^u	0.75	2.5
Tetracycline	$0.7^{f,g}$	7^g	0.8	2.1
Lincomycin	$\sim 0.8^h$	7^h	0.9	2.4
Chloramphenicol	$0.9^i (0.6)^j$	$\sim 6^v$	1.05	2.45
Pilocarpine	$0.9^{k,l}$	$3-5^{k,l,w}$		~ 2
Timolol	$0.6^m (0.35)^n$	$12,^x 9^m$	0.65	2.7, 2.15
Befunolol	0.46^m	10^m	0.5	1.8
Prednisolone acetate	$0.6^{o,p}$	$6, 10^p$	0.7	1.65
Dexamethasone	0.6^o	$14,^o 10^y$	0.65	3
	$0.48^q (0.2)^r$	7^q	0.55	1.45
Dexamethasone phosphate	0.72^s	3.8^s	0.9	1.5
Fluorometholone	$0.7,^o 0.55^t$	$15,^o 12^t$	0.75	3.75

[a] Results of experiments carried out with isotopically labeled drugs are shown in italics; otherwise a bioassay was used. All the data come from rabbits except the values of A placed in brackets, which refer to patients. Values of B are extractable from the data for dexamethasone phosphate,[p] befunolol,[m] and timolol;[m] and are 2.3, 2.0, and 2.1 h^{-1} respectively; [b] BAUM et al. 1974; [c] UTERMANN et al. 1977; [d] VON SALLMANN 1945; [e] PAPAPANOS et al. 1961a; [f] NAKATSUE 1971b; [g] HARDBERGER et al. 1975; [h] KLEINBERG et al. 1979; [i] GREEN and MACKEEN 1976; [j] BEASLEY et al. 1975; [k] SIEG and ROBINSON 1976; [l] LAZARE and HORLINGTON 1975; [m] TAKASE (cited MISHIMA 1981); [n] PHILLIPS et al. 1981; [o] YAMAUCHI et al. 1975; [p] KUPFERMAN and LEIBOWITZ 1976; [q] SHORT et al. 1966; [r] JAIN and BATRA 1979; [s] ROSENBLUM et al. 1967; [t] KUPFERMAN and LEIBOWITZ 1975; [u] BLOOME et al. 1970; [v] BLEEKER and MAAS 1955; [w] SENDELBECK et al. 1975; [x] SCHMITT et al. 1980; [y] KUPFERMAN and LEIBOWITZ 1974b

Table 3. Epithelial and endothelial permeabilities of the cornea[a]

EPITHELIUM

P_{dc} (cm h^{-1})

10^{-1}
- Fluorometholone[b]* | Prednisolone acet.[b]*
- Chloramphenicol[c]**
- Fluorometholone[d]* | Prednisolone acet.[d]*
- Prednisolone PO$_4$[d]*
- Dexamethasone PO$_4$[d]* | Dexamethasone[b]*
- Chloramphenicol[v]

10^{-2}
- Pilocarpine[e,f]
- Propanolol[g]
- Prednisolone[b]*
- Penicillin[h,i,j]* | Sulfacetamide[w]
- Timolol[g,k,l] | TIMOLOL[x]
- Pilocarpine[m]* | Prednisolone PO$_4$[y]
- Hetrazan[n] | CHLORAMPHENICOL[z]

10^{-3}
- Gentamicin[o]
- Atenolol[g]

10^{-4}
- Fluorescein[p]
- Tetracycline[q]

10^{-5}
- FLUORESCEIN[r]
- Streptomycin[s]
- GENTAMICIN[t,u]

P_{ac} (cm h^{-1})

10^{-1}
- Prednisolone PO$_4$[d]*
- Dexamethasone PO$_4$[d]*
- Fluorometholone[d]*
- Prednisolone acet.[d]*
- Penicillin[j]*

10^{-2}
- Gentamicin[aa]*

ENDOTHELIUM

← STROMAL CEILING

k_c (h^{-1})

3
1
- Chloramphenicol
- Lincomycin
- Dexamethasone PO$_4$ | TROPICAMIDE
- Tetracycline | PHENYLEPHRINE
- Penicillin | Fluorometholone
- Prednisolone acet. | Dexamethasone
- Timolol | PILOCARPINE
- Dexamethasone PO$_4$ | CYCLOPENTOLATE
- Fluorescein[bb]*,[cc]
- Befunolol

0.3
- Gentamicin | HOMATROPINE

0.1
- FLUORESCEIN[cc,dd]

sufficiently comprehensive to allow an analysis of this type. The commonest failing was the lack of adequate values in the early period when the concentration is rising, which are essential to the estimate of B. A better yield was achieved from the alternative approach, illustrated in Fig. 8, of using the value of A in connection with measurements of g_{ca}, the corneal–aqueous ratio during the declining phase. A dozen sources provided usable data for the rabbit, though in several cases the number of experimental points or the period of time over which they were collected was less than would be desired. The experimental parameters and the derived coefficients for these experiments are listed in Table 2. The few cases in which B was determinable are from the same set of results and gave values of the coefficients that are in good agreement. The values of k_c from Table 2, as well as those from Table 1 for human eyes, are placed according to their magnitude in the right-hand column of Table 3.

The findings of different experiments with pilocarpine are not consistent. On one hand, the kinetics of the pupil response (Table 1) show a value of k_c within the normal range. On the other, the use of the Ocusert resulted in a steady-state value of r_{ca} (SENDELBECK et al. 1975), which was little different from the value of g_{ca}; application of Eq. (13) indicates a very large value for k_c. This is in accordance with the finding of SIEG and ROBINSON (1976) that there was little concentration difference between the stroma and anterior chamber concentrations while they were dropping, which would suggest the endothelium is very permeable to this drug and consequently its value of k_c should be large.

At the other extreme, the very low values of k_c for scopolamine and atropine shown in Table 1, which are below the scale in Table 3, suggest that the kinetics of these drugs may not be controlled by the stromal reservoir.

Values of k_o also fall out from Fig. 8, and these are listed in Table 2. Little significance should be attached to the differences between them; the accuracy of the figures is heavily dependent on how carefully g_{ca} was measured and the variability of the experimental results was often large. It may also be noted that Eq. (12) requires that the total volume of the cornea should have been collected in the es-

---

[a] When data are from the rabbit, the name of the drug is written in lower case; when from humans, in capitals. When the name of the drug is in italic, it was labeled with a radioisotope. An asterisk against the citation number indicates that experiments were carried out on isolated tissue. When more than one citation is assigned to a drug, the values derived from the data were in good agreement; otherwise the name of the drug is reported at the appropriate levels. For pilocarpine the experimentally determined value of $36\ h^{-1}$ was used for the tear turnover constant rather than $6\ h^{-1}$. Since nearly all the permeability data came from experiments where the fluxes across the entire tissue was measured, the calculated values cannot be greater than that of the stroma, which is indicated in the Table; [b] SCHOENWALD and WARD 1978; [c] GREEN and MacKEEN 1976; [d] HULL et al. 1974a; [e] SIEG and ROBINSON 1976; [f] LAZARE and HORLINGTON 1975; [g] ROS et al. 1978; [h] VON SALLMANN and MEYER 1944; [i] WITZEL et al. 1956; [j] GODBEY et al. 1979; [k] SCHMITT et al. 1980; [l] TAKASE (cited MISHIMA 1981); [m] KROHN 1978; [n] LAZAR et al. 1968; [o] BLOOMFIELD et al. 1978; [p] MAURICE, unpublished; [q] NAKATSUE 1971b; [r] ADLER et al. 1971; [s] BELLOWS and FARMER 1947; [t] UTERMANN et al. 1977; [u] ELLERHORST et al. 1975; [v] LEOPOLD et al. 1950; [w] ROBSON and TEBRICH 1942; [x] PHILLIPS et al. 1981; [y] HULL et al. 1974b; [z] BEASLEY et al. 1975; [aa] KANE et al. 1981; [bb] HALE and MAURICE 1969; [cc] OTA et al. 1974; [dd] JONES and MAURICE 1966.

timate of g_{ca}, and it is possible that this was not always done. Sampling a central area of the cornea would lead to an overestimate of g_{ca} and of k_o.

b) Endothelial Permeability

Up to this point the kinetics of drug movement across the endothelium has been treated in terms of a transfer coefficient, k_c, which is concerned with the fraction of the material in the cornea which leaves it in unit time. Experiments on the isolated tissue yield the value of the permeability constant of the cell layer P_{ac}, which is concerned with the absolute quantity crossing the surface and the concentration gradient across it. Although k_c is a useful working parameter in kinetic theory, it is P_{ac} that more truly describes the properties of the endothelium itself.

A direct measure of P_{ac} is obtained by perfusing both surfaces of the isolated cornea whose epithelium has been scraped off, the transfer of the tracer substance from the solution on one side to that on the other being determined. It could also be established by means of experiments on the intact cornea in vivo after the systemic administration of the tracer by following the concentration changes in the aqueous humor and the central part of the cornea (Sect. D.II.6.a), but the data available for drugs are inadequate for the realization of this analysis except in the case of fluorescein.

In Table 3 the central column displays values of P_{ac} derived from experiments when both surfaces of the deepithelialized cornea were perfused. In these experiments the permeability of the tissue cannot be greater than that of the stroma itself, and this ceiling, as calculated in Sect. B.II.2.d, is shown in Table 3. In the experiments reported by Hull et al. (1974a), the corneal resistance was very close to that of the stroma alone, which makes the endothelial component difficult to distinguish; the values of P_{ac} that result must be regarded with caution, therefore.

To relate k_c to P_{ac} one must note the definition of permeability constant, in the case of the endothelium:

$$\frac{dm_c}{dt} = P_{ac}Q_c(C_a - C_s), \tag{31}$$

where dm_c/dt is the flux of drug across the layer, Q_c is the corneal area, and C_s is the concentration or activity in the tissue fluid. This equation is to be compared with the definition of the transfer coefficient, Eq. (2):

$$\frac{dC_c}{dt} = k_c(r_{ca}C_a - C_c).$$

Writting m_c/V_c for C_c in the latter equation, and V_c/q_c for Q_c in the former, where q_c is the corneal thickness, one obtains:

$$P_{ac} = q_c r_{ca} k_c \tag{32}$$

by comparing the coefficients of C_a.

Active transport by the endothelium is not sufficient to cause a notable concentration unbalance in any substance that has been investigated, so that the equilibrium concentration ratio r_{ca} represents a property of the stroma rather than the cell layer. To determine its value, concentration measurements should be made, in vivo or in vitro, either when C_c has reached an equilibrium or when it is passing through a maximum. These measurements have not been made other than with fluorescein, and it is necessary to assume that a drug is in simple solution in the tissue fluid, so that $r_{ca} = 0.75$. Equation (32) then gives the rough approximation $P_{ac} = 0.03\,k_c$.

The results of Tables 1 and 2 were plotted in the right-hand column of Table 3, on this basis, for comparison with the direct measurements of P_{ac}, and the agreement is reasonable when the same drug appears in both columns. The lipid-insoluble drugs fluorescein and gentamicin give permeability values of the order of magnitude appropriate to their molecular size (MAURICE, to be published a), and there is some degree of correspondence between the lipid solubility of the other drugs and their position in the column.

c) Epithelial Permeability Derivation

The flux of a drug, dm_c/dt, across the epithelial layer is related to its permeability P_{dc} by the equation

$$\frac{dm_c}{dt} = P_{dc}Q_c(C_d - C_s), \tag{33}$$

where C_d and C_s are the concentrations in the tear film and stromal fluid and Q_c is the corneal area. Most often the permeability is so small that C_s may be ignored in comparison with C_d, so that:

$$P_{dc} = \frac{m_o}{Q_c U_d}, \tag{34}$$

where m_o is the total quantity of drug penetrating across the corneal surface and U_d is the corresponding area under the curve for the tear film concentration.

Thus there are two operations required to find the permeability from published experimental data: first, determining m_o, and second, evaluating U_d. Neither operation should present difficulty when the experiments are carried out in vitro on the excised tissue. However, approximations usually have to be incorporated in reducing the published data from in vivo studies because the experimental conditions are not sufficiently defined.

d) Mass Entering the Cornea

In the earliest stages of penetration all the drug is found in the cornea, and the determination of m_o is simple if this tissue has been assayed. In the next stage it accumulates in the aqueous humor without having had time to drain out of the eye to an appreciable extent; usually this fluid is collected and its content can be added to that remaining in the cornea. However, more often in the rabbit, and always in the human, only the levels in the aqueous humor have been determined, and it is necessary to estimate m_o from these alone.

By eliminating k_c from Eq. (8) by means of Eq. (10) it is transformed to:

$$m_o = \frac{C_a V_a k_o (A^{-1} - B^{-1})}{e^{-At} - e^{-Bt}}. \tag{35}$$

If B is established as well as A, the equation may be used in this form. However, as was noted above, this is rarely possible with the available experimental data, and a method of deriving m_o from A alone must be used.

It is evident from Fig. 4 that B must always be considerably larger than A, so that for longer times: $m_o = C_a V_a k_o / A e^{-At}$ or:

$$m_o = \frac{C_A}{A} V_a k_o, \tag{36}$$

where C_A is the intercept of the A component of the C_a curve on the ordinate (Fig. 4). In Table 3, the values of k_o for the drugs listed tend to cluster around 2 h^{-1}. Taking V_a for the rabbit to be 0.25 ml, a figure of 0.5 ml h^{-1} resulted for $V_a k_o$, which was used in every set of experiments where the appropriate value of k_o for a drug was not known.

e) Area Under Tear Curve

In most experiments, a single drop or a series of drops was instilled into the eye. Only very rarely have measurements of the drug concentration in the tear film been made in individual eyes, and in order to estimate the integral $U_d = \int_0^\infty C_d dt$, recourse must be made to average values of tear parameters determined from the general population. As was noted in Sect. B.I.1.b, a single aqueous drop leads to an initial concentration in the tear film which is about one-third of that (C_b g ml^{-1}) in the instilled solution, and this is the value that will be adopted. After the initial concentration of drug in the tear film is established, it leaves the tears at a rate determined by the exponential loss coefficient, α, whose value has been found to be 6 h^{-1} in both rabbits and humans (Sect. B.I.1.a). Equation (18) then leads to the formula $U_d = C_b / 18$ g h^{-1} ml^{-1}. Although this figure can be wide of the mark in an individual case, it is to be hoped that it will be adequate when the average penetration in a number of eyes is being considered.

When a number of drops are given at regular intervals, commonly six times over 30 min, further assumptions have to be made. Immediately after each successive instillation the concentration in the tear fluid may be expected to rise closer to saturation with the instilled solution. The area under the curve in this situation was taken to be the mean of that which would result from total saturation of the tear film over the time from the first to last instillation, and that from noncumulative rises and falls on each application, where the tear concentration dropped with an α of 6 h^{-1} between each application and after the final one.

f) Epithelial Permeability Values

From the above treatment it follows that where a single drop of drug is instilled in the eye, the permeability should be calculated from the formula:

$$P_{dc} = m_o / Q_c U_d = (4.5/A)(C_A/C_b) \text{ cm h}^{-1}$$

for the rabbit eye. The corresponding approximation for the human eye is:

$$P_{dc} = (7/A)(C_A/C_b) \text{ cm h}^{-1}.$$

This allows a number of experimental series to be analyzed and compared to each other and to permeability values established by other techniques. These results are listed on the left-hand side of Table 3. The epithelial permeabilities are generally higher than in a similar list prepared by Mishima (1981) because in that case no account was taken of the initial dilution of a drop by the tears. The exact position of most of the drugs on the scale must be regarded as provisional, not only because of the assumptions that had to be made in deriving U_d, the area under the tear concentration curve, but also on account of the scatter of the experimental values; the difficulty of measuring the small quantities of drug that appear in the anterior chamber, especially when the bioassay of an antibiotic is concerned, often leads to an excessive variability. For several drugs the results of different investigations are in fair agreement, but in others they are quite disparate and are listed separately.

Nonetheless, it is clear that the epithelial permeability covers a very wide range and that this bears a relationship to the lipid solubility, as has already been demonstrated (Fig. 3). The cornea is a considerable barrier to fluorescein and the aminoglycosides, which are lipid-insoluble, while for chloramphenicol and some steroids the permeability of the cornea as a whole was close to that of the stroma alone, showing that the epithelial barrier was negligible.

Another clear indication from Table 3 is that the human epithelium is a considerably greater barrier than that of the rabbit. For each of the three drugs where a comparison is possible the precision of the measurements is low, but they suggest there will be an order of magnitude difference between the species. This conclusion seems also to be true for pilocarpine from a comparison of its penetration into human and rabbit eyes under similar conditions (KROHN 1978). On the other hand, the penetration of prednisolone acetate into the anterior chamber of the two species was not found to be significantly different by LEIBOWITZ et al. (1977), but the epithelium is not an effective barrier to this substance.

A complicating factor in experiments on rabbits is their very low natural blink rate. Furthermore, some workers use anesthetized animals in which blinking may be totally suppressed, others close the lids, and others, again, may stimulate blinking on a regular or occasional basis. This can lead to different rates of loss of drug from the tears. Moreover, differing techniques of instillation can result in different levels of initial saturation of the tear film.

When a drug penetrates well across the epithelial surface, it is not unlikely that the total quantity which enters the cornea is that which was left on its surface after the first blink. In such a case there will be an artificial upper limit imposed on m_o which will correspond to a maximum value for the apparent permeability. This maximum is given by $q_d\alpha$, where q_d is the tear film thickness, and has a value of 5×10^{-3} cm h^{-1}. In fact, there appears to be a cluster of permeability values around that level.

A number of otherwise good reports on the penetration of steroids were neglected because the drug was in the form of a suspension, and there seemed no immediate way of assigning a true tear film concentration. When the epithelial permeability is high, as it is for these substances, its importance as a barrier can be assessed by a direct comparison of the penetration of the drug into eyes where the layer is intact and those where it has been scraped away. Such experiments have been carried out for a number of steroids, and they suggest that the epithelium offers little or no barrier to cortisone, fluorocortisone (LEOPOLD et al. 1955a), prednisone, prednisone acetate (LEOPOLD et al. 1955b), prednisolone acetate (LEOPOLD et al. 1955b; HULL et al. 1974a; KUPFERMAN and LEIBOWITZ 1974a), and fluorometholone (HULL et al. 1974a; KUPFERMAN and LEIBOWITZ 1975). In the case of hydrocortisone (Leopold et al. 1955a), prednisolone (Leopold et al. 1955 b), triamcinolone (Leopold and Kroman 1960), and dexamethasone phosphate (Hull et al. 1974a; Kupferman et al. 1974), an increase in penetration was observed as a result of abrading the epithelium, and this acted as if it was offering a resistance of three to four times that of the stroma alone. These data must be interpreted with caution because of the possibility that the limiting step in penetration is the rate at which the drug dissolves from the crystals (see Sect. B.I.1.b).

III. Conclusions and Recommendations

It has been seen that the distribution of the material that penetrates the epithelium and how this changes with time is generally dominated by the corneal and anterior chamber compartments, and is regulated by the transfer coefficients between them and between the aqueous humor and blood. Other tissues, particularly the iris, have a significant influence on the kinetics of many drugs; nevertheless, a preliminary attempt to fit the experimental data with a two-compartment model is reasonable as a first approximation, and deviations from its predictions will indicate the importance of the additional compartments. Drug exchanges with the iris and lens involve consideration of absorption onto receptors and diffusion in unstirred bodies; their treatment will introduce a higher order of mathematical complexity than adopted in this section and probably require numerical solutions on the computer.

It remains true that the cornea is the most important structure in determining how much drug penetrates into the eye after topical application, and frequently it also regulates how long the material that has penetrated remains in the tissues. The fundamental properties that decide its behavior toward any drug are the permeabilities of its two cell layers and the absorption by the epithelium and stroma. The determination of these properties should be the cornerstone of rational drug design.

A worthwhile first approach to the determinations is the use of the isolated perfused tissue, which can lead to a direct evaluation of the permeability of both cell layers, as well as to the steady-state ratio, r_{ca}.

Epithelial permeabilities are measured by flux determinations across the intact tissue. Endothelial permeabilities can be measured in the same way after the epithelium is removed; however, it is preferable to measure the changes in corneal concentration after perfusion of the posterior surface with a constant concentration of the drug and with exchanges across the anterior surface blocked by air or oil. The technique of Mishima and Trenberth (1968), in which the washout of drug across the endothelium is observed after a depot has been established in the stroma, may also be considered. The steady-state ratios can be obtained similarly, after prolonged perfusion of the posterior surface of the cornea, and previous removal of the epithelium will allow the stromal and epithelial compartments to be distinguished.

The cell layers of the cornea are very susceptible to injury from contact with solid surfaces or to folding or wrinkling during isolation. The effect of damage on permeability is particularly noticeable for the epithelium in the case of those substances to which it offers a high resistance to passage. Special techniques should be employed (MISHIMA and KUDO 1967; DIKSTEIN and MAURICE 1972) to ensure that the cornea does not distort during mounting and that the epithelial surface does not come in contact with solid objects (KLYCE 1972). The normal pressure relationships across the cornea should be maintained during both mounting and the flux measurements.

The values determined in vitro should be confirmed in vivo, and k_o can only be obtained from the living animal. The measurement of epithelial permeability will be established with much more certainty if the concentration of drug in the tear fluids is controlled. Making a reservoir for the fluid over the cornea by raising the lids is recommended, and the surface of the eye should be washed free of the drug after 5 or 10 min of bathing. Various methods of determining k_c and k_o have been noted in the previous pages; it is emphasized that in all circumstances numerous readings should be taken of the corneal and aqueous concentrations over a wide period of time, and preferably these should be continued until they have declined at least one log unit below their maximum value, so that the value of A can be established with precision.

Economy in the use of animals may be effected by adding an inert tracer, whose permeability is well established, to the test drug solution. The permeability of the drug can then be directly related to that of the standard substance. This is particularly valuable in the isolated corneal preparation, where damage to the cell layers can easily occur. Fluorescein is an obvious candidate as a standard and has been so employed by KRUPIN et al. (1974), but it may not be easy to measure in vitro because of its low penetration. Attention should be paid to purity of the drug, and an injectable quality employed. The potentialities of other compounds, particularly those with greater lipid solubilities, will need to be explored.

C. Local Injections

I. Subconjunctival

1. Regurgitation

There are particular concerns in the clinical application of data from about 150 reports on drug injection beneath the conjunctiva. Most experiments were carried out on rabbits, and regurgitation of the drug through the injection hole and its subsequent entry through the cornea from the tears can be very significant in this species. WINE et al. (1964) noted that the penetration of steroid into the globe was modified when the presence of a hole was avoided by injecting into the subconjunctival space of the rabbit by means of a needle passing through the skin of the lids. This was studied in greater detail by CONRAD and ROBINSON (1980) using labeled pilocarpine, and they found that the penetration into the anterior chamber was several hundred times greater when injected in the conventional manner through the conjunctiva. This difference is likely to be considerably smaller for drugs to which the corneal epithelium is a greater barrier than it is to pilocarpine, but it may still be appreciable. The regurgitation can readily be visualized by coloring the injection fluid (MAURICE and OTA 1978), and is very marked in the rabbit even with small injection volumes, but can be prevented by making a needle track through a muscle. The regurgitation can be seen to be much less in humans, but it could become larger if the injection pressure is high or the conjunctiva is torn. Another source of uncertainty is that the passage of fluorescein from the conjunctival depot into the aqueous humor was measured to be more than one order of magnitude greater in the human eye than in the rabbit (MAURICE and OTA 1978).

2. Depot Dynamics

A small injection of iodopyracet labeled with ^{125}I was made beneath the rabbit conjunctiva and its rate of loss from the eye monitored with an external counter (MAURICE and OTA 1978). The disappearance was exponential, and the amount of material present dropped ten times in 30 min, on average. Some qualitative observations on the disappearance of the soluble radiopaque medium showed that it had disappeared in 1 h (LEVINE and ARONSON 1970).

Similar experiments have not been tried with drugs ordinarily used in ophthalmology. However, measurements of the rise in concentration of unlabeled drugs in the blood after their subconjunctival injection have been made and compared with the levels found after intramuscular injection of the same drug. In every case, both in humans (UTERMANN et al. 1977; BRON et al. 1970; PETOUNIS et al. 1978; BOYLE et al. 1971, 1972a, b; UWAYDAH et al. 1976) and rabbits (LITWACK et al. 1969; HAMARD et al. 1975), the blood level after subconjunctival injection quickly rises to a maximum which corresponds to that which would be expected if the same quantity had been injected systemically. In most of the experimental series the transfer from the eye to the blood is virtually complete by the time the first blood measurement is made, and closer examination of the data suggests that at 30 min after the injection there can be only a small fraction of the original dose of drug remaining in the subconjunctival depot. Even though a sizeable bleb may remain at this time, it must be filled with much diluted material. This has been confirmed in the case of pilocarpine by CONRAD and ROBINSON (1980), who collected the bleb after 1 h and found the concentration to be about 1/100 of that in the injected solution.

A reduced rate of take-up of drug by the blood has been claimed when epinephrine is added to the injection fluid, and notable increases in penetration into the anterior chamber have been reported in patients (SAUBERMANN 1956) and in rabbits (SORSBY and UNGAR 1947; LEPRI 1950). It is not evident from the data how much of this increase is a result of slower loss from the depot and how much is due to a reduced absorption of the drug in its passage from the subconjunctival space to the aqueous humor.

Some poorly soluble drugs, particularly steroids, are injected in a crystalline form so that they will be released over a long period. The level in the aqueous humor remains measurable for about 3 weeks after the injection of prednisolone acetate in the rabbit (CASTREN et al. 1964; FAJARDO 1966) and at least 7 days after the injection of hydrocortisone in humans (JAIN and SRIVASTAVA 1978).

3. Aqueous Humor Concentration

The changes in concentration of fluorescein in the anterior chamber of individual subjects were followed after a small subconjunctival injection of the dye (MAURICE and OTA 1978). A considerable coloration was seen within 15 min. This rises to a maximum at 1–2 h and is followed by a steady decline with a decay constant of about 0.4 h^{-1}.

In a number of experimental series, subconjunctival injections have been made in patients at various times before they were operated on for cataract, and their aqueous humor was collected at the time of surgery and analyzed for its drug content. The general run of the separate points is comparable to the curve shown by fluorescein in individual subjects (UTERMANN et al. 1977; HILLMAN et al. 1979; BOYLE et al. 1971, 1972 a, b). Considerable variability is found in the aqueous concentration of a drug at any time, but in each series most values lie within a band having a range of 5 : 1 between its upper and lower concentration limits.

This drug penetration can be expressed as a readily appreciated quantity in the form of the equivalent dilution D, given by m_o/C_a where m_o is the mass injected and C_a is the concentration found in the aqueous humor; the value of D gives the volume of fluid in which the initial injection would have to be diluted in order to give rise to the concentration C_a observed. The results of different workers could best be compared if the maximum value of C_a averaged over many subjects were employed. Sufficient points are generally not available to determine exactly both the time of the maximum and the corresponding average, and it is necessary to assemble those values lying between 30 min and 2–3 h after injection.

The outcome of such calculations is displayed in Table 4. Gentamicin has been the object of several studies, and there are adequate data bases for tobramycin, car-

Table 4. Minimum dilution, $D_{\min}$, after subconjunctival injection of drugs, $D_{\min}$ = mass injected/maximum concentration in aqueous humor [a]

Drug	$D_{\min}$ (ml) Human	Rabbit
Gentamicin	1,000,[b, c] 440,[d] 2,000[e]	2,000,[m, n] 1,500,[o, p] *750*[q, r]
Tobramycin	500[f]	500[s]
Lincomycin	600[g]	1,000[t]
Streptomycin		*500*[u]
Fosfomycin		750[v]
Sisomycin		800[w]
Kanamycin		2,000[x]
Kanendomycin		700[x]
Penicillin G		4,[y] 16,[z] 130,[u] 800,[aa] 3,000,[bb] 5,000,[cc] *6,000*[dd]
Carbenicillin	500[h]	
Cloxacillin	~ 20,000[i]	
Cephalothin	2,000[j]	
Dexamethasone	10[k]	*6,000*,[ee] *1,200*[ff]
Fluorescein	50[l]	2,500[l]

[a] Values in italics were obtained with drugs labeled with radioisotopes; [b] UTERMANN et al. 1977; [c] HILLMAN et al. 1979; [d] MATHALONE and HARDING 1972; [e] FURGIUELE 1970; [f] PETOUNIS et al. 1978; [g] BOYLE et al. 1971; [h] BOYLE et al. 1972a; [i] UWAYDAH et al. 1976; [j] BOYLE et al. 1972b; [k] JAIN and SRIVASTAVA 1978; [l] MAURICE and OTA 1978; [m] FURGIUELE 1967; [n] LITWACK et al. 1969; [o] GOLDEN and COPPEL 1970; [p] KUMING and TOMKIN 1974; [q] OAKLEY et al. 1976; [r] BARZA et al. 1977; [s] OISHI et al. 1975; [t] MELIKIAN et al. 1971; [u] BLOOME et al. 1970; [v] OISHI et al. 1977; [w] FARIS et al. 1980; [x] TAKAHASHI 1971a; [y] PAPAPANOS et al. 1961a; [z] RECORDS 1967; [aa] SORSBY and UNGAR 1947; [bb] ANDREWS 1947; [cc] LEPRI 1950; [dd] OAKLEY et al. 1976; [ee] HAMARD et al. 1975; [ff] AZUMA et al. 1963

benicillin, and lincomycin in humans. There is a fair agreement in the value of D_{min}, which lies in the range 500–2,000 ml in all cases. The differences in the gentamicin figures may result from small differences in technique, but there is no obvious relation between injection volume and D_{min}.

As noted earlier, the penetration of fluorescein in rabbits was found to be very different from that in humans, the equivalent values of D_{min} being 2,500 ml and 50 ml respectively (Maurice and Ota 1978). This disparity is not borne out by the results with antibiotics. A number of experimental series with gentamicin and lincomycin lead to values of D_{min} similar to those found in humans (Table 4). Various workers have published very inconsistent results for penicillin in the rabbit, the values of D_{min} being spread over the range 4–6,000 ml. Part of this variability can possibly be accounted for by a greater regurgitation of the drug into the conjunctival sac in some cases, whence it can cross the epithelium by virtue of its lipid solubility.

4. Entry Pathways

Conrad and Robinson (1980) suggested that for pilocarpine the principal route of penetration into the anterior chamber was across the cornea from the tears when regurgitation through the injection hole in the conjunctiva was possible, and through the general circulation when it was not. In most of the examples cited in Table 4, the importance of the systemic route was excluded by measurements of the drug level in the blood or contralateral eye. Entry through the tears cannot be excluded, but the consistency of the results, the values of D_{min} usually ranging from 500 ml to 2,000 ml in both humans and rabbits, suggests that this is not the main source of entry for most drugs.

Direct penetration into the deeper tissues remains as the obvious pathway, and the first stage must be the saturation of the underlying sclera. It was shown that the diffusion rate of drugs in this tissue was such that the concentration on the inner side should begin to rise about 5 min after the injection of the drug (Maurice and Polgar 1977).

The second stage of penetration, from the sclera into the anterior chamber, could take place via several pathways:
1. Laterally into the stroma of the cornea and across its endothelium
2. Across the trabecular tissue at the angle
3. Through the stroma of the iris and across its anterior surface
4. Into the stroma of the ciliary body and into the freshly secreted aqueous humor
5. Into the vitreous body, principally at the pars plana, and across its anterior hyaloid membrane.

When small volumes of fluorescein are injected subconjunctivally, the diffusion of the dye into the adjacent cornea is seen in the slit lamp. From observations made soon after the injection, Mizuno (1972) was of the opinion that a high proportion of fluorescein penetrated the human anterior chamber from the region of the angle. The concentration changes in the anterior chamber were followed in a few human eyes after fluorescein injection (Maurice and Ota 1978), and described a profile similar to that found after iontophoresis into the cornea, which suggests that route 1. might be dominant. The profiles were not identical, however, and the variation between individuals was greater after subconjunctival injection, indicating that other routes were also being taken. In rabbits, the profiles varied even more among individual animals.

Analysis of the tissues, particularly the cornea and iris, at various times after subconjunctival injection has been carried out in several investigations (ANDREWS 1947; BLOOME et al. 1970; HAMARD et al. 1975; ABEL et al. 1974), and this should also provide a clue as to the origin of the drug appearing in the aqueous humor. For cefazolin (ABEL et al. 1974) the results seem clear cut; the drug concentration in the iris is much lower than in the cornea at all times and is negligible after 2 h. For other drugs, generally a considerably higher concentration is found in the cornea at first, but as time goes on the iris concentration drops less and becomes more important, possibly as a result of drug binding by the pigment.

The distribution of gentamicin in the tissues of the rabbit (BARZA et al. 1977) and monkey (BARZA et al. 1978) eye has been examined in detail 1 h after injection of 0.75 ml or 0.2 ml solution. The bleb spread around the eyeball and the localization is not well defined, but the concentration found in the sclera and cornea in the region of the injection is higher than elsewhere.

5. Vitreous Penetration

The distribution of a drug in the vitreous body after subconjunctival injection will be determined to some extent by where it is able to penetrate the tunics of the eye to the interior, but no information seems to be available on this point. Once within the vitreous body the drug would be subject to the transport and diffusional systems that eliminate it and that develop concentration gradients within the gel, to be described in the next pages. It is to be expected, then, that the distribution of drugs entering from the periocular space would be markedly nonuniform, and this is in accordance with the measurements of ABEL and BOYLE (1976), who found a higher concentration of cefazolin in the anterior than the posterior half of the vitreous after freezing and dividing the eye.

Although there have been a number of measurements of vitreous levels in the rabbit, generally the method of collecting the fluid has not been specified, or it is not made clear, as when collection is through a syringe needle, whence it is forthcoming. The values reported have been variable, ranging from zero to a level equal to that in the aqueous humor (TAKAHASHI 1971a). These data are cited extensively by BARZA (1978), and it is difficult to see how they can be systematized; as a generalization it may be said that the concentration in the vitreous is usually considerably less than that in the aqueous humor.

6. Retrobulbar Injection

The bleb formed by a posterior injection of fluid close to the globe will spread forward, and the bleb from a subconjunctival injection spreads backward, so that there is not a profound difference between the two methods but only a matter of balance. In a few detailed studies that have been carried out, short-term penetration into the sclera was about the same by both methods, and the differences in vitreous penetration are inconsistent. Retrobulbar injection gave a markedly lower level in the cornea (BARZA et al. 1977, 1978; TAKAHASHI 1971a, b) and a correspondingly lower concentration in the aqueous humor.

II. Intravitreal Injection

1. Diffusion in Vitreous

The diffusion of solutes in the vitreous appears to be unrestricted even if they have a large molecular weight. The electrical conductivity of the beef vitreous is the same as that of saline (Maurice 1957), fluorescein spreads as fast as if freely diffusing in water (Cunha-Vaz and Maurice 1967), and dextran appears in the aqueous humor after intravitreal injection as if it were moving in an unrestricted fashion (Maurice, to be published). This lack of resistance to the movement of even large solutes can be accounted for by the low average concentration (0.01%) of collagen in the gel, which implies that the fibrils will be 2 μm apart (Maurice 1959). Even in the region of the lens zonule, the same freedom of movement seems to be permitted. Posterior chamber dynamics suggest that sodium diffusion is unrestricted in this region (Maurice 1957; Kinsey and Reddy 1959).

In general, then, it seems that substances introduced into the vitreous humor will spread both through it and into the anterior chamber at the same rate that they diffuse in free solution. In rabbits, and presumably in humans, unless the vitreous body has become liquefied, any fluid flow through the gel appears to be negligible in comparison with the rate, primarily decided by their molecular weights, at which solutes can spread by their own molecular motion.

2. Loss from the Vitreous Chamber

Once a substance has distributed itself throughout the vitreous by diffusion, it is found that a constant fraction leaves the eye during each hour, so that the loss can be characterized by a single transfer coefficient, k_v. At the same time the ratio of the concentration in the aqueous to that in the vitreous humor maintains a constant value, although both concentrations are falling. Two pathways of exit can be distinguished: first, through the anterior hyaloid membrane into the posterior chamber and thence out of the eye with the aqueous drainage, and second, directly across the retinal surface (Fig. 13). The characteristics of each of these routes of exit will be examined in turn.

a) Loss by the Anterior Chamber

When there is no passage of a tracer out across the retinal surface, it can only leave the vitreous body anteriorly, where it will be carried away by the flow of the aqueous humor or by diffusion across the iris surface. The rate of loss will be controlled by the speed at which it can diffuse through the vitreous body and lens zonule, and this will be determined principally by geometric factors. A simple relationship exists between the rate at which the drug leaves the vitreous body and its concentration in the aqueous humor (Maurice 1959). This is found by equating the rate of loss from the vitreous body to that from the aqueous humor. Thus, because the quantity of drug in the anterior chamber is small compared with that in the vitreous cavity: $k_v C_v V_v = k_o C_a V_a$ so that:

$$k_v = k_o \frac{V_a}{V_v} \frac{C_a}{C_v} \tag{37}$$

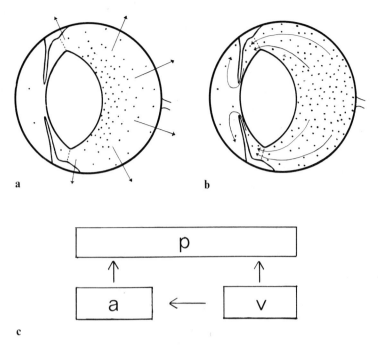

Fig. 13 a–c. Exit pathways from the vitreous body, **a** across the retinal surface and **b** via drainage out of the anterior chamber; **c** represents the compartments concerned: a, anterior chamber; p, plasma; v, vitreous

or, if the diffusional losses across the iris can be neglected:

$$k_v = \frac{f}{V_v} \frac{C_a}{C_v},\qquad(38)$$

where f is the aqueous flow rate. The relationship between k_v and C_a/C_v, for the values of V_v and f pertaining to the rabbit, is graphed as the straight line in Fig. 14. Substances that leave the vitreous humor entirely by the anterior route should have experimental values that plot as points in the neighborhood of this line. Such substances are ^{131}I-serum albumin (MAURICE 1959) and ^{14}C-sucrose (BITO and SALVA-DOR 1972).

An absolute estimate of the rate of loss through the anterior chamber to be expected for substances of different molecular weights present in the rabbit's vitreous humor has been provided by the use of a thermal analog (MAURICE 1959). This calibration is marked on the theoretical linear relationship, and it will be seen that the experimental values lie close enough to the calibration to suggest that the rate of loss is controlled entirely by the slowness of diffusion in the vitreous body. Even the point for hyaluronic acid lies close to the effective molecular weight assigned to it by viscosity measurements, 1.5×10^6 daltons, indicating that this mechanism applies regardless of the size of the solute.

Results with radiolabeled sodium and bromine ions are almost identical to each other (MAURICE 1957; BECKER 1961 a), and give a loss rate of 0.10 h^{-1} and a con-

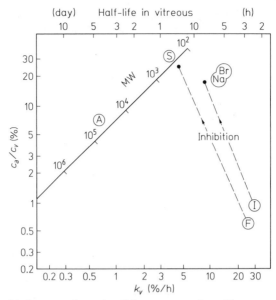

Fig. 14. Relationship between the ratio of the concentration of a tracer substance in the anterior chamber (C_a) to that in the vitreous body (C_v) and its rate of loss from the vitreous (k_v). The *straight line* represents the theoretical relationship for loss entirely by drainage out of the anterior chamber in the rabbit; the molecular weight (MW) calibration was obtained from a thermal diffusion analog (MAURICE 1959). The substances sucrose (S) and albumin (A) fall close to the line, indicating that they leave the vitreous body only by the anterior route. Sodium (Na) and bromide (Br) leave partly by this route but partly across the retina. Fluorescein (F) and iodide (I) leave very much faster and give rise to a very low concentration in the anterior chamber, which corresponds to their loss entirely across the retinal surface. When the transport mechanisms which remove them from the eye are inhibited, they move close to the positions anticipated for nontransported substances. (MAURICE 1976)

centration ratio of 20%. These points lie significantly below the theoretical line, and this is partly because the loss from the anterior chamber by diffusion is not negligible in comparison with the loss by flow for these ions. However, inserting the actual value for k_o in Eq. (37) shows that a substantial proportion of their loss is other than by way of the aqueous humor and is presumably across the retinal surface.

b) Loss Across the Retina

The barrier between the vitreous humor and the retina, shared between the retinal capillaries and the pigment epithelium, is impermeable to materials of high molecular weight such as albumin, but passes others such as small ions. Many substances are actively secreted out of the vitreous body by the retinal structures, which gives the layer highly asymmetric properties. Active mechanisms of removal have been identified for iodide (BECKER 1961 b), iodopyracet (FORBES and BECKER 1960), fluorescein (CUNHA-VAZ and MAURICE 1967), prostaglandin E (BITO and SALVADOR 1972), and indomethacin (MOCHIZUKI 1980). If solutes are transported rapidly across the retina the diffusional path through the vitreous body is short-ened, and the anterior bottleneck between the lens and ciliary body is replaced by a wide surface available for absorption, as is shown by a comparison of Fig. 13a and b. It is to be expected, therefore, that the loss from the eye would be acceler-ated, and this is found to be the case. Thus the rates of removal of fluorescein and iodopyracet are 0.28 and 0.23 h^{-1}, respectively, whereas figures six times smaller would be expected on the basis of their molecular size if they left only by the an-terior route.

Not only is k_v changed but the value of C_a/C_v is also profoundly altered when there is active transport across the retina. For fluorescein the ratio was found to be from 0.3% to 3%, and in the cases of iodopyracet and iodide the quantity in the anterior chamber was below the limits of detection. These points are labeled F and I on Fig. 14, and it is seen that they fall very far from the line that cor-responds to anterior loss; they are displaced both downward and to the right of their appropriate positions.

It is possible to block the transport of these ions by saturation or by competitive or metabolic inhibitors. When transport is blocked, there is a slowing down of the rate of loss from the vitreous chamber and, at the same time, a marked rise in the value of C_a. The plot of k_v and C_a/C_v then moves close to the theoretical line re-presenting the loss by drainage through the anterior chamber (Fig. 14), showing that this has become the major route in the inhibited eye. This is demonstrated in concentration distributions obtained from frozen eyes (CUNHA-VAZ and MAURICE 1967), where the contours show a gradient of fluorescein flow across the retina in the normal and across the vitreous–aqueous interface in the inhibited eye.

3. Drug Kinetics

Direct injection into the vitreous body, as contrasted with other methods of drug administration, gives rise to an initial concentration in the fluid which can be cal-culated with certainty and adjusted to be above the therapeutic level but below that of toxicity. It is evident from the discussion of vitreous dynamics that there are ad-vantages in choosing an antibiotic that leaves the vitreous humor by the anterior rather than the retinal route. Its therapeutic action will be prolonged, its concen-tration will be more uniform throughout the gel, extending unchanged up to the retina, and the anterior segment of the eye will be bathed in the high concentration which is created in the aqueous humor (MAURICE 1976).

There are only a few antibiotics for which k_v and C_a/C_v have both been mea-sured, and the data are often sketchy. The results, in every case from the rabbit, are plotted in Fig. 15. It appears that gentamicin, streptomycin, and sulfacetamide leave the eye predominantly by way of the anterior chamber, and penicillin and novobiocin across the retina.

For several other drugs only the value of k_v has been determined, and this value is sufficient to suggest, but not to establish, by which route loss occurs. These fig-ures, together with those for the antibiotics noted above, are listed as half-lives in Table 5. The penicillins as a group appear to be lost rapidly across the retinal sur-face, and this corresponds to the finding that penicillin G competitively inhibits the active transport of fluorescein (CUNHA-VAZ and MAURICE 1967).

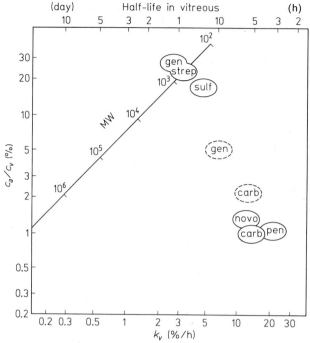

Fig. 15. Relationship of aqueous to vitreous concentration level (C_a/C_v) to rate of loss from the vitreous (k_v) for drugs injected into the vitreous body. Citations to individual values can be obtained from Table 5. Gentamicin (*gen*), streptomycin (*strep*), and sulfacetamide (*sulf*) appear to leave the vitreous by the anterior route, and penicillin (*pen*), carbenicillin (*carb*), and novobiocin (*novo*) across the retina. The *broken outline* corresponds to values in the inflamed eye. *MW*, molecular weight

Table 5. Rate of loss of drugs after injection into vitreous body of rabbit, k_v. Loss route estimated from k_v as explained in the text

Drug	k_v (% h^{-1})	Major route of loss
Gentamicin[a]	3.5	
Streptomycin[b]	3.5	Anterior
Tobramycin[c]	4	chamber
Sulfacetamide[d]	6.5	
Kanamycin[e]	7	
Novobiocin[f]	10	
Methicillin[g]	18	
Penicillin[d]	18	
Carbenicillin[h]	18	
Clindamycin[i]	25	
Dexamethasone[j]	27	
Indomethacin[k]	40	Retina

[a] PEYMAN et al. 1974a; [b] GARDINER et al. 1948; [c] BENNETT and PEYMAN 1974; [d] DUGUID et al. 1947; [e] PEYMAN et al. 1974b; [f] SERY et al. 1957; [g] DAILY et al. 1973; GRANT 1981; [h] SCHENK et al. 1974; BARZA et al. 1982; [i] PAQUE and PEYMAN 1974; [j] GRAHAM and PEYMAN 1974; [k] MOCHIZUKI 1980

A high lipid solubility should be equivalent to an active transport mechanism in leading to a rapid transport across the retinal surface into the blood. This effect has not been established experimentally, but it could account for the rapid loss of steroid from the vitreous.

4. Application to Humans

Experimental data similar to those given above for the rabbit appear to be lacking for the human or monkey. It can only be assumed, therefore, that the materials injected intravitreally in man follow the same general patterns as those found in the rabbit. However, a similarity does exist in the behaviour of fluorescein which passes in negligible quantities into the vitreous body from the blood in any species, and follows similar posterior and anterior chamber dynamics in rabbit and man (CUNHA-VAZ and MAURICE 1969; NAGATAKI 1975).

Because the diameter of the human eye (24 mm) is larger than that of the rabbit (18 mm), diffusion paths are longer in it, and drugs may be expected to leave more slowly when their rate of loss is entirely controlled by diffusion. For drugs that pass out across the retina, their half-lives should increase approximately as the square of the ratio of the diameters, or about 1.7 times. When the loss occurs through the aqueous humor, the ratio is more difficult to estimate because of the irregular geometry of the vitreous body; inspection would suggest that the bottleneck at the lens zonule is more restrictive in the human than in the rabbit, so that the loss may be at least twice as slow.

If the ratio C_a/C_v for the rabbit can be transferred to the human eye, the dilution volume in the aqueous humor, D_{min}, will be about 25 ml for drugs leaving the vitreous through the anterior chamber and 500 ml for those passing out across the retina.

D. Systemic Administration

I. Intraocular Drug Penetration

A drug may be administered systemically in various ways: by ingestion, by intravenous, intramuscular, or intraperitoneal injection, or by absorption across the mucous membranes of the mouth or rectum. In each case it is taken into the bloodstream before it reaches the eye. Here, as in every other tissue of the body, the penetration of the drug is primarily determined by how its chemical activity in the plasma varies with time; this depends upon the coefficients of absorption, excretion, and metabolism in the blood compartment as well as on the extent of binding of the drug by the plasma proteins and formed bodies in the blood. The distribution of the drug in the individual ocular tissues is further modified by factors specific to the eye.

Only rare blood vessels are found in the sclera, although they become more dense around the corneal limbus, and within the globe of the eye only the uvea and retina are well vascularized. The structure and permeability characteristics of the capillaries are different depending on their location (Fig. 1). The tissues of the eye, particularly those essential for the visual function, are well sequestered from the general circulation by various barriers which show high selectivity for the transfer of solutes from blood; this is probably a protective mechanism. In consequence, the concept of the blood–ocular barriers, embracing the blood–aqueous and the blood–retinal or blood–vitreal barriers, has evolved. Many substances are actively transported into the eye and thus evade the barriers, while others, including a number of drugs, are transported out so that their intraocular penetration is particularly restricted. Moreover, it appears that the pigment epithelium can further protect the retina by means of enzymes which metabolize toxic substances brought to it by the blood. Any of these factors may modify the passage of a drug into the eye after systemic administration and its subsequent fate.

1. Structures Related to Entry from Blood

a) Iris and Ciliary Body: The Blood–Aqueous Barrier

Drugs enter into the anterior and posterior chambers principally from the blood circulating in the iris and ciliary body. From the posterior chamber the drug can diffuse freely into the anterior portion of the vitreous body. The structure and physiological nature of the blood–aqueous barrier were described in detail in Sects. B.I.4.b and c.

b) The Choroid and the Pigmented Epithelium of the Retina

The choroid is a highly vascular layer, 0.1–0.2 mm thick in humans, lying immediately inside the sclera and attached to it by a loose tissue, the suprachoroid. In the posterior sector the attachment is firm, but anterior to the equator it is weak (Moses 1965), and in primates the anterior suprachoroid forms part of the uveoscleral or unconventional route of aqueous drainage (see Sect. B.I.4.a).

For the purposes of solute transfer the most important component is the choriocapillaris, a densely packed network of large capillaries forming a single layer on the inner face of the choroid. The surface area of this capillary network in the rabbit is almost two and a half times the surface of the choroid (Baurmann 1930), and the blood flow rate is higher than in other structures in the eye (Alm et al. 1973). Its endothelial cells have abundant fenestrae and, correspondingly, the capillaries are permeable to large electron-dense markers and the extravascular space contains a high concentration of albumin and γ-globulin (Bill 1968). The penetration of fluorescein and other dyes into the space after intravenous injection can be seen to occur within a few seconds (Grayson and Laties 1971).

The pigment epithelium of the retina is a single layer of hexagonal cells lining the outer face of the neural retina. The cells are joined to each other on their apical side by zonulae occludentes (Hogan et al. 1971; Raviola 1977). In the cat, the isolated cell layer has an electrical resistance of up to 3 kΩ cm^2 (Steinberg and Miller 1979), comparable to that of the corneal epithelium, and so its permeability to small ions must be very low. Active transport mechanisms for Na and for Cl, as well as certain amino acids (Steinberg and Miller 1979), have been identified in the isolated pigment epithelium of the frog, and for organic anions in the rabbit (see Sect. C.II.2.b).

c) The Retinal Vessels

In humans and most mammals the arteries and veins run in the superficial layer of the retina over its entire surface and supply a network of capillaries distributed in the inner half of the sensory retina. In the rabbit the vessels run on the retinal surface only above a horizontal strip of myelinated nerve fibers, so that most of the retina is free of vessels.

The endothelial cells of the retinal vessels are joined near their luminal faces by zonulae occludentes, which completely encircle the cells (CUNHA-VAZ 1979). Accordingly, the vascular endothelium of the retinal vessels presents a tight barrier, which does not allow the passage of electron-dense markers. Fluorescein angiography performed as a routine clinical examination shows that the fluorescein contained in the retinal vessels does not leak out into the retina under normal conditions. Furthermore, the endothelium of the retinal capillaries appears to be capable of actively transporting fluorescein out of the vitreous into the blood (CUNHA-VAZ and MAURICE 1967).

Tissues of the neural retina offer little resistance to the diffusion of substances, and electron-dense markers diffuse into the intercellular spaces of the retina after intravitreous injections (SMELSER et al. 1965; PEYMAN et al. 1971).

2. The Blood–Vitreous Barrier

Substances brought to the eye by the bloodstream rapidly equilibrate with the extravascular space of the choroid, and are separated from the retina and the vitreous body by the pigment epithelium, as well as by the endothelial cells of the retinal capillaries – the outer and inner blood–retinal barriers (CUNHA-VAZ 1979). Both these barriers are controlled by tight cellular junctions and form a considerable obstacle to the passage of lipophobic solutes of all sizes, although values for their permeability are hard to come by. The high electrical resistance of the pigment epithelium, corresponding to a permeability of the order of 1×10^{-3} cm h^{-1}, has already been referred to, but an analysis of the loss of radiosodium from the vitreous body of the rabbit suggested that the permeability of the combined barriers should be at least ten times greater than this (MAURICE 1957). Measurements of the penetration of tracers into the vitreous are difficult to analyze in terms of the retinal barrier, because the greater part of the total penetration comes from the posterior aqueous humor. However, regional analysis of the vitreous body in the eyes of both cats (DAVSON et al. 1949) and rabbits (KINSEY 1960; BLEEKER et al. 1968a) which were enucleated and frozen soon after small tracers had been injected into the blood shows a significant penetration near the posterior retina after 30 min or less, long before the tracer could have diffused there from the ciliary body. The level in the posterior part of the vitreous, about 5% of that in the blood after 30 min, leads to a retinal surface permeability of about 2×10^{-2} cm h^{-1}. The easiest way to reconcile this with the much lower pigment epithelium permeability is to assume that it corresponds to the retinal capillaries.

Superimposed on the large obstacle to penetration due to the ultrastructure of the inner and outer barriers is the further restriction that seems to result from the active transport mechanisms resident in the cells. This is exemplified by the behavior of fluorescein, where a concentration in the vitreous body of no more than

1/10,000 that in the plasma can be maintained. Similar outwardly directed transport mechanisms also act on certain drugs, e.g., penicillin and indomethacin (see Sect. C.II. 2.b).

3. Chemical Factors in Drug Penetration

Differences in the penetration of drugs across the blood–ocular barrier must be related to their chemical properties (DAVSON 1969). The difficulty in separating out the effects of a multiplicity of factors has led to only gross distinctions being made between the various compounds. Two of the criteria that have been investigated, molecular weight and lipid solubility, affect the molecules in their passage across the barrier. A third, the binding to the blood proteins, is a property external to the eye and can be measured without reference to it.

a) Binding to Proteins

Drugs are reversibly bound to plasma proteins and only the unbound fraction is in diffusional exchange across the tissue barriers. Thus substances almost completely bound to plasma proteins, e.g., Evans' blue (DAVSON 1969) or naphthylazo-penicillin X (LANGHAM 1951), do not appear in the aqueous humor. Intracameral penetration of various penicillins (RECORDS 1969a) and of tetracyclines (MOOG 1969) was also shown to be dependent on the degree of binding of these drugs to plasma proteins. In principle, the fraction bound by protein is determined by mass action dynamics and should vary with the concentration of drug in the plasma, as well as with the pH. In practice, however, large changes in the concentration within the clinical range do not lead to a detectable change in binding (CURRY 1977).

Measurements of drug binding are available in the literature, but only for a limited number of antibiotics, and often the results of different workers are not in agreement. Determinations of the unbound fraction in the plasma should be made for every drug whose penetration from the blood into the eye is being investigated, and preferably in every experiment carried out, so that binding does not enter as a factor into the ocular kinetics. Many drugs are also bound to tissue proteins and notably to melanin pigments, and this alters distribution of the drug to the tissue (see Sect. B.II.5.c).

b) Molecular Size

Small lipophobic molecules can cross the ciliary epithelium as well as the walls of the iris capillaries and enter the aqueous through these structures. The rate of intracameral entry of such substances is inversely related to their molecular weight, and raffinose (molecular weight 595) enters slowly in relation to small tracers (WELD et al. 1942). BURNS-BELLHORN et al. (1978) observed the entry of a series of graded fluoresceinated dextrans into the anterior chamber of the rat, and found that the amount appearing in the iris and anterior chamber diminished as their size increased; the cut-off point appeared to be with dextran of molecular weight 70,000 and effective radius 6 nm [REFOJO (1982) considers this to be an overestimate]. Consequently, drugs with a large molecular weight will be found in the aqueous at a low concentration after systemic administration, unless they have some degree of lipid solubility.

Although macromolecules cannot cross the cells of the iris capillaries or of the ciliary epithelium, the fenestrated capillaries allow their passage into the ciliary process stroma, whence they move into the anterior chamber through the iris root (VEGGE et al. 1976). Blood proteins are normally found in the aqueous but at a very low concentration, only about 1% of that in the plasma (ZIRM 1980).

c) Lipid Solubility

Compounds may cross the blood–ocular barriers in spite of their large molecular size, and the rate of penetration is correlated with their lipid solubility, as expressed by the partition coefficient between a lipid solvent and water. This has been shown in the anterior chamber using a variety of organic substances, including drugs, e.g., sulfonamides, penicillin, and chloramphenicol, as described in DAVSON (1969). Similarly, lipophobic substances show very poor penetration into the vitreous body, but those which are lipid-soluble can reach appreciable levels (BLEEKER et al. 1968 b). Additional confirmation has been provided by SØRENSEN (1971), who determined the rate of penetration of various substances into the aqueous and vitreous body and showed that it is correlated with their ether/water partition coefficients. Accordingly, intraocular penetration of drugs appears to depend largely on their lipid solubility, and the molecular sieve effect plays a minor role.

The steady-state ratio between the aqueous and blood of patients for a series of tetracyclines of similar molecular weight was measured by MOOG (1969). After correcting for protein binding, he found a good correlation between the level in the anterior chamber and the partition coefficient of the drug between chloroform and water.

d) Active Transport in the Eye

Certain metabolites, such as ascorbic acid (KINSEY and REDDY 1964) and some amino acids (REDDY 1979), have a normal level in the aqueous humor which is higher than that in the plasma, and this is attributed to active transport mechanisms located in the ciliary body. Evidence is lacking for the active transport of any synthetic drug into the eye, however.

A number of organic acids are accumulated by the ciliary body and are transported out of the eye by carrier-mediated transport systems which are sensitive to temperature and to ouabain. These transport systems are similar to those in the renal tubules, liver, and choroid plexus (BÁRÁNY 1976). They are competitively inhibited by a variety of substances, which are thus also likely to be substrates for transport (BITO and DEROUSSEAU 1980). As a result, these substances may reach only a very low concentration in the posterior chamber after systemic administration. The poor efficacy of certain systemically administered drugs, e.g., penicillin (BECKER 1960) and indomethacin (MOCHIZUKI 1980), has been attributed to this transport.

Similar transport systems are present in the retina (BITO and DEROUSSEAU 1980) and are located either in the pigmented epithelium or in the epithelial capillaries, as already mentioned in Sect. C.II.2.b. Drugs which are subject to their action, such as penicillin, penetrate poorly across the retina from the blood and are present at low concentrations in the vitreous humor after systemic administration.

e) Probenecid

Probenecid inhibits the transport of organic acids, particularly penicillins, in the renal tubules; this suppresses their excretion and results in a prolonged high level of the antibiotics in the blood. Its systemic administration slowed the loss of fluorescein from the vitreous in rabbits (CUNHA VAZ and MAURICE 1967). Prior administration of probenecid in rabbits was shown to enhance the intraocular penetration of various penicillins (BARZA and BAUM 1973) and also that of chloramphenicol (BROUGHTON and GOLDMAN 1973). However, the enhanced intraocular penetration was thought (BARZA and BAUM 1973) to be due to a prolonged high blood level of the antibiotics and not to a local inhibition of the excretory mechanisms in the eye. This view is supported by data presented by SALMINEN (1978a) on the penetration of cloxacillin into the rabbit eye, which on kinetic analysis show no significant influence of probenecid on the steady-state aqueous–plasma ratio or the coefficient of entry into the anterior chamber. The influence of systemic probenecid on the rate of loss of actively transported drugs from the rabbit vitreous body is uncertain; GRANT (1981) found that it did not change the rate for methicillin, whereas BARZA et al. (1982) found that it slowed the loss of carbenicillin by a factor of 2 or 3.

4. Drug Distribution in the Eye

a) Aqueous–Plasma Steady-State Ratio

An indication of how well a drug will penetrate into the eye is given by r_{ap}, the ratio of the concentration in the aqueous humor to that of the unbound drug in the blood plasma at steady state, which may be expressed: $r_{ap} = \bar{C}_a / \bar{C}_p$.

In general, the literature reports only the ratio of the aqueous to the total plasma concentration, C'_p, which leads to values of what may be called the apparent aqueous–plasma steady-state ratio, r'_{ap}. Nevertheless, this is of interest in order to compare the bioavailability of different drugs in the anterior segment, as well as to compare the behavior of the human and rabbit eye.

The most accurate estimate of r'_{ap} can be obtained from the equilibrium values, $\bar{C}_a$ and $\bar{C}'_p$, where the latter has been held constant over a long period of time. Most investigators report only concentrations that are changing with time, and the ratio has to be determined from the steady-state condition that occurs transiently while C_a is passing through a maximum, so that $dC_a/dt = 0$. The ratio is then derived from the momentary value of C'_p when the aqueous concentration is at its peak.

The results of such analyses are given in Table 6. It is usually difficult to determine exactly at what time the aqueous concentration is passing through its peak value, and if the blood concentration is falling rapidly in that period, a considerable error in the estimate of r'_{ap} may result. The values in the table can therefore be considered only rough estimates.

b) Dilutions

Although there may be difficulty in determining the exact time when the aqueous humor reaches its peak, usually a good estimate can be made of the maximum value itself. Since the dose given to a patient is accurately known, a fairly precise

Table 6. Minimum dilution volume in anterior chamber of humans, D_{min}, and aqueous to blood steady-state ratio, r'_{ap}, in humans and rabbits for various drugs after systemic administration

Drug	Human		Rabbit
	D_{min} (ml)	r'_{ap} (%)	r'_{ap} (%)[a]
Penicillin G		20[r]	2,[y] 6,[z] 9,[aa] 14,[bb] *26*[cc]
Penicillin V		10[r]	12,[bb] 18[dd]
Ampicillin	1,200,000[b,c]	6,[b] 18[c]	3,[ee] *15*,[ff] 20,[gg] 40[hh]
Tetracycline	1,000,000[d]	15,[d] 17,[s] 20[t]	*10*[ii]
Oxytetracycline		17[s]	25[jj]
Doxycycline	800,000[e]	12[e]	18[jj]
Pyrrolidinomethyl tetracycline	1,000,000[f]	12[s,f]	
Chloramphenicol	1,500,000[d]	52[d]	28,[ee,kk] 33,[ll,mm] 60[nn]
Cephaloridine	450,000[g] 2,000,000[h]	0,[u] 5,[h] 12[g]	3[u,oo]
Cephalothin		0[v]	0,[pp] 3,[h] 8[qq]
Cephalexin	1,250,000[i]	0,[w] 12[i]	20[rr]
Cefaclor	1,500,000[j]	6[j]	
Cefuroxime	750,000[k]	10[k]	
Cefamandole	1,300,000[l]	2[l]	
Tobramycin	350,000[m]	10[m]	
Gentamicin	600,000[n]	4[n]	7[ss,tt]
Rifampicin	280,000[o]		10[o]
Sulfamethoxazole	40,000[p] 90,000[q]	22[p,q]	15[p]
Trimethoprim	180,000[q] 700,000[p]	13[p]	16[p]
Lincomycin		9[x]	20[uu]
Streptomycin			5,[kk,oo] 17[vv]
Dihydrostreptomycin			18[cc]
Kanamycin			0,[m] 4[vv]
Amikacin			8[ww]
Kanendomycin			17[xx]
Erythromycin			18,[ee] 27[yy]
Oleandomycin			70[zz]
Spiramycin			6[nn]
Clindamycin			10[Aa]
Erythromycin			35[kk]
Vancomycin			5[Bb]
Amphotericin B			0[Cc]
Thiosporin			0[Dd]
Dexamethasone			5[Ee]
Methylprednisolone			47[Ff]
Acetazolamide			71[Gg]
Methazolamide			100[Gg]

[a] Values in italics were the results of experiments with radioisotopically labeled drug; [b] MILANO et al. 1971; [c] KUROSE et al. 1965; [d] ABRAHAM and BURNETT 1955; [e] MOOG et al. 1971; [f] MOOG et al. 1969; [g] RILEY et al. 1968; [h] RICHARDS et al. 1972; [i] BOYLE et al. 1970; [j] AXELROD and KOCHMAN 1980; [k] RICHARDS et al. 1979; [l] AXELROD and KOCHMAN 1978; [m] FURGIUELE et al. 1978; [n] UTERMANN et al. 1977; [o] MUSINI et al. 1970; [p] POHJANPELTO et al. 1974; [q] RIEDER et al. 1974; [r] PAPAPANOS et al. 1961 b; [s] MOOG and KNOTHE 1968; [t] KNOTHE et al. 1970; [u] RECORDS 1969 b; [v] RECORDS 1968 b; [w] RECORDS 1971; [x] BECKER 1969; [y] GOLDMAN and KLEIN 1970; [z] VON SALLMANN and MEYER 1944; [aa] KIRISAWA 1954; [bb] TRICHTEL and PAPAPANOS 1961; [cc] BLOOME et al. 1970; [dd] PAPAPANOS et al. 1962; [ee] GOLDMAN et al. 1973; [ff] SALMINEN 1978 b; [gg] KUROSE and LEOPOLD 1965; [hh] FARIS and UWAYDAH 1974; [ii] SALMINEN 1977 a; [jj] KAHAN et al. 1974; [kk] WITZEL et al. 1956; [ll] BLEEKER and MAAS 1955; [mm] BROUGHTON and GOLDMAN 1973; [nn] FURGIUELE et al. 1960; [oo] MIZUKAWA et al. 1965; [pp] RECORDS 1968 a; [qq] MIKUNI et al. 1966; [rr] GAGER et al. 1969; [ss] GOLDEN and COPPEL 1970; [tt] KUMING and TONKIN 1974; [uu] COLES et al. 1971; [vv] HAYASHI 1966; [ww] KASBEER et al. 1975; [xx] TAKAHASHI 1971; [yy] SHORR et al. 1969; [zz] McCOY and LEOPOLD 1959; [Aa] TABBARA and O'CONNOR 1975; [Bb] PRYOR et al. 1962; [Cc] GREEN et al. 1965; [Dd] KUROSE et al. 1964; [Ee] HAMARD et al. 1975; [Ff] LEOPOLD and KROMAN 1960; [Gg] WISTRAND et al. 1960

Table 7. Concentration of various drugs in tissues of rabbit eye as percentage of plasma level 1 h after intravenous injection

	Ampicillin (Salminen 1978 b)	Tetracycline (Salminen 1977 a)	Dexamethasone (Hamard et al. 1975)
Aqueous	20	7	5
Cornea	26	10	20
Sclera	100	100	50
Conjunctiva	130	100	60
Iris and ciliary body	25	35	53
Lens	0	0	2
Vitreous	7	2	5
Choroid and retina	18	40	50

figure for the minimum dilution, D_{min}, can be arrived at by dividing this dose by the maximum concentration in the anterior chamber. Carrying out these calculations with values cited in the literature resulting from the systemic administration of drugs to humans (Table 6) leads to the result that in most cases the value lies not very far from 1,000,000 ml. This volume is the same for drugs as different as chloramphenicol, which has an r'_{ap} of 0.52, and cefamandole, for which it is about 0.04. It is difficult to account for this consistency. That it is fortuitous is suggested by the much higher value found for fluorescein, about 7,000,000 ml, and the low value for sulfamethoxazole, less than 100,000 ml.

The figure of 1,000,000 ml may be compared to the typical volume of D_{min} of about 1,000 ml found for subconjunctival injection (Table 4) and of 25 ml in the case of intravitreal injection in humans. The figures for topical application will be very variable because of the large differences in epithelial permeability. For a single 40 µl drop they might range from a few ml for the steroids to 50,000 ml for gentamicin.

Systemic dilutions were not calculated for the rabbit, since the comparison with humans would be trivial, the result being determined principally by body size.

c) Tissue Distribution

It is of interest in considering the therapeutic action of a drug to know its penetration into the tissues as well as into the humors of the eye. The distribution of some typical drugs 1 h after systemic administration is shown in Table 7 and is evidently controlled to some extent by their chemical identity. How much drug is found in a tissue largely depends on its vascularization, or on its relation to other vascularized tissues and the permeability of intervening barriers.

II. Compartmental Analysis

1. Formulation of Aqueous Humor Dynamics

Ocular physiologists have analyzed the dynamics of the exchange of substances between the blood and the anterior segment of the eye according to the compartmen-

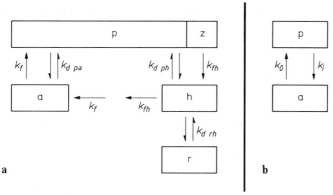

Fig. 16a, b. Compartmental models for aqueous humor dynamics. **a** Two-compartment model: *right-hand side* is for posterior chamber (*h*) and shows the flow and exchange coefficients referred to its volume, according to Eq. (39); *left-hand side* shows the relationships which hold in anterior chamber (*a*) referred to its volume according to Eq. (40). **b** One-compartment simplification corresponding to Eq. (42). *p*, plasma; *z*, ciliary body secretion; *r*, lens and vitreous reservoir; k_f, coefficient of transfer by flow; $k_{d \cdot pa}$, coefficient of transfer by diffusion referred to the anterior chamber volume; $k_{d \cdot ph}$, coefficient of diffusional exchange with the blood referred to the posterior chamber volume; k_{fh}, coefficient of transfer by flow referred to the posterior chamber volume; $k_{d \cdot rh}$, coefficient of diffusional exchange with the posterior reservoir referred to the posterior chamber volume; k_o, coefficient of loss; k_i, coefficient of entry

tal model illustrated in Fig. 16a. The aqueous humor is secreted by the ciliary processes into the posterior chamber and flows in bulk through the pupil into the anterior chamber, whence it is finally drained out of the eye through the outflow channels. In transit through the posterior chamber the aqueous humor bathes the surfaces of the vitreous, lens, and iris epithelium, and carries on diffusional exchanges with these structures. As a first approximation the concentration change in the posterior chamber can be described by the following equation (FRIEDENWALD and BECKER 1955):

$$\frac{dC_h}{dt} = k_{fh}(C_z - C_h) + k_{d \cdot ph}(C_p - C_h) + k_{d.rh}(C_r - C_h), \tag{39}$$

where C_h, C_z, C_p, and C_r are the concentrations, or more precisely the chemical activities, of the substance in the posterior chamber, the fluid secreted by the ciliary processes, the blood plasma, and the posterior reservoir formed by the lens and the vitreous body, and k_{fh}, $k_{d \cdot ph}$, and $k_{d \cdot rh}$ are the coefficients of transfer by flow, diffusional exchange with the blood, and diffusional exchange with the posterior reservoir, all referred to the posterior chamber volume.

The posterior reservoir is unstirred, and simple first-order dynamics, represented by this equation, only apply as an approximation. More rigorous treatments of its exchange with the aqueous have been developed by MAURICE (1957) and KINSEY and REDDY (1964).

Posterior chamber aqueous, concentration C_h, flows through the pupil into the anterior chamber, and anterior aqueous drains out of the eye at the same rate at a concentration C_a. While in the anterior chamber, dissolved substances exchange by diffusion with the blood in the anterior uvea. The concentration changes in the anterior chamber can be represented by (KINSEY and PALM 1955):

$$\frac{dC_a}{dt} = k_f(C_h - C_a) + k_{d \cdot pa}(C_p - C_a), \tag{40}$$

where k_f is the transfer coefficient by flow, i.e., the rate of aqueous flow divided by the anterior chamber volume, and $k_{d \cdot pa}$ is the coefficient of transfer by diffusion referred to the anterior chamber volume (Fig. 16).

The application of this equation requires concurrent determinations of the concentrations of inert tracers in the blood plasma and the posterior and anterior chambers, and a number of such experiments have been carried out in the rabbit. The values of k_f derived by fitting the data to Eq. (40) were found to cluster around $0.8 \, h^{-1}$. From the anterior chamber volume, the rate of aqueous flow in the rabbit was calculated to be about $0.2 \, ml \, h^{-1}$ (KINSEY and REDDY 1964).

When the aqueous humor is stained with fluorescein, both in the human and rabbit eye, bubbles of unstained fluid from the posterior chamber are observed to irrupt at intervals through the margin of the pupil into the anterior chamber; the freshly appearing fluid is known as the pupillary aqueous. After the intravenous injection of fluorescein, it is possible to measure its concentration in the pupillary aqueous as well as the anterior chamber, and Eq. (40) can then be employed to compute values of k_f and $k_{d \cdot pa}$. This technique is applicable to humans (NAGATAKI 1975; ARAIE et al. 1980), and analysis of the results, after correction for the metabolism of the dye to its glucuronide and for the influence of the cornea, led to an average value for k_f of about $0.6 \, h^{-1}$ in the normal eye, and for $k_{d \cdot pa}$ of about one-tenth of this figure. This value is lower than that found from analysis of the concentration changes after the introduction of the dye into the cornea by iontophoresis, about $0.9 \, h^{-1}$ (JONES and MAURICE 1966; BLOOM et al. 1976; COAKES and BRUBAKER 1979).

2. One-Compartment Approximation

In virtually every study of the penetration of a drug its changes in concentration in the posterior chamber have been ignored and only those in the anterior chamber have been reported, making the application of Eq. (40) impossible. GOLDMANN (1951) concluded on theoretical grounds that after intravenous injection the posterior chamber concentration would rise rapidly to a maximum level and thereafter decrease in parallel with the decrease in the blood concentration. In the case of fluorescein the validity of this assumption has received limited verification both in the rabbit and in man (CUNHA-VAZ and MAURICE 1969; NAGATAKI 1975) by measurements of its concentration in the pupillary aqueous.

If the assumption is taken to be generally true, then $C_h = nC_p$ where n is a proportionality constant. Equation (40) is transformed to (PALM 1947):

$$\frac{dC_a}{dt} = (nk_f + k_{d \cdot pa})C_p - (k_f + k_{d \cdot pa})C_a \tag{41}$$

and it may be rewritten as:

$$\frac{dC_a}{dt} = k_i C_p - k_o C_a,\qquad(42)$$

where $k_i = nk_f + k_{d \cdot pa}$ and $k_o = k_f + k_{d \cdot pa}$; k_i is called the coefficient of entry into the anterior chamber and k_o the coefficient of loss from the anterior chamber. In the normal eye, $k_{d \cdot pa}$ was shown to be about 10% of k_f for fluorescein, and therefore k_o may be approximated to k_f for this substance (GOLDMANN 1951).

When $dC_a/dt = 0$, the ratio of the concentration of a drug in the aqueous humor to that in the plasma is given by:

$$r_{ap} = \frac{k_i}{k_o},\qquad(43)$$

where r_{ap} is the steady-state ratio. The relationship of the parameters is displayed in Fig. 17. It will be noted that if one transfer coefficient is determined, the range of possible values for the others is often quite limited. It is also interesting that when the value of r_{ap} is small, the range of values for all the transfer coefficients is very restricted.

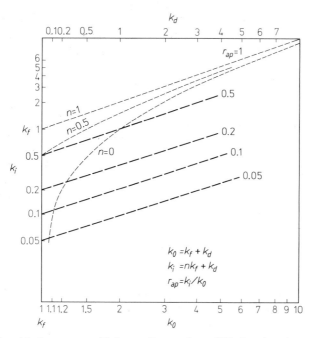

Fig. 17. Relationship between coefficients of entry, loss, diffusional exchange and outflow (k_i, k_o, k_d, and k_f) of the anterior chamber. Admissible values lie between the curves $n=0$, representing the absence of drug in the ciliary secretion, and $n=1$, representing a concentration of drug in the ciliary secretion equal to that in the plasma. The curves are constructed from the first two of the equations listed, which are used in the derivation of Eq. (42). The coefficients are expressed in terms of k_f as unity, making the diagram adaptable to any species. Also shown are a series of *straight lines* corresponding to various values of the aqueous plasma steady-state ratio (r_{ap}), as shown by the third equation listed

3. Changes in Aqueous Concentration

a) Entry from Blood

If the plasma level of the drug were constant from the moment of its administration, Eq. (42) shows that the concentration in the anterior chamber would rise to its steady-state level, $\bar{C}_a$, with a monoexponential course $C_a = \bar{C}_a(1 - e^{-k_o t})$.

However, such a constant blood level can be achieved only under well-controlled experimental conditions, and then with difficulty. Generally, if a drug is given intravenously, its blood level falls rapidly in the 1st h and more slowly thereafter, and if it is injected into a muscle or taken by mouth, the level rises more or less rapidly at first and then falls. In all circumstances the aqueous humor concentration will pass through a maximum; for intravenous injection this maximum will generally occur within the 1st h, but it may be delayed to the 3rd or 4th h for the other routes of delivery.

The analytical solution of the differential Eq. (42) requires that C_p be expressed as a function of time. According to the substance employed and the route by which it is administered, various approximations containing one or more exponential terms have been used to describe the time course of C_p (PALM 1948; GOLDMAN 1951), and the equation has then been solved explicitly [see also Eq. (45)]. Because these descriptions are approximations, at best, and because blood levels are easier to measure than to control, most workers have preferred to follow the plasma concentration by collecting samples of blood at intervals and to solve the equation by numerical methods.

b) Influence of Cornea

In deriving Eq. (42) the exchange between the aqueous humor and the cornea was neglected; this is because in most situations it has been considered to be a minor factor in determining anterior chamber kinetics. When a drug is first brought into the blood, it will enter the cornea from the limbal vessels, as will be described in Sect. D.II.6. This may be thought of as a contribution to the term $k_i C_p$ in Eq. (42), although this contribution will be a very complex function of time. Concurrently, some of the drug which enters the anterior aqueous humor by flow and diffusion will pass across the endothelium in the opposite direction into the central regions of the stroma where the concentration is low. These exchanges may be accounted for, as a first approximation, by considering the cornea as slightly extending the volume of the anterior chamber. ARAIE et al. (1980) calculated, in the case of fluorescein, that ignoring the effect of the cornea would lead to an overestimate of 8% in k_f and 100% in $k_{d \cdot pa}$.

When the drug concentration in the plasma has fallen to a low value and that in the anterior chamber is declining, the influence of the cornea can become very important. Its exchanges with the blood at the limbus and with the aqueous across the endothelium continue, but the direction of the net flux will be reversed. If the rate constant of the drug loss out of the blood is much larger than the transfer coefficient from the cornea to the aqueous, k_c, the cornea will soon replace the blood as the compartment determining the rate of fall of drug concentration in the aqueous humor, following the kinetics described in Sect. B for topical administration. The change from plasma-regulated to cornea-regulated kinetics has not been examined for any drug or tracer; it is too complex a problem to treat generally, depending as it does on the concentration profile in the blood as well as on the ocular kinetic parameters.

4. Kinetics of Intracameral Penetration

The best single measure of how readily a drug will penetrate the anterior chamber is the coefficient of entry, k_i. A dozen papers report data on the intracameral penetration of drugs into the rabbit eye in sufficient detail to allow a kinetic analysis according to Eq. (42). Fewer data are available for the human eye. An example of such a set of data is shown in Fig. 18. The best fit of C_a to the experimental points can be achieved by adjusting the parameters k_i and k_o, and the results of this process are illustrated in the figure; it is greatly simplified by the use of a computer. The results of such computations are displayed in Table 8.

The values of k_o shown in this table are generally considerably lower than those derived from an analysis of topical penetration (Table 2). A smaller discrepancy was found in the case of fluorescein, the k_o for topical administration being 50% greater than that for systemic. The cause of these differences cannot be established at present.

It must be noted that in Eq. (40) the value of C_p, which determines that in Eq. (42), refers to the unbound drug in the blood plasma, whereas published data give the total drug concentration. Consequently, the results of such computations do not give the true coefficient of entry, k_i, but an apparent coefficient of entry, k'_i, corresponding to the apparent aqueous–plasma steady-state ratio, r'_{ap} (see Sect. D.I.4.a).

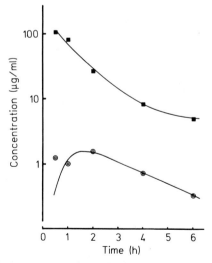

Fig. 18. Serum and aqueous concentrations of cefamandole after intravenous injection of 1 g in a group of cataract patients. *Squares*, serum concentration; *circles*, aqueous concentration. The lines shown are the best fit by a computer, using Eq. (42). (Axelrod and Kochman 1978)

Table 8. Kinetic coefficients of intracameral penetration from the blood of antibiotics in the human and rabbit eye derived from computer and graphic analysis

Antibiotic	r'_{ap} (%)[a]	$k'_i \times 10^{-2}$ (h^{-1})[a]	k_o (h^{-1})[a]	Reference
		HUMAN		
Pyrrolidinomethyltetracycline	12	5.0	0.4	Moog et al. 1969
Tobramycin	9 (10)[b]	4.0 (6.0)	0.4 (0.6)	Furgiuele et al. 1978
Cefamandole	1.6 (1.5)	1.3 (1.2)	0.8 (0.7)	Axelrod and Kochman 1978
Cephaloridine	12 (10)	11 (6.0)	0.9 (0.6)	Riley et al. 1968
		RABBIT		
Penicillin G	1 (2)	0.6 (1.5)	0.6 (0.7)	Goldman and Klein 1970
	– (10)	(8)	(0.8)	Kirisawa 1954
Benzylpenicillin[c]	32 (18)	60 (12)	1.8 (0.66)	Salminen et al. 1969
Cloxacillin	5 (6)	4.5 (6.5)	1.0 (1.1)	Salminen 1978a
Ampicillin	21 (20)	35 (48)	1.7 (2.4)	Kurose and Leopold 1965
Ampicillin	15 (13)	24 (18)	1.7 (1.4)	Salminen 1978b
Doxycycline	18 (18)	15 (17)	0.8 (1.0)	Kahan et al. 1974
Doxycycline	– (18)	(16)	(0.9)	Salminen 1977b
Oxytetracycline	25 (25)	18 (17)	0.7 (0.65)	Kahan et al. 1974
Cephalexin	20 (14)	34 (14)	1.7 (1.0)	Gager et al. 1969
Kanamycin	3 (4)	2.8 (3.8)	1.0 (1.0)	Hayashi 1966

[a] r'_{ap}, apparent aqueous – plasma steady-state ratio; k'_i, apparent coefficient of entry both in reference to the total plasma concentration of the antibiotics; k_o, coefficient of loss from anterior chamber

[b] The values in parentheses are those obtained by simple graphic methods. See Eq. (44)

[c] Where the drug is in italics, radioactive analysis was used, otherwise bioassay

A simple graphic method (GOLDMAN 1951) may be used instead of the computer analysis for extracting k_i' and k_o from curves such as those shown in Fig. 18. By dividing Eq. (42) by C_a and using Eq. (43) one obtains $dC_a/C_a dt = r_{ap} k_o C_p/C_a - k_o$.

As heretofore, writing A for $-dC_a/C_a dt$, it follows:

$$k_o = \frac{A}{1 - r_{ap} C_p/C_a}$$

or since total drug concentration in the plasma, C_p', is being considered:

$$k_o = \frac{A}{1 - r_{ap}' C_p'/C_a} \tag{44}$$

From the experimental curves A, r_{ap}', and C_p'/C_a can be separately determined. It will be noted that, in theory, A can be the slope of the C_a curve at any point, and it does not have to be a constant parameter. A more certain estimate can be achieved, however, if a linear segment of the experimental curve can be chosen, and the ratio C_p'/C_a is best taken from a region when the tangent to the plasma curve is parallel to this segment. The values of k_o reached by this simplified analysis are shown in brackets in Table 8, and the results are in good agreement with those obtained by computer fitting.

5. Penetration into the Vitreous

a) Vitreous Kinetics

Since the vitreous body is unstirred, the exchanges across its boundaries with the blood and aqueous humor are complex and should be expressed, as in heat conduction theory, by a series of exponential terms. Generally after a short period of time a single exponential term predominates, however, and for practical purposes the compartment can be treated as if it were stirred, so that its kinetics can be expressed by a single transfer coefficient, k_v.

In most cases of drug penetration from the systemic circulation a single intravenous injection is given, and to the order of accuracy that is attained in vitreous studies the concentration of the drug in the plasma may be expressed by the equation:

$$C_p = C_o e^{-k_p t}.$$

In this case the vitreous exchanges would be represented by $dC_v/dt = k_v(C_o e^{-k_p t} - C_v)$ and since the initial vitreous concentration is zero:

$$C_v = C_o \frac{k_v}{k_p - k_v} (e^{-k_v t} - e^{-k_p t}). \tag{45}$$

Corresponding to the two routes of loss that can be identified after injection into the vitreous body (see Sect. C.II), the entry of a drug from the systemic circulation can be considered as taking place across the anterior hyaloid membrane from the aqueous humor or across the surface of the retina and pars plana from the blood.

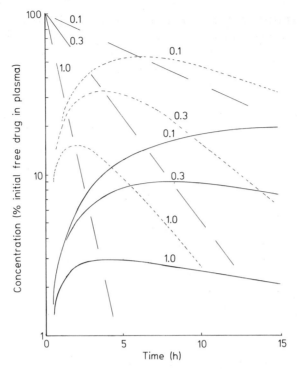

Table 19. Calculated concentration changes in the vitreous body after intravenous administration of a drug according to Eq. (45). The concentration of free drug in the plasma was assumed to fall exponentially with a rate constant of 0.1, 0.3, or 1 h^{-1}, as shown by the *three straight lines*. Vitreous curves were calculated for each of these three cases, and they are shown by *continuous lines* when the drug was assumed to enter from the posterior chamber only, and by *a dashed line* when it was assumed to enter across the entire retinal surface. The curves are based on an unrestricted transfer of drug into the posterior chamber or across the retina and will be lower if this is not the case

The transfer coefficient in either case is determined principally by the rate of diffusion in the vitreous body, and inspection of Fig. 14 suggests a typical value of 0.035 h^{-1} for k_v for the anterior route and 0.25 h^{-1} for the posterior. These extreme values of k_v and three values of k_p, covering the range found experimentally for various drugs, were inserted in Eq. (45), and the corresponding curves for C_p and C_v are shown in Fig. 19.

Three entry patterns can be considered:

1) Entry from the posterior chamber fluid only, the retinal surface being impermeable, which should be the case for lipophobic solutes which are held back at the blood–retinal barrier. The concentration in the posterior aqueous is approximately proportional to that in the plasma but is generally lower by the factor n (see Sect. D.II), so that the continuous curves shown in Fig. 19 will be proportionally lowered. The concentration in the vitreous body will be higher in the anterior than the posterior region before the maximum is reached, but this will be reversed after it is passed.

2) Free entry from the blood across the tissue surfaces, which should occur for certain lipophilic materials, among them the antibiotic chloramphenicol, which have been shown by BLEEKER et al. (1968 b) to be able to reach high concentration in the vitreous. Solutes with lesser fat solubility do not cross the blood-retinal barrier freely, and this may lead to the entry being less than predicted by the broken curves in Fig. 19.

3) Entry from the posterior chamber and active transport out across the retinal surface. The drug entering from the blood will never reach an appreciable concentration in the vitreous except in the most anterior region, as observed directly in the case of fluorescein (CUNHA-VAZ and MAURICE 1967).

b) Drug Penetration

Measurements have rarely been carried out over a long enough period of time and at frequent enough intervals to define the maximum drug concentration in the vitreous after its systemic administration. Because of the low levels found, the gathering of useful data had to await the availability of radio-labeled drugs.

Only tetracycline and doxycycline (SALMINEN 1977 a, b) appear to fit well to the theoretical curves. The value of k_p for these substances, as well as for most drugs tested, is of the order of magnitude of $0.3 \, \text{h}^{-1}$, and the maximum value of C_v appears to be just beyond 3 h, the longest experimental period used. The binding by the plasma has been roughly established for these drugs, and the maximum level measured in the vitreous appears to be in the range of 20%–50% of the calculated free blood concentration at the start of the experiment. The data therefore fit well to the curve that corresponds to these drugs entering from around the entire retinal surface.

Ampicillin also shows a maximum level around 3 h (SALMINEN 1978 b), but penicillin (BLOOME et al. 1970) and cloxacillin (SALMINEN 1978 a) appear to peak at 1 h or less, and these drugs are probably actively transported out of the vitreous humor.

Dexamethasone shows a maximum 2 h after intravenous injection (HAMARD et al. 1975) at a level of 3% of the total steroid in the blood. These workers found considerable metabolic breakdown in the eye, however, and the binding by the plasma was not established, so that it is not possible to draw conclusions as to its route of entry.

6. Penetration into the Cornea and Lens

a) Penetration into the Cornea

The penetration of drugs into the cornea from the blood takes place by two routes: directly from the limbal vessels into the stroma at the corneal periphery, and indirectly into the aqueous humor and then across the corneal endothelium. Some entry from the tears is imaginable for very fat-soluble molecules.

The corneal penetration of lipophobic solutes may be exemplified by the behavior of fluorescein. Figure 20 depicts the fluorescein concentrations in the blood plasma, the aqueous humor, and the central and peripheral cornea after ingestion

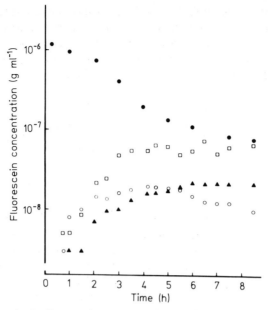

Fig. 20. Changes in the fluorescein concentration in a human subject after oral administration of 5 mg/kg body wt. *Solid circle*, plasma ultrafiltrate; *empty circles*, aqueous humor; *squares*, cornea 2 mm from the limbus; and *triangles*, corneal center. (ARAIE et al. 1980)

of the dye by a normal human volunteer. The concentration increase in the corneal periphery precedes that in the aqueous, but in the corneal center it lags behind it. This indicates that initial entry into the corneal periphery occurs mainly from the limbal vessels, and that into the central part from the aqueous humor (MAURICE 1967 b; SAWA et al. 1981). MAURICE (1969) calculated the steady-state distribution along the cornea of a substance which enters by the two routes. The material entering the cornea from the limbus is lost to the anterior chamber while it diffuses centrally through the tissue, and how far the limbal contribution penetrates depends both on the diffusion coefficient and the endothelial permeability of the substance. The larger the molecular size of the drug, the further it will penetrate toward the center of the cornea. Those with a typical k_c value of 0.7 h^{-1} will drop four times in concentration every 1 mm they penetrate from the limbus.

Very few papers are available which presented the time course of drug entry into the cornea, but the results of SALMINEN (1977 a, 1978 a, b) with tetracycline, ampicillin, and cloxacillin, and of HAMARD et al. (1975) with dexamethasone, indicate that the mode of corneal entry of the antibiotics is similar to that of fluorescein.

If only the central part of the cornea is considered, Eq. (2) applies in the form:

$$\frac{dC_c}{dt} = \frac{P_{ac}}{q}(C_a - C_c/r_{ca}). \tag{46}$$

No data from drugs administered by the systemic route which would allow an estimate of their endothelial permeability are yet available, and it is hoped that in the future the corneal concentration might be determined in the central and peripheral corneas separately. However, values of k_c obtained from topical measurements and their conversion to P_{ac} have been described in Sect. B.II.6.

b) Penetration into the Lens

Systemically administered drugs enter the lens via the ocular humors, which bathe its surfaces. The lens epithelium appears to offer a high resistance to lipophobic substances, and penetration of fluorescein from the aqueous humor is very slow (Sect. B.I.4.a). Systemic antibiotics are usually either undetectable or recoverable only in trace amounts from the lens after systemic administration (Table 7).

More lipid-soluble drugs, such as chloramphenicol (BLEEKER and MAAS 1955), benzylpenicillin (SALMINEN et al. 1969), and tetracycline (SALMINEN 1977a), seem to soak into the lens more rapidly. The systemic injection of rhodamine B, a lipid-soluble dye, quickly stains the cortex of the lens, which then shows in the slit lamp as the most fluorescent structure in the eye. Its use as an analog for lipid-soluble drugs has been suggested (MAURICE et al. 1982).

Although an unstirred body is under consideration in a three-compartment situation, a simple transfer equation was applied to the data of Salminen:

$$\frac{dC_l}{dt} = k_{al}(C_a - r_{al}C_l), \tag{47}$$

where C_1 is the concentration in the lens, k_{al} is the transfer coefficient in reference to the lens volume, and r_{al} is the distribution ratio between the aqueous and the lens. The values arrived at were: k_{al}, 0.9 h^{-1}, r_{al}, 0.32–0.4 for benzylpenicillin, and k_{al} 0.2 h^{-1}, r_{al}, 0.26 for tetracycline. The limitations mentioned above should be borne in mind in interpreting these figures.

The significance of these calculations is that the lens may act as a drug depot within the eye and, when treatment is intermittent, it could return the drug to the aqueous humor and smooth out the variations in drug level between applications. A superficial examination of the figures derived above indicates that the lens could return a notable concentration of a lipophobic drug to the anterior segment after the plasma and aqueous levels had dropped, in the same way that the cornea does under similar circumstances.

III. Conclusions and Recommendations

In the section on topical kinetics there were presented a variety of different methods for determining the transfer coefficients that describe the penetration across the cornea. When it comes to determining the transfer coefficients describing penetration into the eye from the blood, on the other hand, the experimental alternatives are quite limited. The experiments are necessarily carried out on a live animal or a human subject and involve following the level of drug in the blood and measuring how much enters the aqueous and vitreous humors after various time periods. The only way in which they can be varied is by altering the profiles of the plasma drug concentration.

It can be seen from Eq. (44) that only two of the parameters k_i, k_o, and r_{ap} need to be determined in order to derive the third; if k_f is measured or assumed, k_d and

n then follow immediately (Fig. 17). If the method of curve fitting described in Sect. D.II.4 is used, it is not in principle necessary to establish these parameters independently by separate experiments. However, by attempting to maintain a constant concentration of drug in the blood for an extended period, r_{ap} may be established to a given degree of precision with fewer eyes. Similarly, k_i can be determined more efficiently if measurements in the blood and aqueous humor are made during the first hour or two after the administration of the drug, while the level in the eye is still rising. In order to determine the parameters accurately, it is desirable to carry on the measurements for at least 6 h, and if vitreous kinetics are being investigated, for a longer period.

Finally, it must be emphasized that the true value of k_i, and hence the actual barrier presented to the penetration of the drug, cannot be established unless the drug binding by the plasma is determined. Unless the data are available in the literature, the free drug at body temperature should be determined for various concentration levels, either by ultrafiltration or dialysis (NAGATAKI 1975; CUNHA-VAZ and MAURICE 1969).

E. Kinetics in Ocular Disease

Apart from the diagnostic applications of autonomic agents and surface anesthetics, drugs are intended for use in diseased eyes, where their kinetics may be altered by the pathology. The compartmental models presented earlier should remain valid, although the exchange coefficients between compartments will be different. Inflammation can cause large changes in the permeabilities of tissues and can depress active transport systems. On the other hand, unless the disease process has led to the destruction or disorganization of tissues, there is no reason why it should appreciably alter the volume of the compartmental reservoirs – marked edema of the cornea being excepted.

Many groups of diseases will not be discussed in this section. Drugs are used in the treatment of glaucoma only when the rise in pressure is moderate. In these cases the flow rate is not significantly different from normal and the intraocular barriers are not likely to be affected. Cataracts are not likely to have a significant impact on drug movement, even if they affect the diffusional properties of the lens. The extraction of a cataract, however, removes the barrier between the anterior chamber and vitreous body and can have a major influence on kinetics (KRAMER 1976; COBO and FORSTER 1981). Degenerative conditions usually cannot be helped by drugs and have few analogies in experimental animals, so that their study is difficult and not of much value. Models for tumors of the eye are only in the process of development.

The following discussion will be limited to trauma, infection, and immune response, which among them account for much of the treatment with drugs. The reaction of the eye to each of these stimuli has features in common, the inflammatory response, and a corresponding response can be elicited in animals.

I. Inflammation and its Models

After mechanical, thermal, or chemical trauma there is an acute irritative phase of 1–2 h in which the tissues react to the injury either directly or through a neural mechanism (SEARS 1974; JAMPOL et al. 1975; CAMRAS and BITO 1980). The acute response to nociceptive stimuli consists of miosis, hyperemia, disruption of the blood–aqueous barrier, and transient increase in intraocular pressure. This can be followed by the inflammatory response, which is cell mediated. If the response is severe or sustained, permanent functional or structural damage to the eye can result (see Chap. 7).

A variety of chemical and mechanical insults and inflammatory or infective agents have been used in experiments on animal eyes in order to study their effect on drug penetration. For example, a mild reaction in the anterior segment has been caused by paracentesis, a more severe one by acid or alkali burns of the cornea, and a chronic inflammation by the intralamellar injection of clove oil (LEIBOWITZ and KUPFERMAN 1974). In the posterior segment immunogenic uveitis has been provoked by the intravitreal injection of an antigen. Infection of the cornea or vitreous body by standardized doses of bacteria has been used from time to time.

The simple acute reaction has usually given way to the sustained response by the time an eye presents for treatment, and the immediate effects of mild injury, such as paracentesis, on drug kinetics should be of lesser clinical relevance. It should be noted, moreover, that the quality and degree of the acute response may vary according to the species used, the rabbit differing from most others (BITO and KLEIN 1981). Experimental infections are attractive and sometimes comparable to human disease, but the complexity of the process makes interpretation of the results difficult. Uveitis induced by intravitreal or systemically administered (WACKER et al. 1977; DOREY and FAURE 1977; MARAK et al. 1980) antigens is a preferable model, since a more or less stable response of a purely inflammatory nature takes place.

The study of the effects of inflammation in humans would be valuable and the kinetics of fluorescein in the eye can be followed in patients, although the analysis is complicated, especially after its systemic administration, by the leakage of plasma proteins into the aqueous humor (ARAIE et al. 1981). No such observations seem to have been carried out on patients presenting with inflamed eyes, but the effects of the more or less standardized injury resulting from cataract operations have been noted (ARAIE et al. 1981).

II. Effects on Ocular Parameters

1. Permeability

Mild insults to tissues, whether direct or cell-mediated, can increase the permeability of cell layers or of capillaries by opening the junctions between cells, and more severe trauma can destroy the cells themselves.

The barrier offered to the diffusion of lipophobic solutes by the corneal epithelium can be reduced five or ten times in a controlled manner by treatment of the surface of the eye with water (MAURICE 1955), nonionic detergents (MARSH and MAURICE 1971), or acidic drops (KELLER et al. 1980). The endothelial permeability has been reported to rise two to three times on mild trauma (MAURICE 1951, 1955), and the fluorescein permeability was found to be more than doubled 7 days after surgery in patients who had been operated on for cataract (ARAIE et al. 1981).

The blood–aqueous barrier can be broken down as a result of mildly injurious stimuli, with the result that a considerable amount of serum protein enters the anterior chamber. This protein has been reported to enter by way of the posterior chamber in cats (SEIDEL 1918) and in rabbits (NEUFELD and SEARS 1973), but regurgitation from the blood through Schlemm's canal has been identified as an alternative route for a small part after paracentesis in monkeys (RAVIOLA 1974). Numerous microscopic and ultramicroscopic studies (e.g., COLE 1974; LATIES and RAPOPORT 1976; OKISAKA 1976; OHNISHI and TANAKA 1981) have been made to identify the morphological basis for the increased permeability, using pharmacologic and osmotic stimuli as well as paracentesis. The formation of cysts between the pigmented and nonpigmented cell layers at the anterior tips of the ciliary processes is generally seen, and this may progress to a breakdown of the junctional barrier in the nonpigmented cells, the major location for a disrupted blood–aqueous barrier (SHIOSE 1970; VEGGE et al. 1975). Other regions of the epithelial cell layers of the anterior segment and the capillaries of the iris are little affected.

The blood–retinal barriers are rather resistant to a number of mild stimuli, e.g., paracentesis or the local application of histamine, and the permeability of the retinal vessels remains unaltered (CUNHA-VAZ 1979). More severe stress, such as osmotic shock (LATIES and RAPOPORT 1976) or lens extraction accompanied by vitreous loss (TSO and SHIH 1977), can lead to opening of the cell junctions of the vessels and of the pigment epithelium in monkeys. However, the latter workers observed no fluorescein leakage in vivo even in areas where peroxidase was seen later to penetrate the barriers. In the clinic the breakdown of the blood–retinal barriers in inflammatory as well as other pathological conditions is commonly seen (GOLDBERG 1979), and then systemic fluorescein may leak from the choroid into the retina or from the retinal vessels into the retina and vitreous body.

2. Active Transport

After the initial abrupt rise in intraocular pressure related to a disruption of the blood–aqueous barrier and an influx of plasmoid aqueous (SEARS 1961), hypotony or low intraocular pressure follows as a common clinical sign of active uveitis or, better, cyclitis. By an unexplained mechanism the secretion of aqueous humor is suppressed by the inflammatory process. In the dog, O'ROURKE et al. (1969) found a reduction in the rate of loss of albumin and small molecules from the anterior chamber of 50%–60% as a result of uveitis.

After anterior segment surgery a marked increase takes place in aqueous–plasma ratio of both free and bound fluorescein (ARAIE et al. 1981). Undoubtedly, most of this rise must result from increased penetration, but some small part may be due to a reduced flow rate. However, it was not possible to determine changes in the flow rate with certainty, since leakage of protein and bound fluorescein complicates the dynamics and makes their interpretation difficult.

Measurable levels of fluorescein or drugs that are normally excluded from the vitreous body are found in inflammatory as well as degenerative conditions after systemic administration. Often this is the result of a breakdown of the blood–ocular barrier, but sometimes it is not possible to separate this from a failure in the mechanisms which actively transport drugs out of the vitreous body into the blood.

3. Vasomotor Effects

Capillary engorgement is a classic sign of inflammation. In addition to changes in the permeability of the vessels, discussed above, arteriolar vasodilation will result in an increased blood flow through the tissues. Since there is no transfer process within the eye known to be normally rate-limited by blood flow (apart from ascorbic acid secretion), it is not evident how this would affect kinetics.

As discussed previously (Sect. C.II.2), absorption into the blood from the subconjunctival site is normally rapid, but an increased conjunctival blood flow could possibly lead to its being accelerated. However, in both rabbit and monkey eyes after a subconjunctival injection of gentamicin, BARZA et al. (1977, 1978) found no difference in the level of drug in the anterior chamber whether it was infected or normal. Similarly, KUMING and TONKIN (1974) found little difference in the concentration of gentamicin in the primary and secondary aqueous humor of rabbits after its subconjunctival injection. However, these results might represent a balance of opposing effects, since the former workers found that the penetration into the vitreous was much increased in the infected eye.

III. Effects on Drug Kinetics

1. Topical Application

The corneal epithelium is particularly exposed to external insults and can be totally destroyed as a result of infection or trauma. This can lead to a very considerable increase in the penetration of those drugs to which the intact epithelium offers a notable barrier. This is evident from the review of BENSON (1974), who compiled an extensive table summarizing data on topical penetration, including experiments in which the effects of trauma and inflammation were noted.

It appears that general inflammation of the globe as a result of infection or irritation can cause a rise in corneal permeability, e.g., in the case of topical penicillin and lincomycin (NAKATSUE 1971a, b), prednisolone phosphate (KUPFERMAN and LEIBOWITZ 1974c), and dexamethasone phosphate (COX et al. 1972; LEIBOWITZ et al. 1978; HAMARD et al. 1975). In the last paper cited, the rise in aqueous humor concentration could be correlated with a subjective scoring of the degree of inflammation. There was a notable delay in the disappearance of the steroid from the anterior chamber of the inflamed eye, and since it is very improbable that the permeability of the corneal endothelium or the iris capillaries would be lower in this state, this must be a result of the rate of aqueous flow being diminished. The value of A for dexamethasone phosphate fell from its normal value of $0.7\,h^{-1}$ to about $0.3\,h^{-1}$ or less for several days after an immunologic challenge, suggesting that the aqueous flow rate had more than halved. Similarly, BARZA et al. (1981) found that the rate of drop in concentration of gentamicin in the aqueous humor of the inflamed rabbit eye was about one-half of its normal value. The drop in flow rate in itself would lead to a raised concentration in the aqueous humor of topically applied lipophobic drugs even if the corneal permeability was not affected.

Increases in the penetration of lipophobic drugs might be expected not only in inflammatory states but in other clinical conditions which disturb the cell layer, e.g., bullous keratopathy, epithelial edema, and dry eyes, and the degree to which a particular cornea stains with fluorescein is a guide to how much it is affected. On the other hand, the effect of epithelial damage should be low or negligible for lipophilic drugs, which normally penetrate the layer very readily.

Mention may be made of iatrogenic influences on penetration. Tonometry can cause local destruction of cells and a breakdown of the barrier. Certain drugs, notably cocaine, but possibly also the tetracyclines, have an injurious effect on the epithelium. However, the chief agents liable to affect the surface cells are preservatives and wetting agents in commercial eye drops (Burstein 1980). There is a clinical impression that local anesthetics cause a rise in corneal permeability, but this does not seem to be supported by clear-cut evidence.

2. Systemic Penetration

A breakdown of the blood–aqueous barrier will lead to increased values of k_d and r_{ap}. If nothing else was changed this would result in a higher level of drug in the anterior chamber and, as a result of the rise in k_o, would tend to cause a more rapid rise and fall in the concentration, from Eq. (42). Plasma proteins can pass across the broken-down barrier; when a drug is bound by the proteins, this can account for a further increase in its entry. The binding can continue in the anterior chamber, so that the drug may not be effective at the total concentration present.

Values of the ratio of the concentration of the drug in the inflamed eye of a rabbit to the normal eye, after systemic administration, are about 3 for benzylpenicillin (Salminen et al. 1969), 10 for cloxacillin (Salminen 1978a) and tetracycline (Salminen 1977a), 12 for carbenicillin (Barza et al. 1973), and 5 for gentamicin, both after paracentesis (Kuming and Tonkin 1974) and infection (Barza et al. 1981), and 6 for dexamethasone (Hamard et al. 1975).

The applicability of the results to the human eye is uncertain because of a conflict of data in the case of doxycycline. Salminen (1977b) found a tenfold increase in its penetration into the aqueous humor of a rabbit after a simple paracentesis. On the other hand, Tsacopoulos (1969) compared its penetration into the aqueous humor of ten patients with ocular inflammation and ten where was none. He reported a 75% increase in the inflamed eyes; however, if the values of r'_{ap} are calculated and averaged, the increase appears to be only 25%. This may be an illustration of the lack of relevance of the acute reaction of the rabbit eye to that in other species, particularly to the prolonged phase of the inflammatory response, which was referred to at the beginning of this section.

If there is a slowing of the aqueous flow on top of a permeability rise, the peak concentration in the aqueous humor will be further increased, but the rate constants for the exchange with the blood will be somewhat reduced. The drug should remain in the eye at an effective concentration for a longer period; if the animal data are applicable, this time would be doubled. The effects of the drop in k_f appear to predominate over those of the rise in k_d, referred to above.

Barza (1980) has listed details of reports of the effect of inflammation on the penetration of drugs into several tissues of the eye. Generally, there is a large increase in the penetration into the vitreous of the rabbit, but it is not evident whether this is a result of a breakdown of the blood–vitreous barrier or a suppression of the active transport mechanism in the retina that normally excretes the drug.

Saubermann (1956) gives data on the penetration of a variety of drugs into the vitreous body of patients whose eyes had to be enucleated. Generally, quite high levels with respect to the blood were found, but the eyes were in a more or less disorganized condition.

3. Periocular Injection

As noted earlier in this section, inflammation had little influence on the penetration of gentamicin into the anterior chamber after subconjunctival injection. BARZA (1978) has listed a number of results from the literature concerning the penetration of various antibiotics into inflamed eyes after subconjunctival or retrobulbar administration. The results are very variable, and the concentration in the aqueous humor may be either less than or more than in the normal eye, as found by NAKATSUE (1971 a, b, c, d).

4. Intravitreal Injection

Inflammation could both break down the blood–vitreous barrier, so that drugs which normally leave the eye by the anterior route could also pass out across the retinal surface, and inhibit the active transport mechanisms, so that drugs such as penicillin would leave more slowly and toward the anterior segment (see Sect. C.I). There would be a tendency for the drugs belonging to the extreme groups shown in Fig. 15 to move to some intermediate point on the line joining them.

There are adequate experimental data available only for two drugs, gentamicin and carbenicillin, and the average values for the infected eye are shown in Fig. 15. In the former case (KANE et al. 1981), it is apparent that a considerable displacement from the position in the normal eye has taken place, such as to suggest that the drug is being transferred out of the vitreous humor across the retinal surface. This would indicate that a partial breakdown of the blood–vitreous barrier has occurred. Carbenicillin (BARZA et al. 1982), unlike gentamicin, is transported out across the retina, and it leaves the eye slightly slower when it is infected. These workers suggest that the active transport mechanism is partially inhibited by the infection but that a rise in the passive efflux of the drug due to the breakdown of the blood–retinal barrier may compensate for the loss in pump activity.

F. Conclusion

In the previous sections we have analyzed the movement of drugs into and out of the eye in terms of the barriers and reservoirs represented by its component tissues. This analysis was applied to published experimental data, and where possible values have been extracted for transfer coefficients or, in the case of the cornea, the permeabilities of the cell layers. Often the experimental results were insufficient to allow anything other than a very approximate value for these parameters to be established, and in a large number of cases the experiments were not designed in a way to allow any sort of analysis to be attempted. It became evident, however, what data are required for the purpose, and we have made recommendations for designing experimental programs to widen their usefulness.

The study of pharmacokinetics should not be restricted to understanding how the ocular tissues control the penetration, distribution, and persistence of drugs in the eye, but should be extended to correlate this behavior with the chemical properties of the drugs themselves. Only very preliminary steps have been taken in this direction, and we hope that the treatment given in this chapter will provide the groundwork for developing a rational and systematic approach to the goal.

It is clear, however, that although the simple compartmental analysis that has been developed forms a satisfactory basis for the kinetics of many hydrophilic substances, it can only be a first approximation when they exhibit some degree of lipid solubility, which is the case for most drugs. These will penetrate cell membranes, with the result that cellular compartments that were neglected in the simple model, the corneal epithelium, the lens, and the uveal tissue, can become of major importance. Furthermore, there may be nonlinear relationships between the magnitude of the reservoirs and barriers formed by these tissues and the concentration of the drug. In order to characterize the kinetics of each drug, a large body of experimental data will be required, and its analysis will be complex, requiring numerical treatment on a computer.

Fluorescein has proved invaluable in elucidating the kinetics of hydrophilic drugs, and it is possible that its role could be extended by the use of lipid-soluble fluorescent tracers. The concentrations and concentration gradients in all the observable transparent media could then be followed noninvasively in animal or human eyes, and kinetic patterns could be established to which the measurements on therapeutics agents could be related, leading to a considerable economy in experimental material.

References

Abel R, Boyle GL (1976) Dissecting ocular tissue for intraocular drug studies. Invest Ophthalmol 15:216–219

Abel R, Boyle G, Furman M, Leopold IH (1974) Intraocular penetration of cefazolin sodium in rabbits. Am J Ophthalmol 78:779–787

Abraham R, Burnett H (1955) Tetracycline and chloramphenicol studies on rabbit and human eyes. Arch Ophthalmol 54:641–659

Adler CA, Maurice DM, Paterson ME (1971) The effect of viscosity of the vehicle on the penetration of fluorescein into the human eye. Exp Eye Res 11:34–42

Allansmith M, DeRamus A, Maurice D (1979) The dynamics of IgG in the cornea. Invest Ophthalmol Vis Sci 18:947–955

Alm A, Bill A, Young FA (1973) The effects of pilocarpine and neostigmine on the blood flow through the anterior uvea in monkeys. A study with radioactively labelled microspheres. Exp Eye Res 15:31–36

Ambache N (1955) The use and limitations of atropine for pharmacological studies on autonomic effectors. Pharmacol Rev 7:467–494

Anderson JA, Davis WL, Wei CP (1980) Site of ocular hydrolysis of a prodrug, dipivefrin, and a comparison of its ocular metabolism with that of the parent compound, epinephrine. Invest Ophthalmol Vis Sci 19:817–823

Andrews GWS (1947) Distribution of penicillin in the eye after subconjunctival injection. Lancet 6453:594–596

Araie M, Sawa M, Nagataki S, Mishima S (1980) Aqueous humor dynamics in man as studied by oral fluorescein. Jpn J Ophthalmol 24:346–362

Araie M, Sawa M, Takase M (1981) Effect of topical indomethacin on the blood-aqueous barrier after intracapsular extraction of senile cataract – a fluorophotometric study. Jpn J Ophthalmol 25:237–247

Asseff CF, Weisman RL, Podos SM, Becker B (1973) Ocular penetration of pilocarpine in primates. Am J Ophthalmol 75:212–215

Axelrod JL, Kochman RS (1978) Cefamandole levels in primary aqueous humor in man. Am J Ophthalmol 85:342–348

Axelrod JL, Kochman RS (1980) Cefaclor levels in human aqueous humor. Arch Ophthalmol 98:740–742

Azuma I, Abe K, Sakaguchi K (1963) Penetration of steroid hormone into the eye. Acta Soc Ophthalmol Jpn 67:1691–1697

Bárány EH (1976) Organic cation uptake in vitro by the rabbit iris-ciliary body, renal cortex, and choroid plexus. Invest Ophthalmol 15:341–348

Barza M (1978) Factors affecting the intraocular penetration of antibiotics. Scan J Infect Dis [Suppl] 14:151–159

Barza M (1980) Treatment of bacterial infections of the eye. In: Remington JS, Swartz MM (eds) Current clinical topics in infectious diseases McGraw-Hill, New York, pp 158–193

Barza M, Baum J (1973) Penetration of ocular compartments by penicillins. Surv Ophthalmol 18:71–82

Barza M, Baum J, Birkby B, Weinstein L (1973) Intraocular penetration of carbenicillin in the rabbit. Am J Ophthalmol 75:307–313

Barza M, Kane A, Baum JL (1977) Regional differences in ocular concentration of gentamicin after subconjunctival and retrobulbar injection in the rabbit. Am J Ophthalmol 83:407–413

Barza M, Kane A, Baum J (1978) Intraocular penetration of gentamicin after subconjunctival and retrobulbar injection. Am J Ophthalmol 85:541–547

Barza M, Kane A, Baum J (1981) The difficulty of determining the route of intraocular penetration of gentamicin after subconjunctival injection in the rabbit. Invest Ophthalmol Vis Sci 20:509–514

Barza M, Kane A, Baum J (1982) The effects of infection and probenecid on the transport of carbenicillin from the rabbit vitreous. Invest Ophthalmol Vis Sci 22:720–726

Baum JL, Barza M, Shushan D, Weinstein L (1974) Concentration of gentamicin in experimental corneal ulcers. Arch Ophthalmol 92:315–317

Baurmann M (1930) Über das Ciliarfortsatz-Gefäßsystem. Ber Zusammenkunft Dtsch Ophthalmol Ges 48:364–371

Beasley H, Boltralik JJ, Baldwin HA (1975) Chloramphenicol in aqueous humor after topical application. Arch Ophthalmol 93:184–185

Becker B (1960) The transport of organic anions by the rabbit eye. I. In vitro iodopyracet (Diodrast) accumulation by ciliary body-iris preparations. Am J Ophthalmol 50:862–867

Becker B (1961 a) The turnover of bromide in the rabbit eye. Arch Ophthalmol 65:97–99

Becker B (1961 b) Iodide transport by the rabbit eye. Am J Ophthalmol 200:804–806

Becker EF (1969) The intraocular penetration of lincomycin. Am J Ophthalmol 67:963–965

Bellhorn RW (1980) Permeability of blood-ocular barriers of neonatal and adult cat to sodium fluorescein. Invest Ophthalmol Vis Sci 19:870–877

Bellows JG, Farmer CJ (1947) Streptomycin in ophthalmology. Am J Ophthalmol 30:1215–1220

Bennett TO, Peyman GA (1974) Use of tobramycin in eradicating experimental bacterial endophthalmitis. Albrecht Von Graefes Arch Klin Exp Ophthalmol 191:93–107

Benson H (1974) Permeability of the cornea to topically applied drugs. Arch Ophthalmol 91:313–327

Bhattacherjee P (1970) Uptake of ^3H-noradrenaline by the ocular tissues of rabbit. Exp Eye Res 9:73–81

Bhattacherjee P (1971) Distribution of carbonic anhydrase in the rabbit eye as demonstrated histochemically. Exp Eye Res 12:356–359

Bienfang DC (1973) Sector pupillary dilatation with an epinephrine strip. Am J Ophthalmol 75:883–884

Bill A (1965) Movement of albumin and dextran through the sclera. Arch Ophthalmol 74:248–252

Bill A (1968) Capillary permeability to and extravascular dynamics of myoglobin, albumin and gammaglobulin in the uvea. Acta Physiol Scand 73:511–522

Bill A (1971) Aqueous humor dynamics in monkeys (*Macaca irus* and *Cercopithecus ethiops*) Exp Eye Res 11:195–206

Bill A, Phillips CI (1971) Uveoscleral drainage of aqueous humor in human eyes. Exp Eye Res 12:275–281

Bito LZ, De Rousseau CJ (1980) Transport functions of the blood-retinal barrier system and the micro-environment of the retina. In: Cunha-Vaz JG (ed) The blood-retinal barriers, Nato advanced study institutes series, vol 32. Plenum, New York, pp 133–163

Bito LZ, Klein EM (1981) The unique sensitivity of the rabbit eye to x-ray-induced ocular inflammation. Exp Eye Res 33:403–412

Bito LZ, Salvador EV (1972) Intraocular fluid dynamics. III. The site and mechanism of prostaglandin transfer across the blood intraocular fluid barriers. Exp Eye Res 14:233–241

Bleeker GM, Maas EH (1955) The penetration of Aureomycin, Terramycin, and chloramphenicol in the ocular tissues. Ophthalmologica 130:1–8

Bleeker GM, Maas EH (1958) Penetration of penethamate, a penicillin ester, into the tissues of the eye. Arch Ophthalmol 60:1013–1020

Bleeker GM, van Haeringen NJ, Glasius E (1968a) Urea and the vitreous barrier of the eye. Exp Eye Res 7:30–36

Bleeker GM, van Haeringen NJ, Maas ER, Glasius E (1968b) Selective properties of the vitreous barrier. Exp Eye Res 7:37–46

Bloom JN, Levene RZ, Thomas G, Kimura R (1976) Fluorophotometry and the rate of aqueous flow in man. Instrumentation and normal values. Arch Ophthalmol 94:435–443

Bloome M, Golden B, McKee A (1970) Antibiotic concentration in ocular tissues. Penicillin G and dihydrostreptomycin. Arch Ophthalmol 83:78–83

Bloomfield SE, Miyata T, Dunn MW, Bueser N, Stenzel KH, Rubin AL (1978) Soluble gentamicin ophthalmic inserts as a drug delivery system. Arch Ophthalmol 96:885–887

Boberg-Ans J, Grove-Rasmussen KV, Hammarlund ER (1959) Buffering technique for obtaining increased physiological response from alkaloidal eye-drops. Br J Ophthalmol 43:670–675

Boyle GL, Hein HF, Leopold IH (1970) Intraocular penetration of cephalexin in man. Am J Ophthalmol 69:868–872

Boyle GL, Lichtig ML, Leopold IH (1971) Lincomycin levels in human ocular fluids and serum following subconjunctival injection. Am J Ophthalmol 71:1303–1306

Boyle GL, Gwon AE, Zinn KM, Leopold IH (1972a) Intraocular penetration of carbenicillin after subconjunctival injection in man. Am J Ophthalmol 73:754–759

Boyle GL, Abel R Jr, Lazachek GW, Leopold IH (1972b) Intraocular penetration of sodium cephalothin in man after subconjunctival injection. Am J Ophthalmol 74:868–874

Bron AJ, Richards AB, Knight-Jones D, Easty DL, Ainslie D (1970) Systemic absorption of Soframycin after subconjunctival injection. Br J Ophthalmol 54:615–620

Broughton W, Goldman J (1973) The intraocular penetration of chloramphenicol succinate in rabbits. Ann Ophthalmol 5:71–80

Burns-Bellhorn MS, Bellhorn RW, Benjamin JV (1978) Anterior segment permeability to fluorescein-labeled dextrans in the rat. Invest Ophthalmol Vis Sci 17:857–866

Burstein (1980) Cytotoxicity of topically applied drugs, vehicles and preservatives. Surv Ophthalmol 24:15–30

Camras CB, Bito LZ (1980) The pathophysiological effects of nitrogen mustard on the rabbit eye. Exp Eye Res 30:41–52

Castrén JA, Raitta C, Laamanen A (1964) Über das Eindringen eines Depot-corticosteroids in die Vorderkammer und den Glaskörper, und die Verweildauer des Steroids im Auge. Acta Ophthalmol (Copenh) 42:680–684

Chen SC, Nakamura H, Tamura Z (1980) Studies on the metabolites of fluorescein in rabbit and human urine. Chem Pharm Bull (Tokyo) 28:1403–1407

Chrai SS, Robinson JR (1974) Corneal permeation of topical pilocarpine nitrate in the rabbit. Am J Ophthalmol 77:735–739

Chrai SS, Patton TF, Mehta A, Robinson JR (1973) Lacrimal and instilled fluid dynamics in rabbit eyes. J Pharm Sci 62:1112–1121

Coakes RL, Brubaker RF (1979) Method of measuring aqueous humor flow and corneal endothelial permeability using a fluorophotometry nomogram. Invest Ophthalmol Vis Sci 18:288–302

Cobo LM, Forster RK (1981) The clearance of intravitral gentamicin. Am J Ophthalmol 92:59–62

Cogan D, Hirsch E (1944) The cornea: VII. Permeability to weak electrolytes. Arch Ophthalmol 32:276–282

Cole DF (1974) The site of breakdown of the blood-aqueous barrier under the influence of vaso-dilator drugs. Exp Eye Res 19:591–607

Cole DF, Monro PAG (1976) The use of fluorescein-labelled dextrans in investigation of aqueous humour outflow in the rabbit. Exp Eye Res 34:571–585

Coles RS, Boyle GL, Leopold IH (1971) Lincomycin levels in rabbit ocular fluids and serum. Am J Ophthalmol 72:464–467

Conrad JM, Robinson JR (1980) Mechanisms of anterior segment absorption of pilocarpine following subconjunctival injection in albino rabbits. J Pharm Sci 69:875–884

Conrad JM, Reay WA, Polcyn E, Robinson JR (1978) Influence of tonicity and pH on lacrimation and ocular drug bioavailability. J Parenter Drug Assoc 32:149–161

Cox W, Kupferman A, Leibowitz H (1972) Topically applied steroids in corneal disease. I. The role of inflammation in stromal absorption of dexamethasone. Arch Ophthalmol 88:308

Crank J (1975) The mathematics of diffusion. Clarendon, Oxford

Cunha-Vaz JG (1979) Sites and function of the blood-retinal barriers. In: Cunha-Vaz JG (ed) The blood-retinal barriers. Plenum, New York, pp 101–117

Cunha-Vaz JG, Maurice DM (1967) The active transport of fluorescein by the retinal vessels and the retina. J Physiol 191:467–486

Cunha-Vaz JG, Maurice DM (1969) Fluorescein dynamics in the eye. Doc Ophthalmol 26:61–72

Cunha-Vaz JG, Shakib M, Ashton N (1966) Studies on the permeability of the blood-retinal barrier. I. On the existence, development and site of a blood-retinal barrier. Br J Ophthalmol 50:441–453

Curry SH (1977) Drug disposition and pharmacokinetics: with a consideration of pharmacological and clinical relationships, 2nd edn. Blackwell, Oxford

Daily MJ, Peyman GA, Fishman G (1973) Intravitreal injection of methicillin for treatment of endophthalmitis. Am J Ophthalmol 76:343–350

Davson H (1969) The intraocular fluids. In: Davson H (ed) The eye. Academic, New York, pp 67–186

Davson H, Duke-Elder WS, Maurice DM, Ross EJ, Woodin AM (1949) The penetration of some electrolytes and non-electrolytes into the aqueous humor and vitreous body of the cat. J Physiol 108:203–217

Dernouchamps JP, Heremans JF (1975) Molecular sieve effect of the blood-aqueous barrier. Exp Eye Res 31:289–297

Dikstein S, Maurice DM (1972) The metabolic basis to the fluid pump in the cornea. J Physiol 221:29–41

Doane MG, Jensen AD, Dohlman CH (1978) Penetration routes of topically applied eye medications. Am J Ophthalmol 85:383–386

Dorey C, Faure JP (1977) Isolement et charactérisation partielle d'un antigène rétinien responsable de l'uvéo-rétinite autoimmune expérimentale. Ann Immunol (Inst Pasteur) 128C–229–232

Duguid JP, Ginsberg M, Fraser IC, Macaskill J, Michaelson I, Robson JM (1947) Experimental observations on the intravitreous use of penicillin and other drugs. Br J Ophthalmol 31:193–211

Duke-Elder S, Maurice DM (1957) Symbols of ocular dynamics. Br J Ophthalmol 41:702–703

Ehlers N (1965a) The precorneal film. Biomicroscopical, histological and chemical investigations. Acta Ophthalmol [Suppl] (Copenh) 81:1–136

Ehlers N (1965b) On the size of the conjunctival sac. Acta Ophthalmol (Copenh) 43:205–210

Ellerhorst B, Golden B, Nabil J (1975) Ocular penetration of topically applied gentamicin. Arch Ophthalmol 93:371–379

Ellis P, Littlejohn K, Deitrich R (1972) Enzymatic hydrolysis of pilocarpine. Invest Ophthalmol 11:747–751

Ellison SA, Jacobson M, Levine MJ (1981) Lacrimal and salivary proteins. In: Suran A, Gery I, Nussenblatt RB (eds) Proceeding immunology of the eye; workshop III. Immunology Abstracts [Suppl]

Fajardo RV (1966) Subconjunctival injection of methyl-prednisolone. Phillipine J Surg 21:119–122

Faris BM, Uwaydah MM (1974) Intraocular penetration of semisynthetic penicillins. Arch Ophthalmol 92:501–505

Faris BM, Fahd S, Khuri G, Kuraydiyyah I, Uwaydah M (1980) Intraocular penetration of sisomicin in rabbits. Arch Ophthalmol 98:2050–2052

Flynn GL, Yalkowsky SN (1972) Correlation and prediction of mass transport across membranes. I: Influence of alkyl chain length on flux-determining properties of barrier and diffusant. J Pharm Sci 61:838–852

Forbes M, Becker B (1960) The transport of organic anions by the rabbit eye. II. In vivo transport of iodopyracet (Diodrast) Am J Ophthalmol 50:867–873

Friedenwald JS, Becker B (1955) Aqueous humor dynamics. Theoretical considerations. Arch Ophthalmol 54:799–815

Furgiuele FP (1967) Ocular penetration and tolerance of gentamicin. Arch Ophthalmol 64:421–426

Furgiuele FP (1970) Penetration of gentamicin into the aqueous humor of human eyes. Am J Ophthalmol 69:481–483

Furgiuele FP, Sery TW, Leopold IH (1960) Newer antibiotics: their intraocular penetration. Am J Ophthalmol 50:614–622

Furgiuele FP, Smith JP, Baron JG (1978) Tobramycin levels in human eyes. Am J Ophthalmol 85:121–123

Furukawa RE, Polse KA (1978) Changes in tear flow accompanying aging. Am J Optom Physiol Opt 55:69–74

Gager WE, Elsas FJ, Smith JL (1969) Ocular penetration of cephalexin in the rabbit. Br J Ophthalmol 53:403–406

Gardiner PA, Michaelson IC, Rees RJW, Robson JM (1948) Intravitreous streptomycin: its toxicity and diffusion. Br J Ophthalmol 32:449–456

Gerlough TD (1931) The influence of pH on the activity of certain local anesthetics as measured by the rabbit's cornea methods. J Pharmacol Exp Ther 41:307–316

Gladtke E, von Hattingberg HM (1979) Pharmacokinetics: an introduction. Springer, Berlin Heidelberg New York

Godbey REW, Green K, Hull DS (1979) Influence of cetylpyridinium chloride on corneal permeability to penicillin. J Pharm Sci 68:1176–1179

Goldberg M (1979) Diseases affecting the inner blood-retinal barrier. In: Cunha-Vaz JG (ed) The blood retinal barriers, NATO advanced study institutes series. Plenum, New York, pp 309–363

Golden B, Coppel SP (1970) Ocular tissue absorption of gentamicin Arch Ophthalmol 84:792–796

Goldman NJ, Klein JO (1970) Penetration of ampicillin and penicillin G into the aqueous humor. Ann Ophthalmol 2:35–42

Goldman JN, Broughton W, Javed H, Lauderdale V (1973) Ampicillin, erythromycin and chloramphenicol penetration into rabbit aqueous humor. Ann Ophthalmol 5:147–156

Goldmann H (1951) Abflußdruck, Minutenvolumen und Widerstand der Kammerwasserströmung des Menschen. Doc Ophthalmol 5:278–356

Goldstein AM, de Palau A, Botelho SY (1967) Inhibition and facilitation of pilocarpine-induced lacrimal flow by norepinephrine. Invest Ophthalmol 6:498–511

Goodenough DA (1979) Lens gap junctions: a structural hypothesis for nonregulated low-resistance intercellular pathways. Invest Ophthalmol Vis Sci 18:1104–1122

Graham RO, Peyman GA (1974) Intravitreal injection of dexamethasone. Arch Ophthalmol 92:149–154

Grant S (1981) Probenecid and intraocular methicillin. Ann Ophthalmol 13:209–211

Grayson MC, Laties AM (1971) Ocular localization of sodium fluorescein. Arch Ophthalmol 85:600–609

Green K, MacKeen DL (1976) Chloramphenicol retention on and penetration into the rabbit eye. Invest Ophthalmol 15:220–222

Green WR, Bennet JE, Goos RD (1965) Ocular penetration of amphotericin B. Arch Ophthalmol 73:769–775

Gregersen W (1958) The tissue spaces in the human iris and their communication with the anterior chamber by way of the iridic crypts. Acta Ophthalmol 36:819–828

Hale PN, Maurice DM (1969) Sugar transport across the corneal endothelium. Exp Eye Res 8:205–215

Hamard H, Schmitt C, Plazonnet B, Le Douarec JS (1975) Étude de la pénétration oculaire de la dexamethasone. In: DeMailly P, Hamard H, Luton JP (eds) Oeil et cortisone. Masson and Cie, Paris, pp 3–81

Hamashige S, Potts AM (1955) The penetration of cortisone and hydrocortisone into the ocular structures. Am J Ophthalmol 90:211–216

Hansch C, Clayton JM (1973) Lipophilic character and biological activity of drugs II. The parabolic case. J Pharm Sci 62:1–21

Hardberger RE, Hanna C, Goodart R (1975) Effects of drug vehicles on ocular uptake of tetracycline. Am J Ophthalmol 80:133–138

Hayashi H (1966) Penetration of kanamycin into tissues of rabbit eye. III Comparison with streptomycin. Acta Soc Ophthalmol Jpn 70:632–641

Hillman JS, Jacobs SI, Garnett AJ, Kheskani MB (1979) Gentamicin penetration and decay in the human aqueous. Br J Ophthalmol 63:794–796

Hind HW, Goyan FM (1947) A new concept of the role of hydrogen ion concentration and buffer systems in the preparation of ophthalmic solutions. J Am Pharm Assoc 36:33–40

Hirsch M, Renard G, Faure JP, Pouliquen Y (1978) Endothelial cell junctions in the ciliary body microvasculature. A freeze-fracture study in the rabbit. Albrecht Von Graefes Arch Klin Exp Ophthalmol 208:69–76

Hogan MJ, Alvarado JA, Weddell JE (1971) Histology of the human eye. Saunders, Philadelphia

Holly FJ, Lamberts DW (1981) Effect of nonisotonic solutions on tear film osmolality. Invest Ophthalmol Vis Sci 20:236–245

Holm O (1968) A photogrammetric method for estimation of the pupillary aqueous flow in the living human eye. Acta Ophthalmol 46:254–283

Holm O, Krakau CET (1966) Measurements of the flow of aqueous humor according to a new principle. Experientia 22:773

Honegger H (1961) Beitrag zur Frage der Permeationsgeschwindigkeit und Wirkungsdauer von Augensalben am Beispiel des gelösten und kristallinen Chloramphenikol. Klin Monatsbl Augenheilkd 139:38–44

Hull DS, Hine JE, Edelhauser HF, Hyndiuk RA (1974a) Permeability of the isolated rabbit cornea to corticosteroids. Invest Ophthalmol 13:457–459

Hull DS, Edelhauser HF, Hyndiuk RA (1974b) Ocular penetration of prednisolone and the hydrophilic contact lens. Arch Ophthalmol 92:413–416

Iwata S (1973) Chemical composition of the aqueous phase. In: Holly F (ed) International ophthalmology clinics, vol 13. Little, Brown, Boston, pp 29–46

Jain MR, Batra V (1979) Steroid penetration in human aqueous with "Sauflon 70" lenses. Indian J Ophthalmol 11:26–31

Jain MR, Srivastava S (1978) Ocular penetration of hydrocortisone and dexamethasone into the aqueous humor after subconjunctival injection. Trans Opthalmol Soc UK 98:63–65

Jampol LM, Neufeld AH, Sears ML (1975) Pathways for the response of the eye to injury. Invest Ophthalmol 14:184–189

Jones RF, Maurice DM (1966) New methods of measuring the rate of aqueous flow in man with fluorescein. Exp Eye Res 5:208–220

Kahan IL, Papai I, Hammer H (1974) Intraocular penetration of tri-tetracyclines after parenteral and subconjunctival administration. Albrecht Von Graefes Arch Klin Exp Ophthalmol 190:257–265

108   D. M. MAURICE and S. MISHIMA

Kaiser RJ, Maurice DM (1964) The diffusion of fluorescein in the lens. Exp Eye Res 3:156–165

Kane A, Barza M, Baum J (1981) Intravitreal injection of gentamicin in rabbits. Effect of inflammation and pigmentation on half-life and ocular distribution. Invest Ophthalmol Vis Sci 20:593–597

Kasbeer RT, Peyman GA, May DR, Homer PI (1975) Penetration of amicacin into the aphakic eye. Albrecht Von Graefes Arch Klin Exp Ophthalmol 196:85–94

Keller N, Moore D, Carper D, Longwell A (1980) Increased corneal permeability induced by the dual effects of transient tear film acidification and exposure to benzalkonium chloride. Exp Eye Res 30:203–210

Kinsey VE (1960) Ion movement in the eye. Circulation 21:968–987

Kinsey VE, Palm E (1955) Posterior and anterior chamber aqueous humor formation. Arch Ophthalmol 53:330–344

Kinsey VE, Reddy DVN (1959) An estimate of the ionic composition of the fluid secreted into the posterior chamber, inferred from a study of aqueous humor dynamics. Doc Ophthalmol 13:7–40

Kinsey VE, Reddy DVN (1964) Chemistry and dynamics of aqueous humor. In: Prince JH (ed) The rabbit in eye research. Thomas, Springfield, pp 1–102

Kirisawa N (1954) Chemotherapy in ophthalmology. Acta Soc Ophthalmol Jpn 58: 1237–1255

Kishida K, Otori T (1980) A quantitative study on the relationship between transcorneal permeability of drugs and their hydrophobicity. Jpn J Ophthalmol 24:251–259

Kleinberg J, Dea FJ, Anderson JA, Leopold IH (1979) Intraocular penetration of topically applied lincomycin hydrochloride in rabbits. Arch Ophthalmol 97:933–936

Klyce SD (1972) Electrical profiles in the corneal epithelium. J Physiol 226:407–429

Klyce SD (1975) Transport of Na, Cl, and water by the rabbit corneal epithelium at resting potential. Am J Physiol 228:1446–1452

Knothe H, Moog E, Vogel F, Fabricius K (1970) Konzentrationsabläufe des Tetracyclins im Kammerwasser des Menschen nach systemischer Verabreichung. Klin Monatsbl Augenheilkd 156:843–850

Kramer SG (1976) Retinal uptake of topical epinephrine in aphakia. In: Leopold IH, Burns RP (eds) Symposium on ocular therapy. Wiley, New York, pp 73–86

Kramer SG, Potts AM (1969) Iris uptake of catecholamines in experimental Horner's syndrome. Am J Ophthalmol 67:705–713

Kramer SG, Potts AM, Mangnall Y (1972) Autoradiographic localization of catecholamines in the uveal tract. Am J Ophthalmol 74:129–134

Krohn DL (1978) Flux of topical pilocarpine to the human aqueous. Trans Am Soc Ophthalmol 76:502–527

Krupin T, Waltman SR, Becker B (1974) Ocular penetration in rabbits of topically applied dexamethasone. Arch Ophthalmol 92:312–314

Krupin T, Cross DA, Becker B (1977) Decreased basal tear production associated with general anesthesia. Arch Ophthalmol 95:107–108

Kuming BS, Tonkin M (1974) Use of gentamicin sulphate in ophthalmology. I. Absorption of gentamicin into the rabbit aqueous. Br J Ophthalmol 58:609–612

Kupferman A, Leibowitz HM (1974a) Topically applied steroids in corneal disease. IV. The role of drug concentration in stromal absorption of prednisolone acetate. Arch Ophthalmol 91:377–380

Kupferman A, Leibowitz H (1974b) Topically applied steroids in corneal disease. V. Dexamethasone alcohol. Arch Ophthalmol 92:329–330

Kupferman A, Leibowitz H (1974c) Topically applied steroids in corneal disease. VI. Kinetics of prednisolone sodium phosphate. Arch Ophthalmol 92:331–334

Kupferman A, Leibowitz HM (1975) Penetration of fluorometholone into the cornea and aqueous humor. Arch Ophthalmol 93:425–427

Kupferman A, Leibowitz HM (1976) Biological equivalence of ophthalmic prednisolone acetate suspensions. Am J Ophthalmol 182:109–113

Kupferman A, Pratt MV, Suckewer K, Leibowitz HM (1974) Topically applied steroids in corneal disease III. The role of drug derivative in stromal absorption of dexamethasone. Arch Ophthalmol 91:373–376

Kurose Y, Leopold I (1965) Intraocular penetration of ampicillin. I. Animal experiment. Arch Ophthalmol 73:361–365

Kurose Y, Sery TW, Leopold IH (1964) Intraocular penetration of thiosporin. Am J Ophthalmol 57:418–426

Kurose Y, Levy PM, Leopold IH (1965) Intraocular penetration of ampicillin. II. Clinical experiment. Arch Ophthalmol 73:366–369

Langham ME (1951) Factors affecting the penetration of antibiotics into the aqueous humour. Br J Ophthalmol 35:612–620

Laties AM, Rapoport S (1976) The blood-ocular barriers under osmotic stress. Arch Ophthalmol 94:1086–1091

Laurent UBG (1981) Hyaluronate in aqueous humour. Exp Eye Res 33:147–156

Lazare R, Horlington M (1975) Pilocarpine lebels in the eyes of rabbits following topical application. Exp Eye Res 21:281–287

Lazar M, Lieberman TW, Furman M, Leopold IH (1968) Ocular penetration of Hetrazan in rabbits. Am J Ophthalmol 66:215–220

Lee VH, Robinson JR (1979) Mechanistic and quantitative evaluation of precorneal pilocarpine disposition in albino rabbits. J Pharm Sci 68:673–684

Lee VHL, Hui HW, Robinson JR (1980) Corneal metabolism of pilocarpine in pigmented rabbits. Invest Ophthalmol Vis Sci 19:210–213

Leibowitz HM, Kupferman A (1974) Anti-inflammatory effectiveness in the cornea of topically administered prednisolone. Invest Ophthalmol 13:757–763

Leibowitz HM, Berrospi AR, Kupferman A, Restropo GV, Galvis V, Alvarez JA (1977) Penetration of topically administered prednisolone acetate into the human aqueous humor. Am J Ophthalmol 83:402–406

Leibowitz RH, Kupferman A, Stewart RH, Kimbrough RL (1978) Evaluation of dexamethasone acetate as a topical ophthalmic formulation. Am J Ophthalmol 86:418–423

Leopold I, Kroman HS (1960) Methyl and fluoro-substituted prednisolones in the blood and aqueous humor of the rabbit. Arch Ophthalmol 63:943–947

Leopold I, Nichols A, Vogel AW (1950) Penetration of chloramphenicol U.S.P. (Chloromycetin) into the eye. Arch Ophthalmol 44:22–32

Leopold I, Sawyer J, Green H (1955a) Intraocular penetration of locally applied steroids. Arch Ophthalmol 54:916–921

Leopold I, Kroman H, Green H (1955b) Intraocular penetration of prednisone and prednisolone. Trans Am Acad Ophthalmol Otolaryngol 59:771–778

Lepri G (1950) Experimental study of the efficiency of different substances in retarding the absorption of penicillin introduced into the subconjunctival spaces. Br J Ophthalmol 34:425–430

Levine N, Aronson S (1970) Orbital infusion of steroids in the rabbit. Arch Ophthalmol 83:599–607

Levy G (1964) Relationship between elimination rate of drugs and rate of decline of their pharmacologic effects. J Pharm Sci 53:342–343

Levy G (1971) Kinetics of drug action in man. Acta Pharmacol 29:203–210

Litwack K, Pettit T, John BL (1969) Penetration of gentamicin administered intramuscularly and subconjunctivally into aqueous humor. Arch Ophthalmol 82:687–693

Loewenfeld IR, Newsome DA (1971) Iris mechanics I. Influence of pupil size on dynamics of pupillary movements. Am J Ophthalmol 71:347–363

Longwell A, Birss S, Keller N, Moore D (1976) Effect of topically applied pilocarpine on tear film pH. J Pharm Assoc 65:1654–1657

Makoid MC, Robinson JR (1979) Pharmacokinetics of topically applied pilocarpine in the albino rabbit eye. J Pharm Sci 68:435–443

Mandell AI, Stentz F, Kitabachi AE (1978) Dipivalyl epinephrine: a new pro-drug in the treatment of glaucoma. Ophthalmology 85:268–275

Marak GE Jr, Shichi H, Rao NA, Wacker WB (1980) Patterns of experimental allergic uve-itis induced by rhodopsin and retinal rod outer segments. Ophthalmol Res 12:165–176

Maren TH, Jankowska L, Sanyal G, Edelhauser HF (1983) The transcorneal permeability of sulphonamide carbonic anhydrase inhibitors and their effect on aqueous humor secretion. Exp Eye Res 36:457–480

Marsh RJ, Maurice DM (1971) The influence of non-ionic detergents and other surfactants on human corneal permeability. Exp Eye Res 11:43–48

Mathalone MBR, Harden A (1972) Penetration and systemic absorption of gentamicin after subconjunctival injection. Br J Ophthalmol 56:609–612

Matsumoto S, Hayashi K, Tsuchisaka H, Araie M (1981) Pharmacokinetics of surface an-esthetics in the human cornea. Jpn J Ophthalmol 25:335–340

Maurice DM (1951) The permeability to sodium ions of the living rabbit's cornea. J Physiol 112:367–391

Maurice DM (1955) Influence on corneal permeability of bathing with solutions of differing reaction and tonicity. Br J Ophthalmol 39:463–473

Maurice DM (1957) The exchange of sodium between the vitreous body and the blood and aqueous humour. J Physiol 137:119–125

Maurice DM (1959) Protein dynamics in the eye studied with labelled proteins. Am J Oph-thalmol 47:361–367

Maurice DM (1960) The movement of fluorescein and water in the cornea. Am J Ophthal-mol 49:1011–1016

Maurice DM (1967a) The use of fluorescein in ophthalmological research. Invest Ophthal-mol 6:464–477

Maurice DM (1967b) Nutritional aspects of corneal grafts and prostheses. In: Rycroft P (ed) Proceedings of 2nd international corneo-plastic conference, London. Pergamon, Oxford, pp 197–207

Maurice DM (1969) The cornea and sclera. In: Davson H (ed) The eye, vol 1, 2nd edn. Aca-demic, New York, pp 489–600

Maurice DM (1970) The physical state of water in the corneal stroma. In: Langham M (ed) The cornea. Johns Hopkins Press, Baltimore, pp 193–204

Maurice DM (1971) The tonicity of an eye drop and its dilution by tears. Exp Eye Res 11:30–33

Maurice DM (1973) The dynamics and drainage of tears. In: Holly F (ed) International oph-thalmology clinics, vol 13. Little, Brown, Boston, pp 103–116

Maurice DM (1976) Injection of drugs into the vitreous body. In: Leopold I, Burns R (eds) Symposium on ocular therapy, vol 9. Wiley, London, pp 59–72

Maurice DM (1980) Structures and fluids involved in the penetration of topically applied drugs. In: Holly F (ed) Internatinal ophthalmology clinics, vol 20. Little, Brown, Bo-ston, pp 7–20

Maurice DM (to be published a) The cornea and sclera. In: Davson H (ed) The eye, 3rd edn. Academic, New York

Maurice DM (to be published b) Micropharmaceutics of the eye. Ocular Inflammation Ther

Maurice DM, Ota Y (1978) The kinetics of subconjunctival injections. Jpn J Ophthalmol 22:95–100

Maurice DM, Polgar J (1977) Diffusion across the sclera. Exp Eye Res 25:577–582

Maurice DM, Guss RB, Cousins S (1982) Fluorophotometry with rhodamine B. Invest Ophthalmol Vis Sci [ARVO Suppl] 22:180

McCoy GA, Leopold IH (1959) Intraocular penetration of oleandomycin. Am J Opthalmol 48:666–669

McDonald JE, Brubaker S (1971) Meniscus-induced thinning of tear films. Am J Ophthal-mol 72:139–146

Melikian HE, Nowakowski J, Boyle G, Leopold I (1971) Use of subconjunctival hyaluroni-dase. Am J Ophthalmol 71:1313–1316

Miichi H, Nagataki S (1982) Effects of cholinergic drugs and adrenergic drugs on aqueous humor formation in the rabbit eye. Jpn J Ophthalmol 26:425–436

Mikkelson TJ, Chrai SS, Robinson JR (1973) Competitive inhibition of drug protein inter-action in eye fluids and tissues. J Pharm Sci 62:1942–1945

Mikuni M, Oishi M, Hayashi H, Suda S, Imai M (1966) Studies on the ophthalmic use of cephalosporin C-cephalothin. Jpn J Clin Ophthalmol 20:439–444

Milano L, Tieri O, Polzella A, Iura V (1971) La diffusione dell' ampicillina nei fluidi oculari. Boll Oculistica 50:229–237

Mishima S (1965) Some physiological aspects of the precorneal tear film. Arch Ophthalmol 73:233–241

Mishima S (1981) Clinical pharmacokinetics of the eye. Invest Ophthalmol Vis Sci 21:504–541

Mishima S, Hedbys BO (1967) The permeability of the corneal epithelium and endothelium to water. Exp Eye Res 6:10–32

Mishima S, Kudo T (1967) In vitro incubation of rabbit cornea. Invest Ophthalmol 6:329–339

Mishima S, Trenberth SM (1968) Permeability of the corneal endothelium to nonelectrolytes. Invest Ophthalmol 7:34–43

Mishima S, Gasset A, Klyce S, Baum J (1966) Determination of tear volume and tear flow. Invest Ophthalmol 5:264–276

Miyake K, Ohtsuki K (1981) Fluorescence fundusphotography by retrobulbar administration of the dye, photochemical transillumination. Jpn J Ophthalmol 25:280–298

Mizukawa T, Azuma I, Kawaguchi S (1965) Intraocular penetration of new antibiotics, cephalothin and cephaloridine. J Antibiot (Tokyo) 18:525–526

Mizuno K (1972) Vital stain of the anterior chamber. Jpn J Ophthalmol 16:167–173

Mochizuki M (1980) Transport of indomethacin in the anterior uvea of the albino rabbit. Jpn J Ophthalmol 24:363–373

Moog E (1969) Pharmakokinetische Probleme am Auge dargestellt am Beispiel der Tetracycline. Ber Zusammenkunft Dtsch Ophthalmol Ges 70:442–445

Moog E, Knothe H (1968) Der Übertritt verschiedener Tetracycline ins Kammerwasser der Menschen in Abhängigkeit von ihrer Eiweißbindung im Blutserum. Ber Zusammenkunft Dtsch Ophthalmol Ges 69:536–539

Moog E, Knothe H, Vogel F, Fabricius K (1969) Der Übertritt von Pyrrolidinomethyltetracyclin (PMT) in das Kammerwasser des Menschen nach systemischer Verabreichung. Klin Monatsbl Augenheilkd 155:828–836

Moog E, Knothe H, Moller CO (1971) Doxycyclinspiegel in Serum und Kammerwasser beim Menschen. Albrecht Von Graefes Arch klin Exp Ophthalmol 181:246–254

Moses RA (1965) Detachment of ciliary body – anatomical and physical considerations. Invest Ophthalmol 4:935–941

Mosher GL, Mikkelson TJ (1979) Permeability of the N-alkyl-p-aminobenzoate esters across the isolated corneal membrane of the rabbit. Int J Pharmaceutics 2:239–243

Murai Y (1976) Studies of tear flow using sodium pertechnetate TC^{99M}. Jpn J Ophthalmol 20:283–289

Musini A, Cattani F, Bonora F (1970) Emploi de la rifampicine en ophtalmologie. Arch Ophtalmol (Paris) 30:809–816

Nagataki S (1975) Human aqueous humor dynamics. Jpn J Ophthalmol 19:235–249

Nakatsue S (1971a) Intraocular penetration of antibiotics into rabbit eye with purulent virus. I. Penicillin. Acta Soc Ophthalmol Jpn 75:1231–1235

Nakatsue S (1971b) Intraocular penetration of antibiotics into rabbit eye with purulent uveitis. II. Tetracycline. Acta Soc Ophthalmol Jpn 75:1236–1239

Nakatsue S (1971c) Intraocular penetration of antibiotics into rabbit eye. III. Kanamycin. Acta Soc Ophthalmol Jpn 75:1240–1243 Nakatsue S (1971d) Intraocular penetration of antibiotics into rabbit eye with purulent uveitis. IV. Lincomycin. Acta Soc Ophthalmol Jpn 75:1244–1247

Neufeld AH, Sears ML (1973) The site of action of prostaglandin E_2 on the blood-aqueous barrier in the rabbit eye. Exp Eye Res 17:445–448

Newsome DA, Stern R (1974) Pilocarpine adsorption by serum and ocular tissues. Am J Ophthalmol 77:918–922

Oakley DE, Weeks RD, Ellis PP (1976) Corneal distribution of subconjunctival antibiotics. Am J Ophthalmol 81:307–312

O'Brien WJ, Edelhauser HF (1977) The corneal penetration of trifluorothymidine, adenine arabinoside and idoxuridine: a comparative study. Invest Ophthalmol Vis Sci 16:1093–1103

Ohara K (1977) Effects of cholinergic agonists on isolated iris sphincter muscles; a pharmacodynamic study. Jpn J Ophthalmol 21:516–527

Ohnishi Y, Tanaka M (1981) Effects of pilocarpine and paracentesis on occluding junctions between the nonpigmented ciliary epithelial cells. Exp Eye Res 32:635–647

Oishi M, Nishizuka K, Motoyama M, Ogawa T (1975) Intraocular penetration and effect of tobramycin in experimental pseudomonas keratitis. Acta Soc Ophthalmol Jpn 79:1329–1335

Oishi M, Nishizuka K, Motoyama M, Ogawa T (1977) Basic studies on the ophthalmic use of fosfomycin as topical application – stability, ocular disturbance and intraocular penetration. Jpn J Ophthalmol 81:1744–1750

Okisaka S (1976) Effects of paracentesis on the blood-aqueous barrier: a light and electron microscopic study on cynomolgus monkey. Invest Ophthalmol 15:824–834

O'Rourke J, Macri FJ, Berghoffer B (1969) Studies in uveal physiology. Arch Ophthalmol 81:526–533

Ota Y, Mishima S, Maurice DM (1974) Endothelial permeability of the living cornea to fluorescein. Invest Ophthalmol 13:945–949

Palm E (1947) On the passage of ethyl alcohol from the blood into the aqueous humour. Acta Ophthalmol [Suppl] 25:139–164

Palm E (1948) On the phosphate exchange between the blood and the eye. Acta Ophthalmol [Suppl] 32:1–120

Papapanos G, Trichtel F, Papapanu R (1961 a) Über den Penicillinspiegel im Kammerwasser und Glaskörper nach subconjunctivaler, retrobulbärer und iontophoretischer Zufuhr von Penicillin G und V. Albrecht Von Graefes Arch Klin Exp Ophthalmol 163:493–500

Papapanos G, Spitzy KH, Trichtel F (1961 b) Über den Durchtritt von Penicillinen in das Kammerwasser und den Glaskörper des menschlichen Auges. Ophthalmologica 142:519–525

Papapanos G, Trichtel F, Spitzy KH (1962) Die Penicillinkonzentration im Serum, Kammerwasser und Glaskörper nach oraler Penicillinmedikation. Wien Klin Wochenschr 74:439–442

Paque JT, Peyman GA (1974) Intravitreal clindamycin phosphate in the treatment of vitreous infection. Ophthalmol Surg 5:34–39

Patton TF (1977) Pharmacokinetic evidence for improved ophthalmic drug delivery by reduction of instilled volume. J Pharm Sci 66:1058–1059

Patton TF, Robinson JR (1975) Influence of topical anesthesia on tear dynamics and ocular drug bioavailability in albino rabbits. J Pharm Sci 64:267–271

Pavan-Langston D, Dohlman CH, Geary P, Sulzewski D (1973) Intraocular penetration of ARA A and IDU – therapeutic implications in clinical herpetic uveitis. Trans Am Acad Ophthalmol Otolaryngol 77:455–456

Petounis A, Papapanos G, Karageorgiou-Makromihelaki C (1978) Penetration of tobramycin sulphate into the human eye. Br J Ophthalmol 62:660–662

Peyman GA, Spitznas M, Straatsma BR (1971) Peroxidase diffusion in the normal and photocoagulated retina. Invest Ophthalmol 10:181–189

Peyman G, May D, Ericson E, Apple D (1974a) Intraocular injection of gentamicin. Arch Ophthalmol 92:42–47

Peyman G, Nelsen P, Bennett T (1974b) Intravitreal injection of kanamycin in experimentally induced endophthalmitis. Can J Ophthalmol 9:322–327

Phillips CI, Bartholomew RS, Ghulamqadir K, Schmitt CJ, Vogel R (1981) Penetration of timolol eye drops into human aqueous humour. Br J Ophthalmol 65:593–595

Pohjanpelto PEJ, Sarmela TJ, Raines T (1974) Penetration of trimethoprim and sulphamethoxazole into the aqueous humour. Br J Ophthalmol 58:606–608

Polse KA, Keener RJ, Jauregui MJ (1978) Dose-response effects of corneal anesthetics. Am J Optom Physiol Opt 55:8–14

Pryor JG, Apt L, Leopold IH (1962) Intraocular penetration of vancomycin. Arch Ophthalmol 67:607–611

Rae JL (1974) The movement of procion dye in the crystalline lens. Invest Ophthalmol 13:147–150

Raviola G (1974) Effects of paracentesis on the blood-aqueous barrier: an electron microscopic study on *Macaca mulatta* using horseradish peroxidase as a tracer. Invest Ophthalmol 13:828–858

Raviola G (1977) The structural basis of the blood-ocular barriers. The ocular and cerebrospinal fluids. Exp Eye Res [Suppl] 25:27–63

Raviola G, Raviola E (1978) Intercellular junctions in the ciliary epithelium. Invest Ophthalmol Vis Sci 17:958–976

Records R (1967) Subconjunctival injection of the repository penicillins. Arch Ophthalmol 78:380–383

Records R (1968 a) Intraocular penetration of cephalothin. I. Animal studies. Am J Ophthalmol 66:436–440

Records RE (1968 b) Intraocular penetration of cephalothin. II. Human studies. Am J Ophthalmol 66:441–443

Records R (1969 a) The penicillins in ophthalmology. Survey Ophthalmol 13:207–214

Records R (1969 b) Intraocular penetration of cephaloridine. Arch Ophthalmol 81:331–335

Records R (1971) The human intraocular penetration of a new orally effective cephalosporin antibiotic, cephalexin. Ann Ophthalmol 309–313

Reddy VN (1979) Dynamics of transport systems in the eye. Invest Ophthalmol Vis Sci 18:1000–1018

Refojo MF (1982) Molecular shape and effective diffusion radius. Invest Ophthalmol Vis Sci 22:129–130

Richards AB, Bron AJ, Rice NSC, Fells P, Marshall MJ, Jones BR (1972) Intraocular penetration of cephaloridine. Br J Ophthalmol 56:531–536

Richards AB, Bron AJ, McLendon B, Kennedy MRK, Walker SR (1979) The intraocular penetration of cefuroxime after parenteral administration. Br J Ophthalmol 63:687–689

Ridley F (1958) Use of topical antibiotics in ophthalmology. Trans Ophthalmol Soc UK 78:335–358

Rieder J, Ellerhorst B, Schwartz DE (1974) Übergang von Sulfamethoxazol and Trimethoprim in das Augenkammerwasser beim Menschen. Albrecht Von Graefes Arch klin Exp Ophthalmol 190:51–61

Riegelman S, Vaughan DG (1958) A rational basis for the preparation of ophthalmic solutions. Survey Ophthalmol 3:471–492

Riley F, Boyle G, Leopold I (1968) Intraocular penetration of cephaloridine in humans. Am J Ophthalmol 66:1042–1049

Robson JM, Tebrich W (1942) Penetration and distribution of sodium sulphacetamide in ocular tissues of rabbits. Br Med J June 6, 1942:687–690

Rohen JW (1961) Comparative and experimental studies on the iris of primates. Am J Ophthalmol 52:384–396

Ros FE, Innemee HC, van Zwieten PA (1978) Penetration of atenolol in the rabbit eye. Arch Ophthalmol 208:235–240

Rosenblum C, Dengler R, Geoffroy R (1967) Ocular absorption of dexamethasone phosphate disodium by the rabbit. Arch Ophthalmol 77:234–237

Rowland M, Tozer TN (1980) Clinical pharmokinetics: concepts and applications. Lea and Febiger, Philadelphia, pp 124–137

Salminen L (1977 a) Penetration of ocular compartments by tetracyclines. 1. An experimental study with tetracycline. Albrecht Von Graefes Arch klin Exp Ophthalmol 204:189–199

Salminen L (1977 b) Penetration of ocular compartments by tetracyclines. II. An experimental study with doxycycline. Albrecht Von Graefes Arch klin Exp Ophthalmol 204:201–207

Salminen L (1978 a) Cloxacillin distribution in the rabbit eye after intravenous injection. Acta Ophthalmol 56:11–19

Salminen L (1978 b) Ampicillin penetration into the rabbit eye. Acta Ophthalmol 56:977–983

Salminen L, Jarvinen H, Toivanen P (1969) Distribution of tritiated benzylpenicillin in the rabbit eye. Acta Ophthalmol 47:115–121

Saubermann G (1956) Untersuchungen über das Eindringen antibiotischer Substanzen in Kammerwasser und Glaskörper des menschlichen Auges. Bibl Ophthalmol Fasc 46

Sawa M, Araie M, Nagataki S (1981) Permeability of the human corneal endothelium to fluorescein. Jpn J Ophthalmol 25:60–68

Schenk AG, Peyman GA, Paque JT (1974) The intravitreal use of carbenicillin (Geopen) for treatment of pseudomonas endophthalmitis. Acta Ophthalmol 53:707–717

Schmitt CJ, Lotti VJ, LeDouarec JC (1980) Penetration of timiolol into the rabbit eye. Measurement after ocular instillation and intravenous injection. Arch Ophthalmol 98:547–551

Schoenwald RD, Smolen VF (1971) Drug absorption analysis from pharmacological data. II. Transcorneal biophasic availability of tropicamide. J Pharm Sci 60:1039–1045

Schoenwald RD, Ward RL (1978) Relationship between steroid permeability across excised rabbit cornea and octanol water partition coefficients. J Pharm Sci 67:786–788

Schonberg SS, Ellis PP (1969) Pilocarpine inactivation. Arch Ophthalmol 82:351–355

Sears ML (1961) The immediate reaction to ocular trauma. Ophthalmologica 142:558–561

Sears ML (1974) The use of aspirin and aspirin-like drugs in ophthalmology. In: IH Leopold (ed) Symposium on ocular therapy, vol 7. Mosby, St. Louis, chap 10, pp 104–115

Seidel E (1918) Experimentelle Untersuchungen Quelle und den Verlauf der intraokularen Safstromung. Albrecht Von Graefes Arch Klin Exp Ophthalmol 95:1–72

Sendelbeck L, Moore D, Urquhart J (1975) Comparative distribution of pilocarpine in ocular tissues of the rabbit during administration by eyedrop or by membrane-controlled delivery systems. Am J Ophthalmol 80:274–283

Sery TW, Paul SD, Leopold IH (1957) Novobiocin, a new antibiotic. Arch Ophthalmol 57:100–109

Shanthaverrappa TR, Bourne GH (1964) Monoamine oxidase distribution in the rabbit eye. J Histochem Cytochem 12:281–287

Shell JW (1982) Ocular drug delivery systems – a review. J Toxicol Cutaneous Ocular Pathol 1:49–63

Sherman SH, Green K, Laties AM (1978) The fate of anterior chamber fluorescein in the monkey eye. I. The anterior chamber outflow pathways. Exp Eye Res 27:159–173

Shiose Y (1970) Electron microscopic studies on blood-retinal and blood-aqueous barrier. Jpn J Ophthalmol 14:73–87

Shorr N, Mack L, Smith JW (1969) Erythromycin in the aqueous humour. Br J Ophthalmol 53:331–334

Short C, Keates RH, Donovan EF, Wyman M, Murdick PW (1966) Ocular penetration studies. I. Topical administration of dexamethasone. Arch Ophthalmol 75:689–692

Sidikaro J, Jones DB (1981) Concentration of gentamicin in preocular tear film following topical application. Invest Ophthalmol Vis Sci [ARVO Suppl] 20:109

Sieg JW, Robinson JR (1974) Corneal absorption of fluorometholone in rabbits. Arch Ophthalmol 92:240–243

Sieg JW, Robinson JR (1975) Vehicle effects on ocular drug bioavailability. I. Evaluation of fluorometholone. J Pharm Sci 64:931–936

Sieg JW, Robinson JR (1976) Mechanistic studies on transcorneal permeation of pilocarpine. J Pharm Sci 65:1816–1822

Sieg JW, Robinson JR (1977) Vehicle effects on ocular drug bioavailability. II. Evaluation of pilocarpine. J Pharm Sci 66:1222–1228

Smelser GK, Ishikawa T (1962) Investigation on the porosity of the iris. 19th int cong ophthalmol, vol 1, pp 612–623

Smelser GK, Ishikawa T, Pei YF (1965) Electron microscopic studies on intraretinal spaces: diffusion of particulate materials. In: Rohen JW (ed) The structure of the eye 2. Schattauer, Stuttgart, pp 109–120

Smith SE (1974) Dose-response relationships in tropicamide-induced mydriasis cycloplegia. Br J Clin Pharm 1:37–40

Smolen VF (1971) Quantitative determination of drug bioavailability and biokinetic behavior from pharmacological data for ophthalmic and oral administrations of a mydriatic drug. J Pharm Sci 60:354–365

Smolen VF (1973) Optimal control of drug input and response dynamics: a role for biomedical engineering in pharmaceutical science. Am J Pharm Ed 37:107–125

Smolen VF (1978) Bioavailability and pharmacokinetic analysis of drug responding systems. Ann Rev Pharmacol Toxicol 18:495–522

Smolen VF, Siegel FP (1968) Procaine interaction with the corneal surface and its relation to anesthesia. J Pharm Sci 57:378–384

Sørensen N (1971) The penetration of quinine, salicylic acid, PAS, salicyluric acid, barbital and lithium across the vitreous barrier of the rabbit eye. Acta pharmacol Toxicol (Copenh) 29:194–208

Sorsby A, Ungar J (1947) Distribution of penicillin in the eye after subconjunctival injection. Br J Ophthalmol 31:517–528

Steinberg RH, Miller SS (1979) Transport and membrane properties of the retinal pigment epithelium. In: Marmor MF, Zinn KM (eds) The retinal pigment epithelium. Harvard University Press, Cambridge, pp 205–225

Stjernschantz J (1981) Neuropeptides in the eye. In: Sears ML (ed) New directions in ophthalmic research. Yale University Press, New Haven, pp 327–358

Sugaya M, Nagataki S (1978) Kinetics of topical pilocarpine in the human eye. Jpn J Ophthalmol 22:127–141

Susina SV, Hitter FD, Siegel FP, Blake MI (1962) Effect of deuterium oxide on local anesthetic activity of procaine. J Pharm Sci 51:1162–1169

Swan KC, White NG (1942) Corneal Permeability I. Factors affecting penetration of drugs into the cornea. Am J Ophthalmol 25:1043–1058

Swan K, Crisman H, Bailey P (1956) Subepithelial versus subcapsular injections of drugs. Arch Ophthalmol 56:26–33

Szalay J, Nunziata B, Henkind P (1975) Permeability of iridial blood vessels. Exp Eye Res 21:531–543

Tabarra KF, O'Connor GR (1975) Ocular tissue absorption of clindamycin phosphate. Arch Ophthalmol 93:1180–1185

Takahashi T (1971a) Intraocular penetration of kanendomycin. 2. Subconjunctival injection. Acta Soc Ophthalmol Jpn 75:7–12

Takahashi T (1971b) Intraocular penetration of kanendomycin. 3. Retrobulbar injection. Acta Soc Ophthalmol Jpn 75:13–19

Takahashi T (1971c) Intraocular penetration of kanendomycin a4. Systemic administration. Acta Soc Ophthalmol Jpn 75:20–30

Takase M, Komuro S, Nanba H, Araie M (1978) Effects of topical bupranolol hydrochloride on the intraocular pressure. Jpn J Ophthalmol 22:142–154

Trichtel F, Papapanos G (1961) Über den Penicillinspiegel in Serum, Kammerwasser und Glaskörper nach intravenöser und intramuskulärer Injection von Penicillin G und V. Albrecht Von Graefes Arch Klin Exp Ophthalmol 164:42–48

Trolle-Lassen C (1958) Investigations into the sensitivity of the human eye to hypo- and hypertonic solutions as well as solutions with unphysiological hydrogen ion concentrations. Pharm Weekbl [Sci] 93:148–155

Tsacopoulos M (1969) The penetration of Vibramycin (doxycycline) in human aqueous humor. Ophthalmologica 159:418–429

Tso M, Shih C (1977) Experimental macular edema after lens extraction. Invest Ophthalmol 16:381–392

Utermann D, Matz K, Meyer K (1977) Gentamicinspiegel im Kammerwasser des Menschen nach parenteraler, subkonjunktivaler und lokaler Applikation. Klin Monatsbl Augenheilkd 171:579–583

Uwaydah MM, Faris BM, Samara IN, Shammas HF, To'mey KF (1976) Cloxacillin penetration. Am J Ophthalmol 82:114–116

Vegge T, Neufeld AH, Sears ML (1975) Morphology of the breakdown of the blood-aqueous barrier in the ciliary processes of the rabbit eye after prostaglandin E_2. Invest Ophthalmol 14:33–36

Vegge T, Neufeld AH, Sears ML (1976) Movement of a protein tracer (horseradish peroxidase) in the anterior uvea. In: Yamada E, Mishima S (eds) The structure of the eye III. Proceedings of the third international symposium, 1975. Jpn J Ophthalmol 103–110

von Sallmann L (1945) Penetration of penicillin into the eye. Further studies. Arch Ophthalmol 34:195–201

von Sallmann L (1947) Controversial points in ocular penicillin therapy. Trans Am Ophthalmol Soc 45:570–636

von Sallmann L, Meyer K (1944) Penetration of penicillin into the eye. Arch Ophthalmol 31:1–7

Wacker WB, Donoso LA, Kalsaw CM, Yankeelou JA Jr, Organisciak DT (1977) Experimental allergic uveitis. Isolation, characterization, and localization of a soluble uveitopathogenic antigen from bovine retina. J Immunol 119:1949–1957

Wagner JG (1968) Kinetics of pharmacologic response. I. Proposed relationships between response and drug concentration in the intact animal and man. J Theoret Biol 20:173–201

Waltman S, Sears ML (1964) Catechol-O-methyl transferase and monoamine oxidase activity in the ocular tissues of albino rabbits. Invest Ophthalmol 3:601–605

Wei CP, Anderson JA, Leopold I (1978) Ocular absorption and metabolism of topically applied epinephrine and a dipivalyl ester of epinephrine. Invest Ophthalmol Vis Sci 17:315–321

Weld CB, Feindel WH, Davson H (1942) The penetration of sugars into the aqueous humor. Am J Physiol 137:421–425

Wine NA, Gornall AG, Basu PK (1964) The ocular uptake of subconjunctivally injected C^{14} hydrocortisone. I. Time and major route of penetration. Am J Ophthalmol 58:362–366

Wistrand PJ, Rawls JR, Maren TH (1960) Sulphonamide carbonic anhydrase inhibitors and intraocular pressure in rabbits. Acta Pharmacol Toxicol 17:337–355

Witzel SH, Ingrid MD, Fielding IZ, Ormsby HL (1956) Ocular penetration of antibiotics by iontophoresis. Am J Ophthalmol 42:89–95

Yamauchi H, Kito H, Uda K (1975) Studies on intraocular penetration and metabolism of fluorometholone in rabbits: a comparison between dexamethasone and prednisolone acetate. Jpn J Ophthalmol 19:339–347

Yoshida S (1976) Analysis of cycloplegic response to topical tropicamide. Folio Ophthalmol Jpn 11:1009–1011

Yoshida S, Mishima S (1975) A pharmacokinetic analysis of the pupil response to topical pilocarpine and tropicamide. Jpn J Ophthalmol 19:121–138

Zirm M (1980) Proteins in aqueous humor. Adv Ophthalmol 40:100–172

CHAPTER 3

Biotransformation and Drug Metabolism

H. Shichi

A. Introduction

Throughout this chapter, the term "drug" refers to nonbiological or xenobiotic chemicals. The metabolism of "endogenous drugs," such as hormones and neurotransmitters, is not covered.

At least 100,000 foreign chemicals or xenobiotics exist in our environment. Many of these xenobiotic compounds are toxic and cause cancer, mutations, and birth defects. The cells cope with adverse effects of chemicals by detoxifying them metabolically. Most xenobiotic compounds (e.g., drugs and environmental chemicals) are lipid-soluble weak organic acids or bases. After filtration at the renal glomerulus, unmetabolized xenobiotics are reabsorbed by the renal tubular cells. Therefore, once they entered the body, these compounds would remain there indefinitely were it not for drug-metabolizing enzymes of the liver. The compounds must be biotransformed into more polar, hence more water-soluble forms to be excreted rapidly in the urine. The drug-metabolizing enzymes which are responsible for the biotransformation of xenobiotics show several unique features.

First, the enzymes are primarily located in the endoplasmic reticulum of the hepatocyte, where they metabolize a wide variety of foreign as well as endogenous substances by monooxygenation reactions (GRAM et al. 1971). The endoplasmic reticulum vesiculates to microsomes during cell homogenization, and the activities are often called "microsomal monooxygenase" or "mixed function oxidase" activities. In the monooxygenation reactions, one atom of molecular oxygen is incorporated into the substrate (RH) and the other atom is reduced by NAD(P)H to water (HAYAISHI et al. 1955; MASON et al. 1955):

$$RH + O_2 + 2NAD(P)H = ROH + 2NAD(P)^+ + H_2O.$$

Monooxygenase activities contain a carbon monoxide binding cytochrome ($\lambda_{max} = 450$ nm) as the oxygen-activating enzyme (WHITE and COON 1980), and are designated the "cytochrome P-450 mediated monooxygenase system." For the system to function efficiently, the integrity of an electron flow between the cofactor NADPH (or NADH in some cases) and the oxygenated form of cytochrome P-450 is required.

Secondly, the activities of many enzymes involved in drug metabolism are enhanced or induced by aromatic (polycyclic) hydrocarbons (CONNEY 1967), and the inducibility is genetically controlled (NEBERT et al. 1975). Inducers were classified more than a decade ago into two types: phenobarbital-type inducers that induce cytochrome P-450, and 3-methylcholanthrene-type inducers that induce cytochrome P_1-450 (CONNEY 1967). As techniques for separation and assay of cytochrome P-450 have been improved in recent years, it has become evident that an increasing number of compounds are neither like 3-methylcholanthrene nor like phenobarbital, yet they appear to induce their own unique forms of cytochrome P-450.

Thirdly, drug metabolism occurs in two phases (Williams 1959). During phase I (e.g., aryl hydrocarbon hydroxylation), polar groups (e.g., hydroxyl) are introduced into the hydrophobic molecules, thereby providing a site of action for conjugating enzymes (e.g., UDP-glucuronosyltransferase and glutathione S-transferase) of phase II. The conjugated (detoxified) products become sufficiently polar to be excreted from the body. Lastly, inert polycyclic compounds [e.g., benzo(a)-pyrene] are converted or potentiated to highly reactive and therefore harmful products (e.g., epoxide) by phase I reaction. These reactive intermediates may interact with DNA and cellular proteins to cause cancer (chemical carcinogenesis), developmental abnormalities (teratogenesis), and cell death. Therefore, drug metabolism can be harmful rather than beneficial to the cell unless phase II detoxifying enzymes function efficiently. Thus the importance of the cytochrome P-450 monooxygenase system to pharmacology as well as chemical carcinogenesis and toxicology is widely recognized (Heidelberger 1975; Nebert et al. 1975).

In Sect. B of this chapter the current status of our knowledge of drug-metabolizing systems in the liver is reviewed, and to illustrate the importance of ocular metabolism of drugs, some recent findings, mainly from the author's laboratory, are presented in Sect. C. Developmental aspects of drug metabolism (Neims et al. 1976; Dutton 1978) and pharmacogenetics of human diseases (Atlas and Nebert 1976) have been reviewed and are not covered in this chapter. Interrelations between nutrition and drug biotransformation have been reviewed in a recent book (Hathcook and Coon 1978).

B. Hepatic Drug-Metabolizing Systems

I. Microsomal Electron Transport Systems (Phase I Enzymes)

At least two electron transport chains are associated with liver microsomal (i.e., endoplasmic reticulum) membranes. One is composed of NADPH·cytochrome P-450 reductase and cytochrome P-450, while the other consists of NADH (or NADPH)·cytochrome b_5 reductase, cytochrome b_5, and a cyanide-sensitive factor. The cytochrome P-450 and cytochrome b_5 systems interact with each other during electron transport (Fig. 1). In addition to the two major electron transport chains, there is a third microsomal electron transport system, which consists of a single flavoprotein (amine oxidase) and catalyzes the oxygenation of N-alkylamines without the participation of cytochrome P-450 (Ziegler et al. 1973).

$$RCH_2NH_2 \xrightarrow{(O)} RCH_2NHOH \xrightarrow{(O)} RCH{=}NOH \quad \text{oxime}$$

$$\overset{\displaystyle H}{\underset{|}{RCH_2NCH_2R}} \xrightarrow{(O)} \overset{\displaystyle OH}{\underset{|}{RCH_2NCH_2R}} \xrightarrow{(O)} \overset{\displaystyle O^-}{\underset{+}{RCH{=}NCH_2R}} \quad \text{nitrone}$$

$$R_3N \xrightarrow{(O)} R_3N^+ \rightarrow O^- \xrightarrow{H^+} R_3N^+ \rightarrow OH \quad \textit{N-hydroxyammonium ion.}$$

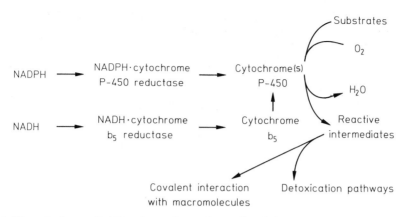

Fig. 1. The cytochrome P-450 and cytochrome b_5 mediated electron transport system of the hepatic endoplasmic reticulum

The microsomal amine oxidase is a flavoprotein with a molecular weight of about 500,000 and contains 7 mol flavine adenine dinucleotide (FAD)/mol protein (ZIEGLER and MITCHELL 1972).

1. Cytochrome P-450

The term "cytochrome P-450" is applied to a group of heme proteins (b-type cytochromes) that distribute in most animals, in plants and microorganisms. The involvement of cytochrome P-450 in the hydroxylation of drugs and steroids was established by the mid 1960s. It was shown that microsomal hydroxylation reactions are inhibited by carbon monoxide and that the action spectrum for the photoreversal of inhibition shows a maximum at 450 nm (ESTABROOK et al. 1963; COOPER et al. 1965). The chromophore, protoheme IX, of cytochrome P-450 has a free sixth ligand position to bind the oxygen. Carbon monoxide inhibits the O_2-activating function of cytochrome P-450 by binding to the sixth ligand position. The active site of cytochrome P-450 is believed to comprise a hydrophobic cleft in the apoprotein in which the heme is located, with the fifth ligand position probably occupied by a thiolate anion contributed by a cysteine residue. Hydrophobic substrates bind to the sixth coordination position of the heme exposed on the surface of the apoprotein. A scheme recently proposed for the mechanism of aromatic hydroxylation catalyzed by liver microsomal cytochrome P-450 is shown in Fig. 2 (WHITE and COON 1980). The 1st step is the binding of substrate to the active site of cytochrome P-450 in the ferric (oxidized) form. Spectral changes are observed upon substrate binding due to perturbations of the spin state of electrons. The next step is one-electron reduction of the substrate-bound heme iron by the electron provided by NADPH. (In the mitochondrial hydroxylation system, electrons are provided by an iron-sulfur redoxin.) In steps 3 and 4 the heme iron in the ferrous state binds an oxygen molecule and is oxidized by intramolecular electron transfer to the oxygen to form a superoxide. The second electron provided probably by NADH through cytochrome b_5 then reduces the superoxide to a peroxide. Step 5

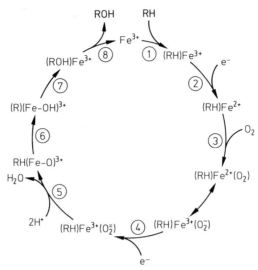

Fig. 2. Proposed mechanism of cytochrome P-450 catalyzed hydroxylation reactions. *RH* and *ROH* represent a substrate and the corresponding product, respectively. *1*, Binding of substrate. *2*, One-electron reduction of substrate. *3*, Binding of oxygen and oxidation of Fe^{2+}. *4*, Reduction of superoxide to peroxide. *5*, Splitting of peroxide to form Fe-oxo complex. *6*, Extraction of hydrogen from substrate. *7*, Hydroxylation of substrate. *8*, Release of hydroxylated product. (White and Coon 1980)

involves splitting of the oxygen species by protons to form water and an iron-oxo complex. The carbon-hydrogen bond on the substrate is then broken by extraction of hydrogen radical by the iron-oxo complex. The alkyl radical then recombines with hydroxyl radical and substrate hydroxylation is completed (steps 6 and 7). The product alcohol attached to the heme iron is then replaced by another substrate, probably because the alcohol has lesser affinity for the enzyme than unaltered substrate. It should be pointed out that the scheme shows only the chromophore function of cytochrome P-450. Additional enzymes which are required to provide electrons to the cycle are present as complexes with cytochrome P-450. Liver microsomal cytochrome P-450 solubilized from membranes with detergent and purified by chromatographic procedures has an apparent molecular weight of 300,000–500,000 and a minimal molecular weight of 55,000–69,000, and contains 1 heme per polypeptide chain (Coon and Persson 1980). The amino terminal sequence of the protein is hydrophobic and similar to the signal peptide, which is believed to lead a newly synthesized polypeptide to penetrate the endoplasmic reticulum membrane from the cytoplasmic side and be cleaved off by a peptidase present on the laminal side of the membrane (Blobel and Doberstein 1975). The presence of such a hydrophobic segment in a mature protein raises a puzzling question concerning its function.

2. NADPH·Cytochrome P-450 Reductase

NADPH · cytochrome P-450 reductase purified from the liver of phenobarbital-treated animals is a protein with a minimal molecular weight of about 75,000, and contains 1 mol each flavine mononucleotide (FMN) and FAD per mol enzyme (MASTERS 1980). The pattern of electron flow from NADPH to P-450 substrate would be NADPH→FAD→FMN→P-450 substrate. Cytochrome c also serves as an electron acceptor for the enzyme and inhibits drug hydroxylations in liver microsomes (GILLETTE et al. 1957). The role of this reductase in drug oxidation was established by the demonstration that specific antibodies raised against NADPH · cytochrome c reductase inhibited the reduction of cytochrome P-450 by NADPH (GLAZER et al. 1971).

3. Cytochrome b_5 and NADH · Cytochrome b_5 Reductase

Cytochrome b_5 is an intrinsic membrane protein with a molecular weight of 16,000, and consists of two peptide domains: a hydrophilic, heme-containing segment (about 80 amino acid residues), and a smaller hydrophobic segment or tail that penetrates the lipid bilayer and binds the cytochrome molecule to the microsomal membrane. Amino acid sequences of the hydrophobic segment of cytochrome b_5 from several species are known (VON JAGOW and SEBALD 1980). The natural electron donor for cytochrome b_5 is NADH · cytochrome b_5 reductase, a tightly membrane-bound flavoprotein with a molecular weight of 45,000 (SPATZ and STRITTMATTER 1973).

Cytochrome b_5, like cytochrome c, has a six-coordinate heme so that it cannot bind oxygen but can only transfer electrons to an appropriate acceptor. Cytochrome b_5 is implicated in NADPH-linked microsomal hydroxylation reactions as an electron donor to cytochrome P-450 (see Figs. 1 and 2). Cytochrome b_5 is also implicated in the reduction of hydroxylamines produced by microsomal amine oxidase (KADLUBAR and ZIEGLER 1974). However, a well-established physiological electron acceptor of cytochrome b_5 is the stearyl CoA desaturase which catalyzes the NADH-dependent desaturation at position 9 of stearyl CoA (OSHINO et al. 1971). Whether cytochrome b_5 and NADH · cytochrome b_5 reductase are essential components for microsomal hydroxylase systems is still a moot point, although strong inhibition of ethylmorphine N-demethylation by stearyl CoA and substrate for fatty acid desaturase occurs, presumably due to channeling of electrons from cytochrome b_5 to the desaturase system rather than to the cytochrome P-450 system (CORREIA and MANNERING 1973).

II. Reactions Catalyzed by the Cytochrome P-450 System

Reactions catalyzed by the cytochrome P-450 system are classified into oxidative reactions and reductive reactions.

1. Oxidative Reactions

The hydroxylation of aromatic hydrocarbons such as benzo(a)pyrene has been most extensively investigated (Fig. 3). The predominant mechanism of hydroxylation is oxygen addition to the carbon-carbon double bond of the aromatic compounds (epoxidation), and subsequent rearrangement of epoxides (arene oxides) to phenols (nonenzymatic) or to diols (enzymatic). Microsomal epoxide hydrase catalyzes the diol formation. Using deuterated substrates, the group on the carbon

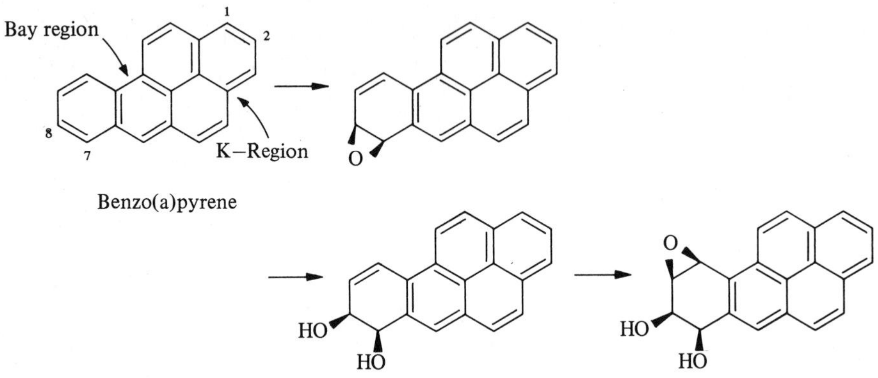

Fig. 3. Hydroxylation of benzo(a)pyrene

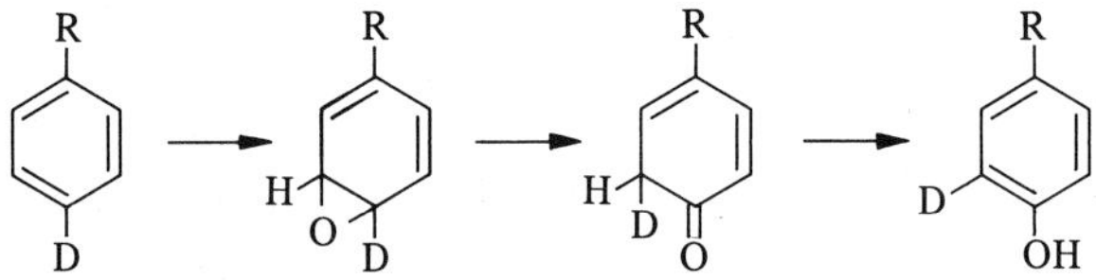

Fig. 4. Migration of hydrogen during hydroxylation (NIH shift)

atom being hydroxylated was found, as shown below, to migrate to an adjacent position during the hydroxylation reaction (Fig. 4).

This migration is known as the "NIH shift" (GUROFF et al. 1967). Cytochrome P-450 monooxygenase responsible for the hydroxylation of aromatic hydrocarbons is called the "aryl hydrocarbon hydroxylase system," and hydroxylates aromatic compounds through an arene oxide intermediate, as well as by direct insertion of an oxygen atom into the aromatic molecule. Rapid rearrangements of arene oxides to phenols are catalyzed by epoxide hydrase (OESCH 1973). Regional selectivity exists in the hydroxylation of benzo(a)pyrene (Fig. 3). Rings in the K region are not hydroxylated. The formation of benzo(a)pyrene 7,8-dihydrodiol is markedly increased in 3-methylcholanthrene-treated microsomes, but is decreased in phenobarbital-treated microsomes (HOLDER et al. 1974). Arene oxides are highly reactive and carcinogenic.

An example of aliphatic hydroxylations catalyzed by the microsomal cytochrome P-450 system is shown in Fig. 5. The reaction does not proceed through the epoxide because of the absence of double bonds. It proceeds probably by a direct insertion of the active oxygen species (COOPER and BRODIE 1955). Hydroxylation occurs frequently on the terminal methyl (ω) or penultimate (ω-1) positions, and primary and secondary alcohols are formed, respectively. However, site selectivity also exists in aliphatic hydroxylations, that is, certain regions of the molecule are hydroxylated selectively by different microsomal preparations (FROMMER et al. 1972). For example, microsomes from phenobarbital-treated rats hydroxylate n-heptane at the 2-, 3-, and 4-positions preferentially to the 1-position. On the other hand, microsomes from benzo(a)pyrene-treated rats prefer hydroxylation at the 3- and 4-positions to the 1- and 2-positions. Site selectivity both in ar-

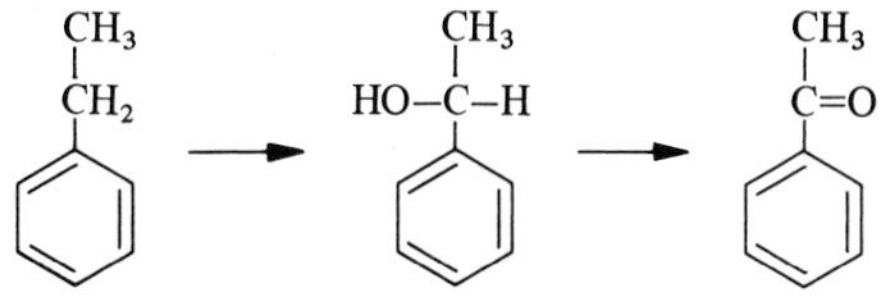

Fig. 5. Hydroxylation of the aliphatic group of ethylbenzene

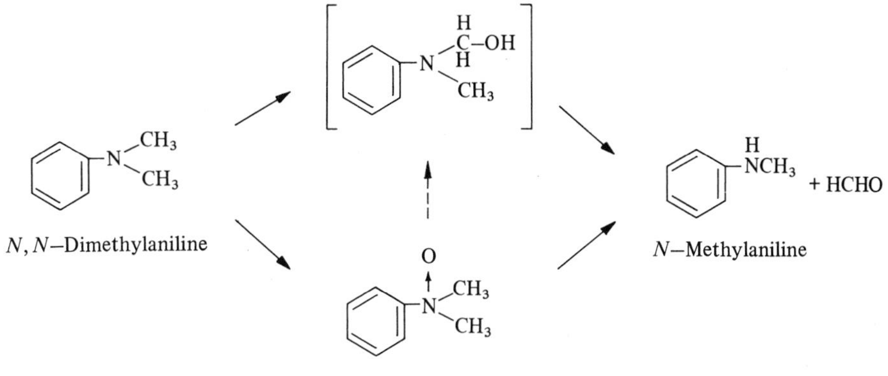

Fig. 6. N-dealkylation of N,N-dimethylaniline. Both N-oxidation and C-oxidation are possible

omatic and aliphatic hydroxylations is ascribed to the effects of inducers which induce different types of cytochrome P-450 and associated enzymes (see Sect. V).

In N-dealkylation (Fig. 6), alkyl substituents, particularly methyl groups, attached to a nitrogen atom are oxidatively removed. Thus removal of alkyl groups from secondary and tertiary amines gives rise to aldehydes and primary and secondary amines. Possibly two different paths exist: a cytochrome P-450-dependent path (McMahon 1966), and a CO-insensitive flavoprotein catalysis (Pettit and Ziegler 1963). The rate of N-dealkylation decreases as the length of the alkyl side chain increases. Dealkylation of tertiary amines may occur either through a carbinolamine intermediate [=NCH(OH)-] or through a tertiary amine N-oxide intermediate ($\equiv$NO). It is not known which intermediate plays a major role in N-dealkylation. If the carbinolamine is more important, the prior formation of the N-oxide may also occur [i.e., $(CH_3)_3NO \rightarrow (CH_3)_2NCH_2(OH)$]. If the reaction produces N-oxide, it is called "N-oxidation." N-oxides are the major products from phenothiazines. Again, there exist two enzymes, a flavoprotein amine oxidase (Ziegler and Pettit 1966) and a cytochrome P-450-dependent enzyme (Hlavica 1971), which catalyze N-oxidation of tertiary amines. The two enzymes can be distinguished by their sensitivity to carbon monoxide.

In N-hydroxylation of amines (e.g., 2-acetylaminofluorene), a primary or secondary amine is directly hydroxylated (Fig. 7). The products (hydroxylamines) are chemically reactive and often more toxic than the parent compound. The hydrox-

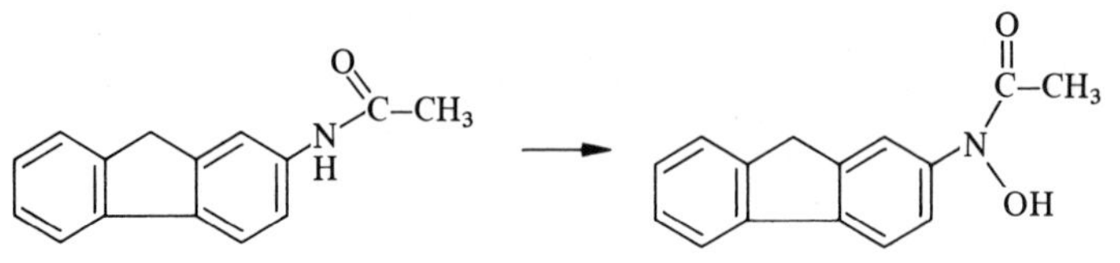

2–Acetylaminofluorene

Fig. 7. *N*-hydroxylation of acetylaminofluorene

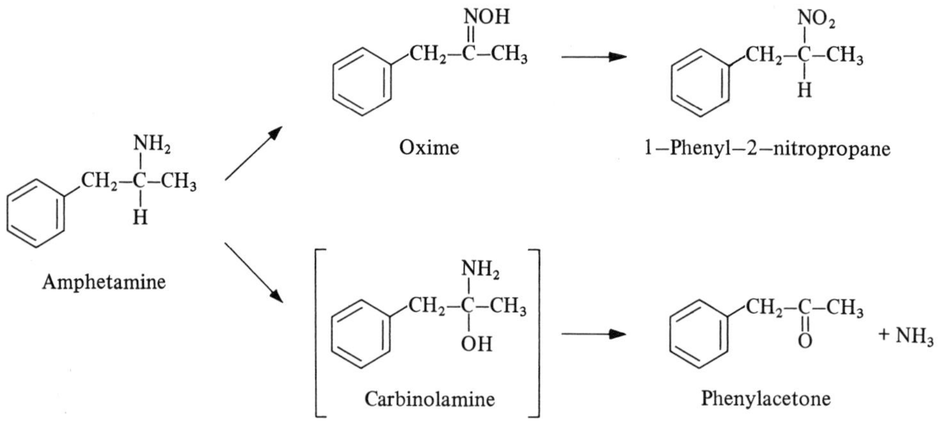

Fig. 8. Metabolism of amphetamine. 1-Phenyl-2-nitropropane is formed by oxidation via the oxime. Phenylacetone is formed by *C*-oxidation and subsequent deamination

ylated compounds exert their toxic effects probably by alkylating cellular macromolecules. The rearrangement of the *N*-hydroxy acetaminophen gives rise to a reactive metabolite (*N*-acetylimidoquinone) which binds to protein or nucleic acid at a position ortho to the ring hydroxyl group (HINSON et al. 1981). Deamination of amphetamine to 1-phenyl-2-nitropropane via the oxime (COUTTS et al. 1976) (Fig. 8) is catalyzed by liver microsomes and NADPH. Phenylacetone, which is also formed by the reaction, with the release of ammonia, is derived from the carbinolamine (BRODIE et al. 1958) rather than from the oxime intermediate.

The oxidative *O*-dealkylation of alkylaryl ethers produces the corresponding aldehyde and the phenol (Fig. 9). Phenacetin (*p*-ethoxyacetanilide) is converted to acetaminophen (*p*-hydroxyacetanilide) (RENSON et al. 1965). The rate of *O*-dealkylation decreases as the length of alkyl chain increases. The reaction probably involves a direct oxidative attack on the leaving alkyl group rather than displacement of the alkoxy group by a hydroxylating species. Different forms of cytochrome P-450 show different capacities to *O*-dealkylate alkoxy compounds. For example, 7-ethoxycoumarin is metabolized more efficiently by liver microsomes (containing cytochrome P-448) from 3-methylcholanthrene-treated rats than by those (containing cytochrome P-450) from phenobarbital-treated rats (ULLRICH et al. 1973).

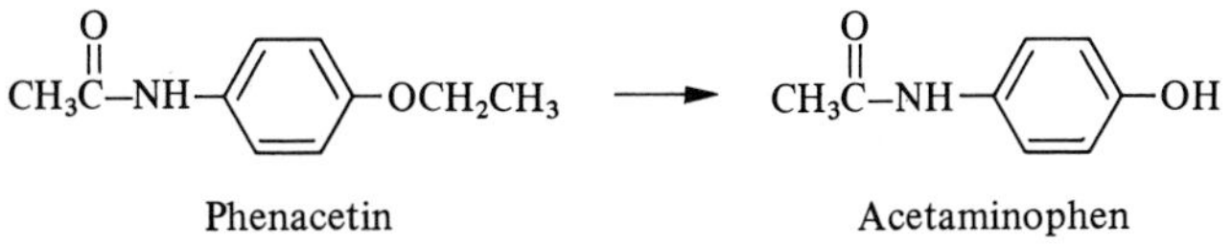

Fig. 9. Oxidative O-dealkylation of phenacetin

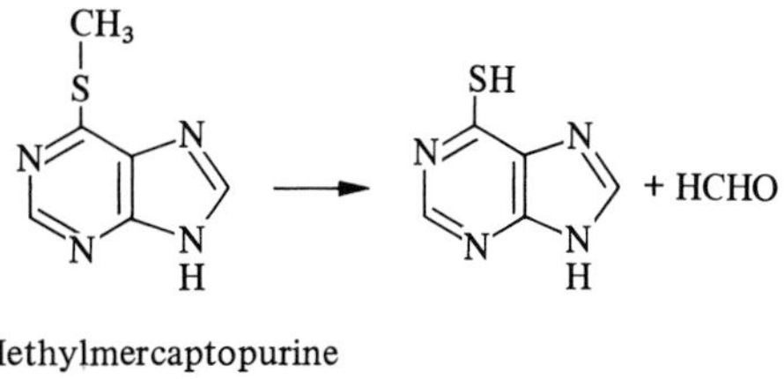

6—Methylmercaptopurine

Fig. 10. Oxidative S-dealkylation of 6-methylmercapto purine

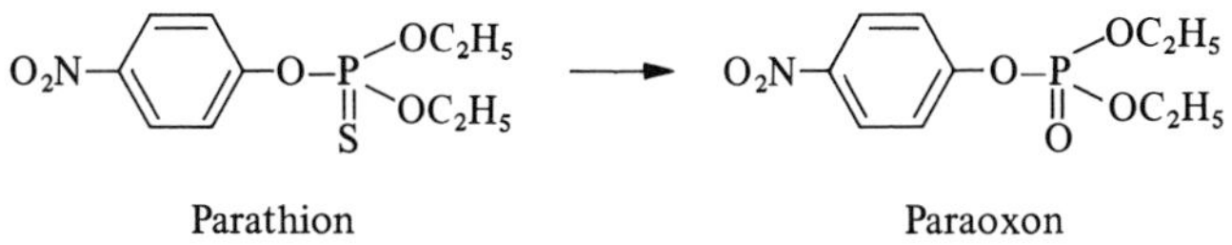

Fig. 11. Desulfuration of parathion to paraoxon

The oxidative S-dealkylation of alkyl thio ethers such as 6-methylmercaptopurine to aldehydes and thiol derivatives occurs in rats (SARCIONE and STUTZMAN 1960) as well as in man (ELION et al. 1962) (Fig. 10). The liver microsomes seem to metabolize a 6-alkylthiopurine only to an alkylsulfinyl purine (alkyl sulfoxide) and the conversion of the alkyl sulfoxide to the aldehyde is catalyzed by a cytoplasmic enzyme (FARBER 1975).

Desulfuration of compounds containing $C=S$ or $P=S$ functional groups occurs by the substitution of oxygen for sulfar and is mediated by the microsomal cytochrome P-450 system. For example, the metabolism of the insecticide parathion to paraoxon (Fig. 11) involves the incorporation of an oxygen atom into paraoxon. Parathion is activated by this reaction to paraoxon, which is a potent inhibitor of cholinesterase and other enzymes having a serine residue at the catalytic site (GAGE 1953). Paraoxon, the $P=O$ analog of parathion, is then hydrolyzed by an aryl phosphatase and detoxified. The covalent binding of sulfur to microsomes occurs during the microsomal desulfuration of parathion and inhibits microsomal monooxygenase activities by decreasing the amount of cytochrome P-450 (KAMATAKI and NEAL 1976).

A number of thioethers and thiocarbamates are metabolized through sulfoxidation to sulfoxides (Fig. 12). For example, thiocarbamate herbicides are oxidized by liver microsomes (and NADPH and O_2) to sulfoxides (HUBBELL and CASIDA 1977). Since the sulfoxide is considerably less toxic than the parent thiocarbamate, the biotransformation represents a detoxication reaction.

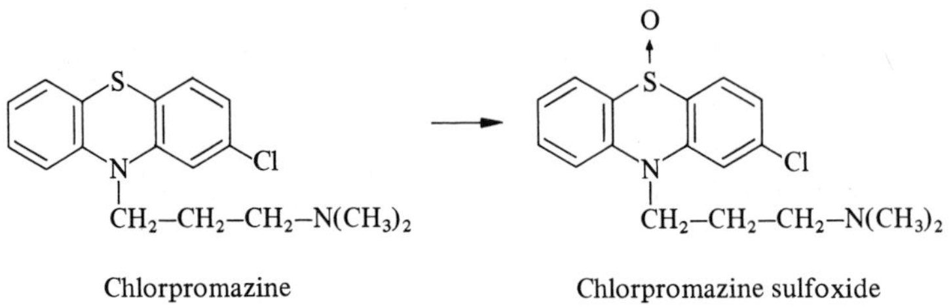

Fig. 12. Sulfoxidation of chlorpromazine to chlorpromazine sulfoxide

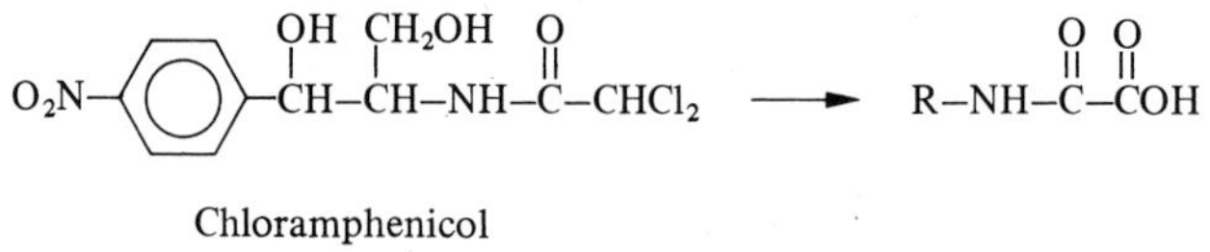

Chloramphenicol

Fig. 13. Oxidative dehalogenation of chloramphenicol

Many pesticides and herbicides are halogenated organic compounds. High resistance to biodegradation is a desirable asset for these chemicals as commercial products. However, their chemically inert nature causes problems for man and animals that ingest the compounds together with food. The microsomal cytochrome P-450 system is one of several enzymes capable of metabolizing halogenated hydrocarbons such as chloramphenicol by oxidative dehalogenation (POHL and KRISHNA 1978) (Fig. 13). Dehalogenation of carbon tetrachloride to carbon dioxide, chloroethanes, chloroform, and trichloroethylene are all mediated by the microsomal enzymes (VAN DYKE and GANDOLFI 1975; POHL et al. 1977).

2. Reductive Reactions

Since the body is generally aerobic, it is questioned whether anaerobic reductions occur in tissues in vivo. Evidence suggests that the majority of the cytochrome P-450 mediated reductive processes occurs in the large intestine and is catalyzed by intestinal bacteria such as *Escherichia coli*.

Halogenated hydrocarbons are metabolized by reductive dehalogenation. Carbon tetrachloride is reductively cleaved to give a chloride ion and the trichloromethyl radical, which is subsequently converted to chloroform (UEHLEKE et al. 1973). Halothane (2-bromo-2-chloro-1,1,1-trifluoroethane) (VAN DYKE and GANDOLFI 1976) and a number of polyhalogenated methanes (WOLF et al. 1975) are all dehydrogenated by the microsomal cytochrome P-450 system under anaerobic conditions. The enzyme activity involved in the reductive dehalogenation of halothane is induced by phenobarbital and polychlorinated biphenyl but not by 3-methylcholanthrene.

Enzyme systems capable of reduction of nitro compounds (Fig. 14) such as nitrobenzene, *p*-nitrobenzoic acid, and chloramphenicol are present in liver microsomes (FOUTS and BRODIE 1957). The reductive reaction is a multistep process ($RNO_2 \rightarrow RN = O \rightarrow RNHOH \rightarrow RNH_2$). It is not known if cytochrome P-450 is involved in all steps of the reductive reaction.

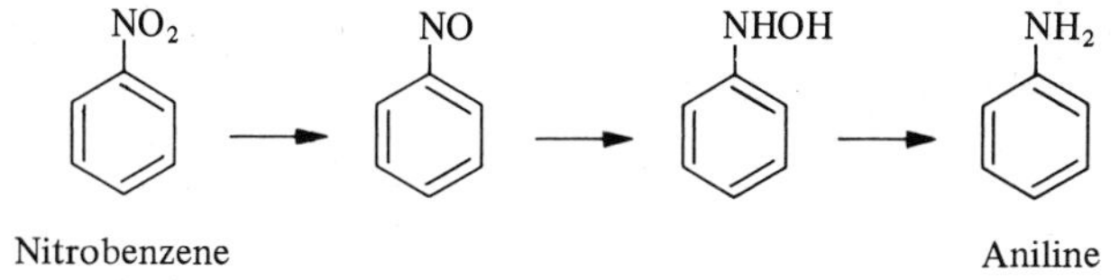

Nitrobenzene   Aniline

Fig. 14. Reduction of nitrobenzene

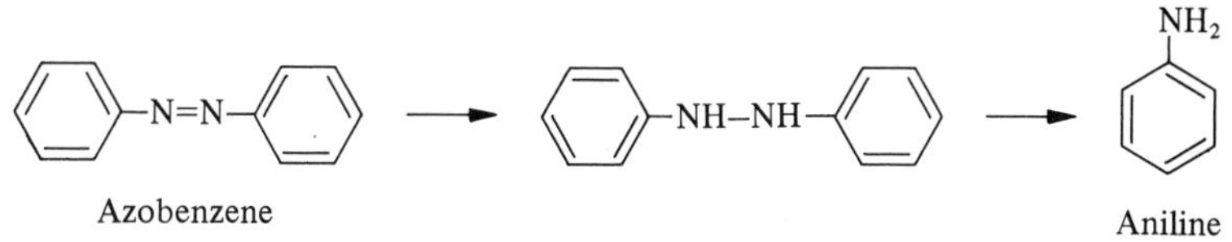

Azobenzene   Aniline

Fig. 15. Reductive cleavage of azobenzene

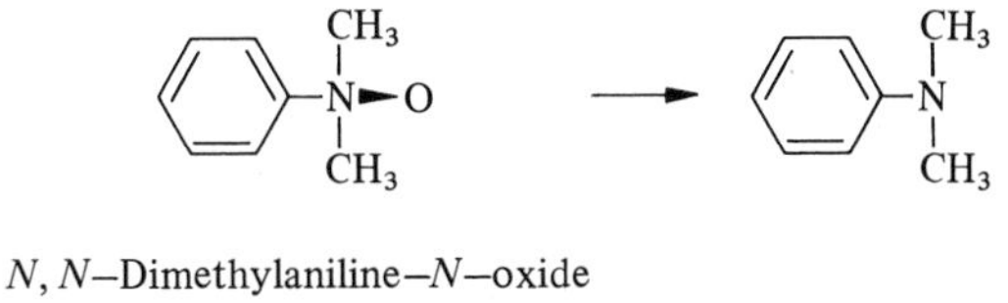

N, N–Dimethylaniline–N–oxide

Fig. 16. Reduction of N,N-dimethylaniline N-oxide

The reductive cleavage of azo compounds (azo reduction, Fig. 15) is mediated either by NADPH · cytochrome c reductase or directly by cytochrome P-450. The relative importance of the two pathways seems to depend on the azo substrate (SHARGEL 1969). The substrates with low oxidation-reduction potentials are reduced by cytochrome P-450, while those with higher potentials are more favored by NADPH · cytochrome c reductase (PETERSON et al. 1977).

Reduction of tertiary amine N-oxides to corresponding tertiary amines (Fig. 16) occurs by three routes: by microsomal enzymes, by a cytosolic enzyme, and by nonenzymatic processes. The cytosolic enzyme copurifies with xanthine oxidase (MURRAY and CHAYKIN 1966). The microsomal activity is considered to be dependent on cytochrome P-450 because reduced cytochrome P-450 itself can reduce tertiary amine N-oxide to tertiary amines in the absence of O_2 (IWASAKI et al. 1977). The lack of substrate specificity suggests that the substrate interacts with the heme moiety of the cytochrome P-450.

III. Conjugation Reactions (Phase II Reactions)

Cytochrome P-450 mediated reactions give rise to products that are much more reactive and therefore potentially more toxic to the cell than the parent compound. For example, the hydrophobic and inert polycyclic compound benzo(a)pyrene is oxidized to a highly reactive epoxide, which is subsequently converted to a diol by epoxide hydrase (OESCH 1973), and the diol undergoes a second oxidation to an extremely carcinogenic diol epoxide (see Fig. 3). The cell detoxifies the reactive products by various conjugation enzymes. Thus drug-metabolizing enzymes convert the hydrophobic substrate to more hydrophilic derivatives to be excreted. If detoxication is defined as a reaction by which hydrophilic substrates are made more water-soluble and more readily excretable, reactions (phase II reactions) catalyzed by various conjugation enzymes are truly detoxication reactions and are distinguished from the preceding oxidative phase I reactions. Phase II conjugation reactions require energy, and include glucuronidation, sulfation, acetylation, methylation, conjugation with amino acids, and conjugation with glutathione. These activities are virtually absent in the fetus and develop perinatally. Phase II conjugation reactions occur both in the microsomes (glucuronidation) and in the cytoplasm (sulfation, glutathione conjugation). Acetylation and acylation (methylation) reactions may decrease the hydrophilicity of the substrate drugs. However, detoxication of the drugs by modifying the reactive (toxic) groups such as amino and hydroxyl groups compensates for the reduction in water solubility of the compounds.

1. Glucuronidation

Glucuronidation is the most important among phase II conjugation reactions in vertebrates. Glucuronides are the major metabolites of many aromatic, aliphatic, and heterocyclic compounds containing, hydroxyl, carboxyl, amino, imino, and sulfhydryl groups. Glucuronide formation is catalyzed by microsomal uridine 5'-diphosphate (UDP) glucuronosyltransferase, which transfers glucuronic acid from UDP-α-D-glucuronic acid to an acceptor to form the β-D-glucuronide (Fig. 17). UDP-glucuronosyltransferase purified to apparent homogeneity from rat liver is a single polypeptide protein with a molecular weight of 59,000 (Gorski and Kasper 1977). An interesting aspect of the enzyme is that the transferase activity of microsomal membrane or of purified enzyme is activated by the carcinogen diethylnitrosamine (Weatherill and Burchell 1978). The activation is selective and activity is enhanced toward certain acceptors (e.g., 2-aminophenol) but not others. The mechanism of activation is not known. Although glucuronidation constitutes the major detoxication reaction, paradoxically, the glucuronidation reaction, when coupled to the aryl hydrocarbon hydroxylase system, may enhance the

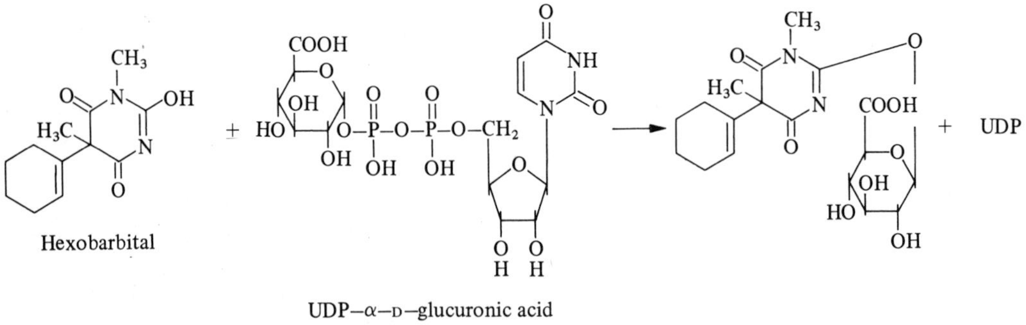

Fig. 17. Formation of hexobarbital glucuronide

carcinogenicity of aromatic hydrocarbons. Quinones of benzo(a)pyrene accumulate in the absence of UDP-glucuronic acid. The quinones are potent inhibitors of both benzo(a)pyrene and benzo(a)pyrene 7,8-dihydrodiol oxidation by the aryl hydrocarbon hydroxylase system (SHEN et al. 1980). Glucuronides formed in the liver and kidney are rapidly secreted into the urine and bile. However, it is worthy of note that glucuronides of drugs in the bile may be hydrolyzed by intestinal or bacterial β-glucuronidase, reabsorbed, and returned to the liver. This may prolong the action of the drug. The N-, S-, and C-glucuronides are also known (DUTTON and BURCHELL 1977). The N- and S-glucuronides are probably formed from UDP-glucuronate by UDP-glucuronosyltransferase. It is not established whether C-glucuronides are formed by the same enzyme.

2. Sulfation

Sulfation or formation of sulfate esters of the structure $ROSO_3$ is another major route of detoxication (Fig. 18). However, it must be recognized that some sulfate esters are more toxic and reactive than their parent compounds. The N, O-sulfate of the carcinogen N-hydroxy-2-acetylaminofluorene is an example. Sulfotransferase catalyzes the transfer of sulfate from 3′-phosphoadenosine 5′-phosphosulfate to the hydroxyl group of various xenobiotics as well as steroids (JAKOBY et al. 1980). The enzyme also catalyzes the formation of N-sulfates (sulfamates) with arylamines (e.g., 2-naphthylamine). Examples of sterol substrates include estrone, dehydroepiandrosterone, and bile salts. Purified arylsulfotransferases have a maximum molecular weight of about 64,000 and a minimum molecular weight of about 35,000, and are probably composed of two subunits (SEKURA and JACOBY 1979). At least three isozymes exist, which have different isoelectric points. Sulfoconjugation of steroids is important for steroid synthesis, not just a means of detoxication. Purified hydroxysteroid sulfotransferases, which also exist in multiple forms having different isoelectric points, are proteins of molecular weight 120,000–180,000 and are composed of subunits (JAKOBY et al. 1980). The hydroxyl group

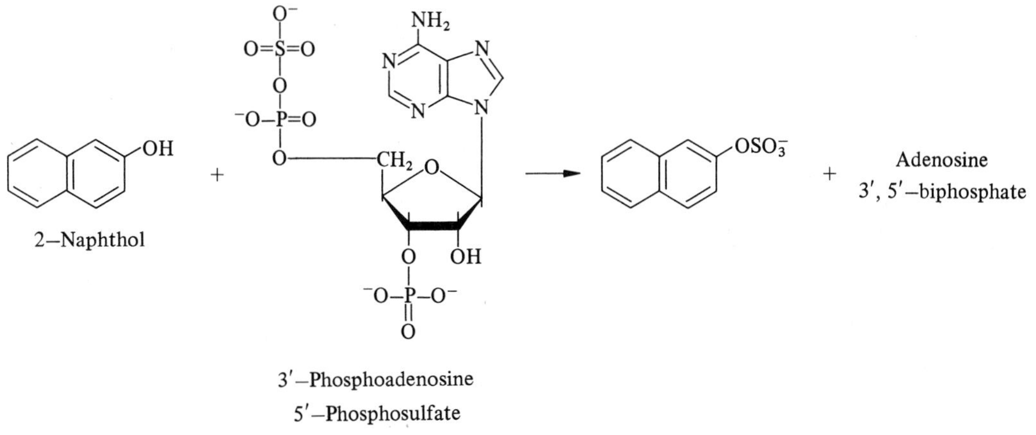

Fig. 18. Sulfation of 2-naphthol

at the 3-position of the hydroxysteroid is preferentially, if not exclusively, sulfated. Bile acids formed in the liver are conjugated with taurine or glycine before excretion into bile. The toxicity of bile salts becomes apparent in cholestasis (i.e., curtailment of bile flow) (Stiehl 1974). Under such conditions, bile salts accumulate in skin and produce pruritus (itching). In the healthy man the amounts of sulfated bile salts in serum and in urine are low or negligible. Sulfate conjugation of bile salts becomes significant in cholestasis. At least two sulfotransferase isozymes exist: kidney enzyme (Chen et al. 1978) and liver enzyme (Chen et al. 1977) have molecular weights of 80,000 and 130,000 respectively, and isoelectric points of 5.3 and 5.8 respectively. These enzymes are distinct from hydroxysteroid and estrogen sulfotransferases. Both aryl and hydroxysteroid sulfotransferases are nonmicrosomal enzymes.

3. Acetylation

Compounds containing amino, hydroxyl, and sulfhydryl groups are acetylated in intact animals. There are not many examples of acetylation of the hydroxyl group. However, aromatic amines are largely metabolized by acetylation in many tissues of most animal species (Williams 1959). Endogenous substrates for N-acetyltransferases include 5-hydroxytryptamine and histamine. The soluble enzyme acetyl CoA:arylamine N-acetyltransferase catalyzes the transfer of acetyl group from acetyl CoA to an acceptor substrate.

$$CH_3CO \cdot SCoA + RNH_2 \rightarrow RNHCOCH_3 + CoASH$$

N-acetyltransferase from rabbit liver has a molecular weight of 26,500–37,000 (Cohen et al. 1973; Schulte et al. 1974). The enzyme has a broad substrate specificity, although reactive acceptors must have an amino group attached directly to unsaturated rings or by way of a carbonyl group. Thus the enzyme acetylates isoniazid, p-aminobenzoic acid, aminofluorene, 4-aminoantipyrine, aniline, and p-aminosalicylic acid, but is not active with glucosamine, pyridoxamine, phenylalanine, or glutamine.

A hereditary polymorphism exists in the rate of drug N-acetylation in man (Evans et al. 1960). Based on the rate of acetylation of drugs such as isoniazid and other arylamine and hydrazine drugs, persons are classified as rapid acetylators or slow acetylators. The acetylation polymorphism (an autosomal dominant trait) is determined by two alleles (r and R). Slow acetylators are homozygous for a recessive allele (rr) and rapid acetylators are either homozygous (RR) or heterozygous (Rr). Slow acetylators usually retain higher serum levels of administered drug (e.g., isoniazid) than rapid acetylators. Therefore, the polymorphism has important consequences in drug therapy. Furthermore, the fact that arylamine carcinogens are acetylated by the polymorphic N-acetyltransferase suggests the possibility that genetic differences in acetylating capacity may determine man's susceptibility to chemical carcinogenicity of arylamines (Glowinski et al. 1978). Animals capable of N-acetylation convert arylhydroxamic acids to their carcinogenic metabolites arylhydroxylamines.

$$\underset{\substack{\displaystyle | \\ OH}}{\overset{\displaystyle \overset{O}{\underset{||}{C-R}}}{Ar-N}} \xrightarrow{\text{Enzyme}} Ar-NHOH + Enzyme \overset{O}{\underset{||}{-C-R}}$$

Arylhydroxamic acid   Arylhydroxylamine

$$\downarrow \qquad \overset{O}{\underset{||}{}}$$

$$(Ar-NHO-C-R) \rightarrow \rightarrow \text{Nucleic acid adducts}$$
Acyloxyarylamine

Evidence suggests that N-acyloxylarylamines formed from arylhydroxylamines are probably involved in the induction of extrahepatic tumors (KING and ALLABEN 1978).

4. Conjugation with Amino Acids

Conjugation of aromatic carboxyl group with the α-amino group of amino acids is an acylation reaction. The body seems to use this mechanism when glucuronidation capacity is low, as at birth in man. Conjugation with amino acids requires ATP to activate the carboxyl group of aromatic compounds, and is catalyzed by ATP-dependent acid: CoA ligases (AMP).

$$RCOO^- + ATP^{4-} + CoASH \rightleftharpoons RCOSCoA + AMP^{2-} + PPi^{3-}$$

$$RCOSCoA + R'NH_2 \rightarrow RCONHR' + CoASH$$

Overall: $RCOO^- + ATP^{4-} + R'NH_2 \rightarrow RCONHR' + AMP^{2-} + PPi^{3-}$, where $RCOO^-$ is aromatic acid and $R'NH_2$ represents amino acid. The second reaction (conjugation) is catalyzed by acyl-CoA:amino acid N-acyltransferases, also known as amino acid acylases. Typical reactions include hippurate synthesis from benzoate and glycine and taurocholate formation from cholate and taurine. Both acid:CoA ligases (KILLENBERG et al. 1971) and acyl-CoA: amino acid N-acyltransferases (LAU et al. 1977) are mitochondrial enzymes and have been purified only partially. Acid:CoA ligases have a broad substrate specificity and activate C_4–C_{12} straight chan fatty acids, benzoate, vinyl acetate, branched chain, hydroxy, and unsaturated fatty acids, but not salicylate and p-aminosalicylate (JENCKS 1974). Two types of acyl-CoA:amino N-acyltransferase activity are identified in liver microsomes of rhesus monkeys and humans (WEBSTER et al. 1979): one uses fatty acyl-CoA substrates, and the other prefers phenylacetyl-CoA to acyl-CoA substrate. Acyl-CoA:amino acid N-acyltransferases in mammals conjugate benzoic acids with glycine rather than L-glutamate, whereas the enzyme in man and the Old World monkey synthesizes L-glutamate conjugates of arylacetic acids.

Hydroxylated C_{24} steroid acids formed as degradation products of cholesterol in mammalian liver are collectively known as bile acids. These potentially toxic compounds are removed from the liver as conjugates with either glycine or taurine. Bile acids in normal bile or urine are in conjugated form; unconjugated acids which are formed by intestinal bacteria are reabsorbed and reconjugated by hepatocytes. Distinct bile acid:CoA ligase and bile acid-CoA:amino acid N-acyltransferase specific for steroid acids are present in the liver microsomes (Killenberg 1978). Both taurine and glycine serve as amino acid acceptors with purified rat liver N-acyl-transferase. In general, the amino acid substrate affinity in vitro is consistent with the composition of conjugates in bile. In the guinea pig and man, however, glycine conjugates predominate in bile despite a greater affinity of N-acyltransferase for taurine (Vessey 1978). The discrepancy may be attributed to a limited intrahepatic pool of taurine in the guinea pig and man.

5. Methylation

S-Adenosyl-L-methionine-dependent methyltransferases catalyze biological N- and O-methylation reactions (Fig. 19). Catechol O-methyltransferase is of primary importance not only for extraneuronal inactivation of endogenous catecholamines (dopamine, norepinephine, epinephrine) as well as for the further metabolism of oxidized metabolites of catecholamine, but also in the detoxication of catechol drugs (isoproterenol, α-methyldopa, L-dopa) used in the treatment of hypertension, asthma, and Parkinson's disease (Guldberg and Marsden 1975). Catechol O-methyltransferase is a widely distributed cytosolic enzyme which exists in two forms (molecular weights 24,000 and 47,000), and requires Mg^{2+} for activity (Huh and Friedhoff 1979). The enzyme shows high specificity for catechol but a broad specificity concerning substitutents on the aromatic nucleus. Ascorbate, which has an enediol structure similar to catechol, is also methylated by catechol O-methyltransferase.

Of particular importance for N-methylation is histamine N-methyltransferase, which catalyzes the transfer of a methyl group from S-adenosyl-L-methionine to histamine to form 1-methyl-4-(β-aminoethyl) imidazole (or 1-methylhistamine)

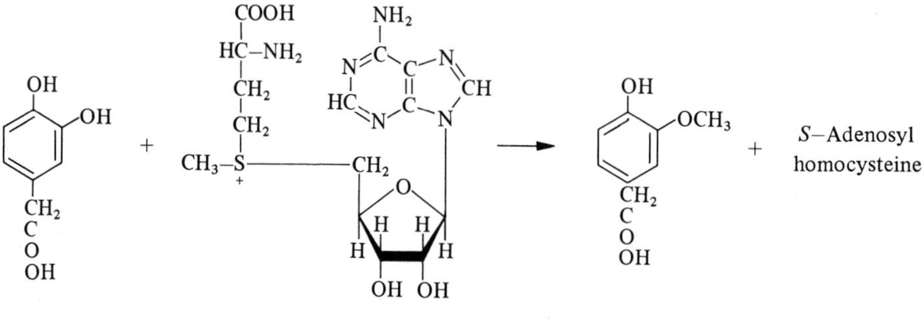

3, 4–Dihydroxyphenylacetic acid   S–Adenosylmethionine

Fig. 19. O-Methylation of 3,4-dihydroxyphenylacetic acid

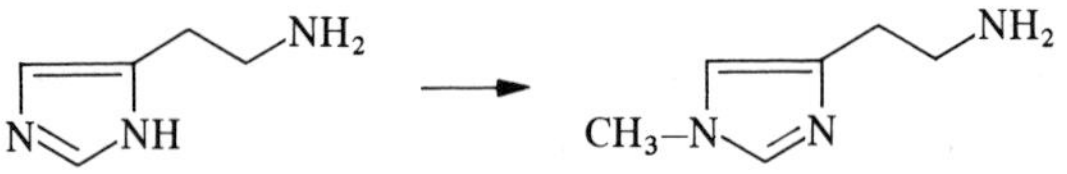

Histamine

Fig. 20. N-Methylation of histamine

(Fig. 20). The methylated histamine is the initial product of histamine metabolism in the brain, and is further oxidized (by diamine oxidase) and reduced (by aldehyde dehydrogenase) to 1-methylimidazole-4-acetic acid (SCHWARTZ et al. 1971). The enzyme occurs in the cytoplasm, requires no particular metal ion for activity, and has high specificity for histamine and S-adenosyl-L-methionine as the methyl donor (BROWN et al. 1959). Indolamine N-methlytransferase catalyzes the transfer of a methyl group from S-adenosyl-L-methionine to the amino group of a variety of indolamines (AXELROD 1962). In view of a lack of substrate specificity, the enzyme may play a role in the detoxication of xenobiotic amines.

Methyl transfer from S-adenosyl-L-methionine to the sulfur atom of thiols is catalyzed by microsomal thiol S-methyltransferase. The importance of this enzyme for detoxication is evident. Exposure to toxic sulfur compounds is unavoidable in our industrial society. The simplest thiol, hydrogen sulfide, is as toxic as hydrogen cyanide when inhaled, since it binds to cytochrome oxidase and other heme proteins. Hydrogen sulfide is detoxified by two-step methylation to dimethyl sulfide (WEISIGER and JAKOBY 1979):

$$H_2S \xrightarrow{\text{S-adenosylmethionine}} CH_3SH \xrightarrow{\text{S-adenosylmethionine}} (CH_3)_2S.$$

In addition to a number of drugs and environmental chemicals, substrates for this enzyme also arise from disulfide interchange reactions catalyzed by thioltransferase (AXELSSON et al. 1978): $GSH + XSSY \rightarrow GSSY + XSH$). It should be noted that glutathione (GSH) and cysteine do not serve as substrates for the S-methyltransferase.

6. Conjugation with Glutathione

Glutathione S-transferase (Fig. 21) is principally a cytosolic enzyme, although a microsomal enzyme is also known (MORGENSTERN et al. 1982). The enzyme conjugates a variety of aromatic hydrocarbons, aryl amines, organohalides, etc. with glutathione. The products are more water-soluble than the parent compounds and are either excreted as biliary glutathione conjugates or further metabolized to mercapturic acids. Perhaps the most important role of this enzyme in drug detoxication is inactivation of toxic epoxide (arene oxide) intermediates produced by aromatic hydroxylation reactions. Although substrates for conjugation are varied, one property common to the compounds is the presence of an electrophilic center that reacts with the nucleophilic SH group of glutathione. Multiple forms (isozymes) with different isoelectric points are known for rat liver enzyme (JAKOBY and HABIG 1980). On the basis of the order of elution from carboxymethyl-cellulose columns, isozymes $E(pI = 10)$, D, C, B, A, $AA(pI = 7.3)$ were defined. These isozymes are proteins with a molecular weight of about 47,000 and are composed of two subunits of similar molecular weight. Beside glutathione conjugation with electrophilic aromatic compounds, the enzyme catalyzes a variety of reactions involving glutathione. Organic nitrate esters are reduced to alcohols and inorganic nitrite (HEPPEL and HILMOE 1950): $[GSH + CH_2(ONO_2)CH(ONO_2)CH_2(ONO_2) \rightarrow GSNO_2 + CH_2(ONO_2)CHOHCH_2(ONO_2)]$. $GSNO_2$ undergoes reaction with a second molecule of GSH to form nitrite $(GSNO_2 + GSH \rightarrow GSSG + HNO_2)$. The enzyme catalyzes the positional isomerization of double bonds. An example is the isomer-

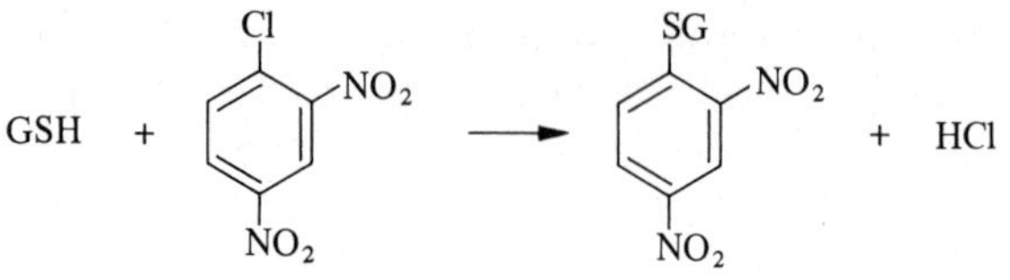

$$GSH \quad + \quad \text{[1-Chloro-2,4-dinitrobenzene structure]} \quad \longrightarrow \quad \text{[SG-dinitrobenzene structure]} \quad + \quad HCl$$

1–Chloro–2, 4–dinitrobenzene

Fig. 21. Conjugation of glutathione with 1-chloro-2, 4-dinitrobenzene

$$R \cdot X \ + \ HSCH_2CHCONHCH_2CO_2H$$
$$| \qquad\qquad$$
$$NHCOCH_2CH_2CHCO_2H$$
$$|$$
$$NH_2$$

Glutathione S—transferases

$$R \cdot S \ CH_2CHCONHCH_2CO_2H$$
$$|$$
$$NHCOCH_2CH_2CHCO_2H$$
$$|$$
$$NH_2$$

γ—Glutamyltranspeptidase

$$R \cdot S \ CH_2CHCONHCH_2CO_2H$$
$$|$$
$$NH_2$$

Aminopeptidase

$$R \cdot SCH_2CHCO_2H \qquad N—\text{Acetyltransferase} \qquad R \cdot SCH_2CHCO_2H$$
$$| \qquad\qquad\qquad\qquad\qquad\qquad\qquad\qquad | $$
$$NH_2 \qquad\qquad\qquad\qquad\longrightarrow\qquad\qquad\qquad NHCOCH_3$$

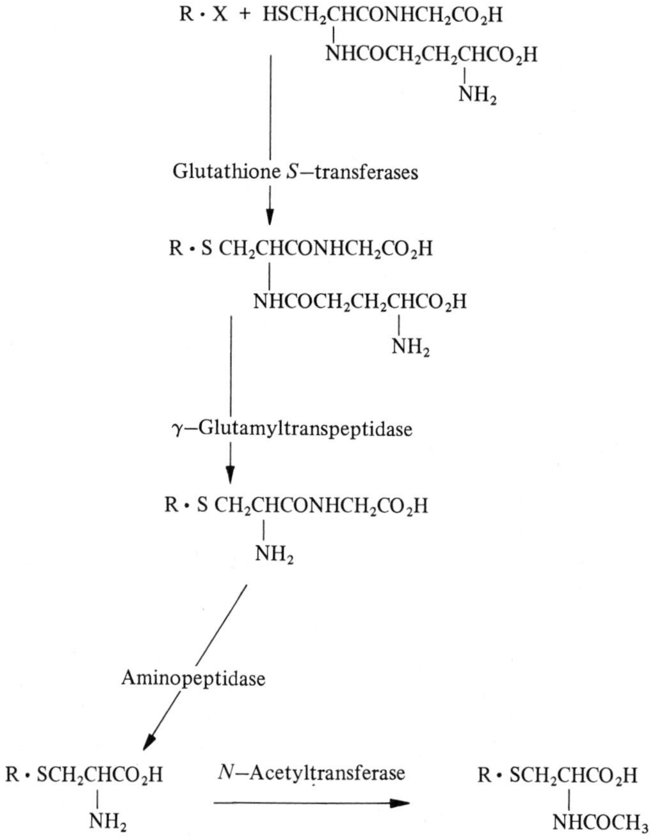

Mercapturic acid

Fig. 22. Formation of mercapturate from glutathione conjugate

ization of maleylacetoacetic acid to fumarylacetoacetic acid (Keen and Jakoby 1978). The reaction does not consume GSH and proceeds probably with the formation of a glutathonyl adduct and subsequent regeneration of free GSH. Another reaction catalyzed by the enzyme is thiolysis of p-nitrophenyl acetate by GSH to p-nitrophenol and an acetyl thiol ($GSCOCH_3$) (Keen and Jakoby 1978). The enzyme shows glutathione peroxidase activity which is not dependent on selenium and therefore distinct from the selenium enzyme (Prohaska and Ganther 1977).

Finally, glutathione S-transferase B is identified as ligandin, a soluble protein which binds various organic anions such as bilirubin (HABIG et al. 1974). Bilirubin, a poorly soluble toxic compound is carried by albumin in the blood, but in the hepatocyte the compound may be bound to glutathione transferase B and stored.

The formation of mercapturates from glutathione conjugates involves three enzymes: γ-glutamyltranspeptidase, aminopeptidase, and N-acetyltransferase (Fig. 22). γ-Glutamyltranspeptidase and aminopeptidase are associated with the cell membrane, while the other enzyme, N-acetyltransferase, is a microsomal enzyme (TATE 1980). Therefore, N-acetyltransferase involved in mercapturate formation is different from the cytosolic N-acetyltransferase discussed in the preceding section (Sect. III.B.3). The aminopeptidase (which has a molecular weight of about 95,000) consists of two identical subunits and hydrolyzes a variety of dipeptides but not tripeptides or tetrapeptides (MCINTYRE and CURTHOYS 1982). Although a number of xenobiotics are excreted as mercapturic acids, there is no evidence for the formation of significant amounts of mercapturates of endogenous compounds in mammals.

IV. Induction of Drug-Metabolizing Enzymes

One of the interesting features of drug-metabolizing enzymes is the inducibility of enzyme activities by aromatic hydrocarbons. Although a large number of monooxygenases are induced by inducers, it has been generally accepted that only two types of cytochrome P-450 are induced by different inducers: cytochrome P-450 induced typically by phenobarbital, and cytochrome P_1-450 induced typically by 3-methylcholanthrene (CONNEY 1967). However, recent evidence indicates that at least six forms of cytochrome P-450 exist: four forms of phenobarbital-induced P-450 and two forms of P-450 induced by 3-methylcholanthrene or 2,3,7,8-tetrachlorodibenzo-p-dioxin (TCDD) (NEBERT et al. 1981). The number of inducible forms of cytochrome P-450 will undoubtedly increase as the techniques of identification are improved. In an extreme model (NEBERT 1979b), organisms are able to induce as many forms of P-450 as inducers. Most of these forms may not be distinguishable spectrally, but have slightly different amino acid sequences in the polypeptide. Since Nebert's most recent model for the induction of cytochrome P-450 and drug-metabolizing enzymes (NEBERT et al. 1981) is perhaps the most provocative and deserves particular attention, it is briefly discussed here.

Following intraperitoneal injections of aromatic hydrocarbons (e.g., 3-methylcholanthrene), cytochrome P_1-450 is induced in the inbred C57/BL6 (B6) mouse strain but not in the inbred DBA/2 (D2) mouse strain. This responsiveness to aromatic hydrocarbons is designated "the Ah locus." The Ah (responsive)/Ah (nonresponsive) heterozygote is responsive, indicating a mendelian autosomal dominant trait. Although cytochrome P_1-450 induced by different inducers appears to be a single species by spectral identification, numerous enzyme activities are induced. Thus the induction of at least 20 monooxygenase activities is known to be closely associated with the Ah locus (NEBERT and JENSEN 1979). Examples are aryl hydrocarbon [benzo(a)pyrene] hydroxylase, zoxazolamine 6-hydroxylase, naphthalene monooxygenase, and acetaminophen N-hydroxylase. The inducibility of zoxazolamine 6-hydroxylase can be used to determine the Ah allele phenotype (Nebert 1979a). Zoxazolamine causes muscle paralysis in experimental animals. For example, mice are pretreated with aromatic hydrocarbons to induce zoxazolamine 6-hydroxylase activity and then injected with zoxazolamine (250 mg/kg body wt.). Responsive strains are able to metabolize and detoxify the drug efficiently and are paralyzed for less than 30 min, while nonresponsive strains are paralyzed for almost 2 h. On the other hand, there are cytochrome P-450 mediated monooxygenase activities which are not associated with the Ah locus. These include the basal as well as induced activities for metabolism of pentobarbital, hexobarbital, aniline, ethylmorphine, estrogen, and testosterone. The induction of neither NADPH-cytochrome P-450 reductase nor epoxide hydrolase is associated with the Ah locus. For phase II conjugation enzymes, UDP-glucuronosyltransferase is associated with the Ah, but cytosolic glutathione S-transferase is not. Another notable point about the Ah locus is that the difference between the Ah (responsive) and the Ah (nonresponsive) is not attributed to differences in structural genes. Unlike most of the inducers, TCDD can induce monooxygenase activities in nonresponsive mice if given in a dose 15 times higher than that required to induce the activities in responsive mice (Poland et al. 1974). This was interpreted to suggest that the nonresponsive mice have a defective (low-affinity) Ah receptor but intact structural genes. Thus the cytosolic receptor (with high affinity for TCDD) is regarded as the major product of the Ah regulatory genes. The receptor binds not only TCDD but a variety of other aromatic hydrocarbons, and appears to control at least two dozen monooxygenase activities. All nonresponsive mouse strains so far examined are deficient in the high-affinity Ah receptor.

The process of enzyme induction is initiated by the entry of xenobiotic inducer into the cell and the specific binding to the cytosolic Ah receptor. The apparent translocation of the inducer–receptor complex into the nucleus is then followed by nuclear responses such as the activation of numerous structural genes and subsequent synthesis of enzymes. The genetic regulation of the induction process has been explained by the Davidson–Britten model (Davidson and Britten 1973) with modifications (Fig. 23). Consider that the effectors (receptor–inducer complexes) α, β, and γ represent receptors complexed with different types of inducers, e.g., TCDD, isosafrole, and phenobarbital, respectively. This assumption is made although specific cytosolic receptors for the latter two inducers are not yet known. The effector binds to a sensor site to the $5'$ end of an integrator gene set. The transcription of the gene set results in the production of hypothetical activator message (RNA), which is capable of turning on structural genes on the same chromosome as well as on other chromosomes. The formation of activator message RNA may be a gene amplification process. Binding of the activator message RNA to specific acceptor sites (the promotor regions to the $5'$ end of structural genes) results in the synthesis of mRNA and consequently the synthesis of enzyme proteins. Such a model could explain the existence of structural gene mutants. For example, in a mutant mouse which has been treated with 3-methylcholanthrene, aryl hydrocarbon hydroxylase may be induced but other hydroxylases may not be induced despite the presence of receptor. The model could also explain the induction of apparently the same form of P-450 by different inducers. Both activator message Mc derived from the Ah-related gene set (I^{α}) and activator message Mc from the pheno-

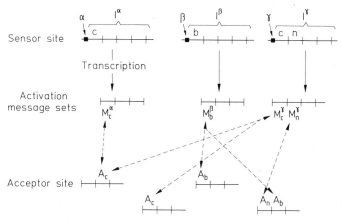

Fig. 23. Nebert's model for inducer-elicited gene expression for drug-metabolizing enzymes (NEBERT et al. 1981). α, β, and γ: receptor–inducer complex. a, b, c, n: gene; I, gene set; M, activator message; A, promotor region of structural gene. For example, binding of inducer (e.g., 3-methylcholanthrene) to site α activates the Ah-related gene set (I^{α}) which turns of synthesis of activator message RNA M_c^{α}. M_c^{α} then binds to the promotor region (A_c) of structural gene and facilitates synthesis of mRNA for cytochrome P-450 synthesis

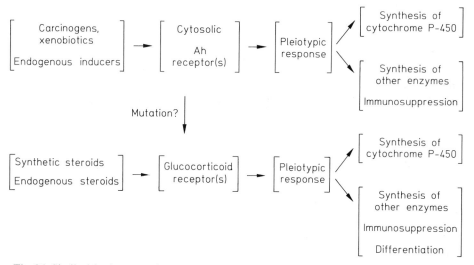

Fig. 24. Similarities between the Ah receptor system and the glucocorticoid receptor system (NEBERT et al. 1981)

barbital-related gene set (I^{γ}) would bind to the promotor region (Ac) of structural gene (Fig. 23). The subsequent formation of the same mRNA leads to the synthesis of the same form of cytochrome P-450 protein.

In the proposed model, the cytosolic receptor is assumed to be the regulatory gene product of the Ah genes. But why receptor? Although we cannot answer the question at the present, there seems some evolutionary reason to assume that nature has selected the receptor as the regulatory product. Striking similarities are noted in properties between the Ah receptor and the glucocorticoid receptor (Fig. 24) (Nebert et al. 1981). Both receptors, upon binding ligands (xenobiotics or steroids), show pleiotypic responses which lead to the induction of enzymes (including cytochrome P-450) and immunosuppression. The close similarities make us wonder if the glucocorticoid receptor developed as a mutated Ah receptor, or vice versa, during evolution.

C. Ocular Drug Metabolism

Drug-metabolizing systems similar to those in the liver are also present in various nonhepatic tissues (Gram 1980). The eye is no exception in this respect. The presence of cytochrome P-450 is spectrally identified in the retinal pigmented epithelium (Shichi 1969). However, only scanty information is available on ocular drug metabolism, although much is known of the absorption, distribution, and clinical usefulness of ophthalmic drugs (Zimmerman et al. 1980). Various drugs show diverse side effects on the eye. To mention a few, anti-inflammatory steroids increase intraocular pressure (IOP). Narcotics such as morphine and marijuana may lower IOP (Goodman and Gilman 1975). Phenothiazines (e.g., chlorpromazine) cause abnormal corneal and lens pigmentation and pigmentary retinopathy (Smith 1974). Chloroquine accumulation is causative of the retinopathy in chloroquine-treated arthritis patients and others (Bernstein 1967). These adverse effects of drugs will persist indefinitely unless the eye possesses mechanisms to detoxify and remove these compounds. Information about genetic differences in ocular drug metabolism and toxicity is largely lacking. An example is steroid-induced "glaucoma," possibly a pharmacogenetic disorder. About 5% of the United States population is homozygous for the recessive allele causing elevated IOP induced by corticosteroid ophthalmic medication (Armaly 1968).

A systematic study of ocular drug metabolism was virtually nonexistent when we initiated our work. Discussion below is mainly based on our findings and concerns first the genetic regulation in the eye of the phase I enzyme aryl hydrocarbon hydroxylase (one of the cytochrome P-450 mediated monooxygenases), then deals with the distribution of both phase I enzyme (aryl hydrocarbon hydroxylase) and phase II enzyme (UDP-glucuronosyltransferase) in ocular tissues. Finally, a possible significance of the tissue distribution of drug-metabolizing enzymes for ocular functions is discussed with particular reference to acetaminophen toxicity.

I. Aryl Hydrocarbon Hydroxylase Induction in the Eye

The genetic expression of the Ah locus seems to be systemic, for it occurs not only in the liver but also in lung, kidney, intestine, placenta, skin, eye, and testis (Gram 1980). Aryl hydrocarbon hydroxylase activity in the eye is induced by polycyclic aromatic compounds such as β-naphthoflavone, 3-methylcholanthrene, and TCDD (Shichi et al. 1975). The genetic regulation of the inducibility is clearly demonstrated in Fig. 25, which illustrates the relationship between the β-naphthoflavone-inducible hydroxylase ativity in the eye and in liver microsomes of B6

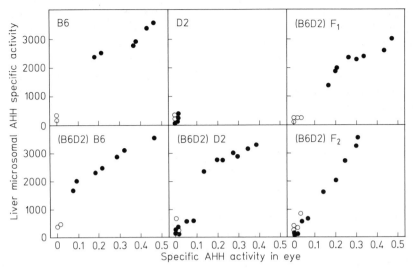

Fig. 25. Relationship between genetic variance and aryl hydrocarbon hydroxylase (*AHH*) induction in the eye and in liver microsomes of β-naphthoflavone-treated B6 and D2 mouse strains, F_1 and F_2 offspring, and progeny from backcrosses. *Empty circle*, not treatment; *solid circle*, β-naphthoflavone pretreatment. (SHICHI et al. 1976)

(responsive) and D2 (nonresponsive) inbred mice and of progeny derived from the various genetic crosses. The hydroxylase activity is inducible in the eye and liver microsomes from the responsive B6, all (B6D2)F1 progeny, and all offspring from (B6D2)F1 × B6 backcross. However, a bimodal distribution is seen in the progeny from (B6D2)F1 × D2 backcross and the F1 × F1 intercross. These results indicate that the expression of the hydroxylase inducibility in the eye is, as in the liver, an autosomal dominant mendelian trait.

II. Tissue Distribution of Drug-Metabolizing Enzymes in the Eye

Distribution of aryl hydrocarbon hydroxylase (phase I enzyme) and UDP-glucuronosyltransferase (phase II enzyme) in ocular tissues is shown in Table 1 (DAS and SHICHI 1981). Since the animal was not pretreated with polycyclic hydrocarbon inducers, the activities are basal (not induced) activities. The enzyme activities are primarily associated with the structures of the ciliary body and pigmented epithelium of the choroid. Little activity is detected in the cornea, retina, or lens. Drug-metabolizing activities may be concentrated in the epithelial cells of the cornea and lens, however. The metabolism of benzo(a)pyrene by the lens epithelium has been reported (GOOS et al. 1981). While the enzyme activities of the choroid alone have not been investigated, the activities are unquestionably associated with the retinal pigmented epithelium. When cultured chick embryonic pigmented epithelial cells are treated with benzo(a)anthracene, aryl hydrocarbon hydroxylase and UDP-glucuronosyltransferase activities are fully induced (SHICHI et al. 1976). Furthermore, of various subcellular fractions prepared from the inducer-treated cells, the microsomal fraction shows the highest activities of these enzymes and contains appreciable amounts of cytochrome P-450 (SHICHI and NEBERT 1980). It is worthy of note that the hydroxylase activity of the ciliary body is almost 20 times higher than that of the pigmented epithelium-choroid. The ciliary body contains a complete set of enzymes for mercapturate synthesis (DAS and SHICHI 1981). Low levels of glutathione S-transferase are present in the lens (AWASTHI et al. 1980). One may wonder whether the specialized location of drug-metabolizing enzymes in the eye is suggestive of their physiological functions. The blood vessels which enter the eye can be divided into two distinct systems – retinal and uveal. Retinal circulation is an important but restricted channel that provides nutrients directly to the inner layers of the retina. The uveal circulation accounts for as much as 88% of the entire ocular blood flow (FRIEDMAN et al. 1964, 1965; BILL 1975) and supports the functions of the ciliary body and iris in the anterior uvea and the pigmented epithelium of the choroid in the posterior uvea. It is significant that drug-metabolizing enzymes are associated with these tissues, which are in contact with the ocular blood barrier uveal blood supply. This part of the "ocular" circulation is outside the barrier. Polycyclic aromatic hydrocarbons which are brought in the blood to the posterior uvea will be removed by adsorption to the melanin granules in the choroid (MEIR-RUGE and CERLETTI 1966; POTTS 1964). If the level of polycyclic compounds in the blood exceeds the capacity of the ocular blood barrier melanin granules, however, the compounds will pass through the barrier to enter the pigmented epithelium. It is therefore reasonable to assume that the drug-metabolizing enzymes of this tissue metabolize the xenobiotic compounds and detoxify the blood nutrients to be provided for the photoreceptor cells. On the other hand, the major function of the ciliary epithelium is aqueous humor formation by metabolically regulated action on the plasma filtrate of blood present in the stroma of the ciliary processes. The melanin granules of the pigmented epithelia of the ciliary processes will serve as the primary adsorbents of polycyclic compounds (YAMASHITA et al. 1981), as in the case of the pigmented epithelium of the choroid. When the melanin granules of this outer cell layer are saturated by adsorbed compounds, the drug-metabolizing enzymes of the ciliary epithelium will become of critical importance.

Table 1. Distribution of aryl hydrocarbon hydroxylase, uridine 5′-diphosphate-glucuronosyltransferase, and γ-glutamyl transpeptidase in various ocular tissues

Tissues	Enzyme activities (units per mg protein)[a]		
	Aryl hydrocarbon hydroxylase	UDP-glucuronosyl-transferase	γ-Glutamyl transpeptidase
Retina	0.03	6	400
Lens	Not detectable	5	3
Cornea	0.02	8	320
Iris	0.15	23	640
Pigmented epithelium-choroid	0.31	84	430
Ciliary body	5.74	396	3,850

[a] Tissue homogenates were used for assay of enzymic activities. One unit of activity is the amount of enzyme protein that produces 1 pmol product/min. Enzyme activities given here are specific activities, i.e., units per milligram enzyme protein per minute

III. Drug Toxicity – An Experimental Approach

As mentioned earlier, polycyclic hydrocarbons [e.g., benzo(a)pyrene] are converted or potentiated to highly reactive and therefore harmful products (e.g., epoxides) by phase I monooxygenases (PELKONEN and NEBERT 1982). The intermediates may react with DNA and cellular proteins to cause cancer (chemical carcinogenesis), developmental abnormalities, and cell death. Therefore, drug metabolism can be harmful rather than beneficial to the cell unless phase II detoxication enzymes function efficiently. A survey of the responsiveness of several mouse strains points to a possible correlation between the drug-metabolizing capacity of the pigmented epithelium and hereditary retinal degeneration (SHICHI et al. 1976). Polycyclic inducer-responsive mouse strains such as C3H/HeJ, C57BL/6J le rd, and CBA/J develop retinal degeneration, whereas nonresponsive DBA/2J, ARK/J, and 129/J inbred strains do not (Table 2). Although many factors must contribute to retinal degeneration in mice, aryl hydrocarbon hydroxylase and other cytochrome P-450 mediated monooxygenases inducible in the pigmented epithelium may be one of the factors. The eyes of nonresponsive strains of mouse are not vulnerable probably because they do not have high capacity to convert xenobiotics to reactive intermediates. Cytotoxic metabolites produced in responsive strains may cause retinal degeneration by labilizing the lysosomes of the pigmented epithelium. It has been suggested that the degeneration of photoreceptor cells in some animals may be caused by the breakdown of retinal and pigmented epithelial lysosomes by membrane-disrupting agents (READING 1970). It may be interesting to investigate whether the mouse strains with retinal dystrophy contain normal levels of phase II detoxication enzymes in the pigmented epithelium.

If the function of a drug-metabolizing and detoxifying system in the ciliary body is to detoxify the serum for aqueous humor production, the failure of the sys-

Table 2. Correlation between aryl hydrocarbon hydroxylase inducibility and retinal degeneration in mice

	Aryl hydrocarbon hydroxylase activity [pmol benzo(a)pyrene hydroxylated/mg protein/min]				Retinal degeneration[a]
	Liver microsomes		Eye		
	Control	Induced	Control	Induced	
C3H/HeJ	330	1,870	0.08	0.36	+
C57BL/6J le rd	310	2,020	0.09	0.41	+
CBA/J	340	1,520	0.09	0.38	+
C57/BL/6J be	290	1,490	0.09	0.37	±[b]
DBA/2J	190	170	0.07	0.07	−
AKR/J	380	330	0.08	0.08	−
129/J	340	350	0.08	0.08	−

Plus indicates morphological defect in the retina and minus indicates normal appearance
[a] Retinas of 4–6 week old mice were examined
[b] Morphological signs of retinal degeneration were seen in about 10% of animals examined

tem will result in the damage of the avascular tissues of the eye by reactive metabolites of xenobiotics contained in the aqueous. This is indeed found to be the case when large doses of acetaminophen are administered to polycyclic inducer-responsive mice (e.g., B6) (Shichi et al. 1978, 1980). Responsive and nonresponsive mice which have been pretreated with 3-methylcholanthrene are injected with large doses (1 g/kg body wt.) of acetaminophen. Lens opacity develops within 6 h after administration of the drug. The cornea remains clear and the retina and pigmented epithelium are normal. Acetaminophen-caused acute cataract is closely correlated to the Ah (responsive) locus. Thus lens opacification is observed in 3-methylcholanthrene-pretreated responsive inbred strains such as A/J, CBA/J, and C3H/HeJ, but not in similarly treated nonresponsive inbred strains such as RF/J, AKR/J, SJL/J, and SWR/J. After administration of radiolabeled acetaminophen to the responsive animal, covalent binding of acetaminophen metabolites to the lens is demonstrated. The glutathione level of the lens remains virtually unchanged for at least 4 h following acetaminophen injection, whereas hepatic glutathione concentration decreases markedly in less than 1 h. Acetaminophen is known to be detoxified as conjugates with glucuronate and sulfate (Ruchirawa et al. 1981) and glutathione (Mitchell et al. 1973). It awaits further studies to see whether the lens epithelium of responsive mice does not have sufficient capacities to detoxify acetaminophen metabolites, especially as glutathione conjugates. Although acetaminophen is generally considered a safe drug, liver necrosis is caused by overdosage (Jollow et al. 1974). Since an injection of large doses of acetaminophen into responsive mice is often fatal, the animals were fed low concentrations of the drug over a length of time. Feeding of low concentrations of acetaminophen to polycyclic hydrocarbon-pretreated responsive mice also results in irreversible cataract formation in otherwise healthy animals (Shichi et al. 1980). In these animals, not only lens opacity but tissue degeneration in the ciliary body and iris, anterior synechiae, and an invasion of inflammatory cells are also observed. The location of tissue damage indicates that cytotoxic metabolites can be secreted with the aqueous humor into the posterior chamber and flow into the anterior chamber. Whatever the mechanism of tissue degeneration, the acetaminophen toxicity to the anterior segment of the eye clearly illustrates the importance of a drug-detoxifying system of the ciliary body.

D. Concluding Remarks

A large body of information is available on drug metabolism and detoxication in the liver. Studies in other tissues have been markedly stimulated in recent years and led to our realization that drug-metabolizing activities are usually associated with the epithelial cells and may be beneficial as well as detrimental to the cell. Phase I enzymes convert xenobiotic compounds to chemically reactive intermediates which are capable of binding covalently to DNA, proteins, and cell membranes, and are detrimental to cellular functions. In normal conditions, however, the oxidized intermediates are detoxified by phase II conjugation enzymes as well as reducing enzymes. Both phase I and phase II enzymes are induced by polycyclic inducers. The levels of these enzymes vary depending on developmental stages, and are also affected by nutritional factors. Therefore, tissue susceptibility to chemical carcinogenesis and other degenerative effects may be determined by a subtle interplay of differences in responsiveness of these phase I and phase II enzymes to inducers, age, and nutritional factors.

Compared to what is known about other nonhepatic tissues, our knowledge of drug metabolism in ocular tissues is very limited. In view of the fact that a variety of drugs and chemicals affect visual acuity, IOP, etc., the importance of drug-metabolizing and detoxifying enzymes in the uvea (at the level of the blood–ocular barrier) is evident. For example, autocoids like the prostaglandins and leukotrienes may be synthesized by the ocular tissues and released into the aqueous after trauma and in inflammatory conditions (see Chaps. 7 and 10b). The ciliary body has a high capacity to accumulate organic acids and perhaps to metabolize these. To study the accumulation and metabolism of autocoids under conditions as nearly physiological as possible, a perfusion system for an enucleated eye (TAZAWA and SEAMAN 1972; MACRI and CEVARIO 1973) may be especially useful. In such a system, drugs and chemicals may be introduced into the ciliary body from the long posterior ciliary artery, and the levels of compounds (and their metabolites) accumulated in the ciliary body and those secreted into the aqueous humor can be determined. Such a system may also make it possible to investigate the induction of drug-metabolizing enzymes in the ciliary body and other tissues by perfusing the isolated eye with polycyclic inducers.

Finally, an understanding of the distribution and function of drug-metabolizing enzymes in the eye should be helpful for drug designing. For example, γ-glutamyl dopa was tested for its renal vasodilator activity (WILK et al. 1978). γ-Glutamyl dopa is converted to dopamine in the kidney as a result of the sequential action of γ-glutamyltranspeptidase and aromatic L-amino acid decarboxylase, two enzymes highly concentrated in the kidney. The concentration of dopamine in the kidney after a dose of γ-glutamyl dopa was almost five times higher than after an equivalent dose of L-dopa. γ-Glutamyl dopa may also be useful as a prodrug in the ciliary body, since this tissue has high γ-glutamyltranspeptidase activities (REDDY and UNAKAR 1973; ROSS et al. 1973; DAS and SHICHI 1979).

References

Armaly MF (1968) Genetic factors related to glaucoma. Ann NY Acad Sci 151:861–875

Atlas SA, Nebert DW (1976) Pharmacogenetics and human disease. In: Parke DV, Smith RL (eds), Drug metabolism – from microbe to man. Taylor and Francis, London, pp 393–430

Awasthi YC, Saneto RP, Srivastava SK (1980) Purification and properties of bovine lens glutathione S-transferase. Exp Eye Res 30:29–39

Axelrod J (1962) The enzymatic N-methylation of serotonin and other amines. J Pharmacol Exp Ther 138:28–33

Axelsson K, Eriksson S, Mannervik B (1978) Purification and characterization of cytoplasmic thiol transferase (glutathione:disulfide oxidoreductase) from rat liver. Biochemistry 17:2978–2984

Bárány EH (1973) The liver-like anion transport system in rabbit kidney, uvea and choroid plexus. II. Efficiency of acidic drugs and other anions as inhibitors. Acta Physiol Scand 88:491

Bernstein HN (1967) Chloroquine ocular toxicity. Survey Ophthalmol 12:415–447

Bill A (1975) Blood circulation and fluid dynamics in the eye. Physiol Rev 55:383–417

Blobel G, Doberstein B (1975) Transfer of proteins across membranes. I. Presence of pro-
teolytically processed and unprocessed nascent immunoglobulin light chains on membrane bound ribosomes of murine myeloma. J Cell Biol 67:835–851

Brodie BB, Gillett JR, Ladu BN (1958) Enzymatic metabolism of drugs and other foreign
compounds. Ann Rev Biochem 27:427–454

Brown DD, Tomchick R, Axelrod J (1959) Distribution and properties of a histamine-
methylating enzyme. J Biol Chem 234:2948–2950

Chen L-J, Bolt RJ, Admirand WH (1977) Enzymatic sulfation of bile salts. Partial purification and characterization of an enzyme from rat liver that catalyzes the sulfation of
bile salt. Biochim Biophys Acta 480:219–227

Chen L-J, Imperato TJ, Bolt RJ (1978) Enzymatic sulfation of bile salts. II. Studies on bile
salt sulfotransferase from rat kidney. Biochim Biophys Acta 522:443–451

Cohen SN, Baumgarter R, Steinberg MS, Weber WW (1973) Changes in the physiochemical
characteristics of rabbit liver N-acetyltransferase during post-natal development.
Biochim Biophys Acta 304:473–481

Conney AH (1967) Pharmacological implications of microsomal enzyme induction. Pharmacol Rev 19:317–366

Coon MJ, Persson AV (1980) Microsomal cytochrome P-450: A central catalyst in detoxication reactions. In: Jakoby WB (ed). Enzymatic basis of detoxication. Academic Press,
New York

Cooper DY, Levin S, Narasimhulu S, Rosenthal O, Estabrook RW (1965) Photochemical
action spectrum of the terminal oxidase systems. Science 147:400–402

Cooper JR, Brodie BB (1955) Enzymatic oxidation of pentobarbital and thiopental. J Pharmacol Exp Ther 120:75–83

Correia MA, Mannering GJ (1973) DPNH synergism of TPNH-dependent mixed function
oxidase reactions. Drug Metab Dispos 1:139–149

Coutts RT, Dawson GW, Beckett AH (1976) In vitro metabolism of 1-phenyl-2-(n-propy-
lamino) propane (n-propylamphetamine) by rat liver homogenates. J Pharm Pharmacol
28:815–821

Das ND, Shichi H (1979) Gamma-glutamyl transpeptidase of bovine ciliary body: Purification and properties. Exp Eye Res 29:109–121

Das ND, Shichi H (1981) Enzymes of mercapturate synthesis and other drug-metabolizing
reactions-specific localization in the eye. Exp Eye Res 33:525–533

Davidson EH, Britten RJ (1973) Organization, transcription, and regulation in the animal
genome. Q Rev Biol 48:565–613

Dutton GJ (1978) Developmental aspects of drug conjugation, with special reference to glucuronidation. Ann Rev Pharmacol Toxicol 18:17–35

Dutton GJ, Burchell B (1977) Newer aspects of glucuronidation. Prog Drug Metab 2:1–70

Elion GB, Callahan SW, Hitchings GH, Rundles RW, Laszlo J (1962) Experimental, clinical and metabolic studies of thiopurines. Cancer Chemother Rep 16:197–202

Estabrook RW, Cooper DY, Rosenthal O (1963) The light reversible carbon monoxide inhibition of the steroid C21-hydroxylase systems of the adrenal cortex. Biochem J
338:741–755

Evans DAP, Manley KA, McKusick VA (1960) Genetic control of isoniazid metabolism in
man. Br Med J 2:485–491

Farber TM (1975) Enzymatic S-de-ethylation and the mechanisms of S-dealkylation. Proc
Soc Exp Biol Med 149:13–18

Fouts JR, Brodie BB (1957) The enzymatic reduction of chloramphenicol, p-nitrobenzoic
acid and other aromatic nitro compounds in mammals. J Pharmacol Exp Ther 119:197–
207

Friedman E, Kopald HH, Smith TR, Mimura S (1964) Retinal and choroidal blood flow
determined with krypton-85 anesthetized animals. Invest Ophthalmol 3:539–547

Friedman E, Smith TR, Mimura-Oak S (1965) Estimation of retinal blood flow in animals.
Invest Ophthalmol 4:1122–1128

Frommer U, Ullrich V, Staudinger H, Orrenius S (1972) The monooxygenation of n-heptane by rat liver microsomes. Biochim Biophys Acta 280:487–494

Gage JC (1953) A cholinesterase inhibitor derived from O,O-diethyl O-p-nitrophenyl trio-phosphate *in vivo*. Biochem J 54:426–430

Gillette JB, Brodie BB, Ladu BN (1957) The oxidation of drugs by liver microsomes: on the role of TPNH and oxygen. J Pharmacol Exp Ther 119:532–540

Glazer RI, Schenkman JB, Sartorelli AC (1971) Immunochemical studies on the role of reduced nicotinamide adenine dinucleotide phosphate cytochrome c (P-450) reductase in drug oxidation. Mol Pharmacol 7:683–688

Glowinski IB, Radtke HE, Weber WW (1978) Genetic variation in N-acetylation of carcinogenic arylamines by human and rabbit liver. Mol Pharmacol 14:940–949

Goodman LS, Gilman A (eds) (1975) The pharmacological basis of therapeutics, 5th edn. Macmillan, New York

Goos CMAA, Hukkelhoven MWAC, Vermorken AJM, Henderson PT Bloemendal H (1981) Metabolism of benzo(a)pyrene in bovine lens epithelium. Exp Eye Res 33:345–350

Gorski JP, Kasper CB (1977) Purification and properties of microsomal UDP-glucuronosyl-transferase from rat liver. J Biol Chem 252:1336–1343

Gram TE (ed) (1980) Extrahepatic drugs and other foreign compounds. SP Medical and Scientific, New York

Gram TE, Schroeder DH, Davis DC, Reagan RL, Guarino AM (1971) Further studies on the submicrosomal distribution of drug-metabolizing components in liver: localization in fractions of smooth microsomes. Biochem Pharmacol 20:2885–2893

Guldberg HC, Marsden CA (1975) Catechol-O-methyltransferase: pharmacological aspects and physiological role. Pharmacol Rev 27:135–206

Guroff G, Daly JW, Jerina DM, Renson J, Witkop B, Udenfriend S (1967) Hydroxylation-induced migration: the NIH shift. Science 157:1524–1530

Habig WH, Pabst MJ, Fleischner G, Gatmaitan F, Arias IM, Jakoby WB (1974) The identity of glutathione S-transferase B with ligandin, a major binding protein of liver. Proc Natl Acad Sci USA 71:3879–3882

Hathcock JN, Coon J (eds) (1978) Nutrition and drug interactions. Academic, New York

Hayaishi O, Katagiri M, Rothberg S (1955) Mechanism of the pyrocatechase reaction. J Am Chem Soc 77:5450–5451

Heidelberger C (1975) Chemical carcinogenesis. Ann Rev Biochem 44:79–121

Heppel LA, Hilmore RJ (1950) Metabolism of inorganic nitrite and nitrite esters. II. The enzymatic reduction of nitroglycerin and erythritol tetranitrate by glutathione. J Biol Chem 183:129–138

Hinson JA, Pohl LR, Monks TJ, Gillett JR (1981) Acetaminophen-induced hepatotoxicity. Life Sci 29:107–116

Hlavica P (1971) Hepatic mixed function amine oxidases. An allosteric system. Xenobiotica 1:537–538

Holder G, Yagi H, Dansette P, Jerina DM, Levin W, Lu AYH, Conney AH (1974) Effects of inducers and epoxide hydrase on the metabolism of benzo(a)pyrene by liver microsomes and a reconstituted system: analysis by high pressure liquid chromatography. Proc Natl Acad Sci USA 71:4356–4360

Hubbell JP, Casida JE (1977) Metabolic fate of the N,N-dialkylcarbamoyl moiety of thiocarbamate herbicides in rats and corn. J Agric Food Chem 25:404–413

Huh MM, Friedhoff AJ (1979) Multiple molecular forms of catechol-O-methyltransferase. J Biol Chem 254:299–308

Iwasaki K, Noguchi H, Kato R, Imai Y, Sato R (1977) Reduction of tertiary amine N-oxide by purified cytochrome P-450. Biochem Biophys Res Commun 77:1143–1149

Jakoby WB, Habig W (1980) Glutathione transferases In: Jakoby WB (ed) Enzymatic basis of detoxication, Vol. 2. Academic, New York, pp 63–94

Jakoby WB, Sekura RD, Lyon ES, Marcus CJ, Wang J-L (1980) Sulfotransferases In: Jakoby WB (ed) Enzymatic basis of detoxication, Vol. 2. Academic, New York, pp 199–228

Jencks WP (1974) Acyl activation In: Boyer PO (ed) The enzymes, Vol. 6, 3rd edn. Academic, New York, pp 373–385

Jollow DJ, Thorgeirsson SS, Potter WZ, Hashimoto M, Mitchell JR (1974) Acetaminophen-induced hepatic necrosis. VI. Metabolic disposition of toxic doses of acetaminophen. Pharmacology 12:251–271

Kadlubar FF, Ziegler M (1974) Properties of an NADH-dependent *N*-hydroxylamine reductase isolated from pig liver microsomes. Arch Biochem Biophys 162:83–92

Kamataki T, Neal RA (1976) Metabolism of diethyl *p*-nitrophenyl phosphorothionate (parathion) by a reconstituted mixed-function oxidase enzyme system: studies of the covalent binding of the sulfur atom. Mol Pharmacol 12:933–944

Keen JH, Jakoby WB (1978) Glutathione transferases. Catalysis of nucleophilic reactions of glutathione. J Biol Chem 253:5654–5657

Killenberg P (1978) Measurement and subcellular distribution of chololyl-CoA synthetase and bile and bile acid-CoA:amino acid *N*-acyltransferase activities in rat liver. J Lipid Res 19:24–31

Killenberg PG, Davidson ED, Webster LT (1971) Evidence for a medium-chain fatty acid: coenzyme A ligase (adenosine monophosphate) that activates salicylate. Mol Pharmacol 7:260–268

King CM, Allaben WT (1978) The role of arylhydroxamic acid *N-O*-acyltransferase in carcinogenicity of aromatic amines. In: Aitio A (ed) Conjugation reactions in drug biotransformation. Elsevier/North-Holland Biomedical, Amsterdam, pp 431–441

Lau EP, Haleg BE, Barden RF (1977) Photoaffinity labeling of acyl CoA:glycine *N*-acyltransferase with *p*-azidobenzoyl-coenzyme A. Biochemistry 16:2581–2585

Macri FJ, Cevario SJ (1973) The induction of aqueous humor formation by the use of Ach + eserine. Invest Ophthalmol 123:910–916

Mason HS, Fowlks WL, Peterson E (1955) Oxygen transfer and electron transport by the phenolase complex. J Am Chem Soc 77:2914–2915

Masters BSS (1980) The role of NADPH-cytochrome c (P-450) reductase in detoxication. In: Jakoby WB (ed) Enzymatic basis of detoxication, Academic, New York

McIntyre T, Curthoys NP (1982) Renal catabolism of glutathione. Characterization of a particulate rat renal dipeptidase that catalyzes the hydrolysis of cysteinylglycine. J Biol Chem 257:11915–11921

McMahon RE (1966) Microsomal dealkylations of drugs: substrate specificity and mechanism. J Pharm Sci 55:457–466

Meir-Ruge W, Cerletti A (1966) The significance of the melanin-bearing choroid in the retina. In: Biochemistry of the eye. Karger, Basel, pp 521–525

Mitchell JR, Jollow DJ, Potter WZ, Gilette JR, Brodie BB (1973) Acetaminophen-induced hepatic necrosis. IV. Protective role of glutathione. J Pharmacol Exptl Therap 187:211–217

Morgenstern R, Guthenberg C, Depierre JW (1982) Purification of microsomal glutathione *S*-transferase. Acta Chem Scand 36:257–259

Murray KN, Chaykin S (1966) The reduction of nicotinamide *N*-oxide by xanthine oxidase. J Biol Chem 241:3468–3473

Nebert DW (1979 a) Genetic differences in the induction of monooxygenase activities by polycyclic aromatic compounds. Pharmacol Ther 6:395–417

Nebert DW (1979 b) Multiple forms of inducible drug-metabolizing enzymes. A reasonable mechanism by which any organism can cope with adversity. Mol Cell Biochem 27:27–46

Nebert DW, Jensen NM (1979) The Ah locus: genetic regulation of the metabolism of carcinogens, drugs, and other environmental chemicals by cytochrome P-450-mediated monooxygenases. CRC Crit Rev Biochem 6:401–437

Nebert DW, Robinson JR, Niwa A, Kumaki K, Poland AP (1975) Genetic expression of aryl hydrocarbon hydroxylase activity in the mouse. J Cell Physiol 85:393–414

Nebert DW, Eisen HJ, Negishi M, Land MA, Hjelmeland LM (1981) Genetic mechanisms controlling the induction of polysubstrate monooxygenase (P-450) activities. Ann Rev Pharmacol Toxicol 21:431–462

Neims AH, Warner M, Loughnan PM, Aranda JV (1976) Developmental aspects of the hepatic cytochrome P-450 monooxygenase system. Ann Rev Pharmacol Toxicol 16:427–445

Oesch F (1973) Mammalian epoxide hydrases: inducible enzymes catalysing the inactivation of carcinogenic and cytotoxic metabolites derived from aromatic and olefinic compounds. Xenobiotica 3:305–340

Oshino N, Imai Y, Sato R (1971) A function of cytochrome b_5 in fatty acid desaturation by rat liver microsomes. J Biochem 69:155–167

Pelkonen O, Nebert DW (1982) Metabolism of aromatic hydrocarbons: etiologic role in carcinogenesis. Pharmacol Rev 34:189–222

Peterson FJ, Mason RP, Holtzman JL (1977) Microsomal azo reduction: role of cytochrome P-450 and NADPH cytochrome c reductase. Pharmacologist 19:210

Pettit FH, Ziegler DM (1963) The catalytic demethylation of N,N-dimethylaniline-N-oxide by liver microsomes. Biochem Biophys Res Commun 13:193–197

Pohl LR, Krishna G (1978) Study of the mechanism of metabolic activation of chloramphenicol by rat liver microsomes. Biochem Pharmacol 27:335–341

Pohl LR, Bhooshan B, Whittaker NF, Krishna G (1977) Phosgene: a metabolite of chloroform. Biochem Biophys Res Commun 79:684–691

Poland AP, Glover E, Robinson JR, Nebert DW (1974) Genetic expression of aryl hydrocarbon hydroxylase activity. Induction of monooxygenase activities and cytochrome P-450 formation by 2,3,7,8-tetrachlorodibenzo-p-dioxin in mice genetically "nonresponsive" to other aromatic hydrocarbons. J Biol Chem 249:5599–5606

Potts AM (1964) Further studies concerning the accumulation of polycyclic compounds on uveal melanin. Invest Ophthalmol 3:399–404

Prohaska JR, Ganther HE (1977) Glutathione peroxidase activity of glutathione-S-transferase purified from rat liver. Biochem Biophys Res Commun 76:437–445

Reading HW (1970) Biochemistry of retinal dystrophy. J Med Genetics 7:277–284

Reddy VN, Unakar NJ (1973) Localization of gamma-glutamyl transpeptidase in rabbit lens, ciliary process and cornea. Exp Eye Res 17:405–408

Renson J, Weissback H, Udenfriend S (1965) On the mechanism of oxidative cleavage of aryl-alkyl ethers by liver microsomes. Mol Pharmacol 1:145–148

Ross LL, Barber L, Tate SS, Meister A (1973) Enzymes of the gamma-glutamyl cycle in the ciliary body and lens. Proc Nat Acad Sci USA 70:2211–2214

Ruchirawa M, Aramphongphan A, Tanphaichitr V, Bandittanukool W (1981) The effect of thiamine deficiency on the metabolism of acetaminophen (paracetamol). Biochem Pharmacol 30:1901–1906

Sarcione EJ, Stutzman L (1960) A comparison of metabolism of 6-mercaptopurine and its 6-O-methyl analog in the rat. Cancer Res 20:387–392

Schulte EH, Schloot W, Goedde HW (1974) Purification of human liver serotonin-isoniazid N-acetyltransferase by preparative polyacrylamide-electrophoresis and determination of molecular weight. Z Naturforsch 29:661–666

Schwartz JC, Pollard H, Bischoff S, Rehault MC, Verdiere-Sahuque M (1971) Catabolism of ³H-histamine in the rat brain after intracisternal administration. Eur J Pharmacol 16:326–335

Sekura RD, Jakoby WB (1979) Phenol sulfotransferases. J Biol Chem 254:5658–5663

Shargel LD (1969) Influence of electron carrier systems in microsomal metabolism of drugs. Thesis, George Washington University

Shen AL, Fahl WE, Wrighton SA, Jefcoate CR (1980) Inhibition of benzo(a)pyrene and benzo(a)pyrene-7,8-dihydrodiol metabolism by benzo(a)pyrene quinones. Cancer Res 39:4123–4129

Shichi H (1969) Microsomal electron transfer system of bovine retinal pigment epithelium. Exp Eye Res 8:60–68

Shichi H, Nebert DW (1980) Drug metabolism in ocular tissues. In: Gram TE (ed) Extrahepatic metabolism of drugs and other foreign compounds. SP Medical and Scientific, New York, pp 333–363

Shichi H, Atlas SA, Nebert DW (1975) Genetically regulated aryl hydrocarbon hydroxylase induction in the eye: functional significance of the drug-metabolizing enzyme system for the retinal pigmented epithelium-choroid. Exp Eye Res 21:557–567

Shichi H, Tsunematsu Y, Nebert DW (1976) Aryl hydrocarbon hydroxylase induction in retinal pigmented epithelium: possible association of genetic differences in a drug-metabolizing enzyme system with retinal degeneration. Exp Eye Res 23:165–176

Shichi H, Gaasterland DE, Jensen NM, Nebert DW (1978) Ah locus: genetic differences in susceptibility to cataracts induced by acetaminophen. Science 200:539–541

Shichi H, Tanaka M, Jensen NM, Nebert DW (1980) Genetic differences in cataract and other ocular abnormalities induced by paracetamol and naphthalene. Pharmacology 20:229–241

Smith MB (1974) Handbook of ocular pharmacology. Publishing Sciences Group, Acton, Massachusetts

Spatz L, Strittmatter P (1973) A form of reduced nicotinamide adenine dinucleotide-cytochrome b_5 reductase containing both catalytic site and additional hydrophobic membrane binding segment. J Biol Chem 248:793–799

Stiehl A (1974) Bile salt sulphates in cholestasis. Eur J Clin Invest 4:59–63

Tate SS (1980) Enzymes of mercapturic acid formation. In: Jakoby WB (ed) Enzymatic basis of detoxication. Academic, New York, pp 95–120

Tazawa Y, Seaman AJ (1972) The electroretinogram of the living extracorporeal bovine eye. The influence of anoxia and hypothermia. Invest Ophthalmol 11:691–698

Uehleke H, Hellmer KH, Tarabelli S (1973) Binding of 14C-carbon tetrachloride to microsomal proteins *in vitro* and formation of $CHCl_3$ by reduced liver microsomes. Xenobiotica 3:1–11

Ullrich V, Frommer U, Weber P (1973) Differences in the *O*-dealkylation of 7-ethoxycoumarine after pretreatment with phenobarbital and 3-methylcholanthrene. Hoppe-Seylers Z Physiol Chem 354:514–520

Van Dyke RA, Gandolfi AJ (1975) Characterization of a microsomal dechlorination system. Mol Pharmacol 11:809–817

Van Dyke RA, Gandolfi AJ (1976) Anaerobic release of fluoride from halothane. Relationship to the binding of halothane to hepatic cellular constituents. Drug Metab Dispos 4:40–44

Vessey DA (1978) The biochemical basis for the conjugation of bile acids with either glycine or taurine. Biochem J 174:621–626

Von Jagow G, Sebald W (1980) B-type cytochromes. Ann Rev Biochem 49:281–314

Weathrill PJ, Burchell B (1978) Reactivation of a pure defective UDP-glucuronosyltransferase from homozygous Gunn ral liver. FEBS Lett 87:207–211

Webster LJ, Siddiqui UA, Lucas SV, Strong JM, Mieyal JJ (1976) Identification of separate acyl-CoA:glycine and acyl-CoA:L-glutamine *N*-acyltransferase activities in mitochondrial fractions from liver of rhesus monkey and man. J Biol Chem 251:3352–3358

Weisiger RA, Jakoby WB (1979) Thiol *S*-methyltransferase from rat liver. Arch Biochem Biophys 196:631–637

White RE, Coon MJ (1980) Oxygen activation by cytochrome P-450. Ann Rev Biochem 49:315–356

Wilk S, Mizoguchi H, Orlowski M (1978) γ-Glutamyl dopa: a kidney-specific dopamine precursor. J Pharmacol Exp Ther 206:227–232

Williams RT (1959) The metabolism of aromatic amines. Detoxication mechanisms, 2nd edn. Wiley, New York

Wolf CR, King LJ, Parke DV (1975) Anaerobic dechlorination of trichlorofluoromethane by liver microsomal preparations *in vitro*. Biochem Soc Trans 3:175–177

Yamashita H, Uyama M, Sears ML (1981) Comparative study by electron microscopy of response to urea between ciliary epithelia of albino and pigmented rabbits. A function of the ciliary pigmented epithelium. Jpn J Ophthalmol 25:313–320

Ziegler DM Mitchell CH (1972) Microsomal oxidase. IV. Properties of a mixed-function amine oxidase isolated from pig liver microsomes. Arch Biochem Biophys 150:116–125

Ziegler DM, Pettil FH (1966) Microsomal oxidases. I. The isolation and dialkylarylamine oxygenase activity of pork liver microsomes. Biochemistry 5:2932–2938

Ziegler DM, McKee EM, Poulsen LL (1973) Microsomal flavoprotein-catalyzed *N*-oxidation of arylamines. Drug Metab Dispos 1:314–321

Zimmerman TJ, Leader B, Kaufman HE (1980) Advances in ocular pharmacology. Ann Rev Pharmacol Toxicol 20:415–428

CHAPTER 4

Cholinergics

P. L. KAUFMAN, T. WIEDMAN, and J. R. ROBINSON

A. Chemistry Related to Biological Activity

I. Cholinergic Neurotransmission

Cholinergic drugs can exert biological activity by modifying the normal mechanism of ACh-mediated autonomic neurotransmission in several ways (Fig. 1; KOELLE 1975a): interference with transmitter synthesis (hemicholinium); prevention of transmitter release (botulinum toxin); displacement of transmitter from axonal terminal (carbachol); mimicry of transmitter at postsynaptic receptor (methacholine, carbachol, nicotine); blockade of transmiter at postsynaptic receptor (atropine, D-tubocurarine, hexamethonium); inhibition of enzymatic breakdown of transmitter (anticholinesterases).

Cholinergic drugs are classified on the basis of these mechanisms of action. Those which imitate the transmitter ACh are referred to as "direct-acting," and those which inhibit ACh metabolism are called "indirect-acting." Since the action of both types is referable to ACh, one might expect similarities between drugs of the two classes, and in fact some drugs possess the ability to act by both mechanisms and are referred to as "mixed-acting."

Drugs which imitate ACh may act at either or both of the two major types of cholinoceptive sites, muscarinic and nicotinic, the latter being subdivided into N_1 and N_2 types. This classification is based on differences in the relative potency of various agonists and antagonists. Generally, muscarinic receptors are located in smooth muscle and glands, and are also stimulated by muscarine and inhibited by atropine. N_1 nicotinic receptors are found in autonomic ganglionic synapses and are stimulated by dimethylphenylpiperazine and inhibited by hexamethonium and D-tubocurarine. N_2 nicotinic receptors are located in striated muscles and are stimulated by phenyltrimethylammonium and inhibited by decamethonium or D-tubocurarine. Nicotine itself acts at both types of nicotinic sites to produce stimulation in low doses, blockade in high doses [see LANGLEY (1898) for a historically interesting application of the ganglionic blocking action of nicotine].

The indirect-acting drugs bind AChE, the enzyme responsible for metabolizing ACh. This class of drugs has been subdivided into reversible and irreversible inhibitors, based on the ease with which hydrolysis of the enzyme-inhibitor complex occurs (KOELLE 1975b).

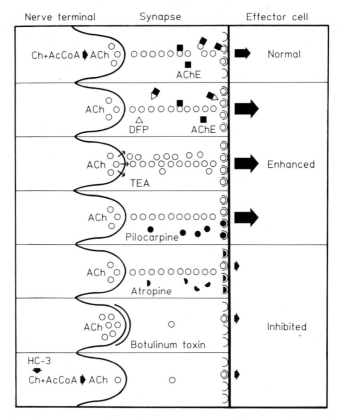

Fig. 1. Cholinergic neurotransmission (schematic, muscarinic). Acetylcholine (*ACh*) is synthesized in the postganglionic parasympathetic nerve terminal via acetylation of choline (*Ch*) by acetylcoenzyme A (*AcCoA*), a reaction catalyzed by the enzyme choline acetyltransferase (*ChAc*). Acetylcholine is released in response to nerve impulses reaching the terminal, traverses the synaptic cleft, and binds to the postjunctional muscarinic receptor on the effector cell membrane, triggering the intracellular reactions culminating in the physiological response of the effector cell. Acetylcholine is inactivated by hydrolysis in a reaction catalyzed by acetylcholinesterase (*AChE*). Direct-acting agonists (e. g., pilocarpine, carbachol) activate the postjunctional receptor in the same manner as ACh. Some indirect agonists (anticholinesterases) bind AChE, protecting ACh from enzymatic hydrolysis. Others [e. g., carbachol, tetraethylammonium (*TEA*)] promote the release of ACh from the nerve terminal. Competitive antagonists (e.g., atropine, scopolamine) bind to the postjunctional receptor, blocking it from ACh, but do not activate it. Hemicholinium-3 (*HC-3*) interferes with ACh synthesis by blocking the transport system by which Ch accumulates in the nerve terminal, while botulinum toxin prevents ACh release by the terminal. Ganglionic blocking agents (e. g., hexamethonium) are competitive antagonists of ACh at the postjunctional nicotinic receptor in parasympathetic ganglia, reducing impulse frequency in the postganglionic neuron. (Adapted from KOELLE 1975a)

II. Direct-Acting Agonists

1. Muscarinic Agents

Ophthalmic drugs which activate muscarinic receptors include pilocarpine, methacholine, carbachol, and aceclidine. Their structures, along with those of ACh

Table 1. Structures of cholinergic drugs

Direct agonists

Acetylcholine

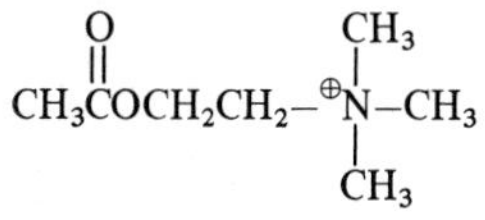

$$CH_3\overset{\overset{\textstyle O}{\|}}{C}OCH_2CH_2-\overset{\overset{\textstyle CH_3}{|}}{\overset{\oplus}{N}}-CH_3$$
$$|$$
$$CH_3$$

Methacholine

$$CH_2\overset{\overset{\textstyle O}{\|}}{C}OCHCH_2-\overset{\overset{\textstyle CH_3}{|}}{\overset{\oplus}{N}}-CH_3$$
$$\underset{\textstyle CH_3}{|} \quad \underset{\textstyle CH_3}{|}$$

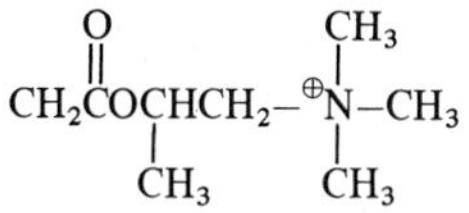

Carbamylcholine
(carbachol)

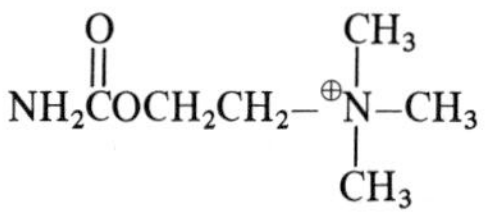

$$NH_2\overset{\overset{\textstyle O}{\|}}{C}OCH_2CH_2-\overset{\overset{\textstyle CH_3}{|}}{\overset{\oplus}{N}}-CH_3$$
$$|$$
$$CH_3$$

Pilocarpine

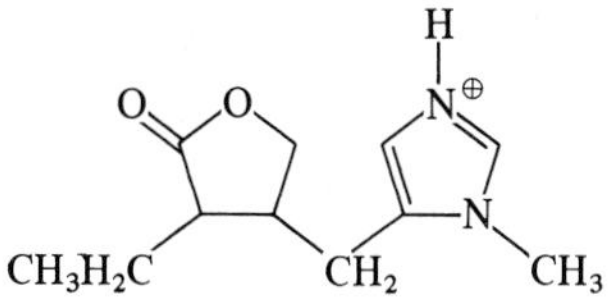

Muscarine

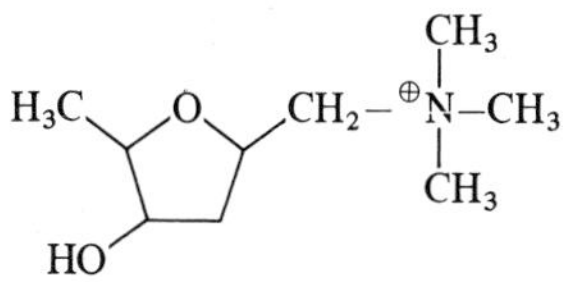

Aceclidine

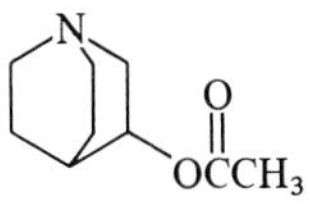

Indirect agonists: anticholinesterase agents

Carbamates

Physostigmine

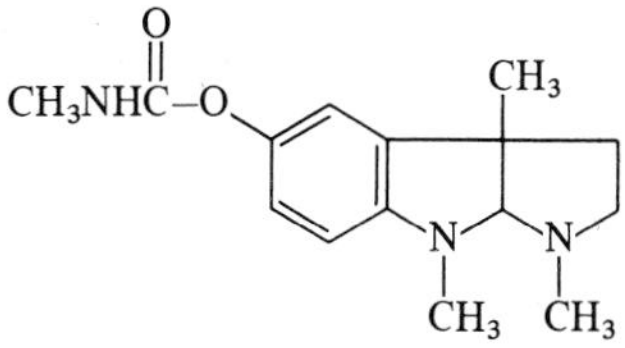

Table 1 (continued)

Indirect agonists:
anticholinesterase agents

Neostigmine

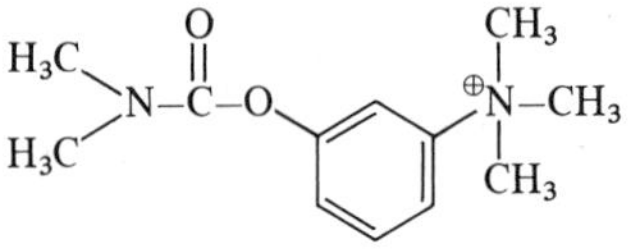

Demecarium

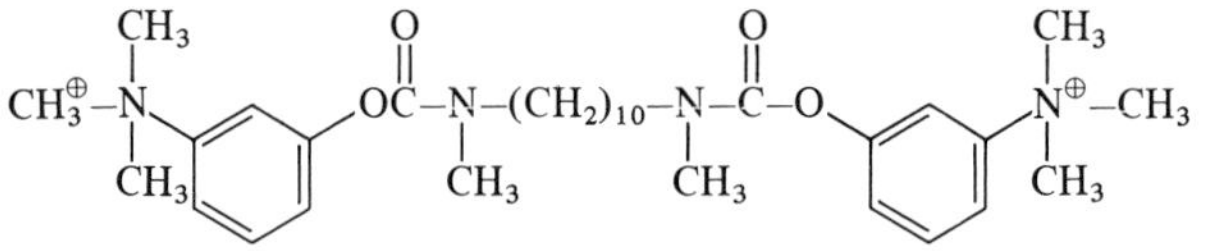

Organophosphorous
compounds

Diisopropylphosphoro-
fluoridate

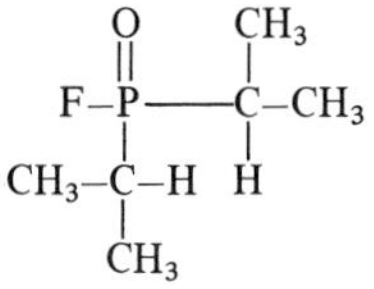

Diethoxyphosphinyl-
thiocholine iodide

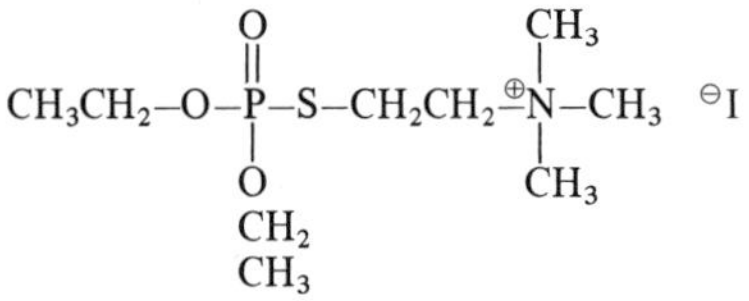

and muscarine, are shown in Table 1. Acetylcholine, muscarine, and pilocarpine are naturally occurring, ACh in nerve terminals and the other two from plant sources. Methacholine, carbachol, and aceclidine are synthetic compounds (KOELLE 1975c).

The relative activity of these compounds may reflect in part the testing method used: in vivo, in situ, or in vitro. In vivo testing, as the name implies, involves administration of the compound to a test animal with subsequent measurement of some biological response. In this case it is not possible to delineate activity of the compound at the receptor site, because of uncontrolled variables such as the rate of absorption, distribution, metabolism, and excretion. However, this method is directly applicable to a clinical setting, and as such, the dose required reflects the overall activity in producing the measured biological response. In situ experimental methods are the most commonly used. This involves application of drug to an isolated tissue section and measurement of the biological response. A well-controlled method yields good results of comparison of activities among different drugs. A problem that might arise is that since ACh and some other cholinergic agonists are metabolized by AChE, their ability to activate the receptor will appear diminished in relation to other drugs in the class being studied, which are more resistant to the enzyme. However, the addition of an AChE inhibitor can correct for this effect.

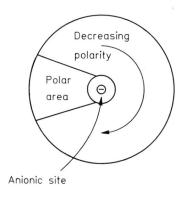

Fig. 2. Proposed models of muscarinic receptors. (Triggle and Triggle 1976)

One must, of course, use caution in comparing results obtained from different tissues due to the possibility of dissimilarity of receptor sites occupied and susceptibility to activation. In vitro testing involves evaluation of drugs with isolated muscarinic receptors. Progress in isolation techniques has been slow due to the lack of a tissue possessing a rich supply of receptors (Heilbronn 1975). Triggle and Triggle (1976) have summarized present procedures. The use of isolated receptors in the study of drug binding reduces artifacts that may arise in the use of tissue samples, but drug affinity for the active site may not reflect its ability to elicit a biological response.

Structure-activity relationships of muscarinic agents have been discussed in detail elsewhere (Brimblecombe 1974; Carrier 1972; Moran and Triggle 1971; Shefter 1971; Triggle and Triggle 1976), and investigations still continue in this area. The functional groups common to these compounds which appear to be important in binding to the receptor all contain nitrogen and oxygen. It is believed that there exists an anionic site on the receptor which interacts with the nitrogen-containing group through ion-pairing. Generally, quaternary ammonium groups are more active than the corresponding tertiary groups, although notable exceptions exist. The oxygen-containing group probably interacts in a polar region through hydrogen binding. Finally, there is a certain degree of hydrophobic interaction with the receptor and drug, which also contributes to a drug's affinity. Proposed models for the receptor are shown in Fig. 2.

2. Nicotinic Agents

Since activation of nicotinic receptors causes stimulation of postganglionic neurons, both sympathetic and parasympathetic, and a response of opposing functions, these drugs are not used clinically. All muscarinic agonists can act on nicotinic receptors, but the dose required for an effect is generally greater by two to three orders of magnitude. Considerably more is known about nicotinic receptors than about muscarinic receptors. Information about the former is a result of the rich source of these receptors in the Torpedo californica electric organ (DE ROBERTIS et al. 1970), which, along with snake venoms that bind with great affinity and specificity to the nicotinic receptor, has led to its isolation. A comparison of isolation methods has been reviewed, as has an evaluation of the activity of its binding or ion channels after incorporation into lipid vesicles (LINDSTROM et al. 1980). Detailed discussions of structure-activity relationships have been provided by TRIGGLE and TRIGGLE (1976), CARRIER (1972), and BRIMBLECOME (1974).

III. Indirect-Acting Agonists: Anticholinesterases

1. Carbamates

Ophthalmic drugs in the category of carbamates include physostigmine, neostigmine, and demecarium, the structures of which may be found in Table 1. Physostigmine is a naturally occurring compound found in Calabar beans, also known as Esere nuts; hence eserine is an alternate name for physostigmine. Neostigmine and demecarium are synthetic drugs (KARCZMAR 1970).

Technically, carbachol is a carbamate and thus has the ability to inhibit AChE. However, it is usually classified as a direct-acting agonist instead of a mixed-acting agonist because in the dose range used its primary mode of action is on muscarinic receptors.

Carbamates are now known to be irreversible inhibitors; however, until recently they were considered reversible (KOELLE 1975b). The potency of irreversible inhibitors is based on the rate of inhibition rather than the degree of association, as is the case with reversible inhibitors, and thus, unfortunately, potencies of carbamates are still reported in terms of I_{50} or PI_{50}.

Experimental determination of inhibitor potency may be accomplished by similar techniques as with drug-receptor interactions. However, since cholinesterases (ChEs) are readily purified (HOPFF et al. 1975), in vitro methods are preferred. Caution must be exercised when experimentally determining inhibition kinetics, since enzymes are very sensitive to conditions of temperature, pH, and concentration of ions (USDIN 1970).

The portion of ChE which is responsible for hydrolysis contains an anionic and esteratic site. Figure 3 depicts the suggested sequence of events resulting from interaction of carbamates with ChE (USDIN 1970; CARRIER 1972; BRIMBLECOMBE 1974; KOELLE 1975b). Binding to the enzyme occurs as a result of interaction of the quaternary ammonium group with the carbonyl group of glutamic acid, with subsequent stabilization of the complex through hydrophobic interaction. A classic S_N1 reaction takes place, with the oxygen of the serine group attacking the carbon atom of the carbamate, and thus the enzyme is complexed with the inhibitor. The hydrogen atom, which was transferred from the serine to the histadine residue, participates in acid hydrolysis of the inhibitor. The enzyme is then restored by hydrolysis of the bond between the carbamate and the serine residue (USDIN 1970).

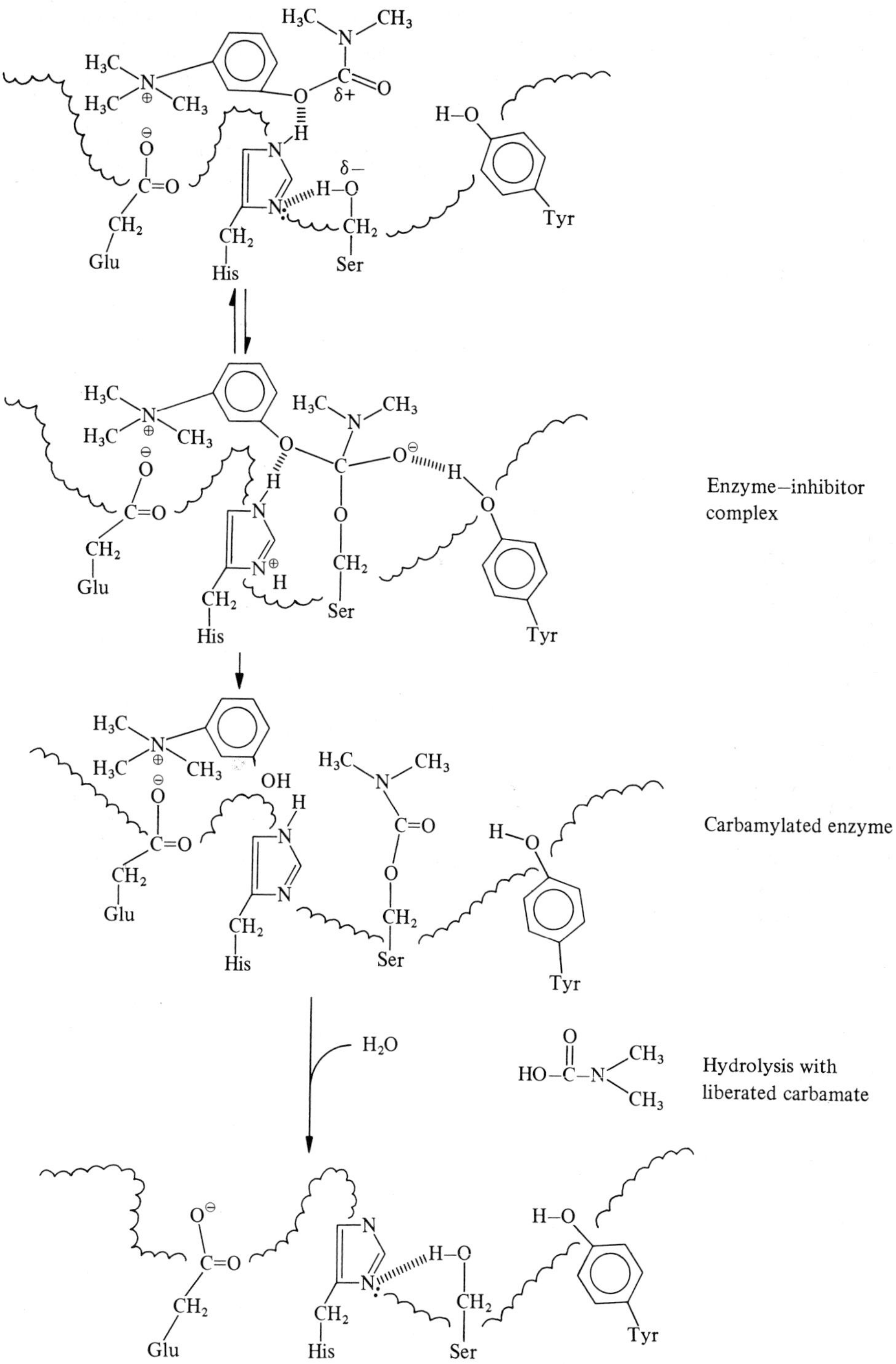

Fig. 3. Sequence of events for the interaction of carbamates with cholinesterase. (Adapted from KOELLE 1975 b, and TRIGGLE and TRIGGLE 1976)

Methacholine and carbachol are considerably more resistant to hydrolysis by AChE than either carbamates or ACh (KOELLE 1975c; HAVENER 1978). With methacholine, the β-methyl group causes steric hindrance and reduces the complexation step (BRIMBLECOMBE 1974). Alternatively, with carbachol, which is a combination of a carbamate and ACh, the lack of an electron-withdrawing group such as the benzene group on carbamates causes a significant reduction in the rate of carbamylation.

2. Organophosphorous Compounds

The organic phosphorous compounds used in ophthalmology include diisopropyl-phosphorofluoridate (DFP) and diethoxyphosphinylthiocholine iodide (echothiophate iodide). Both are synthetic drugs and their structures are shown in Table 1. The mechanism of phosphorylation of AChE is identical to that of carbamylation; however, the former is more resistant to hydrolysis and thus yields a longer duration of action.

B. Ocular Anatomy/Physiology Relevant to Cholinergic Mechanisms: Acute Effects of Cholinergic Drugs

I. Lacrimation

The optical integrity and normal function of the eye are dependent upon an adequate supply of fluid covering its surface. This moist layer (a) maintains an optically uniform corneal surface; (b) lubricates the ocular surface and flushes foreign matter from the cornea and conjunctiva; (c) transfers oxygen, nutrients, and metabolites to and from the cornea; and (d) provides antibacterial protection to the ocular surface (MILDER 1981).

The tear film is composed of three layers. A superficial oily layer, derived from the meibomian glands and the accessory sebaceous glands of Zeis, reduces the rate of evaporation of the underlying aqueous layer and forms a barrier along the lid margins that retains the lid margin tear strip and prevents its overflow onto the skin. The middle watery tear fluid layer, secreted by the lacrimal gland and the accessory glands of Krause and Wolfring, is important in transfer of material to and from the cornea. The inner mucoid layer, elaborated by the goblet cells of the conjunctiva, is important in the normal wetting of the cornea and maintenance of the integrity of the tear film as a whole (MILDER 1981; LEMP et al. 1970, 1971). Details of the location, innervation, and anatomic structure of the various glandular tissues contributing to the tear film have been described by MILDER (1981).

The complex neurogenic control of the secretion of tears may be best understood in terms of JONES's (1966) concept of basal and reflex secretion. The basal secretors are the accessory lacrimal glands of Krause and Wolfring, together with the mucous and sebaceous glands; these structures provide all three layers of the tear film. Reflex production of tears is provided by the lacrimal gland, which secretes only watery fluid. Reflex secretion may be of peripheral sensory origin through fifth nerve stimulation (cornea, conjunctiva, skin, nose), or of central sensory origin (retinal, psychogenic).

The control of basal tear secretion is unclear, but the efferent neural pathway mediating reflex larcrimation is clearly parasympathetic. Electrical stimulation of these neurons causes lacrimation (BOTELHO et al. 1966, 1969; MCEWEN and GOODNER 1969; ARENSON and WILSON 1971). Denervation causes a decrease in neurogenic lacrimation, but has no apparent effect on basal secretion rate (WHITEWELL 1958; SEARS and SELKER 1967). Similarly, by acting on muscarinic receptors, cholinomimetics stimulate and cholinolytics inhibit lacrimation (EMMELIN and STRÖMBLAD 1956; DE HAAS 1960; BROGDANSKI et al. 1961; CHIANG and LEADERS 1971; CASHIN et al. 1972; BERTACCINI et al. 1972).

The mechanism by which neurogenic lacrimation occurs is thought to be similar to that in other exocrine glands. Cholinergic stimulation causes an initial depolarization and a subsequent hyperpolarization of the secretory cell membranes, due to changes in permeability to potassium (PAROD and PUTNEY 1978 a, b; PUTNEY et al. 1977), calcium (PAROD and PUTNEY 1980; PUTNEY et al. 1978), and sodium (IWATUSKI and PETERSEN 1978; PAROD et al. 1980). This in turn initiates a sequence of events resulting in degranulation of secretory cell membranes and constriction of the excretory ducts and lobules, causing secretion of tears onto the conjunctival surface (TANGKRISANAVINONT and PHOLPRAMOOL 1979; EHLERS 1977).

The composition of tears produced by cholinomimetics differs from that produced by basal secretions, due to increased flow rate. ALEXANDER and VAN LENNEP (1972), using a micropuncture technique with rats, found that potassium concentration was more than three times greater with low flow rates than with high flow rates. However, THAYSEN and THORN (1954), working with humans, found no change in potassium levels, while other investigators (KIKKAWA 1968; 1970; YOSHIMURA and HOSOKAWA 1963), working with rabbits, determined that potassium increased slightly with increased flow rates. These discrepancies may be explained by species differences, but it is more likely that sampling of tears from the cul-de-sac does not allow for the normal occurrence of ion exchange across the conjunctiva. Other investigators (BROMBERG 1981; HERZOG et al. 1976; KERYER and ROSSIGNOL 1976; DARTT and BOTELHO 1979) have found that cholinergic stimulation causes an increase in protein secretion over and above the rate of basal lacrimal secretion.

II. Cornea

The cornea is the principal refracting element of the eye. Its optical clarity is essential for normal vision. The cornea must function without a vascular supply in a relatively deturgesced state in the face of aqueous environments on both its surfaces. A variety of structural and metabolic specializations allow it to meet these requirements. Cholinergic processes have been implicated in maintaining normal corneal physiology and anatomy, but their role is unclear.

Corneal epithelium has one of the highest concentrations of ACh of all body tissues (20–40 μg/gm) (WILLIAMS and COOPER 1965; HOWARD et al. 1973; MINDEL et al. 1979; FITZGERALD and COOPER 1971; VON BRÜCKE 1938; VON BRÜCKE et al. 1949; HELLAUER 1950; PESIN and CANDIA 1982). Most if not all of the ACh resides within the epithelial cells and not in the nerve endings (GNÄDINGER et al. 1973; STEVENSON and WILSON 1974; MINDEL and MITTAG 1977). The epithelial cells also contain the enzymes required for ACh synthesis [choline acetyltransferase (ChAc);

GNÄDINGER et al. 1973; WILLIAMS and COOPER 1965; VAN ALPHEN 1957; MINDEL and MITTAG 1976; HOWARD et al. 1973] and hydrolysis (AChE; WILLIAMS and COOPER 1965; HOWARD et al. 1973; GNÄDINGER et al. 1967; PETERSEN et al. 1965). The effects of corneal denervation on corneal epithelial ACh content have been variable, ranging from no change to total loss (FITZGERALD and COOPER 1971; OLSEN and NEUFELD 1979; VON BRÜCKE et al. 1949).

Given the substantial concentrations of ACh and related synthesizing and degradative enzymes in the corneal epithelium, a transmitter function has been considered likely. Suggestions concerning a role for corneal ACh have included pain reception (FITZGERALD and COOPER 1971), ion transport (STEVENSON and WILSON 1975), or control of mitotic rate (CAVANAGH 1975). If ACh were acting as a transmitter in the cornea, one might expect the tissue to contain cholinergic receptors (FOGLE and NEUFELD 1979). However, there is controversy on this point. Some workers (OLSEN and NEUFELD 1979; MITTAG 1979) found the rabbit cornea lacking in both muscarinic and nicotinic cholinergic receptors; others (CAVANAGH and COLLEY 1981) found muscarinic receptors present in this species, noted that ACh stimulated cGMP accumulation, and felt that this pathway might influence proliferation during healing of corneal epithelial defects. The use of topical cholinergic drugs on both short- and long-term bases has not led to clinically apparent epithelial alteration.

Endogeneous ACh appears to have a stimulatory effect on both sodium and chloride transport and chloride permeability in the frog cornea (PESIN and CANDIA 1982). 4-(1-Naphthylvinyl)pyridine (NVP), an inhibitor of ChAC, reduces ACh concentration in frog corneal epithelium and inhibits both Na^+ and Cl^- transport. Atropine, a muscarinic antagonist, and nicotine, a nicotinic agonist, inhibit both Na^+ and Cl^- transport (PESIN and CANDIA 1982). If in the frog the epithelium is devoid of muscarinic and nicotinic cholinergic receptors, these compounds may act directly on the transport systems (PESIN and CANDIA 1982; see Sect. B. III).

The role of cholinergically regulated ionic transport and permeability in maintaining normal corneal physiology and transparency is uncertain (GNÄDINGER et al. 1973; WILLIAMS and COOPER 1965; VAN ALPHEN 1957; HOWARD and WILSON 1973; PETERSEN et al. 1965; STEVENSON and WILSON 1975), as is a definite understanding of the complete role of cholinergic processes in the cornea (FOGLE and NEUFELD 1979).

III. Lens

The transparent crystalline lens provides the mammalian eye with the ability to image objects at varying distances sharply on the retina, i.e., it provides the eye with a variable focusing mechanism (see Sect. B. IV). Like the cornea, the lens exists in an avascular environment, relying on the surrounding intraocular fluids and its own transport mechanisms for its metabolic needs.

Choline acetyltransferase appears not to be present in mammalian lenses (MINDEL and MITTAG 1976). Acetylcholinesterase is present in calf (MICHON and KINOSHITA 1967), rabbit (DE ROETTH 1966; FURMAN et al. 1969), and human (DE ROETTH 1966; LEOPOLD and FURMAN 1971) lens capsule/epithelium preparations; the cortex and nucleus do not contain the enzyme (MICHON and KINOSHITA 1967;

FURMAN et al. 1969). Echothiophate applied topically to the eye in vivo completely inhibits AChE activity in rabbit and human lens capsule/epithelium (DE ROETTH 1966), and physostigmine abolishes the AcheE activity of calf lenses in vitro (MICHON and KINOSHITA 1967).

Pilocarpine, physostigmine, demecarium, and echothiophate cause increased hydration and altered cation balance in cultured rabbit lenses (HARRIS et al. 1959; MICHON and KINOSHITA 1968 a). Demecarium and echothiophate also caused anterior or posterior subcapsular vacuoles (MICHON and KINOSHITA 1968 a). Echothiophate- and demecarium-induced increased efflux of ^{86}Rb from the lens, interpreted as increased lens permeability, preceded the gain in lens water, and was noted even when the water gain was prevented by a hyperosmotic environment (MICHON and KINOSHITA 1968 b). Cation transport as judged by the ability of the lens to accumulate ^{86}Rb was normal (MICHON and KINOSHITA 1968 b). These investigators suggest that the alteration in lens permeability is a primary effect of the drugs and that this increased permeability initiates the shift of lens cations, the gain in lens water, and the appearance of subcapsular vacuoles (MICHON and KINOSHITA 1968 b). Topical DFP decreases and atropine increases mitosis and DNA synthesis in rabbit lens epithelium (BITO et al. 1965). Changes in the concentration of lens metabolites and oxygen consumption have also been observed after in vivo or in vitro treatment with pilocarpine or ChE inhibitors (MICHON and KINOSHITA 1968 b; MÜLLER et al. 1956; HÄRKÖNEN and TARKKANEN 1970) in a variety of mammalian species, including humans.

The lenticular physiological roles, if any, played by ACh and AChE are totally unknown. At one extreme is the possibility that the lenticular cholinergic system is entirely vestigial; i.e., since the lens, like the skin, is embryologically derived from surface ectoderm (DUKE-ELDER and COOK 1963), one might expect it to possess at least a rudimentary cholinergic system. On the other hand, the cholinergic system might somehow help regulate lens permeability to various ions, which might in turn be crucial in maintaining the proper ionic milieu for lenticular protein synthesis. It is also conceivable that the physiological substrate for lenticular AChE is not ACh; certainly other esters may be fair game for this enzyme.

IV. Pupillary Movement and Accommodation

The two iris smooth muscles effect pupillary movement. Simply stated, the parasympathetically innervated sphincter pupillae constricts the pupil, while the sympathetically innervated dilator pupillae dilates it. As the amount of light reaching the retina increases, more impulses are carried via optic nerve fibers to the oculomotor nerve nucleus, causing increased parasympathetic neural tone to the sphincter, while the sympathetic tone to the dilator decreases. The result is contraction of the sphincter, relaxation of the dilator, and overall constriction of the pupil. When the retinal light stimulation decreases, the neuromuscular responses are reversed and the pupil dilates.

The ability of the eye to focus on objects at different distances is controlled by the parasympathetically innervated ciliary muscle. When the object of regard moves nearer, parasympathetic neuronal tone to the muscle increases, and the muscle contracts. This moves the main mass of the ciliary body forward and in-

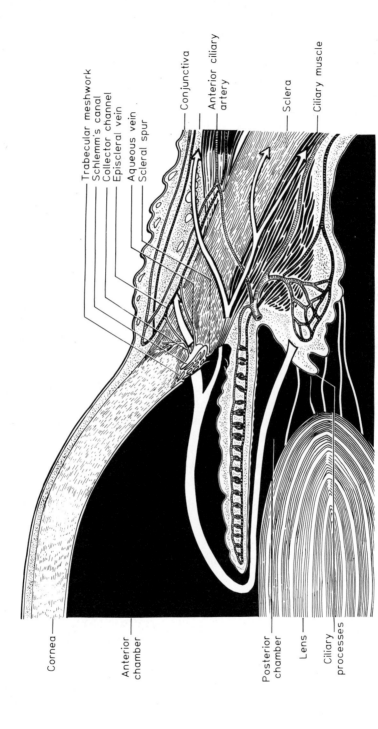

Fig. 4. Schematic representation of the primate anterior ocular segment. *Arrows* indicate aqueous humor flow pathways. Aqueous humor is formed by the ciliary processes, enters the posterior chamber, flows through the pupil into the anterior chamber, and exits at the chamber angle via the trabecular and uveoscleral routes.

ward, lessening the tension on the zonular suspensory ligaments, and allowing the elastic lens to become more spherical (Fig. 4). This in turn increases the refractive power of the lens, focusing the image of the near object on the retina (accommodation). When the object of regard recedes, parasympathetic neuronal input to the ciliary muscle decreases, the muscle relaxes, the ciliary ring moves posterolaterally, and the zonular ligaments tighten, stretching and thinning the lens to decrease its refractive power and bring the image of the distant object into focus on the retina.

It should be noted that both iris smooth muscles and the ciliary muscle appear to be sympathetically innervated, and that the iris dilator muscle appears also to be parasympathetically innervated (RICHARDSON 1964; EHINGER 1966; NOMURA and SMELSER 1974; LATIES and JACOBOWITZ 1966; NISHIDA and SEARS 1968 a, b). The sympathetic responses of the ciliary muscle appear to be weakly relaxant (VAN ALPHEN et al. 1962, 1965; TÖRNQVIST 1966; CASEY 1966; MOSES 1981 b), and for the purposes of this discussion may be ignored. The functions of the apparent sympathetic innervation to the iris sphincter muscle and the parasympathetic innervation to the dilator are unclear; the possibilities of sympathetic vascular innervation and the putative role of ACh in mediating postganglionic sympathetic neurotransmission (BURN and RAND 1962) must be considered.

The acute responses of the pupillary and accomodative mechanisms to muscarinic cholinergic agonists and antagonists are as anticipated from the neuromuscular anatomy. Thus topically or systemically applied muscarinic agonists produce pupillary constriction, cyclotonia, and accommodation; anticholinergics produce pupillary dilation, loss of the pupillary light reflex, cycloplegia, and paralysis of accommodation.

V. Aqueous Humor Formation, Removal, and Composition; Blood-Aqueous Barrier

1. Basic Anatomy and Physiology

a) Aqueous Humor Formation and Drainage

Figure 4 schematically illustrates the basic anatomy of the primate anterior ocular segment and the normal pathways of aqueous humor flow. Aqueous enters the posterior chamber from the ciliary processes as a consequence of hydrostatic and osmotic gradients between the posterior chamber and the ciliary process vasculature and stroma (BÁRÁNY 1963; SEARS 1981; MOSES 1981 a; BILL 1975), and active ionic transport across the ciliary epithelium (KINSEY 1971; MAREN 1974). The aqueous then flows around the lens and through the pupil into the anterior chamber, and leaves the eye by passive bulk flow via two pathways at the anterior chamber angle:

1. Through the trabecular meshwork, across the inner wall of Schlemm's canal, and thence into collector channels, aqueous veins, and the general venous circulation – the trabecular or conventional route.
2. Across the iris root and the anterior face of the ciliary muscle, through the connective tissue between muscle bundles, into the suprachoroidal space, and thence out through the sclera – the posterior, unconventional, or uveoscleral route (BILL 1975).

In different monkey, species, the trabecular route accounts for perhaps 45%–70% of the total drainage of aqueous humor, the uveoscleral pathway draining the remainder (BILL 1971a). In the normal human eye, the importance of the uveoscleral pathways has not been well quantitated, but in elderly eyes with posterior segment tumors it accounts for 5%–20% of total aqueous humor drainage (BILL and PHILLIPS 1971). There is relatively little uveoscleral drainage of aqueous humor in the cat (BILL 1966a), and virtually none in the rabbit (BILL 1966b).

The chamber angle tissues offer a certain normal resistance to fluid outflow. Intraocular pressure (IOP) builds up, in response to the inflow of aqueous, to the level sufficient to drive fluid across that resistance at the same rate it is produced by the ciliary body; this is the steady-state IOP. In the glaucomatous eye, this resistance is unusually high, causing elevated IOP. Although the precise distribution of this resistance within the chamber angle tissues is unsettled, the general consensus is that in the normal monkey and the normal and glaucomatous human eye, most of the resistance lies across and within the trabecular meshwork (GOLDMANN 1951; BÁRÁNY 1955; GRANT 1963), perhaps in the cribriform region adjacent to the inner wall of Schlemm's canal (LÜTJEN-DRECOLL 1973; BILL and SVEDBERGH 1972; BILL 1975). This region consists of several layers of endothelial cells enmeshed in a matrix of glycosaminoglycans, proteoglycans, and other macromolecules (MIZOKAMI 1977; SCHACHTSCHABEL et al. 1977).

Putative cholinergic nerve terminals are present in the posterior portion of the cynomolgus monkey trabecular meshwork, apparently just anterior to the insertion of the longitudinal ciliary muscle fibers (NOMURA and SMELSER 1974). However, these muscle fibers or their tendons may extend anterior to the scleral spur and well into the trabecular meshwork, inserting in the subendothelial region adjacent to the inner wall of Schlemm's canal (ROHEN et al. 1981; LÜTJEN-DRECOLL et al. 1981). Therefore, it is unclear exactly what structure(s) these putative cholinergic terminals innervate, whether they are truly functional cholinergic nerve endings, or what their functional significance in terms of regulating aqueous outflow might be.

b) Aqueous Humor Composition/Blood-Aqueous Barrier

The blood-aqueous barrier is a functional concept, rather than a discrete structure, invoked to explain the degree to which various solutes are relatively restricted in travel from the ocular vasculature into the aqueous humor. The capillaries of the ciliary processes and choroid are fenestrated, but the retinal pigmented epithelia and the nonpigmented ciliary epithelia respectively are joined to each other by tight junctions (zonulae occludentes) and constitute an effective barrier to intermediate and high-molecular-weight substances, e. g., proteins (BILL 1975, 1981; SEARS 1981). The iris has no similar epithelium between its vasculature and the aqueous humor, but its stromal capillaries are of the nonfenestrated, impermeable type (BILL 1975, 1981; SEARS 1981). Finally, the ciliary processes possess the ability actively to transport a variety of organic and inorganic compounds and ions out of or exclude them from the eye – i. e., to move them from the aqueous/vitreous to the blood against a concentration gradient. These systems satisfy all the criteria for active transport – saturability, energy-dependence, Michaelis-Menten kinetics, etc. (BECKER 1960, 1961); BÁRÁNY 1972, 1973a, b, 1974, 1975, 1976; FORBES and

BECKER 1960; STONE 1979 a, b). The physiological role of these outward-directed systems is unknown, but at least some of them may serve to rid the eye of or protect it from potentially injurious metabolites or autacoids (BITO 1972 a, b; BITO and SALVADOR 1972, 1976; BITO et al. 1976). Inward-directed (blood to eye) transport systems also exist for certain substances (e. g., ascorbate, amino acids, sodium (BECKER 1967; REDDY et al. 1962; KINSEY and REDDY 1962; REDDY 1967; WÅLINDER and BILL 1969 a, b; KINSEY 1947), which may be crucial to the normal metabolism of the non-blood-perfused ocular tissues. Thus, for our purposes here, one may say that the blood-aqueous barrier is comprised of the tight junctions of the nonpigmented ciliary epithelium and the iris vasculature, and the outward-directed active transport systems of the ciliary processes. Of course, a more universal concept of the blood-aqueous barrier must deal with the movement of smaller molecules, lipid-soluble substances, and water into the eye (SEARS 1981).

2. Acute Effects of Cholinergic Drugs

a) Conventional (Trabecular) Outflow

In primates the iris root inserts into the ciliary muscle and the uveal meshwork just posterior to the scleral spur, while the ciliary muscle inserts at the scleral spur and the posterior inner aspect of the trabecular meshwork (HOGAN et al. 1971; ROHEN et al. 1967). The influence of these two contractile, cholinergically innervated structures on resistance to aqueous humor outflow has long been a source of speculation. Voluntary accommodation (human; ARMALY and BURIAN 1958), electrical stimulation of the third cranial nerve (cat; ARMALY 1959 a, b, c), topical, intracameral, or systemically administered cholinergic agonists (monkey and human; MOSES 1981 a; BÁRÁNY 1965), and in enucleated eyes (monkey and human) pushing the lens posteriorly with a plunger through a corneal fitting (VAN BUSKIRK and GRANT 1973) all decrease outflow resistance, while ganglionic blocking agents and cholinergic antagonists increase resistance (BÁRÁNY 1965; HARRIS 1968; SCHIMEK and LIEBERMAN 1961; BÁRÁNY and CHRISTENSEN 1967; GALIN 1961). Furthermore, the resistance-decreasing effect of intravenous pilocarpine in monkeys is virtually instantaneous, implying that the effect is mediated by an arterially perfused structure or structures (BÁRÁNY 1967). These findings collectively suggested that iris sphincter and/or ciliary muscle contraction physically alters meshwork configuration so as to decrease resistance, while muscle relaxation deforms it so as to increase resistance (MOSES 1981 a; BÁRÁNY 1967). However, not all the experimental evidence supported this strictly mechanical view of cholinergic and anticholinergic effects on meshwork function. Thus in monkeys intravenous atropine rapidly reverses some but not all of the pilocarpine-induced resistance decrease (BÁRÁNY 1962, 1966 a), and topical pilocarpine causes a much greater resistance decrease per diopter of induced accommodation than does systemic pilocarpine (monkey; BÁRÁNY 1966 a) or voluntary accommodation (human; SHAFFER 1961). While several explanations for these latter findings could be advanced, the possibility of a resistance-decreasing pharmacologic effect directly on the endothelium of the trabecular meshwork or Schlemm's canal was especially intriguing (BÁRÁNY 1962, 1966 a).

A means of distinguishing secondary mechanical effects of drugs from primary pharmacologic ones was achieved with the development of techniques in the living

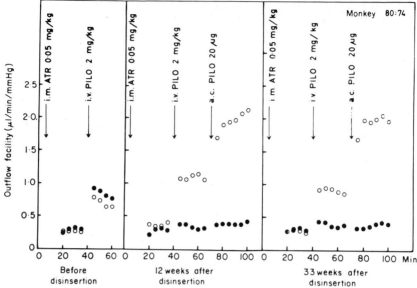

Fig. 5. Outflow facility and facility responses to intravenous and intracameral pilocarpine hydrochloride (*i.v. PILO, a.c. PILO*) before and after unilateral ciliary muscle disinsertion in a typical bilaterally iridectomized cynomolgus monkey. Intramuscular atropine sulfate (*i.m. ATR*) was given before each perfusion to minimize systemic effects of intravenous pilocarpine. Note absence of facility increase following intravenous and intracameral pilocarpine in the iridectomized and disinserted eye (*solid circles*), as opposed to the large facility increases in the opposite iridectomized-only eye (*open circles*). (KAUFMAN and BÁRÁNY 1976a)

monkey eye for totally removing the iris at its root (KAUFMAN and LÜTJEN-DRE-COLL 1975), and for disinserting the anterior end of the ciliary muscle over its entire circumference and retrodisplacing it to a more posterior position on the inner scleral wall (KAUFMAN and BÁRÁNY 1976a). In these preparations, the ciliary muscle retains its normal morphology and its contractibility in response to pilocarpine, and the meshwork exhibits its normal light and electron microscopic appearance (LÜTJEN-DRECOLL et al. 1977). Aniridia has no effect on IOP, resting outflow resistance, or resistance responses to intravenous or intracameral pilocarpine (KAUFMAN 1979). After total iris removal and ciliary muscle disinsertion, however, there is virtually no acute resistance response to either intravenous or intracameral pilocarpine (Fig. 5; KAUFMAN and BÁRÁNY 1976a), and no response to topical pilocarpine given at 6-h intervals for 18–24 h (KAUFMAN and BÁRÁNY 1976b). It thus seems virtually certain that the acute resistance-decreasing action of pilocarpine, and presumably of other cholinomimetics, is mediated entirely by drug-induced ciliary muscle contraction, with no direct pharmacologic effect on the meshwork itself. The inability of atropine to reverse the pilocarpine-induced facility increase in normal eyes rapidly and completely could be due to mechanical hysteresis of the meshwork; ciliary muscle contraction forces a rapid structural change on the meshwork, but muscle relaxation cannot itself reverse this change; elasticity of the meshwork is involved and its effects may be exerted slowly (KAUFMAN and BÁRÁNY 1976b). The variation in the relative magnitude of pilocarpine-induced accommodation and resistance decrease when the drug is administered by different routes might reflect differences in bioavailability of the drug to different regions of the muscle. No information is available regarding the possible existence of very slowly developing (weeks or longer) primary cholinomimetic effects on meshwork function, but there seems little reason to postulate such a phenomenon.

Light and electron microscopic studies of the trabecular meshwork and Schlemm's canal have demonstrated pilocarpine-induced alterations in the size and shape of the intertrabecular spaces and in various characteristics, including vacuolization, of the inner canal wall endothelium (MOSES 1981a; HOLMBERG and BÁRÁNY 1966; FORTIN 1925, 1929; ROHEN 1964; UGA 1968; HEINE 1900; ASAYAMA 1902; ALLAN and BURIAN 1965; FLOCKS and ZWENG 1957). However, these alterations are considered to be secondary to pilocarpine-induced ciliary muscle contraction and augmented transtrabecular outflow (GRIERSON et al. 1978). Furthermore, we have no idea what structural alteration in the meshwork accounts for the ciliary-muscle-contraction-induced decrease in resistance to passive bulk fluid outflow. Whether opening entirely new channels, decreasing the resistance of some or all existing channels, widening Schlemm's canal, or some other alteration is critical is unknown, as is the means by which ciliary muscle traction on the meshwork brings about the critical change. In short, we are rather ignorant of the physics behind the physiology.

b) Unconventional (Uveoscleral) Outflow

When the ciliary muscle contracts in response to exogenous pilocarpine, the spaces between the muscle bundles are essentially obliterated (BÁRÁNY and ROHEN 1965; ROHEN et al. 1967). Conversely, during atropine-induced muscle relaxation, the spaces are widened (Fig. 6; BÁRÁNY and ROHEN 1965). If mock aqueous humor containing ^{131}I-albumin or ^{125}I-albumin (which under resting conditions leave the anterior chamber essentially completely by bulk flow via the trabecular and uveoscleral drainage routes) is perfused through the anterior chamber, autoradiographs may be made to show qualitatively the distribution of the flow (BILL 1967; BILL and PHILLIPS 1971). In the pilocarpinized eye, radioactivity is present in the iris stroma, the iris root, the region of Schlemm's canal and the surrounding sclera, and the very anteriormost portion of the ciliary muscle. In the atropinized eye, radioactivity is found in all these tissues but additionally throughout the entire ciliary muscle and even further posteriorly in the choroid/sclera (Fig. 7; BILL 1967; BILL and PHILLIPS 1971). In other perfusion experiments quantifying uveoscleral drainage, pilocarpinized eyes demonstrate but a fraction of the uveoscleral flow in atropinized eyes (BILL 1967, 1969; BILL and WÅLINDER 1966).

Thus, to generalize in the primate eye, pilocarpine (and presumably all cholinergic agonists) augments aqueous humor drainage via the trabecular route, and diminishes drainage via the uveoscleral route. In most instances in the human, the former apparently exceeds the latter, and the net result is enhanced aqueous drainage and decreased IOP (MOSES 1981a; KAUFMAN 1979). In the normal monkey eye, where drainage via the trabecular and uveoscleral routes are more nearly equal, pilocarpine may induce a slight rise in IOP, perhaps by inhibiting uveoscleral drainage more than increasing trabecular drainage (BILL 1967; BILL and WÅLINDER 1966).

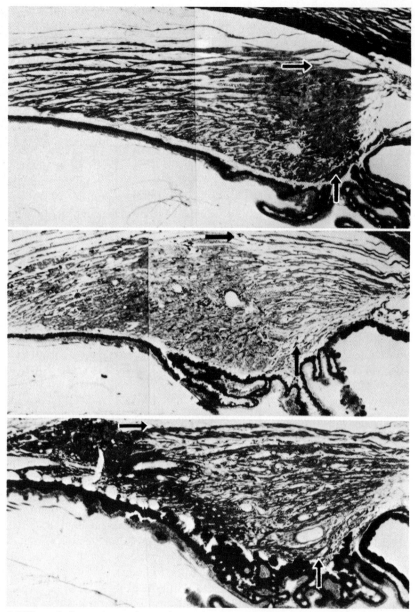

Fig. 6. Effect of pilocarpine and atropine on intramuscular spaces within the ciliary muscle of the vervet monkey. *Top*, intracameral heavy pilocarpine solution; crowding of muscle bundles within the anterior part of the longitudinal muscle. Zone of localized contraction indicated by *arrows*. *Middle*, intramuscular pilocarpine followed by intracameral heavy atropine solution (atropine allowed to act for 3 min); loose arrangement of anterior longitudinal muscle bundles. *Arrows* indicate boundary between zone of localized relaxation and other, contracted, parts of muscle. *Bottom*, same protocol as *middle*, but atropine allowed to act for 10 min. The zone of loosely-arranged muscle bundles reaches far toward the posterior region. Only the posterior extremity of the muscle appears intensely contracted. *Arrows* indicate boundary between contracted and relaxed muscle portions. Heidenhain's Azan stain, × 63. (BÁRÁNY and ROHEN 1965)

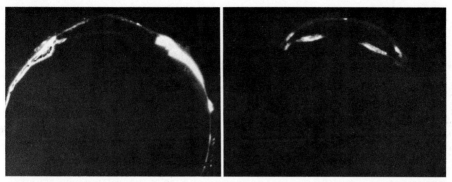

Fig. 7. The effect of ciliary muscle contraction on the passage of radioactively labeled protein through the ciliary muscle in a cynomolgus monkey. *Left*, anterior chamber perfused with a mixture of 5 µg/ml pilocarpine and 10 µg/ml atropine. *Right*, anterior chamber perfused with 5 µg/ml pilocarpine only. Both perfusion solutions contain equal amounts of radioactive albumin. Posterior passage of fluid is blocked in the pilocarpine-only eye, with visible radioactivity restricted to the miotic iris and the scleral tissue near Schlemm's canal. (BILL 1967)

c) Aqueous Humor Formation and Composition; Blood-Aqueous Barrier

The effects of cholinergic drugs on aqueous humor formation and composition, and on the blood-aqueous barrier, are unclear, with conflicting results arising from various studies. In general, cholinergic drugs cause vasodilation, and this appears to hold true also for the primate anterior segment (GARTNER 1944; WILKE 1974; ALM et al. 1973), resulting in increased blood flow to the iris, ciliary processes, and ciliary muscle (ALM et al. 1973; JAMES and CALKINS 1957). These responses are apparently mediated by muscarinic receptors in the arterioles of the anterior uvea (ALM et al. 1973), receptors perhaps associated with facial parasympathetic nerve terminals (RUSKELL 1971). Congestion in the iris and ciliary body are well-recognized clinical side effects of topical cholinomimetics, especially the anti-ChEs (KOLKER and HETHERINGTON 1976). The presence of flare (Tyndall effect, indicating increased protein concentration) and/or the detection of cells in the aqueous humor by biomicroscopy indicates that these agents can also cause breakdown in the blood-aqueous barrier and perhaps frank inflammation (KOLKER and HETHERINGTON 1976). Pilocarpine increases barrier permeability to iodide (BECKER 1962) and inulin (SWAN and HART 1940). Cholinergic-drug-induced vasodilation might disrupt the tight junctions in anterior uveal blood vessels, perhaps contributing to barrier breakdown (SHABO et al. 1976). Cholinergic drugs may alter the aqueous humor concentration of inorganic ions (BITO et al. 1965) and the movement of certain amino acids from the blood into the aqueous humor (perhaps consequent to changes in the rate of aqueous humor formation), and may also influence the outward-directed transport systems of the ciliary processes (WÅLINDER 1966; WÅLINDER and BILL 1969 b).

The ultrafiltration component of aqueous humor formation is pressure-sensitive, decreasing with increasing IOP. This phenomenon is quantifiable and is termed "pseudofacility," because a pressure-sensitive decrease in inflow will appear as an increase in outflow when techniques such as tonography and constant pressure perfusion are used to measure outflow (MOSES 1981 a; BÁRÁNY 1963; 1966 a, b; BILL and BÁRÁNY 1966; BILL 1971 b). Under certain conditions, pilocarpine may increase pseudofacility (BÁRÁNY 1963; GAASTERLAND et al. 1975). Using a variety of species, conditions, and experimental techniques, cholinergic agents or parasympathetic nerve stimulation have been reported to increase, decrease, or not alter the aqueous humor formation rate and to slightly increase the episcleral venous pressure (KUPFER 1973; GAASTERLAND et al. 1975; WÅLINDER and BILL 1969 a, b; UUSITALO 1972 a, b; BERGGREN 1965, 1970; STJERNSCHANTZ 1976; MACRI and CEVARIO 1973, 1974; LIU and CHIOU 1981; CHIOU et al. 1980; GREEN and PADGETT 1979; NAGATAKI and BRUBAKER 1980; BILL 1967; BILL and WÅLINDER 1966). These apparently confusing results may indicate that cholinergic drug effects on these parameters are extremely dependent on species- and technique-related factors and on the ambient neurovascular milieu. In any event, the effects on the rate of aqueous humor formation and episcleral venous pressure are probably not responsible for the drug-induced decrease in IOP which forms the basis of pilocarpine's therapeutic efficacy in chronic glaucoma; the latter resides in its ability to decrease outflow resistance via its effect on the ciliary muscle. However, the importance of cholinergic drug effects on aqueous humor formation and composition in terms of the ultimate therapeutic efficacy and toxicity of these drugs awaits determination.

VI. Retina

Cholinergic photoreceptor cells may be present in goldfish and turtle retinas (SCHWARTZ and BOK 1979; SARTHY and LAM 1979; LAM 1972), but apparently not in mammals (ROSS et al. 1975; ROSS and McDOUGAL 1976; NIEMEYER 1978; MASLAND and AMES 1976; MASLAND and MILLS 1979). However, most vertebrate retinas contain high levels of ChAc and AChE in the inner plexiform layer, where cholinergic synapses are located (BAUGHMAN and BADER 1977; GRAHAM 1974; HEBB 1955; SARTHY and LAM 1979; ROSS et al. 1975; ROSS and McDOUGAL 1976; NICHOLS and KOELLE 1967, 1968; RAVIOLA and RAVIOLA 1962; NEAL and GILROY 1975; REALE et al. 1971; VOGEL et al. 1977; MASLAND and AMES 1976; MASLAND and MILLS 1979). Acetylcholine is synthesized by a relatively small fraction of the cells in the inner nuclear and ganglion cell layers immediately adjacent to the inner plexiform layer (MASLAND and MILLS 1979); these are probably amacrine cells (NICHOLS and KOELLE 1967; MASLAND and MILLS 1979). Some ganglion cells, primarily those with on-center or directionally sensitive receptive fields, possess ACh receptors (MASLAND and AMES 1976), and cholinergic input contributes to the response to light of many retinal ganglion cells (MASLAND and AMES 1976; MASLAND and MILLS 1979). However, ACh-sensitive ganglion cells also receive input via neurotransmitters other than ACh, and these other neurotransmitters can produce a substantial part of the cell's response to light, even in the presence of adequate cholinergic blockade (MASLAND and AMES 1976; MASLAND and MILLS 1979). Furthermore, the grosser characteristics of receptive fields, such as center-surround organization, are not selectively affected by application of cholinergic agents to the retina (MASLAND and AMES 1976). The precise identity and role of the ACh-synthesizing cells and ACh-mediated neurotransmission in the mammalian retina remain unknown, and have been the source of much speculation (MASLAND and MILLS 1979).

VII. Oculorotary and Respiratory Skeletal Muscles

The six extraocular muscles responsible for rotation of the globe, and the levator palpebra superioris, responsible for elevation of the upper eyelid, are of the striated skeletal type, with ACh serving as the neurotransmitter at the neuromuscular junction. Details of the specific neuromuscular anatomy and physiology have been well summarized elsewhere (BURDE 1981). Topical application of direct-acting muscarinic agonists, ChE inhibitors, or competitive antagonists to the intact human eye, as in the treatment of glaucoma or uveitis, appears to have no clinically discernible effects on the extraocular muscles or the levator.

Systemically administered ChE inhibitors are useful in the diagnosis and treatment of myasthenia gravis, a disease which was formerly postulated as due to deficient release of ACh at skeletal neuromuscular junctions in response to neuronal impulses, but is now thought to be consequent to decreased numbers of available ACh receptors on the postsynaptic membrane, in turn due to an autoimmune reaction against the ACh receptor (DRACHMAN 1978a, b). Ptosis and diplopia, due respectively to impaired function of the levator palpebrae superioris and oculorotary muscles, are prominent manifestations (WALSH and HOYT 1969). The beneficial effects of ChE inhibitors are due to protection of that ACh which is released, enhancing muscular responses (DRACHMAN 1978b).

Topically administered ChE inhibitors may be used to reduce the magnitude of accommodative esotropia. Classically, this is ascribed to peripheral enhancement of ACh-mediated accommodation, lessening the centrally originating neuronal tone and its associated stimulation of convergence required for a given amount of accommodation (A), but it has been clearly demonstrated that the effect of anti-ChE in strabismus is to reduce the amount of accommodative convergence (AC) required, i.e., lessen the AC/A ratio (or slope) (SLOAN et al. 1960). Topical ChE inhibitors can, under appropriate conditions, enhance the in vitro responses of the oculorotary muscles to ACh (BUNKE and BITO 1981), and a plausible argument may be made that such enhancement should play a role in the therapeutic effect of ChE inhibitors in accommodative insufficiency.

Botulinum toxin injected directly into an extraocular muscle of a rhesus monkey produces reversible denervation and weakness of the muscle, resulting in a persistent strabismus, presumably related to weakening and atrophy of the injected muscle and unopposed contraction and perhaps subsequent contracture of the antagonist muscle (SCOTT et al. 1973). This technique may prove useful clinically as a pharmacologic alternative to the surgical treatment of strabismus, i.e., to weaken the muscle overacting in the affected field of gaze (SCOTT 1980).

Succinylcholine (SCh) binds to the N_2 nicotinic receptors of the postjunctional skeletal muscle cell membrane to produce a sustained depolarization lasting several minutes, during which time the muscle is refractory to neuronal impulses. Succinylcholine is often given systemically to produce muscle relaxation before tracheal intubation in patients undergoing general anesthesia (MILLER and SAVARESE 1981). Initially, of course, the skeletal muscles fasciculate and contract upon depolarization, and then are silent. There is simultaneous cocontraction of all the extraocular muscles, transiently and abruptly raising the IOP (HOFMANN and HOLZER 1953). If intraocular surgery is undertaken in these circumstances, extrusion of intraocular contents may occur, with disastrous consequences. The depolarizing event is transient, and, from a practical point of view, of no consequence if the eye is unopened.

Succinylcholine is normally metabolized rapidly by nonspecific plasma ChE. Some people have a genetically determined qualitative abnormality of this enzyme, rendering it ineffective against SCh, while others may have decreased levels of qualitatively normal enzme, due to liver disease, pregnancy, or various drugs. In such patients, particularly those with the qualitative genetic enzyme abnormality, SCh may produce prolonged apnea, due to paralysis of the diaphragm and intercostal muscles, necessitating ventilatory assistance. This problem may also occur in patients receiving ChE inhibitors topically in the eye for treatment of glaucoma or strabismus (MILLER and SAVARESE 1981). Plasma and erythrocyte ChE levels are significantly depressed following topical ocular administration of ChE inhibitors, due to systemic drug absorption through the lacrimal drainage system (DE ROETTH et al. 1965; WAHL and TYNER 1965; ELLIS and LITTLEJOHN 1974). Normally, this has no adverse consequences, but in the SCh-paralyzed anesthetized patient it could be devastating (PANTUCK 1966; GESZTES 1966). Nonspecific plasma ChE also catalyzes the hydrolysis of various noncholine esters, including certain local anesthetics (e. g., procaine, tetracaine) (ELLIS and LITTLEJOHN 1974). The depression of plasma ChE levels resulting from topical ocular application of ChE inhibitors significantly decreases the rate of hydrolysis of such anesthetics in the plasma, theoretically increasing the risk of systemic toxicity from large local anestethic doses (ELLIS and LITTLEJOHN 1974). Finally, individuals exposed to ChE inhibitors during their everyday lives (e. g., farm workers exposed to anti-ChE insecticides) may encounter adverse systemic reactions when treated topically with ChE inhibitors, due to the additive systemic drug dosages.

C. Longer-Term Effects of Cholinergic Drugs or Altered Cholinergic Neurotransmission

I. Cholinergic Sensitivity in Ocular Smooth Muscles

1. Physiologically and Pharmacologically Induced Alterations

Continuous stimulation of the anterior segment of the eye with high levels of ACh, induced by continuous light exposure (cats, rats; BITO and DAWSON 1970; BITO et al. 1971; CLAESSON and BÁRÁNY 1978) or topical ChE inhibitors (rabbits, dogs, monkeys; BITO and DAWSON 1970) BITO et al. 1967; BITO 1968; BITO and BANKS 1969; BITO and BAROODY 1979) causes marked subsensitivity of the pupillary response to cholinergic agonists. Conversely, decreased cholinergic stimulation by continuous exposure to darkness (cats; BITO and DAWSON 1970; BITO et al. 1971; rats; CLAESSON and BÁRÁNY 1978), ciliary ganglionectomy (cats; BITO and DAWSON 1970), or intravitreal injection of hemicholinium-3 (cats; BITO and DAWSON 1970) results in increased cholinergic sensitivity of the iris. Intermediate over- or understimulation results in intermediate sub- or supersensitivity (BITO and DAWSON 1970; BITO et al. 1971). Studies of binding of ^3H-quinuclidinylbenzilate (^3H-QNB), a muscarinic receptor antagonist, in the cat iris (RAINA and BITO 1979) and rabbit iris-ciliary body (MITTAG 1980) have shown that functional sensitivity of the iris sphincter is inversely correlated with the tissue density of high-affinity muscarinic receptors. These findings are all consistent with the concept that tissue sensitivity to cholinergic drugs is inversely related to the average local concentration of agonist – the higher the agonist concentration, the less the sensitivity, and vice-versa – possibly because agonist concentration regulates receptor density on the tissue cell membrane (BITO and DAWSON 1970). KLOOG et al. (1979 a, b) reported that ^3H-N-methyl-4-piperidylbenzilate (^3H-NMPB), a muscarinic receptor antagonist, binds to a distinct site in albino rabbit irides and to two sites in pigmented cat and rabbit irides. The two ^3H-NMPB binding sites in pigmented irides of rabbits have different dissociation constants and binding capacities. The high-affinity ^3H-NMPB binding site in pigmented cat and rabbit irides was identical to the ^3H-NMPB binding site in albino rabbit irides. The presence of another high-capacity, low-affinity binding site in pigmented irides but not in albino irides suggests that these binding sites are present on or in the melanocytes of the pigmented iris (AKESSON et al. 1983). This latter site will, of course, influence biological responses.

In the rat iris, alterations in sensitivity begin within hours and perhaps sooner after altering environmental lighting. Adaptation is largely but not completely achieved within several days. These data probably indicate that the receptor population involved has a half-life of 1–2 days, and that strong excitation prevents the formation of new receptors without accelerating the decay of already formed ones, while lack of excitation accelerates the formation of new receptors, again without affecting the removal of those already present (CLAESSON and BÁRÁNY 1978). The effect of cholinergic treatment on cholinergic sensitivity of the ciliary muscle has also been studied. Topical administration of pilocarpine eye drops thrice daily for 2 weeks (monkeys) causes no alteration in sensitivity of the outflow resistance response to intramuscular pilocarpine; accommodative responses were not reported (BÁRÁNY 1977). However, continuous pilocarpine treatment via a pericorneally sutured sustained release membrane delivery system causes marked subsensitivity of the accommodative and resistance responses to pilocarpine and carbachol within a few days (BÁRÁNY 1977). Topical echothiophate induces profound subsensitivity of both the accommodative (KAUFMAN and BÁRÁNY 1975; KAUFMAN 1978) and resistance (KAUFMAN and BÁRÁNY 1976c) responses to pilocarpine within a few days. Recovery begins shortly after short treatment periods with pilocarpine or echothiophate are discontinued, but after long-term echothiophate treatment, several weeks to many months are required before sensitivity returns to normal (Figs. 8 and 9; KAUFMAN and BÁRÁNY 1975; KAUFMAN 1978; KAUFMAN and BÁRÁNY 1976c). The apparent discrepancy between the comparatively short recovery time after altered environmental lighting and the protracted recovery after long-term treatment with irreversible ChE inhibitors is easily explained: alteration of local ACh concentration in the former case would be essentially immediate, while in the latter case it would depend on the rate of synthesis of new enzyme protein and would therefore be much more gradual.

The data indicate that although continuous exposure to high levels of any cholinergic agonist induces subsensitivity to all agonists, subsensitivity to some agonists is more profound than to others. Closer analysis of both in vivo physiological and in vitro receptor binding data suggest that differential partial agonism may not alone explain differing agonist potencies in the subsensitive eye, and that there may

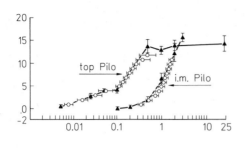

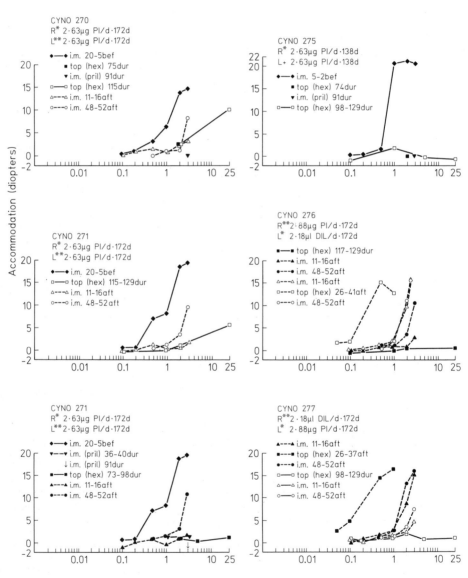

Accommodation (diopters)

Pilocarpine HCl (mg or mg/kg)

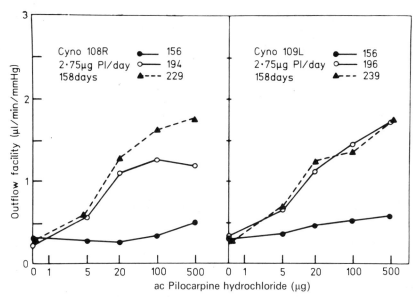

Fig. 9. Pilocarpine dose-outflow facility response relationship during and after topical echothiophate iodide (*PI*) treatment for two cynomolgus (*Cyno*) monkey eyes: *R*, right; *L*, left. *Each panel* shows all the curves for one eye. *Each curve* was obtained at one perfusion experiment, and numbered according to days after PI treatment was started. Thus, *in each panel*, the *156-day curve* was obtained 2 days before stopping treatment. *Each point* represents the average of the three highest facility values obtained after that anterior chamber (*ac*) pilocarpine dose. Facility at 0 µg pilocarpine represents average facility after intramuscular hexamethonium bromide (10–20 mg/kg) but before pilocarpine. (KAUFMAN and BÁRÁNY 1976c)

well be two or more distinct populations of relevant muscarinic receptors in the iris sphincter and ciliary muscles; two receptor populations certainly exist in terms of high and low affinity for binding ligands (BITO et al. 1971; RAINA and BITO 1979; MITTAG 1980; BÁRÁNY 1977; BÁRÁNY et al. 1982; ZLOCK et al. 1983). In the cynomolgus monkey, long-term (months) topical treatment with echothiophate ZLOCK et al. 1983) and short-term (single application to 1 week) topical treatment with carbachol or pilocarpine (BÁRÁNY et al. 1982) cause a decrease

← ――

Fig. 8. Pilocarpine dose-accommodation response relationship in echothiphate-treated eyes. *Abscissa*, pilocarpine hydrochloride dose in mg or mg/kg body wt; *ordinate*, accommodation (diopters); + denotes iris present throughout experiments; **, iris removed 4 days after discontinuing echothiophate or control solution; *, aniridic throughout experiments; *PI*, topical echothiophate iodide; *DIL*, control solution; *d*, day(s); *solid symbols*, right eye; *open symbols*, left eye (symbols sometimes displaced laterally or vertically for clarity); *i.m.*, intramuscular pilocarpine hdrochloride; *top*, topical pilocarpine hydrochloride; (*hex*), intramuscular hexamethonium bromide; (*pril*), retrobulbar prilocaine hydrochloride; *bef*, number of days before starting topical echothiophate; *dur*, number of days after starting echothiophate (during treatment); *aft*, number of days after discontinuing echothiophate or control solution. *Upper left panel* shows arithmetic and geometric mean curves for nonechothiophate-treated eyes. (KAUFMAN 1978)

in the concentration off muscarinic receptors on the ciliary muscle. Other studies have suggested that changes in receptor affinity (EHLERT et al. 1980), or even changes beyond the receptor (KORCZYN 1979), rather than changes in receptor density on target tissue membranes may be involved, despite the binding data cited and despite arguments (BITO and DAWSON 1970; BÁRÁNY 1977) that such alternatives are not readily compatible with the physiological data. Species and experimental methodological differences may contribute to the uncertainty in this area. More specific characterization of cholinergic modulation of cholinergic receptors and its relevance to sub- and supersensitivity in the iris and ciliary muscle is needed.

The physiological findings suggest that whatever molecular mechanisms are involved will have a definite bearing on potentially important clinical questions. Would patients receiving long-term cholinergic drug treatment for glaucoma eventually become refractory to therapy? How could drug-induced refractoriness be clinically distinguished from progression of the disease? Would certain agonists be more likely to induce profound refractoriness than others? Could the problem be alleviated by periodically switching from one cholinomimetic to another, or by alternating periods of cholinomimetic therapy and abstinence? Would the obvious clinical advantages of low-dose sustained release systems over pulsed topical eye drop delivery be offset by a greater tendency to induce subsensitivity (as in BÁRÁNY 1977)? Would the induced subsensitivity be as reversible in the diseased human eye as it apparently was in the healthy animal eye? Could noniatrogenic abnormalities in cholinergic systems be causally related to glaucoma? These questions will be difficult to answer, especially since the parameter of greatest clinical interest, IOP, is influenced by so many different anatomic structures and physiological processes. Clinical experience to date with sustained release pilocarpine delivery systems does not appear consistently to demonstrate a progressive loss of IOP-lowering efficacy analogous to the experimental results in the monkey (BÁRÁNY 1977), although some late therapeutic failures certainly occur (CHEN and LEE 1976).

2. Disease-Induced Alterations

Cholinergic supersensitivity is manifested clinically by the phenomenon of Adie's syndrome (WALSH and HOYT 1969). Patients with this condition have anisocoria, with the larger pupil reacting poorly to light. The near reaction, however, is extensive, although slow and tonic (i. e., it outlasts the near vision effort for some time). Tonicity of accommodation may also occur; patients may find it difficult to shift their gaze from far to near or the reverse. The tonic pupil constricts more than the normal pupil in response to appropriate concentrations of topically applied cholinergic drugs (2.5% methacholine, ADLER and SCHEIE 1940; 0.0625%–0.125% pilocarpine, COHEN and ZAKOV 1975; YOUNGE and BUSKI 1976; BOURGEN et al. 1978); i.e., it is supersensitive. Histological studies of three patients with this condition (RUTNER 1947; LIEGL and KÖHN 1962; HARRIMAN and GARLAND 1967 cited by WALSH and HOYT 1969) have demonstrated almost complete loss of ganglion cells in the ciliary ganglion and mild iris atrophy. Small unmyelinated axons were plentiful in the ganglion; they seemed to pass through the ganglion without synapsing. There were degenerated axons but also many normal-appearing axons in the postganglionic ciliary nerves. None of the patients exhibited related abnormalities in the oculomotor nerves, brain, brain stem, or spinal cord. Apparently, the syndrome is related to damage to the postganglionic parasympathetic fibers in the orbit destined for the iris and ciliary muscle, presumably followed by vigorous regeneration. Collaterals would theoretically sprout primarily from the accommodation fibers (which in rhesus monkeys normally outnumber the pupil fibers by > 30:1; WARWICK 1954), reinnervating the ciliary muscle and the iris. Thus, while the light reflex is lost, the pupil still constricts when the patient looks at a near object (LOWENSTEIN and LOWENFELD 1965; LOWENFELD and THOMPSON 1967).

The plasticity of the autonomic nervous system was elegantly demonstrated in LANGLEY'S (1898) historic experiments. Using cats, he apposed the central end of the severed vagus nerve and the peripheral end of the severed cervical sympathetic chain (proximal to the superior cervical ganglion). After a suitable waiting period, he showed that electrical stimulation of the vagus produced typical sympathetic responses in the eye, which could be blocked by intravenous nicotine.

3. Surgically Induced Alterations

The histological findings, the physiological and pharmacologic responses, and the pathophysiological mechanism proposed for Adie's syndrome are all consistent with the principles of parasympathetic denervation (diminished responses to physiological stimuli requiring intact innervation and enhanced responsiveness to exogenous pharmacologic stimuli, the latter perhaps related to increased receptor density or affinity on the muscle cell membrane), and with experimental findings in the monkey following surgical extirpation of the ciliary ganglion. Thus ciliary ganglionectomy produces partial degeneration of the pupillary sphincter and ciliary muscles, and supersensitivity of pupillary and accommodative responses to exogenous pilocarpine (ARMALY 1968; KAUFMAN 1982, unpublished data).

Another possible ocular example of denervation supersensitivity in the parasympathetic nervous system occurs after panretinal scatter photocoagulation (PRP) with xenon arc or argon laser light. This is the indicated treatment for certain stages of diabetic retinopathy (DIABETIC RETINOPATHY STUDY RESEARCH GROUP 1978) and perhaps other vasoproliferative retinopathies. Prepresbyopic patients undergoing PRP sometimes suffer permanent postphotocoagulation cycloplegia of sufficient magnitude to interfere seriously with near visual activities (ROGELL 1979). Although the pathophysiology of this phenomenon is not understood, two studies equivocally suggest that the pupillary sphincter muscle may be somewhat supersensitive to topical pilocarpine following peripheral iris photocoagulation (VOLK et al. 1979; LOBES and BOURGON 1978), perhaps implicating PRP-induced parasympathetic denervation of the anterior segment. If this proves to be the case, it may be possible to devise a photocoagulation strategy to prevent its occurrence.

II. Cholinergic Toxicity

1. Lens (Cataractogenesis)

Chronic topical application of long-acting ChE inhibitors to human eyes for the treatment of certain cases of glaucoma or accommodative esotropia can cause a characteristic type of anterior and posterior subcapsular lens opacity (Axelsson and Holmberg 1966; Shaffer and Hetherington 1966; de Roetth 1966; Tarkkanen and Karjalainen 1966; Axelsson 1968; Morton et al. 1970). At least one report suggests that pilocarpine may also be cataractogenic, although much less so than ChE inhibitors, but that it may exert some protective effect in the event of subsequent exposure to a ChE inhibitor (Levene 1969). Attempts to induce cataracts in subprimate mammals in vivo by topical application of ChE inhibitors have been unsuccessful (Härkönen and Tarkkanen 1970; Axelsson 1969). However, twice-daily topical application of echothiophate for 2.5–14 weeks to the eyes of vervet or cynomolgus monkeys consistently induces anterior and posterior subcapsular cataracts strongly resembling those attributed to ChE inhibitors in the human (Fig. 10; Kaufman and Axelsson 1975; Kaufman et al. 1977a). The microradiographic and light and electron microscopic characteristics of echothiophate-induced cataracts in the monkey have been described (Philipson et al. 1979). When atropine is administered topically to monkeys simultaneously with echothiophate, cataractogenesis is prevented entirely or is of much delayed onset and diminished severity (Kaufman et al. 1977b). Chemical interaction between the drugs does not occur (Kaufman et al. 1977b).

Despite several in vitro studies demonstrating biochemical and morphological alterations in subprimate mammalian lenses exposed to ChE inhibitors (Bito et al. 1965; de Roetth 1966; Härkönen and Tarkkanen 1970; Michon and Kinoshita 1967; 1968a, b; Müller et al. 1956), the mechanism of ChE-inhibitor cataractogenesis and its inhibition by atropine is unknown. That atropine is inhibitory at a dose that at least partially prevents echothiophate-induced accommodation may indicate that a cholinergic effect, either mechanical (e. g., accommodation itself; van Heyningen 1975) or biochemical (e. g., a cholinergically induced, atropine-inhibitable change in aqueous humor composition; Wålinder and Bill 1969b), is involved. However, a direct toxic effect of echothiophate on the lens still cannot be ruled out. Atropine inhibits the incorporation of ^{32}P from labeled $DF^{32}P$ in the nuclear, mitochondrial, microsomal, and supernatant fractions of rat liver (Ågren and Ramachandran 1964). If atropine has a similar action in the lens, it might protect the lens against a toxic cataractogenic effect of ChE inhibitors.

To rule out the possible mechanism of mechanical stress due to sustained intense accommodation, cynomolgus monkeys with a surgically disinserted and retrodisplaced ciliary muscle in one eye were chronically treated topically with echothiophate. The disinserted eyes are relatively hyperopic and do not accomodate in response to pilocarpine or echothiophate (Kaufman et al. 1979, 1983a). The disinserted and nondisinserted eyes all developed typical echothiophate cataracts, with no differences in topography or severity of cataracts in the two types of eye. Thus accommodative mechanical stress on the lens plays no role in the pathophysiology of echothiophate cataractogenesis in primates (Kaufman et al. 1983a), and the mechanism by which ChE inhibitors cause cataracts in vivo remains unknown. The possible roles of other anterior segment cholinergic mechanisms might be explored in ciliary ganglionectomized, ganglion-blocked, or hemicholinium-treated monkeys. Ciliary ganglionectomy itself is not cataractogenic in monkeys followed up for up to 6 months postsurgically (Kaufman, unpublished data).

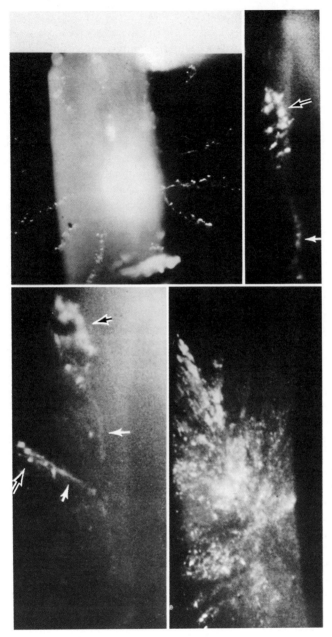

Fig. 10. Echothiophate cataractogenesis in a cynomolgus monkey, Cyno 271, right eye iridectomized, left eye untouched, both eyes echothiophate-treated (63 µg twice daily). *Top left and right* and *bottom left*, right eye after 45 days. *Top left*, radially oriented posterior sub-capsular chains of vacuoles in midperiphery at approximately clock-hourly intervals. *Top right*, chain of vacuoles (*black/white arrow*) is continuous with radial boundary line (*white arrow*) of central wedge of opacities. *Bottom left*, adjacent chains of vacuoles (*black/ white arrows*) continuous with adjacent boundary lines (*white arrows*), delimiting a wedge of opacities. *Bottom right*, left eye after 122 days, showing anterior subcapsular opacities. Note central network and radially oriented peripheral opacities. (KAUFMAN et al. 1977a)

2. Iris/Ciliary Muscle/Trabecular Meshwork

It was assumed that cholinergic subsensitivity was a strictly physiological/pharmacologic phenomenon in accordance with prevailing concepts of regulation of tissue sensitivity to autonomic agonists. However, rabbits receiving topical DFP unilaterally in vivo exhibited increased resting outflow resistance in the DFP-treated eye as compared to the untreated opposite eye, whether resistance was determined in vivo or after enucleation (AURICCHIO and DIOTALLEVI 1959a, b). Also, resting resistance after ganglionic blockade tended to be higher in the echothiophate-treated eyes of unilaterally echothiophate-treated monkeys (KAUFMAN and BÁRÁNY 1976 c). Although secondary phenomena, such as obstruction of the outflow channels by debris released during a drug-induced inflammatory reaction, or by iridial occlusion of the chamber angle (angle closure), could be responsible, the possibility arose that ChE inhibitors themselves or high levels of ACh and perhaps other direct-acting cholinomimetics might have a direct effect on the outflow pathways.

Histological and ultrastructural studies of monkey eyes treated topically in vivo with echothiophate (LÜTJEN-DRECOLL and KAUFMAN 1979) or sustained release pilocarpine delivery systems (LÜTJEN-DRECOLL 1981) indeed revealed significant tissue damage to trabecular meshwork, iris sphincter, and ciliary muscle, stroma, and epithelium (Fig. 11). Although the time course of these alterations has not been carefully defined, they were detectable within a few days after starting pilocarpine and were still present 6 months after stopping echothiophate (LÜTJEN-DRECOLL and KAUFMAN, work in preparation). The pathophysiology of the changes is unknown. They might be due to cellular effects of pilocarpine, ACh, or echothiophate itself, to inhibition of enzymes other than ChEs within the tissues, or to altered aqueous humor composition (BITO et al. 1965; WÅLINDER and BILL 1969 b). An altered mechanical state of the meshwork or ciliary muscle, perhaps due to sustained intense contraction of the muscle, might also play a role. Continuous contraction of the ciliary muscle might also cause chronic obstruction of uveoscleral drainage (BILL 1967), perhaps preventing removal of protein and toxic metabolites from the ciliary body. In short, simple down-regulation of receptor density may not be the only mechanism involved in loss of tissue sensitivity to cholinergic drugs in the anterior segment.

The structural changes in the ciliary muscle and trabecular meshwork might partly explain some of the physiological and clinical findings in animal and human eyes chronically treated with long-acting ChE inhibitors or sustained delivery pilocarpine systems: that is, (a) the subsensitivity of the accommodative and outflow facility response to cholinergic agonists in pilocarpine- and echothiophate-treated monkeys (BÁRÁNY 1977; KAUFMAN and BÁRÁNY 1975, 1976c; KAUFMAN 1978); (b) the tendency for resting outflow facility after ganglionic blockade to be lower in the echothiophate-treated eyes of unilaterally echothiophate-treated monkeys (KAUFMAN and BÁRÁNY 1976c); (c) the decreased outflow facility of living and enucleated rabbit eyes treated in vivo with DFP as compared to their untreated opposite eyes (AURICCHIO and DIOTALLEVI 1959a, b); and (d) the gradual loss of the resistance and IOP-lowering effect of ChE inhibitors and pilocarpine in some glaucomatous human eyes.

Preliminary studies of the mechanism of the cholinergically induced structural alterations in the chamber angle tissues indicate that with echothiophate there is

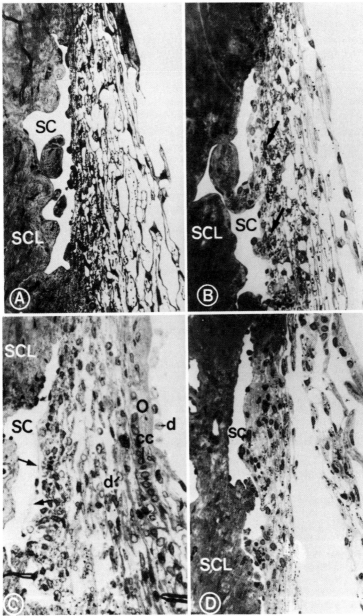

Fig. 11 a–d. Echothiophate (PI)induced structural alterations in trabecular meshwork and Schlemm's canal of cynomolgus monkeys. **a**, Monkey 225, right eye, 54 days' diluent; meshwork and inner canal wall appear normal: *SC*, Schlemm's canal; *SCL*, sclera. **b**, Monkey 225, left eye, 54 days' PI: *arrows* indicate thickened cribriform meshwork. **c**, Monkey 110, left eye, 115 days' PI: *arrows* indicate separation of inner wall endothelium from first sub-endothelial cell layer; *d*, degenerating trabecular and corneal endothelial cells; *O*, operculum; *cc*, subopercular endothelial cell clusters. **d**, Monkey 280, left eye, 215 days' PI. Cribriform and corneoscleral meshwork are dense and collapsed. Light micrograph, semithin sagittal sections, Richardson's stain; × 160. (LÜTJEN-DRECOLL and KAUFMAN 1979)

avulsion of the ciliary muscle tendons, leading to collapse and densification of the trabecular meshwork, in turn resulting in underperfusion of the meshwork by aqueous humor and consequent accumulation of extracellular material in the mesh. Atropine is at least partially protective, suggesting that a mechanism mediated at least in part by a muscarinic receptor somewhere in the anterior segment is involved (with the caveat noted in the lens section), rather than a nonmuscarinic toxic effect of ACh. Ciliary muscle disinsertion is also protective if the resulting scar tissue expands the posterior portion of the meshwork, suggesting that a toxic effect of echothiophate directly on the meshwork is not responsible for the alterations, since such surgery should not diminish echothiophate concentrations in the aqueous humor or the meshwork. Collectively, these findings indicate that at least the meshwork alterations relate to the mechanical consequences of ciliary muscle contraction (LÜTJEN-DRECOLL and KAUFMAN, work in preparation). However, the entire story is far from complete.

Acknowledgment. This work was supported in part by National Eye Institute grants EY00137 and EY2698. Ms. Bernadette Bull expertly executed the typing and editing. Permission to borrow freely from KAUFMAN (to be published) was granted by Academic Press Inc. for portions of the text dealing with aqueous humor outflow.

References

Adler FH, Scheie H (1940) The site of the disturbance in tonic pupils. Trans Am Ophthalmol Soc 38:183–192

Ågren G, Ramachandran BV (1964) The effect of pyridinium aldoximes and atropine on the incorporation of $DF^{32}P$ in rat liver cell fractions. Acta Physiol Scand 60:95–102

Akesson C, Swanson C, Patil PN (1983) Muscarinic receptors of rabbit irides. Naunyn-Schmiedebergs Arch Pharmacol 322:104–110

Alexander JH, van Lennep EW (1972) Water and electrolyte secretion by the exorbital lacrimal gland of the rat studied by micropuncture and catheterization techniques. Pflügers Arch 337:299–309

Allan L, Burian HM (1965) The valve action of the trabecular meshwork. Studies with silicone models. Am J Ophthalmol 59:382–389

Alm A, Bill A, Young FA (1973) The effects of pilocarpine and neostigmine on the blood flow through the anterior uvea in monkeys. A study with radioactively labelled microspheres. Exp Eye Res 15:31–36

Arenson MS, Wilson H (1971) The parasympathetic secretory nerves of the lacrimal gland of the cat. J Physiol 217:201–212

Armaly MF (1959a) Studies on intraocular effects of the orbital parasympathetic pathway. I. Technique and effects on morphology. Arch Ophthalmol 61:14–29

Armaly MF (1959b) Studies on intraocular effects of the orbital parasympathetics. II. Effects on intraocular pressure. Arch Ophthalmol 62:117–124

Armaly MF (1959c) Studies on intraocular effects of the orbital parasympathetic pathway. III. Effect on steady state dynamics. Arch Ophthalmol 62:817–827

Armaly MF (1968) Degeneration of ciliary muscle and iris sphincter following resection of the ciliary ganglion. Trans Am Ophthalmol Soc 66:475–502

Armaly MF, Burian HM (1958) Changes in the tonogram during accommodation. Arch Ophthalmol 60:60–68

Asayama J (1902) Zur Anatomie des Ligamentum Pectinatum. Albrecht von Graefes Arch Ophthalmol 53:113–128

Auricchio G, Diotallevi M (1959a) La resistenza al deflusso in occhi di coniglio dopo prolungato trattamento con diisopropilfluorofosfato. Ann Ottalmol e Clin Ocul 85:493–496

Auricchio G, Diotallevi M (1959 b) Uteriori ricerchi sull' influenza esercitata dal DFP sulla al deflusso in occhi di coniglio. Ann Ottalmol e Clin Ocul 85:567–570

Axelsson U (1968) Glaucoma, miotic therapy, and cataract. I. The frequency of anterior subcapsular vacuoles in glaucoma eyes treated with echothiophate (phospholine iodide), pilocarpine, or pilocarpine-eserine, and in non-glaucomatous untreated eyes with common senile cataract. Acta Ophthalmol 46:83–98

Axelsson U (1969) Glaucoma miotic therapy and cataract. VI. Experimental studies on the guinea pig eye. Acta Ophthalmol 47:1–11

Axelsson U, Holmberg Å (1966) The frequency of cataract after miotic therapy. Acta Ophthalmol 44:421–429

Bárány EH (1955) Resistance to aqueous outflow. In: Newell FW (ed) Glaucoma, transactions of the first conference. Josiah Macy Jr Foundation, New York, pp 112–113

Bárány EH (1962) The mode of action of pilocarpine on outflow resistance in the eye of a primate (*Cercopithecus ethiops*). Invest Ophthalmol 1:712–727

Bárány EH (1963) A mathematical formulation of intraocular pressure as dependent on secretion, ultrafiltration, bulk outflow, and osmotic reabsorption of fluid. Invest Ophthalmol 2:584–590

Bárány EH (1965) Relative importance of autonomic nervous tone and structure as determinants of outflow resistance in normal monkey eyes (*Cercopithecus ethiops* and *Macaca irus*). In: Rohen JW (ed) The structure of the eye, 2nd symposium. Schattauer, Stuttgart, pp 223–236

Bárány EH (1966 a) The mode of action of miotics on outflow resistance. A study of pilocarpine in the vervet monkey, *Cercopithecus ethiops*. Trans Ophthalmol Soc UK 86:539–578

Bárány EH (1966 b) Pseudofacility and uveo-scleral outflow routes. Some non-technical difficulties in the determination of outflow facility and rate of formation of aqueous humor. Glaucoma symposium, Tutzing Castle, Karger, Basel, pp 27–51

Bárány EH (1967) The immediate effect on outflow resistance of intravenous pilocarpine in the vervet monkey, *Cercopithecus ethiops*. Invest Ophthalmol 6:373–380

Bárány EH (1972) Inhibition by hippurate and probenecid of in vitro uptake of iodipamide and *o*-iodohippurate – composite uptake system for iodipamide in choroid plexus, kidney cortex, and anterior uvea of several species. Acta Physiol Scand 86:12–27

Bárány EH (1973 a) The liver-like anion transport system in rabbit kidney, uvea, and choroid plexus. I. Selectivity of some inhibitors, direction of transport, possible physiological substrates. Acta Physiol Scand 88:412–429

Bárány EH (1973 b) The liver-like anion transport system in rabbit kidney, uvea, and choroid plexus. II. Efficiency of acidic drugs and other anions as inhibitors. Acta Physiol Scand 88:491–504

Bárány EH (1974) Bile acids as inhibitors of the liver-like anion transport system in the rabbit kidney, uvea, and choroid plexus. Acta Physiol Scand 92:195–203

Bárány EH (1975) In vitro uptake of bile acids by choroid plexus, kidney cortex, and anterior uvea. I. The iodipamide sensitive transport systems in the rabbit. Acta Physiol Scand 93:250–268

Bárány EH (1976) Organic cation uptake in vitro by the rabbit iris-ciliary body, renal cortex, and choroid plexus. Invest Ophthalmol 15:341–348

Bárány EH (1977) Pilocarpine-induced subsensitivity to carbachol and pilocarpine of ciliary muscle in vervet and cynomolgus monkeys. Acta Ophthalmol 55:141–163

Bárány EH, Christensen RE (1967) Cycloplegia and outflow resistance. Arch Ophthalmol 77:757–760

Bárány EH, Rohen JW (1965) Localized contraction and relaxation within the ciliary muscle of the vervet monkey (*Cercopithecus ethiops*). In: Rohen JW (ed) The structure of the eye, 2nd symposium. Schattauer, Stuttgart, pp 287–311

Bárány EH, Berrie CP, Birdsall NJM, Burgen ASV, Hulme EC (1982) The binding properties of the muscarinic receptors of the cynomolgus monkey ciliary body and the response to the induction of agonist subsensitivity. Br J Pharmacol 77:731–739

Baughman RW, Bader CR (1977) Biochemical characterization and cellular localization of the cholinergic system in the chicken retina. Brain Res 138:469–485

Becker B (1960) The transport of organic anions by the rabbit eye. I. In vitro iodopyracet (Diodrast) accumulation by ciliary body-iris preparations. Am J Ophthalmol 50:862–867

Becker B (1961) Iodide transport by the rabbit eye. Am J Physiol 200:804–806

Becker B (1962) The measurement of rate of aqueous flow with iodide. Invest Ophthalmol 1:52–58

Becker B (1967) Ascorbate transport in guinea pig eyes. Invest Ophthalmol 6:10–15

Berggren L (1965) Effect of parasympathomimetic and sympathomimetic drugs on secretion in vitro by the ciliary processes of the rabbit eye. Invest Ophthalmol 4:91–97

Berggren L (1970) Further studies on the effect of autonomic drugs on in vitro secretory activity of the rabbit eye ciliary processes. Acta Ophthalmol 48:293–302

Bertaccini G, Impicciatore M, Mossini F (1972) Action of some N-methyl derivatives of histamine on salivary and lacrimal secretion of the cat. Biochem Pharmacol 21:3076–3078

Bill A (1966a) Formation and drainage of aqueous humor in cats. Exp Eye Res 5:185–190

Bill A (1966b) The routes for bulk drainage of aqueous humor in rabbits with and without cyclodialysis. Doc Ophthalmol 20:157–169

Bill A (1967) Effects of atropine and pilocarpine on aqueous humor dynamics in cynomolgus monkeys (Macaca irus). Exp Eye Res 6:120–125

Bill A (1969) Effects of atropine on aqueous humor dynamics in the vervet monkey (Cercopithecus ethiops). Exp Eye Res 8:284–291

Bill A (1971a) Aqueous humor dynamics in monkeys (Macaca irus and Cercopithecus ethiops). Exp Eye Res 11:195–206

Bill A (1971b) Effects of long-standing stepwise increments in eye pressure on the rate of aqueous humor formation in a primate (Cercopithecus ethiops). Exp Eye Res 12:184–193

Bill A (1975) Blood circulation and fluid dynamics in the eye. Pharmacol Rev 55:383–417

Bill A (1981) Ocular circulation. In: Moses RA (ed) Adler's physiology of the eye. Clinical application, 7th ed. Mosby, St. Louis, chap. 6, pp 184–203

Bill A, Bárány EH (1966) Gross facility, facility of conventional routes, and pseudofacility of aqueous humor outflow in the cynomolgus monkey. The reduction in aqueous humor formation rate caused by moderate increments in intraocular pressure. Arch Ophthalmol 75:665–673

Bill A, Phillips CI (1971) Uveoscleral drainage of aqueous humor in human eyes. Exp Eye Res 12:275–281

Bill A, Svedbergh B (1972) Scanning electron microscopic studies of the trabecular meshwork and the canal of Schlemm – an attempt to localize the main resistance to outflow of aqueous humor in man. Acta Ophthalmol 50:295–320

Bill A, Wålinder P-E (1966) The effects of pilocarpine on the dynamics of aqueous humor in a primate (Macaca irus). Invest Ophthalmol 5:170–175

Bito LZ (1968) The absence of sympathetic role in anti-ChE-induced changes in cholinergic transmission. J Pharmacol Exp Ther 161:302–309

Bito LZ (1972a) Accumulation and apparent active transport of prostaglandins by some rabbit tissues in vitro. J Physiol 221:371–387

Bito LZ (1972b) Comparative study of concentrative prostaglandin accumulation by various tissues of mammals and marine vertebrates and invertebrates. Comp Biochem Physiol 43:65–82

Bito LZ, Banks N (1969) Effects of chronic cholinesterase inhibitor treatment. I. The pharmacological and physiological behavior of the anti-ChE-treated (Macaca mulatta) iris. Arch Ophthalmol 82:681–686

Bito LZ, Baroody RA (1979) Gradual changes in the sensitivity of rhesus monkey eyes to miotics and the dependence of these changes on the regimen of topical cholinesterase inhibitor treatment. Invest Ophthalmol Vis Sci 18:794–801

Bito LZ, Dawson MJ (1970) The site and mechanism of the control of cholinergic sensitivity. J Pharmacol Exp Ther 175:673–684

Bito LZ, Salvador EV (1972) Intraocular fluid dynamics. III. The site and mechanism of prostaglandin transfer across the blood intraocular fluid barriers. Exp Eye Res 14:233–241

Bito LZ, Salvador EV (1976) Effects of anti-inflammatory agents and some other drugs on prostaglandin biotransport. J Pharmacol Exp Ther 198:481–488

Bito LZ, Davson H, Snider N (1965) The effects of autonomic drugs on mitosis and DNA synthesis in the lens ephthelium and on the composition of the aqueous humor. Exp Eye Res 4:54–61

Bito LZ, Hyslop A, Hyndman J (1967) Antiparasympathomimetic effects of cholinesterase inhibitor treatment. J Pharmacol Exp Ther 157:159–169

Bito LZ, Dawson MJ, Petrinovic L (1971) Cholinergic sensitivity: normal variability as a function of stimulus background. Science 172:583–585

Bito LZ, Davson H, Salvador EV (1976) Inhibition of in vitro concentrative prostaglandin accumulation by prostaglandins, prostaglandin analogues, and by some inhibitors of organic anion transport. J Physiol 256:257–271

Botelho SY, Hisada M, Fuenmayor N (1966) Functional innervation of the lacrimal gland in the cat. Arch Ophthalmol 16:581–588

Botelho SY, Goldstein AM, Hisada M (1969) The effects of autonomic nerve impulses and autonomic drugs on secretion by the lacrimal gland. In: Botelho SY, Brooks FP, Shelley WB (eds) Exocrine glands: proceedings of a satellite symposium of the 25th international congress of physiological sciences. University of Pennsylvania Press, Philadelphia, pp 227–245

Bourgon P, Pilley SFJ, Thompson HS (1978) Cholinergic supersensitivity of the iris sphincter in Adie's tonic pupil. Am J Ophthalmol 85:373–377

Brimblecombe RW (1974) Drug actions at peripheral muscarinic sites. In: Brimblecombe RW (ed) Drug actions on cholinergic systems. University Park Press, Baltimore, pp 19–42

Brogdanski DF, Silser F, Brodie BB (1961) Comparative action of reserpine, tetrabenazine and chlorpromazine on central parasympathetic activity: effects on pupillary size and lacrimation in rabbit and on salivation in dog. J Pharmacol Exp Ther 132:176–182

Bromberg BB (1981) Autonomic control of lacrimal protein secretion. Invest Ophthalmol Vis Sci 20:110–116

Bunke A, Bito LZ (1981) Gradual increase in the sensitivity of extraocular muscles to acetylcholine during topical treatment of rabbit eyes with isoflurophate. Am J Ophthalmol 92:259–267

Burde RM (1981) The extraocular muscles. Anatomy, physiology, and pharmacology. In: Moses RA (ed) Adler's physiology of the eye. Clinical application, 7th edn. Mosby St. Louis, chap. 5, pt 1, pp 84–121

Burn JH, Rand MJ (1962) A new interpretation of the adrenergic fiber. Adv Pharmacol 1:1–30

Carrier O Jr (1972) Cholinergic drugs. In: Carrier O Jr (ed) Pharmacology of the peripheral autonomic nervous system. Year Book Medical Publishers, Chicago, pp 34–73

Casey WJ (1966) Cervical sympathetic stimulation in monkeys and the effects on outflow facility and intraocular volume. A study in the East African vervet (Cercopithecus aethiops). Invest Ophthalmol 5:33–41

Cashin CH, Holten TM, Szinai SS (1972) Synthesis and anticholinergic properties of 1-adamant-1-yl-1-phenyl-3-N-pyrrolidino-1-propranolol hydrochloride. J Medicinal Chem 15:853–854

Cavanagh HD (1975) Herpetic ocular disease: therapy of persistent epithelial defects. Int Ophthalmol Clin 15:67–88

Cavanagh HD, Colley AM (1981) β-Adrenergic and muscarinic binding in corneal epithelium. Invest Ophthalmol Vis Sci 20 [ARVO suppl]:37

Chen T-T, Lee P-F (1976) Clinical experience on Ocusert – pilocarpine system – a long-term evaluation. Invest Ophthalmol 15 [ARVO suppl]:48

Chiang TS, Leaders FF (1971) Antagonism of aceclidine-induced tremor, analgesia, hypothermia, salivation, and lacrymation of some pharmacological agents. Arch Int Pharmacodyn Ther 189:295–302

Chiou GC, Liu HK, Trzeciakowski J (1980) Studies of action mechanism of antiglaucoma drugs with a newly developed cat model. Life Sci 27:2445–2451

Claesson H, Bárány E (1978) Time course of light induced changes in pilocarpine sensitivity of rat iris. Acta Physiol Scand 102:394–398

Cohen DN, Zakov ZN (1975) The diagnosis of Adie's pupil using 0.0625% pilocarpine solution. Am J Ophthalmol 79:883–885

Dartt DA, Botelho SY (1979) Protein in rabbit lacrimal gland fluid. Invest Ophthalmol Vis Sci 18:1207–1209

de Haas EBH (1960) Lacrimal gland response to parasympathomimetics after parasympathetic denervation. Arch Ophthalmol 64:34–43

De Robertis E, Fizer de Plazas S, La Torre JL, Lunt GS (1970) Proteo lipid cholinergic receptor isolated from the central nervous system and electric tissue. In: Heilbronn E, Winters A (eds) Drugs and cholinergic mechanisms in the CNS. Försvarets Forskningsanstalt, Stockholm, pp 505–520

de Roetth A Jr (1966) Lens opacities in patients on phospholine iodide therapy. Am J Ophthalmol 62:619–628

de Roetth A Jr, Dettbarn W-D, Rosenberg , Wilensky JG, Wong A (1965) Effect of phospholine iodide on blood cholinesterase levels of normal and glaucoma subjects. Am J Ophthalmol 59:586–592

Diabetic Retinopathy Study Research Group (1978) Photocoagulation treatment of proliferative diabetic retinopathy: the second report of diabetic retinopathy study findings. Ophthalmology (Rochester) 85:82–106

Drachman DB (1978 a) Myasthenia gravis (first of two parts). N Engl J Med 298:136–142

Drachman DB (1978 b) Myasthenia gravis (second of two parts). N Engl J Med 298:186–193

Duke-Elder S, Cook C (1963) The development of the surface ectoderm. In: Duke-Elder S (ed) System of ophthalmology, vol 3, pt 1. Normal and abnormal development: embryology. Mosby, St. Louis, chap 5, pp 127–138

Ehinger B (1966) Adrenergic nerves to the eye and to related structures in man and in the cynomolgus monkey (Macaca irus). Invest Ophthalmol 5:42–52

Ehlers N (1977) Pharmacology of the conjunctival sac. In: Dikstein S (ed) Drugs and ocular tissues. Karger, New York, pp 23–56

Ehlert FJ, Kokka N, Fairhurst AS (1980) Altered [^3H]quinuclidinyl benzilate binding in the striatum of rats following chronic cholinesterase inhibition with diisopropylfluorophosphate. Mol Pharmacol 17:24–30

Ellis PP, Littlejohn K (1974) Effects of topical anticholinesterases on procaine hydrolysis. Am J Ophthalmol 77:71–75

Emmelin NG, Strömblad BCR (1956) Sensitization of the lacrimal gland by treatment with a parasympatholytic agent. Acta Physiol Scand 36:171–174

Fitzgerald GG, Cooper JR (1971) Acetylcholine as a possible sensory mediator in rabbit corneal epithelium. Biochem Pharmacol 20:2741–2748

Flocks M, Zweng HC (1957) Studies on the mode of action of pilocarpine on aqueous outflow. Am J Ophthalmol 44:380–388

Fogle JA, Neufeld AH (1979) The adrenergic and cholinergic corneal epithelium. Invest Ophthalmol Vis Sci 18:1212–1215

Forbes M, Becker B (1960) The transport of organic anions by the rabbit eye. II. In vivo transport of iodopyracet (Diodrast). Am J Ophthalmol 50:867–875

Fortin EP (1925) Canel de Schlemm y ligamento pectineo. Arch Ophthalmol 4:454–459

Fortin EP (1929) Action du muscle ciliaire sur la circulation de l'oeil; insertion du muscle ciliaire sur la paroi du canal de Schlemm. Signification physiologique et pathologique. CR Soc Biol 102:432–434

Furman M, Lazar M, Leopold IH (1969) Cholinesterase isoenzymes in rabbit ocular tissue homogenates. Doc Ophthalmol 26:185–191

Gaasterland D, Kupfer C, Ross K (1975) Studies of aqueous humor dynamics in man. IV. Effects of pilocarpine upon measurements in young normal volunteers. Invest Ophthalmol 14:848–853

Galin MA (1961) Mydriasis provocative test. Arch Ophthalmol 66:353–355

Gartner S (1944) Blood vessels of the conjunctiva. Arch Ophthalmol 32:464–476

Gesztes T (1966) Prolonged apnea after suxamethonium injection associated with eye drops containing an anticholinesterase agent. Br J Anaesthesiol 38:408–409

Gnädinger M, Walz D, von Hahn HP, Grun F (1967) Acetylcholine-splitting activity of abraded and cultivated corneal epithelial cells. Exp Eye Res 6:239–242

Gnädinger M, Heimann E, Markstein R (1973) Choline acetyltransferase in corneal epithelium. Exp Eye Res 15:395–399

Goldmann H (1951) L'origine de l'hypertension oculaire dans le glaucome primitif. Ann Ocul (Paris) 184:1086

Graham LT (1974) Comparative aspects of neurotransmitters in the retina. In: Davson H, Graham LT (eds) The Eye, vol 6. Academic, New York, pp 283–342

Grant WM (1963) Experimental aqueous perfusion in enucleated human eyes. Arch Ophthalmol 69:783–801

Green K, Padgett D (1979) Effect of various drugs on pseudofacility and aqueous formation in the rabbit eye. Exp Eye Res 28:239–246

Grierson I, Lee WR, Abraham S (1978) Effects of pilocarpine on the morphology of the human outflow apparatus. Br J Ophthalmol 62:302–313

Härkönen M, Tarkkanen A (1970) Effect of phospholine iodide on energy metabolites of the rabbit lens. Exp Eye Res 10:1–7

Harris LS (1968) Cycloplegic-induced intraocular pressure elevations. Arch Ophthalmol 79:242–246

Harris JE, Gruber L, Hoskinson G (1959) The effect of methylene blue and certain other dyes on cation transport and hydration of the rabbit lens. Am J Ophthalmol 47:387–395

Havener WH (1978) Autonomic drugs. In: Havener WH (ed) Ocular pharmacology, 4th edn. Mosby, St. Louis, pp 218–328

Hebb CO (1955) Choline acetylase in mammalian and avian sensory systems. QJ Exp Physiol Cogn Med Sci 40:176–186

Heilbronn E (1975) Biochemistry of cholinergic receptors. In: Waser PG (ed) Cholinergic mechanisms. Raven, New York, pp 343–364

Heine L (1900) Die Anatomie des akkommodierten Auges – mikroskopische Fixierung des Akkommodationspaltes. Albrecht von Graefes Arch Klin Exp Ophthalmol 49:1–7

Hellauer HF (1950) Sensibilität und Acetylcholingehalt der Hornhaut verschiedener Tiere und des Menschen. Z Vergl Physiol 32:303–310

Herzog V, Sies H, Miller F (1976) Exocytosis in secretory cells of rat lacrimal gland. Peroxidase release from lobules and isolated cells upon cholinergic stimulation. J Cell Biol 70:692–706

Hofmann H, Holzer H (1953) Die Wirkung von Muskelrelaxantien auf den intraocularen Druck. Klin Monatsbl Augenheilkd 123:1–16

Hogan MJ, Alvarado JA, Weddell JE (1971) Histology of the human eye. An atlas and textbook. Saunders, Philadelphia, pp 205:303–309

Holmberg Å, Bárány EH (1966) The effect of pilocarpine on the endothelium forming the inner wall of Schlemm's canal: an electron microscopic study in the monkey *Cercopithecus aethiops*. Invest Ophthalmol 5:53–58

Hopff WH, Riggio G, Waser PG (1975) Progress in isolation of acetylcholinesterase. In: Waser PG (ed) Cholinergic mechanisms. Raven, New York, pp 293–298

Howard RO, Wilson WS, Dunn BJ (1973) Quantitative determination of choline acetylase, acetylcholine, and acetylcholinesterase in the developing rabbit cornea. Invest Ophthalmol 12:418–425

Iwatsuki N, Petersen OH (1978) Membrane potential, resistance, and intercellular communication in the lacrimal gland: effects of acetylcholine and adrenaline. J Physiol 275:507–520

James RG, Calkins JP (1957) Effect of certain drugs on iris vessels. Arch Ophthalmol 57:414–417

Jones LT (1966) The lacrimal secretory system and its treatment. Am J Ophthalmol 63:47–60

Karczmar AG (1970) History of research with anticholinesterase agents. In: Radouco-Thomas C, Karczmar AG (eds) Anticholinesterase agents, International encyclopedia of pharmacology and therapeutics, sect 13, vol 1. Pergamon, Oxford, pp 1–44

Kaufman PL (1978) Anticholinesterase-induced cholinergic subsensitivity in primate accommodative mechanism. Am J Ophthalmol 85:622–631

Kaufman PL (1979) Aqueous humor dynamics following total iridectomy in the cynomolgus monkey. Invest Ophthalmol Vis Sci 18:870–875

Kaufman PL (to be published) Aqueous humor outflow: In: Zadunaisky JA, Davson H (eds) Current topics in eye research. Academic Press, New York

Kaufman PL, Axelsson U (1975) Induction of subcapsular cataracts in aniridic vervet monkeys by echothiophate. Invest Ophthalmol 14:863–866

Kaufman PL, Bárány EH (1975) Subsensitivity to pilocarpine in primate ciliary muscle following topical anticholinesterase treatment. Invest Ophthalmol 14:302–306

Kaufman PL, Bárány EH (1976a) Loss of acute pilocarpine effect on outflow facility following surgical disinsertion and retrodisplacement of the ciliary muscle from the scleral spur in the cynomolgus monkey. Invest Ophthalmol 15:793–807

Kaufman PL, Bárány EH (1976b) Residual pilocarpine effects on outflow facility after ciliary muscle disinsertion in the cynomolgus monkey. Invest Ophthalmol 15:558–561

Kaufman PL, Bárány EH (1976c) Subsensitivitiy to pilocarpine of the aqueous outflow system in monkey eyes after topical anticholinesterase treatment. Am J Ophthalmol 82:883–891

Kaufman PL, Lütjen-Drecoll E (1975) Total iridectomy in the primate in vivo: surgical technique and postoperative anatomy. Invest Ophthalmol 14:766–771

Kaufman PL, Axelsson U, Bárány EH (1977a) Induction of subcapsular cataracts in cynomolgus monkeys by echothiophate. Arch Ophthalmol 95:499–504

Kaufman PL, Axelsson U, Bárány EH (1977b) Atropine inhibition of echothiophate cataractogenesis in monkeys. Arch Ophthalmol 95:1262–1268

Kaufman PL, Rohen JW, Bárány EH (1979) Hyperopia and loss of accommodation following ciliary muscle disinsertion in the cynomolgus monkey: physiologic and scanning electron microscopic studies. Invest Ophthalmol Vis Sci 18:665–673

Kaufman PL, Erickson KA, Neider MW (1983a) Echothiophate cataracts in monkeys: occurrence despite loss of accommodation induced by retrodisplacement of ciliary muscle. Arch Ophthalmol 101:125–128

Kaufman PL, Polansky JR, Southren AL, Anderson DR (1983b) Aqueous humor dynamics: outflow. In: Vision research – a national plan. 1983–1987. The 1983 report of the national advisory eye council. Report of the glaucoma panel. US-DHHS. (NIH pub. no. 83–2474), vol 2, pt 4, chap 3, pp 41–53

Keryer G, Rossignol B (1976) Effect of carbachol on ^{45}Ca uptake and protein secretion in rat lacrimal gland. Am J Physiol 230:99–104

Kikkawa T (1968) Studies on the mechanism of tear secretion. 1. On the salt and water secretion from the lacrimal gland and its secretions. Acta Soc Ophthalmol Jap 72:1005–1009

Kikkawa T (1970) Secretory potentials in the lacrimal gland of the rabbit. Jap J Ophthalmol 14:247–262

Kinsey VE (1947) Transfer of ascorbic acid and related compounds across the blood-aqueous barrier. Am J Ophthalmol 30:1262–1266

Kinsey VE (1971) Ion movement in ciliary processes. In: Bittar EE (ed) Membranes and ion transport, vol 3. Wiley, New York

Kinsey VE, Reddy DVN (1962) Transport of amino acids into the posterior chamber of the rabbit eye. Invest Ophthalmol 1:355–362

Kloog Y, Sachs DI, Korczyn AD, Heron DS, Sokolovsky M (1979a) Muscarinic acetylcholine receptors in cat iris. Biochem Pharmacol 28:1505–1511

Kloog Y, Heron DS, Korczyn AD, Sachs DI, Sokolovsky M (1979b) Muscarinic acetylcholine receptors in albino rabbit iris-ciliary body. Mol Pharmacol 15:581–587

Koelle GB (1975a) Neurohumoral transmission and the autonomic nervous system. In: Goodman LS, Gilman A (ed) The pharmacological basis of therapeutics, 5th edn. MacMillan, New York, chap 2, pp 404–444

Koelle GB (1975b) Anticholinesterase agents. In: Goodman LS, Gilman A (eds) The pharmacological basis of therapeutics, 5th edn. MacMillan, New York, chap 22, pp 445–466

Koelle GB (1975c) Parasympathomimetic agents. In: Goodman LS, Gilman A (eds) The pharmacological basis of therapeutics, 5th edn. MacMillan, New York, chap 22, pp 467–476

Kolker AE, Hetherington J Jr (1976) Becker-Shaffer's diagnosis and therapy of the glaucomas, 4th edn. Mosby, St. Louis, pp 78–87, 325–334

Korczyn AD, Kloog Y, Heron DS, Sachs DI, Sokolovsky M (1979) Muscarinic receptor binding following denervation or decentralization of the iris. Invest Ophthalmol Vis Sci 18 [ARVO suppl]:189

Kupfer C (1973) Clinical significance of pseudofacility. Am J Ophthalmol 75:193–204

Lam DMK (1972) Biosynthesis of acetylcholine in turtle photoreceptors. Proc Natl Acad Sci US 69:1987–1991

Langley JN (1898) On the union of cranial autonomic (visceral) fibers with the nerve cells of the superior cervical ganglion. J Physiol 23:240–270

Laties AM, Jacobowitz D (1966) A comparative study of the autonomic innervation of the eye in monkey, cat, and rabbit. Anat Rec 156:383–395

Lemp MA, Holly FJ, Iwata S, Dohlman CH (1970) The precorneal tear film. 1. Factors in spreading and maintaining a continuous tear film over the corneal surface. Arch Ophthalmol 83:89–94

Lemp MA, Dohlman CH, Kuwabara T, Holly FJ, Carroll JM (1971) Dry eye secondary to mucus deficiency. Trans Am Acad Ophthalmol Otolaryngol 75:1223–1227

Leopold IH, Furman M (1971) Cholinesterase isoenzymes in human ocular tissue homogenates. Am J Ophthalmol 72:460–463

Levene RZ (1969) Echothiophate iodide and lens changes. In: Leopold IH (ed) Symposium on ocular therapy, vol 4. Mosby, St. Louis, pp 45–52

Liegl O, Köhn K (1962) Zur Pathogenese der Pupillotonie. Beobachtungen an einer Choroiditis carcinomatosa. Klin Monatsbl Augenheilkd 140:327–328

Lindstrom J, Anhott R, Einarson B, Engel A, Osame M, Montal M (1980) Purification of acetylcholine receptors, reconstitution into lipid vesicles, and study of agonist-induced cation channel regulation. J Biol Chem 255:8340–8350

Liu HK, Chiou GCY (1981) Continuous, simultaneous, and instant display of aqueous humor dynamics with a micro-spectrophotometer and a sensitive drop counter. Exp Eye Res 32:583–592

Lobes LA Jr, Bourgon P (1978) Pupillary abnormalities following argon laser ablation for proliferative diabetic retinopathy. Invest Ophthalmol 17 [ARVO suppl]:224

Lowenfeld IE, Thompson HS (1967) The tonic pupil: a re-evaluation. Am J Ophthalmol 63:46–87

Lowenstein O, Lowenfeld IE (1965) Pupillotonic pseudotabes (syndrome of Markus-Weill and Reys-Holmes-Adie). A critical review of the literature. Surv Ophthalmol 10:129–185

Lütjen-Drecoll E (1973) Structural factors influencing outflow facility and its changeability under drugs. Invest Ophthalmol 12:280–294

Lütjen-Drecoll E (1981) Ultrastructural changes in the monkey eye following long-term treatment with pilocarpine. Invest Ophthalmol Vis Sci 20 [ARVO suppl]:30

Lütjen-Drecoll E, Kaufman PL (1979) Echothiophate-induced structural alterations in the anterior chamber angle of the cynomolgus monkey. Invest Ophthalmol Vis Sci 18:918–929

Lütjen-Drecoll E, Kaufman PL, Bárány EH (1977) Light and electron microscopy of the anterior chamber angle structures following surgical disinsertion of the ciliary muscle in the cynomolgus monkey. Invest Ophthalmol Vis Sci 16:218–225

Lütjen-Drecoll E, Futa R, Rohen JW (1981) Ultrahistochemical studies on tangential sections of the trabecular meshwork in normal and glaucomatous eyes. Invest Ophthalmol Vis Sci 21:563–573

Macri FJ, Cevario SJ (1973) The induction of aqueous humor formation by the use of acetylcholine and eserine. Invest Ophthalmol 12:910–916

Macri FJ, Cevario SJ (1974) The dual nature of pilocarpine to stimulate or inhibit the formation of aqueous humor. Invest Ophthalmol 13:617–619

Maren TH (1974) HCO$_3^-$ formation in aqueous humor: mechanism and relation to the treatment of glaucoma. Invest Ophthalmol 13:179–483

Masland RH, Ames A III (1976) Response to acetylcholine of ganglion cells in the isolated mammalian retina. J Neurophysiol 39:1220–1235

Masland RH, Livingstone CH (1976) Effect of activity on the synthesis and release of acetylcholine by an isolated mammalian retina. J Neurophysiol 39:1210–1219

Masland RH, Mills JW (1979) Autoradiographic identification of acetylcholine in the rabbit retina. J Cell Biol 83:159–178

McEwen WK, Goodner EK (1969) Secretion of tears and blinking. In: Davson H (ed): The eye, vol 3. Academic, London, pp 341–378

Michon J Jr, Kinoshita JH (1967) Cholinesterase in the lens. Arch Ophthalmol 77:804–808

Michon J Jr, Kinoshita JH (1968 a) Experimental miotic cataract. I. Effects of miotics on lens structure, cation content, and hydration. Arch Ophthalmol 79:79–86

Michon J Jr, Kinoshita JH (1968 b) Experimental miotic cataract. II. Permeability, cation transport, and intermediary metabolism. Arch Ophthalmol 79:611–616

Milder B (1981) The lacrimal apparatus. In: Moses RA (ed) Adler's physiology of the eye. Clinical application, 7th Edn, Mosby, St. Louis, chap 2, pp 16–37

Miller RD, Savarese JJ (1981) Pharmacology of muscle relaxants, their antagonists, and monitoring of neuromuscular function. In: Miller RD (ed) Anesthesia, vol 1. Churchill Livingstone, New York, chap 17, pp 487–538

Mindel JS, Mittag TW (1976) Choline acetyltransferase in ocular tissues of rabbits, cats, cattle, and man. Invest Ophthalmol 15:808–814

Mindel JS, Mittag TW (1977) Variability of choline acetyltransferase in ocular tissues of rabbits, cats, cattle and humans. Exp Eye Res 24:25–33

Mindel JS, Szilagyi PI, Zadunaisky JA, Mittag TW, Orellana J (1979) The effects of blepharorrhaphy induced depression of corneal cholinergic activity. Exp Eye Res 29:463–468

Mittag TW (1979) On the presence of acetylcholine receptors in ocular structures of the rabbit. Invest Ophthalmol Vis Sci 18 [ARVO suppl]:189

Mittag TW (1980) Receptors in iris and ciliary body. Proc Int Soc Eye Res 1:114

Mizokami K (1977) Demonstration of masked acidic glycosaminoglycans in normal human trabecular meshwork. Jap J Ophthalmol 21:57–71

Moran JF, Triggle DJ (1971) Multiple ligand binding sites at the cholinergic receptor. In: Triggle DJ, Moran JF, Barnard EA (eds) Cholinergic ligand interactions. Academic, London, pp 119–136

Morton WR, Drance SM, Fairclough M (1970) Effect of echothiophate iodide on the lens. Am J Ophthalmol 68:1003–1010

Moses RA (1981 a) Intraocular pressure. In: Moses RA (ed) Adler's physiology of the eye. Clinical application, 7th edn. Mosby, St. Louis, chap 8, pp 227–254

Moses RA (1981 b) Accommodation. In: Moses RA (ed) Adler's physiology of the eye. Clinical application, 7th edn. Mosby, St. Louis, chap 11, pp 304–325

Müller HK, Kleifeld O, Hockwin O, Dardenne U (1956) Der Einfluß von Pilocarpin und Mintacol auf den Stoffwechsel der Linse. Ber Dtsch Ophthalmol Ges 60:115–120

Nagataki S, Brubaker RF (1982) The effect of pilocarpine on aqueous humor formation in humans. Arch Ophthalmol 100:818–821

Neal MJ, Gilroy J (1975) High affinitiy choline transport in the isolated rat retina. Brain Res 93:548–551

Nichols CW, Koelle GB (1967) Acetylcholinesterase method for demonstration in amacrine cells of rabbit retina. Science 155:477–478

Nichols CW, Koelle GB (1968) Comparison of the localization of acetylcholinesterase and non-specific cholinesterase activities in mammalian and avian retinas. J Comp Neurol 133:1–16

Niemeyer G (1978) Cholinergic antagonists fail to block S potentials in the cat retina. Invest Ophthalmol Vis Sci 17 [ARVO suppl]:385

Nishida S, Sears ML (1969 a) Fine structural innervation of the dilator muscle of the iris of the albino guinea pig studied with permanganate fixation. Exp Eye Res 8:292–296

Nishida S, Sears ML (1969 b) Dual innervation of the iris sphincter muscle of the albino guinea pig. Exp Eye Res 8:467–469

Nomura T, Smelser GK (1974) The identification of adrenergic and cholinergic nerve endings in the trabecular meshwork. Invest Ophthalmol 13:525–532

Olsen JS, Neufeld AH (1979) The rabbit cornea lacks cholinergic receptors. Invest Ophthalmol Vis Sci 18:1216–1225

Pantuck EJ (1966) Echothiophate iodide eye drops and prolonged response to suxamethonium. Br J Anaesthesiol 38:406–407

Parod RJ, Putney JW Jr (1978 a) An alpha-adrenergic receptor mechanism controlling potassium permeability in the rat lacrimal gland acinar cell. J Physiol 281:359–369

Parod RJ, Putney JW Jr (1978 b) The role of calcium in the receptor mediated control of potassium permeability in the rat lacrimal gland. J Physiol 281:371–381

Parod RJ, Putney JW Jr (1980) Stimulus-permeability coupling in rat lacrimal gland. Am J Physiol 239:G106–G113

Parod RJ, Leslie BA, Putney JW Jr (1980) Muscarinic and alpha-adrenergic stimulation of Na and Ca uptake by dispersed lacrimal cells. Am J Physiol 239:G99–G105

Pesin SR, Candia OA (1982) Acetylcholine concentration and its role in ionic transport by the corneal epithelium. Invest Ophthalmol Vis Sci 22:651–659

Petersen RA, Lee K-J, Donn A (1965) Acetylcholinesterase in the rabbit cornea. Arch Ophthalmol 73:370–377

Philipson B, Kaufman PL, Fagerholm P, Axelsson U, Bárány EH (1979) Echothiophate cataracts in monkeys. Electron microscopy and microradiography. Arch Ophthalmol 97:340–346

Putney JW Jr, Parod RJ, Marier SH (1977) Control by calcium of exocytosis and membrane permeability to potassium in the rat lacrimal gland. Life Sci 20:1905–1912

Putney JW Jr, Van de Walle CM, Leslie BA (1978) Stimulus-secretion coupling in the rat lacrimal gland. Am J Physiol 235:C188–C198

Raina MK, Bito LZ (1979) Correlation between muscarinic receptor concentration, measured by ^3H-quinuclidinyl benzilate binding, and in vivo cholinergic sensitivity of cat eyes. Invest Ophthalmol Vis Sci 18 [ARVO suppl]:189

Raviola E, Raviola G (1962) Richerche istochemiche sulla retina di coniglio nel corso dello sviluppo postnatale. Z Zellforsch 56:552–572

Reale EL, Luciano L, Spitznas M (1971) The fine structural localization of acetylcholinesterase activity in the retina and optic nerve of rabbits. J Histochem Cytochem 19:85–96

Reddy DVN (1967) Distribution of free amino acids and related compounds in ocular fluids, lens, and plasma of various mammalian species. Invest Ophthalmol 6:478–483

Reddy DVN, Kinsey VE, Skrentny BA, Hopkins EK (1962) Transport of alpha-aminoisobutyric acid into ocular fluids and lens. Invest Ophthalmol 1:41–51

Richardson KC (1964) The fine structure of the albino rabbit iris with special reference to the identification of adrenergic and cholinergic nerves and nerve endings in its intrinsic muscles. Am J Anat 114:173–205

Rogell GD (1979) Internal ophthalmoplegia after argon laser panretinal photocoagulation. Arch Ophthalmol 97:904–905

Rohen JW (1964) Handbuch der mikroskopischen Anatomie des Menschen. Springer, Berlin Heidelberg New York, pp 217–221

Rohen JW, Lütjen E, Bárány EH (1967) The relation between the ciliary muscle and the trabecular meshwork and its importance for the effect of miotics on aqueous outflow resistance. Albrecht Von Graefes Arch Klin Exp Ophthalmol 172:23–47

Rohen JW, Futa R, Lütjen-Drecoll E (1981) The fine structure of the cribriform meshwork in normal and glaucomatous eyes as seen in tangential sections. Invest Ophthalmol Vis Sci 21:574–585

Ross CD, McDougal DB (1976) The distribution of choline acetyltransferase activity in vertebrate retina. J Neurochem 26:521–526

Ross D, Cohen AI, McDougal DB (1975) Choline acetyltransferase and acetylcholinesterase in normal and biologically fractionated mouse retinas. Invest Ophthalmol 14:756–761

Ruskell GL (1971) Facial parasympathetic innervation of the choroidal blood vessels in monkeys. Exp Eye Res 12:166–172

Ruttner F (1947) Die tonische Pupillenreaktion: klinische und anatomische Untersuchungen. Mschr Psychiat Neurol 114:265–330

Sarthy PV, Lam DMK (1979) Endogenous levels of neurotransmitter candidates in photoreceptor cells of the turtle retina. J Neurochem 32:455–561

Schachtschabel DP, Bigalke B, Rohen JW (1977) Production of glycosaminoglycans by cell cultures of the trabecular meshwork of the primate eye. Exp Eye Res 24:71–80

Schimek R, Lieberman WJ (1961) The influence of Cyclogyl and Neo-synephrine on tonographic studies of miotic control in open angle glaucoma. Am J Ophthalmol 51:781–784

Schwartz IR, Bok D (1979) Electron microscopic localization of α-bungarotoxin I^{125} binding sites in the outer plexiform layer of the goldfish retina. J Neurocytol 8:53–66

Scott AB (1980) Botulinum toxin injection into extraocular muscles as an alternative to strabismus surgery. Ophthalmology 87:1044–1049

Scott AB, Rosenbaum A, Collins CC (1973) Pharmacologic weakening of extraocular muscles. Invest Ophthalmol 12:924–927

Sears ML (1981) The aqueous. In: Moses RA (ed) Adler's physiology of the eye. Clinical application, 7th edn. Mosby, St. Louis, chap 7, pp 204–226

Sears ML, Selker RG (1967) Denervation supersensitivity of the lacrimal gland. Am J Ophthalmol 63:481–483

Shabo AL, Maxwell DS, Kreiger AE (1976) Structural alterations in the ciliary process and the blood-aqueous barrier of the monkey after systemic urea injections. Am J Ophthalmol 81:162–172

Shaffer RN (1961) In: Newell FW (ed) Glaucoma, transactions of the 5th conference. Josiah Macy Jr Foundation, New York, pp 234–237

Shaffer RN, Hetherington J Jr (1966) Anticholinesterase drugs and cataracts. AM J Ophthalmol 62:613–618

Shefter E (1971) Structural variations in cholinergic ligands. In: Triggle DJ, Moran JF, Barnard EA (eds) Cholinergic ligand interactions. Academic, London, pp 83–117

Sloan LS, Sears ML, Jablonski M (1960) Convergence accommodation relationships. Arch Ophthalmol 63:283–306

Stevenson RW, Wilson WS (1974) Drug-induced depletion of acetylcholine in the rabbit corneal epithelium. Biochem Pharmacol 23:3449–3457

Stevenson RW, Wilson WS (1975) The effect of acetylcholine and eserine on the movement of Na^+ across the corneal epithelium. Exp Eye Res 21:235–244

Stjernschantz J (1976) Effect of parasympathetic stimulation on intraocular pressure, formation of aqueous humor and outflow facility in rabbits. Exp Eye Res 22:639–645

Stone RA (1979a) The transport of para-aminohippuric acid by the ciliary body and by the iris of the primate eye. Invest Ophthalmol Vis Sci 18:807–818

Stone RA (1979b) Cholic acid accumulation by the ciliary body and by the iris of the primate eye. Invest Ophthalmol Vis Sci 18:819–826

Swan K, Hart W (1940) A comparative study of the effects of mecholyl, doryl, eserine, pilocarpine, atropine, and epinephrine on the blood-aqueous barrier. Am J Ophthalmol 23:1311–1319

Tangkrisanavinont V, Pholpramool C (1979) Extracellular free calcium and fluid secretion by the rabbit lacrimal gland in vivo. Pfluegers Arch 382:275–277

Tarkkanen A, Karjalainen K (1966) Cataract formation during miotic treatment for chronic open-angle glaucoma. Acta Ophthalmol 44:932–939

Thaysen JH, Thorn NA (1954) Excretion of urea, sodium, potassium and chloride in human tears. Am J Physiol 178:160–164

Törnqvist G (1966) Effect of cervical sympathetic stimulation on accommodation in monkeys. An example of a beta-adrenergic, inhibitory effect. Acta Physiol Scand 67:363–372

Triggle DJ, Triggle CR (1976) Chemical pharmacology of the synapse. Academic, London, pp 291–398, 602–629

Uga S (1968) Electron microscopy of the ciliary muscle. II. On the fine structure of the anterior terminal portion of the ciliary muscle. Acta Soc Ophthalmol Jpn 72:1019–1025

Usdin E (1970) Reactions of cholinesterases with substrate inhibitors and reactivators. In: Radouco-Thomas C, Karczmar AG (eds) Anticholinesterase agents. International encyclopedia of pharmacology and therapeutics, Sect. 13, vol 1. Pergamon, Oxford, pp 47–354

Uusitalo R (1972 a) Effect of sympathetic and parasympathetic stimulation on the secretion and outflow of aqueous humor in the rabbit eye. Acta Physiol Scand 86:315–326

Uusitalo R (1972 b) The action of physostigmine, morphine, cyclopentolate and homatropine on the secretion and outflow of aqueous humor in the rabbit eye. Acta Physiol Scand 86: 239–249

van Alphen GWHM (1957) Acetylcholine synthesis in corneal epithelium. Arch Ophthalmol 58:449–451

van Alphen GWHM, Robinette SL, Macri FJ (1962) Drug effects on ciliary muscle and choroid preparations in vitro. Arch Ophthalmol 68:81–93

van Alphen GWHM, Kern R, Robinette S (1965) Adrenergic receptors of the intraocular muscles. Comparison to cat, rabbit, and monkey. Arch Ophthalmol 74:253–259

Van Buskirk EM, Grant WM (1973) Lens depression and aqueous outflow in enucleated primate eyes. Am J Ophthalmol 76:632–640

van Heyningen R (1975) What happens to the human lens in cataract? Sci Am 233:70–81

Vogel Z, Maloney GJ, Ling A, Daniels MP (1977) Identification of synaptic acetylcholine receptor sites in retina with peroxidase-labeled α-bungarotoxin. Proc Natl Acad Sci USA 74:3268–3272

Volk CR, Wirtschafter JD, Summers CG (1979) Temporary denervation of the cat iris sphincter muscle: an experimental model of the "tonic pupil" syndrome. Invest Ophthalmol Vis Sci 18 [ARVO suppl]:280

von Brücke H (1938) Die Behandlung der Trigeminusneuralgie durch Alkoholinjektion ins Ganglion Gasseri. Arch f. Klin Chirurg 192:328–353

von Brücke H, Hellauer HF, Umrath K (1949) Azetylcholin und Aneuringehalt der Hornhaut und seine Beziehungen zur Nervenversorgung. Ophthalmologica 117:19–35

Wahl JW, Tyner GS (1965) Echothiophate iodide: the effect of 0.0625% solution on blood cholinesterase. Am J Ophthalmol 60:419–427

Wålinder P-E (1966) Influence of pilocarpine on iodopyracet and iodide accumulation by rabbit ciliary body – iris preparations. Invest Ophthalmol 5:378–385

Wålinder P-E, Bill A (1969 a) Aqueous flow and entry of cycloleucine into the aqueous humor of vervet monkeys (Cercopithecus ethiops). Invest Ophthalmol 8:434–445

Wålinder P-E, Bill A (1969 b) Influence of intraocular pressure and some drugs on aqueous flow and entry of cycloleucine into the aqueous humor of vervet monkeys (Cercopithecus ethiops). Invest Ophthalmol 8:446–458

Walsh FB, Hoyt WF (1969) Clinical neuro-ophthalmology, 3rd edn. Williams and Wilkins, Baltimore, pp 496–501, 1277–1297

Warwick R (1954) The ocular parasympathetic nerve supply and its mesencephalic sources. J Anat 88:71–93

Whitewell J (1958) Denervation of the lacrimal secretion. Br J Ophthalmol 42:518–525

Wilke K (1974) Early effects of epinephrine and pilocarpine on the intraocular pressure and the episcleral venous pressure in the normal human eye. Acta Ophthalmol 52:231–241

Williams JD, Cooper JR (1965) Acetylcholine in bovine corneal epithelium. Biochem Pharmacol 14:1286–1289

Yoshimura H, Hosokawa K (1963) Studies on the mechanism of salt and water secretion from the lacrimal gland. Jpn J Physiol 13:303–318

Younge BR, Buske ZJ (1976) Tonic pupil. A simple screening test. Can J Ophthalmol 11:295–299

Zlock D, Erickson K, Kaufman P, Brasier A, Polansky J (1983) Cholinergic rx results in a decreased content of muscarinic receptors in ciliary muscle. Invest Ophthalmol Vis Sci 24 (ARVO Suppl): 199

Autonomic Nervous System: Adrenergic Agonists

M. L. SEARS

A. Introduction

Increased understanding of the adrenergic nervous system has occurred because of the availability of radiolabeled catecholamines of high specific activity and the development of biochemical and histofluorescent methods for measuring catecholamines and the biological responses to them with a high degree of sensitivity. Interest in applying the tools of contemporary adrenergic pharmacology to the eye stems from several sources:

1. The uveal tract, especially the iris, is a place of very rich noradrenergic innervation, and the eye and its fluid chambers are suited for investigation of basic mechanisms.
2. The adrenergic nervous system participates in several ocular regulatory and neurotransmitter mechanisms.
3. A possible role for adrenergic dysregulation exists in certain disease states.
4. Adrenergic compounds are relied upon in the treatment of glaucoma.

The basic anatomy, physiology, and pharmacology of the three important endogenous catecholamines, dopamine, epinephrine, and norepinephrine, and their relationships to the separate tissue functions of the eye and adnexal tissues comprised the subject of an extensive review (SEARS 1975). For the sake of brevity and to avoid repetition, the present chapter presumes knowledge of the basic information contained in that review and covers the literature bearing on the subject from 1975 to the end of 1982. Many publications concerned with the ocular pharmacology of adrenergic agonists are clinical and deal with ocular blood flow, intraocular pressure, or therapy for glaucoma; some deal with neurotransmission in the retina; a few papers treat the physiology of the lacrimal gland; and a few report an adrenergic presence in the cornea and lens. References to other ocular tissue functions are scattered. The current chapter will reflect the foregoing distribution.

B. Cellular Sites and Mechanism of Adrenergic Action

The conceptual background for understanding adrenoceptor function is based on AHLQUIST's (1948) classification of adrenoceptors into two types, α and β. α-Receptors have been considered to be excitatory (causing e.g., mydriasis and vasoconstriction) and β-receptors inhibitory for smooth muscle; however, β-receptor-mediated "glandular" secretion is stimulatory, as are the β-adrenergic effects on heart muscle. β-Receptors were later resolved into two subtypes, β_1 and β_2 (LANDS et al. 1967). The former predominate in cardiac tissue, the latter in smooth muscle, the lung, and glandular tissue.

Table 1. Partial list of compounds with presynaptic α_2- and postsynaptic (α_1-)activity arranged in order of potency as determined in peripheral tissues innervated by norepinephrine (modified from LANGER et al. 1980, p. 204)

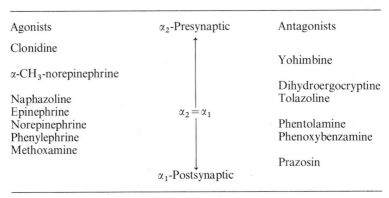

Agonists	α_2-Presynaptic	Antagonists
Clonidine		
		Yohimbine
α-CH$_3$-norepinephrine		
		Dihydroergocryptine
Naphazoline		Tolazoline
Epinephrine	$\alpha_2 = \alpha_1$	
Norepinephrine		Phentolamine
Phenylephrine		Phenoxybenzamine
Methoxamine		
		Prazosin
	α_1-Postsynaptic	

Pharmacologic analysis on a molecular level supports the idea that there are also presynaptic adrenergic receptors (LANGER 1973). These receptors act to modify the release of neurotransmitters. There are presynaptic receptors for a wide variety of drugs as well as presynaptic autoreceptors that are sensitive to endogenous transmitters. Furthermore, although (ophthalmic) therapeutic drugs have a classic postsynaptic action, they could act at presynaptic receptors to modify the release of transmitter. LANGER (1974) first summarized evidence to indicate that presynaptic and postsynaptic α-receptors are not identical. α-Adrenoreceptors were subdivided again into α_1- and α_2-subtypes. Initially, the α_1-subtype was designated postsynaptic, e.g., mediating vasoconstriction, and the α_2, presynaptic, modulating the release of norepinephrine. However, pharmacologic characterization defined the α_1-adrenoreceptor as being stimulated by phenylephrine but blocked by prazosin and the α_2-adrenoreceptor as being stimulated by clonidine but blocked by yohimbine (Table 1). By this definition α_2-adrenoreceptors would also include postsynaptic platelets, fat cells, and vessels. Indeed, they may carry α-receptors all over their surface. α_2-Agonists decrease (by feedback mechanisms) and antagonists increase release of the transmitter, norepinephrine. The inhibition of neurotransmission by agonists implies that feedback inhibition is a natural phenomenon. Released norepinephrine may diffuse to the same or nearby neurons to inhibit further release of norepinephrine. Presynaptic receptors can be activated by agonists different from the transmitter itself and can modulate the release of norepinephrine. Thus there are facilitating (angiotensin II) and inhibiting (muscarine, dopamine, prostaglandins) influences upon presynaptic α_2-receptors. β-Receptors at prejunctional sites that exert positive feedback control of noradrenergic transmission (LANGER and DUBOCOVICH 1978) are also a reality. These are usually of the β_2-type and may thus respond to circulating epinephrine to augment neural release of norepinephrine. Therefore, adrenergic effects, α or β, on pre- as well as postsynaptic receptors, must be considered in analyzing endogenous mechanisms or the action of exogenously administered adrenergic drugs. Radioligand-binding analyses have quantified the affinities of these receptors for various drugs, and bring the question of the functional importance of these receptors into focus.

Indeed, the clinical significance of these receptors for ophthalmic physiology and therapeusis has not been determined. Applications of the concept of presynaptic α_2-receptors to the eye tissues have been few (SMITH et al. 1979; MURRAY and LEOPOLD 1980, 1981; MITTAG et al. 1982). One recent example is the demonstration that α-methyldopa, administered to the cat intracerebroventricularly, produced mydriasis that was blocked by yohimbine but not by prazosin. The metabolite α-methylnorepinephrine is actually the α_2-agonist, since the effect was prevented by inhibiting the enzymatic decarboxylation of α-methyldopa (GHEREZSHIHER et al. 1982). Selective α_2-adrenoreceptor agonists decrease ocular blood flow (BILL and HEILMANN 1975) and may affect intraocular pressure (INNEMEE et al. 1981; INNEMEE and VAN ZWIETEN 1982), but studies of the site and mechanism have not been carried out and the duration of the effects on intraocular pressure effects is short. α-Antagonists can facilitate the release of endogenous norepinephrine, perhaps to reduce intraocular pressure by the reduction of aqueous inflow via β-receptors coupled to adenylate cyclase. These effects may be small. It has been proposed that timolol or other β-adrenergic antagonists may reduce blood pressure, in part at least, by blocking the presynaptic mechanism (β_2-mediated and facilitating) that promotes release of norepinephrine. Similarly, it has been suspected that part of the action of timolol to reduce intraocular pressure may be on a presynaptic β_2-receptor, but the equivalent effects of the drug in the normal eyes and in the affected contralateral eyes of patients with postganglionic Horner's syndrome (WENTWORTH and BRUBAKER 1981) make this supposition unlikely.

C. Modulation and Interaction of Receptor Types

Information about adrenergic receptors has developed in stages. First, physiological response to agonists were classified. Then agonist-induced biochemical changes in the secondary intracellular messengers were studied. More recently, radioligand techniques have been used to characterize, quantify, and discover coupling or regulatory mechanisms for adrenergic receptors. In the course of this evolution a broader definition of a receptor has developed. The receptor is frequently thought of as a protein in the cell membrane with which a chemical mediator interacts. This interaction is usually closely coupled to a biochemical effector. The cell membrane receptors become residents in the cell membrane with finite numbers and bind a ligand with a certain (high) affinity and specificity. Often, however, these resident molecules bind ligands with no measurable associated biological function or response. Radioligand techniques are easy to perform but the results may have little to do with adrenergic receptors (MOTULSKY and INSEL 1982). The hazards due to careless work are abundant in the literature. Furthermore, presynaptic receptors – or others, for that matter – may be unimportant physiologically (although they could prove useful sites for therapeutic drugs). The presence of several different types of α- and β-, pre- and postsynaptic, adrenergic receptors closely located within the separate ocular tissues adds complexity to the analysis of physiological and pharmacologic responses. Thus interactions are complex and, where the effects are modest and selectivity of agonists is of a low order, interpretations are very difficult. Of course, interactions and modulations do occur among the α-receptors, but documentation in ocular tissues is awaited. Interactions may well take place between α- and β-receptors, and this type of interaction could be of a very important regulatory nature. For example, in the membranes of kidney cells it has been shown that stimulation of α-receptors causes a specific decrease in the affinity of isoproterenol for the β-receptors (WOODCOCK and JOHNSTON 1980). Ocular studies are required.

D. Sensitivity

The relative sensitivities of the adrenoreceptors to the three commonly studied catecholamines epinephrine (E), norepinephrine (NE), and isoproterenol (I) are:

$$\alpha_1, E \gtrless NE > I; \alpha_2, E \simeq NE > I; \beta_1, I > E = NE; \beta_2, I \gtrless E > NE.$$

There are many examples of drugs that select receptors (see Table 2). Phenylephrine is considered to be a pure α-stimulator, while isoproterenol is considered to be virtually exclusively a β-stimulator, nonselective.

Subsensitivity and supersensitivity are phenomena that have been established for ocular as well as systemic tissues. Subsensitivity is usually linked to chronic stimulation of receptors (as by chronic drug treatment), and supersensitivity is usually linked to receptor blockade or defective neurotransmission. FLEMING (1975) developed a new classification of these responses, into deviation and nondeviation super- or subsensitivity. Deviation supersensitivity is based on an impair-

Table 2. Drugs that select receptors (modified from GOODMAN and GILMAN 1980)

| | | β | α | | Clinical action | |
		CH—CH—NH			α-Receptor NP	β-Receptor BC
Dopamine	3—OH, 4—OH	H	H	H	P	
Isoproterenol	3—OH, 4—OH	OH	H	$CH(CH_3)_2$		B, C
Metaproterenol	3—OH, 5—OH	OH	H	$CH(CH_3)_2$		B
Terbutaline	3—OH, 5—OH	OH	H	$C(CH_3)_3$		B
Metaraminol	3—OH	OH	CH_3	H	P	
Phenylephrine	3—OH	OH	H	CH_3	N, P	
Tyramine	4—OH	H	H	H		
Hydroxy-amphetamine	4—OH	H	CH_3	H	N, P	C
Methoxamine	2—OCH_3, 5—OCH_3	OH	CH_3	H	P	
Albuterol	3—CH_2OH, 4—OH	OH	H	$C(CH_3)_3$		B

N, nasal decongestant; P, pressor; B, bronchodilator; C, cardiac

ment of the site of loss of agonist such that an increased concentration of agonist at the receptor site causes increased responses, e.g., inhibition of uptake mechanism by cocaine. Nondeviation supersensitivity develops more slowly and shows an increased response to ordinary concentrations of agonists at the receptors, e.g., surgical or chemical denervation, receptor blockade, prevention of release of transmitter). Supersensitive (augmented) increases in the outflow of aqueous humor (SEARS and SHERK 1963, 1964; SEARS 1966a; FLACH et al. 1981) and subsensitivity of pupillary responses (BITO and DAWSON 1970) have been demonstrated and attempts made to apply these concepts to therapy. Supersensitivity denervation induced by chemical means, either guanethidine (for review see GREVE 1977; NAGASUBRAMANIAN et al. 1976; HITCHINGS and GLOVER 1982) or 6-hydroxydopamine (for review see DIAMOND 1976; KITAZAWA et al. 1975) is popular therapy for glaucoma in some quarters in England, France, and the United States. The effect is again to reduce by about tenfold the requirement for topical epinephrine. The top of the dose–response curve, the maximum pressure-reducing effect, remains the same; that is, there is no increased effect. The idea of subsensitivity fits the unacceptability of the inordinately high doses of topical pharmacologic agents used in ophthalmology. Drug delivery systems styled upon rates of penetration and of decay represent a welcome and timely approach to the problem of "clinical" subsensitivity (SHELL 1982, Chap. 2). Ordinary sensitivity of an effector organ is very likely determined by the degree of either neural or humoral tone. Regulation of the quality and quantity of receptors by exogenous or endogenous factors is an important topic in the physiology and pharmacology of the eye which is likely to be clarified in the near future. Thus the appropriate application of the concepts of supersensitivity or subsensitivity for ocular pharmacotherapy can utilize basic physiological mechanisms.

E. Stereoisomerism

Uptake characteristics of various organs from various species for L- and D-norepinephrine have shown that rabbit, rat, and guinea pig iris exhibit membranal and/or granular preference for the dextrorotatory form. Both D- and L-epinephrine and D- and L-norepinephrine, however, are equivalent inhibitors of amine uptake$_2$, a process that proceeds at high amine concentrations (IVERSEN 1967). Stereospecificity studies in the eye are otherwise few.

It is generally known that dextrorotatory substitution on the α-carbon of catecholamines usually yields activity greater than the levorotatory isomer in the central nervous system. Several physiological studies (SEIDEHAMEL et al. 1975; POTTER and ROWLAND 1978; ROWLAND 1980) indicate that D-isomers of isoproterenol, epinephrine, and norepinephrine can lower intraocular pressure in rabbits, as can the D-isomers of salbutamol and soterenol (SEIDEHAMEL et al. 1975). Low but functional degrees of contamination with the active levorotatory form must be ruled out in these studies. In other species, monkey and human, D-isoproterenol was ineffective (KASS et al. 1976). The possibility that a low incidence of side effects will prevail with D-isomers has prompted continued study, but the paucity of data prevails. A study of isomeric activity ratios is a useful technique, but these have not been employed to differentiate receptors in the eye (PATIL and LAPIDUS 1972).

F. Storage, Release, and Degradation

I. Monoamine Oxidase

It is widely accepted that the principal mechanism of inactivation of catecholamines at the neuroeffector junction in most varieties of normal smooth muscle involves reuptake into the prejunctional neuron and binding in intraaxonal storage granules (IVERSEN 1967). Processes of enzymatic inactivation are generally found to be unimportant. Surprisingly, in this regard, potentiating effects after monoamine oxidase (MAO) inhibition have been found on mydriasis in the rabbit (ZELLER et al. 1975; COLASANTI and BÁRÁNY 1979; BALACCO-GABRIELI 1971 a, b). In vivo topical application of the inhibitor pargyline lowers intraocular pressure in the normal rabbit eye but not in the sympathetically denervated eye, suggesting a mediation of the pargyline effect through adrenergic nerves (BAUSHER 1976) rather than extraneuronally. On the other hand, HOYNG and VAN ALPHEN (1981) suggested that a transient hypertensive effect of tranylcypromine was mediated by the

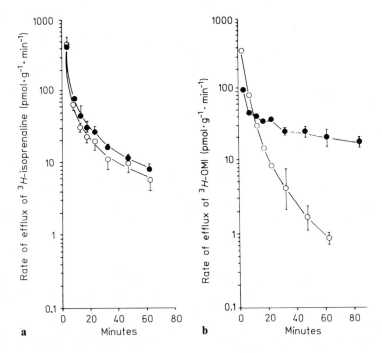

Fig. 1 a, b. Efflux of **a** ^3H-isoprenaline and **b** ^3H-OMI from rabbit irides initially exposed to 1.5 μmol/l ^3H-isoprenaline for 120 min and then washed out with amine-free solution containing 10 μmol/l U-0521 (to prevent any formation of ^3H-OMI during washout). *Ordinates:* rate of efflux (in pmol · min^{-1}; log scale); *abscissae:* minutes after onset of washout. Shown are geometric means ($\pm$ SE as *vertical bars*) for efflux from albino (O; $n=4$) and from pigmented irides ($\bullet$; $n=4$). Note that catechol-O-methyltransferase was not inhibited during the initial loading of the tissue (PATIL and TRENDELENBURG 1982, p. 163)

stimulated synthesis and release of prostaglandins. Since tranylcypromine, although an MAO inhibitor, apparently releases norepinephrine, the transient hypertensive effect may simply be contraction of extraocular muscle. Intraocular pressure in the eyes of rabbits and also of glaucoma patients fell after therapy with pargyline (MEHRA et al. 1974; ZELLER et al. 1975). If pargyline is solely an MAO inhibitor, these results are puzzling in view of the dominance of uptake mechanisms in determining steady state. One possible explanation is that pigment granules can accumulate norepinephrine (PATIL 1972; PATIL and TRENDELENBURG 1982) (Fig. 1). Norepinephrine not normally metabolized and accumulated in this way is bound, relatively protected, and might be slowly released to affect intraocular pressure. The effect upon intraocular pressure of amines that act by displacement of endogenously stored norepinephrine, such as tyramine, administered together with MAO inhibitors has not been reported. This could be an area for therapeutic possibilities in otherwise resistant cases. Only one report has dealt with the chemistry of the two forms of MAO, A and B, in ocular tissues (BAUSHER 1976). Inhibition curves using specific inhibitors support the presence of A and B enzyme forms, with the following ratios of A/B activity: iris-ciliary body, 40/60; superior cervical ganglion, 90/10; pineal gland, 13/87. In ocular tissue, the enzymes have a very largely extraneuronal location (WALTMAN and SEARS 1964). Accordingly, no significant differences in activity were observed between iris-ciliary body preparations from normal or denervated animals with substrates specific for A or B forms or with substrates deaminated by both A and B forms (BAUSHER 1976).

II. Catechol-O-methyltransferase

In vitro studies, using tissues highly sensitive to catecholamines, also suggest a possible regulatory role for catechol-O-methyltransferase (TRENDELENBURG et al. 1971). A study of the effects of inhibition of catechol-O-methyltransferase did indeed indicate that, combined with epinephrine treatment, such inhibition prolonged the mydriasis obtained with epinephrine alone. Interestingly, epithelial cells were protected against the toxic effects of epinephrine in culture. Metabolism of pigment was not affected (KREJCI and KREJOCOVA 1974).

Dose–response curves for mydriasis and decrease in intraocular pressure with topical epinephrine were determined in normal and sympathetically denervated rabbit eyes (BAUSHER and SEARS 1976). Topical pretreatment with the catechol-O-methyltransferase inhibitor U-0521 potentiated the effects of epinephrine on both the pupil and pressure in the denervated eye only. These observations suggested that in absence of normal reuptake mechanisms O-methylation could be important in the termination of drug action. The rabbit iris seems to have an intracellular but extraneuronal (WALTMAN and SEARS 1964) mechanism to O-methylate catecholamines. This O-methylating system can function as a site of loss for catecholamines, but it is a system in which the corticosterone-sensitive uptake$_2$ process for catecholamines (TRENDELENBURG 1980) is probably not involved (PATIL and TRENDELENBURG 1982). Storage and release mechanisms have been given earlier (SEARS and GILLIS 1967; SEARS 1973, 1975).

G. Pharmacokinetics

I. Penetration

The corneal epithelium impedes the penetration of instilled amines, being more permeable to lipophilic than to lipophobic compounds. Relative permeabilities of this cell layer have been given (MISHIMA 1981). On a scale rating epinephrine as unity (1×10^{-4} cm h^{-1}), examples of relative epithelial permeability were pilocarpine 10, timolol 14, and dipivalyl epinephrine 53. This last compound is a pivalic acid diester of epinephrine which can reduce intraocular pressure in the eyes of rabbits and humans (MCCLURE 1975). It was brought to the attention of ophthalmologists and pharmacologists via a contract with the National Eye Institute (SEARS 1971) after a report of the capacity of lipophilic derivatives of norepinephrine to cross the blood–brain barrier (CREVELING et al. 1969). A dose of ester $^{1}/_{10}$–$^{1}/_{20}$ of the dose of topical epinephrine produces the same effect (KABACK et al. 1976; KRIEGL-STEIN and LEYDHECKER 1978). About nine times more epinephrine is found in ocular tissues after topical dipivefrin treatment than after topical epinephrine (ANDERSON et al. 1980). The effectiveness is related to the presence of a larger intraocular amount of the active drug. The cornea, especially the epithelium, accounts for most of the hydrolysis (ANDERSON et al. 1980). The capacity of the iridial stores for catecholamines are vast and the uptake mechanism avid, so that a large amount of the drug is found protected, unmetabolized in the eye.

II. Distribution and Accumulation

After topical application of catecholamines to the cornea about 1% of the administered drug is found within the ocular contents (SEARS 1971). The concentration of catecholamines is considerably higher in the iris and ciliary body than it is in the anterior chamber. Very little of the exogenously administered catecholamine is found in metabolite form. Rather, the bulk of the administered dose is protected by the avid uptake mechanisms within the iris and ciliary body. The distribution of radioactivity in the iris, ciliary processes, and choroid corresponds exactly to the distribution of adrenergic nerves (KRAMER et al. 1972). After carotid infusion only small amounts of radioactivity are found associated with metabolites; i.e., infused catechols are rapidly taken up and protected (KRAMER and POTTS 1971). Only very minute amounts of catecholamines are therefore available to the receptor. This may well account for the degree of supersensitivity denervation that occurs after superior cervical sympathetic ganglionectomy (see SEARS 1975 for review), and also for the large quantity of exogenous catecholamine that is required to produce a physiological response when applied to the normally innervated eye (SEARS 1975; KAUFMAN and BÁRÁNY 1981).

Of possible clinical importance with respect to the issue of cystoid macular edema is the observation that after topical application of ^{14}C-epinephrine the choroidal concentration of epinephrine was two and a half times greater in aphakic than in phakic eyes (KRAMER 1980).

III. Duration

MISHIMA (1981) has clearly indicated that the duration of the effect of a drug depends upon the least effective dose, upon the dose applied, and also, obviously, upon the rate at which the drug is eliminated. In the case of certain autonomic drugs, this rate may be "determined" by pupillary responses. The rate of elimination for pilocarpine, for example, was found to be 0.3–0.4/h. The least effective dose may be found by an extrapolation of the dose–response relationship (MISHIMA 1981). For the design of a therapeutic regimen MISHIMA (1981) introduced the idea of the rate at which a drug effect disappears. The slope of the regression line relating drug concentration and agonist duration, defined as the interval between peak effect and termination of action, gives the rate of effect disappearance K, and the intercept gives the least effective drug concentration, C_{min}. It is now possible to determine T, the duration of the effect of a drug applied topically with a concentration C, by the formula $T = \ln (C/C_{min})K$. The frequency of instillation required to maintain an effect may then be ascertained (MISHIMA 1981; MISHIMA et al. 1983).

IV. Action of Drugs on Intraocular Pressure

The determinants of the steady state level of intraocular pressure are net aqueous inflow, resistance to outflow, and episcleral venous pressure. The latter is influenced by drugs hardly at all. Furthermore, it turns out that the linear relationship between intraocular pressure and the reduction in pressure after drugs has its intercept at about 9 mmHg (MISHIMA 1981), a reasonable value for episcleral venous pressure (cf. GOLDMANN 1950; LINNER 1956; SEARS 1966 b). This indicates that the relationship of the drug dose to its hypotensive effect can be effectively analyzed by utilizing the reduction ratio of the outflow pressure (MISHIMA 1981). Reduction ratios of the outflow pressure and the apparent outflow resistance are similar in the case of pilocarpine and epinephrine, indicating that the hypotensive effects of these drugs result from a drop in outflow resistance (see also KRONFELD 1967). The reduction ratios of outflow pressure and aqueous inflow for timolol, for example, are similar, indicating that the fall in eye pressure after timolol is a consequence of reduced inflow (MISHIMA 1981). Similar simple calculations can sometimes be made to indicate clearly the site of effect of other adrenergic agents. The expected effectivity of a drug dose can be compared to the actual clinical response; e.g., did acetazolamide provide the expected 50% reduction in outflow pressure?

H. Tissue Functions

I. Lacrimal Gland

The lacrimal gland is innervated by both parasympathetic and sympathetic components of the autonomic nervous system. Details have previously been summarized (SEARS 1975). The effects of the cholinergic system in increasing the flow and electrolyte content of lacrimal fluid are known. Adrenergic secretory effects have been difficult to disentangle from vascular effects (BOTELHO et al. 1973, 1976). Data from use of tissue slices, however, have shed new light on lacrimal gland physiology. In acinar cells of the lacrimal glands of rats there is an α-adrenergic receptor activation of which leads to an increase in membrane permeability to potassium (PAROD and PUTNEY 1978). Apparently, activation of either α-adrenergic or muscarinic receptors can stimulate potassium release. Secretion of peroxidase from rat lacrimal tissue as well as potassium release occurs with stimulation of α-adrenergic or cholinergic receptors. β_1-Receptors can regulate lacrimal flow in the intact rabbit gland independent of cholinergic receptors (BOISSIER et al. 1976; ABERG et al. 1979). Protein secretion may also be dependent upon a β-adrenergic receptor (FRIEDMAN et al. 1981). These responses were studied and interpreted by BROMBERG (1981) to mean that parasympathetic tone may regulate flow rate and electrolyte content and that sympathetic tone regulates the macromolecular content of lacrimal fluid. Considerably more work is needed to explain the regulatory mechanisms for the protein secretion accomplished by the lacrimal gland, but interest has developed in this important area (SAPSE et al. 1969; BROEKHUYSE 1974; FORD et al. 1976; HERZOG et al. 1976; KERYER and ROSSIGNOL 1976; LITTLE et al. 1969; VAN HAERINGEN et al. 1978; DARTT and BOTELHO 1979).

The catecholamine content of the lacrimal fluid from normal and glaucomatous patients has been compared (ZABUREVA and KISELEVA 1977). Lacrimal fluid of glaucoma patients was found to have a reduced content of catechols.

II. Cornea and Lens

The demonstration of β-adrenergic receptors in the rabbit cornea by radioligand techniques (NEUFELD et al. 1978) and the synthesis of cAMP in bovine and human corneal epithelia after stimulation by β-adrenergic agents (WALKENBACH et al. 1980) are among observations that indicate an adrenergic presence in the cornea (NEUFELD et al. 1978). The attempt to develop a regulatory link between these biochemical events and biological phenomena has not yet been entirely successful.

A circadian rhythm for corneal epithelial mitosis has been described (GOLOLOBOVA 1958; KOSICHENKO 1960). There is apparently no diurnal variation in the basal (or adrenergically) stimulated production of cAMP by corneal tissue (FOGLE et al. 1980). There is indeed a transient decrease in the corneal epithelial mitotic rate (FRIEDENWALD and BUSCHKE 1944; MISHIMA 1957) upon degeneration release of norepinephrine from sympathetic nerves 20 h after ganglionectomy (SEARS et al. 1966), which is not surprisingly associated with an increased production of cyclic adenosine monophosphate (cAMP) (BUTTERFIELD and NEUFELD 1977), but the likelihood of an endogenous adrenergic regulatory mechanism for circadian fluctuations in corneal epithelial mitosis has not been proved.

A circadian rhythm exists for corneal thickness (FUJITA 1980) and is unchanged in phase and amplitude when sleep–wake cycles are reversed. Attempts have been made to relate corneal thickness and deturgescence to biochemical events of an adrenergic nature. The amphibian corneal epithelium transports chloride ions from solutions bathing the inner (aqueous humor) side to the tear surface (ZADUNAISKY 1966). Chloride transport across the amphibian cornea can be stimulated by a variety of substances, including adrenaline and dibutyryl cyclic adenosine monophosphate (DBcAMP) (CHALFIE et al. 1972; KLYCE and WONG 1977), prostaglandins (BEITCH et al. 1974), and the calcium ionophore A23187 (CANDIA et al. 1977). Adenosine activates adenylate cyclase and increases chloride transport through a receptor different from the one described for epinephrine and prostaglandins in the corneal epithelium (SPINOWITZ and ZADUNAISKY 1979). Increased transepithelial (stroma to tears) chloride transport is stimulated by β-adrenergic agents, appropriately β-blocked, and is associated with increased cAMP production (KLYCE et al. 1973) and with increased light transmission (CHALFIE et al. 1972), but the specific relationship of these phenomena to the endogenous regulation of corneal deturgescence (DIKSTEIN 1973) is unproved. The corneal epithelium is further said to contain two receptor pathways for synthesis of cAMP and chloride transport. The β-adrenergic pathway is located on the anterior surface of the apical cells with a greater density than the serotonergic pathway, which is apparently located deeper within the epithelium (NEUFELD et al. 1982). The physiological consequence of the stimulation of chloride transport by these two pathways is unclear.

Taking these laboratory and clinical observations together, a conservative posture is in order with respect to the extrapolation of results from the use of radioligand binding to the importance of associated cellular biochemical events that may occur. Often saturation data are not provided for the ligands studied (PAGE and NEUFELD 1978), so that characterization of the adrenergic receptor is incomplete. The cells used to characterize the receptor should preferably be from a homogeneous population, and data on the affinities of the receptor for several agonists and on cellular factors that dynamically influence the affinities and the numbers of receptors will help to establish the functional importance of those receptors. Assays done with radioligands are of limited use for the study of the dynamics of receptors. For example, biophysical studies utilizing fluorescence polarization have been done to study the β-receptor in frog corneal epithelia. In this type of study two different populations were found in addition to a nonspecific binding component (CHERKSEY and ZADUNAISKY 1981).

Except for the documented membrane-stabilizing (anesthetic) effect of propranolol, pathophysiological consequences for the cornea after the topical use of the adrenergic compounds are unknown. Prolonged use of topical epinephrine does cause a decrease in density of β-adrenergic receptors associated with decreased cAMP production and decreased chloride transport. Also, an increase in β-adrenergic receptor density is found after topical timolol, but is not paralleled by an increased potential for the synthesis of cAMP (CANDIA and NEUFELD 1978). The sensitivity of increased or decreased density of receptors may well be determined, however, by the excitable state of those receptors. Reactivity could depend upon the action of other modulators or transmitters.

Commercially prepared epinephrine can cause endothelial toxicity, but the corneal damage is related to the buffer capacity of the epinephrine solution (EDELHAUSER et al. 1982).

Of potential clinical importance is the observation that collagenase activity in cultured rabbit corneas may be inhibited by cAMP (BAUM and SILBERT 1978).

β-Adrenergic receptors are present in the lens epithelium and stimulation of these suppresses the mitotic activity (SALLMAN and GRIMES 1971, 1974).

III. Iris

For a detailed discussion of the influence of the adrenergic nervous system upon the intrinsic muscles of the eye, the reader is referred to an earlier review (SEARS 1975). Although the reactions of the pupil are conditioned by the state of the whole nervous system and do not depend on the activity of an isolated reflex, valuable information regarding types of receptors and drug receptor mechanisms can be obtained from studies of the isolated perfused eye (BEAVER and RIKER 1962) and from isolated iris strips (CLARK 1937; BEAN and BOHR 1941; QUILLIAM 1949; RUEGG and HESS 1953, WALTER et al. 1954; DUYFF 1958; SCHAEPPI et al. 1966). In this way a more precise quantitative evaluation of the neuroeffector junction may be carried out.

The isolated perfused eye (BEAVER and RIKER 1962) has not often been used, but this preparation has the advantage of not injuring the intimate relation between the sphincter muscle fibers and Bruch's membrane (myoepithelial contractile layer of the dilator muscle), and permits the muscle to be suspended and to contract in its physiological position. Although drugs are not usually delivered from the arterial side, neurohumors could reach the iris in such a manner. There is a rich adrenergic innervation on the anterior surface of the dilator muscle (EHINGER 1966). The plexus of the pupillary margin forms the adrenergic innervation to the sphincter. Cholinergic and adrenergic innervation to the sphincter has been demonstrated in the rat (NILSSON 1964; MALMFORS 1965), cat (EHINGER 1967), and guinea pig (NISHIDA and SEARS 1969 b).

The presence of adrenergic and cholinergic fibers in both sphincter (OCHI et al. 1968; NISHIDA and SEARS 1969 b; GELTZER 1969) and dilator muscles (HÖKFELT and NILSSON 1965; MALMFORS 1965; RICHARDSON 1968; HÖKFELT 1966, 1967; EHINGER 1967; ERÄNKÖ 1967) complicates the pharmacologic analysis of the pupillary muscles. Furthermore, distribution of α- and β-adrenergic responses is unequal (SCHAEPPI and KOELLA 1964 a, b; SCHAEPPI et al. 1966). Quantitative aspects of these receptor activities have not been fully explored because of technical difficulties. (The maximum tension developed by the iris muscles of smaller animals is less than 70 mg.) A sphincter muscle strip from a larger animal has proved helpful (DJAHANGUIRI 1963; PATIL 1969). Bovine iris sphincter appears to have a negligible number of excitatory α-receptors and many β-adrenergic inhibitory receptors (BEAN and BOHR 1941; POOS 1927). The presence of adrenergic inhibitory effects in the iris sphincter of cat (SCHAEPPI and KOELLA 1964 a, b; VAN ALPHEN et al. 1964) and rabbit (VAN ALPHEN et al. 1965) has been well documented. During mydriasis there is active relaxation of sphincter muscle fibers (JOSEPH 1921).

Further studies of the neural control of the isolated cat iris have been made in atropine-pretreated and in parasympathetically denervated preparations (SCHAEPPI et al. 1966). The first and second peaks of electrically induced mydriasis were selectively suppressed by α- and β-block respectively. The first peak was attributed to active dilator contraction and the second to β-adrenergic sphincter relaxation. Pupillary width in the cat is controlled by β-induced relaxation of the sphincter and contraction of the sphincter induced by acetylcholine and α-reception. The β-effects are tuned to higher frequencies of stimulation than are the α-effects. In the dilator muscle (SCHAEPPI and KOELLA 1964), β-activity and acetylcholine are found to cause relaxation, whereas α-receptors mediate contraction of the dilator muscle. In the human, mydriatic action is mediated by α-receptors (TURNER and SNEDDON 1968; MAPSTONE 1970), whereas in the mouse both α- and β-stimuli appear to act in the same direction (FRIEDENWALD 1934).

The action of sympathomimetic amines can vary with temperature. In the isolated iris dilator muscle of rabbits, β- and α-adrenergic receptors are present. α-Receptor responses are greater at lower temperatures and β-receptor responses are greater at high temperatures. Alteration of receptor sensitivity, interconversion of receptors, or changes induced by a diffusible modulating substance are potential elements in a local environment that determines the sensitivity of an adrenergic receptor to a drug (MATHENY and AHLQUIST 1974).

The sensitivity of the dilator can also be changed by variations in light. Constant light enhances the mydriatic response of the rabbit iris (dilation) to adrenergic agonists (COLASANTI and TROTTER 1976).

The iris has also been used to study influences upon the rate of maturation of adrenergic receptors and uptake and storage mechanisms (HOFFMAN and GIACOBINI 1980). DAVIES and NAVARATNAM (1979) found that receptors may very well mature before the capacity of their associated nerve terminals to release transmitter develops. In the development of the human iris an adrenergic dilator response occurs before the iris can respond to amphetamine by release of norepinephrine. In the neonatal rat iris, norepinephrine synthesis and storage systems have not fully developed, so that α-adrenergic receptors apparently develop before the nerve terminals with which they are associated, and, develop even when sympathetic innervation is disrupted (DAVIES and NAVARATNAM 1981). Clinical investigations gave comparable results (LAOR et al. 1977).

A study of the mydriasis induced by clonidine indicated that clonidine inhibition of parasympathetic tone may involve a central adrenergic inhibitory action (KOSS and SAN 1976).

Employing the iris, an interesting series of reports about the mediation of the neurotransmitter-induced responses in smooth muscle have appeared. The loss of ^{32}P from triphosphoinositide (the TPI effect) after norepinephrine stimulation has been found to be an indicator of denervation supersensitivity (ABDEL-LATIF et al. 1979). The TPI effect is associated with calcium influx (AKHTAR and ABDEL-LATIF 1978).

Denervation supersensitivity to both cholinergic and adrenergic drugs was produced after inhibition of axoplasmic flow in autonomic nerves by intravitreal injection of either colchicine or vinblastine in cats (HAHNENBERGER 1976).

An important series of papers studying the mechanics of mydriasis in detail have appeared; in these it was concluded that safe mydriasis (in patients whose eyes have occludable iridocorneal angles) is produced by phenylephrine, with subsequent miosis induced by thymoxamine (MAPSTONE 1977), an α-adrenergic blocker.

J. Blood Flow

Proportionately the largest avascular mass of tissue in an organ anywhere in the body is contained in the eye. No blood vessels are found in the cornea, lens, vitreous, or chamber angle (the iridocorneal angle containing the trabecular meshwork and Schlemm's canal). Even those vessels found in the essentially avascular sclera are merely in transit. In sharp contrast to these tissues stands the retina, with the highest metabolic rate of any tissue and demands for a large blood supply. Furthermore, the eye is almost continually cooled by exposure to the atmosphere. For these reasons a very high rate of blood flow is maintained to ensure a constant composition of the interstitial tissues and fluids of the eye, as well as a constant workable temperature.

The anatomy and physiology of the vascular system is complex (ALM 1983; SEARS 1975; BILL 1975, 1980). Two circulations supply the ocular tissues: uveal and retinal. The former is densely innervated and the latter autoregulated. The intraocular retinal vessels of the human, cat, rabbit, and rat do not have an adrenergic innervation (LATIES 1967), but sympathetic stimuli cause extraocular vasoconstriction of the retinal vascular tree (DOLLERY et al. 1963; FRAYSER and HICKAM 1965).

Stimulation of the cervical sympathetic chain produces intense uveal vasoconstriction in rabbits and cats. α-Receptors are present (BILL 1962, 1965; COLE and RUMBLE 1970a, b). Uveal vessels respond to norepinephrine (WUDKA and LEOPOLD 1956) but not to isoproterenol (BILL 1962; COLE and RUMBLE 1970b; MORGAN et al. 1981). There are probably no vascular β-receptors, although MALIK et al. (1976) did show regional increases in blood flow to the pig eye after isoproterenol. Demonstration of sympathetic vasodilator nerves to the uvea is lacking. Acetylcholine does lower uveal vascular resistance, but the source of innervation for an acetylcholine-sensitive receptor is unknown. Increases in uveal blood flow are probably caused by peptidergic fibers (STJERNSCHANTZ and BILL 1980). Other vasodilators cause an increase in uveal blood flow only if they do not cause a large decrease in systemic arterial pressure. Stimuli triggering the generalized sympathetic response of vasoconstriction would be expected to prevent sudden changes in ocular blood volume, and in some instances could cause an increase in blood flow to the eye.

The purpose of a responsive vascular bed must be to maintain a high rate of nutrient flow to the retina via the choriocapillaris. Rates of 12 ml/g per minute have been estimated (TROKEL 1964, 1965; FRIEDMAN and SMITH 1965). The choriocapillaris is a rich vascular bed located for the greatest part in a single plane that equilibrates with a small volume of (retinal) tissue having a Qo_2 of 31. The retina itself receives about 2 ml/g per minute; however, one group of investigators reported a flow rate of 8 ml/g per minute for combined retina and choroid (FRIEDMAN and SMITH 1965). The ciliary body has an even higher rate of flow (BECKER and LINNER 1952; BILL 1967), 20 ml/g per minute, but extracts oxygen much less efficiently than the retina. Neurohumorally directed shifts in the distribution of blood flow within the uvea (HENKIND 1965; COLE 1966) could be of importance in the regulation of aqueous formation and intraocular pressure.

Recent studies of blood flow employing the radiolabeled microsphere technique indicate that topical epinephrine in the monkey (ALM 1980) can reduce anterior uveal blood flow for as long as 6 h. The effects of epinephrine on the posterior segment could not be documented. In the rabbit (MORGAN et al. 1981) recovery of reduced blood flow begins after 3 h. In neither case is ciliary body blood flow (or flow to the ciliary processes) reduced drastically enough (30%) to affect aqueous inflow. In cats, clonidine (now known to be an α_2-adrenergic agonist) reduces blood flow in the iris by 30% and the ciliary body by 42% after intravenous administration (BILL and HEILMAN 1975). These effects (reduction of ocular perfusion) are undesirable in patients with glaucoma, who may already have disease of the small blood vessels (BENGTSSON 1981). Pharmacologic studies of blood flow to the optic nerve are sorely needed. More studies of ocular blood flow under the influences of systemic drugs are required. Large numbers of publications report the lack of an effect of β-antagonists on blood flow, an unsurprising result in view of the apparent absence of vascular β-receptors in the eye (cf. MALIK et al. 1976).

β-Antagonists (ARAIE and TAKASE 1981) and β-agonists do alter iridial permeability, and the effect of the latter has been shown to be age dependent (SZALAY 1980). Apparently, the permeability of the venous endothelia is increased (SZALAY et al. 1980).

K. Intraocular Pressure

The finding that intraocular pressure might be reduced significantly by topically applied timolol, a nonselective β-adrenergic blocker, has caused a major revolution and scramble in ocular pharmacology. New investigations have been pursued and have led to the conclusions that stimulation of the ciliary epithelial adenylate cyclase complex can reduce intraocular pressure and net aqueous inflow (GREGORY et al. 1981a, b; SEARS 1980; SEARS et al. 1981; SEARS and MEAD 1983) and that timolol may lower intraocular pressure by a mechanism other than β-blockade (NEUFELD 1979, 1981; GREGORY et al. 1981). Furthermore, the recognition that the adenylate cyclase receptor complex within the secretory ciliary epithelia of the eye can influence intraocular pressure has led to a new therapeutic approach (CAPRIOLI and SEARS 1983; CAPRIOLI et al., to be published; SEARS et al., to be published).

In the 1960s and the following years it was shown that several β-adrenergic blockers can lower intraocular pressure, but the dramatic effect of timolol in lowering intraocular pressure (VAREILLES et al. 1977) by means of a reduction in aqueous humor inflow (YABLONSKI et al. 1978; COAKES and BRUBAKER 1978) provided genuine excitement for clinicians and researchers. In 1958 synthesis of the first β-adrenergic blocker, dichloroisoproterenol (DCI), an analog of isoproterenol, was accomplished (POWELL and SLATER 1958). SEARS and BÁRÁNY (1960; SEARS 1965) were the first to study this β-blocker and reported its failure to block the α-adrenergic effects of degeneration release of norepinephrine upon eye pressure after sympathetic ganglionectomy. DCI had intrinsic properties: the drug itself lowered eye pressure. It did so in the sympathetically denervated eyes of rabbits and in normal human eyes to a modest degree (SEARS, unpublished), its mild effect being similar to that of the β-blockers later to be developed. In 1967, for example, a slight reduction in intraocular pressure was found in patients with glaucoma treated for systemic hypertension with β-adrenergic-blocking drugs (PHILLIPS et al. 1967). It was then shown that topical propanolol could reduce eye pressure (BUCCI et al. 1968). The very modest effects, however, taken together with its local anesthetic (membrane-stabilizing) properties made propanolol unsuitable for topical use. In the ensuing years propranolol and other β-blockers were tried (BONOMI and CARLI 1972), but not until the use of timolol did expectations rise for the β-blockers as antiglaucomatous drugs. Timolol was first shown to have an effect upon intraocular pressure in rabbits (VAREILLES et al. 1977) that had developed long-term elevations of pressure of 30–35 mmHg after α-chymotrypsin-induced glaucoma (SEARS and SEARS 1974). On the basis of these laboratory investigations timolol maleate was approved for human investigational studies in the United States (MERCK REPORTS 1974, 1977). Then clinical studies done in France, Germany, Switzerland,

and the United States showed that timolol produced a dramatic decrease in the intraocular pressures of normal volunteers (KATZ et al. 1976) and of patients with chronic open-angle glaucoma (ZIMMERMAN and KAUFMAN 1977a, b; BISCHOFF 1978; KRIEGLSTEIN 1978; NIELSEN 1978; PLANE et al. 1978). Thus for the clinician a very potent, useful topical agent has been developed for the treatment of glaucoma. For the laboratory scientist, the paradox that adrenergic agonists and antagonists act in the same direction to reduce intraocular pressure remained. Attempted resolutions of this paradox have been discussed elsewhere (SEARS et al. 1981; SEARS and MEAD 1983; Chap. 5b). It is quite possible that effective β-blockers lower intraocular pressure by additional mechanisms not directly related to their β-blocking activity. Interestingly, in the original paper describing intraocular pressure reduction by timolol (VAREILLES et al. 1977), low doses of timolol that did not affect intraocular pressure were able to interfere with the inhibitory effect of isoproterenol on the rise of intraocular pressure induced by the water load test in rabbits. Similar findings have been recorded in humans (SILVERSTONE and SEARS, unpublished) with low doses of timolol that have no intraocular pressure effect but that do block the pressure reduction ordinarily induced by topical catecholamines.

The use of adrenergic agonists to reduce intraocular pressure dates at least as far back as 1900, when DARIER tried subconjunctival injections of adrenaline. HAMBURGER (1923) applied the drug topically in the treatment of glaucoma patients. It was largely a result of the work of GOLDMANN (1951) that it was accepted that topical epinephrine lowered intraocular pressure by reducing aqueous humor formation. Then WEEKERS et al. (1955), who were the first to show that isoproterenol lowered intraocular pressure, and GARNER et al. (1959) reported that not all the pressure reduction by epinephrine could be accounted for by a decrease in inflow. BALLINTINE (1960) and BECKER et al. (1961), using tonography, measured increased outflow facility. Studies of denervation supersensitivity and degeneration release in the rabbit, where pseudofacility is unimportant, supported the idea that outflow of aqueous was increased by epinephrine and that the increase was mediated by an α-receptor (SEARS and BÁRÁNY 1960; EAKINS 1963; EAKINS and EAKINS 1964; SEARS and SHERK 1963, 1964; ROSSER and SEARS 1968).

These and other clinical observations, especially by GRANT (1955, 1969), prompted the description of the reduction in ocular pressure after topical application of the mixed adrenergic agonist, epinephrine, by phases (SEARS 1966a; SEARS and NEUFELD 1975): first, an α-adrenoreceptor effect; secondly, an intermediate phase, lasting several hours and comprising a β-adrenoreceptor effect; and finally, a long-term effect, not fully accepted by all, of progressive increases in outflow (BALLINTINE and GARNER 1961), related to mucopolysaccharide metabolism in the outflow channels (SEARS 1966a; HAYASAKA and SEARS 1978) or perhaps to gradual loss of agonist from its former pigment-binding site (PATIL and TRENDELENBURG 1982). This hypothesis did not completely address cellular mechanisms, but did tend to explain many clinical observations (see above).

In the field of aqueous humor dynamics two concepts with potential clinical application appeared:

1. Pseudofacility (BÁRÁNY 1963), defined as a pressure-sensitive part of aqueous humor formation, appears as "facility" when manometric or tonometric estimates of aqueous outflow are made.

2. Uveoscleral flow, a pressure-independent outflow, occurs via convincingly demonstrated unconventional paths (BILL 1965, 1971).

Both concepts operated to diminish enthusiasm for and reliance upon manometric measurements of gross outflow facility and to prompt a fresh clinical interest in noninvasive measurements of inflow in the undisturbed eye, especially using improved methods for photofluorometry (JONES and MAURICE 1966). Study of pseudofacility was done in the monkey eye (BILL and BÁRÁNY 1966) and in the human eye (KUPFER and SANDERSON 1968). In the monkey, under general anesthesia, pseudofacility measured large (30% and more). Measurements under acute experimental conditions, i.e., single-dose experiments, indicated even in the human that as much as 20% of total gross facility might be pressure (tonometer) sensitive. The lower the tonographic outflow facility, the greater a percentage of it would then be represented by pseudofacility, an idea (site) of possible importance for the regulation of pressure in the glaucoma eye, where outflow facility is reduced. No studies of the phenomenon have appeared recently and there is still no information about pseudofacility in patients either in steady state or on chronic drug treatment. By contrast, a great number of publications have appeared manifesting confidence in the results obtained using improved photofluorometry after JONES and MAURICE (1966). For example, these showed the anticipated reduction in inflow obtained with systemically administered carbonic anhydrase inhibitors and comparable reductions after topical use of timolol (YABLONSKI et al. 1978). The enthusiasm generated by these demonstrations diminished considerably when these techniques were applied to analyze the relatively small effects seen even after pharmacologic doses of either α- or β- or mixed adrenergic agonists. An excellent attempt has been made to review the body of data (MISHIMA 1982). Numerous reports of the pharmacologic effect of the adrenergic compounds on intraocular pressure, inflow, or outflow in several species (rabbit, cat, subhuman primates, and man) have shown inexplicable differences or have been found to be in conflict (see POTTER 1981). Some but not all of the confusion can be explained by failure to disentangle vascular from steady state effects, and by the administration of different doses of the same drug by different routes, these then reaching different unknown targets in unknown amounts, their effects being measured at different times and by different techniques. Fluorometric determinations of aqueous flow done after topical fluorescein (YABLONSKI and GRAY 1983) of after iontophoresis (JONES and MAURICE 1966) have sources of error different from others done after oral or intravenous fluorescein (ARAIE and TAKASE 1981) or after posterior chamber fluorescein (MIICHI and NAGATAKI 1982) or after an intravitreal plant of fluorescein-labeled dextran (MAURICE 1983). This latter may allow determinations over a more prolonged period of time and take posterior chamber dynamics into account, and may disentangle multiple phases (i.e., increases, then decreases) and perhaps demonstrate the relatively small changes in flow induced by catecholamines that otherwise would go undetected (MAURICE 1983). The most likely explanation for the flow effects after topical epinephrine, a mixed β-agonist, is that flow may increase slightly and transiently, then decrease over a more prolonged period of time (Table 3).

Within these severe limitations and on the basis of the body of published data, the following interpretations seem justified:

Table 3. Fluorometric studies of aqueous flow after topical catecholamines

Topical fluorescein		Other routes	
WEEKERS et al.[a](1955)	↓	GOLDMANN[f] (1951)	↓
NAGATAKI[a] (1977)	↓	TAKASE[b] (1976)	↓
TOWNSEND and BRUBAKER (1980)	↑	ARAIE and TAKASE[c] (1981)	↓
HIGGINS and BRUBAKER[a] (1980)	↑	MIICHI and NAGATAKI[d] (1982)	↓
SCHENKER et al. (1981)	↑	MAURICE[e] (1983)	↑↓
NAGATAKI and BRUBAKER (1981)	↑		
BRUBAKER and GAASTERLAND (to be published)	↔		

Flow increases ↑, decreases ↓, ↔ no change
[a] See comments by BRUBAKER and GAASTERLAND (1983) or MISHIMA (1982). Flow probably increases slightly then decreases
[b] Rhesus monkey
[c] Flow was reduced with epinephrine, but increased by metaproterenol, a beta agonist
[d] Posterior chamber fluorescein
[e] Rabbit vitreous; fluorescein-dextran
[f] Systemic fluorescein

1. There are no β-receptors for vascular tissue in the eye (BILL 1962; COLE and RUMBLE 1970 b; MORGAN et al. 1981) in all likelihood.
2. α-Adrenergic vascular effects are transient and are not drastic enough to reduce blood flow to its limiting rate for aqueous humor inflow (and therefore are unimportant for the steady state regulation of intraocular pressure).
3. Early moderate-sized α-effects on true outflow can be convincingly demonstrated (SEARS and SHERK 1963; EAKINS and EAKINS 1964; KRONFELD 1964; LORENZETTI 1971; ROSSER and SEARS 1968; BILL 1969; TOWNSEND and BRUBAKER 1980; KAUFMAN and BÁRÁNY 1981).
4. Reductions in intraocular pressure after topical epinephrine last longer than the eye is white, so probably β-adrenergic reception is involved. These *may* in part be mediated by small increases in outflow: isoproterenol-induced increases in outflow could not be blocked by β-blockers (GNADINGER and BÁRÁNY 1964; BÁRÁNY 1966). Indeed, a response of markedly reduced inflow (GREGORY et al. 1981 b; SEARS et al. 1981; SEARS and MEAD 1983; CAPRIOLI and SEARS 1983) occurs after activation of adenylate cyclase in the ciliary processes. Therefore, it is more reasonable to postulate that the modest effects of catecholamines, mediated by the β-receptor and coupled to the enzyme adenylate cyclase act in the same direction to reduce net aqueous inflow (see below).

   To avoid the pharmacodynamic complexities of in vivo studies, laboratory investigations to characterize the interaction between drug and β-receptor in the ciliary epithelium, the tissue secreting the aqueous humor, have been done. In a well-controlled, in vitro, cell-free system, the drug concentration at the receptor can be determined. It has been possible to quantify the drug–receptor relationship (GREGORY et al. 1981). β-Adrenergic receptors were studied in crude particulate preparations of the ciliary processes of rabbit eyes by a direct ligand-binding assay using ^{125}I-hydroxybenzylpindolol (BROMBERG et al. 1980) and by examining the kinetic

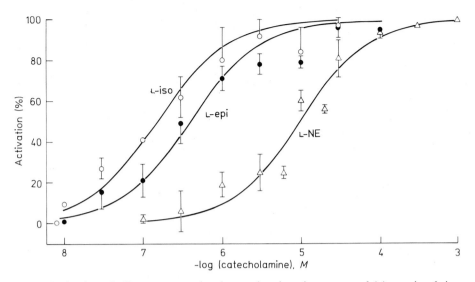

Fig. 2. Activation of ciliary process adenylate cyclase by L-isoproterenol (o), L-epinephrine (●), and L-norepinephrine (△) (Courtesy of D. GREGORY)

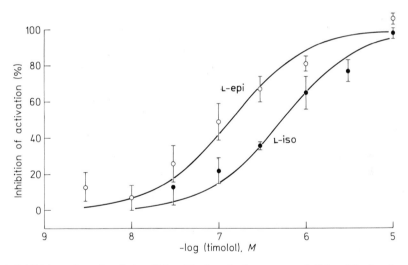

Fig. 3. Inhibition of L-epinephrine (0.1 mM; o) and L-isoproterenol (0.1 mM; ●) activation of ciliary process adenylate cyclase by timolol (Courtesy of D. GREGORY)

and regulator properties of adenylate cyclase linked to the β-adrenergic receptors (GREGORY et al. 1981) (Figs. 2 and 3).

High-affinity binding sites for ^{125}I-hydroxybenzylpindolol were found in the same particulate membrane fractions of homogenized ciliary processes as adenylate cyclase activity (Figs. 4 and 5). Stimulation of adenylate cyclase activity by catecholamines (WAITZMAN and WOODS 1971) was completely blocked by several β-adrenergic antagonists, but not by phenoxybenzamine, an α-blocker (NEUFELD et

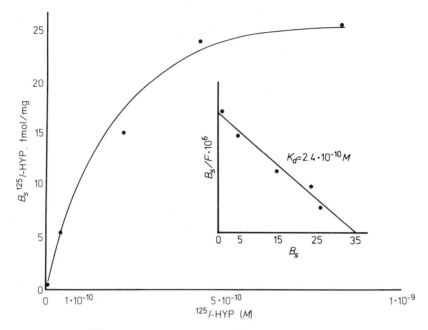

Fig. 4. Binding of ^{125}I-hydroxybenzylpindolol (^{125}I-HYP) to crude particulate fraction from homogenized ciliary processes. B_s, specific binding (total binding minus binding in the presence of an excess, 0.15–0.30 nM, of unlabeled hydroxybenzylpindolol); F, concentration of unbound ^{125}I-HYP (BROMBERG et al. 1980, p. 205)

al. 1972; NEUFELD and SEARS 1974). The K_d is comparable to that for β-adrenergic receptors of other tissues (Table 4). NEUFELD and PAGE (1977) found a higher K_d, possibly a reflection of a technique that included nonspecific binding sites. K_{act} for stimulation of enzyme activity was of the order expected for a β-adrenergic-receptor-linked adenyl cyclase, and K_I's for inhibition of L-epinephrine stimulation were similar to binding constants for these β-antagonists in other systems. Similar results to those of GREGORY et al. (1981 a) have been obtained in membrane preparations from sheep eyes (TROPE and CLARK 1982; TROPE et al. 1982), in monkey (BHARGAVA et al. 1980), in rabbit (VIRTANEN et al. 1983), and human (NATHANSON 1981 a; MITTAG and TORMAY 1981). The potency order of agonist activation indicates that ciliary processes contain a predominance of β_2-adrenergic receptors (NATHANSON 1980, 1981 a). Finally, binding constants determined by the direct ligand-binding technique and by the assay for adenylate cyclase agree, except for L-alprenolol (Fig. 6). The agreement certainly suggests that the two techniques measure the interaction between β-adrenergic ligands and the β-receptor of the ciliary processes (GREGORY et al. 1981).

On a molecular level, stimulation of the β-adrenergic receptor leads to activation of membrane-bound adenyl cyclase and to an accelerated rate of production of intracellular cAMP. This cellular response can now be used to analyze the effects of adrenergic drugs and the effects of stimulation of the ciliary epithelial adenylate cyclase receptor complex on eye pressure.

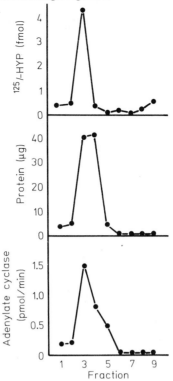

Fig. 5. Distribution of ^{125}I-hydroxybenzylpindolol (^{125}I-HYP) binding sites, protein, and adenylate cyclase in particulate membrane fractions from homogenized ciliary processes. ^{125}I-HYP concentration is $2.4 \times 10^{-10} M$ (BROMBERG et al. 1980, p. 206)

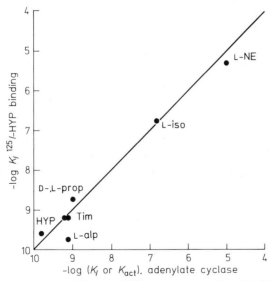

Fig. 6. Correlation of K_I from inhibition of ^{125}I-hydroxybenzylpindolol (HYP) binding with K_{act} and K_I from adenylate cyclase assays. The *line* is the line of identity. L-NE, L-norepinephrine; L-iso, L-isoproterenol; Tim, timolol; L-alp, L-alprenolol (GREGORY et al. 1981 a)

Table 4. Binding constants for β-adrenergic agonists and antagonists (Gregory et al. 1981a; original data from Bromberg et al. 1980)

	^{125}I-HYP binding	Adenylate cyclase
Antagonists		
D-, L-hydroxybenzylpindolol	0.24 nM [a]	0.18 nM [c]
L-alprenolol	0.18 nM [b]	0.74 nM [c]
D-, L-propranolol	1.90 nM [b]	1.10 nM [c]
L-timolol	0.63 nM [b]	0.41 nM [c]
Agonists		
L-isoproterenol	0.17 μM [b]	0.14 μM [d]
L-epinephrine	–	0.36 μM [d]
L-norepinephrine	5.10 μM [b]	9.00 μM [d]

HYP, hydroxybenzylpindolol

[a] K_d determined by Scatchard analysis of ^{125}I-HYP-binding data.

[b] K_I determined from inhibition of ^{125}I-HYP binding using the equation:

$$K_I = \frac{K_d \cdot I_{50}}{K_d + [L]}$$

where K_d is the binding constant for ^{125}I-HYP, $[L]$ is the concentration of ^{125}-HYP, and I_{50} is the concentration of antagonist which gives 50% inhibition of ^{125}I-HYP binding.

[c] K_I determined from inhibition of L-epinephrine stimulation of adenylate cyclase using the equation:

$$K_I = \frac{K_{act} \cdot I_{50}}{K_{act} + [A]},$$

where K_{act} is the activation constant for epinephrine, $[A]$ is the concentration of L-epinephrine (0.1 mM), and I_{50} is the concentration of antagonist which half inhibits stimulation by 0.1 mM L-epinephrine.

[d] K_{act} is the concentration of agonist which half-maximally stimulates adenylate cyclase.

It turns out that diverse adrenoreceptor stimulation of the ciliary processes can increase cAMP (Waitzman and Woods 1971; Neufeld et al. 1972; Neufeld and Sears 1974; Čepelík and Černohorský 1981), but not necessarily in direct relation to an agent's hypotensive action (Rowland and Potter 1979; Boas et al. 1981). This observation is not necessarily surprising considering that the determinants for cAMP destruction reside intracellularly, and not in the aqueous, and that the cascade of intracellular amplifying biochemical events occurs after even small increases in the second messenger. Selective β-agonism (Langham and Diggs 1974; Wettrell et al. 1977; Potter and Rowland 1978), especially $β_2$-stimulation, is probably an effective mechanism for lowering intraocular pressure (Colasanti and Trotter 1981). After all, β-adrenergic receptors present in the iris, ciliary body, and ciliary processes are predominantly $β_2$. It has been suggested that $β_2$-antagonists be used to lower intraocular pressure (IPS 339). Only equivocal results have been achieved with this equivocally specific blocker, as with butoxamine, a reputed $β_2$-antagonist (Nathanson 1981b). Salbutamol, among other β-agonists, gives puzzling results (Langham and Diggs 1974; Potter and Rowland 1978;

MIICHI and NAGATAKI 1982; MISHIMA 1982) and also can cause an external ocular hyperemia.

In analyzing the effects of adrenergic agents, it still might be fruitful to ask: Is the accelerated production of cAMP stimulated by *nonadrenergic* agents associated with increased or decreased intraocular pressure, inflow or outflow? The answer is provided by examining the effect of classic stimulators of the adenylate cyclase receptor complex (SEARS 1978, 1982). Stimulation of the adenylate cyclase receptor complex by cholera toxin gives very suggestive physiological, chemical, and anatomic evidence for the pressure-regulating role of the adenylate cyclase receptor complex in the ciliary process tissue of the eye. Exquisitely low doses of cholera toxin (2.4×10^{-11} mol delivered by close arterial injection or 10^{-11} mol by intravitreal injection) lowered intraocular pressure dramatically by reducing net aqueous inflow (GREGORY et al. 1981 b; SEARS et al. 1981) (Fig. 7). The fall in intraocular pressure was not accounted for by a drop in blood flow, which actually increased (Fig. 8), and could not be explained by any increases in outflow (GREGORY et al. 1981 b). Activation of adenylate cyclase could be demonstrated directly by measuring the rate of conversion of $\alpha^{32}P$-adenosine triphosphatase to ^{32}P-cAMP in the particulate fraction of a broken cell preparation (Fig. 9), or indirectly by measuring cAMP produced by intact processes (Fig. 10). Still other agents, acting to stimulate the production of cAMP at an accelerated rate, reduce eye pressure by reducing net aqueous humor flow. These agents include several commercial preparations of the gonadotropin hormones, expecially human chorionic gonadotropin and follicle-stimulating hormone (SEARS and MEAD 1983) (Fig. 11), but not the gonadal hormones, that actually inhibit cAMP production, e.g., progesterone (FINIDORI-LEPICARD et al. 1981). Furthermore, compounds that act directly to stimulate the catalytic unit of adenylate cyclase (Fig. 12) without the intervening step of a cell surface receptor, like organic fluorides (SEARS 1982; SEARS and MEAD 1983), and forskolin (CAPRIOLI and SEARS 1983; CAPRIOLI et al., to be published) (Fig. 13) also lower intraocular pressure (Table 5) by reducing net flow (Fig. 14) (Table 6). Thus the adenylate cyclase receptor complex in the secretory tissue of the eye, the ciliary processes, when activated, reduces the net rate of aqueous inflow and the level of intraocular pressure (Fig. 15). This must also be the action of the β-adrenergic agonists (Table 3), albeit slight to moderate (GOLDMANN 1951; EAKINS 1963; GAASTERLAND et al. 1973; TAKASE 1976; TOWNSEND and BRUBAKER 1980; ARAIE and TAKASE 1981; MIICHI and NAGATAKI 1982). [See also summary table of manometric determinations of flow in HIGGINS and BRUBAKER (1980). To these could be added the paper of HARRIS et al. (1970), who found that low doses of topical epinephrine may have been associated with reductions in inflow and larger doses with increases in outflow.] Small early increases in flow detected by fluorometry are possibly related to muscular action, i.e., relaxation of the ciliary muscle and increased uveoscleral flow. The later prolonged decreases in flow (MAURICE 1983) undoubtedly reflect a reduction in net flow mediated via the adenyl cyclase receptor complex in the ciliary processes.

The component parts of the adenylate cyclase receptor complex are present in the secretory ciliary epithelium. Data on the roles of most of the components of the second messenger system have been given: β-receptor protein; adenylate cyclase activity; guanyl nucleotide binding protein (N) with guanosine triphosphatase

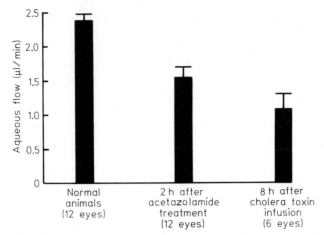

Fig. 7. Aqueous flow in normal, acetazolamide-treated, and cholera-toxininfused rabbits. Acetazolamide-treated animals received 100 mg acetazolamide (50 mg/ml) intravenously (marginal ear vein) only 2 h before measurements of aqueous flow made to confirm suppression of flow values by method described. Aqueous flow was determined 6–8 h after infusion with 2.1 µg cholera toxin in 10 ml 0.85% NaCl (2.4×10^{-11}mol) through right internal maxillary artery. Flow values in treated groups are significantly different from those in controls ($P < 0.01$) (Sears et al. 1981)

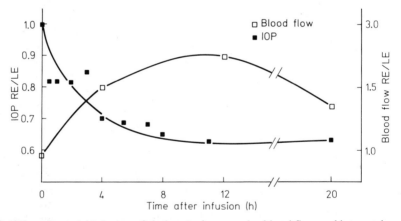

Fig. 8. Effect of arterial infusion of cholera toxin on ocular blood flow and intraocular pressure (*IOP*). Blood flow at each interval is mean of values from four rabbits. IOP was measured in ten additional animals by applanation tonometry. Rates of blood flow can be grouped according to preinfusion, pre-IOP-reduction, IOP-reduction, and early recovery periods (Sears et al. 1981)

(GTP) activity, i.e., GTP hydrolysis is a signal that terminates activity (Fig. 16); phosphodiesterase activity; dependence on magnesium (Gregory et al. 1981 a); and the probable presence of cAMP-dependent kinases (Coca-Prados et al. 1983). Lipids are important in the microenvironment of the adenylate cyclase enzyme receptor system. After agonists are bound to the β-adrenergic receptor, methylation

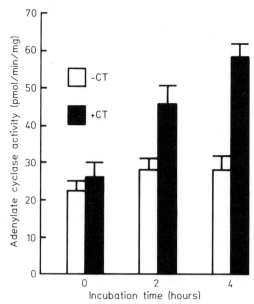

Fig. 9. Activation of adenyl cyclase in intact ciliary processes by cholera toxin (*CT*) in vitro. Ciliary processes were incubated with 25 µg/ml CT at 30 °C in Hank's balanced salt solution. At intervals indicated, the processes were washed three times with Hank's solution and homogenized in 0.5 ml homogenizing medium, and washed particulate fractions were prepared. Adenyl cyclase activity in each washed particulate fraction was assayed. Assay conditions were 1.0 m*M* adenosine triphosphate, 1.0 m*M* cyclic adenosine monophosphate, 5.0 m*M* MgSO₄, 2.0 m*M* dithiothreitol, 10 m*M* creatine phosphate, 60 units/ml creatine kinase, and 0.5 mg/ml bovine serum albumin (pH 7.5) (SEARS et al. 1981)

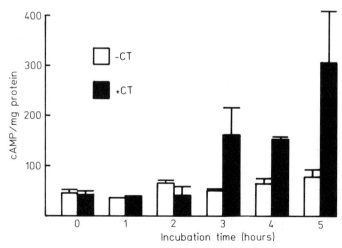

Fig. 10. Production of cyclic adenosine monophosphate (*cAMP*) by intact ciliary processes incubated with cholera toxin (*CT*) (25 µg/ml) at 30 °C in Hank's balanced salt solution containing 10 m*M* theophylline. At intervals shown the ciliary processes were homogenized in trichloroacetic acid and cAMP was assayed (SEARS et al. 1981)

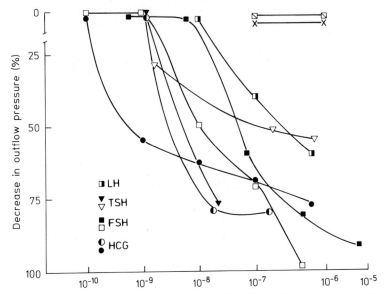

Fig. 11. A summary dose–response curve showing the effects of several commercial glyco-peptide preparations upon ocular outflow pressure in the rabbit, reflecting the time of peak response (usually about 16 h). *Each point* represents the mean of five to eight eyes. *LH*, luteinizing hormone; *TSH*, thyroid-stimulating hormone; *FSH*, follicle-stimulating hormone; *HCG*, human chorionic gonadotropin. Progesterone (×) and quingestanol (□) given to animals observed for 24 h had no effect at doses plotted (Modified from SEARS and MEAD 1983)

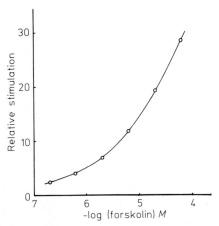

Fig. 12. Dose–response curve for stimulation of rabbit adenylate cyclase by forskolin. Relative stimulation = ratio of activity in presence of forskolin to basal activity. Maximal relative stimulation by 4 mM sodium fluoride and 100 µM isoproterenol was 9.6 and 2.5 respectively (BAUSHER et al. 1983)

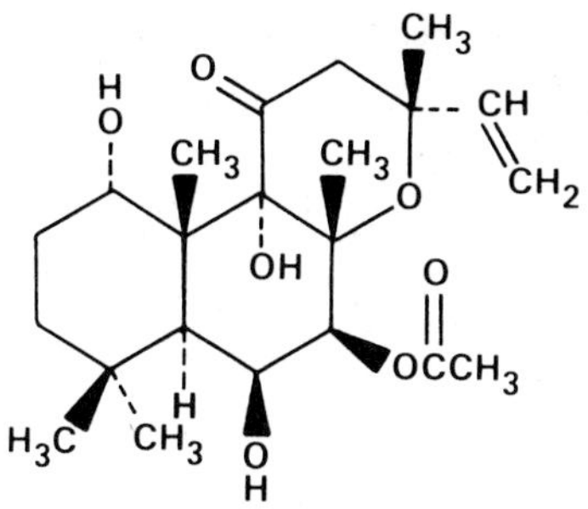

Fig. 13. Structure of forskolin

Table 5. Topical forskolin and intraocular pressure in rabbits, monkeys, and man (modified from CAPRIOLI and SEARS, 1983)

Species (n)	Forskolin (%)	Onset[a] (h)	Peak effect (h)	Decrease in outflow pressure[b] (%)	Duration[a] (h)
Rabbit (20)	0.1	2	4.6 ± 0.8	23 ± 4	2
(20)	1.0	2	3.8 ± 0.3	51 ± 5	14
(20)	4.0	2	4.1 ± 0.3	45 ± 5	22
Monkey (10)	1.0	1	3.0 ± 0.6	39 ± 7	> 7
Human (10)	1.0	1	2.0 ± 0.4	70 ± 16	> 5

[a] Of statistically significant effect ($p < 0.01$)
[b] Values are expressed as mean ± SEM. Statistically significant for all groups ($p < 0.005$). Outflow pressure equals (intraocular pressure minus episcleral venous pressure)

Table 6

Aqueous flow	µl/min[a]	Relative[b] reductions
Controls	2.4 ± 0.09 (12)	100% (20)
Acetazolamide	1.6 ± 0.12 (12)	41% (8)
Cholera toxin	1.1 ± 0.15 (6)	
Forskolin		46% (16)
Forskolin plus acetazolamide		72% (8)

The number in parentheses indicates the number of eyes
[a] Bolus method (GREGORY et al. 1981)
[b] Fluorescein-dextran method

of phospholipids in the cell membrane occurs (HIRATA et al. 1979). Attempts to identify this system in the ciliary epithelium have not yet been reported.

Stimulation of catalytic adenyl cyclase after hormonal signals from membrane receptors requires the presence of a specific protein in the plasma membrane, the N protein. Cholera toxin proved useful in the identification of this protein. The N protein binds GTP and couples the activated receptor to the cyclase, thereby mediating the synthesis of cAMP induced by cholera toxin. It is believed that cholera

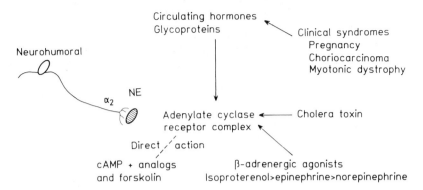

Fig. 14. Summary of activators of ciliary epithelial adenylate cyclase mediated directly or via the β-adrenergic receptor, receptors for gonadotropins, especially hCG and FSH, or ganglioside binding of cholera toxin. (Modified from Sears and Mead 1983)

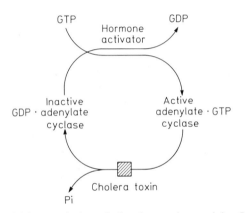

Fig. 15. Simplified model for regulation of adenylate cyclase activity. Hormone-induced insertion of guanosine triphosphate (*GTP*) is required for the activation of adenyl cyclase. Hydrolysis of bound GTP turns the reaction off. Cholera toxin interferes with this hydrolysis (presumably acting to adenosine diphosphate ribosylate the protein binding GTP, thereby inactivating the GTPase reaction. *GDP*, guanosine diphosphatase; *Pi*, phosphate. (From Selinger and Cassel 1981)

toxin enzymatically catalyzes adenosine diphospho-ribosylation of the N protein nicotinamide adenine dinucleotide (NAD) + acceptor N protein → ADP-ribose-acceptor N protein + nicotinamide), thereby inhibiting the GTPase activity associated with the N protein, to stimulate cAMP synthesis (Fig. 15). Activation of adenylate cyclase by an endogenous adenosine diphospho-ribosyltransferase could occur (Sears et al. 1981, see p. 126) by a process similar to that catalyzed by exogenous cholera toxin. If so, reduced aqueous flow may be the physiological reflection of an intraepithelial chemical process in which the GTP-binding N protein has been ADP-ribosylated (Fig. 16). Substantiation of this idea will, at least, require the isolation of a protein from the ciliary epithelia that has ADP-ribosyltransferase activity and is capable of activating adenylate cyclase, as in the case of the turkey

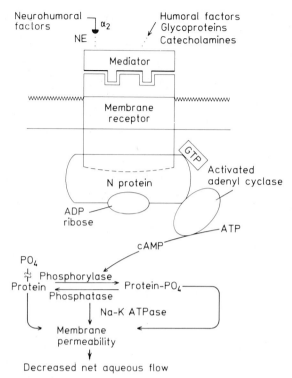

Fig. 16. When mediators act on a membrane-bound β-receptor, the catalytic moiety of the adenylate cyclase complex is activated via the coupling protein, N, that binds guanosine triphosphate (GTP). When the N coupling protein is in this ribosylated state, an associated GTPase is inhibited, an effect that keeps adenyl cyclase activated. (The regulatory role of the guanine nucleotide may include an amplifying effect by GTP and a dampening effect by guanosine diphosphate.) Cyclic adenosine monophosphate ($cAMP$) is now produced at an accelerated rate and activates or deactivates a phosphorylation system which may directly regulate membrane permeability or indirectly regulate the rate of formation of aqueous humor by altering the rate at which sodium is presented to an Na-K-ATPase pump. NE, norepinephrine; ADP, adenosine diphosphate; ATP, adenosine triphosphate (Modified from Sears et al. 1981)

erythrocyte (Moss and Vaughn 1978). Investigation of substrate competition for a ADP-ribosylating enzyme may form another approach in the future development of knowledge about either endogenous or exogenous stimulators or inhibitors that can alter aqueous humor formation and intraocular pressure.

How the adenylate cyclase complex in the ciliary processes acts to reduce aqueous inflow is not known. Cholera toxin induces watery diarrhea by stimulating an intestinal epithelial adenylate cyclase, with consequent efflux of sodium and water into the lumen of the intestine (Finkelstein 1973). Cholera toxin increases the production of cerebrospinal fluid by the choroid plexus and increases endolymph production in the inner ear (Feldman and Brusilow 1976; Epstein et al. 1977; Cramer et al. 1978). In all these instances stimulation of adenylate cyclase activity with accelerated production of cAMP in the epithelial cell causes the move-

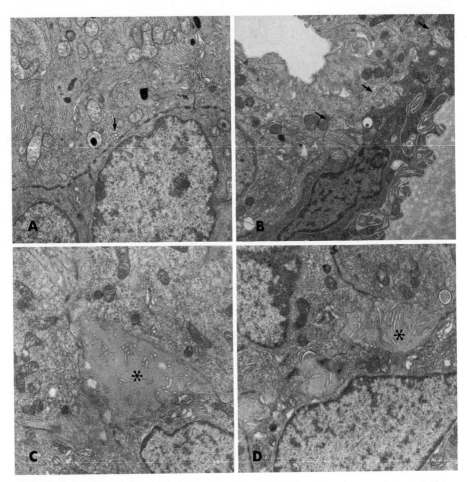

Fig. 17 a–d. Ciliary channels (*arrows*) in **a** anterior portion of ciliary process of normal albino rabbit and **b** iridial processes of normal albino rabbit. Fluid accumulation in ciliary channels between apices of pigment epithelium and nonpigment epithelium 1 h after topical application of 1% forskolin indicated by *asterisks:* **c** ciliary process, **d** iridial process. Note intact intercellular junctions. (**a–d** × 5,500) (Courtesy of Dr. K. Kondo)

ment of water from the basal to the apical portion of the cell and thence into the lumen. The cell polarity of the secretory *ciliary* epithelium is "reversed" because the optic vesicle invaginates during development of the eye. The cell polarity may explain the difference in the directional movement of fluid produced by the epithelia of these different organs. The path for this fluid movement from the apices of the nonpigmented epithelium may be via the intercellular "ciliary" channels into which numerous microvilli project from the apical parts of pigmented epithelial and nonpigmented epithelial cells. This area provides a potential space into which water and metabolites may be secreted. This channel is prominently seen between the two ciliary epithelial layers in man, and in the iridial processes (Fig. 17 b) and in the anterior part of the ciliary processes (Fig. 17 a) in the rabbit, and can be enlarged by

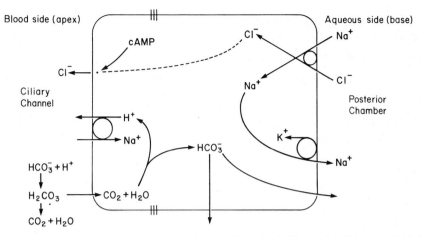

Fig. 18. A model for two-way transport in the nonpigmented ciliary epithelia that includes a cAMP-mediated increase in apical permeability to chloride in response to a secretory stimulus and a bicarbonate-dependent (perhaps sodium-coupled) mechanism for movement of water into the posterior chamber according to FRIEDENWALD, BECKER, and MAREN. |||, zonula occludens

stimulation of adenylate cyclase (Fig. 17c, d) before intraocular pressure decreases. [Interestingly, enlargement of these channels was previously described (UENO 1976) after isoproterenol but the author's attention was drawn to an apparent increase in SER.] It was recently described in more detail after cholera toxin (MISHIMA et al. 1982a, b) and after forskolin (SEARS et al., to be published). Importantly, the increase in the ciliary space is not accompanied by any disruption in the gap, desmosomal, or zonula occludens junctions. The fluid may find its way from the ciliary channels into the stroma of the ciliary processes across the pigmented epithelial cell layer (FUJITA et al., to be published; KONDO and SEARS, to be published).

The source of the fluid within the ciliary channels is not absolutely certain. It is barely possible that the interapical fluid represents a "transudate" across the pigmented epithelium. The increased blood flow that follows stimulation of ciliary process adenylate with cholera toxin, isoproterenol, or forskolin would dilute the colloidal osmotic power of the ciliary stroma (already 70% of the plasma) to favor resorption of fluid into the ciliary capillaries. Furthermore, if the fluid in the ciliary channels were the result of an increased hydrostatic pressure, one might expect to find increased aqueous flow and intraocular pressure, but the reverse occurs. The polarity of the nonpigmented epithelium (apex toward the pigmented epithelium and the blood) suggests that the fluid results from absorption across the basolateral or basal surfaces of the nonpigmented epithelium with secretion from the apices of this cell layer into the ciliary channels. Evidence from other solute and water secreting epithelia (FRIZZELL et al. 1979) such as rabbit ileum and colon, frog stomach and cornea, dogfish rectal gland, among others, indicates that apical exit is enhanced by increased production of cAMP. An increase in the apical permeability to chloride and water occurs after an accelerated production of cAMP (FRIZZELL et al. 1979; KLYCE and WONG 1977) (Fig. 18).

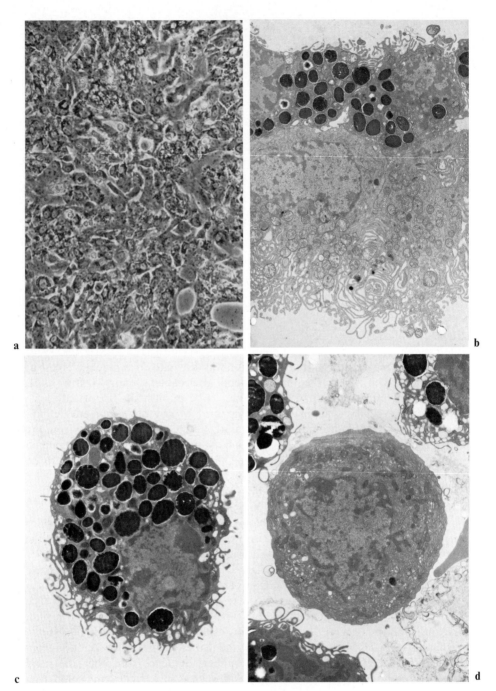

Fig. 19a–d. a Low-power (× 250) phase contrast micrograph of cultured human epithelia from fetal ciliary processes. **b** Stage of progressive digestion of epithelia (× 3900). **c** Pigmented epithelial cell (× 4500). **d** Nonpigmented epithelial cell (× 4600). (Coca-Prados et al. 1983)

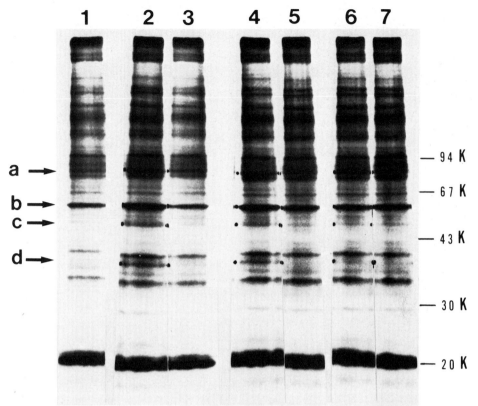

Fig. 20. Protein phosphorylation stimulated by equimolar amounts $(10^{-6}M)$ of: isoproterenol (*lane 2*), epinephrine (*lane 4*), and norepinephrine (*lane 6*). Bands *a–d* correspond to proteins with increased ^{32}P incorporation in response to β-adrenergic agonists. *Lane 3*, isoproterenol plus timolol $(10^{-5}M)$ *lane 5*, epinephrine plus timolol; *lane 7*, norepinephrine plus timolol; *lane 1*, control, no drugs added. Molecular weights correspond to protein markers run on the same gel (COCA-PRADOS et al. 1983)

The sum of the forces for the movement of aqueous humor from the stroma into the posterior chamber and from the posterior chamber into the ciliary channels will determine a total "net" flow. The secretion of a substance against its concentration gradient across an animal cell plasma membrane frequently involves the coupling of that movement to the electrochemical gradient of sodium. Thus the opposing processes may be further regulated by membrane-bound Na-K ATPase activity. Whether this enzyme is a substrate for phosphorylases activated by cAMP is an issue under study. cAMP-dependent protein kinase activity has been demonstrated within the pigmented epithelial cell layer (COCA-PRADOS et al. 1983) (Figs. 19, 20, and 21). Identification and further studies of the phosphorylated proteins in the nonpigmented epithelial layer will be important. Here the energetics and enzyme systems for transport are known to be present (COLE 1966; SHIOSE and SEARS 1966; SHIMIZU et al. 1967; TSUKAHARA and MAEZAWA 1978).

Excellent reviews of the effects of adrenergic drugs upon intraocular pressure have been given and will not be repeated (POTTER 1981; MISHIMA 1982). "More

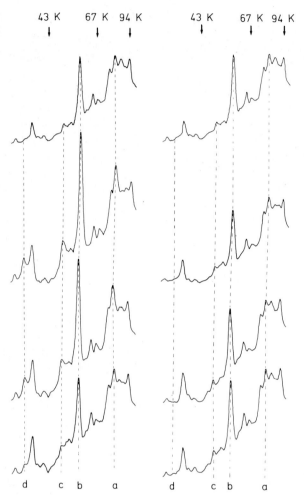

Fig. 21. Densitometer tracing of ^{32}P-orthophosphate-labeled proteins from Fig. 20. *Arrows* indicate protein markers, *dashed lines* positions of bands a, b, c, and d where changes in incorporation of ^{32}P occurred. For convenience only the 94 K–34 K region of the gel is displayed. *Top trace:* control; *second trace: left*, isoproterenol; *right*, timolol plus isoproterenol; *third trace: left*, epinephrine; *right*, timolol plus epinephrine; *bottom trace: left*, norepinephrine; *right*, timolol plus norepinephrine (COCA-PRADOS et al. 1983)

refined clinical methods are required" (MISHIMA 1982) as well as more uniform protocols for proper elucidation of adrenergic effects. A summary emerges which indicates that α-adrenoreceptors can mediate increases in true outflow while β-adrenoreceptors mediate changes in flow. α-Effects are probably α_1, but analyses of subclasses of receptors have just begun. β-Effects appear to be largely mediated by β_2-receptors. Pure α-antagonists may be without effect on the steady state determinants of intraocular pressure (LEE et al. 1981). Timolol, an effective nonselective β-blocker in a tissue concentration approximating its K_d, lowers neither intraocular pressure nor inflow, yet in concentrations two or more orders of magnitude higher exerts its effect on these parameters (UNGRICHT 1982). The site of action for the effects of α-reception on outflow is probably trabecular, and is modest in comparison to the increases produced via the ciliary muscle by cholonomimetics. The site of action for the β-agonist-induced reduction in inflow is probably the ciliary epithelium, possibly the nonpigmented epithelium. Early after drug application (presumably in a nonirritated eye) the inflow may rise slightly, then later a (modest) decrease in flow occurs (MAURICE 1983). Uveoscleral flow is increased by adrenergic agonists (BILL 1969, 1970, 1971; SCHENKER et al. 1981).

Studies of the modes of adrenergic effects on intraocular pressure have led to increased understanding of the importance of the adenylate cyclase receptor complex in the ciliary processes for the regulation of intraocular pressure via aqueous flow. These findings may promote development of compounds which activate the enzyme as new hypotensive agents. Furthermore, the development of new information about the component parts of the β-receptor adenylate cyclase complex in the eye may finally enable investigators to follow a molecular approach to the pathophysiology of glaucoma. β-Adrenergic receptors are dynamic protein components of the cell surface membrane. They have their own turnover mediating a variety of physiological phenomena. It is quite plausible that glaucoma or subsets of the glaucoma syndrome reflect variations in quality or quantity of β-adrenergic receptors. Changes in β-receptors with aging have already been noted (WEISS et al. 1980). It is even possible that autoantibodies to these cell surface receptors may develop, as in myasthenia gravis (autoantibodies to the acetylcholine receptor), or as in some forms of diabetes mellitus (insulin autoantibodies). Defects in coupling of the receptor to the enzyme, or in the enzyme itself, may also exist. Variation in the sensitivity of receptors to changes in lighting, for example, is a finding that indicates that controls of a humoral or neural nature may regulate the β-receptor, and therefore that these influences are themselves subject to alterations. The future is bright for increased understanding of the adrenergic regulatory phenomena related to intraocular pressure and the glaucoma syndromes.

There still is not enough knowledge to enable development of a recipe for determining the pressure level at which therapy for glaucoma should be initiated. Provocative tests utilizing aqueous humor dynamics have lost popularity because they cannot predict functional loss. Clinical examinations of the optic papilla are being pursued in an attempt to develop predictive parameters for tissue loss. Others are interested in documenting early functional loss by means of computer-directed perimetry, psychophysical tests, or laser scanning of the retina for scotomata, in the hopes that such loss will be reversible. Some doubt that lowering intraocular pressure will reverse field loss or even arrest it. Tissue factors or "susceptibility" as primary events of a "metabolic" nature make several ophthalmologists (BENGTSSON 1981) doubt either the philosophic validity or the practical value of therapy aimed at reducing pressure. By this concept elevated pressure would be only a sign, perhaps an aggravating factor, but not a cause of glaucoma.

The reduction of intraocular pressure remains the only feasible therapeutic modality at the time of writing, however. In this regard, therapeutic possibilities are now, in 1983, more numerous than ever. Topical timolol, the mechanism of which is unknown, is very popular because it is without effects on the pupil or accommodation and only infrequently produces local irritating effects in comparison to the adrenergic agonists, like epinephrine, or its pivalic acid ester. Timolol, when used in patients without pulmonary defects or disease, without cardiac arrhythmias or cardiac disease or defects, and, if avoided in children, has a remarkably low incidence of side effects. The pivalic acid diester of epinephrine reaches the top of the dose–response curve at one-tenth the dose of epinephrine, a slight advantage, but, like epinephrine, is also associated with local irritating effects (WANDEL and SPINAK 1981). In a few years we will learn whether the long-term incidence of these local side effects is less than in the case of epinephrine. Systemic side effects of the derivitized ester are likely to be reduced because of better ocular penetration. A popular treatment, not replete with rationale, has been the combined use of timolol and epinephrine. Most patients treated with either drug are unlikely to have a substantial long-term increased reduction in intraocular pressure when the other is added to the therapeutic regime (KOREY et al. 1982). A similar interpretation can be given to the interesting report (OHRSTROM 1982) of a dose–response study of oral timolol combined with topical epinephrine. These thorough studies show how failure to apply important basic information on a drug-receptor level frequently handicaps the clinician and promotes the inadequacy of certain clinical approaches.

Tachyphylaxis or tolerance are important shortcomings of therapy with the β-adrenergic agonists (LANGHAM 1975). Furthermore, adrenergic effects are modest and there are side effects. In this regard, the use of forskolin, a diterpene, to lower intraocular pressure is promising because the cell surface receptor is bypassed. There is apparently no tolerance, i.e., no downregulation of receptors (CAPRIOLI and SEARS 1983). These compounds interact directly with the catalytic unit of the enzyme, adenylate cyclase. The rationale of this approach to therapy is supported by the evidence presented above for the central influential role of the adenylate cyclase complex in the ciliary processes (SEARS 1982).

The reader is referred to other works and texts for a detailed consideration of adrenergic therapy and toxicology in glaucoma (KOLKER and HETHERINGTON 1976; HEILMANN and RICHARDSON 1978; CHANDLER and GRANT 1979; HAVENER 1974).

L. Other Interactions

I. Guanyl Cyclase

Although a diversity of cellular activities can be influenced by cyclic guanosine monophosphate (cGMP), the biological importance of cGMP has not yet been defined (GOLDBERG and HADDOX 1977). cGMP formation in intact tissues can be stimulated by hormones and other compounds such as sodium nitroprusside and nitrosamines. Guanylate cyclase is associated with both supernatant and particulate fractions of homogenates of tissues. (The forms differ from one another and no particular form has been purified from mammalian tissue.) The ciliary processes are especially rich in guanyl cyclase activity. GREGORY (personal communication) has studied the relative activities of adenylate and guanylate cyclase activities from washed particulate preparations of homogenized rabbit ciliary processes and found the rates to be 61.3 ± 11.4 and 32.4 ± 3.4 (8) pmol/min per milligram protein respectively. About 40% of total guanylate cyclase activity is found in the supernatant. The ocular function of this enzyme is not known. KRUPIN et al. (1977) found an increased intraocular pressure in the eyes of rabbits after topical sodium nitroprusside or sodium azide, both activators of the enzyme. The work has not been confirmed. Further investigations of this enzyme activity are needed to evaluate its importance.

II. Steroids and Adrenergics

Steroids cause a direct, reversible, noncompetitive inhibition of adenylate cyclase activity both in bovine corneal epithelia and in the particulate fraction of epithelia from rat kidneys (WALKENBACH and LEGRAND 1982). The finding of mixed-type kinetics is consistent with a diffuse action rather than specific enzyme inhibition. In this regard, it is interesting that both SPAETH (1980) and KASS et al. (1977) reported that increased responsiveness to corticosteroids and to epinephrine tended to be present in the same patients, and the latter suggested cyclic nucleotides as a possible common pathway. An action upon the cell surface membrane receptors to block the action of increased adenylate cyclase activity to reduce aqueous flow could underlie the steroid-provoked rise in intraocular pressure. In this connection, it is of potential importance to note that LINNER (1959) observed an early rise in intraocular pressure after steroids, as did WEINREB et al. (1979) more recently. Inhibition of the flow-reducing tendency of activated adenylate cyclase might be one pathway whereby steroids act acutely to increase intraocular pressure. On the other hand, HARRIS and SCHWARTZ (1983) found in vitro enhanced cyclase activity with steroid pretreatment.

III. Adrenergics and Prostaglandins

The rate at which norepinephrine is released from neurones depends mainly on the frequency of action potentials, but local controls of norepinephrine release by norepinephrine, dopamine, angiotensin, acetylcholine, and prostaglandins, especially of the E variety, have been demonstrated. Nerve stimulation or degeneration release of norepinephrine is followed by an increase in synthesis and release of prostaglandin E. The latter then inhibits the amount of norepinephrine released and its effect on postsynaptic receptors. Contrariwise, inhibition of prostaglandin E synthesis and release leads to increased norepinephrine release and potentiation of the response to norepinephrine. (Prostaglandin F may enhance adrenergic neurotransmission.) These interactions have, in a few instances, been studied in ocular functions.

Prostaglandins may mediate some of the α-effects to keep intraocular pressure low (HOYNG et al. 1982). After chemical or surgical sympathetic denervation, the eye exhibits supersensitivity to the effects of α-adrenoreceptor stimulation and prostaglandin release is accentuated (UNGER 1979). This increased sensitivity to α-adrenoreceptor-dependent prostaglandin release is also manifested by an increased iridial sensitivity to laser-induced irritation (UNGER et al. 1981). The degeneration hyperemia consequent to the release of norepinephrine from dying sympathetic ganglion cell axons is caused by prostaglandins because the reaction can be blocked by indomethacin, and must be norepinephrine dependent because prior depletion of the nerves by blockade of biosynthesis eliminates the reaction (NEUFELD et al. 1973). Thus synthesis and release of prostaglandins occur upon α-adrenoreceptor stimulation and the locus of action of the former can be postsynaptic. The response of the blood–aqueous barrier to the damaging effects of prostaglandins can be attenuated by α-agonists at a postsynaptic level (BENGTSSON 1977). (The effects of α-melanocyte-stimulating hormone appear to be mediated by β-adrenergic activity.) Prostaglandin E can affect the lacrimal secretion of water and electrolytes via a β-adrenergic receptor (PHOLPRAMOOL 1979). The mechanism of the adrenergic induction of prostaglandin synthesis and release was studied in isolated rabbit iris-ciliary bodies, where phenylephrine caused prostaglandin release. Concomitant esterification of arachidonic acid suggested that, after α-adrenergic stimulation, activation of certain lipases supplies arachidonic acid for prostaglandin synthesis (ENGSTROM and DUNHAM 1982).

The development of subsensitivity occurs after repeated application of topical norepinephrine to the rabbit eye. It was concluded that prostaglandins mediate the reduced hypotensive response to topical norepinephrine because flurbiprofen, a cyclooxygenase inhibitor of prostaglandin synthesis, blocked the subsensitivity (DUFFIN et al. 1981).

Prostaglandins can also act at a presynaptic locus to decrease the calcium-dependent release of norepinephrine in irides that are field stimulated (NEUFELD and PAGE 1975).

IV. Adrenergics and Ocular Pigment

Intraocular melanin is found in the pigmented epithelium of the iris, ciliary body, and retina, and in the melanocytes of the uveal tract (MIESCHER 1923). The latter comprise a pseudosyncytium of branching cells, stimulated by the sympathetics (GLADSTONE 1969). Sympathetic cells and melanocytes originate from the neural crest. The pigmented cells of the posterior surface of the iris arise from those neuroectodermal cells that separate from the outer wall of the optic cup before pigment migration. Cells from the neural crest, stellate-shaped melanophores, travel into the iris and choroid. They can be followed by a dopa staining technique (MORONE 1953; BERNHEIMER 1964). In the congenital absence of sympathetic input the iris remains hypopigmented because the chromatophores fail to migrate. Injuries during or after birth can also account for lack of pigmentation. Recovery can take place up to the age of 2 years. In the adult the depigmentation may be more subtle, and suggests some kind of trophic sympathetic influence on the melanocytes. It has been observed by BRINI (1973) that damage to the sympathetic nerve terminals of the iris by 6-hydroxydopamine could also produce hypochromia.

After either decentralization or denervation the activity of ocular tyrosinase decreases (LATIES and LERNER 1975). Months later iris tyrosinase activity is roughly 70% of normal. As the melanin of the iris is slowly depleted by ordinary metabolic processes, the iris gradually loses color. Tyrosinase, the rate-limiting enzyme active in the production of melanin, is apparently dependent upon sympathetic innervation. In lower animals direct innervation of melanocytes has been reported (JACOBOWITZ and LATIES 1968), but in mammals evidence for close contact with adrenergic terminals is apparent (FEENEY and HOGAN 1961; EHINGER and FALCK 1970).

A rapid mechanism for color change is not present in mammals, but in lower animals rapid color changes are indeed under direct neural control. Consistent with these observations is the demonstration of direct innervation of certain melanocytes in fish. In frogs, changes in skin color can be influenced by endocrine secretions (McGuire 1970). Lightening, which represents an aggregation of melanophores, is mediated by an α-receptor and can be provoked by melatonin, phenylephrine, and acetylcholine. Darkening, or a dispersion of melanophores, is mediated by β-reception and may be provoked by melanocyte-stimulating hormone, adrenocorticotropic hormone, caffeine, isoproterenol, and cAMP itself.

Of recent interest is the topical use of selective adrenergic antagonists to determine whether iris pigmentation in newborn rabbits could be inhibited. The topical administration of an α-adrenergic antagonist, thymoxamine, was associated with iris hypochromia. Similar treatment with β-antagonists was not associated with iris hypochromia. Apparently, the adrenergic influence on iris stromal melanogenesis is mediated by an α-receptor (Odin and O'Donnell 1982).

Alterations in β-adrenergic receptor number and function and in the responsiveness of adenylate cyclase to hormones have been observed in tumors. Phorbol myristate acetate is a potent tumor promoter, and by uncoupling the β-adrenergic receptor from adenylate cyclase induces a loss of responsiveness to catecholamines (Garte and Belman 1980). Whether these findings can be tied together with the clinical observation that ocular melanomas are not reported in eyes of patients with Horner's syndrome is a problem the answer to which may merit further pursuit.

M. Retina

Retinal tissue has been used to study neuronal processing, and popular candidates for mediators have been catecholamines. Catecholamine-containing fibers were found in the retina (see Sears 1975, for review) and a dopamine-responsive adenylate cyclase identified (Brown and Makman 1973; Bucher and Schorderet 1975; Joo and Wollemann 1980). It has turned out that adenylate cyclase activity in the vertebrate retina is not distributed evenly. Activity is four times greater in the inner retina than in the layer of photoreceptor cells. Multiple influences are present, however, and these differ in different locations (De Vries et al. 1982; Ferrendelli et al. 1982). The retinal dopamine receptors have not yet been biochemically characterized. By indirect methods, D_1 dopamine receptors (coupled to adenylate cyclase) but not D_2 (uncoupled or coupled to inactive adenylate cyclase) have been found to characterize the retina (Iversen et al. 1980). In the human retina, amacrine cells of the inner nuclear layer and in the inner plexiform layer are apparently dopaminergic as defined by the methods of uptake, localization, synthesis, and release (Frederick et al. 1982). In the cynomolgous monkey dopaminergic "inter-amacrine" neurons have been described (Holmgren 1982; Taylor 1982). If dopaminergic receptors are contained in these neurons, they are probably linked to adenylate cyclase (DeMello et al. 1982). Calcium probably modulates the agonist–receptor interaction (Van Buskirk and Dowling 1982). Embryogenetic studies (De Mello et al. 1982; Negishi et al. 1982 a, b), modulation by opiates (Barbaccia et al. 1982), the effect of benzodiazepines (Kamp and Morgan 1982), the light-enhanced dopamine reactions (Proll and Morgan 1982; Proll et al. 1982; Morgan and KAMPF 1982; PARKINSON and RANDO 1983), and the serotonin-stimulated release of dopamine (KATO et al. 1982) have all pointed to the probable importance of dopamine as an interneuronal modulator of retinal transmission (KRAMER 1971). In this connection, morphological and electrophysiological studies conducted in the brain have indicated that neurotransmitter release from the dendritic portion of neurones does occur (STJÄRNE et al. 1981). Neural processing was formerly thought to be unidirectional. Anatomic and physiological data indicate that neurotransmitters can be released from the dendritic end of a neuronal cell. By dendrites, dopaminergic neurons could modify or process information on its way to adjacent cells. Dendrodendritic excitatory and inhibitory synapses exist in the olfactory bulb. Dendrites involved in local circuits have been found in the cerebral cortex and in the retina. Physiological and chemical studies support the existence of dopaminergic receptors on nerve terminals in the substantia nigra (SHEPERD 1978). Dopamine, probably released from dendrites, is involved in a lateral inhibition of the nigral dopaminergic neurons. It may also be involved in the regulation of activity of nigral efferent neurons other than dopaminergic-containing cells. Knowledge of what actually transpires in the dendrites of retinal neurons will require the direct measurement of electrical events.

The use of chemical denervation (MARC 1982), isolated retinas (GLICKMAN et al. 1982), and cultured amacrine cells (LASATER and DOWLING 1982) have all been used in an attempt to qualify and quantify the responses of the amacrines, interneurons, and ganglion cells to amines, amino acids, and peptides. Acetylcholine, phosphorus, and γ-aminobutyric acid, but not dopamine, can apparently be released from amacrine cells to affect the membranes of ganglion cells that have receptors for these compounds (GLICKMAN et al. 1982). The complexities of the retinal anatomy and chemistry are proving to be profound, but progress has been made (cf DOWLING 1970). It is of no small clinical interest that visual hallucinations can be produced by either L-dopa or by haloperidol (FRAUNFELDER 1982) and perhaps by many butyrophenones. These drugs are apparently more potent at D_2 sites, however, so their action may be central.

Retinal α_2 (prejunctional) receptors have been described in bovine retinas by the technique of radioligand inhibition of drug binding to retinal membranes, but α_1-receptors were not found (BITTIGER et al. 1980). This finding is, of course, of great interest because of the inhibiting action of dopamine on α_2-adrenoreceptors. A recording of the presynaptic electrical events would be useful.

Retinomotor pigment migration occurs in response to changes in environmental lighting. Apparently, cellular movements of the retinal pigmented epithelia optimize light reception for the photoreceptor. When retinas from teleosts are placed in culture, treatments which increase intracellular cAMP cause the retinal pigmented epithelium and the cone photoreceptors to assume and maintain a dark-adapted retinomotor position. cGMP is without effect (BURNSIDE and BASINGER 1983).

Cyclic guanosine monophosphate is produced and found in rod photoreceptors. Increased levels of cGMP can be found in the retinas of animals with certain inherited diseases. It is possible that an ineffective phosphodiesterase may account for the finding. Recent studies in culture indicate that elevation of cGMP levels can produce degeneration alterations in rod photoreceptors (ULSHAFER et al. 1980).

Roles proposed for the effects of cyclic nucleotide metabolism upon the retina and the retinal pigmented epithelium in normal and diseased states are manifold and beyond the scope of this chapter (for reviews see MILLER 1981; SEARS et al. 1981).

Acknowledgment. The typing, editing, and referencing of this chapter were completed through the untiring skills of Mrs. Susan Fleischmann O'Hara, to whom the author is indebted.

References

Abdel-Latif AA, Luke B (1981) Sodium ion and the neurotransmitter-stimulated 32P labelling of phosphoinositides and other phospholipids in the iris muscle. Biochim Biophys Acta 673:64–74

Abdel-Latif AA, Green K, Smith JP (1979) Sympathetic denervation and the triphosphoinositide effect in the iris smooth muscle: a biochemical method for the determination of alpha adrenergic receptor denervation supersensitivity. J Neurochem 32:225–228

Aberg G, Adler G, Wikberg J (1978) Inhibition and facilitation of lacrimal flow by β-adrenergic drugs. Acta Ophthalmol (Copenh) 57:225–235

Ahlquist RP (1948) A study of the adrenotropic receptors. Am J Physiol 153:586–600

Akhtar RA, Abdel-Latif AA (1978) Calcium ion requirement for acetylcholine-stimulated breakdown of triphosphoinositide in rabbit iris smooth muscle. J Pharmacol Exp Ther 204:655–668

Alexander JH, van Lennep EW, Young JA (1972) Water and electrolyte secretion by the exorbital lacrimal gland of the rat studied by micropuncture and catheterization techniques. Pflügers Arch 337:299–309

Alm A (1980) The effect of topical 1-epinephrine on regional ocular blood flow in monkeys. Invest Ophthalmol Vis Sci 19:487–491

Alm A (1983) Microcirculation of the eye. In: Mortillaro NA (ed) The physiology and pharmacology of the microcirculation, vol. 1. Academic Press, New York, pp 299–359 (in press)

Anderson JA, Davis WL, Wei C-P (1980) Site of ocular hydrolysis of a prodrug, dipivefrin, and a comparison of its ocular metabolism with that of the parent compound, epinephrine. Invest Ophthalmol Vis Sci 19:817–823

Araie M, Takase M (1981) Effects of various drugs on aqueous humor dynamics in man. Jpn J Ophthalmol 25:91–111

Araie M, Sawa M, Nagataki S, Mishima S (1980) Aqueous humor dynamics in man as studied by oral fluorescein. Jpn J Ophthalmol 24:346–362

Araie M, Takase M, Sakai Y, Ishii Y, Yokoyama Y, Kitagawa M (1982) Beta adrenergic blockers: ocular penetration and binding to the uveal pigments. Jpn J Ophthalmol 26:248–263

Ashburn FS, Gillespie JE, Kass MA, Becker B (1979) Timolol plus maximum tolerated antiglaucoma therapy: a one year follow-up study. Surv Ophthalmol 23:389–394

Balacco-Gabrieli C (1971a) Preliminary observations of the action of an MAO inhibitor (pargyline) on iris motility. Boll Soc Ital Biol Sper 47:33–35

Balacco-Gabrieli C (1971b) Preliminary observations on the action of an MAO inhibitor (iproniazid) on iris motility. Boll Soc Ital Biol Sper 47:36–38

Ballintine EJ (1960) In: Newell FW (ed) Glaucoma: transactions of the fifth conference. Josiah Macy Jr Foundation, New York p 249

Ballintine EJ, Garner LL (1961) Improvement of the coefficient of outflow in glaucomatous eyes. Arch Ophthalmol 66:314–317

Bárány EH (1963) A mathematical formulation of intraocular pressure as dependent on secretion, ultrafiltration, bulk outflow and osmotic reabsorption of fluid. Invest Ophthalmol 2:584–590

Bárány EH (1966) Adrenergic effects on outflow facility. In: Paterson G, Miller SJH, Paterson GD (eds) Drug mechanisms in glaucoma. The Gilston Glaucoma Symposium. Churchill, London

Bárány EH (1973) The liver-like anion transport system in rabbit kidney uvea and choroid plexus. I. Selectivity of some inhibitors, direction of transport, possible physiological substrates. Acta Physiol Scand 88:412–429

Barbaccia ML, Lucchi L, Kobayashi H, Spano PF, Govoni S, Trabucchi M (1982) Modulation of dopamine turnover in rat retina by opiates: effects of different pharmacological treatments. Pharmacol Res Commun 14:541–550

Baum JL, Silbert AM (1978) Aspects of corneal wound healing in health and disease. Trans Ophthalmol Soc UK 98:348–351

Bausher LP (1976) Identification of A and B forms of monoamine oxidase in the iris-ciliary body, superior cervical ganglion, and pineal gland of albino rabbits. Invest Ophthalmol 15:529–537

Bausher LP, Sears ML (1976) Potentiation of the effects of topical epinephrine on the pupil and intraocular pressure in the sympathetically denervated rabbit eye by a catechol-O-methyltransferase inhibitor. Invest Ophthalmol 15:854–857

Bausher LP, Gregory DS, Sears ML (1983) Forskolin activates adenylate cyclase in ciliary processes. Invest Ophthalmol Vis Sci [Suppl] 24:4

Bean JW, Bohr DF (1941) Effects of adrenalin and acetylcholine on isolated iris muscle in relation to pupillary regulation. Am J Physiol 133:106–111

Beaver WT, Riker WF (1962) The quantitative evaluation of autonomic drugs on the isolated eye. J Pharmacol Exp Ther 138:48–56

Becker B, Linner E (1952) Ascorbic acid as a test substance for measuring relative changes in the rate of plasma flow through the ciliary processes. III. The effect of preganglionic section of the cervical sympathetic in rabbits on the ascorbic acid content of the aqueous humor at varying plasma levels. Acta Physiol Scand 26:79–85

Becker B, Pettit TH, Gay AJ (1961) Topical epinephrine therapy of open-angle glaucoma. Arch Ophthalmol 66:219–225

Beitch BR, Beitch I, Zadunaisky JA (1974) The stimulation of chloride transport by prostaglandins and their interaction with epinephrine, theophylline, and cyclic AMP in corneal epithelium. J Membr Biol 19:381–396

Bengtsson B (1981) Aspects of the epidemiology of chronic glaucoma. Acta Ophthalmol [Suppl] (Copenh) 146

Bengtsson E (1977) Interaction of adrenergic agents with α-melanocyte-stimulating hormone and infrared irradiation of the iris in the rabbit eye. Invest Ophthalmol Vis Sci 16:209–217

Bentley PJ, McGahan MC (1982) A pharmacological analysis of chloride transport across the amphibian cornea. J Physiol (Lond) 325:481–492

Bernheimer H (1964) Über das Vorkommen von Katecholaminen und von 3,4-Dihydroxyphenylalanin (Dopa) im Auge. Arch Exp Pathol Pharmakol 247:202–213

Bhargava G, Makman MH, Katzman R (1980) Distribution of β-adrenergic receptors and isoproterenol-stimulated cyclic AMP formation in monkey iris and ciliary body. Exp Eye Res 31:471–477

Bill A (1962) Autonomic nervous control of uveal blood flow. Acta Physiol Scand 56:70–81

Bill A (1965) The aqueous humor drainage mechanism in the cynomolgus monkey (Macaca irus) with evidence for unconventional routes. Invest Ophthalmol 4:911–919

Bill A (1969) Early effects of epinephrine on aqueous humor dynamics in vervet monkeys (Cercopithecus ethiops). Exp Eye Res 8:35–43

Bill A (1970) Effects of norepinephrine, isoproterenol and sympathetic stimulation on aqueous humor dynamics in vervet monkeys. Exp Eye Res 10:31–46

Bill A (1971) Aqueous humor dynamics in monkeys (Macaca irus and Cercopithecus ethiops). Exp Eye Res 11:195–206

Bill A (1975) Blood circulation and fluid dynamics in the eye. Physiol Rev 55:383–417

Bill A (1980) Ocular circulation. In: Moses RA (ed) Adler's physiology of the eye. Mosby, St. Louis, Chap. 7

Bill A, Bárány EH (1966) Gross facility, facility of conventional routes and pseudofacility of aqueous humor outflow in the cynomolgus monkey. Arch Ophthalmol 75:665–673

Bill A, Heilmann K (1975) Ocular effects of clonidine in cats and monkeys (Macaca irus). Exp Eye Res 21:481–488

Bischoff P (1978) Erfahrungen mit Timolol in der Glaukom-Therapie. Klin Monatsbl Augenheilkd 173:202–207

Bito LA, Dawson MJ (1970) The site and mechanism of the control of cholinergic sensitivity. J Pharmacol Exp Ther 175:673–684

Bittiger H, Heid J, Wigger N (1980) Are only alpha$_2$-adrenergic receptors present in bovine retina? Nature 287:645–647

Boas RS, Messenger MJ, Mittag TW, Podos SM (1981) The effects of topically applied epinephrine and timolol on intraocular pressure and aqueous humor cyclic-AMP in the rabbit. Exp Eye Res 32:681–690

Boissier J-R, Advenier CH, Ho S (1976) Sécrétion lacrymale chez le lapin et récepteurs β-adrénergiques. J Pharmacol 7:241–250

Bonomi L, Carli A (1972) Sugli effetti dell'instillazione di propranololo sulla dinamica dell'umore acqueo in occhi umani glaucomatosi. Minerva Oftal 14:28–32

Botelho SY, Goldstein AM, Martinez EV (1973) Norepinephrine-responsive β-adrenergic receptors in rabbit lacrimal gland. Am J Physiol 224:1119–1122

Botelho SY, Martinez EV, Pholpramool C, van Prooyen HC, Janssen JT, DePalau A (1976) Modification of stimulated lacrimal gland flow by sympathetic nerve impulses in rabbit. Am J Physiol 230:80–84

Brini A (1973) Hypochromia of the rabbit iris induced by 6-hydroxydopamine. Invest Ophthalmol 12:312–313

Broekhuyse RM (1974) Tear lactoferrin: a bacteriostatic and complexing protein. Invest Ophthalmol 13:550–554

Bromberg BB (1981) Autonomic control of lacrimal protein secretion. Invest Ophthalmol Vis Sci 20:110–116

Bromberg BB, Gregory DS, Sears ML (1980) Beta adrenergic receptors in ciliary processes of the rabbit. Invest Ophthalmol Vis Sci 19:203–207

Brown JH, Makman MH (1973) Influence of neuroleptic drugs and apomorphine on dopamine-sensitive adenylate cyclase of retina. J Neurochem 21:477–479

Brubaker RF, Gaasterland D (to be published) The effect of isoproterenol on aqueous humor formation in humans

Bucci MG, Missiroli A, Pecori Giraldi J, Virno M (1968) Local administration of propranolol in the glaucoma therapy. Boll Ocul 47:51–60

Bucher MB, Schorderet M (1975) Dopamine- and apomorphine-sensitive adenylate cyclase in homogenates of rabbit retina. Naunyn Schmiedebergs Arch Pharmacol 288:103–107

Burnside B, Basinger S (1983) Retinomotor pigment migration in the teleost retinal pigment epithelium. II. Cyclic-3′,5′-adenosine monophosphate induction of dark-adaptive movement in vitro. Invest Ophthalmol Vis Sci 24:16–23

Butterfield LC, Neufeld AH (1977) Cyclic nucleotides and mitosis in the rabbit cornea following superior cervical ganglionectomy. Exp Eye Res 25:427–433

Candia OA, Neufeld AH (1978) Topical epinephrine causes a decrease in density of beta-adrenergic receptors and catecholamine-stimulated chloride transport in the rabbit cornea. Biochim Biophys Acta 543:403–408

Candia OA, Montoreano R, Podos SM (1977) Effect of the ionophore A23187 on chloride transport across isolated frog cornea. Am J Physiol 233:F94–101

Caprioli J, Sears M (1983) Forskolin lowers intraocular pressure in rabbits, monkeys and man. Lancet I:958–960

Caprioli J, Sears M, Bausher L, Gregory D (to be published) Forskolin lowers intraocular pressure by reducing aqueous flow. Invest Ophthalmol Vis Sci

Čepelík J, Černohorský M (1981) The effects of adrenergic agonists and antagonists on the adenylate cyclase in albino rabbit ciliary processes. Exp Eye Res 32:291–299

Chalfie M, Neufeld AH, Zadunaisky JA (1972) Action of epinephrine and other cyclic AMP-mediated agents on the chloride transport of the frog cornea. Invest Ophthalmol 11:644–650

Chandler PA, Grant WM (eds) (1979) Glaucoma, 2nd edn. Lea and Febiger, Philadelphia

Cherksey BD, Zadunaisky JA (1981) Membrane beta receptors: interaction with cytoskeleton in chloride secreting systems. Ann NY Acad Sci 372:309–331

Clark SL (1937) Innervation of the intrinsic muscles of the eye of the cat. J Comp Neurol 66:307–320

Coakes RL, Brubaker RF (1978) The mechanism of timolol in lowering intraocular pressure in the normal eye. Arch Ophthalmol 96:2045–2048

Coca-Prados M, Kondo K, Sears M (1983) Protein phosphorylation in cultured human ciliary epithelia in response to activators of adenylate cyclase, cyclic AMP and analogues. In: Krieglstein GK, Leydhecker HW (eds) Glaucoma update II. International glaucoma symposium, Carmel, California, 22–27 October 1982. Springer, Berlin Heidelberg New York

Cohen KL, van Horn DL, Edelhauser HF, Schultz RO (1979) Effect of phenylephrine on normal and regenerated endothelial cells in cat cornea. Invest Ophthalmol Vis Sci 18:242–249

Colasanti BK, Bárány EH (1979) Potentiation of the mydriatic effect of norepinephrine in the rabbit after MAO inhibition. Invest Ophthalmol Vis Sci 18:200–203

Colasanti BK, Trotter RR (1976) Alterations in adrenergic sensitivity of the rabbit iris after variation of environmental lighting conditions. Invest Ophthalmol 15:44–47

Colasanti BK, Trotter RR (1981) Effects of selective beta$_1$ and beta$_2$ adrenoreceptor agonists and antagonists on intraocular pressure in the cat. Invest Ophthalmol Vis Sci 20:69–76

Cole DF (1966) Aqueous humor formation. Doc Ophthalmol 21:116–238

Cole DF, Monro PAG (1976) The use of fluorescein-labelled dextrans in investigation of aqueous humour outflow in the rabbit. Exp Eye Res 23:571–585

Cole DF, Rumble R (1970a) Effects of catecholamines on circulation in the rabbit iris. Exp Eye Res 9:219–232

Cole DF, Rumble R (1970b) Responses of iris blood flow to stimulation of the cervical sympathetic in the rabbit. Exp Eye Res 10:183–191

Cramer H, Hammers R, Maier P, Schindler H (1978) Cyclic 3′,5′-adenosine monophosphate in the choroid plexus: stimulation by cholera toxin. Biochem Biophys Res Commun 84:1031–1037

Creveling CF, Daly JW, Tokuyama T, Witkop B (1969) Labile lipophilic derivatives of norepinephrine capable of crossing the blood-brain barrier. Experientia 25:26–27

Darier A (1900) De l'extrait de capsule surrénales en thérapeutique oculaire. Lab Clin Ophthalmol 6:141

Dartt LA, Botelho SY (1979) Protein in rabbit lacrimal gland fluid. Invest Ophthalmol Vis Sci 18:1207–1209

Davies DC, Navaratnam Y (1979) Development of adrenoceptive and cholinoceptive responsiveness in the neonatal rat iris. Exp Eye Res 29:203–210

Davies DC, Navaratnam V (1981) Differentiation of α-adrenergic responsiveness in the neonatal rat iris after decentralization or extirpation of the superior cervical ganglion. Brain Res 213:119–216

Demailly P, Lehner MA, Duperré J (1976) A new beta blocker in the treatment of chronic glaucoma: timolol maleate. Bull Soc Ophtalmol Paris 76:801–802

De Mello MC, Ventura AL, Paes-de-Carvalho R, Klein WL, De Mello FG (1982) Regulation of dopamine and adenosine-dependent adenylate cyclase systems of chicken embryo retina cells in culture. Proc Natl Acad Sci USA 79:5708–5712

De Vries GW, Campau KM, Ferrendelli JA (1982) Adenylate cyclases in the vertebrate retina: distribution and characteristics in rabbit and ground squirrel. J Neurochem 38:759–765

Diamond JG (1976) 6-hydroxydopamine in treatment of open angle glaucoma. Arch Ophthalmol 94:41–47

Dikstein S (1973) Efficiency and survival of the corneal endothelial pump. Exp Eye Res 15:639–644

Djahanguiri B (1963) Action d'amine dérivées du catéchol sur le muscle iridien de bovidé. Arch Int Pharmacodyn Ther 142:276–278

Dollery CT, Hill DW, Hodge JV (1963) The response of normal retinal blood vessels to angiotensin and noradrenaline. J Physiol (Lond) 165:500–506

Dowling JE (1970) Organization of vertebrate retinas. Invest Ophthalmol 9:655–680

Dowling JE, Ehinger B (1978) The interplexiform cell system. I. Synapses of the dopaminergic neurons of the goldfish retina. Proc. R Soc Lond [Biol] 201:7–26

Duffin RM, Christensen RE, Bergamini MVW (1981) Suppression of adrenergic adaptation in the eye with a prostaglandin synthesis inhibitor. Invest Ophthalmol Vis Sci 21:756–759

Duyff JW (1958) Kinetics of receptor occupation. Acta Physiol Pharmacol Neerl 7:239–254

Eakins KE (1963) Effect of intravitreous injections of norepinephrine, epinephrine, and isoproterenol on the intraocular pressure and aqueous humor dynamics of rabbit eyes. J Pharmacol Exp Ther 140:79–84

Eakins KE, Eakins HMT (1964) Adrenergic mechanisms and the outflow of aqueous humor from the rabbit eye. J Pharmacol Exp Ther 144:60–65

Edelhauser HF, Hyndiuk RA, Zeeb A, Schulte RO (1982) Corneal edema and the intraocular use of epinephrine. Am J Ophthalmol 93:327–333

Ehinger B (1966) Ocular and orbital vegetative nerves. Acta Physiol Scand [Suppl] 268

Ehinger B (1967) Double innervation of the feline iris dilator. Arch Ophthalmol 77:541–545

Ehinger B, Falck B (1970) Innervation of iridic melanophores. Z Zellforsch Mikrosk Anat 105:538–542

Engstrom P, Dunham EW (1982) Alpha adrenergic stimulation of prostaglandin release from rabbit iris ciliary body in vitro. Invest Ophthalmol Vis Sci 22:757–767

Epstein MH, Feldman AM, Brusilow SW (1977) Cerebrospinal fluid production: stimulation by cholera toxin. Science 196:1012–1013

Eränkö O, Räisänen L (1965) Fibers containing both noradrenaline and acetylcholinesterase in the nerve net of the rat iris. Acta Physiol Scand 63:505–506

Eränkö O (1967) Histochemistry of nervous tissues: catecholamines and cholinesterases. Ann Rev Pharmacol 7:203–222

Feeney L, Hogan MJ (1961) Electron microscopy of the human choroid. II. The choroidal nerves. Am J Ophthalmol 51:200–211

Feldman AM, Brusilow SW (1976) Effects of cholera toxin on cochlear endolymph production. Model for endolymphatic hydrops. Proc Natl Acad Sci USA 73:1761–1764

Ferrendelli JA, Campau KM, DeVries GW (1982) Adenylate cyclases in vertebrate retina: enzymatic characteristics in normal and dystrophic mouse retina. J Neurochem 38:753–758

Finidori-Lepicard J, Schorderet-Slatkine S, Hanoune J, Baulieu EE (1981) Progesterone inhibits membrane-bound adenylate cyclase in Xenopis laevis oocytes. Nature 292:255–256

Finkelstein RA (1973) Cholera. CRC Crit Rev Microbiol 2:553–623

Flach AJ, Peterson JS, Wood I, Roizen MF (1981) Degeneration of nerve terminals in cats following systemic epinephrine: depletion of tissue norepinephrine correlated with ultrastructural changes. Exp Eye Res 32:389–394

Fleming WW (1975) Supersensitivity in smooth muscle. Introduction and historical perspective. Fed Proc 34:1960–1970

Flower RJ, Blackwell GJ (1979) Anti-inflammatory steroids induce biosynthesis of a phospholipase A_2 inhibitor which prevents prostaglandin generation. Nature 278:456–459

Fogle JA, Neufeld AH (1979) The adrenergic and cholinergic corneal epithelium. Invest Ophthalmol Vis Sci 18:1212–1215

Fogle JA, Yoza BK, Neufeld AH (1980) Diurnal rhythm of mitosis in rabbit corneal epithelium. Albrecht von Graefes Arch Klin Exp Ophthalmol 213:143–148

Ford LC, DeLance RJ, Petty RW (1976) Identification of a nonlysosomal bactericidal factor (beta lysin) in human tears and aqueous humor. Am J Ophthalmol 81:30–33

Fraunfelder FT (1982) Drug-induced ocular side effects and drug interactions. 2nd edn. Lea and Febiger, Philadelphia

Frayser R, Hickam JB (1965) Effect of vasodilatator drugs in the retinal blood flow in man. Arch Ophthalmol 73:640–642

Frederick JM, Rayborn ME, Laties AM, Lam DM, Hollyfield JG (1982) Dopaminergic neurons in the human retina. J Comp Neurol 210:65–79

Friedenwald JS (1934) Retinal vascular dynamics. Am J Ophthalmol 17:387–395

Friedenwald JS, Buschke W (1958) The effects of excitement of epinephrine and sympathectomy on the mitotic activity of the corneal epithelium in rats. Am J Physiol 141:689–694

Friedman E, Smith TR (1965) Estimation of retinal blood flow in animals. Invest Ophthalmol 4:1122–1128

Friedman Z, Lowe M, Selinger Z (1981) Beta adrenergic receptors stimulated peroxidase secretion from rat lacrimal gland. Biochem Biophys Acta 675:40–45

Frizzell RA, Field M, Schultz SG (1979) Sodium coupled chloride transport by epithelial tissues. Am J Physiol 236:F1–F8

Fujita S (1980) Diurnal variation in human corneal thickness. Jpn J Ophthalmol 24:444–456

Fujita H, Kondo K, Sears M (to be published) Hypothesis on the formation of aqueous humor with special regard to the role of the nonpigmented epithelium of the ciliary processes. Internat Ophthalmol

Gaasterland D, Kupfer C, Ross K, Gabelnick HL (1973) Studies of aqueous humor dynamics in man. 3. Measurements in young normal subjects using norepinephrine and isoproterenol. Invest Ophthalmol 12:267–279

Garner LL, Johnstone WW, Ballintine EJ, Carrol ME (1959) Effect of 2% levorotatory epinephrine on the intraocular pressure of the glaucomatous eye. Arch Ophthalmol 62:230–238

Garte SJ, Belman S (1980) Tumour promoter uncouples β-adrenergic receptor from adenyl cyclase in mouse epidermis. Nature 284:171–173

Geltzer A (1969) Autonomic innervation of the cat iris. An electron microscopic study. Arch Ophthalmol 81:70–83

Gherezshiher T, Christensen HD, Koss MC (1982) Studies on the mechanism of methyl-dopa-induced mydriasis in the cat. Naunyn Schmiedebergs Arch Pharmacol 320:58–62

Gladstone RM (1969) Development and significance of heterochromia of the iris. Arch Neurol 21:184–191

Glickman RD, Adolph AR, Dowling JE (1982) Inner plexiform circuits in the carp retina: effects of cholinergic agonists, GABA and substance P on the ganglion cells. Brain Res 234:81–99

Gnädinger MC, Bárány EH (1964) Die Wirkung der β-adrenergischen Substanz Isoprenalin auf die Ausfluß-Fazilität des Kaninchenauges. Albrecht von Graefes Arch Ophthalmol 167:483–492

Goldberg ND, Haddox MR (1977) Cyclic GMP metabolism and involvement in biological regulation Annu Rev Biochem 46:823–896

Goldmann H (1950) Der Druck im Schlemm'schen Kanal bei Normalen und bei Glaukoma simplex. Experientia 6:110–111

Goldmann H (1951) L'origine de l'hypertension oculaire dans le glaucome primitif. Ann Ocul (Paris) 184:1086

Gololobova MT (1958) Changes in mitotic activity in rats in relation to the time of day or night. Bull Exp Biol Med 46:1143–1146

Goodman LS, Gilman A (eds) (1980) The pharmacological basis of therapeutics, 6th edn. MacMillan, New York, p 642

Grant WM (1955) Physiological and pharmacological influences upon intraocular pressure. Pharmacol Rev 7:143–182

Grant WM (1969) Action of drugs on movement of ocular fluids. Annu Rev Pharmacol 9:85–94

Gregory DS, Bausher LP, Bromberg BB, Sears ML (1981a) The beta adrenergic receptor and adenyl cyclase of rabbit ciliary processes. In: Sears ML (ed) New directions in ophthalmic research. Yale University Press, New Haven, pp 127–148

Gregory DS, Sears ML, Bausher L, Mishima H, Mead A (1981b) Intraocular pressure and aqueous flow are decreased by cholera toxin. Invest Ophthalmol Vis Sci 20:371–381

Greve EL (ed) (1977) Symposium on medical therapy in glaucoma, Amsterdam, 15 May 1976. Doc Ophthalmol 12

Hahnenberger RW (1976) Influence of intraocular colchicine and vinblastine on the cat iris. Acta Physiol Scand 98:425–432

Hamburger K (1923) Experimentelle Glaukomtherapie. Klin Monatsbl Augenheilkd 7:810–811

Harris L, Galin M, Lerner R (1970) The influence of low-dose 1-epinephrine on aqueous outflow facility. Ann Ophthalmol 2:455–458

Harris MA, Schwartz B (1983) Dexamethasone-induced stimulation of beta-adrenergic sensitive adenylate cyclase in ciliary process epithelium. Invest Ophthalmol Vis Sci [Suppl] 24:5

Havener WH (1974) Ocular pharmacology. Mosby, St. Louis

Hayasaka S, Sears M (1978) Effects of epinephrine, indomethacin, acetylsalicylic acid, dexamethasone, and cyclic AMP on the in vitro activity of lysosomal hyaluronidase from the rabbit iris. Invest Ophthalmol Vis Sci 17:1109–1113

Hedden WL Jr, Dowling JE (1978) The interplexiform cell system. II. Effects of dopamine on goldfish retinal neurones. Proc R Soc Lond [Biol] 201:7–26

Hedqvist P (1973) Autonomic neurotransmission. In: Ramwell PW (ed) The prostaglandins, vol 1. Plenum, New York

Heilmann K, Richardson KT (1978) Glaucoma. Conceptions of a disease. Pathogenesis, diagnosis, therapy. Saunders, Philadelphia

Henkind P (1965) Circulation in the iris and ciliary processes. Br J Ophthalmol 49:6–10

Herzog V, Sies H, Miller F (1976) Exocytosis in secretory cells of rat lacrimal gland. J Cell Biol 70:692–706

Higgins RG, Brubaker RF (1980) Acute effect of epinephrine on aqueous humor formation in the timolol-treated normal as measured by fluorophotometry. Invest Ophthalmol Vis Sci 19:420–423

Hirata F, Strittmatter WJ, Axelrod J (1979) β-Adrenergic receptor agonists increase phospholipid methylation, membrane fluidity, and β-adrenergic receptor-adenylate cyclase coupling. Proc Natl Acad Sci USA 76:368–372

Hitchings RA, Glover D (1982) Adrenaline 1% combined with guanethidine 1% versus adrenaline 1%: a randomized prospective double-blind cross-over study. Br J Ophthalmol 66:247–249

Hökfelt T (1966) Electron microscopic observations on nerve terminals in the intrinsic muscles of the albino rat iris. Acta Physiol Scand 67:255–256

Hökfelt T (1967) Ultrastructural studies on adrenergic nerve terminals in the albino rat iris after pharmacological and experimental treatment. Acta Physiol Scand 69:125–126

Hökfelt T, Nilsson O (1965) The relationship between nerves and smooth muscle cells in the rat iris. II. The sphincter muscle. Z Zellforsch Mikrosk Anat 66:848–853

Hoffman DW, Giacobini E (1980) Characteristics of norepinephrine uptake in developing peripheral nerve terminals. Brain Res 201:57–70

Hoffman DW, Marchi M, Giacobini E (1980) Norepinephrine uptake in aging adrenergic nerve terminals. Neurobiol Aging 1:65–68

Holmgren I (1982) Synaptic organization of the dopaminergic neurons in the retina of the cynomolgus monkey. Invest Ophthalmol Vis Sci 22:8–24

Hoyng PF, van Alphen GW (1981) Behavior of IOP and pupil size after topical tranylcypromine in the rabbit eye. Doc Ophthalmol 51:225–234

Hoyng PH, van Alphen GW, Haddeman E (1982) Does prostacyclin mediate alpha adrenergic induced hypotension? Doc Ophthalmol 53:159–171

Innemee HC, van Zwieten PA (1982) The role of beta$_2$-adrenoceptors in the IOP-lowering effect of adrenaline. Albrecht von Graefes Arch Klin Exp Ophthalmol 218:297–300

Innemee HC, de Jonge A, van Meel JCA, Timmermans PB, van Zwieten PA (1981) The effect of selective α_1- and α_2-adrenoceptor stimulation on intraocular pressure in the conscious rabbit. Naunyn Schmiedebergs Arch Pharmacol 316:294–298

Iversen LL (1967) The uptake and storage of noradrenaline in sympathetic nerves. Cambridge University Press, London

Iversen LL, Quik M, Emson PC, Dowling JE, Watling KJ (1980) Further evidence for the existence of multiple receptors for dopamine in the central nervous system. In: Pepeu G, Kuhar MJ, Enna SJ (eds) Receptors for neurotransmitters and peptide hormones. Raven, New York, pp 193–202

Jacobowitz D, Laties AM (1968) Direct adrenergic innervation of a teleost melanophore. Anat Rec 162:501–504

Jones RF, Maurice DM (1966) New methods of measuring the rate of aqueous flow in man with fluorescein. Exp Eye Res 5:208–220

Joo I, Wollemann M (1980) The effect of catecholamines and of their inhibitors on the solubilized adenylate cyclase activity of bovine retina. Exp Eye Res 31:659–663

Joseph DR (1921) The inhibitory influence of the cervical sympathetic nerve upon the sphincter muscle of the iris. Am J Physiol 55:279–280

Kaback MB, Podos SM, Harbin TS Jr, Mandell A, Becker B (1976) The effects of dipivalyl epinephrine on the eye. Am J Ophthalmol 81:768–772

Kamp CW, Morgan WW (1982) Benzodiazepines suppress the light response of retinal dopaminergic neurons in vivo. Eur J Pharmacol 77:343–346

Kass MA, Reid TW, Neufeld AH, Bausher LP, Sears ML (1976) The effect of d-isoproterenol on intraocular pressure in the rabbit, monkey and man. Invest Ophthalmol 15:113–118

Kass MA, Shin DH, Cooper DG (1977) The ocular hypotensive effect of epinephrine in high and low corticosteroid responders. Invest Ophthalmol Vis Sci 16:530–531

Kato S, Teranishi T, Kuo CH, Negishi K (1982) 5-Hydroxytryptamine stimulates [^3H]dopamine release from the fish retina. J Neurochem 39:493–498

Katz IM (1978) Beta blockers and the eye: an overview. Ann Ophthalmol 10:847–850

Katz IM, Berger ET (1979) Effects of iris pigmentation on response of ocular pressure to timolol. Surv Ophthalmol 23:395–398

Katz IM, Hubbard WA, Getson AJ (1976) Intraocular pressure decrease in normal volunteers following timolol ophthalmic solution. Invest Ophthalmol 14:489–492

Kaufman PL, Barany EH (1981) Adrenergic drug effects on aqueous outflow facility following ciliary muscle retrodisplacement in the cynomolgus monkey. Invest Ophthalmol 20:644–651

Keryer G, Rossignol B (1976) Effect of carbachol on ^{45}Ca uptake and protein secretion in rat lacrimal gland. Am J Physiol 230:99–104

Kitazawa Y, Nose H, Horie T (1975) Chemical sympathectomy with 6-hydroxydopamine in the treatment of primary open angle glaucoma. Am J Ophthalmol 79:98–103

Klyce SD, Wong RKS (1977) Site and mode of adrenaline action of chloride transport across the rabbit corneal epithelium. J Physiol (Lond) 266:777–799

Klyce SD, Neufeld AH, Zadunaisky JA (1973) The activation of chloride transport by epinephrine and Db cyclic AMP in the cornea of the rabbit. Invest Ophthalmol 12:127–139

Klyce SD, Palkama KA, Härkönen M, Marshall WS, Huhtaniitty S, Mann KP, Neufeld AH (1982) Neural serotonin stimulates chloride transport in the rabbit corneal epithelium. Invest Ophthalmol Vis Sci 23:181–192

Kolker AE, Hetherington J Jr (1976) Becker and Shaffer's diagnosis and therapy of the glaucomas, 4th edn. Mosby, St. Louis

Kondo K, Sears M (to be published) Influence of drugs upon the ciliary channels.

Korey MS, Hodapp E, Kass MA, Goldberg I, Gordon M, Becker B (1982) Timolol and epinephrine: long-term evaluation of concurrent administration. Arch Ophthalmol 100:742–745

Kosichenko LP (1960) The character of the 24-h periodicity of mitosis in the corneal epithelium of various laboratory animals. Bull Exp Biol Med 49:617–619

Koss MC, San LC (1976) Analysis of clonidine-induced mydriasis. Invest Ophthalmol 15:566–570

Kramer SG (1971) Dopamine: a retinal neurotransmitter. I. Retinal uptake, storage and light-stimulated release of H^3-dopamine in vivo. Invest Ophthalmol 10:438–452

Kramer SG (1980) Epinephrine distribution after topical administration to phakic and aphakic eyes. Trans Am Ophthalmol Soc 78:947–982

Kramer SG, Potts AM (1971) Catecholamine metabolite formation in the iris and ciliary body in vivo. Am J Ophthalmol 72:939–946

Kramer SG, Potts AM, Mangnall Y (1972) Autoradiographic localization of catecholamines in the uveal tract. 1. Light microscopic study. Am J Ophthalmol 74:129–133

Krejci L, Krejocova H (1973) Combined effects of corticosteroids and antiglaucoma drugs on corneal epithelium. A comparative tissue culture study. Ophthalmol Res 5:186–192

Krejci L, Krejocova H (1974) Changes in pupil diameter and effects on corneal tissue cultures from topically administered N-butyl gallate (COMT inhibitor) and epinephrine. Ophthalmol Res 6:15–22

Krieglstein GK (1978) Die Wirkung von Timolol-Augentropfen auf den Augeninnendruck bei Glaucoma simplex. Klin Monatsbl Augenheilkd 172:667–685

Krieglstein GK, Leydhecker W (1978) The dose-response relationships of dipivalyl epinephrine in open-angle glaucoma. Albrecht von Graefes Arch Klin Ophthalmol 205:141–146

Krieglstein GK, Langham ME, Leydhecker W (1978) The peripheral and central neural actions of clonidine in normal and glaucomatous eyes. Invest Ophthalmol Vis Sci 17:149–158

Kronfeld PC (1964) Dose-effect relationships as an aid in the evaluation of ocular hypotensive drugs. Invest Ophthalmol 3:258–265

Kronfeld PC (1967) The efficacy of combination of ocular hypotensive drugs. Arch Ophthalmol 78:140–146

Krupin T, Weiss A, Becker B, Holmberg N, Fritz C (1977) Increased intraocular pressure following topical azide or nitroprusside. Invest Ophthalmol Vis Sci 16:1002–1007

Kupfer C, Sanderson P (1968) Determination of pseudofacility in the eye of man. Arch Ophthalmol 80:194–196

Langer SZ (1973) The regulation of transmitter release elicited by nerve stimulation through presynaptic feed-back mechanism. In: Usdin E, Snyder SH (eds) Frontiers in catecholamine research. Pergamon, New York, pp 543–549

Langer SZ (1974) Presynaptic regulation of catecholamine release. Biochem Pharmacol 23:1793–1800

Langer SZ, Dubocovich ML (1978) Recent advances in the pharmacology of adrenoceptors, 1st edn. Elsevier/North Holland Biomedical, New York, pp 181–189

Langer SZ, Briley MS, Raisman R (1980) Regulation of neurotransmission through presynaptic receptors and other mechanisms: possible clinical relevance and therapeutic potential. In: Pepeu G, Kuhar MJ, Enna SJ (eds). Receptors for neurotransmitters and peptide hormones. Raven, New York, pp 203–212

Langham ME (1975) Adrenergic tachyphylaxis in animal and human eyes. Exp Eye Res 20:174–175

Langham ME (1977) The aqueous outflow system and its response to autonomic receptor agonists. Exp Eye Res [Suppl] 311:322

Langham ME, Diggs E (1974) Beta adrenergic responses in the eyes of rabbits, primates and man. Exp Eye Res 19:281–295

Langham ME, Krieglstein GK (1976) The biphasic intraocular pressure response of conscious rabbits to epinephrine. Invest Ophthalmol 15:119–127

Laor N, Korczyn AD, Nemet P (1977) Sympathetic pupillary activity in infants. Pediatrics 59:195–198

Lasater EM, Dowling JE (1982) Carp horizontal cells in culture respond selectively to 1-glutamate and its agonists. Proc Natl Acad Sci USA 79:936–940

Laties AM (1967) Central retinal artery innervation. Arch Ophthalmol 77:405–409

Laties AM (1974) Ocular melanin and the adrenergic innervation to the eye. Trans Am Ophthalmol Soc 72:560–605

Laties AM, Lerner A (1975) Iris colour and relationship of tyrosinase activity to adrenergic innervation. Nature 255:152–153

Lee DA; Brubaker RF, Nagataki S (1981) Effect of thymoxamine on aqueous humor formation in the normal human eye as measured by fluorophotometry. Invest Ophthalmol Vis Sci 21:805–811

Leopold IH, Murray DL (1979) Ocular hypotensive action of labetalol. Am J Ophthalmol 88:427–431

Leydhecker HCV (1977) Sympathomimetics and sympatholytics in the treatment of glaucoma. Klin Monatsbl Augenheilkd 171:538–546

Linner E (1956) Further studies of the episcleral venous pressure in glaucoma. Am J Oph-
    thalmol 41:646–651
Linner E (1959) Adrenocortical steroids and aqueous humor dynamics. Doc Ophthalmol
    13:210–224
Little JM, Centifanto YM, Kaufman HE (1969) Immunoglobulins in tears. Am J Ophthal-
    mol 68:898–905
Lorenzetti OJ (1971) Dose-dependent influence of topically instilled adrenergic agents on
    intraocular pressure and outflow facility in the rabbit. Exp Eye Res 12:80–87
Malik AB, van Heuven WAJ, Satler LF (1976) Effects of isoproterenol and norepinephrine
    on regional ocular blood flows. Invest Ophthalmol Vis Sci 15:492–495
Malmfors T (1965) The adrenergic innervation of the eye as demonstrated by fluorescence
    microscopy. Acta Physiol Scand 65:259–267
Mandell AI, Stentz F, Kitabchi AE (1978) Dipivalyl epinephrine: a new pro-drug in the
    treatment of glaucoma. Ophthalmology (Rochester) 85:268–275
Mapstone R (1970) Safe mydriasis. Br J Ophthalmol 54:690–692
Mapstone R (1977) Dilating dangerous pupils. Br J Ophthalmol 61:517–524
Marc RE (1982) Spatial organization of neurochemically classified interneurons of the gold-
    fish retina. I. Local patterns. Vision Res 22:589–608
Masuda K, Izawa Y, Mishima S (1975) Prostaglandins and glaucomatocyclitic crisis. Jpn
    J Ophthalmol 19:368–375
Matheny JL, Ahlquist RP (1974) Adrenoceptor alteration by temperature in iris dilator
    muscle of rabbit. Arch Int Pharmacodyn Ther 209:197–203
Maurice D (1983) A simple method for measuring aqueous flow in the rabbit. Invest Oph-
    thalmol Vis Sci [Suppl] 24:5
McClure DA (1975) The effect of a pro-drug of epinephrine (dipivalyl epinephrine) in glau-
    coma. General pharmacology, toxicology and clinical experience. In: Higuchi T, Stella
    V (eds) Pro-drugs as novel drug delivery systems. Amer Chemical Society, Washington
    D.C. pp 224–236
McGuire J (1970) Adrenergic control of melanocytes. Arch Dermatol 101:173–180
Mehra KS, Roy PN, Singh R (1974) Pargyline drops in glaucoma. Arch Ophthalmol
    92:453–454
Melikian HE, Lieberman TW, Leopold LH (1971) Ocular pigmentation and pressure and
    outflow response to pilocarpine and epinephrine. Am J Ophthalmol 72:70–73
Merck, Sharp & Dohme Research Laboratories Report (1974) Timolol maleate ophthalmic
    solutions. Ocular studies in animals, 18 December 1974
Merck, Sharp & Dohme Research Laboratories Report (1977) Timolol maleate ophthalmic
    solutions. Preclinical evaluation, 15 September 1977
Miescher G (1923) Pigmentgenese im Auge nebst Bemerkungen über die Natur des Pigment-
    korns. Arch Mikrosk Anat Entwicklungsgesch 97:326–396
Miichi H, Nagataki S (1982) Effects of cholinergic drugs and adrenergic drugs on aqueous
    humor formation in the rabbit eye. Jpn J Ophthalmol 26:425–436
Miller WH (ed) (1981) Molecular mechanisms of photoreceptor transduction. Academic,
    New York
Mishima H, Sears M, Bausher L, Gregory G (1982a) Ultracytochemistry of cholera-toxin
    binding sites in ciliary processes. Cell Tissue Res 223:241–253
Mishima H, Bausher L, Sears M, Gochu M, Ono H, Gregory D (1982b) Fine structural
    studies of ciliary processes after treatment with cholera toxin or its B subunit. Graefe's
    Arch Clin Exp Ophthalmol 219:272–278
Mishima S (1957) The effects of the denervation and the stimulation of the sympathetic and
    trigeminal nerve on the mitotic rate of the corneal epithelium in the rabbit. Jpn J Oph-
    thalmol 1:65–73
Mishima S (1981) Clinical pharmacokinetics of the eye. Invest Ophthalmol Vis Sci 21:504–
    541
Mishima S (1982) Ocular effects of beta adrenergic agents. Surv Ophthalmol 27:187–208
Mishima S, Takase M, Araie M, Kitazawa Y (1983) Beta adrenergic agonists and antago-
    nists: clinical pharmacokinetics. In: Krieglstein G, Leydhecker HW (eds) Glaucoma up-

date II. International glaucoma symposium, Carmel, California, 22–27 October 1982. Springer, Berlin Heidelberg New York

Mittag T, Tormay A (1981) Adrenergic receptors in iris-ciliary body direct ligand binding studies. Invest Ophthalmol Vis Sci [Suppl] 20:198

Mittag T, Tormay A, Messenger M (1982) The ocular hypotensive response to pirbuterol and nylidrin: receptor mechanisms in the rabbit eye. Invest Ophthalmol Vis Sci [Suppl] 22:91

Morgan TR, Green K, Bowman K (1981) Effects of adrenergic agonists upon regional ocular blood flow in normal and ganglionectomized rabbits. Exp Eye Res 32:691–697

Morgan WW, Kamp CW (1982) Postnatal development of the light response of the dopaminergic neurons in the rat retina. J Neurochem 39:283–285

Morone G (1953) Indagini sull' attività aminossidasica dell' iride dopo la resezione del simpatico cervicale. Riv Otoneurooftalmol 28:317–322

Moss J, Vaughn M (1978) Isolation of an avian erythrocyte protein processing ADP-ribosyltransferase activity and capable of activating adenyl cyclase. Proc Natl Acad Sci USA 75:3621–3624

Motulsky HJ, Insel PA (1982) Adrenergic receptors in man. Direct identification, physiologic regulation and clinical alterations. N Engl J Med 307:18–29

Murray DL, Leopold IH (1980) Evidence for more than one type of alpha-adrenergic receptor in rabbit eyes. Invest Ophthalmol Vis Sci [Suppl] 19:66

Murray DL, Leopold IH (1981) Alpha-adrenergic receptors and intraocular pressure. Invest Ophthalmol Vis Sci [Suppl] 20:105

Nagasubramanian S, Tripathi RC, Poinoosawmy D, Gloster J (1976) Low concentration guanethidine and adrenaline therapy of glaucoma. Trans Ophthalmol Soc UK 96:179–183

Nagataki S (1977) Effects of adrenergic drugs on aqueous humor dynamics in man. Acta Soc Ophthalmol Jpn 81:1795–1800

Nagataki S, Brubaker RF (1981) Early effect of epinephrine on aqueous formation in the normal human eye. Ophthalmology (Rochester) 88:278–282

Nathanson JA (1980) Adrenergic regulation of intraocular pressure: identification of beta$_2$-adrenergic-stimulated adenylate cyclase in ciliary process epithelium. Proc Natl Acad Sci USA 77:7420–7424

Nathanson JA (1981 a) Human ciliary process adrenergic receptor: pharmacological characterization. Invest Ophthalmol Vis Sci 21:798–804

Nathanson JA (1981 b) Effects of a potent and specific beta$_2$-adrenoceptor antagonist on intraocular pressure. Br J Pharmacol 73:97–100

Negishi K, Teranishi T, Kato S (1982 a) Growth zone of the juvenile goldfish retina revealed by fluorescent flat mounts. J Neurosci Res 7:321–330

Negishi K, Teranishi T, Kato S (1982 b) New dopaminergic and indoleamine-accumulating cells in the growth zone of goldfish retinas after neurotoxic destruction. Science 216:747–749

Neufeld AH (1979) Experimental studies on the mechanism of action of timolol. Surv Ophthalmol 23:363–370

Neufeld AH (1981) Epinephrine and timolol: how do these drugs lower intraocular pressure? Ann Ophthalmol 13:1109–1111

Neufeld AH, Page ED (1975) Regulation of adrenergic neuromuscular transmission in the rabbit iris. Exp Eye Res 20:549–561

Neufeld AH, Page ED (1977) In vitro determination of the ability of drugs to bind to adrenergic receptors. Invest Ophthalmol Vis Sci 16:1118–1124

Neufeld AH, Sears ML (1974) Cyclic AMP in ocular tissues of the rabbit, monkey and human. Invest Ophthalmol 14:688–689

Neufeld AH, Jampol LM, Sears ML (1972) Cyclic-AMP in the aqueous humor: the effects of adrenergic agents. Exp Eye Res 14:242–250

Neufeld AH, Chavis RM, Sears ML (1973) Degeneration release of norepinephrine causes transient ocular hyperemia mediated by prostaglandins. Invest Ophthalmol 12:167–175

Neufeld AH, Zawistowski KA, Page ED, Bromberg BB (1978) Influences on the density of beta adrenergic receptors in the cornea and iris-ciliary body of the rabbit. Invest Ophthalmol Vis Sci 17:1069–1075

Neufeld AH, Ledgard SE, Jumblatt MM, Klyce SD (1982) Serotonin-stimulated cyclic AMP synthesis in the rabbit corneal epithelium. Invest Ophthalmol Vis Sci 23:193–198

Nielsen NV (1978) Timolol: hypotensive effect used alone and in combination for treatment of increased intraocular pressure. Acta Ophthalmol (Copenh) 56:504–509

Nilsson O (1964) The relationship between nerves and smooth muscle cells in the rat iris. I. The dilatator muscle. Z Zellforsch Mikrosk Anat 64:166–171

Nishida S, Sears ML (1969a) Fine structural innervation of the dilator muscle of the iris of the albino guinea pig studied with permanganate fixation. Exp Eye Res 8:292–296

Nishida S, Sears ML (1969b) Dual innervation of the iris sphincter muscle of the albino guinea pig. Exp Eye Res 8:467–469

Ochi J, Konishi M, Yoshikawa H, Sano Y (1968) Fluorescence and electron microscopic evidence for the dual innervation of the iris sphincter muscle of the rabbit. Z Zellforsch Mikrosk Anat 91:90–95

Odin L, O'Donnell FE Jr (1982) Adrenergic influence on iris stromal pigmentation: evidence for alpha-adrenergic receptors. Invest Ophthalmol Vis Sci 23:528–530

Ohrstrom A (1982) Dose response of oral timolol combined with adrenaline. Br J Ophthalmol 66:242–246

Page ED, Neufeld AH (1978) Characterization of α and β-adrenergic receptors in membranes prepared from the rabbit iris before and after development of supersensitivity. Biochem Pharmacol 27:953–958

Parkinson D, Rando RR (1983) Effect of light on dopamine turnover and metabolism in rabbit retina. Invest Ophthalmol Vis Sci 24:384–388

Parod RJ, Putney JW Jr (1978) An alpha adrenergic receptor mechanism controlling potassium permeability in the rat lacrimal gland acinar cell. J Physiol (Lond) 281:359–369

Patil PN (1969) Adrenergic receptors of the bovine iris sphincter. J Pharmacol Exp Ther 166:299–307

Patil PN (1972) Cocaine binding by the pigmented and the nonpigmented iris and its relevance to the mydriatic effect. Invest Ophthalmol 11:739–746

Patil PN, LaPidus JB (1972) Stereoisomerism in adrenergic drugs. In: Reviews of physiology, biochemistry, and experimental pharmacology, vol 66. Springer, Berlin Heidelberg New York, pp 213–260

Patil PN, Trendelenburg U (1982) The extraneuronal uptake and metabolism of ^3H-isoprenaline in the rabbit iris. Naunyn Schmiedebergs Arch Pharmacol 318:158–165

Phillips CJ, Howitt G, Rowland J (1967) Propranolol as ocular hypotensive agent. Br J Ophthalmol 51:222–226

Pholpramool C (1979) Secretory effect of prostaglandins on the rabbit lacrimal gland in vivo. Prostaglandins Med 3:185–192

Plance C, Sole P, Ourgaud AG, Hamard H, Vidal R (1978) Double-observer comparison of timolol maleate and pilocarpine in open angle glaucoma. Proc int symp glaucoma XIII, International congress of ophthalmology, Kyoto, Japan, pp 41–48

Poos F (1927) Pharmakologische und physiologische Untersuchungen an den isolierten Irismuskeln. Arch Exp Pathol Pharmakol 126:307–351

Potter DE (1981) Adrenergic pharmacology of aqueous humor dynamics. Pharmacol Rev 33:133–153

Potter DE, Rowland JM (1978) Adrenergic drugs and intraocular pressure: effects of selective β-adrenergic agonists. Exp Eye Res 27:615–625

Powell CE, Slater IH (1958) Blocking of inhibitory adrenergic receptors by dichloro analog of ispoproterenol. J Pharmacol Exp Ther 122:480–488

Proll MA, Morgan WW (1982) Adaptation of retinal dopamine neuron activity in light-adapted rats to darkness. Brain Res 241:359–361

Proll MA, Kamp CW, Morgan WW (1982) Use of liquid chromatography with electrochemistry to measure effects of varying intensities of white light on DOPA accumulation in rat retinas. Life Sci 30:11–19

Quilliam JP (1949) A quantitative method for the study of the reactions of the isolated cat's iris. J Physiol (Lond) 110:237–247

Radius R, Langham ME (1973) Cyclic AMP and the ocular responses to norepinephrine. Exp Eye Res 17:219–229

Richardson KC (1968) Cholinergic and adrenergic axons in methylene blue-stained rat iris: an electron microscopical study. Life Sci 7:509–604

Ritch R, Hargette NA, Podos SM (1978) The effect of 1.5% timolol maleate on intraocular pressure. Acta Ophthalmol (Copenh) 56:6–10

Ross RA, Drance SM (1970) Effect of topically applied isoproterenol on aqueous dynamics in man. Arch Ophthalmol 83:39–46

Rosser MJ, Sears ML (1968) Further studies on the mechanism of the increased outflow of aqueous humor from the eyes of rabbits twenty-four hours after cervical sympathetic ganglionectomy. J Pharmacol Exp Ther 164:280–289

Rowland JM, Potter DE (1979) Effects of adrenergic drugs on aqueous cAMP and cGMP and intraocular pressure. Albrecht von Graefes Arch Klin Exp Ophthalmol 212:67–77

Rowland JM, Potter DE (1980a) Adrenergic drugs and intraocular pressure: suppression of ocular hypertension induced by water loading. Exp Eye Res 30:93–104

Rowland JM, Potter DE (1980b) Adrenergic drugs and intraocular pressure: the hypertensive effect of epinephrine. Ophthalmol Res 12:221–229

Rowland JM, Potter DE (1981) Steric structure activity relationships of various adrenergic agonists: ocular and systemic effects. Current Eye Res 1:25–35

Ruegg JC, Hess WR (1953) Die Wirkung von Adrenalin, Noradrenalin und Acetylcholin auf die isolierten Irismuskeln. Helv Physiol Pharmacol Acta 11:216–230

Sallman L von, Grimes P (1971) Isoproterenol-induced changes of cell proliferation in rat lens epithelium. Invest Ophthalmol 10:943–947

Sallman L von, Grimes P (1974) Effects of isoproterenol and cyclic AMP derivatives on cell division in cultured rat lenses. Invest Ophthalmol 13:210–218

Salminen L, Aaltonen H, Jantti V (1980) Mydriatic effect of low dose phenylephrine. Ophthalmic Res 12:235–239

Sapse AT, Bonavida B, Stone W, Sercaz EE (1969) Proteins in human tears. I. Immuno-electrophoretic patterns. Arch Ophthalmol 81:815–919

Schachtschabel DO, Bigalke B, Rohen JW (1977) Production of glycosaminoglycans by cell cultures of the trabecular meshwork of the primate eye. Exp Eye Res 24:71–80

Schaeppi U, Koella WP (1964a) Adrenergic innervation of cat iris sphincter. Am J Physiol 207:273–278

Schaeppi U, Koella WP (1964b) Innervation of the cat iris dilator. Am J Physiol 207:1411–1416

Schaeppi U, Rubin R, Koella WP (1966) Electrical stimulation of the isolated cat iris. Am J Physiol 210:1165–1169

Schenker HI, Yablonski ME, Podos SM, Linder L (1981) Fluorophotometric study of epinephrine and timolol in human subjects. Arch Ophthalmol 99:1212–1216

Sears DE, Sears ML (1974) Blood aqueous barrier and alpha chymotrypsin glaucoma in rabbits. Am J Ophthalmol 77:378–383

Sears ML (1965) Adrenergic receptors. Arch Ophthalmol 74:150–151

Sears ML (1966a) The mechanism of action of adrenergic drugs in glaucoma. Invest Ophthalmol 5:115–119

Sears ML (1966b) Pressure in the canal of Schlemm and its relation to the site of resistance to outflow of aqueous humor in the eyes of Ethiopian green monkeys. Invest Ophthalmol 5:610–623

Sears ML (1971) Development of drugs useful in treatment of glaucoma and their evaluation in both animals, and man, NIH Contract NO1-EY-1-2512

Sears ML (1973) Adrenergic supersensitivity of the scorbutic iris. Trans Am Ophthalmol Soc 71:536–557

Sears ML (1975) Catecholamines in relation to the eye. In: Astwood E, Greep R (eds) Handbook of physiology. American Physiological Society, Washington DC, pp 553–590

Sears ML (1978) Perspectives in glaucoma research. Friedenwald lecture. Invest Ophthalmol Vis Sci 17:6–22

Sears ML (1980) The aqueous. In: Moses RA (ed) Adler's physiology of the eye, 7th edn. Mosby, St. Louis, pp 204–226

Sears ML (1982) Perspectives in the medical treatment of glaucoma. In: Krieglstein GK, Leydhecker W (eds) Medikamentöse Glaukomtherapie. Bergmann, Munich

Sears ML, Bárány EH (1960) Outflow resistance of rabbit eye. Effect of cervical sympathectomy and adrenergic inhibitors. Arch Ophthalmol 64:839–848

Sears ML, Gillis CN (1967) Mydriasis and the increase in outflow of aqueous humor from the rabbit eye after cervical ganglionectomy in relation to the release of norepinephrine from the iris. Biochem Pharmacol 16:777–782

Sears ML, Neufeld AH (1975) Adrenergic modulation of the outflow of aqueous humor. Invest Ophthalmol 14:83–86

Sears M, Mead A (1983) A major pathway for the regulation of intraocular pressure. In Ophthalmol 6:201–212

Sears ML, Sherk TE (1963) Supersensitivity of the aqueous outflow resistance in rabbits after sympathetic denervation. Nature 197:387–388

Sears ML, Sherk TE (1964) The trabecular effect of noradrenalin in the rabbit eye. Invest Ophthalmol 3:157–163

Sears ML, Mizuno K, Cintron C, Alter A, Sherk T (1966) Changes in outflow facility and content of norepinephrine in iris and ciliary processes of albino rabbits after cervical ganglionectomy. Invest Ophthalmol 5:312–318

Sears ML, Gregory D, Bausher L, Mishima H, Stjernschantz J (1981) A receptor for aqueous humor formation. In: Sears ML (ed) New directions in ophthalmic research. Yale University Press, New Haven, chap 10, pp 163–183

Sears M, Caprioli J, Kondo K, Bausher L (to be published) A mechanism for the control of aqueous humor formation. In: Drance S, Neufeld AH (ed) Applied pharmacology in the medical treatment of the glaucomas. Grune & Stratton, New York

Seidehamel RJ, Dungan KW, Hickey TE (1975) Specific hypotensive and antihypertensive ocular effects of d-isoproterenol in rabbits. Am J Ophthalmol 79:1018–1025

Selinger Z, Cassel D (1981) Role of guanine nucleotides in hormonal activation of adenylate cyclase. In: Dumont JE, Greengard P, Robison GA (eds) Advances in cyclic nucleotide research. Raven Press, New York, pp 15–22

Shannon RP, Mead A, Sears ML (1976) The effect of dopamine on the intraocular pressure and pupil of the rabbit eye. Invest Ophthalmol 15:371–380

Shell W (1982) Pharmacokinetics of topically applied ophthalmic drugs. Surv Ophthalmol 26:207–218

Shepherd GM (1978) Microcircuits in the nervous system. Sci Am 238:92–102

Shimizu H, Riley MV, Cole DF (1967) The isolation of whole cells from the ciliary epithelium together with some observations on the metabolism of the two cell types. Exp Eye Res 6:141–151

Shiose Y (1970) Electron microscopic studies on blood-retinal and blood-aqueous barrier. Jpn J Ophthalmol 14:73–87

Shiose Y, Sears ML (1966) Fine structural localization of nucleoside phosphatase activity in the ciliary epithelium of albino rabbits. Invest Ophthalmol 5:152–165

Smith BR, Murray DL, Leopold IH (1979) Topical prazosin lowers intraocular pressure. Invest Ophthalmol Vis Sci [Suppl] 18:24

Spaeth GL (1980) The effect of autonomic agents on the pupil and the intraocular pressure of eyes treated with dexamethasone. Br J Ophthalmol 64:426–429

Spinowitz BS, Zadunaisky JA (1979) Action of adenosine on chloride active transport of isolated frog cornea. Am J Physiol 237:F121–F127

Stjärne L, Hedqvist P, Lagercrantz H, Wennmalm A (eds) (1981) Chemical neurotransmission, 75 years. Academic, London

Stjernschantz J, Bill A (1980) Vasomotor effects of facial nerve stimulation: noncholinergic vasodilation in the eye. Acta Physiol Scand 109:45–50

Szalay J (1980) Effect of beta adrenergic agents on blood vessels of the rat iris. II. Morphological modifications of the vessel wall. Exp Eye Res 31:299–311

Szalay J, Fliegenspan J, Zaager A, Tobin G, Cross S (1980) Effect of beta-adrenergic agents on blood vessels of the rat iris. I. Permeability to carbon particles. Exp Eye Res 31:289–297

Takase M (1976) Effects of topical isoproterenol and propranolol on flow-rate of aqueous in rhesus monkey. Acta Soc Ophthalmol Jpn 80:379–383

Taylor IH (1982) Electron microscopy of aminergic retinal neurons. Acta Ophthalmol [Suppl] (Copenh) 152:1–40

Terenghi G, Polak JM, Probert L, McGregor GP, Ferri GL, Blank MA, Butler JM, Unger WG, Zhang S, Cole DF, Bloom SR (1982) Mapping quantitative distribution and origin of substance P and VIP containing nerves in the uvea of guinea pig eye. Histochemistry 75:399–417

Townsend DJ, Brubaker RF (1980) Immediate effect of epinephrine on aqueous formation in the normal human eye as measured by fluorophotometry. Invest Ophthalmol Vis Sci 19:256–266

Trendelenburg U (1980) A kinetic analysis of extraneuronal uptake and metabolism of catecholamines. In: Reviews of Physiology, Biochemistry, and Pharmacology, vol 87. Springer, Berlin Heidelberg New York, pp 33–115

Trendelenburg U, Höhn D, Graefe KH, Pluchino S (1971) The influence of block of catechol-O-methyltransferase on the sensivitity of isolated organs to catecholamines. Naunyn Schmiedebergs Arch Pharmakol 271:59–92

Trokel S (1964) Measurement of ocular blood flow and volume by reflective densitometry. Arch Ophthalmol 71:88–92

Trokel S (1965) Quantitative studies of choroidal blood flow by reflective densitometry. Invest Ophthalmol 4:1129–1140

Trope GE, Clark B (1982) Beta adrenergic receptors in pigmented ciliary processes. Br J Ophthalmol 66:788–792

Trope GE, Clark B, Titinchi SJS (1982) Identification of beta-adrenergic receptors in the pigmented mammalian iris-ciliary diaphragm. Exp Eye Res 34:153–157

Tsukahara S, Maezawa N (1978) Cytochemical localization of adenyl cyclase in the rabbit ciliary body. Exp Eye Res 26:99–106

Turner P, Sneddon JM (1968) Alpha receptor blockade by thymoxamine in the human eye. Clin Pharmacol Ther 9:45–49

Ueno K (1976) The effect of beta and alpha adrenergic drugs on the ciliary body of the rabbit eye: an electron microscopical study. Folia Ophthalmol Jpn 27:1012–1015

Ulshafer RJ, Garcia CA, Hollyfield JG (1980) Sensitivity of photoreceptors to elevated levels of cGMP in the human retina. Invest Ophthalmol Vis Sci 19:1236–1241

Unger WG (1979) Prostaglandin mediated inflammatory changes induced by alpha adrenoceptor stimulation in the sympathectomized rabbit eye. Albrecht von Graefes Arch Klin Exp Ophthalmol 211:289–300

Unger WG, Butler JM, Cole DF (1981) Prostaglandin and an increased sensitivity of the sympathectically denervated rabbit eye to laser-induced irritation of the iris. Exp Eye Res 32:699–707

Ungricht AL (1982) Retention of timolol in the ocular tissues of the rabbit. Thesis, Yale University

Van Alphen GWH, Robinette SL, Macri FJ (1964) The adrenergic receptors of the intraocular muscles of the cat. Int J Neuropharmacol 2:259–272

Van Alphen GWH, Kern R, Robinette SL (1965) Adrenergic receptors of the intraocular muscles. Arch Ophthalmol 74:253–259

Van Buskirk R, Dowling JE (1982) Calcium alters the sensitivity of intact horizontal cells to dopamine antagonists. Proc Natl Acad Sci USA 79:3350–3354

Van Haeringen NJ, Ensink FTE, Glasius E (1978) The peroxidase-thiocyanate-hydrogen-peroxidase system in tear fluid and saliva of different species. Exp Eye Res 28:343–347

Vareilles P, Silverstone DL, Plazonnet B, LeDouarec J-C, Sears ML, Stone CA (1977) Comparison of the effects of timolol and other adrenergic agents on intraocular pressure in rabbit. Invest Ophthalmol Vis Sci 16:987–996

Virtanen J, Raij K, Uusitalo R, Uusitalo H, Palkama A (1983) Adenylate cyclase activity and beta-adrenergic receptors in isolated rabbit ciliary epithelium. Invest Ophthalmol Vis Sci [Suppl] 24:5

Waitzman MB, Woods WD (1971) Some characteristics of an adenyl cyclase preparation from rabbit ciliary body tissue. Exp Eye Res 12:99–111

Walkenbach RJ, LeGrand RD (1982) Inhibition of adenylate cyclase activity in the corneal epithelium by anti-inflammatory steroids. Exp Eye Res 34:161–168

Walkenbach RJ, LeGrand RD, Barr RE (1980) Characterization of adenylate cyclase activity in bovine and human corneal epithelium Invest Ophthalmol Vis Sci 19:1080–1086

Walter WG, van Gemert AGM, Duyff JW (1954) Kinetics of pupillary dilation induced by administration of l-epinephrine. Acta Physiol Pharmacol Neerl 3:309–324

Waltman S, Sears M (1964) Catechol-O-methyltransferase and monoamine oxidase activity in the ocular tissues of albino rabbits. Invest Ophthalmol 3:601–605

Wandel T, Spinak M (1981) Toxicity of dipivalyl epinephrine. Ophthalmology (Rochester) 88:259–260

Weekers R, Projot E, Gustin J (1952) Recent advances and future prospects in the medial treatment of ocular hypertension. Br J Ophthalmol 38:742–746

Weekers R, Delmarcelle Y, Gustin J (1955) Treatment of ocular hypertension by adrenaline and diverse sympathomimetic amines. Am J Ophthalmol 40:666–672

Wei C, Anderson JA, Leopold I (1978) Ocular absorption and metabolism of topically applied epinephrine and a dipivalyl ester of epinephrine. Invest Ophthalmol Vis Sci 17:315–321

Weinreb RN, Polansky JR, Kramer SG (1979) Acute intraocular pressure response to steroids in glaucoma. Invest Ophthalmol Vis Sci [Suppl] 18:41

Weiss B, Greenberg LH, Cantor E (1980) Denervation supersensitivity in β-adrenergic receptors as a function of age. In: Pepeu G, Kuhar MJ, Enna SJ (eds) Receptors for neurotransmitters and peptide hormones. Raven, New York

Wentworth WO, Brubaker RF (1981) Aqueous humor dynamics in a series of patients with third neuron Horner's eye syndrome. Am J Ophthalmol 92:407–415

Wettrell K, Wilke K, Pandolfi M (1977) Effect of adrenergic agonists and antagonists on repeated tonometry and episcleral venous pressure. Exp Eye Res 24:613–619

Wikberg JES (1979) Synthesis of [^3H]-acetylcholine in the rabbit lacrimal gland and its release by electrical field stimulation. Acta Physiol Scand 105:108–113

Woodcock EA, Johnston CI (1980) α-Adrenergic receptors modulate β-receptor affinity in rat kidney membranes. Nature 286:159–160

Wudka E, Leopold IH (1956) Experimental studies of the choroidal vessels. IV. Pharmacologic observations. Arch Ophthalmol 55:857–885

Yablonski ME, Gray JR (1983) Use of the fluorotron master to measure aqueous flow. Invest Ophthalmol Vis Sci [Suppl] 24:88

Yablonski ME, Zimmermann TJ, Waltman SR, Becker B (1978) A fluorophotometric study of the effect of topical timolol on aqueous humor dynamics. Exp Eye Res 27:135–142

Zabureva TV, Kiseleva ZM (1977) Catecholamine content of the lacrimal fluid of healthy people and glaucoma patients. Ophthalmologica 175:339–344

Zadunaisky JA (1966) Active transport of chloride in frog cornea. Am J Physiol 211:506–512

Zeller EA, Shoch D, Cooperman SG, Schnipper RI (1967) Enzymology of the refractory media of the eye. IX. On the role of monoamine oxidase in the regulation of aqueous humor dynamics of the rabbit eye. Invest Ophthalmol 6:618–623

Zeller EA, Knepper PA, Shoch D (1975) Differential effects of inhibitors of monoamine oxidase types A and B on the adrenergic system of the rabbit iris. Invest Ophthalmol 14:155–159

Zimmerman TJ, Kaufman HE (1977a) Timolol: a beta-adrenergic blocking agent for the treatment of glaucoma. Arch Ophthalmol 95:601–604

Zimmerman TJ, Kaufman HE (1977b) Timolol: Dose response and duration of action. Arch Ophthalmol 95:605–609

Autonomic Nervous System: Adrenergic Antagonists

V. J. Lotti, J. C. LeDouarec, and C. A. Stone

A. Introduction

Until recently, the primary interest in adrenergic antagonists in ocular pharmacology was as tools for the elucidation of the physiological role of adrenergic mechanisms in the eye. The discovery of the intraocular-pressure (IOP)-lowering effect of oral propranolol in 1967 (Phillips et al. 1967) and the successful clinical utilization of topical timolol in treating glaucoma (Heel et al. 1979) has provided one impetus for a large number of animal and clinical studies on adrenergic blocking agents, particularly with regard to their effects upon IOP and aqueous humor dynamics. More recently, some attention has also been given to the effects on IOP of agents having α-adrenergic or both α- and β-adrenergic blocking properties.

In the present chapter, the ocular pharmacology of adrenergic antagonists is reviewed. Attention is focused upon the ocular pharmacology of β-adrenergic antagonists, particularly with respect to their mode and mechanism of action in lowering IOP. A brief review of α-adrenergic antagonists is also included.

B. Beta-Adrenergic Antagonists

A large number of drugs possessing β-adrenergic blocking properties have been described. Many of these agents also possess other properties, namely, intrinsic sympathomimetic action, membrane-stabilizing activity, and cardioselectivity. The chemical structures and pharmacologic properties of the β-adrenergic blockers most widely employed in ocular pharmacology and referred to in the present chapter are given in Table 1.

I. Animal Pharmacology

1. Intraocular Pressure

The effects on IOP of a variety of β-adrenergic antagonists, administered both systemically and locally, in normal animals as well as animals made experimentally hypertensive, have been reported. The vast majority of the studies in normal (conscious or anesthetized) animals have utilized rabbits as the test animal and are summarized in Table 2.

Table 1. Chemical structures and pharmacologic properties of β-adrenergic blockers[a]

Generic name	Chemical structure	Cardio-selec-tivity	Partial agonist activity (ISA[c])	Mem-brane-stabi-lizing activity
Alprenolol	OCH$_2$CHOHCH$_2$NHCH(CH$_3$)$_2$ —CH$_2$CH=CH$_2$	−	+	+
Atenolol	OCH$_2$CHOHCH$_2$NHCH(CH$_3$)$_2$ CH$_2$CONH$_2$	+	−	−
Bupranolol[b]	OCH$_2$CHOHCH$_2$NHCH(CH$_3$)$_2$ Cl— CH$_3$	−	−	+
Butoxamine	OCH$_3$ —CHOHCHNHC(CH$_3$)$_3$ CH$_3$ OCH$_3$	−	−	
Metoprolol	OCH$_2$CHOHCH$_2$NHCH(CH$_3$)$_2$ CH$_2$CH$_2$OCH$_3$	+	−	+
Oxprenolol	OCH$_2$CHOHCH$_2$NHCH(CH$_3$)$_2$ —OCH$_2$CH=CH$_2$	−	+	+
Pindolol	OCH$_2$CHOHCH$_2$NHCH(CH$_3$)$_2$ N H	−	+	+

Table 1 (continued)

Generic name	Chemical structure	Cardio-selectivity	Partial agonist activity (ISA[c])	Membrane-stabilizing activity
Practolol	$OCH_2CHOHCH_2NHCH(CH_3)_2$ $NHCOCH_3$	+	+	−
Propranolol	$OCH_2CHOHCH_2NHCH(CH_3)_2$	−	−	+
Sotalol	$CHOHCH_2NHCHCH_3$ CH_2CH_3 $NHSO_2CH_3$	−	−	−
Timolol	$-OCH_2CHOHCH_2-\overset{H}{N}-C(CH_3)_3$	−	−	−

[a] EVANS et al. (1979)
[b] KRIEGLSTEIN (1978)
[c] Intrinsic sympathomimetic activity

a) Systemic Administration to Normal Rabbits

SEARS and BÁRÁNY (1960) first demonstrated that the intravenous or subcutaneous administration of the β-adrenergic blocking agent dichloroisoproterenol (6–11 mg/kg) lowered IOP in anesthetized rabbits. Several investigators have since reported that propranolol (0.05–0.5 mg/kg), administered intravenously to anesthetized or conscious rabbits, produces a 2–6 mmHg decrease in IOP which lasts 2–6 h (VIRNO et al. 1969; VALE and PHILLIPS 1970; TAKATS et al. 1972; GOS et al. 1975; STANKIEWICZ et al. 1978). Similar effects upon IOP in normotensive rabbits have been reported following intravenous injection of pindolol (0.5 mg/kg) (STANKIEWICZ et al. 1978).

In contrast to the above studies, higher doses of propranolol (5–10 mg/kg) given intravenously apparently had no demonstrable effect upon IOP or pupil size of

Table 2. Studies of the effect of β-adrenergic blockers on normal intraocular pressure in the rabbit

β-Adrenergic blocker	Experimental conditions	Additional parameters measured	Route of administration (dose)	Reference
Dichloroisoproterenol	Anesthetized animals Manometry	C, BP, pupil	s.c., i.v. (6–11 mg/kg)	SEARS and BÁRÁNY (1960)
Propranolol	Conscious animals Tonometry	Pupil	i.v. (10 mg/kg)	LANGHAM (1965)
	Anesthetized animals Manometry	C, BP, pupil	i.v. (5 mg/kg)	HENDLEY and CROMBIE (1967)
	Anesthetized animals Exper. hypertension by laminaria	BP	i.v. (0.2–0.4 mg/kg)	VIRNO et al. 1969
	Conscious animals Tonometry		i.v. (0.05–0.5 mg/kg)	VALE and PHILLIPS (1970)
	Anesthetized animals Manometry	C, F	i.v. (0.3 mg/kg)	TAKATS et al. (1972)
	Conscious animals Tonometry		Topical (0.5%)	NORTON and VIERNSTEIN (1972)
	Conscious animals Tonometry	Pupil	i.v. (5 mg/kg)	LANGHAM et al. (1973)
	Tonometry	C	i.v., topical, subconjunctival (0.1 mg/kg, 2%)	GOS et al. (1975)
	Conscious animals Tonometry Exper. hypertension (water load, α-chymotrypsin)	Aqueous and plasma levels	Topical (0.01–2%)	VAREILLES et al. (1977)
	Conscious animals Tonometry	Na/K in aqueous	i.v. (0.5 mg/kg)	STANKIEWICZ et al. (1978)
	Conscious animals Tonometry Exper. hypertension (glucose infusion, β-methasone)	Pupil	Topical (1%)	BONOMI et al. (1979)

Drug	Conditions	Measurement	Dose/Route	Reference
Timolol	Conscious animals, Tonometry; Exper. hypertension (water load, α-chymotrypsin)	Pupil	Topical (0.01–1.5%)	Vareilles et al. (1977)
	Conscious animals, Tonometry	Pupil	Topical (0.01–0.5%)	Radius et al. (1978)
	Conscious animals, Tonometry; Exper. hypertension (glucose infusion, β-methasone)	Pupil	Topical (1%)	Bonomi et al. (1979)
	Anesthetized animals	BP, HR	Topical (0.5%, 4%)	Bartels et al. (1980)
	Conscious animals, Tonometry	F, C	Topical (1%)	Vareilles and Lotti (1981)
Pindolol	Conscious animals	Na/K in aqueous	i.v. (0.5 mg/kg)	Stankiewicz et al. (1978)
	Conscious animals, Tonometry; Exper. hypertension (glucose infusion, β-methasone)	Pupil	Topical (1%)	Bonomi et al. (1979)
Bupranolol	Conscious animals	Ocular penetration	Topical (1%)	Komuro et al. (1979)
Atenolol Butadrine Sotalol Oxprenolol Practolol Metoprolol	Conscious animals, Tonometry; Exper. hypertension (glucose infusion, β-methasone)	Pupil	Topical (1%)	Bonomi et al. (1979)

C, aqueous outflow facility; F, aqueous production; BP, blood pressure; HR, heart rate

normotensive conscious or anesthetized rabbits (LANGHAM 1965; HENDLEY and CROMBIE 1967; LANGHAM et al. 1973).

b) Topical Administration to Normal Rabbits

Administered topically, sotalol (1%) and oxprenolol (1%) are reported to result in a small but significant (2–3 mmHg) decrease in IOP in normotensive rabbits (BONOMI et al. 1979). However, no significant changes in IOP in normal rabbits were reported after topical administration of propranolol (0.01%–1%), butadrine (1%), metroprolol (1%), atenolol (1%), pindolol (1%), or practolol (1%) (NORTON and VIERNSTEIN 1972; VAREILLES et al. 1977; BONOMI et al. 1979).

Data in the literature on the effects of topically administered timolol upon IOP in normal rabbits are somewhat contradictory. VAREILLES et al. (1977), studying concentrations of timolol ranging from 0.01%–1%, reported small (2–3 mmHg) decreases in IOP, which although significant were not consistent from experiment to experiment. A similar small decrease in IOP (2 mmHg) was observed 1 h after instillation of timolol (1%) by BONOMI et al. (1979). In anesthetized rabbits, in which control IOP was somewhat depressed (≈ 15 mmHg), timolol (0.5% and 4%) had no significant effect upon IOP or arterial blood presure (BARTELS et al. 1980).

In contrast to the results of VAREILLES et al. (1977), RADIUS et al. (1978) observed a dose-related decrease in IOP in normal rabbits after topical administration of timolol (0.01%–0.5%). The pressure fall (30% of control; ≈ 8 mmHg), which was much more profound than reported by others, was maximal at a concentration of 0.125%, peaked at 1 h, and persisted for more than 8 h. This effect of timolol was maintained after twice-daily instillation of timolol (0.5%) for 1 week and was not associated with changes in pupil size.

On the basis of the information provided it is difficult to explain the differences observed in the effect of topically administered timolol on IOP in normal rabbits as reported by VAREILLES et al. (1977) and RADIUS et al. (1978). It should be noted, however, that in the studies of RADIUS et al. a local anesthetic was employed (proparacaine, 0.5%) and the IOP of untreated control eyes ($\approx 28–29$ mmHg) was considerably higher than those used in the study of VAREILLES et al. (1977) (18–20 mmHg), who did not employ a local anesthetic.

c) Topical Administration to Ocular Hypertensive Rabbits

The IOP-lowering effects of topically administered β-adrenergic blockers are generally more pronounced and consistent in rabbits with experimentally elevated IOP than in normotensive animals. Table 3 summarizes the existing data obtained with these and other agents under various experimental conditions.

Although ROWLAND and POTTER (1980a) reported a lack of activity for timolol and only minimal activity for propranolol (-2 mmHg) in rabbits with water-load-induced increase in IOP, other investigators reported marked effects of timolol and propranolol in this and other models of ocular hypertension. VAREILLES et al. (1977, 1980) and BONOMI et al. (1979), using buphthalmic rabbits or several techniques to elevate IOP of normal rabbits artificially (water load, glucose infusion, α-chymotrypsin, and β-methasone), demonstrated IOP-lowering effects for these agents which ranged in magnitude from 5–11 mmHg and persisted for 4 h and longer. Both of the latter authors agree that the potency of timolol as an ocular hypotensive agent in these models is somewhat greater than that of propranolol

Table 3. Effect of topically administered β-adrenergic antagonists upon experimentally elevated intraocular pressure (IOP) in rabbits

β-Adrener-gic blocker	Concentration tested	Experimental model	IOP-lower-ing effect[a] (effective con-centration)	Reference
Propranolol	0.5%–1.5%	Water load	+(1.5%)	VAREILLES et al. (1977)
	2%	Water load	+	ROWLAND and POTTER (1980a)
	2%	α-Chymotrypsin	+	VAREILLES et al. (1977)
	1%	Glucose infusion	+	BONOMI et al. (1979)
	0.25%–1%	β-Methasone	+(0.5%)	BONOMI et al. (1979)
	0.01%–1%	Buphthalmia	+(0.5%)	VAREILLES et al. (1980)
	0.2–0.4 mg/kg i.v.	Laminaria	+(0.4 mg/kg)	VIRNO et al. (1969)
Timolol	0.1%–1.5%	Water load	+(0.5%)	VAREILLES et al. (1977)
	2%	Water load	−	ROWLAND and POTTER (1980a)
	0.5% & 1.5%	α-Chymotrypsin	+(0.5%)	VAREILLES et al. (1977)
	1%	Glucose infusion	+	BONOMI et al. (1979)
	0.25%–1%	β-Methasone	+(0.25%)	BONOMI et al. (1979)
	0.001%–1%	Buphthalmia	+(0.01%)	VAREILLES et al. (1980)
Metoprolol	2%	Water load	−	ROWLAND and POTTER (1980b)
	1%	Glucose infusion	+	BONOMI et al. (1979)
	0.25%–1%	β-Methasone	+(1%)	BONOMI et al. (1979)
Oxprenolol	0.01%–1%	Water load	−	SCHMITT et al. (1981a)
	1%	Glucose infusion	+	BONOMI et al. (1979)
	0.25%–1%	β-Methasone	+(1%)	BONOMI et al. (1979)
Practolol	0.01%–1%	Water load	−	SCHMITT et al. (1981a)
	1%	Glucose infusion	+	BONOMI et al. (1979)
Butoxamine	2%	Water load	−	ROWLAND and POTTER (1980a)
Alprenolol	0.1%–1%	Water load	+	SCHMITT et al. (1981a)
Sotalol	2%	Glucose infusion	+	BONOMI et al. (1979)
Pindolol	2%		+	
Butadrine	2%		+	
Atenolol	2%		+	
Sotalol	0.25%–1%	β-Methasone	+(0.25%)	BONOMI et al. (1979)
Pindolol	0.25%–1%		+(0.25%)	
Butadrine	0.25%–1%		+(1%)	
Atenolol	0.25%–1%		+(0.25%)	

[a] + denotes effective in lowering IOP, − denotes ineffective in lowering IOP

(Table 3). Of the nine β-adrenergic antagonists investigated by BONOMI et al. (1979), potency and duration of action comparisons indicated an order of activity: timolol ≃ sotalol > pindolol ≃ oxprenolol ≃ practolol ≃ propranolol > atenolol ≃ butadrine ≃ metroprolol. In additional studies, VAREILLES et al. (1977) further demonstrated that the action of timolol in α-chymotrypsin-treated rabbits is maintained after three instillations a day for 8 days, indicating a lack of tolerance development.

As shown in Table 3, apart from timolol and propranolol, there is disagreement as to the IOP effects of several other β-adrenergic blocking agents, depending upon the experimental model of ocular hypertension employed. In particular, although metroprolol (1%), oxprenolol (1%), and practolol (1%) are effective in lowering elevated IOP produced by glucose infusion or β-methasone (Bonomi et al. 1979), these agents are reported to be ineffective, at equal or higher concentrations, in lowering IOP in the water load assay (Rowland and Potter 1980a; Schmitt et al. 1981a). It should be noted that metroprolol, oxprenolol, and practolol effectively lower IOP when administered topically to man (Krieglstein 1979; Boger 1979).

In rabbit models of experimental hypertension, no clear distinction is obvious between the IOP effects of β_1-selective antagonists (metroprolol, practolol, and atenolol), β_2-selective antagonists (butoxamine), and nonselective agents (timolol, propranolol, oxprenolol, alprenolol, sotalol, or pindolol). However, only in the glucose infusion model, in which concentration response curves were not conducted, was the hypotensive activity of the β_1-selective agent practolol (1%) comparable to that of nonselective β-adrenergic blockers (Bonomi et al. 1979). Also, as previously mentioned, the β_1-selective agents practolol (1%) and metroprolol (2%) were ineffective in the water load assay (Rowland and Potter 1980a; Schmitt et al. 1981a). Furthermore, based upon potency and duration of action, metroprolol and atenolol were among the weakest hypotensive agents tested in the β-methasone model (Bonomi et al. 1979). In general, there thus appear to be some indications that the hypotensive effects of nonselective β-adrenergic antagonists in rabbit models of experimental hypertension may be more consistent or pronounced than β_1-selective agents. In accordance with this view, the decrease in IOP produced in normotensive rabbits by topical administration of β_1- and β_2-adrenergic agonists is similarly more pronounced with agents having predominantly β_2-adrenergic-stimulating properties (Potter and Rowland 1978).

d) Effects on Intraocular Pressure in Other Species

Few studies have been conducted on the IOP effects of β-adrenergic antagonists in species other than the rabbit. In conscious normotensive cats, topical instillations of timolol (2% and 4%) and the β_2-selective antagonist H 35/25 (2% and 4%) are reported to produce decreases in IOP (≈ 2 and 5 mmHg) which persist for at least 6 h (Colasanti and Trotter 1981). Dose–response studies showed that lower concentrations (1%) of both agents were essentially ineffective in lowering IOP, and the pressure-lowering responses to a higher concentration (8%) were less (≈ 2 mmHg) than those observed at a 4% concentration. The pressure responses to timolol and H 35/25 in cats were diminished in sympathectomized eyes or eyes rendered subsensitive to cholinomimetics (chronic echothiophate treatment), suggesting that adrenergic and cholinergic inputs are required for mediation of the action of these drugs in this species.

Additional investigations by Colasanti and Trotter (1981) showed that the β_1-selective antagonist atenolol (4%–8%) was ineffective in lowering IOP in conscious cats, and that the ability of the β_1-selective agonist CGP7760B to reduce

IOP was modest in comparison to the β_2-selective agonist salbutamol (4% and 12%). The data suggest that, as indicated in rabbits, the β-adrenergic receptors mediating pressure changes in cat eyes are predominantly β_2 in nature.

The above studies in cats suggest that this species may represent a fair animal model for evaluation of the effects of β-adrenergic antagonists on IOP. However, the necessity of using high concentrations of drugs compared to those used in the rabbit and man and the restricted effective drug concentration range (2%–4%) producing linear, significant pressure reductions with the agents thus far examined may limit the utility of this model. Additionally, atenolol, an agent which is effective in lowering IOP in man following acute instillation (BOGER 1979), is apparently ineffective in normotensive cats.

In anesthetized cats, timolol (0.1 mg/kg) administered intravenously also reduced IOP (by 4.8 mmHg) in the majority of eyes (6 of 8) examined (HELAL et al. 1979). In contrast, in the enucleated arterially perfused cat eye, perfusion of timolol (0.1 µg/ml/30 min) did not significantly affect IOP (MACRI et al. 1980).

Sotalol (2%) is reported to have no effect upon IOP in conscious owl monkeys (LAMBLE and LAMBLE 1977).

It is obvious from the studies described in the present section that demonstration of the IOP-lowering effect of β-adrenergic antagonists is best shown in rabbits with experimentally induced ocular hypertension. Of the models studied to the present time, only the rabbit water load, glucose infusion, and β-methasone models have been examined with a variety of agents. As pointed out previously, obvious inexplicable discrepancies exist in the activity of common β-adrenergic blockers studied in these assays by several different investigators. Only in the studies of BONOMI et al. (1979), using the rabbit glucose infusion and β-methasone models of ocular hypertension, have all of the β-antagonists investigated been effective in significantly lowering IOP. There is a clear need for further investigations on the action of β-adrenergic antagonists upon IOP under different experimental conditions, as well as in animal species other than the rabbit.

2. Aqueous Humor Dynamics

As will be discussed later (Sect. B.II.2), the effect of β-adrenergic blockers upon aqueous humor dynamics has been more extensively examined in man than animals. SEARS and BÁRÁNY (1960) first reported that dichloroisoproterenol (6–11 mg/kg) administered subcutaneously or intravenously to anesthetized rabbits decreased IOP decreased outflow resistance. Later, also in anesthetized rabits, TAKATS et al. (1972) reported that propranolol (0.3 mg/kg) given intravenously decreased IOP, decreased facility of outflow, and decreased the formation of aqueous humor. The effect of intravenous propranolol (0.1 mg/kg) upon outflow facility in rabbits was confirmed by Gos et al. (1975), who attributed the reduction in facility to a reflex reaction of the eye to a decreased aqueous secretion. Earlier studies by HENDLEY and CROMBIE (1967) using a higher dose level of propranolol intravenously (5 mg/kg) found no effect of propranolol upon the outflow of aqueous humor in anesthetized rabbits.

The finding of STANKIEWICZ et al. (1978) that the fall in IOP after intravenous propranolol (0.5 mg/kg) in rabbits was correlated with a reduction in sodium and potassium content of the aqueous humor supported a suppressive effect of propranolol on secretory activity of the ciliary body. Intravenous propranolol is also reported to increase the penetration of intravenously administered fluorescein into the aqueous humor of rabbits (Reina et al. 1978). The above results indicate that intravenously administered propranolol lowers IOP in rabbits primarily by reducing aqueous humor secretion.

Vareilles and Lotti (1981) studied the effects of topically administered timolol upon IOP, aqueous humor flow (IOP recovery rate method), and outflow facility (constant pressure perfusion method). In unanesthetized rabbits timolol (1%) reduced IOP, reduced aqueous humor flow, and had no effect upon outflow facility. The latter results suggested that in rabbits a reduction in aqueous humor is primarily responsible for the IOP-lowering response to local instillation of timolol.

The effects of β-adrenergic blockers upon aqueous humor dynamics have also been studied in species other than the rabbit. In anesthetized cats, intravenously administered timolol (0.01 mg/kg) produced a transient elevation in aqueous humor formation followed by a subsequent decrease below control values (Helal et al. 1979). The inhibition of aqueous humor formation was related to a reduction in IOP. Similarly, in anesthetized cats, timolol infused intracamerally at concentrations of 0.005%, 0.025%, and 0.15% reduced aqueous humor formation rates by 28%, 56%, and 71% respectively, but did not significantly affect aqueous humor outflow (Liu et al. 1980; Chiou et al. 1980). In vervet anesthetized monkeys, propranolol (5 mg/kg) administered intravenously had no apparent effect upon aqueous humor formation or facility of outflow (Bill 1970). In contrast, topically instilled propranolol (2%) produced a reduction in flow rate of rhesus monkeys (Takase 1976).

The above studies indicate that in the rabbit and cat a reduced rate of aqueous humor formation plays a major role in the lowering of IOP produced by β-adrenergic antagonists. The ocular hypotensive action of β-adrenergic blockers in man is similarly believed to result mainly from a reduction in aqueous humor (see Sect. B.II.2).

3. Interactions with Beta-Adrenergic Receptors in the Eye

a) Presence of Beta-Adrenergic Receptors

Several lines of investigation provide evidence that specific β-adrenergic receptors are present in ocular structures associated with the aqueous humor dynamics in the rabbit and other species. The membrane-bound enzyme adenylate cyclase, which is coupled to the function of β-adrenoceptors in various biological systems (Sutherland and Robison 1966), is present in the ciliary process, iris-ciliary body, sclera-trabecular ring, and aqueous humor of the rabbit, monkey, and human. Activation of adenylate cyclase in these tissues by isoproterenol and other catecholamines has also been demonstrated (Waitzman and Woods 1971; Neufeld et al. 1972; Neufeld and Sears 1974; Nathanson 1980; Gregory et al. 1981; Schmitt et al. 1981a). The data of Nathanson (1980) additionally show an enrichment of μ-adrenergic-sensitive adenylate cyclase activity in epithelial cell fractions of rabbit ciliary process compared to ciliary body, iris, and ciliary vascular tissue. Cytochemical localization studies using electron microscopy also strongly suggest that the adenylate cyclase activity of rabbit ciliary process is distributed predominantly on the plasma membrane of nonpigmented epithelial cells (TSUKAHARA and MAEZAWA 1978a).

Recent studies using radioligand binding techniques provide additional evidence for the presence of β-adrenergic receptors in the eye. High-affinity, specific binding or ^3H-dihydroalprenolol and ^{125}I-hydroxybenzylpindolol to membrane fractions of rabbit iris-ciliary body and isolated ciliary processes, respectively, have been described which can be displaced by catecholamines with the expected order of potency (isoproterenol > epinephrine > norepinephrine) (NEUFELD and PAGE 1977; BROMBERG et al. 1980). In the former studies, utilizing iris-ciliary body preparations, propranolol (K_d 4 nM) and timolol (K_d 6 nM) exhibited a high order of potency in displacing ^3H-dihydroalprenolol binding. Similarly, in the latter study using isolated ciliary processes, l-alprenolol (K_d 0.18 nM), timolol (K_d 0.63 nM), and propranolol (K_d 1.93 nM), but not the α-adrenergic blocker phentolamine (K_d > 50 µM), were capable of displacing ^{125}I-hydroxybenzylpindolol. Significantly, BROMBERG et al. (1980) were able to associate ^{125}I-hydroxybenzylpindolol binding and adenylate cyclase with the same membrane fractions.

Consistent with current concepts of receptor mechanisms, chronic ocular instillation of timolol (1% twice daily for 4 days) increases the density of β-adrenergic receptors in membranes of rabbit iris-ciliary bodies as measured by specific binding of ^3H-dihydroalprenolol (NEUFELD et al. 1978).

Recently, β-adrenergic receptors have been localized in the ciliary process and episcleral blood vessels of the rabbit and rat eye by in vivo histochemical methodology utilizing the fluorescent analog of propranolol, 9-aminoacridinepropranolol (9-AAP) (TSUKAHARA and MAEZAWA 1978b; LAHAV et al. 1978; DAFNA et al. 1979). Pretreatment with propranolol decreased 9-AAP fluorescence in the structures. The localization of β-adrenergic receptors in the ciliary process of the rabbit eye has also been demonstrated using light microscopic radioautography after instillation of ^{14}C-bupranolol (TSUKAHARA et al. 1980).

b) Blockade of Beta-Adrenergic Receptors

A variety of animal studies have demonstrated the ability of at least some β-adrenergic blockers to act as antagonists of β-adrenergic receptors in the eye. Determined on the basis of the ability of β-adrenergic blockers to antagonize various effects of isoproterenol, β-adrenergic blockade has been demonstrated in rabbits, cats, and monkeys in vitro, as well as after systemic or topical administration (Table 4). These effects have included the antagonism of the actions of isoproterenol in decreasing IOP, increasing water permeability in the ciliary epithelium, or elevating cAMP levels in aqueous humor and ocular tissues of rabbits, depressing aqueous formation in the isolated cat eye, and increasing aqueous outflow and formation in vervet monkeys. In the quantitative studies thus far undertaken with more than one β-adrenergic antagonist, timolol, topically instilled in vivo, was at least ten times more potent than propranolol or oxprenolol in antagonizing the ability of topically instilled isoproterenol to induce elevations of aqueous humor cAMP in rabbits (SCHMITT et al. 1981a). Similarly, in vitro timolol ($K_i = 0.6$ nM) was approximately seven times more potent than propranolol ($K_i = 4$ nM) in blocking isoproterenol-stimulated synthesis of cAMP in rabbit iris-ciliary body tis-

Table 4. β-Adrenergic blockers as antagonists of isoproterenol responses on intraocular pressure (IOP) and related ocular systems

Agent tested	Experimental conditions	Isoproterenol response	Route of administration (dose)	Reference
Propranolol	Conscious rabbit, sedated rhesus monkey	IOP	i.v. (5–10 mg/kg)	LANGHAM (1965); LANGHAM and DIGGS (1974)
Propranolol	Anesthetized vervet monkeys	F, C	i.v. (5 mg/kg)	BILL (1970)
Propranolol	Conscious rabbit	IOP	i.v. (0.2 mg/kg)	BHATTACHERJEE (1971)
Timolol	Conscious rabbit (water load model)	IOP	Topical (0.00001%–1.0%)	VAREILLES et al. (1977)
Propranolol Sotalol	Rabbit Ciliary epithelium	Permeability	In vitro (10^{-5} M)	GREEN and GRIFFIN (1978)
Bupranolol	Rabbit	Aqueous cAMP	i.v. (5 mg/kg)	TAMURA et al. (1978)
Timolol	Cat Isolated perfused eye	F	In vitro (0.1 µg/ml)	MACRI et al. (1980)
Timolol Propranolol	Conscious rabbit Iris-ciliary body	IOP, aqueous cAMP cAMP	Topical (0.5%–4%) In vitro (10^{-9}–10^{-5} M)	BARTELS et al. (1980)
Propranolol Timolol IPS 339 H 35/25 Atenolol Practolol	Rabbit Ciliary epithelium	cAMP	In vitro (10^{-9}–5×10^{-7} M) In vitro (10^{-9}–10^{-7} M) In vitro (10^{-9}–10^{-6} M) In vitro (10^{-7}–10^{-3} M) In vitro (10^{-6}–10^{-3} M) In vitro (10^{-5}–10^{-3} M)	NATHANSON (1980)
Propranolol Timolol Oxprenolol Alprenolol Practolol	Conscious rabbit (water load model)	Aqueous cAMP, IOP	Topical (0.0001%–1%)	SCHMITT et al. (1981 a)

C, aqueous humor outflow; F, aqueous humor production

sue (BARTELS et al. 1980). However, using rabbit ciliary process tissue, timolol ($K_i = 2.5\,nM$) and propranolol ($K_i = 1.4\,nM$) are reported to be essentially equipotent (NATHANSON 1980), and timolol ($K_i = 0.4\,nM$), propranolol ($K_i = 1.1\,nM$) (GREGORY et al. 1981).

In the above study of NATHANSON (1980), in addition to the nonselective β-adrenergic antagonists timolol and propranolol, the β_2-selective antagonists IPS 339 ($K_i = 3.2\,nM$) and H 35/25 ($K_i = 430\,nM$) also exhibited a high order of activity in antagonizing isoproterenol-stimulated cAMP production. In contrast, the β_1-selective adrenergic antagonist atenolol ($K_i = 11\,\mu M$) and practolol ($K_i = 21\,\mu M$) were considerably less active in the latter regard. The data strongly suggest that β_2-adrenergic receptor subtypes are predominantly involved in mediation of isoproterenol stimulation of cAMP production in the rabbit ciliary process. In vivo and in vitro studies with selective and nonselective β-adrenergic agonists in elevating cAMP in aqueous humor or ciliary process tissue of rabbits are in agreement with this view (ROWLAND and POTTER 1979; NATHANSON 1980). Unpublished data (SCHMITT) have also demonstrated that β_1-selective antagonists, practolol ($K_i > 300\,nM$), metroprolol ($K_i > 1\,\mu M$), and atenolol ($K_i > 300\,mM$) are ineffective in displacing ^3H-dihydroalprenolol from rabbit iris-ciliary body tissue, further indicating that only β_2-adrenergic receptors are present in these ocular structures.

In in vitro studies using iris-ciliary body tissues (BARTELS et al. 1980) or ciliary process (NATHANSON 1980; GREGORY et al. 1981), the K_i's for timolol (0.6, 2.5, 0.4 nM, respectively) and propranolol (4, 1.4, 1.1 nM, respectively) in antagonizing isoproterenol-activated cAMP synthesis are not markedly different from the K_d values reported for timolol (0.63 nM) and propranolol (1.93 nM) in displacing ^{125}I-hydroxybenzylpindolol from membranes of rabbit ciliary processes (BROMBERG et al. 1980). These concentrations of the two agents are substantially exceed in the aqueous humor of rabbits following ocular instillation of 1% solutions to rabbits (see SCHMITT et al. 1981b; Sect. B.I.3).

Intravenous administration of propranolol (5 mg/kg) and topically instilled timolol (0.5%) has also been reported to antagonize the IOP-lowering effect of the β-adrenergic agonists salbutamol and albuterol in rhesus monkeys and rabbits, respectively (LANGHAM and DIGGS 1974; RADIUS et al. 1978). In cats, pretreatment with timolol (4%) completely antagonizes the IOP-lowering effect of salbutamol, and pretreatment with the β_1-selective antagonist atenolol (8%) similarly abolishes the decrease in IOP produced by the β_1-selective agonist CGP7760B (COLASANTI and TROTTER 1981).

Of the five β-adrenergic blockers studied by SCHMITT et al. (1981a) (Table 4), it should be noted that, when instilled topically, only timolol and oxprenolol and not propranolol, practolol, or alprenolol were effective in antagonizing isoproterenol's action in lowering IOP in the water load assay and stimulating aqueous cAMP production. The possible significance of these findings will be discussed in Sect. B.I.4.b. It should also be mentioned that intravenously administered propranolol (5 mg/kg) was ineffective in blocking the IOP decrease and elevation of aqueous cAMP in response to topical isoproterenol in rabbits (NEUFELD et al. 1972). Similarly, GNADINGER and BÁRÁNY (1964) reported that intravenous nethalide (10 mg/kg) did not antagonize the outflow facility increase produced by subconjunctivally or intravitreally injected isoproterenol in rabbits.

4. Mechanisms of Action on Intraocular Pressure

a) Site of Action

The previously described studies demonstrate that topically administered β-adrenergic antagonists lower IOP in normotensive rabbits and/or rabbits with experimentally elevated IOP. The IOP reduction produced by these agents appears to be mainly the result of a reduction in aqueous humor inflow. The latter actions of these agents are generally considered to be the result of a local action of the drug upon the eye. However, the possibility of a general systemic (e.g., lowering of blood pressure) and/or central nervous system site of action partly contributing to the IOP response is indicated by the findings that unilateral instillation of timolol to rabbit and man significantly reduces IOP in the contralateral eye (VAREILLES et al. 1977; RADIUS et al. 1978; ZIMMERMAN and KAUFMAN 1977 b).

In the above studies, the IOP response in the contralateral eye of rabbits acutely instilled with timolol was uniformly less than the treated eye. It thus appears likely that the IOP responses in the treated eyes are largely the result of a local action on the eye rather than of a general systemic or CNS effect. However, the possibility of such an extraocular locus of action for the IOP response in the untreated eye cannot be excluded.

Systemically administered propranolol (1 mg/kg) and pindolol (0.125 mg/kg) can produce modest hypotension (≈ 10 mmHg) in conscious rabbits (DURAO and RICO 1977). Furthermore, topical administration of timolol (0.5% and 4%) to anesthetized rabbits produces significant bradycardia (BARTELS et al. 1980). The latter findings indicate that significant amounts of timolol can enter the circulation, and suggest the possibility that the consensual response to timolol could be in part due to a systemic action of the drug on sites outside the eye.

The concentrations of timolol achieved in plasma (≈ 600 nM) after topical application of 0.5% solutions to rabbits are some 200 times or more than the K_i for this agent in inhibiting isoproterenol-stimulated cAMP in isolated ciliary process and iris-ciliary body or displacing ^{125}I-hydroxybenzylpindolol from membranes of rabbit ciliary processes (see Sect. B.I.3.b and VAREILLES et al. 1977). It is thus also possible that the consensual IOP responses of timolol could be partly the result of a local action of the drug upon the contralateral eye after its absorption into the blood.

b) Mode of Action

Although existing data support a local ocular action of timolol, and most likely other β-adrenergic blocking agents, the question as to whether their ocular hypotensive activity in animals is directly related to an ability to block classical β-adrenergic receptors as defined on extraocular tissues is yet to be resolved. The evidence that blockade of such receptors may be involved comes from several observations discussed in detail in previous sections. These include:

1. A number of structurally unrelated agents having β-adrenergic blocking properties are capable of lowering IOP
2. β-Adrenergic receptors are present in ocular structures associated with aqueous humor dynamics.

3. Some β-adrenergic blockers in vitro and in vivo are capable of antagonizing various actions of isoproterenol which influence IOP and aqueous humor dynamics.
4. The actions of β-adrenergic blockers upon 1, 2, and 3 appear, in general, to exhibit characteristics of an action upon β_2-, as opposed to β_1, adrenergic systems described in extraocular tissues.
5. Other pharmacologic activities shared by a number of β-adrenergic antagonists, such as intrinsic sympathomimetic activity, membrane-stabilizing activity, or local anesthetic activity, are lacking in timolol, one of the most effective and widely studied agents upon IOP and related ocular systems (SCRIABINE et al. 1973).

In spite of the evidence cited above, several observations have raised questions as to whether the ocular hypotensive activity of this class of agents is directly related to their ability to block classic β-adrenergic receptors. Apart from the obvious, often-stated anomaly that both β-adrenergic agonists and antagonists lower IOP and have similar effects upon aqueous humor dynamics, the additional evidence in this regard is summarized below.

VAREILLES et al. (1977) first noted that, in rabbits, much higher concentrations of timolol were needed to reduce water-load-induced elevation of IOP (minimal effective concentration 0.5%) than were required to antagonize the inhibitory effects of isoproterenol in the same assay (minimal effective concentration 0.001%). Furthermore, the concentrations of timolol in aqueous humor following instillation of 0.5% solutions in rabbits were considerably above ($\approx 1,000$ times) that required to block β-adrenergic receptors in other tissues. On the basis of these facts, the latter authors suggested that the β-receptors concerned with pressure regulation in the eye may differ fundamentally from those in other tissues.

More recently, SCHMITT et al. (1981 a), in an extension of the studies of VAREILLES et al. (1977), could find little relationship between the ability of timolol, propranolol, alprenolol, oxprenolol, and practolol to antagonize the IOP-lowering effect of isoproterenol in water-loaded rabbits and their ability to lower IOP themselves in the same assay. Additionally, the ability of these β-adrenergic blocking agents, administered topically, to antagonize isoproterenol-induced elevation of aqueous humor cAMP was not correlated with their ocular hypotensive activity. Of the agents examined, timolol exhibited hypotensive activity and antagonized the actions of isoproterenol on IOP and cAMP, whereas practolol was inactive in all respects. However, although propranolol and alprenolol effectively lowered IOP, they exhibited little or no activity in antagonizing either the effects of isoproterenol on IOP or cAMP. In contrast, oxprenolol had little or no ocular hypotensive activity but yet was very active in antagonizing both actions of isoproterenol. The varied results obtained with these agents could not be readily explained on the basis of their relative ability to penetrate into the eye, since all the agents had equal or greater access to the aqueous humor as timolol following ocular instillation in rabbits (SCHMITT et al. 1981 b).

BONOMI et al. (1979) observed that the effectiveness of various β-adrenergic antagonists in lowering IOP in rabbit models of experimental ocular hypertension did not correlate with their peripheral β-blocking potencies judged by inhibition of isoproterenol tachycardia. On a similar line, SEARS (1979) reported that preliminary studies with his co-workers indicate that the β-adrenergic binding and blocking potencies of propranolol, timolol, and pindolol do not appear to parallel their IOP-lowering effects (see also GREGORY et al. 1981).

Collectively, the above studies provide some indications that the receptors at which β-adrenergic blocking agents act in the rabbit eye to lower IOP may have different characteristics or properties from those of the classic β-adrenergic receptors described in other tissues. The increasing application of new receptor and enzyme technology in ocular pharmacology will undoubtedly facilitate resolution of the existing complex questions relating to the mechanism of action of β-adrenergic antagonists in the eye.

5. Ocular Penetration and Distribution

In comparison to the number of studies conducted on the pharmacologic effects of β-adrenergic blockers, few studies have appeared concerning the intraocular penetration and distribution of these drugs. In the studies that have been reported, most have measured total radioactivity after instillation of radiolabeled compounds or have used spectrofluorometric techniques which do not permit distinction between parent compounds and metabolites in the ocular tissues or fluids. Using the latter methodology the ocular penetration of ^{14}C-labeled timolol, propranolol, atenolol, metoprolol, and bupranolol has been determined after topical instillation in rabbits (VAREILLES et al. 1977, 1978; ROS et al. 1978 b, 1979; KOMURO et al. 1979; SCHMITT et al. 1980; HUSSAIN et al. 1980).

With one exception (ROS et al. 1979), the concentration of drugs and/or the experimental conditions employed in the above studies were sufficiently different to preclude direct comparisons of ocular penetration or distribution of the various β-adrenergic antagonists studied. In general however, all authors agree that each of the above β-adrenergic blockers rapidly penetrates into the eyes, reaching peak levels in ocular tissues and fluids within 30 min after instillation, and have a relative distribution of cornea > iris-ciliary body > aqueous humor > lens.

Of the four β-adrenergic blockers (atenolol, metoprolol, timolol, and propranolol) examined by ROS et al. (1979), only the former two agents were studied at the same concentration (4%). After instillation of ^{14}C-atenolol, which is considerably less lipophilic than ^{14}C-metroprolol, radioactivity levels in the nictitating membrane were much higher, and peak levels in aqueous humor were attained later than with ^{14}C-metoprolol, indicating poorer ocular penetration. ROS et al. (1979) also made comparisons of the relative ocular penetration and distribution of atenolol (4%), metoprolol (4%), timolol (0.5%), and propranolol (1%), assuming a linear arithmetical relationship between the concentration instilled and ocular tissue levels. The validity of such an assumption is questionable, however, especially in view of the data of SCHMITT et al. (1980) showing that the concentration of timolol instilled and the aqueous humor levels attained exhibit a linear logarithmic relationship.

In the studies of SCHMITT et al. (1980), using ^{14}C-timolol (1.5%), the distribution of radioactivity in 15 ocular and extraocular tissues and fluids of the rabbit was compared after ocular instillation and intravenous injection of a similar dose (100 μl). Levels of radioactivity in ocular tissues and fluids were considerably greater after instillation than after intravenous injection, whereas in extraocular tissues the levels were similar after both routes of administration. The data provided strong support for the use of timolol by the topical route in the treatment of glaucoma.

In the same study, aqueous humor and serum levels after topical and intravenous administration of the same dose of timolol were determined by means of liquid scintillation (LSC) and gas liquid chromatography (GLC). Evaluation of the data disclosed the following relationships: topically, GLC levels $\geqq$ LSC levels in aqueous humor; LSC levels > GLC levels in serum; and intravenously, LSC levels > GLC levels in both fluids. Since LSC measures total radioactivity and GLC measures untransformed timolol only, it was concluded that, following instillation, only timolol was present in aqueous humor, whereas timolol as well as metabolites were present in serum. The apparent lack of metabolism of timolol in aqueous humor may explain in part the long duration of action of timolol after ocular instillation in rabbits and man (VAREILLES et al. 1977; ZIMMERMAN and KAUFMAN 1977a, b). Binding to pigment and other structures is an important factor.

Comparison of the data obtained by GLC and LSC also indicated that, following intravenous administration, timolol was metabolized extensively and metabolites appeared in serum and aqueous humor.

There is only one report on the comparative ocular penetration of β-adrenergic blockers using gas chromatographic techniques to measure parent compounds (SCHMITT et al. 1981 b). Aqueous humor and serum levels of timolol, propranolol, oxprenolol, alprenolol, and practolol were measured following ocular instillation of 1% solutions in rabbits. Octanol/buffer partition ratios were also determined. No apparent relationship was found between the peak levels of the agents in aqueous humor and their octanol/buffer partition ratios. However, peak aqueous humor levels of timolol (461 ng/100 mg) and practolol (919 ng/100 mg), whose partition ratios were less than unity, occurred somewhat later (1 h) than propranolol (859 ng/100 mg) (10 min), oxprenolol (1,771 ng/100 mg) (10 min), or alprenolol (1,004 ng/100 mg) (30 min), whose partition ratios exceeded unity. Peak levels in serum of timolol (8 ng/100 µl), propranolol (4.2 ng/100 µl), oxprenolol (11.5 ng/100 µl), and alprenolol (4.5 ng/100 µl) were achieved within 10 min and reduced to less than 15% within 4 h. Peak serum levels of practolol (7 ng/100 µl) occurred somewhat later (30 min) and remained high (48%) 7½ h later. The lower extent of metabolism of practolol in serum presumably accounted for its slower elimination from this fluid.

It is obvious from the above studies that the previously mentioned high order of activity of topically administered timolol and the lack of activity of practolol, oxprenolol, propranolol, or alprenolol, either in lowering experimentally elevated IOP or in antagonizing responses to isoproterenol in the eye, cannot be explained on the basis of their relative penetration into the rabbit eye.

6. Other Ocular Pharmacology

As shown by the existence of adenylate cyclase and its stimulation by catecholamines, histochemical localization using 9-AAP, radio-autographic localization using ^{14}C-bupranolol, and/or specific binding of ^{3}H-dihydroalprenolol, evidence is provided for the existence of β-adrenergic receptors in the cornea, sclera, iris, choroid, and limbal conjunctiva of the rabbit, monkey, rat bovine, and man (Neufeld and Sears 1974; Page and Neufeld 1978; Tsukahara and Maezawa 1978a, b; Neufeld et al. 1978; Lahav et al. 1978; Dafna et al. 1979; Mochizuki 1979; Bartels et al. 1980; Tsukahara et al. 1980; Walkenbach et al. 1980).

a) Cornea

In rabbit, bovine, or human cornea, timolol and propranolol are capable of inhibiting catecholamine-stimulated cAMP (Bartels et al. 1980; Walkenbach et al. 1980). Chronic instillation of timolol (1%, twice daily for 4 days) is also reported to cause an increase in the density of β-adrenergic receptors in rabbit corneal tissue (Neufeld et al. 1978). Curiously, the increase in receptor density was not associated with an altered ability to synthesize cAMP.

In isolated rabbit and frog cornea, timolol (10^{-5} M) and propranolol (10^{-5} M) also inhibit the stimulation of chloride transport induced by isoproterenol (Montoreano et al. 1976; Candia et al. 1979). In frog cornea timolol alone (10^{-5} M) did not change the electrical parameters of the cornea, nor did it block stimulation caused by the calcium ionophore A23187 (Candia et al. 1979).

Applied topically to the eyes of rabbits, propranolol (0.2%) and alprenolol (0.1%), but not timolol (1%), exhibit marked local anesthetic activity (Bartch and Knopf 1970; Vareilles et al. 1978).

b) Iris/Pupil

Using contractile responses of isolated muscle strips and appropriate agonists and antagonists, the presence and distribution of α- and β-adrenergic receptors in sphincter, dilator, and ciliary muscles of the rabbit, cat, monkey, and man have been described by van Alphen et al. (1965) and van Alphen (1976). In rabbit irides, ^3H-dihydroalprenolol exhibits high-affinity specific binding which is displaced by agonists and antagonists with potencies corresponding to β-adrenergic receptors (propranolol > isoproterenol ≧ epinephrine > norepinephrine > phentolamine) (Page and Neufeld 1978). And in vitro, the contractile relaxation and increase in cAMP level of the rabbit spincter pupillae muscle produced by isoproterenol is blocked by pretreatment with propranolol (3×10^{-6} M) (Mochizuki 1979).

Abdel-Latif and Smith (1976) investigated the in vitro effects of DL-propranolol and sotalol on the synthesis of glycerolipids by rabbit iris muscle. At concentrations of 0.03–0.5 mM, propranolol, an amphiphilic cationic drug, appeared to inhibit phosphatidate phosphohydrolase and enhance the availability of Ca^{2+} in muscle, thus redirecting de novo synthesis of phospholipids. Sotalol, which possesses a more polar group in its chemical structure, was devoid of similar effects, indicating that the effect of propranolol on phospholipid metabolism in the iris is not related to β-adrenergic blockade.

Various β-adrenergic blockers have been shown not to alter pupil size of rabbits when administered intravenously or topically over a wide dosage range (Hendley and CROMBIE 1967; LANGHAM et al. 1973; VAREILLES et al. 1978; RADIUS et al. 1978; BONOMI et al. 1979; ROWLAND and POTTER 1980 a).

c) Lacrimal System

The acute intravenous administration of propranolol (0.3–10 mg/kg) or metroprolol (3–30 mg/kg) or the chronic oral administration of propranolol (40.1 mg/kg/day) or practolol (330 mg/kg/day) has no discernible effect upon tear flow in conscious rabbits measured by modified Schirmer techniques (BOISSIER et al. 1976; ABERG et al. 1979). Similarly, in anesthetized rabbits, tear flow from the cannulated excretory ducts is not changed after intraarterial injection of sotalol (3 mg/kg) (BOTELHO et al. 1973). However, administered intravenously, propranolol, metoprolol, pindolol, penbutolol, practolol, and atenolol are all effective in blocking the increase in tear flow produced by isoproterenol in rabbits (BOISSIER et al. 1976; ABERG et al. 1979).

II. Clinical Pharmacology

The clinical literature concerning the action of β-adrenergic blockers upon IOP and their use in the treatment of ocular hypertension and glaucoma has grown dramatically in the past few years. An extensive review of the literature in this regard is beyond the scope of the present chapter. For the latter, the reader is referred to some recent reviews (BOGER 1979; HEEL et al. 1979; ZIMMERMAN et al. 1980). The following section is included with the intention of providing a few corollaries between the animal pharmacology and what has been described in man.

1. Intraocular Pressure

A variety of β-adrenergic antagonists are reported to lower IOP when administered topically or systemically to normal volunteers or glaucomatous patients (BOGER 1979). In contrast to the absence or minimal effects upon IOP of most β-adrenergic blockers applied topically to normotensive rabbits (see Sect. B.I.1), in normotensive patients topically instilled β-adrenergic antagonists including timolol, propranolol, pindolol, bupranolol, and befunolol produce pronounced and consistent IOP-lowering effects (MUSINI et al. 1971; KATZ et al. 1976; COAKES and BRUBAKER 1978; S. E. SMITH et al. 1979; TAKASE and ARAIE 1980). The latter observations appear to represent a significant difference in the IOP responses to β-adrenergic antagonists in man and rabbits.

As indicated in rabbits with experimental ocular hypertension, in normal or glaucomatous patients the potency of timolol appears to be greater than that of most other β-adrenergic antagonists (ROS et al. 1978 a; BOGER 1979; TAKASE and ARAIE 1980). Dose–response studies by ZIMMERMAN and KAUFMAN (1977 b) demonstrated that timolol (0.1–1%) produces IOP-lowering effects which last at least 24 h. Comparative studies in normal volunteers indicated that the ratio of hypotensive potency of propranolol, befunolol, bupranolol, and timolol was 1:2.5:5:11 (TAKASE and ARAIE 1980).

Although there are indications that β_2-adrenergic receptors may be predominantly involved in responses to β-adrenergic blockers in the rabbit eye (see Sects.

B.I.1.c and B.I.3.b), the lack of adequate data relating to dose–response, ocular penetration, and metabolism in man precludes elucidation of the possible roles of β-adrenergic receptor subtypes (B_1 vs β_2) in the action of these agents in the human eye. Dose–response data are of particular importance in this regard, since all β_1-selective agents studied in man may have sufficient β_2-adrenergic blocking activity to be manifested at the concentration employed. The significance of an apparently diminished IOP response over time to the β_1-selective adrenergic agent atenolol, but not to the nonselective β-adrenergic antagonist timolol, is yet to be determined (PHILLIPS et al. 1977; WETTRELL and PANDOLFI 1977; BRENKMAN 1978; BOGER 1980).

2. Aqueous Humor Dynamics

Administered topically to open-angle glaucoma patients in acute studies, neither timolol (0.25–0.5%), propranolol (1%), bupranolol (0.5%), nor pindolol increases the facility of aqueous humor outflow (ZIMMERMAN et al. 1977; SONNTAG et al. 1978; TIERI and POLZELLA 1975; KRIEGLSTEIN et al. 1977; BONOMI and STEINDLER 1975). Other long-term studies demonstrated only a slight increase in outflow (AIRAKSINEN 1979). These findings, together with fluorimetric studies demonstrating a definite decrease in the rate of aqueous humor formation, strongly indicate that the major action by which β-adrenergic blocking agents lower IOP in man is by reducing aqueous flow (YABLONSKI et al. 1978; COAKES and BRUBAKER 1978). Additional electrooculogram studies in normal volunteers may indirectly support this view (MISSOTTEN and GOETHALS 1977). As mentioned previously (Sect. B.I.2), β-adrenergic antagonists appear to lower IOP mainly by reducing aqueous formation also in rabbits and cats. The mechanism is unknown.

CRISTINI and GIOVANNI (1979), using rheographic methods to measure the quantity of blood flow in the eye, have reported that instillation of timolol (0.25%) in glaucomatous patients markedly increases blood flow. The maximal effect upon blood flow preceded the maximal lowering of IOP. It was implied that this hemodynamic action of timolol may act as a trigger for its pressure-lowering action, although how the two observations might functionally relate to each other or to a reduction in aqueous humor secretion was not discussed. Further evidence for an action of timolol upon vasculature in the eye is provided by the finding that timolol (0.5%) produces apparent iridial vasodilation as indicated by the appearance of increased peripupillary dye leakage (fluorescein angiography) after its instillation in glaucomatous patients (KOTTOW 1980).

3. Beta-Adrenergic Receptor Blockade in the Eye

In comparison to animals, few studies on the acute interaction of selective β-adrenergic agonists and β-adrenergic blockers in the eye of man have been reported. Topical pretreatment with oxprenolol (1%) was observed to inhibit the peripheral side effects (tachycardia) induced by isoproterenol (4%), but not isoproterenol's ocular hypotensive action (BIETTIE et al. 1977). The findings of these single-dose studies are in contrast to the ability of oxprenolol to antagonize the IOP-lowering effects of isoproterenol in the rabbit water load assay (SCHMITT et al. 1981 a).

Studies on the interaction of timolol and epinephrine are contradictory and difficult to interpret in view of the nonselective α- and β-agonist activity of epinephrine (GOLDBERG et al. 1980).

4. Mechanisms of Action

a) Site of Action

As observed in rabbits, administered to one eye of man β-adrenergic blockers such as timolol (0.5%–1.5%) and pindolol (15) significantly reduce IOP in the contralateral untreated eye (although to a lesser extent than the treated eye) (ZIMMERMAN and KAUFMAN 1977b; S. E. SMITH et al. 1979). The asymmetry of the response in the treated versus untreated eyes and the lack of effect of timolol on blood pressure (ZIMMERMAN et al. 1980) suggest primarily a local rather than a general systemic or CNS site of action for the IOP response in the treated eye. However, systemic absorption and an extraocular site of action of the drug in the untreated eye cannot be excluded, since systemically administered β-adrenergic blockers lower IOP and apparently sufficient timolol and pindolol are absorbed after topical instillation to reduce resting heart rate and exercise tachycardia slightly (ZIMMERMAN et al. 1979; S. E. SMITH et al. 1979; AFFRIME et al. 1980). Additionally, as noted above, topically instilled oxprenolol (1%) is capable of antagonizing the tachycardia induced by topical isoproterenol (4%) (BIETTI et al. 1977).

b) Mode of Action

Although not established, the mediation of the IOP-lowering effect of β-adrenergic antagonism in man via blockade of β-adrenergic receptors is suggested by the fact that a number of structurally different agents having β-adrenergic blocking properties are capable of lowering IOP, and that this effect cannot be related to other common pharmacologic actions, such as intrinsic sympathomimetic, membrane-stabilizing, or local anesthetic activity (HEEL et al. 1979; ZIMMERMAN et al. 1980). However, there is no strong evidence either supporting or refuting the concept that these agents lower IOP directly as a result of their ability to block classical β-adrenergic receptors as described in peripheral tissues. Moreover, the apparent contradiction that both β-adrenergic antagonists and agonists such as isoproterenol lower IOP and reduce aqueous flow in man and animals (WETTRELL 1977) may indicate a yet undefined mechanism unrelated to classical β-adrenergic blockade.

5. Ocular Penetration

Using gas chromatographic techniques to measure parent compound, the systemic availability of timolol following ocular instillation in healthy volunteers and glaucoma patients has been determined (AFFRIME et al. 1980; ALVAN et al. 1980). Plasma levels measured after acute or chronic (5-day) instillation of 2 drops of timolol (0.25% and 0.5%) were low, usually undetectable, and did not exceed 10 ng/ml (32 nM). Urinary excretion varied between 14 μg and 60 μg (total drug) during 24 h. In the studies of AFFRIME et al. (1980), the expected decreases in IOP observed in normal subjects were accompanied by small and in most cases clinically insignificant systemic effects upon exercise tachycardia, resting pulse, blood pressure, or forced expiratory volume. Interestingly, ALVAN et al. (1980) estimated that 12% –88% of the dose administered ocularly appeared in the paper tissue used to collect overflow from the eye. The volume delivered topically was 60 µl.

Comparisons of plasma levels achieved in man and rabbits (Sect. B.I.3) are difficult in view of differences in blood volume, dosage, measurement intervals, and other considerations. Recent unpublished observations (PHILLIPS et al., to be published) indicate that aqueous humor levels 1–2 h after instillation of timolol (0.5%) in patients about to undergo cataract extraction (150 ng/100 mg maximum) are not markedly different from levels observed in rabbits (247 ± 51 ng/100 mg) (VAREILLES et al. 1977).

The ocular and cardiovascular effects of topical pindolol (4 drops of 1% solution) were also determined in normal volunteers (S. E. SMITH et al. 1979). Using less specific spectrofluorimetric methods, much higher concentrations of pindolol (6.8 µM peak) were found in plasma than were previously found with timolol, even though the total dosages of both agents were similar (≈ 0.8 mg timolol; 1.13 mg pindolol). The instillation of pindolol was associated with a minimal reduction in resting pupil diameter and light reflex responses. As with timolol (see above), topical instillation of pindolol also somewhat reduced resting heart rate and exercise tachycardia.

C. Alpha-Adrenergic Antagonists

Although the vast majority of animal and clinical investigations have centered around the ocular pharmacology of β-adrenergic antagonists, the latter research has prompted renewed interest in the action of α-adrenergic antagonists in the eye. In comparison to β-adrenergic antagonists, only a limited number of α-adrenergic antagonists have been examined. Particular attention has been given to the effect upon IOP of new agents such as prazosin, which is considered to be a selective α_1-adrenergic antagonist, and labetalol, which possesses both α- and β-adrenergic blocking properties.

I. Animal Pharmacology

1. Selective Alpha-Adrenergic Antagonists

α-Adrenergic blocking agents such as dibenamine, phentolamine, phenoxybenzamine, thymoxamine, and prazosin have been shown to lower the IOP of normal and experimentally ocular hypertensive rabbits when given systemically or topically (SEARS and BÁRÁNY 1960; KOSTYUCHENKOV 1970; BURBERI et al. 1970; LANGHAM et al. 1973; BONOMI and TOMAZZOLI 1977; B. R. SMITH et al. 1979). Among the various agents in this class, only the action of prazosin upon IOP in rabbits has been examined in any detail.

B. R. SMITH et al. (1979) reported that topical ocular application of concentrations of 0.0001%–0.1% prazosin reduced IOP in normotensive rabbits. The maximal effect of 0.1% occurred at 2 h (-6 to -7 mmHg) and persisted for 6–8 h. Substantial ocular toxicity or pupillary changes were not observed. The IOP-lowering effect of prazosin was still observed in both eyes of unilaterally sympathectomized rabbits, although the effect in sympathectomized eyes was less than the normal eyes. The authors concluded that the ability of prazosin to lower IOP in sympathectomized eyes suggests that its action upon IOP is not due to blockade of endogenous catecholamines in these eyes.

A 0.1-mg topical dose (1%) of prazosin in rabbits effected an early decrease (1 h) in arterial blood pressure and in both normal IOP and IOP artificially elevated by water-loading (ROWLAND and POTTER 1980 b). The late drug effects (6 h) were a suppression of elevated IOP but not of normal IOP. A lack of synchrony between the blood pressure changes and IOP changes observed by these authors supported earlier preliminary results of B. R. SMITH et al. (1979), and indicated that the IOP-lowering effects of prazosin were not due to a reduction in systemic blood pressure.

Using a lower concentration of prazosin (0.01%), KRUPIN et al. (1980) demonstrated a decrease in IOP in normal rabbits without significant changes in blood pressure or pulse rate. Futhermore, the latter authors reported that the same concentration of prazosin did not alter outflow facility, episcleral venous pressure, or ocular blood flow. Tonography showed a 27% decrease in the rate of aqueous humor formation and a reduced level of aqueous ascorbate in the posterior chamber, indicating a decreased entry rate of water into the eye. Earlier studies (SEARS and BÁRÁNY 1960) reported that intravenously administered dibenamine (25 mg/kg) in rabbits increased outflow resistance, did not change flow and also opposed, virtually abolished, the resistance-lowering effect of ganglionectomy.

The presence of α-adrenergic receptors in rabbit iris-ciliary bodies is indicated by radioligand binding studies demonstrating that ^3H-dihydroergocryptine binds to membrane preparations and is displaced by adrenergic agents with the expected order of potency (phentolamine > epinephrine $\geq$ norepinephrine > isoproterenol = propranolol) (NEUFELD and PAGE 1977). Consistent with the known action of prazosin as a postsynaptic α-adrenergic receptor blocking agent, topical prazosin prevents the mydriatic action of phenylephrine. Significantly, the IOP-lowering effects of topical prazosin in rabbits is prevented by systemic pretreatment with the α-adrenergic blocker phentolamine, but not with propranolol or atropine (KRUPIN et al. 1980).

Perhaps the latter suggest that the IOP-lowering effects of prazosin in rabbits are due, at least in part, to a reduction in aqueous humor formation unrelated to a fall in systemic blood pressure. The role of α-adrenergic blockade in the ocular effects of prazosin, although indicated, has not yet been established. As is the case with β-adrenergic agents, the anomaly of having both agonists and antagonists with the same ocular action exists with α-adrenergic agents as well.

2. Alpha- and Beta-Adrenergic Antagonists (Labetalol)

Labetalol is a unique adrenergic antagonist in that it exhibits both α- and β-adrenergic blocking properties (FARMER et al. 1972). Labetalol, administered topically (0.1%–1%), produces a dose-related long-lasting (up to 6 h) decrease in IOP (up to −7 mmHg) in normal rabbits, and at a concentration of 1% prevents the increase in IOP after water-loading without affecting pupil diameter (MURRAY et al. 1979). Tonographic studies by the same authors indicated that the IOP decrease was not mediated through an increase in facility of aqueous outflow.

In further studies on the mechanism of action of labetalol upon IOP in rabbits, LEOPOLD and MURRAY (1979) showed that labetalol, topically applied to rabbits at a concentration (1%) which significantly reduced IOP, had no effect on arterial or venous blood pressure. At the same concentration it also failed to block the IOP responses to isoproterenol or norepinephrine. The hypotensive action of labetalol was neither blocked nor potentiated by the α-adrenergic blocker phenoxybenzamine; however, timolol did reduce the action of labetalol. These observations suggested to the latter authors that labetalol's ocular hypotensive effect may occur through some mechanism other than α- or β-adrenergic blockade. Their additional observations that cervical sympathectomy reduced the hypotensive response to labetalol indicated that intact sympathetic nerve endings are necessary for labetalol to act.

II. Clinical Pharmacology

Topically applied thymoxamine (0.1%–1%) induces miosis in humans and has been advocated as a safe agent for reversing mydriasis produced for diagnostic purposes (TURNER and SNEDDON 1968; MAPSTONE 1970; SMALL et al. 1976; WAND and GRANT 1976; BONOMI and TOMAZZOLI 1977). This agent is also reported to be effective in the therapy of angle-closure glaucoma (RUTKOWSKI et al. 1973). The usefulness of this agent in treatment of closed angle glaucoma is controversial. PATERSON and PATERSON (1972) and WAND and GTANT (1976) report a lack of effect of this agent (1% and 0.5% respectively) upon IOP in open-angle glaucoma patients, whereas (BONOMI and TOMAZZOLI (1977) report some IOP-lowering effect of thymoxamine (1%) in these patients. The latter two authors agreed that thymoxamine does not affect the facility of aqueous outflow, although PATERSON and PATERSON (1972) reported a reduction in outflow facility after instillation of thymoxamine.

There have been clearly fewer clinical investigations of the potential utility of topically administered α-adrenergic blocking agents than of β-adrenergic antagonists. The recent animal pharmacology on prazosin and labetalol (see above) will undoubtedly precipitate additional investigations on the potential utility of α-adrenergic blockers in open-angle glaucoma.

References

Abdel-Latif AA, Smith JP (1976) Effects of DL-Propranolol on the synthesis of glycerolipids by rabbit iris muscle. Biochem Pharmacol 25:1697–1704

Aberg G, Adler G, Wikberg J (1979) Inhibition and facilitation of lacrimal flow by β-adrenergic drugs. Acta Ophthalmol 57:225–235

Affrime MB, Lowenthal DT, Tobert JA, Shirk J, Eidenson B, Cook T, Onesti G (1980) Dynamics and kinetics of ophthalmic timolol. Clin Pharmacol Ther 27:471–477

Airaksinen PJ (1979) The long-term hypotensive effect of timolol maleate compared with the effect of pilocarpine in simple and capsular glaucoma. Acta Ophthalmol 57:425–434

Alvan G, Calissendorff B, Seideman P, Widmark K, Widmark G (1980) Absorption of ocular timolol. Clin Pharm 5:95–100

Bartels SP, Roth HO, Jumblatt MM, Neufeld AH (1980) Pharmacological effects of topical timolol in the rabbit eye. Invest Ophthalmol Vis Sci 19:1189–1197

Bartsch W, Knopf K-W (1970) Eine modifizierte Methode zur Prüfung der Oberflächenanästhesie an der Kaninchen-Cornea: demonstriert am Beispiel von Cocain, Procain, Propranolol, Alprenolol, INPEA and Verapamil. Arzneimittelforsch (Drug Res) 20:1140–1143

Bhattacherjee P (1971) Effects of catecholamines on the ocular tension of normal and sympathetically denervated rabbit eyes. Exp Eye Res 12:13–24

Bietti GB, Bucci MG, Pecosolido N (1977) Lokales Oxprenolol bei der Behandlung verschiedener Glaukomformen. Klin Monatsbl Augenheilkd 170:824–830

Bill A (1970) Effects of norepinephrine, isoproterenol and sympathetic stimulation on aqueous humour dynamics in vervet monkeys. Exp Eye Res 10:31–46

Boger WP III (1979) The treatment of glaucoma: role of β-blocking agents. Drugs 18:25–32

Boissier J-R, Advenier C, Ho S (1976) Sécrétion lacrymale chez le lapin et récepteurs β-adrenergiques. J Pharmacol 7 2:241–250

Bonomi L, Steindler P (1975) Effect of pindolol on intraocular pressure. Br J Ophthalmol 59:301–303

Bonomi L, Tomazzoli L (1977) Thymoxamine and intraocular pressure. Albrecht von Graefes Arch Klin Exp Ophthalmol 204:95–100

Bonomi L, Perfetti S, Noya E, Bellucci R, Massa F (1979) Comparison of the effects on nine beta-adrenergic blocking agents on intraocular pressure in rabbits. Albrecht Von Graefes Arch Klin Exp Ophthalmol 210:1–8

Botelho SY, Goldstein AM, Martinez EV (1973) Norepinephrine-responsive beta-adrenergic receptors in rabbit lacrimal gland. Am J Physiol 224:1119–1122

Brenkman RF (1978) Long-term hypotensive effect of atenolol 4% eye drops. Br J Ophthalmol 62:287–291

Bromberg BB, Gregory DS, Sears ML (1980) Beta-adrenergic receptors in ciliary processes of the rabbit. Invest Ophthalmol Vis Sci 19:203–207

Burberi P, Piccinelli D, Silvestrini B (1970) Effects of systemically administered drugs on intraocular pressure in rabbits. Arzneimittel-Forsch (Drug Res) 20:1142–1147

Candia OA, Podos SM, Neufeld AH (1979) Modification by timolol of catecholamine stimulation of chloride transport in isolated corneas. Invest Ophthalmol Vis Sci 18:691–695

Chiou GCY, Liu HK, Trzeciakowski J (1980) Studies of action mechanism of antiglaucoma drugs with a newly developed cat model. Life Sci 27:2445–2451

Coakes RL, Brubaker RF (1978) The mechanism of timolol in lowering intraocular pressure in the normal eye. Arch Ophthalmol 96:2045–2048

Colasanti BK, Trotter RR (1981) Effects of selective beta$_1$- and beta$_2$-adrenoreceptor agonists and antagonists on intraocular pressure in the cat. Invest Ophthalmol Vis Sci 20:69–76

Cristini G, Giovanni A (1979) Pressure lowering effect of timolol with reference to its topical vascular action. Albrecht Von Graefes Arch Klin Exp Ophthalmol 211:325–328

Dafna Z, Lahav M, Melamed E (1979) Localization of β-adrenoceptors in the anterior segment of the albino rabbit eye using a fluorescent analog of propranolol. Exp Eye Res 29:327–330

Durao V, Rico JMGT (1977) Modification by indomethacin of the blood pressure lowering effect of pindolol and propranolol in conscious rabbits. Eur J Pharmacol 43:377–381

Evans DB, Fox R, Hauck FP (1979) β-Adrenergic receptor blockers as therapeutic agents. In: Hess HJ (ed) Annual reports in medicinal chemistry. Academic, New York, chap 9, pp 81–90

Farmer JB, Kennedy I, Levy GP, Marshall RJ (1972) Pharmacology of AH 5158; a drug which blocks both α- and β-adrenoceptors. Br J Pharmacol 45:660

Gnädinger MC, Bárány EH (1964) Die Wirkung der β-adrenergischen Substanz Isoprenalin auf die Ausfluß-Fazilität des Kaninchenauges. Albrecht Von Graefes Archiv Ophthalmol 167:483–492

Goldberg I, Ashburn FS Jr, Palmberg PF, Kass MA, Becker B (1980) Timolol and epinephrine – a clinical study of ocular interactions. Arch Ophthalmol 98:484–486

Gos R, Stankiewicz A, Stanislaw R, Kudinski W (1975) Experimental investigations on the influence of propranolol on the intraocular pressure in rabbits. Klin Oczna 45:4, 322

Green K, Griffin C (1978) Adrenergic effects on the isolated rabbit ciliary epithelium. Exp Eye Res 27:143–149

Gregory DS, Bausher LP, Bromberg BB, Sears ML (1981) The beta-adrenergic receptor and adenyl cyclase of rabbit ciliary processes. In: Sears ML (ed) New directions in ophthalmic research. Yale University Press, New Haven, pp 127–148

Heel RC, Brogden RN, Speight TM, Avery GS (1979) Timolol: a review of its therapeutic efficacy in the topical treatment of glaucoma. Drugs 17:38–55

Helal J, Macri FJ, Cevario SJ (1979) Timolol inhibition of aqueous humor production in the cat. Gen Pharmacol 10:377–380

Hendley ED, Crombie AL (1967) The 24-hour ganglionectomy effect in rabbits: the influence of adrenergic blockade, adrenalectomy and carotid ligation. Exp Eye Res 6:152–164

Hussain A, Hirai S, Sieg J (1980) Ocular absorption of propranolol in rabbits. J Pharm Sci 69:737–738

Katz IM, Hubbard WA, Getson AJ, Gould AL (1976) Intraocular pressure decrease in normal volunteers following timolol ophthalmic solution. Invest Ophthalmol Vis Sci 15:489–492

Komuro S, Nanba H, Takase M (1979) Studies of bupranolol therapy for glaucoma. 1. Ocular penetration and hypotensive effect. Acta Soc Ophthalmol Jap 83:537–541

Kostyuchenkov VN (1970) Effect of phentolamine on the ophthalmotone. Farmakol Toksikol 33:569–572

Kottow MH (1980) Effects of topical timolol on iris vessels. Glaucoma 2:383–388

Krieglstein GK (1979) Response of the intraocular pressure to various β-blocking agents. In: Krieglstein GK, Leydhecker W (eds) Glaucoma update, Springer, Berlin Heidelberg New York, pp 179–189

Krieglstein GK, Sold-Darseff J, Leydhecker W (1977) The intraocular pressure response of glaucomatous eyes to topically applied bupranolol: a pilot study. Albrecht Von Graefes Arch Klin Exp Ophthalmol 202:81–86

Krupin T, Feitl M, Becker B (1980) Effect of prazosin on aqueous humor dynamics in rabbits. Arch Ophthalmol 98:1639–1642

Lahav M, Melamed E, Dafna Z, Atlas D (1978) Localization of beta receptors in the anterior segment of the rat eye by a fluorescent analogue of propranolol. Invest Ophthalmol Vis Sci 17:645–651

Lamble JW, Lamble AP (1977) Effects of catecholamines on the intraocular pressure of conscious owl monkeys. Invest Ophthalmol Vis Sci 16:628–633

Langham ME (1965) The response of the pupil and intraocular pressure of conscious rabbits to adrenergic drugs following unilateral superior cervical ganglionectomy. Exp Eye Res 4:381–389

Langham ME, Diggs E (1974) β-Adrenergic responses in the eyes of rabbits, primates and man. Exp Eye Res 19:281–295

Langham ME, Simjee S, Josephs S (1973) The alpha and beta-adrenergic responses to epinephrine in the rabbit eye. Exp Eye Res 15:75–84

Leopold IH, Murray DL (1979) Ocular hypotensive action of labetalol. Am J Ophthalmol 88:427–431

Liu HK, Chiou GCY, Garg LC (1980) Ocular hypotensive effects of timolol in cat eyes. Arch Ophthalmol 98:1467–1479

Macri FJ, Cevario S-J, Helal J (1980) Timolol inhibition of isoproterenol action – 1. Effects on aqueous humor production and IOP. Gen Pharmacol 11:207–211

Mapstone R (1970) Safe mydriasis. Br J Ophthalmol 54:690–692

Missotten L, Goethals M (1977) Timolol reduces the standing potential of the eye. Ophthalmic Res 9:321–323

Mochizuki M (1979) The beta-adrenergic effects and cyclic AMP in the sphincter pupillae of the albino rabbit. Acta Soc Opthalmol Jpn 83:9, 1517–1523

Montoreano R, Candia OA, Cook P (1976) α- and β-Adrenergic receptors in regulation of ionic transport in frog cornea. Am J Physiol 230:1487–1493

Murray DL, Podos SM, Wei C, Leopold IH (1979) Ocular effects in normal rabbits of topically applied labetalol. Arch Ophthalmol 97:723–726

Musini A, Fabbri B, Bergamaschi M, Mandelli V, Shanks RG (1971) Comparison of the effect of propranolol, lignocaine, and other drugs on normal and raised intraocular pressure in man. Am J Ophthalmol 72:773–781

Nathanson JA (1980) Adrenergic regulation of intraocular pressure: identification of β_2-adrenergic-stimulated adenylate cyclase in ciliary process epithelium. Proc Natl Acad Sci USA 77:7420–7424

Neufeld AH, Page ED (1977) In vitro determination of the ability of drugs to bind to adrenergic receptors. Invest Ophthalmol Vis Sci 16:1118–1124

Neufeld AH, Sears ML (1974) Cyclic-AMP in ocular tissues of the rabbit, monkey, and human. Invest Ophthalmol Vis Sci 13:475–477

Neufeld AH, Jampol LM, Sears ML (1972) Cyclic-AMP in the aqueous humor: the effects of adrenergic agents. Exp Eye Res 14:242–250

Neufeld AH, Zawistowski KA, Page ED, Bromberg BB (1978) Influences on the density of β-adrenergic receptors in the cornea and iris-ciliary body of the rabbit. Invest Ophthalmol Vis Sci 17:1071–1075

Norton AL, Viernstein LJ (1972) The effect of adrenergic agents on ocular dynamics as a function of administration site. Exp Eye Res 14:154–163

Page ED, Neufeld AH (1978) Characterization of α- and β-adrenergic receptors in membranes prepared from the rabbit iris before and after development of supersensitivity. Biochem Pharmacol 27:953–958

Paterson GD, Paterson G (1972) Drug therapy of glaucoma. Br J Ophthalmol 56:288–294

Phillips CI, Howitt G, Rowlands DJ (1967) Propranolol as ocular hypotensive agent. Br J Ophthalmol 51:222–226

Phillips CI, Gore SM, MacDonald MJ, Cullen PM (1977) Atenolol eye drops in glaucoma: a double-masked, controlled study. Br J Ophthalmol 61:349–353

Phillips CI, Bartholomew RS, Kazi G, Schmitt CJ, Vogel R (to be published) Penetration of timolol eye drops into human aqueous humor.

Potter DE, Rowland JM (1978) Adrenergic drugs and intraocular pressure: effects of selective β-adrenergic agonists. Exp Eye Res 27:615–625

Radius RL, Diamond GR, Pollack IP, Langham ME (1978) Timolol: a new drug for management of chronic simple glaucoma. Arch Ophthalmol 96:1003–1008

Reina RA, Gorgone G, Ragusa C (1978) Effect of propranolol on ciliary permeability and aqueous humor outflow. Boll Soc Ital Biol Sper 54:1–4

Ros FE, Dake CL, Nagelkerke NJD, Greve EL (1978a) Metoprolol eye drops in the treatment of glaucoma: a double-blind single-dose trial of a beta$_1$-adrenergic blocking drug. Albrecht Von Graefes Arch Klin Exp Ophthal 206:247–254

Ros FE, Innemee HC, van Zwieten PA (1978b) Penetration of atenolol in the rabbit eye. Albrecht Von Graefes Arch Klin Exp Ophthalmol 208:235–240

Ros FE, Innemee HC, van Zwieten PA (1979) Ocular penetration of beta-adrenergic blocking agents: an experimental study with atenolol, metoprolol, timolol, and propranolol. Doc Ophthalmol 48:291–301

Rowland JM, Potter DE (1979) Effects of adrenergic drugs on aqueous cAMP and cGMP and intraocular pressure. Albrecht Von Graefes Arch Klin Exp Ophthalmol 212:65–75

Rowland JM, Potter DE (1980a) Adrenergic drugs and intraocular pressure: suppression of ocular hypertension induced by water loading. Exp Eye Res 30:93–104

Rowland JM, Potter DE (1980b) The effects of topical prazosin on normal and elevated intraocular pressure and blood pressure in rabbits. Eur J Pharmacol 64:361–363

Rutkowski PC, Fernandez JL, Galin MA, Halasa AH (1973) Alpha adrenergic blockade in the treatment of angle closure glaucoma. Trans Am Acad Ophthalmol Oto-Laryngol 77:137–142

Schmitt CJ, Lotti VJ, Le Douarec JC (1980) Penetration of timolol into the rabbit eye: measurements after ocular instillation and intravenous injection. Arch Ophthalmol 98:547–551

Schmitt C, Lotti VJ, Le Douarec JC (1981a) Beta-adrenergic blockers: lack of relationship between antagonism of isoproterenol and lowering of intraocular pressure in rabbits. In: Sears ML (ed) New directions in ophthalmic research. Yale University Press, New Haven, Chap 9, pp 147–162

Schmitt C, Lotti VJ, Le Douarec JC (1981 b) Penetration of five β-adrenergic antagonists into the rabbit eye after ocular instillation. Albrecht Von Graefes Arch Klin Exp Ophthalmol 217:167–174

Scriabine A, Torchiana ML, Stavorski JM, Ludden CT, Minsker DH, Stone CA (1973) Some cardiovascular effects of timolol, a new beta-adrenergic blocking agent. Arch Int Pharmacodyn Ther 205:76

Sears ML (1979) Mechanism of adrenergic treatment of glaucoma. In: Krieglstein GK, Leydhecker W (eds) Springer Berlin Heidelberg New York, pp 153-157

Sears ML, Bárány EH (1960) Outflow resistance and adrenergic mechanisms. Arch Ophthalmol 64:839–848

Small S, Stewart-Jones JH, Turner P (1976) Influence of thymoxamine on changes in pupil diameter and accommodation produced by homatropine and ephedrine. Br J Ophthal 60:132–134

Smith BR, Murray DL, Leopold IH (1979) Influence of topically applied prazosin on the intraocular pressure of experimental animals. Arch Ophthalmol 97:1933–1936

Smith SE, Smith SA, Reynolds F, Whitmarsh VB (1979) Ocular and cardiovascular effects of local and systemic pindolol. Br J Ophthalmol 63:63–66

Sonntag JR, Brindley GO, Shields MB (1978) Effect of timolol therapy on outflow facility. Invest Ophthalmol Vis Sci 17:293–296

Stankiewicz A, Gos R, Kuligowa H, Cukrowski H, Rosiek S (1978) Mechanism of the hypotensive effect of beta-adrenolytic drugs on rabbit eye. Klin Oczna 48:305–306

Sutherland EW, Robison GA (1966) The role of cyclic – 3′-5′ AMP in response to catecholamines and other hormones. Pharmacol Rev 18:145–161

Takase M (1976) Effects of topical isoproterenol and propranolol on flow-rate of aqueous in rhesus monkey. Acta Soc Ophthalmol Jpn 80:379–384

Takase M, Araie M (1980) Comparison of ocular hypotensive effect and adverse reaction of topically applied beta-blockers. Jpn J Clin Ophthalmol 34:557–561

Takáts I, Szilvássy I, Kerek A (1972) Intraocular Druck und Kammerwasserzirkulations-Untersuchungen an Kaninchenaugen nach intravenöser Verabreichung von Propranolol (Inderal). Albrecht Von Graefes Arch Klin Exp Ophthalmol 185:331–342

Tamura T, Osada E, Ueno K (1978) Effect of bupranolol hydrochloride (KL 255) on cyclic AMP level of aqueous humor, iris and ciliary body of albino rabbit. Acta Soc Ophthalmol Jpn 82:517–521

Tieri O, Polzella A (1975) Emploi clinique et méchanisme d'action du propranololum. Ophthalmologica 170:36–42

Tsukahara S, Maezawa N (1978 a) Cytochemical localization of adenyl cyclase in the rabbit ciliary body. Exp Eye Res 26:99–106

Tsukahara S, Maezawa N (1978 b) The localization of beta-adrenoceptor sites in rat ocular tissues. Acta Soc Ophthalmol Jpn 82:6, 464–469

Tsukahara S, Yoshida K, Nagata T (1980) A radioautographic study on the incorporation of ^{14}C-bupranolol (beta-blocking agent) into the rabbit eye. Histochemistry 68:237–244

Turner P, Sneddon JM (1968) Alpha receptor blockade by thymoxamine in the human eye. Clin Pharmacol Ther 9:45–49

Vale J, Phillips CI (1970) Effect of DL- and D-propranolol on ocular tension in rabbits and patients. Exp Eye Res 9:82–90

van Alphen GWHM (1976) The adrenergic receptors of the intraocular muscles of the human eye. Invest Ophthalmol Vis Sci 15:502–505

van Alphen GWHM, Kern R, Robinette SL (1965) Adrenergic receptors of the intraocular muscles: comparison to cat, rabbit and monkey. Arch Ophthal 74:253–259

Vareilles P, Lotti VJ (1981) Effect of timolol on aqueous humor dynamics in the rabbit. Ophthalmic Res 13:72–79

Vareilles P, Silverstone D, Plazonnet B, Le Douarec J-C, Sears ML, Stone CA (1977) Comparison of the effects of timolol and other adrenergic agents on intraocular pressure in the rabbit. Invest Ophthalmol Vis Sci 16:987–996

Vareilles P, Schmitt C, Lotti VJ, Le Douarec JC (1978) Etude experimentale du timolol: un nouvel hypotenseur oculaire. J Fr Ophthalmol 12:717–721

Vareilles P, Conquet P, Lotti VJ (1980) Intraocular pressure responses to antiglaucoma agents in spontaneous buphthalmic rabbits. Opthalmic Res 12:296–302

Virno M, Giraldi JP, Marinosch F, Missiroli A (1969) Indagine sul meccanismo d'azione di due agenti ipotensivi endoculari: l'ergotamina e il propanololo. Boll Ocul 48:907–919

Waitzman MB, Woods WD (1971) Some characteristics of adenyl cyclase preparation from rabbit ciliary process tissue. Exp Eye Res 12:99–111

Walkenbach RJ, LeGrand RD, Barr RE (1980) Characterization of adenylate cyclase activity in bovine and human corneal epithelium. Invest Ophthalmol Vis Sci 19:1080–1086

Wand M, Grant WM (1976) Thymoxamine hydrochloride: effects of the facility of outflow and intraocular pressure. Invest Ophthalmol Vis Sci 15:400–403

Wettrell K (1977) Beta-adrenoceptor antagonism and intraocular pressure: a clinical study on propranolol, practolol and atenolol. Acta Ophthalmol Supp 134:1–54

Wettrell K, Pandolfi M (1977) Effect of topical atenolol on intraocular pressure. Br J Ophthalmol 61:334–338

Yablonski ME, Zimmerman TJ, Waltman SR, Becker B (1978) A fluorophotometric study of the effect of topical timolol on aqueous humor dynamics. Exp Eye Res 27:135–142

Zimmerman TJ, Kaufman HE (1977a) Timolol: a β-adrenergic blocking agent for the treatment of glaucoma. Arch Ophthalmol 95:601–604

Zimmerman TJ, Kaufman HE (1977b) Timolol: dose response and duration of action. Arch Ophthalmol 95:605–607

Zimmerman TJ, Harbin R, Pett M, Kaufman HE (1977) Timolol and facility of outflow. Invest Ophthalmol Vis Sci 16:623–624

Zimmerman TJ, Kass MA, Yablonski ME, Becker B (1979) Timolol maleate: efficacy and safety. Arch Ophthalmol 97:656–658

Zimmerman TJ, Leader B, Kaufman HE (1980) Advances in ocular pharmacology. Ann Rev Pharmacol Toxicol 20:415–428

CHAPTER 6

Carbonic Anhydrase: Pharmacology of Inhibitors and Treatment of Glaucoma

B. R. FRIEDLAND and T. H. MAREN

A. History

Carbonic anhydrase inhibitors have an established place in the treatment of glaucoma. This role is based on over three decades of research on the anatomy and physiology of aqueous humor secretion, as well as the pharmacology and distribution of the sulfonamide carbonic anhydrase inhibitors in the eye.

In his 1949 Proctor Lecture, FRIEDENWALD questioned "whether more effort might not profitably be directed toward a reduction in the formation of aqueous in cases of glaucoma." He went on to propose that the ciliary body acted to separate protons and electrons at the boundaries within cells. This "redox" function of a secretory epithelium produced gradients of OH^- ion which could be buffered by CO_2, forming bicarbonate, and balanced by sodium. Friedenwald suggested these ideas prior to KINSEY's (1953) measurement of high $NaHCO_3$ production or turnover in aqueous humor, and before WISTRAND (1951), under the direction and tutelage of Bárány, discovered carbonic anhydrase in the rabbit uveal tract. MELDRUM and ROUGHTON (1933) had already shown the presence of carbonic anhydrase in red cells, as well as in pancreas; it was a logical step to consider carbonic anhydrase in other tissues. After 1935, it was known (MANN and KEILIN 1940) that sulfanilamide was a carbonic anhydrase inhibitor, and that this explained the presence of an acidosis in patients taking the drug for its antibacterial properties (SOUTHWORTH 1937). However, it remained for ROBLIN and CLAPP (1950) to develop more powerful carbonic anhydrase inhibitors. DAVENPORT (1945) showed that, in intact red cells, more than 99% of the enzyme had to be inhibited before a physiological effect was seen. Later these same principles were shown to hold for renal and ocular systems as well (MAREN 1963a).

By 1954 a powerful carbonic anhydrase inhibitor, acetazolamide, was available, having first been shown to be nontoxic in large doses and with chronic administration (MAREN et al. 1954a). This surprised everyone, especially ROUGHTON (1935) and DAVIES (1951), who had predicted "a speedy death" if much of the body's carbonic anhydrase were inhibited. The renal effect of a single dose of acetazolamide in promoting the urinary excretion of Na^+, K^+, and HCO_3^- was established, and it was shown that titratable acid and NH_4^+ disappeared from the urine (MAREN et al. 1954b). FRIEDENWALD (1955a) described this diuresis as an "alkaline flood," because the major anion component of the urine was bicarbonate. However, the key factor in preventing toxicity was that these urinary changes did not persist. The metabolic acidosis sets into play a mechanism for HCO_3^- reabsorption unrelated to carbonic anhydrase, and thus unaffected by inhibiton (Maren 1956).

In addition to Friedenwald's speculations on charge separation in the ciliary body, and Wistrand's discovery of the enzyme in rabbit uvea, Kinsey (1953) discovered that rabbit aqueous humor contained high amount of bicarbonate, more in the posterior than in the anterior chamber. The stage was set for Friedenwald's resident, Becker (1954), to give acetazolamide to patients with glaucoma, and achieve a fall in intraocular pressure.

In his final years, Friedenwald (1955a, b) reviewed the data showing that acetazolamide reduced aqueous flow in man and rabbits (both from tonographic and fluorescein photometry data), and this reduced intraocular pressure. He commented on Becker's study (1955a) showing the drug's equal effect on nephrectomized and normal rabbits; this answered the question of a direct ocular effect of acetazolamide or an indirect one "via the matabolic disturbance resulting from the alkaline diuresis." Becker (1955b) also showed a fall in posterior aqueous HCO_3^- concentration after 6 h of carbonic anhydrase inhibition in both rabbits and guinea pigs.

As will become apparent, the rate of HCO_3^- production and not its actual concentration is of primary importance in delineating the role of carbonic anhydrase in aqueous humor formation. The choice of the rabbit (as opposed to cat or dog) as the animal model for this research turned out to be a lucky selection for the proper theories to develop, since the measured HCO_3^- concentration in the posterior chamber of rabbit is high.

The next step showed clearly that carbonic anhydrase was involved in the rate of accumulation of HCO_3^- in the aqueous. Kinsey and Reddy (1959) showed that the extremely rapid entry of labeled HCO_3^- into the posterior chamber was greatly reduced by acetazolamide's inhibition of carbonic anhydrase. The actual labeled HCO_3^- entry was so rapid under normal circumstances that it could not be measured.

The basic aspects of a HCO_3^- accumulating system also were present in the elasmobranch uvea; this organ contained carbonic anhydrase and the HCO_3^- entry could be inhibited by acetazolamide. This discovery (Maren 1963b; Maren et al. 1975) was notable for two reasons: it established the bicarbonate-accumulating system as a fundamental pattern through all vertebrates (reviewed in Maren 1977a), even to the type of high-activity carbonic anhydrase present in the elasmobranch ciliary folds (Maren et al. 1980); and, more importantly, the ocular HCO_3^- entry mechanism was inhibited by acetazolamide in the absence of a renal effect, since elasmobranchs lack kidney carbonic anhydrase and there is no renal response to the drug (Hodler et al. 1955). Acidosis inhibited secretion (mimicking acetazolamide), while alkalosis reduced the effect of the drug, implying that the newly formed aqueous humor is alkaline (Wistrand and Maren 1960).

Some confusion appeared in the literature when various authors (Becker 1959; Cole 1979; reviewed by Kinsey 1971) attempted to reconcile the concentration of ions in the posterior or anterior chamber fluid of various species with the role of carbonic anhydrase in the rates of ion movement, and thus aqueous humor formation. For example, certain primates, including man, have Cl^- rather than HCO_3^- excess in the posterior chamber (Becker 1957, 1959), and this was taken to imply that the bicarbonate-accumulating mechanism previously described was not at work for primates. However, this matter was resolved by measurement in dog and monkey of the isotopic movement of Na^+, Cl^-, and HCO_3^- from plasma to aqueous. These species have little or no HCO_3^- excess in the posterior chamber, yet acetazolamide has its normal reductive effect on flow and pressure (BECKER, 1959; GELATT et al. 1979), while reducing HCO_3^- and Na^+ entry in equimolar amounts (MAREN 1976a; see Sect. C.IV below). Although transport of the sodium portion of this system is reduced by inhibition of Na^+-K^+-ATPase (by ouabain), the linkage between HCO_3^- and Na^+ is shown by the fact that when ouabain and acetazolamide are given together (GARG and OPPELT 1970), the effect on aqueous flow is no greater than for each drug alone. The nature of this relationship is not understood, and is an exciting subject for future work.

Evidence supporting carbonic anhydrase dependent bicarbonate transport comes from work begun in the early 1960s showing that all carbonic anhydrase inhibitors, at the proper dose, had the same effect on aqueous humor secretion, even though they differed in many physical and chemical properties (WISTRAND et al. 1960b). The specificity of the aryl-sulfonyl unsubstituted compounds as carbonic anhydrase inhibitors built upon the original work of MANN and KEILIN (1940), and has recently been reviewed (MAREN 1976b).

B. Pharmacology of the Clinically Used Carbonic Anhydrase Inhibitors

There are four compounds utilized as carbonic anhydrase inhibitors in the treatment of glaucoma: acetazolamide, methazolamide, ethoxzolamide, and dichlorphenamide (Table 1). Their common feature is a free sulfonamide group ($-SO_2NH_2$) linked to an aromatic ring (MAREN 1976b). Salient pharmacologic and chemical features will be briefly described, following an earlier review of this subject (MAREN 1967). All the compounds used clinically are potent carbonic anhydrase inhibitors with about the same range of activity, except ethoxzolamide, which is five to ten times more active against the enzyme. This comparison of potency (Table 1) is based on inhibitory activity against carbonic anhydrase in vitro, as described by the inhibition dissociation constant (K_I). The important differences among the drugs are based on physico-chemical properties (pK_a, lipid solubility, plasma protein binding) which affect their body distribution.

Acetazolamide, the first drug of this group synthesized, was introduced originally for its action on renal carbonic anhydrase. It is less diffusible than methazolamide and ethoxzolamide (HOLDER and HAYES 1965). Indeed, its high plasma binding and high degree of ionization make acetazolamide a less than ideal compound for penetration of ocular tissues from the systemic circulation. Unlike methazolamide, it is actively secreted into the renal tubules of the dog and passively reabsorbed by nonionic diffusion (WEINER et al. 1959). This appears to be the case in the rabbit (WISTRAND 1959) and, from plasma decay curves, in man (MAREN and ROBINSON 1960). Thus, for a given plasma level of acetazolamide, a larger proportion of the dose is inhibitory for renal carbonic anhydrase than with methazol-

Table 1. Chemical–pharmacologic properties of clinically used carbonic anhydrase inhibitors (adapted from WISTRAND et al. 1960b)

Name	Structure	$K_I{}^a$ $\times 10^9\,M$	pK_{a_1}	% Union- ized pH 7.4	Ether parti- tion coeff. pH 7.4	% Plasma un- bound (man)	$t_{1/2}$ Plas- ma (h) man
Ethoxzol- amide		1	8.1	83	140	4	6
Acetazol- amide		6	7.4	50	0.14	5	4
Methazol- amide		8	7.2	39	0.62	45	15
Dichlor- phen- amide		18	8.3	89	11	–	2

[a] K_I is against human red cell carbonic anhydrase C in barbital buffer at $0\,°C$. Determined by method described in MAREN and WILEY (1968), EI System

amide. Entry into the ocular tissues appears to be passive and dependent on diffusivity (WISTRAND 1959).

The plasma half-life of acetazolamide in man is about 4 h (MAREN 1967; LEHMANN et al. 1969). It is hemodialyzable, and has an acetazolamide to urea nitrogen ratio of 0.16, probably as a consequence of its high degree of plasma binding (VAZIRI et al. 1980).

Figures 1 and 2 show the renal effects of oral acetazolamide in the dog, which are identical to those in man. Note also that drug appears nearly quantitatively in urine. Initially there is loss of Na^+, K^+, and HCO_3^-; H^+ and NH_4^+ disappear from urine; Cl^- is unaffected. As Fig. 2 shows, none of these changes continue; it is this fortunate feature which makes clinical use of this class of drugs possible. The specific renal effects include alkalinization of the urine, with net HCO_3^- loss initially being 1–5 mEq/kg, depending on the dose and dosage interval (MAREN et al. 1954b). The mild metabolic acidosis that develops with acetazolamide therapy in the 1,000 mg/day (in man) range is a consequence of the initial bicarbonate loss. Continued enzyme inhibition at the level of the distal tubule represses a return to normal urinary acidification, and thus prevents complete recovery from the acidosis. On the other hand, bicarbonate reabsorption independent of carbonic anhydrase insures that there is no further loss of this ion or deepening acidosis (MAREN 1974a).

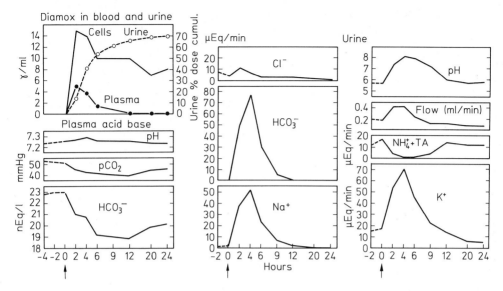

Fig. 1. Pharmacologic and renal effects of acetazolamide in the dog. Single oral dose 5 mg/kg. *TA*, titratable acidity. (MAREN et al. 1954b)

The result of these varied forces is seen in Fig. 2. Note that by dose 4 urinary composition is normal despite high concentration of drug in plasma and urine.

The renal effect is the major difference between clinically comparable doses of methazolamide and acetazolamide, but methazolamide will also cause inhibition of renal carbonic anhydrase, with a concomitant acidosis, at doses ≥ 4 mg/kg (MAREN et al. 1977; STONE et al. 1977).

Additional systemic effects secondary to the mild metabolic acidosis generally seen with acetazolamide include a $\sim 10\%$ net deficit of both sodium and potassium, which does not progress (MAREN et al. 1954b; HANLEY and PLATTS 1961). There are also changes in citrate excretion, which is increased initially and later falls (CRAWFORD et al. 1959).

The plasma levels achieved with a given dose of acetazolamide generally vary only by a factor of 1.5–2, and correlate closely with intraocular pressure (LEHMANN et al. 1969; FRIEDLAND et al. 1977; BERSON et al. 1980; YAKATAN et al. 1978). The first of these studies gives important and comprehensive data on the pharmacokinetics of acetazolamide in man, and defines the plasma concentration (5–10 μg/ml total drug) and dose interval (6–8 h) for optimal treatment of glaucoma. Figure 3a shows the relation between plasma concentration and outflow pressure. A later study by FRIEDLAND et al. (1977) gives similar data for doses between 63 mg and 500 mg. The relationships between free drug in plasma, enzyme inhibition, and ocular effect are discussed in Sect. C.VI below. Figure 3b gives an interesting overall view of the kinetic movement of acetazolamide in man, from oral absorption to enzyme inhibition to ocular effect to renal excretion (WISTRAND 1974).

An important consideration with respect to acetazolamide is that the dose–response curve for the ocular effect is not very far removed from that for the kidney

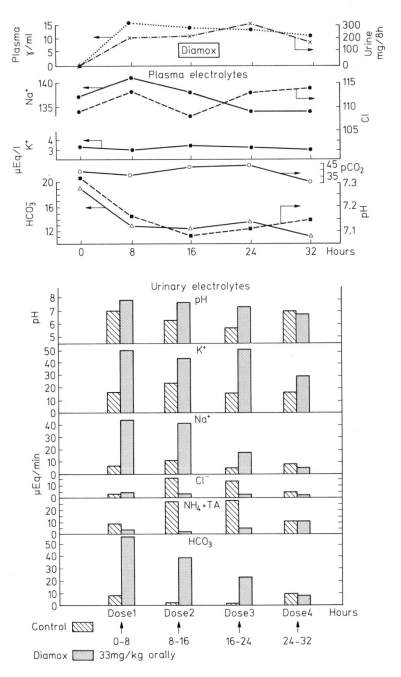

Fig. 2. The effect of sustained carbonic anhydrase inhibition on body electrolytes. *TA*, titratable acidity. (MAREN et al. 1954 b)

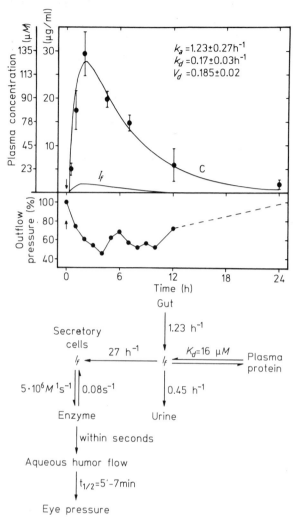

Fig. 3a. Plasma concentration and effect on outflow pressure following 500 mg acetazolamide orally at zero time. *Top curve* shows means and standard errors from ten patients with glaucoma, *bottom curve* in five patients. *C* denotes total drug concentration, I_f unbound concentration in plasma. k_a is first-order absorption constant; k_d is first-order decay constant; V_d is volume of distribution in l/kg (LEHMAN et al. 1969). **b** Scheme of the kinetics of body distribution, enzyme inhibition, and ocular effects following acetazolamide in man. The various rate constants are taken from the literature. The opposing rate constants for enzyme inhibition correspond to the dissociation constant; $K_I = 1.6 \times 10^{-8} M$. This does not include the red cell compartment; see HOLDER and HAYES (1965). (WISTRAND 1974)

(Fig. 4). Methazolamide, which is not secreted by the kidney, has a wider discrimination of dose–response between the eye and the kidney (Fig. 5); doses can be chosen so that the tissue level in the ciliary body is high enough to inhibit >99% of the carbonic anhydrase present. This is discussed further in Sect. C.VI below. Similar percentage inhibition in the kidney is without physiological effect because

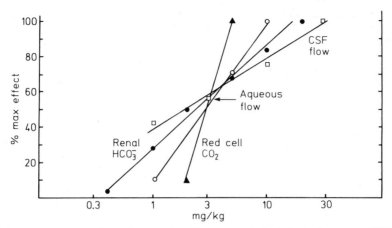

Fig. 4. Dose–response studies of acetazolamide in several physiological systems. *CSF*, cerebrospinal fluid. (MAREN 1979)

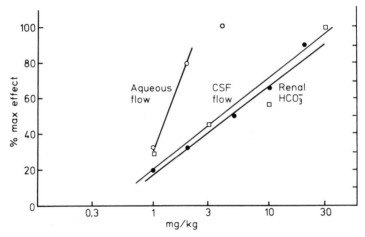

Fig. 5. Dose–response study of methazolamide in eye and kidney. *CSF*, cerebrospinal fluid. (MAREN 1979)

the actual concentration of enzyme in the kidney is some ten times greater than that in the ciliary process (MAREN et al. 1977). These data show clearly that a lowering of intraocular pressure can be achieved by 25–50 mg methazolamide, with little or no lowering of plasma HCO_3^- concentration.

Figure 6 shows absorption distribution and excretion of methazolamide in man. The drug is well absorbed and gives sustained plasma levels. Only 25% appears unchanged in the urine; its metabolic fate is still unknown. It is not actively taken up or secreted by the kidney. Binding to red cells reflects quantitatively the carbonic anhydrase present.

Methazolamide is much less plasma bound than acetazolamide (Table 1), and because of its pK_a and water and lipid solubility has a faster diffusivity into ocular

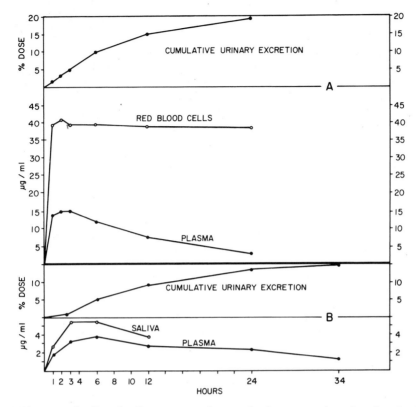

Fig. 6. Plasma, red cell, and saliva concentrations, and urinary excretion of methazolamide, following single oral doses in man. *A*, dose of 7.5 mg/kg; *B*, dose of 2.5 mg/kg. (MAREN et al. 1977)

and other tissues (WISTRAND et al. 1960b; HOLDER and HAYES 1965). These properties make methazolamide a more ideal drug for use as an ocular carbonic anhydrase inhibitor. Further details of its pharmacology are given by MAREN et al. (1977) and by BAYNE et al. (1981).

There appears to be slightly less intraocular-pressure-lowering effect for a 50-mg dose of methazolamide than for 250 mg acetazolamide (DAHLEN et al. 1978; STONE et al. 1977), but this may be a consequence of the metabolic acidosis present with all eye-effective doses of acetazolamide (EPSTEIN and GRANT 1979; DAHLEN et al. 1978). Metabolic acidosis causes a fall in intraocular pressure independent of carbonic anhydrase inhibition (WISTRAND and MAREN 1960; KRUPIN et al. 1977). If there is a correlation between acidosis and side effects, as suggested by some authors (EPSTEIN and GRANT 1979) but disputed by others (ALWARD and WILENSKY 1980), then ophthalmologists must decide whether the additional fall in intraocular pressure afforded in the presence of metabolic acidosis is worth the associated unpleasant effects (cf. Sects. C.V and VI).

It has recently been confirmed that there is a clear dose–resonse curve for the effect of acetazolamide on intraocular pressure in the nephrectomized rabbit between 1 mg/kg (no effect) and 15 mg/kg (full effect). At 5 mg/kg there is a 3-

mmHg pressure drop with no alteration in acid–base chemistry. At 15–50 mg/kg there is some respiratory acidosis, which appears to add to the pressure-lowering effect (FRIEDMAN et al. 1982), as shown many years ago (WISTRAND and MAREN 1960). It should be mentioned, however, that large clinical doses of acetazolamide do not produce a respiratory acidosis in man (unless there is pulmonary disease), as it does in rabbits and dogs (BIRZIS et al. 1958).

Ethoxzolamide is also a weak organic acid and is slightly secreted by the renal tubules. About 40% is excreted unchanged in the dog. It has a higher in vitro activity (K_I) against carbonic anhydrase than the other drugs discussed. However, this effect is vitiated by its high plasma binding (Table 1). The diffusibility of ethoxzolamide appears high, with rapid entry into the anterior chamber and subsequent fall in intraocular pressure (WISTRAND et al. 1960b); this would be predicted from the high lipid solubility of this compound. For other aspects of its pharmacology, see MAREN (1967). Dichlorphenamide has a K_I in the range of $7 \times 10^{-8} M$ (Table 1) and other properties which make it the least acceptable candidate for ocular carbonic anhydrase inhibition. It exhibits a mixed pharmacology with the thiazide diuretics as a result of its chloruretic activity (BEYER and BAER 1961). This is a potentially hazardous property, because unlike the pure metabolic acidosis induced by acetazolamide, methazolamide, or ethoxzolamide, the continued loss of chloride in the urine can contribute to continued potassium loss in the urine, with resultant hypokalemia characteristic of other thiazide diuretics. The two sulfonamide groups do nothing to enhance the carbonic anhydrase inhibiting activity, and indeed are the structural basis for the unwanted chloruretic effect. Clearly, this compound is not the best for decreasing intraocular pressure, and furthermore, it is associated with a higher incidence of side effects, particularly headache.

C. Physiology of Ocular Carbonic Anhydrase Inhibition

I. Aqueous Humor Dynamics

The highly vascularized ciliary processes produce aqueous humor by a serial mechanism of ultrafiltration and secretion. The capillaries of the ciliary process are fenestrated and permit a protein-rich filtrate to enter the stroma of the processes by ultrafiltration. This stromal pool is then substrate for the transporting ciliary epithelia. The epithelial cells of the processes are arranged in a double layer and the epithelia of each layer are not in register. The structure of the outer pigmented cell layer resembles retinal pigmented epithelium, while the inner layer of nonpigmented epithelia is remarkably similar to choroid plexus and renal proximal tubule (reviewed in MAREN 1980; RECTOR 1981). The ciliary processes of rabbits contain about 0.3 μM carbonic anhydrase of high-activity C-type (WISTRAND and GARG 1979). This is about one-tenth that in the kidney or choroid plexus (MAREN 1967).

The aqueous humor produced enters the posterior chamber (volume 50 µl in rabbit and man), then flows forward between lens and iris to enter the anterior chamber (about 250 µl volume), where it leaves the eye by a pressure-dependent mechanism at the iridocorneal angle via the trabecular meshwork to Schlemn's canal, and then either into intrascleral and episcleral veins or directly into aqueous veins. A small proportion of the fluid leaves the anterior chamber by a pressure-independent mechanism, "uveoscleral flow," passing posteriorly through the base of the iris into the ciliary body (BILL 1975). In its passage the composition of aqueous is influenced by diffusional exchanges across the vitreous, ciliary body, iris, and lens, and also by metabolic events in these structures.

II. Aqueous Flow

The fluid turnover rate is quite constant among mammals: 1% of the total volume per minute. In man the formation rate has been represented at 2 µl/min with plasma flow rate of 75 ml/min (BILL 1975). Aqueous flow rates have been measured by numerous methods, and there is considerable agreement among authors that maximally effective doses of carbonic anhydrase inhibitors reduce aqueous humor flow by 40%–60% in man and various animal species. These rates have been measured by:

1. Dilation techniques measuring, for example, rates of loss of anterior chamber fluorescein (JONES and MAURICE 1966), chemicals such as inulin after perfusion into the posterior (OPPELT 1967; GARG and OPPELT 1970) and anterior chamber (MACRI et al. 1965), or isotopically labeled protein (BILL 1975)
2. The turnover of systemically administered substances in the posterior and anterior chamber, such as ascorbate (BECKER 1956), p-aminohippuric acid (KINSEY et al. 1955), urea (KINSEY et al. 1960), iodide (BECKER 1961, 1962), iodopyracet (FORBES and BECKER 1961)
3. Fluorescein appearance times in the anterior chamber (LINNER and FRIEDENWALD 1957)
4. Photogrammetric methods (HOLM and WIEBERT 1968)
5. Constant rate or constant pressure perfusion techniques or tonography (BECKER 1954; BECKER and CONSTANT 1955)
6. Changes in the steady-state concentration of endogenous ascorbate or phosphate in anterior and posterior chambers (CONSTANT and FALCH 1963).

Each method has its own strengths and shortcomings beyond the scope of this discussion. However, results with all of these diverse methods indicate that the fall in intraocular pressure seen with carbonic anhydrase inhibition is caused by decreased aqueous humor flow.

III. Relation to Pressure

The total eye pressure (at constant volume) is: $(P - P_v) = F \cdot R$ where P_v is the episcleral venous pressure (about 8 mmHg in man), F is the aqueous flow (2 µl/min), and R is the outflow resistance, or $1/C$. C is outflow facility in µl/min/mmHg outflow pressure (DAVSON 1969). R has a value of about 4. This equation can be expanded to include uveoscleral flow and the pressure-dependent part of aqueous humor formation, i.e., pseudofacility (MOSES 1980). Several investigations of carbonic anhydrase inhibition have indicated no striking effect on any of these factors except for flow, which is halved in both normal and glaucomatous man (LINNER 1956; KUPFER et al. 1971; AZUMA 1973).

There has, however, been considerable discussion about the effect of sulfonamides on C; clearly there is no initial effect, but there is some evidence that in normal animals or man C may decrease to adjust to the lower inflow (Friedenwald 1966 b; Becker and Constant 1955). Such homeostasis is fortunately absent in nearly all glaucomatous patients, thus permitting continued pressure lowering. This matter is well reviewed by Wistrand (1964). Possibly related to compensatory changes in C is the vexing question of rabbits initially resistant to the ocular hypotensive effect of the sulfonamides. Kinsey et al. (1955 b) correlated this phenomenon with salt depletion and restored responsiveness with aldosterone, but Wistrand (1964) could not reach the same conclusion. Long-term changes of C in normal animals or man and effects of salt on C remain to be studied.

IV. Chemical Mechanisms of Flow

The composition of aqueous humor, as measured by analysis of steady-state concentrations in the anterior and posterior chambers, varies among species (summarized in Maren 1967). This finding has led to some confusion about the mechanism of aqueous humor formation (Maren 1974 b). Fortunately, the rabbit has been the animal most widely used in the study of aqueous humor dynamics. Rabbits show a large excess (16 mM) of bicarbonate in the posterior chamber, which falls with carbonic anhydrase inhibition (Becker 1955 c). The rate of bicarbonate turnover in rabbit posterior chamber aqueous (Kinsey and Reddy 1959) with ^{14}C-bicarbonate (see Sect. C.I) is extremely rapid, with a turnover of less than 10 s. After acetazolamide injection, posterior chamber turnover was slowed at least 10- to 15-fold, while plasma turnover remained unchanged (Fig. 7). Analysis of these data (Maren 1967) showed that the bicarbonate accumulated in the posterior chamber was formed from CO_2, catalyzed by carbonic anhydrase, and not due to ionic transport of bicarbonate.

Recent studies (Zimmerman et al. 1976 a, b; Maren 1976 a, 1977 b) of ionic accession rates in dog and monkey again show that HCO_3^- formation in newly formed aqueous humor does occur and is inhibited by acetazolamide. Contrary to the case in the rabbit (Fig. 7), HCO_3^- formation in these two species was not too rapid to measure; the half-time to equilibrium in dog was about 7 min (Fig. 8). Following carbonic anhydrase inhibition the equivalent time was lengthened to 18 min. Figure 8 shows that chloride accession is not altered by acetazolamide, but sodium accession is reduced about 30%. The data in Fig. 8 are converted to the critical ion accession rates in Table 2; in row 3 we may see how sodium transport is matched by chloride and bicarbonate. Note that $Cl^- + HCO_3^-$ rates approach that of sodium; this is important evidence that the HCO_3^- rates do represent real movement, not isotope exchange. About 36% of Na^+ entry is matched by HCO_3^- formation under normal conditions. When carbonic anhydrase is inhibited, the molar transports of these two ions decline about equivalently – 1.9 mM/min for Na^+ and 1.6 mM/min for HCO_3^-. Under these conditions aqueous humor flow falls by about 50%. In some way not yet understood, fluid flow and Na^+ transport seem to be linked to HCO_3^- formation. It is important to realize that even though the observed HCO_3^- concentration in the posterior aqueous of dog (Table 2), monkey (Maren 1977 b), and presumably man (Becker 1959) is not very much higher than in plasma (by contrast to the case in rabbit or the smooth dogfish; Maren 1967), the cal-

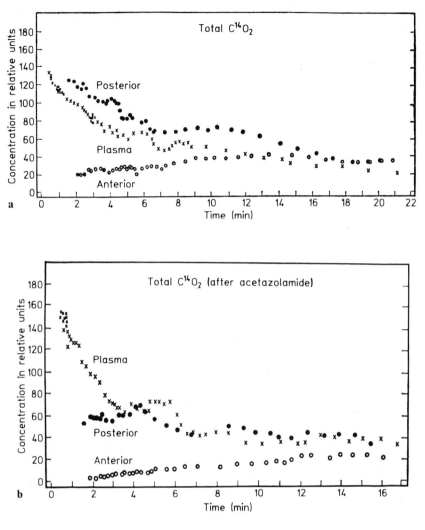

Fig. 7 a, b. Accumulation of HCO_3^- in aqueous from blood CO_2 and its inhibition by acetazolamide. ^{14}C-labeled bicarbonate and CO_2 were injected at zero time, and total [14]CO_2 concentration determined in the fluids at times shown. **a**, normal rabbit; **b** acetazolamide (50 mg/kg i.v.) given 15 min before zero time. In the normal rabbit, total CO_2 is partitioned in its physiological ratios between posterior aqueous and plasma within 1 min. Figure 6B shows that with 50 mg/kg acetazolamide, there is a profound delay in the accumulation of total CO_2 in the posterior aqueous. (KINSEY and REDDY 1959)

culated concentration in "nascent" posterior aqueous humor of dog is two and a half times that in plasma, and this is reduced to the level of plasma when the enzyme is inhibited (column 4 Table 2). Reciprocally, nascent Cl^- concentration is low, and rises with inhibition, while Na^+ concentration in nascent fluid is the same as plasma (column 4, Table 2).

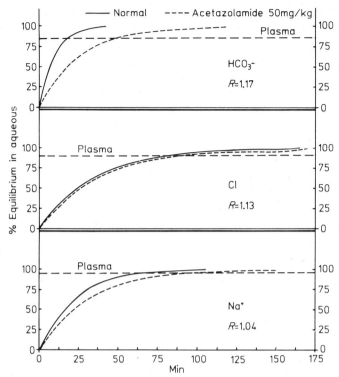

Fig. 8. Accession of ions from plasma to posterior chamber of dog following intravenous injection of the isotope at zero time. R is the distribution ratio posterior aqueous/plasma at equilibrium. (Maren 1976 a)

Table 2. Entry of ions to posterior aqueous of dog: normal values and those following carbonic anhydrase inhibition (CAI)[a, b]

	Plasma (mM)	k_{in}(min^{-1})	Accession rate (mM/min)[c]	Calculated concentration nascent fluid (mM)[d]	Measured fluid concentration (mM)	
					Posterior	Anterior
Na$^+$						
Control	152	0.044	6.7	149	153	153
CAI	156	0.031	4.8	149	152	151
Cl$^-$						
Control	117	0.028	3.3	73	132	128
CAI	117	0.027	3.2	100	130	129
HCO$_3^-$						
Control	22	0.109	2.4	53	26	25
CAI	21	0.039	0.8	25	24	24

[a] Data from Maren (1977 b); Zimmerman et al. (1976 a, b)
[b] Aqueous flow is 9 µl/min in control and 6.4 µl/min during inhibition, as calculated from sodium accession rates. CAI by 50 mg/kg acetazolamide i.v. 1 h before isotope
[c] Product of first and second columns
[d] Product of third column and Volume posterior chamber ($=0.2$ ml)/Aqueous flow

As mentioned before, experiments giving ouabain and acetazolamide together (GARG and OPPELT 1970; KOLKER and HETHERINGTON 1976) showed no additive effect on flow or ion transport. There are transient shifts in blood–aqueous potential induced by carbonic anhydrase inhibition (MILLER 1962; COLE 1966, 1979), which are enhanced by acidosis and reduced by alkalosis, and might be related to reduced bicarbonate and sodium transfer. Studies of dimethyloxazolidinedione distribution after carbonic anhydrase inhibition (CONSTANT 1962) suggest a pH-partitioning role at the blood–aqueous barrier. To date, there have been no measurements of intraocular pH shifts which would support an indirect relationship between carbonic anhydrase and Na^+–K^--ATPase via intracellular buffering, although there has been much speculation in this area (COLE 1979; COTLIER 1979).

V. Relation to Systemic Effects

Systemic acidosis, both respiratory and metabolic, lower intraocular pressure and enhance the pressure-lowering effect of acetazolamide, while alkalosis reduces the effect of carbonic anhydrase inhibition (WISTRAND and MAREN 1960). Systemic acidosis alone reduces aqueous humor production (LANGHAM and LEE 1957; KRUPIN et al. 1977). There is some controversy concerning the effect of respiratory acidosis, with hypercarbia also causing a rise in intraocular pressure (PETOUNIS et al. 1980). The somewhat larger effect of acetazolamide than of (small doses of) methazolamide on intraocular pressure is probably a result of the metabolic acidosis associated with dosages used clinically (cf. Sect. C.II). Some authors (BIETTI et al. 1975) have attempted to explain the pressure-lowering effect of acetazolamide solely on the basis of systemic metabolic acidosis. BENEDIKT et al. (1974) and SÖSER et al. (1980) have shown clearly that the pressure fall cannot be caused by the acidosis because the metabolic acidosis mediated by renal carbonic anhydrase lags behind the drop in intraocular pressure by several hours. Indeed, this conclusion was implicit in the data of BECKER (1955b), who showed reduction in eye pressure in the nephrectomized rabbit and also that the effect preceded any appreciable renal loss of bicarbonate. Finally, the renal effect of acetazolamide is blocked by metabolic acidosis (MAREN et al. 1954b), but the ocular effect, as noted above, is augmented.

VI. Pharmacology of the Inhibitors Related to Ocular Effect and Enzyme Inhibition

The pressure-lowering effect is primarily ocular, and not systemic, because intracarotid injection of acetazolamide causes a pressure fall on the ipsilateral side (WISTRAND 1957). Intraocular pressure drops almost immediately after intravenous inhibition, long before systemic metabolic acidose develops secondary to the renal effect. As noted above, acetazolamide works in the nephrectomized animal, and when the renal effect is blocked by NH_4Cl (BECKER 1955b); systemic metabolic acidosis may add to the local effect, but the two are readily separable. It might be argued that the ocular effect is secondary to respiratory acidosis, but this seems unlikely since elevation of pCO_2 is very small in the normal breathing mammal. Such

Table 3. Transcorneal permeability of sulfonamides (Maren et al. 1983)

	Ether part coeff. at pH 7.2	pK$_a$	Transcorneal rate constant (k $\times$ 10^3/h)		Solubility (mM)		In vivo transcorneal Rate at ph 7.8 Col. 4 $\times$ col. 6 (μM/h)	Conc. in ciliary body 2 h after dose (μmol/kg)
			In vitro	In vivo	Water	pH 7.8		
Acetazol-amide	0.14	7.4	0.4	2	2	8	16	–
Ethoxzol-amide	140	8	40	250	0.04	0.04	10	1
Methazol-amide	0.6	7.4	1	5	5	14	70	13
Trifluor-methazol-amide[a]	6	6.6	3	10	8	120	1,200	55

[a] CF_3—CO—N= replaces CH_3—CO—N= in methazolamide (Table 1)

hypercapnia does not in itself lower pressure (Petounis et al. 1980). However, attempts to induce a pressure-lowering effect with topical or subconjunctival injection of acetazolamide have been unsuccessful (Green and Leopold 1954; Becker 1955b; Foss 1955; Kimura 1978). Azuma (1960) did achieve bilateral pressure reduction with unilateral 15 mg/kg subconjunctival acetazolamide and assumed that systemic absorption caused the effect.

It therefore seemed likely that the failure of acetazolamide and certain other drugs of this class to lower pressure topically was due to chemical and/or pharmacologic factors, principally failure to penetrate the cornea and other structures well and to reach the ciliary body. Indeed, exploration of a series of sulfonamides showed a 400-fold range of corneal penetration rate constants in vitro or in vivo, with acetazolamide at the low end and ethoxzolamide at the high, in agreement with lipid solubilities (Table 3). However, for delivery of pharmacologically active concentrations into the eye, water solubility was also built into the molecule; results with such a compound are shown in Table 3. Trifluormethazolamide reaches the anterior chamber at 100 times the rate of acetazolamide, and intraocular pressure and flow are lowered in the rabbit and cat (Maren et al. 1983; Stein et al. 1983). Trifluormethazolamide requires relatively long application and is chemically unstable, so that intensive further research is under way to find a clinically acceptable carbonic anhydrase inhibition for the treatment of glaucoma.

Of major interest is the relation between the potential chemical rates of HCO_3^- production in the ciliary process and the actual transport numbers. Estimates of the chemical rates may be made, since we know the substrates for the reaction ($CO_2 + OH$), the secretory volume (roughly), the uncatalyzed and catalyzed rate constants for the reaction, the concentration of carbonic anhydrase present, and the kinetic parameters [turnover number (TON) = k_{cat}, and K_m] of the enzyme. Figure 9 summarizes these considerations, which are given in more detail by Maren (1976a). These uncatalyzed and catalyzed rates are put in the context of the ob-

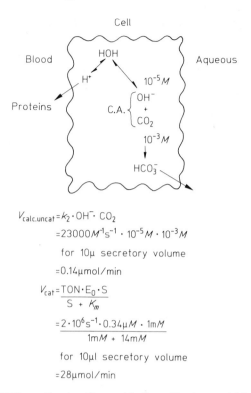

$$V_{calc.uncat} = k_2 \cdot OH^- \cdot CO_2$$
$$= 23000 M^{-1} s^{-1} \cdot 10^{-5} M \cdot 10^{-3} M$$

for 10μ secretory volume

$$= 0.14 \mu mol/min$$

$$V_{cat} = \frac{TON \cdot E_0 \cdot S}{S + K_m}$$

$$= \frac{2 \cdot 10^6 s^{-1} \cdot 0.34 \mu M \cdot 1mM}{1mM + 14mM}$$

for 10μl secretory volume

$$= 28 \mu mol/min$$

Fig. 9. Model for HCO_3^- formation in ciliary epithelium. (See text and MAREN 1976a). *TON*, turnover number; E_o, enzyme concentration in ciliary processes; *S*, CO_2 conc; $V_{calc.uncat}$, calculated uncatalyzed rate; V_{cat}, calculated catalyzed rate; *CA*, carbonic anhydrase

served physiological rates (from Table 2) in Table 4. The top row shows that the chemically calculated catalytic rate (V_{cat}) is 60 times greater than the observed rate (V_{obs}). When the calculated uncatalyzed rate ($V_{calc.uncat}$) is subtracted from V_{obs}, the remainder is the true catalytic rate in vivo ($V_{obs\,cat}$), which is nearly 100 times less than the chemical V_{cat}. Thus it appears that there is an excess or reserve of enzyme concentration to about this degree.

Inhibition studies add greatly to this kinetic analysis. For many years it has been recognized that the physiological effects of carbonic anhydrase inhibition in many organs are only apparent when more than 99% of the enzyme is inactivated (MAREN 1967). The eye is no exception, as presaged very early by FRIEDENWALD (1955a, b). This phenomenon is shown by Fig. 10; the dose required for full intraocular effect of methazolamide is about 3 mg/kg in the rabbit. For this dose the fractional inhibition of the enzyme (*i*) is calculated as shown, where I_f is the free drug concentration in fluid in contact with the enzyme, and K_I is the dissociation constant between enzyme and inhibitor. I_f may usually be taken as unbound drug in plasma; an exception is a highly charged ionic drug such as benzolamide, which does not traverse the ciliary process from its unbound concentration in plasma and has a very weak effect on aqueous humor dynamics (WISTRAND et al. 1960). A good

Table 4. Chemical and physiological rates of HCO_3^- formation in dog eye ($\mu mol/min$)

	1 V_{cat} [a]	2 V_{obs}	3 $V_{calc.\,uncat}$ [a]	4 $V_{obs\,cat}$ [d]
Normal	28	0.48 [b]	0.14	0.34
$i=0.99$	0.28	0.42 [c]	0.14	0.28
$i=0.999$	0.028	0.17 [b]	0.14	0.03

V_{cat}, chemically calculated catalytic rate; V_{obs}, observed rate; $V_{calc.\,uncat}$, calculated uncatalyzed rate; $V_{obs\,cat}$, true catalytic rate

[a] From Fig. 2 and the entered values of i
[b] From data of Table 2 for HCO_3^-, column 3 (mM/min), adjusted for posterior chamber volume of 0.2 ml
[c] Calculated from column 1 minus column 3. Note also no effect of $i=0.99$ in Fig. 10
[d] Column 2 minus column 3

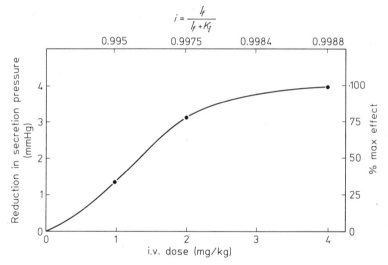

Fig. 10. Relations between dose, fractional inhibition of carbonic anhydrase, and reduction in aqueous humor secretion 30 min after intravenous injection of methazolamide in rabbits. The concentrations shown in the graph are free drug (unbound to plasma protein) (I_f) in plasma. $K_I = 2 \times 10^{-8}$ M. (Maren et al. 1977)

model is that of methazolamide, because the unbound concentration in plasma approaches that in aqueous humor, and I_f is estimated with some certainty; as shown in Fig. 10 it is about 12 μM at the top of the dose–response curve. K_I is given in Table 1, or more accurately from the inhibition of the ciliary process enzyme itself, as in Maren et al. (1977); the tissue enzyme has properties very close to that of the human red cell carbonic anhydrase C (or II), which is the prototypic secretory or transport enzyme in mammalian species.

Figure 10 shows that when $i=0.99$, there is no physiological effect, and that full effect is achieved when i approaches 0.999. It will be recognized that this is to be expected if there is indeed a 100-fold excess of enzyme, as we have shown independently by the rate analysis given above. Table 4 shows the rates at the different levels of inhibition. This indicates in a different way that when $i = 0.99$, the residual catalyzed rate plus the uncatalyzed rate are almost enough to sustain normal secretion, but when $i = 0.999$, the residual catalyzed rate is negligible. Remarkably, the observed rate at this high level of inhibition is nearly identical to the calculated uncatalyzed rate.

The data in Fig. 10 agree fairly well with those in man. Methazolamide (50 mg every 12 h) generates plasma concentrations (unbound) of 8–12 μM, which lowers pressure 3.2 mmHg in patients with ocular hypertension (MAREN et al. 1977). In the case of acetazolamide, the much higher plasma binding (95%) means that a higher dose of drug should be necessary for full effects – usually 250–500 mg or about 4–7 mg/kg. The corresponding unbound concentration in plasma is about 4 μM (LEHMAN et al. 1969; MAREN et al. 1977), which is unaccountably low for full effect. This might lead one to suspect that this drug has a higher free concentration in the ciliary process than in plasma, but this was not found in the rabbit (WISTRAND et al. 1960b). In the same context is the surprising finding that as little as 63 mg acetazolamide, administered orally, lowers pressure within 1–2 h in man – here the unbound plasma concentration is only 1 μM (FRIEDLAND et al. 1977). This is confirmed by MERTÉ et al. (1977). In the case of ethoxzolamide, K_I is less than for the other drugs (Table 1), but plasma binding is very high so that the effective dose is still about 100 mg. A quantitative analysis of the activity of nine sulfonamides for the lowering of intraocular pressure in the rabbit is available (WISTRAND et al. 1960).

D. Clinical Uses of Carbonic Anhydrase Inhibitors

I. Glaucoma

Short-term administration of carbonic anhydrase inhibitors to reduce intraocular pressure by reduction of aqueous humor formation is often very effective in secondary glaucomas because the outflow channels for aqueous are the sites of pathology that may make them unresponsive to medications acting on outflow. Examples of these are: contusion angle deformities, tumors, and inflammations. These drugs may be useful before operation for congenital glaucoma by reducing intraocular pressure and corneal edema to improve visualization of the chamber angle for goniotomy.

In angle-closure glaucoma, carbonic anhydrase inhibitors are also useful as a preoperative medication (KOLKER and HETHERINGTON 1976). Since patients are often nauseated or even vomiting, parenteral therapy may be required. Acetazolamide can be given as an i.v. injection of 250 mg. Pressure begins to fall within a few minutes, and the effect lasts 2–4 h. As the pressure falls and the iridial and ciliary muscles recover from the ischemia of high pressure, outflow facility can again respond to drugs like topical pilocarpine. The purpose of all medications in angle-closure attacks is to buy time for iridectomy, the procedure and treatment of choice.

In modern day cataract surgery, rises in intraocular pressure are often seen early in the postoperative course. Some of these eyes may suffer from either transient effects of α-chymotrypsin, or from precise tight microscopic wound closure. Carbonic anhydrase inhibition can be useful to tide the patient over these few days.

The major use of carbonic anhydrase inhibitors has been as an adjunct in the long-term treatment of primary open-angle glaucoma. The practice is to add orally administered carbonic anhydrase inhibitors to topical preparations of pilocarpine and/or timolol and/or epinephrine.

Normalization of intraocular pressure may well avert the risk of further visual field loss that would arise were the eye to be subjected to higher pressures. Furthermore, it is agreed that the resistance to outflow is increased at higher eye pressures because of trabecular compression. It is therefore quite likely that outflow resistance may fall (improve) under conditions of reduced intraocular pressure. In this way medications like pilocarpine that act to reduce outflow resistance ordinarily may exhibit a synergistic effect when a carbonic anhydrase inhibitor is added to the therapeutic program.

Adrenergic agents can act directly upon the secretion of aqueous humor and may be additive to the effect of carbonic anhydrase inhibition, indicating another path or mechanism of action, e.g., epinephrine or the β-blockers, atenolol (MacDonald et al. 1977), timolol (Scharrer and Ober 1979; Berson and Epstein 1981), and bupranolol (Stiegler 1979), which also reduce secretion. The data of Berson and Epstein (1981) show that both timolol and acetazolamide act solely by reducing secretion, but surprisingly the effects on pressure are not fully additive. On the other hand, Scharrer and Ober (1979) and Dailey et al. (1982) suggest an additive effect; the discrepancies may be based on differences in experimental design.

It is important again to stress the usefulness of methazolamide in the 1–2 mg/kg/day range (low dose) when the additive nature of the role of these medications is considered. Despite many studies addressing the pressure-lowering effects of methazolamide (Maren et al. 1977; Stone et al. 1977; Dahlen et al. 1978; Merkle 1980), careful clinical comparison of methazolamide to acetazolamide as an added drug in miotic regimens has not been reported. However, it appears that in long-term therapy, low-dose methazolamide will prove a useful replacement for acetazolamide, with less risk or discomfort of side effects and less or no acidosis. Of course, the development of a topically active carbonic anhydrase inhibitor will eliminate the unwanted side effects seen when these drugs are given orally.

II. Miscellaneous Uses and Effects

Acetazolamide has been used to study changes in outflow pressure in ocular hypertensives and in glaucoma patients (Linner 1978; Nissen et al. 1976), in an attempt to differentiate these conditions in early stages. It is unlikely, however, that this approach will predict the tissue susceptibility to visual field loss, the information both the patient and the ophthalmologist want.

Another area which may have practical significance relates the effects of acetazolamide on retinal blood flow to the standing potential in the human electroretinogram (Yonemura and Kawasaki 1979). Since Stanescu and Michiels (1975) showed a rise in amplitude of the electroretinogram b wave after administration of acetazolamide, various explanations have been presented, related either to rapid pCO_2 or intraocular pressure shifts affecting retinal blood flow. There are no reported toxic effects of carbonic anhydrase inhibition on retinal function in mammals (see, however, the discussion of retinal toxicity in freshwater fish following sulfonamide inhibitors, MAREN 1967). YONEMURA and KAWASAKI (1979) feel that the b wave enhancement by acetazolamide can be used to quantify differences in retinal pigmented epithelial responses between normal and diabetic patients with retinopathy, but further clinical work is needed.

E. Urolithiasis with Carbonic Anhydrase Inhibitors

There is evidence to link acetazolamide treatment with urinary tract stones in a moderate number of cases (PERSKY et al. 1956; SHAH et al. 1958; GORDON and SHEPS 1957; DAVIES 1959; MACKENZIE 1960; PARFITT 1969; PEPYS 1970; RUBENSTEIN and BUCY 1975).

Recently, a retrospective case control study (KASS et al. 1981) has attempted to quantify this association, and to separate the risk of carbonic anhydrase inhibitor therapy from the high incidence of urolithiasis in the older population exposed to the drug (LANDES 1976). The incidence of stones in the acetazolamide group was 11 times greater than in the matched no-acetazolamide group, and 15 times greater than that in the treated group prior to acetazolamide therapy. The rate was 24 per 1,000 people per year of therapy; however, after the 1st year, the cumulative risk of stone formation did not rise appreciably, suggesting that most persons at risk of urolithiasis from acetazolamide develop stones within the first 15 months of therapy. This finding is in line with modern concepts indicating that in some patients and in some localities there are "stone formers," a definite subset of the population. Such people appear at greater risk in this situation.

The mechanisms behind this relate the metabolic acidosis induced by acetazolamide and the associated depression of renal citrate excretion (CRAWFORD et al. 1959; CONSTANT and BECKER 1959). When this occurs, more calcium is freed to form insoluble salts, particularly urate and carbonate. However, no evidence of renal stones was found in the long-term, high-dose toxicity studies in animals which led to the introduction of acetazolamide into medicine (MAREN et al. 1954a).

The problem is complicated by questions of diet, vitamin D and possibly parathyroid metabolism, as suggested by the following studies. HARRISON and HARRISON (1955) induced renal stones in rats only when they were injected with vitamin D and fed a high-calcium, high-phosphate diet. EVANS and MACPHERSON (1956) suggested that vitamin D and acetazolamide were synergistic factors in stone formation, but they were unable to prevent stones in rats by alkalinizing the urine. GILL and VERMEULEN (1962) were unable to produce stones in the rat by decreasing urinary citrate with acetazolamide. GYÖRY et al. (1970) have suggested that urinary citrate excretion is not as important as the shifts in magnesium and urinary pH induced by the underlying metabolic acidosis, and that diet manipulation, at least in the rat, can decrease the risk of nephrocalcinosis.

TAKEMOTO (1978) was able to diminish significantly the incidence of stone formation in a population of 26 glaucoma patients by giving potassium citrate 8–10 g/day or sodium citrate 4–6 g/day. This regimen partially corrected the metabolic acidosis in these patients, raising plasma bicarbonate from 16 ± 3 mM in patients receiving 250–750 mg acetazolamide per day to 19 ± 2.5 mM. It is noteworthy, however, that urinary citrate increased four fold during this treatment, to nearly normal levels. Since the correction of acidosis was not complete, it must be concluded that the beneficial effect on stone formation was due to the citrate itself.

These findings, however, still indicate that if metabolic acidosis and citrate lowering is avoided, stone formation will be abolished. MAREN et al. (1977) showed that low doses of methazolamide, which effectively do reduce intraocular pressure (STONE et al. 1977; DAHLEN et al. 1978), do not cause metabolic acidosis or the concomitant reduction in urinary citrate. However, urolithiasis has been reported with the higher doses of methazolamide, i.e., 100 mg three times a day (SHIELDS and SIMMONS 1976) or 200 mg twice a day (ELLIS 1973).

F. Other Toxic Effects

In addition to the apparent increased incidence of nephrolithiasis associated with acetazolamide therapy, there are a number of distressing side effects which have been reported. These include numbness and tingling, malaise, anorexia, nausea, and gastrointestinal distress and depression (BECKER 1960; GRANT 1973; EPSTEIN and GRANT 1979). Becker noted that 60% of all compliance failures from intolerance to carbonic anhydrase inhibitors, particularly acetazolamide, were related to these side effects.

Diminished libido has been documented in 39 cases, with 3 reported reversible cases of impotence (WALLACE et al. 1979). All four drugs have been responsible, even low-dose methazolamide (50 mg twice daily). There was no direct dose–response relationship, although in a few cases diminishing the dose ameliorated this side effect.

Another curious complaint has been loss of taste for carbonated beverages and a strange "metallic taste" reported by some patients but not universally present. Normally one cannot taste the CO_2 present dissolved in carbonated beverages, as it is rapidly converted to H_2CO_3 and thence to HCO_3^- by hydration mediated by carbonic anhydrase, either in the red cells or in the taste buds themselves. This hydration step is more rapid than the rate of nerve conduction. Carbonic anhydrase inhibition slows the hydration step to the uncatalyzed rate, which is slower than nerve conduction. The ingested CO_2 can then be sensed by the taste buds (SWENSON and MAREN 1978). The effect is slight or absent at the low (25 mg) methazolamide dose (MAREN et al. 1977).

EPSTEIN and GRANT (1977, 1979) have attempted to quantify the complaints of a large group of glaucoma patients into a "malaise symptom complex" consisting of malaise, fatigue, depression, anorexia, weight loss, and diminished libido. They sought relationships between side effects and the changes in serum composition seen in patients taking either acetazolamide or methazolamide, and did report a correlation with systemic acidosis. However, it must be realized that acidosis may simply be concomitant with high plasma concentration. Recently, ALWARD and WILENSKY (1981) presented data suggesting that all patients who comply with a standard dosage regimen (250 mg four times daily) of acetazolamide develop systemic acidosis, while those not taking the medication regularly have more normal serum CO_2-combining power. It is necessary to point out that some patients receiving low-dose methazolamide (DAHLEN et al. 1978; STONE et al. 1977) who lacked either the acidosis or renal citrate depletion did develop the side effects described. The factors leading to the development of uncomfortable side effects appear to be complex. Much of the work only compares the tolerance to various carbonic anhydrase inhibitors (GARRISON et al. 1967). The treatment of systemic acidosis with sodium chloride, sodium citrate, and sodium bicarbonate to ameliorate side effects has been attempted (DRAEGER 1963; EPSTEIN and GRANT 1979). However, there is little concrete evidence that the doses given actually reverse the acidosis; also it may be a sodium-related effect, since sodium chloride is equally effective in some patients (LEOPOLD et al. 1955). Some authors have tried to treat this symptom complex with potassium. However, careful studies have shown no evidence of potassium depletion with carbonic anhydrase inhibitors alone, in the absence of thiazide diuretics (SPAETH 1967). It is worth remembering that dichlorphenamide has thiazide chloriuretic properties, and as such is prone to cause hypokalemia. In general, little progress has been made in diminishing the symptoms in susceptible patients taking standard regimens of acetazolamide or methazolamide (DAHLEN et al. 1978). There is apparently a lower incidence of these side effects with lower doses of methazolamide (STONE et al. 1977).

The physiology of this train of symptoms is not understood, especially since patients with renal tubular acidosis and related metabolic alterations do not have similar complaints. Metabolic acidosis alone, when induced in humans to this degree, causes no such symptom complex. It is likely that a mild degree of total body Na^+ depletion occurs, as has been noted in dogs (MAREN 1968). The mild metabolic acidosis might pose a potential risk if superimposed in three special disease categories:

1. Diabetes with superimposed ketosis or susceptibility to ketoacidosis (GRANT 1973)
2. Hepatic insufficiency. Here the obligatory urinary alkalinization causes decreased ammonia trapping and excretion, leading to a concomitant rise in plasma NH_3 (OWEN et al. 1960)
3. Chronic obstructive pulmonary disease where CO_2 elimination is impaired and a gradient develops between arterial blood CO_2 and pulmonary alveolar CO_2 (BLOCK and ROSTAND 1978).

These more serious instances will be discussed below.

An earlier comparative study (GARRISON et al. 1967), which unfortunately did not include methazolamide, did find a high proportion of malaise-related side effects with dichlorphenamide, fewer with acetazolamide, and fewest with ethoxzolamide, when each compound was given for 10 days in a double-masked manner with known acetazolamide as a positive control. A more recent study to compare side effects (LICHTER et al. 1978) used a relatively high dose of methazolamide (50 mg every 6 h) and comparably high doses of acetazolamide tablets and sequels. It had previously been suggested that such sequels were well tolerated (GARNER et al. 1963). Acetazolamide sequels were slightly better tolerated than high-dose methazolamide. The final suggestion of LICHTER et al. (1978) was to develop a sustained low-dose release form of methazolamide to improve compliance and tolerance.

Patients with chronic obstructive pulmonary disease (Block and Rostand 1978) can develop severe CO_2 retention, which is exacerbated by the standard doses of carbonic anhydrase inhibitors. High doses of these drugs should never be given to this class of patients, for the risk of CO_2 narcosis and death is too great. The basis for this effect is the inhibition of red cell carbonic anhydrase. While normal patients can compensate for this effect, this is not the case in the presence of pulmonary disease or deep anesthesia. Low doses (50 mg twice daily) of methazolamide may be used with caution, and measurement of arterial blood gases is suggested when such patients are started on carbonic anhydrase inhibitors.

Liver disease is a contraindication to the systemic use of carbonic anhydrase inhibitors. Such patients may develop "flapping tremor" and hallucinations. The probable basis for this reaction is the diversion of renal NH_3 into the bloodstream following urinary alkalinization. This reaction was observed very early in the development of these drugs, and fortunately further instances of toxicity have been avoided (see Maren 1967).

Rare side effects from this class of drug include those common to the sulfonamides, namely the blood dyscrasias and other allergic reactions such as skin rash. There are probably no more than 20 reported dyscrasia cases in the literature, although thrombocytopenia and aplastic anemia have been reported for both methazolamide and acetazolamide (Langlois 1966; Wisch et al. 1973; Rentiers et al. 1970; Werblin et al. 1979). The effect is idiosyncratic; checking white blood counts will not detect susceptible patients.

Liver failure as a result of drug hypersensitivity and hepatitis has been reported (Kristinnson 1967), but it is extremely rare.

Carbonic anhydrase inhibitors should be avoided in pregnant women, since a characteristic forelimb deformity has been seen in offspring of rodents following drug at days 10–11 of pregnancy (Layton and Hallsey 1965; Hallsey and Layton 1969). The matter has been reviewed and potential risks in pregnant women have been outlined (Maren 1971). The defect now appears to be peculiarly characteristic of this class of drugs, since all carbonic anhydrase inhibitors of sufficient potency cause the lesion, and only such drugs yield the specific morphological response (Maren and Ellison 1972). The mechanism of the effect is not known; acidosis has been ruled out (Ellison and Maren 1972).

A rare and curious side effect, believed to be sulfonamide-related, is the transient myopia sometimes seen as an idiosyncratic reaction to acetazolamide (Galin et al. 1962) or ethoxzolamide (Beasley 1962). Such a reaction had been previously noted for sulfonamides and described as a sensitivity, with ciliary body edema, since it occurred most often in patients who had already received the drug. The responses to acetazolamide in the one patient exhibiting this sensitivity were not consistent. It is an extremely rare phenomenon and is almost certainly unrelated to lens carbonic anhydrase inhibition, since acetazolamide enters the lens poorly (Friedland and Maren 1981).

Finally, there is one reported case of hirsutism in a 2½-year-old girl treated for congenital glaucoma (Weiss 1974). There was no evidence of virilism and the hair growth regressed when treatment was stopped. The author presumed the cause to be secondary to some interaction between acetazolamide and some unnamed function of the adrenal glands and acid–base metabolism – leading to an androgenic effect which would not be noticed in the adult. Despite that speculation, there have been no other reported cases in which to test the hypothesis.

It is important to point out that the antibacterial and the carbonic anhydrase inhibiting sulfonamides are not closely linked in structure. The underlying chemistries and structure–activity relationships are quite dissimilar (MAREN 1976 b).

There are no overlapping activities in any system, and there is no reason to suspect overlapping sensitivities between the two classes of drugs.

G. Summary

A remarkable series of scientific coincidences and observations led to the introduction of the carbonic anhydrase inhibitors for the treatment of glaucoma. The use of these compounds rests on a reasonably solid physiological and biochemical base. The secretion of aqueous humor depends in part on the synthesis of HCO_3^- from CO_2, and this reaction is catalyzed by carbonic anhydrase. Fluid and sodium transport may be linked to HCO_3^- production. When the enzyme is inhibited, fluid, HCO_3^- and Na movement are all reduced. The result is a fall in intraocular pressure. There is no effect upon outflow, and there is no evidence that the sulfonamides which inhibit carbonic anhydrase have any other pharmacologic action.

The chief drug in use, acetazolamide, is well absorbed from the gut and is excreted unchanged. It acts for about 6 h, and at the doses necessary for reduction of IOP, there is action on the kidney leading to excretion of HCO_3^-, Na, and K, and metabolic acidosis. Despite this effect, patients have been maintained on constant dosage for many years. Although serious toxicity is rare, there are many complaints from patients, usually of a psychological or neurological type, and compliance is often poor. Methazolamide has a somewhat different and more favorable pharmacology and reaches the ciliary processes better than acetazolamide, and so may be used in lower doses that have few renal effects and less toxicity. Neither drug is effective by topical administration because penetration through the cornea is poor relative to what is required for inhibition of carbonic anhydrase at the secretory site.

With these drugs there is no pharmacologic effect until over 99% of enzyme in the ciliary processes is inhibited. Thus only very powerful inhibitors are effective, and relatively high plasma levels must be maintained for pressure-lowering. It is possible to correlate all of these factors into a satisfying model which connect the basic science to the clinical control of eye pressure.

References

Alward PD, Wilensky JT (1981) Determination of acetazolamide compliance in patients with glaucoma. Arch Ophthalmol 99:1973–1976

Azuma I (1960) Studies on the mechanism of intraocular pressure lowering effect of acetazolamide (Diamox). Folia Ophthalmol Jpn 11:65–77

Azuma I (1973) Graphical expression of the intraocular pressure dynamics. Jpn J Ophthalmol 17:310–322

Bayne WF, Tao FT, Rogers G, Chu LC, Theeuwes F (1981) Time course and disposition of methazolamide in human plasma and red blood cells. J Pharm Sci 70:75–81

Beasley FJ (1962) Transient myopia and retinal edema during ethoxzolamide (Cardrase) therapy. Arch Ophthalmol 68:490–491

Becker B (1954) Diamox and the therapy of glaucoma. Am J Ophthalmol 38:16–17

Becker B (1955a) The mechanism of the fall in intraocular pressure induced by the carbonic anhydrase inhibitor, Diamox. Am J Ophthalmol 39:177–184

Becker B (1955b) The effects of the carbonic anhydrase inhibitor, acetazolamide, on the composition of aqueous humor. Am J Ophthalmol 40:129–136

Becker B (1956) The effects of acetazolamide on ascorbic acid turnover. An application of the theory of aqueous humor dynamics. Am J Ophthalmol 41:522–529

Becker B (1957) The chemical composition of human aqueous humor, effects of acetazolamide. Arch Ophthalmol 57:793–800

Becker B (1959) Carbonic anhydrase and the formation of aqueous humor. The Friedenwald memorial lecture. Am J Ophthalmol 47:342–361

Becker P (1960) Use of methazolamide (Neptazane) in the therapy of glaucoma: comparison with acetazolamide (Diamox). Am J Ophthalmol 49:1307–1311

Becker B (1961) Iodide transport by the rabbit eye. Am J Physiol 200:804–806

Becker B (1962) The measurement of aqueous flow with iodide. Invest Ophthalmol 1:52–58

Becker B, Constant MA (1955) Experimental tonography. The effect of the carbonic anhydrase inhibitor acetazolamide on aqueous flow. Arch Opthalmol 54:321–329

Benedikt O, Zirm M, Harnoncourt K (1974) Die Beziehungen zwischen metabolischer Azidose und intraokulärem Druck nach Carboanhydrasehemmung mit Acetazolamid. Albrecht Von Graefes Arch Klin Exp Ophthalmol 190:247–255

Berson FG, Epstein DL (1981) Separate and combined effects of timolol maleate and acetazolamide in open-angle glaucoma. Am J Ophthalmol 92:788–791

Berson FG, Epstein DL, Grant WM, Hutchinson BT, Dobbs P (1980) Acetazolamide dosage forms in the treatment of glaucoma. Arch Ophthalmol 98:1051–1054

Beyer KH, Baer JE (1961) Physiological basis for the action of newer diuretic agents. Pharm Rev 13:517–562

Bietti G, Virno M, Pecon-Geraldi J, Pellegrino N (1975) Acetazolamide, metabolic acidosis, and intraocular pressure. Am J Ophthalmol 80:360–369

Bill A (1975) Blood circulation and fluid dynamics in the eye. Physiol Rev 55:383–417

Birzis L, Carter CH, Maren TH (1958) Effect of acetazolamide on CSF pressure and electrolytes in hydrocephalus. Neurology 8:522–528

Block ER, Rostand RA (1978) Carbonic anhydrase inhibition in glaucoma: hazard or benefit for the chronic lunger? Surv Ophthalmol 23:169–172

Cole DF (1966) Aqueous humor formation. Doc Ophthalmol 21:116–238

Cole DF (1979) Ciliary processes. In: Heilman K, Richardson KT (eds) Glaucoma – conceptions of a disease. Saunders, Philadelphia, pp 44–53

Constant MA (1962) The distribution of 5,5-dimethyl-2,4-oxazolidinedione (DMO). II. Studies of the effect of carbonic anhydrase inhibitors and of plasma levels. Invest Ophthalmol 1:609–617

Constant MA, Becker B (1960) The effect of carbonic anhydrase inhibitors on urinary excretion of citrate by humans. Am J Ophthalmol 49:929–934

Constant MA, Falch J (1963) Phosphate and protein concentrations of intraocular fluids. I. Effect of carbonic anhydrase inhibition in young and old rabbits. Invest Ophthalmol 2:332–343

Cotlier E (1979) Bicarbonate ATP-ase in ciliary body and a theory of Diamox effect on aqueous humor formation. Int Ophthalmol 1:123–128

Crawford MA, Milne MD, Scribner BH (1959) The effects of changes in acid base balance on urinary citrate in the rat. J Physiol (Lond) 149:413–423

Dahlen K, Epstein DL, Grant WM, Hutchinson BT, Prien EL, Krall JM (1978) A repeated dose-response study of methazolamide in glaucoma. Arch Ophthalmol 96:2214–2218

Dailey RA, Brubaker RF, Bourne WM (1982) The effects of timolol maleate and acetazolamide on the rate of aqueous formation in normal human subjects. Am J Ophthalmol 93:232–237

Davenport HW (1945) The inhibition of carbonic anhydrase by thiophene-2-sulfonamide and sulfanilamide. J Biol Chem 158:567–571

Davies DW (1959) Acetazolamide with renal complications. Brit Med J 1:214–215

Davies RE (1951) The mechanism of hydrochloric acid production by the stomach. Biol Rev 26:87–120

Davson H (1969) The intraocular fluids. In: Davson H (ed) The eye, Vol I, 2nd edn, Academic, New York

Draeger J, Grüttner R, Theilmann W (1963) Avoidance of side-reactions and loss of drug efficacy during long-term administration of carbonic anhydrase inhibitors by concomitant supplemental electrolyte administration. Br J Ophthalmol 47:457–468

Ellis PP (1973) Urinary calculi with methazolamide therapy. Doc Ophthalmol 34:137–142

Ellison AC, Maren TH (1972) The effects of metabolic alterations on teratogenesis. Johns Hopkins Med J 130:87–94

Epstein DL, Grant WM (1977) Carbonic anhydrase inhibitor side effects: serum chemical analysis. Arch Ophthalmol 95:1378–1382

Epstein DL, Grant WM (1979) Management of carbonic anhydrase inhibitor side effects. In: Leopold IH, Burns RP (eds) Symposium on ocular therapy, vol. 2 Wiley, New York, pp 51–64

Evans BM, Macpherson CR (1956) Some observations on acetazolamide induced nephrocalcinosis in the rat. Br J Exp Pathol 37:533–540

Forbes M, Becker B (1961) The transport of organic anions by the rabbit ciliary body. Am J Ophthalmol 51:1047–1051

Foss RH (1955) Local application of Diamox. An experimental study of its effect on the intraocular pressure. Am J Ophthalmol 39:336–339

Friedenwald JS (1949) The formation of the intra-ocular fluid. Am J Ophthalmol 32:9–27

Friedenwald JS (1955a) Carbonic anhydrase inhibition and aqueous flow. Am J Ophthalmol 39:59–64

Friedenwald JS (1955b) Current studies on acetazolamide (Diamox) and aqueous humor flow. Am J Ophthalmol 40:139–146

Friedland BR, Maren TH (1981) The relation between carbonic anhydrase activity and ion transport in elasmobranch and rabbit lens. Exp Eye Res 33:545–561

Friedland BR, Mallonee J, Anderson DR (1977) Short-term dose response characteristics of acetazolamide in man. Arch Ophthalmol 95:1809–1812

Friedman Z, Krupin T, Becker B (1982) Ocular and systemic effects of acetazolamide in nephrectomized rabbits. Invest Ophthalmol 23:209–213

Galin MA, Baras I, Zweifach P (1962) Diamox-induced myopia. Am J Ophthalmol 54:237–243

Garg LC, Oppelt WW (1970) The effect of ouabain and acetazolamide on the transport of sodium and chloride from plasma to aqueous humor. J Pharmacol Exp Ther 175:237–247

Garner LL, Carl EF, Ferwerda JR (1963) Advantages of sustained release therapy with acetazolamide in glaucoma. Am J Ophthalmol 55:323–327

Garrison L, Roth A, Rundle H, Christensen RE (1967) A clinical comparison of three carbonic anhydrase inhibitors. Trans Pac Coast Otolaryngol Ophthalmol Soc 48:137–145

Gelatt KN, Gum GG, Williams LW, Gwin RM (1979) Ocular hypotensive effects of carbonic anhydrase inhibitors in normotensive and glaucomatous beagles. Am J Vet Res 40:334–345

Gill WB, Vermeulen (1962) Causation of stone by two co-acting agents – Diamox and operative insult upon urinary tract. J Urol 88:103–109

Gordon EE, Sheps SG (1957) Effect of acetazolamide on citrate excretion and formation of renal calculi. Report of a case and study of five normal subjects. N Engl J Med 256:1215–1219

Grant WM (1973) Antiglaucoma drugs. Problems with carbonic anhydrase inhibitors. In: Leopold IH (ed) Symposium on ocular therapy, vol 6 Mosby, St. Louis, pp 19–38

Green H, Leopold IH (1955) Effects of locally administered Diamox. Am J Ophthalmol 40:137–139

Győry AZ, Edwards KDG, Robinson J, Palmer AA (1970) The relative importance of urinary pH and urinary content of citrate, magnesium, and calcium in the production of nephro calcinosis by diet and acetazolamide in the rat. Clin Sci 39:605–623

Hallesy DW, Layton WM (1969) Forelimb deformity of rats given dichlorphenamide during pregnancy. Proc Soc Exp Biol Med 126:6–8

Hanley T, Platts MM (1956) Diminishing effect of carbonic anhydrase inhibitor acetazolamide on urinary bicarbonate excretion. J Appl Physiol 9:279–286

Harrison HE, Harrison HC (1955) Inhibition of urine citrate excretion and the production of renal calcinosis in the rat by acetazolamide (Diamox) administration. J Clin Invest 34:1662–1670

Hodler J, Heinemann HO, Fishman AP, Smith HW (1955) Urine pH and carbonic anhydrase activity in the marine dogfish. Am J Physiol 183:155–162

Holder L, Hayes S (1965) Diffusion of sulfonamides in aqueous buffers and into red cells. Mol Pharmacol 1:266–279

Holm O, Wiebert O (1968) The effect of systemically given acetazolamide (Diamox) on the formation of aqueous humor in the human eye measured with a new photogrammetric method. Acta Ophthalmol (Copenh) 46:1243–1246

Jones RF, Maurice DM (1966) New methods of measuring the rate of aqueous flow in man with fluorescein. Exp Eye Res 5:208–220

Kass MA, Kolker AE, Gordon M, Goldberg I, Gieser DK, Krupin T, Becker B (1981) Acetazolamide and urolithiasis. Ophthalmology 88:261–265

Kimura R (1978) Effect of long-term subconjunctival administration of Diamox (acetazolamide) on the ocular tension in rabbit. Albrecht Von Graefes Arch Klin Exp Ophthalmol 205:221–227

Kinsey VE (1953) Comparative chemistry of aqueous humor in posterior and anterior chambers of rabbit eyes. Arch Ophthalmol 50:401–417

Kinsey VE (1971) Ion movement in ciliary processes. In: Bittar EE (ed) Membranes and ion transport, vol. 3. Wiley, New York, pp 185–209

Kinsey VE, Reddy DVN (1959) Turnover of carbon dioxide in the aqueous humor and the effect thereon of acetazolamide. AMA Arch Ophthalmol 62:78–83

Kinsey VE, Camacho E, Cavanaugh GA, Constant MA (1955a) Diamox and intraocular fluid dynamics. Am J Opthalmol 40:147–148 (abstract)

Kinsey VE, Camacho E, Cavanaugh GA, Constant MA, McGinty DA (1955b) Dependence of IOP-lowering effect of acetazolamide on salt. Arch Ophthal 53:680–685

Kinsey VE, Reddy DVN, Skrentny BA (1960) Intraocular transport of ^{14}C-labelled urea and the influences of Diamox on its rate of accumulation in aqueous humors. Am J Ophthalmol 50:1130–1141

Kolker AE, Hetherington J (1976) Medications that decrease the rate of aqueous formation. In: Becker-Shaffer's diagnosis and therapy of the glaucomas, 4th edn. Mosby, St. Louis, pp 336–353

Kristinnson A (1967) Fatal reaction to acetazolamide. Br J Ophthalmol 51:348–349

Krupin T, Oestrich CJ, Bass J, Podos SM, Becker B (1977) Acidosis, alkalosis, and aqueous humor dynamics in rabbits. Invest Ophthalmol 16:997–1001

Kupfer C, Gaasterland D, Ross K (1971) Studies of aqueous humor dynamics in man. II. Measurements in young normal subjects using acetazolamide and L-epinephrine. Invest Ophthalmol 10:523–533

Landes RR (1976) Incidence and management of ureteral calculi in general hospital patients: a nationwide survey. In: Finlayson B, Thomas WC (eds) Colloquium on renal lithiasis. University Presses of Florida, Gainesville, pp 249–276

Langham ME, Lee PM (1957) Action of Diamox and ammonium chloride on the formation of aqueous humor. Br J Ophthalmol 41:65–92

Langlois (1966) Diamox et thrombocytopénie. Arch Ophthal (Paris) 26:701–705

Layton WM, Hallesy DW (1965) Deformity of forelimb in rats: association with high doses of acetazolamide. Science 149:306–308

Lehmann B, Linner E, Wistrand PJ (1969) The pharmacokinetics of acetazolamide in relation to its use in the treatment of glaucoma and its effects as an inhibitor of carbonic anhydrases. In: Rospe G (ed) Schering workshop in pharmakokinetics, advances in the biosciences 5. Pergamon, New York, pp 197–217

Leopold IH, Eisenberg IJ, Yasuma J (1955) Experience with Diamox in glaucoma. Am J Ophthalmol 39:885–888

Lichter PR, Newman LP, Wheeler NC, Beall OV (1978) Patient tolerance to carbonic anhydrase inhibitors. Am J Ophthalmol 85:495–502

Linner E (1956) Further studies of the episcleral venous pressure in glaucoma. Am J Ophthalmol 41:646–651

Linner E (1978) Ocular hypertension. II. A carbonic anhydrase test for early detection of glaucoma. Acta Ophthalmol 56:179–189

Linner E, Friedenwald TS (1957) The appearance time of fluorescein as an index of aqueous flow. Am J Ophthalmol 44:225–229

Macdonald MJ, Crane SM, Cullen PM, Phillips CI (1977) Comparison of ocular hypotensive effects of acetazolamide and atenolol. Br J Opthalmol 61:345–348

Mackenzie AR (1960) Acetazolamide induced renal stone. J Urol 84:453–455

Macri FJ, Dixon RL, Rall DP (1965) Aqueous humor turnover rates in the cat. I. Effect of acetazolamide. Invest Ophthalmol 4:927–934

Mann T, Keilin D (1940) Sulfanilamide as a specific inhibitor of carbonic anhydrase. Nature 146:164–165

Maren TH (1956) Carbonic anhydrase inhibition. IV. The effects of metabolic acidosis on the response to Diamox. Bull Johns Hopkins Hosp 98:159–183

Maren TH (1963 a) The relation between enzyme inhibition and physiological response in the carbonic anhydrase system. J Pharmacol Exptl Therap 139:140–153

Maren TH (1963 b) Ionic composition of cerebrospinal fluid and aqueous humor of the dogfish, *Squalus acanthias*. Comp Biochem Physiol 5:201–215

Maren TH (1967) Carbonic anhydrase: chemistry, physiology, and inhibition. Physiol Rev 47:595–781

Maren TH (1968) Renal carbonic anhydrase and the pharmacology of sulfonamide inhibitors. In: Herken H (ed) Diuretica. Springer, Berlin Heidelberg New York, pp 195–256 (Handbook of experimental pharmacology, vol. 24)

Maren TH (1971) Teratology and carbonic anhydrase inhibition. Arch Ophthalmol 85:1–2

Maren TH (1974 a) Chemistry of the renal reabsorption of bicarbonate. Can J Physiol Pharmacol 52:1041–1050

Maren TH (1974 b) HCO_3^- formation in aqueous humor: mechanism and relation to the treatment of glaucoma. Invest Ophthalmol 13:479–484

Maren TH (1976 a) The rates of movement of Na^+, Cl^-, and HCO_3^- from plasma to posterior chamber: effect of acetazolamide and relation to the treatment of glaucoma. Invest Ophthalmol 13:356–364

Maren TH (1976 b) Relations between structure and biological activity of sulfonamides. Annu Rev Pharmacol Toxicol 16:309–327

Maren TH (1977 a) Physiology and chemistry of cerebrospinal fluid, aqueous humor and endolymph in *Squalus acanthias*. J Exp Zool 199:317–324

Maren TH (1977 b) Ion secretion into the posterior aqueous humor of dogs and monkeys. Exp Eye Res [Suppl] 25:245–247

Maren TH (1979) Theodore Weicker Oration: An historical account of CO_2 chemistry and the development of carbonic anhydrase inhibitors. Pharmacologist 20:303–321

Maren TH (1980) Cerebrospinal fluid, aqueous humor, and endolymph. In: Mountcastle VB (ed) Medical physiology, 14th edn. Mosby, St. Louis, pp 1218–1252

Maren TH, Ellison AC (1972) The teratological effect of certain thiadiazoles related to acetazolamide, with a note on sulfanilamide and thiazide diuretics. Johns Hopkins Med J 130:95–104

Maren TH, Robinson B (1960) The pharmacology of acetazolamide as related to cerebrospinal fluid and the treatment of hydrocephalus. Bull Johns Hopkins Hosp 106:1–24

Maren TH, Wiley CE (1968) The *in vitro* activity of sulfonamides against red cell carbonic anhydrases. J Med Chem 11:228–232

Maren TH, Mayer E, Wadsworth BC (1954 a) Carbonic anhydrase inhibition. I. The pharmacology of Diamox, 2-acetylamino-1,3,4-thiadiazole 5-sulfonamide. Bull Johns Hopkins Hosp 95:199–243

Maren TH, Wadsworth BC, Yale EK, Alonso, LG (1954 b) Carbonic anhydrase inhibition. III. Effects of Diamox on electrolyte metabolism. Bull Johns Hopkins Hosp 95:277–321

Maren TH, Wistrand P, Swenson ER, Talalay AR (1975) The rates of ion movement from plasma to aqueous humor in the dogfish, *Squalus acanthias*. Invest Ophthalmol 14:662–673

Maren TH, Haywood JR, Chapman SK, Zimmerman TJ (1977) The pharmacology of methazolamide in relation to the treatment of glaucoma. Invest Ophthalmol 16:730–742

Maren TH, Friedland BR, Rittmaster R (1980) Kinetic properties of primitive vertebrate carbonic anhydrases. Comp Biochem Physiol 67B:69–74

Maren TH, Jankowska L, Sanyal G, Edelhauser HF (1983) The transcameral permeability of sulfonamide carbonic anhydrase inhibitors and their effect on aqueous humor secretion. Exp Eye Res 36:457–480

Meldrum NU, Roughton FJW (1933) Carbonic anhydrase: its preparation and properties. J Physiol (Lond) 80:113–142

Merkle W (1980) Untersuchungen über die Wirkung von Methazolamid auf den intraokulären Druck. Klin Monatsbl Augenheilkd 176:181–185

Merté HJ, Heilman K, Hallwich I (1977) Untersuchungen über die Wirkung von verschiedenen Dosierungen von Acetazolamid (Diamox) auf den intraokolären Druck. Klin Monatsbl Augenheilkd 170:473–479

Miller JE (1962) Alterations of the blood-aqueous potentials in the rabbit. Invest Ophthalmol 1:59–62

Moses RA (1980) Intraocular pressure. In: Moses RA (ed) Adler's physiology of the eye, 7th edn. Mosby, St. Louis, Chap. 8, p 227

Nissen OI, Kjer D, Olsen L (1976) A comparison between an acetazolamide test and weight tonography in pathological and apathological circulation of the aqueous humor. Invest Ophthalmol 15:844–848

Oppelt WW (1967) Measurement of aqueous humor formation rates by posterior-anterior chamber perfusion with inulin. Normal values and the effect of carbonic anhydrase inhibition. Invest Ophthalmol 6:76–88

Owen EE, Tyor MP, Flanagan JF, Berry JN (1960) The kidney as a source of blood ammonia in patients with liver disease: the effect of acetazolamide. J Clin Invest 39:288–294

Parfitt AM (1969) Acetazolamide and sodium bicarbonate induced nephrocalcinosis and nephrothiasis, relationship to citrate and calcium excretion. Arch Int Med 24:736–740

Pepys MB (1970) Acetazolamide and renal stone formation. Lancet 1:837

Persky L, Chambers D, Potts A (1956) Calculus formation and ureteral colic following acetazolamide (Diamox) therapy. JAMA 161:1625–1626

Petounis AD, Chandreli S, Vaulaluka-Sekioti A (1980) Effect of hypercapnea on human intraocular pressure during general anesthesia following acetazolamide administration. Br J Ophthalmol 64:422–425

Rector FC (1981) Acid-base renal physiology. In: Brenner BM, Rector FC (eds) The kidney, 2nd edn. Saunders, Philadelphia, pp 286–298

Rentiers PK, Johnson AC, Buskard N (1970) Severe aplastic anemia as a complication of acetazolamide therapy. Can J Ophthalmol 5:337–342

Roblin RO Jr, Clapp JW (1950) The preparation of heterocyclic sulfonamides. J AM Chem Soc 72:4890–4892

Roughton FJW (1935) Recent work on carbon dioxide transport by the blood. Physiol Rev 15:241–296

Rubenstein MA, Bucy JG (1975) Acetazolamide-induced renal calculi. J Urol 114:610–612

Scharrer A, Ober M (1979) Timolol and acetazolamide in the treatment of increased intraocular presure. Albrecht Von Graefes Arch Klin Exp Ophthalmol 212:129–134

Shah A, Constant MA, Becker B (1958) Urinary excretion of citrate in humans following administration of acetazolamide (Diamox). Arch Ophthalmol 59:536–540

Shields MB, Simmons RJ (1976) Urinary calculus during methazolamide therapy. Am J Ophthalmol 81:622–624

Söser M, Ogriseg M, Kessler B, Zirm H (1980) New findings concerning changes in intraocular pressure and blood acidosis after peroral application of acetazolamide. Klin Monatsbl Augenheilkd 176:88–92

Southworth H (1937) Acidosis associated with the administration of para-amino-benzene sulfonamide (Prontylin). Proc Soc Exp Biol Med 36:58–61

Spaeth GL (1967) Potassium, acetazolamide, and intraocular pressure. Arch Ophthalmol 78:578–582

Stanescu B, Michiels J (1975) The effects of acetazolamide on the human electroretinogram. Invest Ophthalmol 14:935–937

Stein A, Pinke R, Krupin T, Glabb E, Podos SM, Serle J, Maren TH (1983) The effect of topically administered carbonic anhydrase inhibitors on aqueous humor dynamics in rabbits. Am J Ophthalmol 95:222–228

Stiegler G (1979) Bupranolol eyedrops in glaucoma therapy. Klin Monatsbl Augenheilkd 174:267–275

Stone RA, Zimmerman TJ, Shin DH, Becker B, Kass MA (1977) Low-dose methazolamide and intraocular pressure. Am J Ophthalmol 83:674–679

Swenson ER, Maren TH (1978) A quantitative analysis of CO_2 transport at rest and during maximal exercise. Respir Physiol 35:129–159

Takemoto M (1978) Prophylaxis for acetazolamide induced urolithiasis: clinical study. Jpn J Urol 69:963–987

Vaziri ND, Saiki J, Barton CH, Rajudin M, Ness R (1980) Hemodialyzability of acetazolamide. South Med J 73:422–423

Wallace TR, Fraunfelder FT, Petursson GJ, Epstein DC (1979) Decreased libido – a side effect of carbonic anhydrase inhibitor. Ann Ophthalmol 11:1563–1566

Weiner IM, Washington TA, Mudge GH (1959) Studies on the renal excretion of salicylate in the dog. Bull Johns Hopkins Hosp 105:284–297

Weiss IS (1974) Hirsutism after chronic administration of acetazolamide. Am J Ophthalmol 78:327–331

Werblin TP, Pollack IP, Liss RA (1979) Aplastic anemia and agranulocytosis in patients using methazolamide for glaucoma. JAMA 241:2817–2818

Wisch N, Fischbein FI, Siegel R, Glass JL, Leopold I (1973) Aplastic anemia resulting from the use of carbonic anhydrase inhibitors. Am J Ophthalmol 75:130–132

Wistrand PJ (1951) Carbonic anhydrase in the anterior uvea of the rabbit. Acta Physiol Scand 24:144–148

Wistrand PJ (1957) Local action of the carbonic anhydrase inhibitor, acetazolamide, on the intraocular pressure in cats. Arch Pharmacol Toxicol 14:27–37

Wistrand PJ (1959) The effect of carbonic anhydrase inhibitor on intra-ocular pressure with observations on the pharmacology of acetazolamide in the rabbit. Acta Pharmacol Toxicol 16:171–193

Wistrand PJ (1964) Intraocular pressure and resistance to aqueous outflow. Effects of carbonic anhydrase inhibition, salt depletion, adrenalectomy and fluoro-cortisone. Exp Eye Res 3:141–155

Wistrand P (1974) Pharmacokinetics and pharmacodynamics of acetazolamide in relation to its use in the treatment of glaucoma. In: Teorell T, Dedrick RL, Condliffe PG (eds) Pharmacology and pharmacokinetics. Plenum, New York, pp 191–194

Wistrand PJ, Garg LC (1979) Evidence of a high activity C type of carbonic anhydrase in human ciliary processes. Invest Ophthalmol 18:802–806

Wistrand PJ, Maren TH (1960) The effect of carbonic anhydrase on intraocular pressure of rabbits with different blood CO_2 equilibria. Am J Ophthalmol 50:291–297

Wistrand PJ, Nechay BR, Maren TH (1960a) Effect of carbonic anhydrase inhibition on cerebrospinal and intraocular fluids in the dog. Acta Pharmacol Toxicol 17:315–336

Wistrand PJ, Rawls JA, Maren TH (1960b) Sulfonamide carbonic anhydrase inhibitors and intra-ocular pressure in rabbits. Acta Pharmacol Toxicol 17:337–355

Yakatan GJ, Frome EL, Leonhard RG, Shah AC, Doluisio JT (1978) Bioavailability of acetazolamide tablets. J Pharm Sci 67:252–256

Yonemura D, Kawasaki K (1979) New approaches to ophthalmic electrodiagnosis by retinal oscillatory potential, drug induced responses from retinal pigment epithelium and cone potential. Doc Ophthalmol 48:163–222

Zimmerman TJ, Garg LC, Vogh BP, Maren TH (1976a) The effect of acetazolamide on the movement of anions into the posterior chamber of the dog eye. J Pharmacol Exp Therap 196:510–515

Zimmerman TJ, Garg LC, Vogh BP, Maren TH (1976b) The effect of acetazolamide on the movement of sodium into the posterior chamber of the dog eye. J Pharmacol Exp Therap 199:510–517

CHAPTER 7

Autacoids and Neuropeptides

J. Stjernschantz

A. Introduction

This chapter deals with the ocular effects of agents classified as autacoids or neuro-peptides. The oldest representative of the autacoids is histamine. Other agents are 5-hydroxytryptamine and members of the prostaglandin group, as well as products of the lipoxygenase pathway in the metabolism of arachidonic acid. The plasma kinins and the renin-angiotensin system are discussed in connection with this group too. The term "neuropeptide" is used to indicate peptides assumed to be involved directly or indirectly in neurotransmission, and peptides with hormonal activity se-creted by neural elements. Of the neuropeptides, substance P and neurotensin can be considered as gut-brain peptides, whereas the enkephalins have been found pri-marily in the central nervous system. Somatostatin, thyrotropin-releasing hor-mone, and luteinizing-hormone-releasing hormone are hypothalamic peptides regulating the adenohypophysis. Antidiuretic hormone and oxytocin are neurohy-pophyseal hormones, and the melanocyte-stimulating hormones have classically been associated with the intermediate lobe of the hypophysis. However, the melanocyte-stimulating hormones have also been found in other parts of the brain. Vasoactive intestinal polypeptide, glucagon, and gastrin/cholecystokinin are pri-marily gastrointestinal polypeptides, although they have been found in various parts of the nervous system.

The physiological and pathophysiological significance of some of the agents of these groups is dubitable, while that of others, e. g., histamine, the prostaglandins and substance P is clearer. The latter agents are interesting from a pathophysiolog-ical point of view, since they may be involved in the acute reaction of the eye to injury, or later in inflammation. Several neuropeptides have been found in the ret-ina, but their function remains unknown. The text vis-à-vis these is therefore most-ly descriptive. It should be pointed out that in the text the peptides have often been referred to by using their names instead of using the expression "positive im-munoreactivity" or "biological activity." It is wise to keep in mind the problems caused by cross-reactivity in immunological techniques, as well as the problems caused by impurities in biological assays in this respect.

B. Prostaglandins, Prostacyclin, Thromboxane, and Lipoxygenase Products

I. General Background

The prostaglandins constitute a group of oxygenated fatty acids with a wide range of biological activity. They have been found in almost all mammalian tissues and have been shown to be involved in normal physiological as well as pathophysiological processes. The prostaglandins are derived from 20-carbon essential fatty acids which contain three, four, or five double bonds [8,11,14-eicosatrienoic acid (dihomo-γ-linolenic acid), 5,8,11,14-eicosatetraenoic acid (arachidonic acid), and 5,8,11,14,17-eicosapentaenoic acid]. In man and higher animals, PGE_2 and $PGF_{2\alpha}$, derived from arachidonic acid, are the most abundant prostaglandins. The precursors are stored esterified mainly as components of the phospholipids in cell membranes, and are released enzymatically by phospholipase A_2 by a variety of stimuli. The precursor, mostly arachidonic acid, is then rapidly oxygenated either through a cyclooxygenase or lipoxygenase pathway. In many cells both pathways exist.

In the cyclooxygenase pathway arachidonic acid is metabolized by a complex microsomal enzymatic system. In the first reaction arachidonic acid is oxygenated to the cyclic endoperoxide PGG_2 by prostaglandin cyclooxygenase. Prostaglandin G_2 is then converted to PGH_2 by prostaglandin hydroperoxidase. During this enzymatic conversion an oxidant is released from the hydroperoxy group that is involved in cooxygenation phenomena. The oxidant released has the ability to act on a wide variety of organic compounds, including proteins, and the prostaglandin hydroperoxidase is therefore thought to have a destructive effect on cells. Since the oxidant also affects enzymes in the biosynthesis of prostaglandins, reducing agents will enhance prostaglandin synthesis. This enzyme may be involved in the damage seen during inflammation. The endoperoxide PGH_2 is isomerized enzymatically or nonenzymatically to PGD_2, PGE_2, or $PGF_{2\alpha}$. It can also be converted by thromboxane synthetase to thromboxane A_2 (TxA_2), an extremely short-lived compound with strong vascular effects causing, e. g., platelet aggregation and contraction of aortic smooth muscle, or by prostacyclin synthetase to prostacyclin (PGI_2), another relatively short-lived compound having opposite effects. The metabolism of arachidonic acid is outlined in Fig. 1. Thromboxane A_2 does not contain a cyclopentane but an oxane ring, and is therefore actually not a prostaglandin. The PGE und PGF series are generally referred to as primary prostaglandins to emphasize their abundant occurrence (especially PGE_2 and $PGF_{2\alpha}$). In contrast to this, PGA, PGB, and PGC are unlikely to occur naturally. Inactivation of the prostaglandins and probably PGI_2 is initiated by prostaglandin 15-OH-dehydrogenase. Many organs efficiently inactivate prostaglandins, e. g., the lungs, kidneys, liver, spleen, and intestine.

In the lipoxygenase pathway arachidonic acid is metabolized to hydroperoxyeicosatetraenoic acids (HPETEs). These hydroperoxides can further be metabolized to analogous alcohols [hydroxyeicosatetraenoic acids (HETEs)] through peroxidatic reduction. 5-Hydroperoxyeicosatetraenoic acid can be converted through epoxide formation to leukotriene A_4, which is subsequently converted to

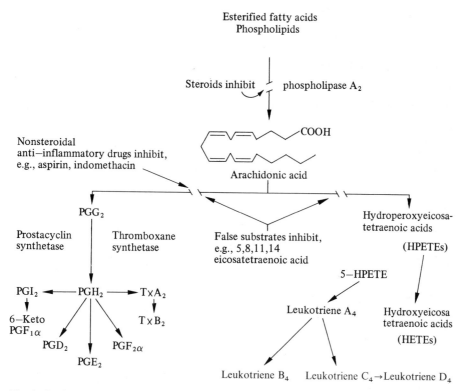

Fig. 1. Cyclooxygenase pathway leading to conventional prostaglandins, prostacyclin, and thromboxane, and lipoxygenase pathway leading to hydroperoxyeicosatetraenoic acids and their derivatives in arachidonic acid metabolism. PGI_2, prostacyclin; TxA_2, thromboxane A_2; TxB_2, thromboxane B_2

leukotriene B_4 or to leukotriene C_4 by glutathione-S-transferase. Leukotriene C_4 can further be converted to leukotriene D_4 through the action of γ-glutamyltranspeptidase. Many of the HETEs and leukotrienes, particularly leukotriene B_4, are strong chemotactic agents for polymorphonuclear leukocytes, and may be involved in inflammatory reactions. Leukotriene D_4 has been identified as a slow-reacting substance in anaphylaxis (SRS-A). Several other compounds in the lipoxygenase pathway have recently been found, but the function of these is unknown. The lipoxygenase pathway in the metabolism of arachidonic acid is also outlined in Fig. 1.

The inhibitory effect of glucocorticoids on the synthesis of prostaglandins is the result of interference with phospholipase A_2 (FLOWER and BLACKWELL 1979), i.e., the release of precursor from esterified lipid stores. This is likely to be mediated through a receptor in the cytosol and the synthesis of a new protein. Consequently, glucocorticoids are potent anti-inflammatory agents. They can suppress both cyclooxygenase and lipooxygenase pathways. By contrast, most nonsteroidal anti-inflammatory agents, like aspirin or indomethacin, interfere with the cyclocygenase step directly but will not prevent the synthesis of lipooxygenase products.

False substrate, e. g., 5,8,11,14-eicosatetraenoic acid, interferes with both the cyclooxygenase and lipooxygenase pathways. For more detailed information on the general pharmacology and metabolism of prostaglandins, PGI_2, thromboxane, and lipooxygenase products the reader is referred to recent review articles, e. g., by Kuehl and Egan (1980), Moncada et al. (1980), and Borgeat and Sirois (1981).

II. Occurrence and Biosynthesis in the Eye

The research on prostaglandins in the eye started with the classic studies by Ambache of an unknown smooth-muscle-stimulating substance extracted from rabbit irides, named irin (Ambache 1955, 1956, 1957). Irin was suggested to be an unsaturated hydroxy fatty acid (Ambache 1959). Ängard and Samuelsson (1964) isolated $PGF_{2\alpha}$ from sheep irides. Ambache's group demonstrated the presence of PGE_2 and $PGF_{2\alpha}$ in irides of cats and rabbits, utilizing thin-layer chromatography (Ambache et al. 1966; Ambache and Brummer 1968). Prostaglandins of the F type in the rabbit iris were also reported by Waitzman et al. (1967). Van Dorp et al. (1967) reported that PGE_1 and $PGF_{1\alpha}$ could be synthesized by isolated pig iris from dihomo-γ-linolenic acid in the presence of glutathione and hydroquinone as reducing agents. Christ and van Dorp (1972) showed that the rabbit iris has marked ability to synthesize prostaglandins, and later Bhattacherjee and Eakins (1974) demonstrated that arachidonic acid was converted to PGE-like activity by isolated microsomal fractions from the rabbit anterior uvea and conjunctiva. Microsomes isolated from the retina and the cornea seemed to possess only a slight ability for this conversion. ^{14}C-Arachidonic acid has been shown to be incorporated both into neutral lipids, and phospholipids, e. g., phosphatidylcholine, phosphatidylethanolamine, and phosphatidylinositol in the rabbit iris (Abdel-Latif and Smith 1979).

In a recent study microsomes isolated from the rabbit iris-ciliary body were reported to convert arachidonic acid to PGE_2, $PG_{2\alpha}$, PGD_2, thromboxane B_2 (TxB_2), the inactive end product of thromboxane synthesis, and 6-keto-$PGF_{1\alpha}$, the end product of PGI_2 metabolism, in the presence of epinephrine as cofactor (Kass and Holmberg 1979). The synthesis of all the products could be prevented by indomethacin, blocking the cyclooxygenase step, and the synthesis of TxB_2 in addition to imidazole, which blocks TxA_2 synthesis. Microsomes from the rabbit conjunctiva and cornea also synthesized prostaglandins from arachidonic acid but to a lesser extent, whereas microsomes from the sclera, retina-choroid, and lens synthesized little if any prostaglandin. Incubation of ciliary body-iris microsomes with 8,11,14-eicosatrienoic acid resulted in the formation of $PGF_{1\alpha}$, PGD_1, and PGE_1. Similar results were reported by Bhattacherjee et al. (1979). They found that the chopped rabbit iris-ciliary body converted arachidonic acid mainly to PGE_2 and $PGF_{2\alpha}$, whereas the chopped rabbit conjunctiva converted it to PGE_2, $PGF_{2\alpha}$, PGI_2, and TxA_2 in the absence of cofactors. In the presence of epinephrine, the iris-ciliary body and conjunctiva converted arachidonic acid to PGD_2, PGE_2, $PGF_{2\alpha}$, PGI_2, and TxA_2. The biosynthesis of the prostaglandins could be blocked by indomethacin and the synthesis of TxA_2 could be blocked by either imidazole or indomethacin.

Microsomes isolated from the bovine iris-ciliary body have been reported to convert prostaglandin endoperoxides to PGI_2 but not to TxA_2 (Kulkarni et al.

1977). The PGI_2 conversion was sensitive to tranylcypramine, an inhibitor of PGI_2 synthesis. Microsomes isolated from human irides have been reported to synthesize TxA_2, PGI_2, PGE_2, $PGF_{2\alpha}$, and PGD_2 (KULKARNI and EAKINS 1977); KULKARNI 1981). The TxA_2 synthesis could be blocked by imidazole as well as by compound N 0164, and the PGI_2 formation by tranylcypramine. Normal aqueous humor in man and rabbit has been reported to contain less than 2 ng/ml prostaglandin activity (EAKINS et al. 1972a, b; COLE and UNGER 1973; MILLER et al. 1973; CAMRAS et al. 1977; SAKATA and YOSHIDA 1979; YAMAUCHI et al. 1979). In normal human tears less than 0.1 ng/ml PGE activity was found (DHIR et al. 1978). The value increased significantly in patients with vernal conjunctivitis or trachoma.

Preliminary data indicate that the iris and the conjunctiva in many species, at least in the rat, guinea pig, rabbit, and cat, have the ability to synthesize compounds of the lipoxygenase pathway, 12-HETE being predominant (BHATTACHER-JEE et al. 1980). However, in albino rabbits and kittens this ability seemed to be lacking.

It is evident in many mammalian species that the conjunctiva and the anterior uvea, the latter in man as well, possess the ability to synthesize prostaglandins, PGI_2, thromboxane, and lipoxygenase products. In the cornea, sclera, choroid, retina, and lens this ability is weaker or totally lacking, at least as far as the cyclooxygenase products are concerned. So far there has been no publication on the lipoxygenase pathway in human ocular tissues. SAKATA and YOSHIDA (1979), using an immunofluorescence method, found that PGE was localized to the cytoplasm of mesenchymal cells in the fibrous stroma of the rabbit iris. The number of these cells increased remarkably after iridectomy or in inflamed irises.

III. Elimination

Very little prostaglandin 15-OH-dehydrogenase activity has been found in ocular tissues as compared to the lungs and kidneys (EAKINS et al. 1974). Brain tissue also seems to be virutally devoid of enzymes required for the inactivation of prostaglandins (WOLFE 1975). On the blood side of the blood-ocular barrier, the prostaglandins are eliminated mainly by the circulation. If, however, prostaglandins were released into the vitreous or aqueous humor, they would reach the avascular tissues, the lens, the cornea, and the trabecular meshwork, with possible adverse effects because of slow inactivation and removal. They may also have negative effects in the retina (WALLENSTEIN and BITO 1978). This is prevented by a transport system of prostaglandins across the blood-ocular barriers, preferentially in the ciliary processes and/or at the posterior side of the iris, but probably also in the retinachoroid (BITO 1972a, b, 1973; BITO and SALVADOR1 1972; EHINGER 1973; BITO and WALLENSTEIN 1977). A comparable transport system has earlier been demonstrated for organic anions in the ciliary processes of the rabbit eye (BECKER 1960; FORBES and BECKER 1960). When a mixture of ^3H-PGE_1 and ^{14}C-sucrose was injected intravitreously in rabbits, the half-life of the former in the vitreous was about 3 h while that of ^{14}C was around 15 h (BITO and SALVADOR 1972). None of the ^3H activity could be detected in the aqueous humor in contrast to the ^{14}C activity, indicating that the prostaglandin was transported out from the eye and never reached the anterior chamber, since less than 3% of the ^3H activity could be traced to intraocular tissues. When both agents were injected simultaneously into the anterior chamber, the clearance of each was essentially identical. Thus, once in the anterior chamber, the prostaglandins can be eliminated by the bulk outward flow of aqueous humor. It has been suggested that there is a saturable carrier-mediated transport system of prostaglandins across the blood-ocular barrier (BITO and WALLENSTEIN 1977). Such a transport system has been demonstrated in the vagina (BITO 1975) and in the brain (BITO et al. 1976). Perhaps prostaglandins are thus transported from the intraocular fluids, i.e., the vitreous and the posterior chamber aqueous, into the blood to be removed for inactivation. Autoradiography shows that there is an accumulation in the retina too, after intravitreal injection of ^3H-PGE$_1$ (BHATTACHERJEE 1974). The ability of the iris-ciliary body to accumulate radioactive prostaglandin in vitro has been demonstrated to be widely distributed and was found in invertebrates (squid), elasmobranchs (dogfish and skate), and teleosts (flounder, scup, sea bass, and sea robin), as well as in cats, rabbits, and rats (BITO 1972 b). In the latter species the iris-ciliary body accumulates at least PGE$_1$, PGF$_{1\alpha}$, PGF$_{2\alpha}$, and PGA$_1$ (BITO 1972 a, b). Recent studies indicate that a similar transport system in the anterior uvea may exist also for PGI$_2$, 6-keto-PGF$_{1\alpha}$, and TxB$_2$ (DIBENEDETTO and BITO 1980). The prostaglandin transport system can effectively be blocked, e.g., by probenecid, bromcresol green or high doses of indomethacin (about 30 times the dose required to block the synthesis of prostaglandins) (BITO and WALLENSTEIN 1977). No reports so far have been published concerning the inactivation of lipoxygenase products in the eye.

IV. Effects in the Eye

The prostaglandins can exert numerous effects in the eye. However, a considerable species difference exists, the rabbit eye being particularly susceptible. The effects of exogenously administered prostaglandins are also linked to the route of delivery. Moreover, differences between individual prostaglandins exist. Generally, the order of potency with regard to most of the intraocular effects in PGE$_1$ > PGE$_2$ > PGF$_{2\alpha}$ > PGF$_{1\alpha}$ (EAKINS 1977). Very little is known about the effects of TxA$_2$ and PGI$_2$ in the eye, and the same is true of the leukotrienes as well as other products of the lipoxygenase pathway.

1. Blood Flow

The effect of prostaglandins on ocular blood flow has been dealt with only in a few studies. STARR (1971 a), using implanted thermocouples in the anterior chamber of the rabbit, demonstrated that close arterial infusion of PGE$_{1-2}$ induced increased blood flow in the iris. Prostaglandins F$_{1\alpha-2\alpha}$ had only a weak effect, but both PGE$_{1-2}$ and PGF$_{1\alpha-2\alpha}$ significantly inhibited vasoconstriction induced by norepinephrine. Intracameral infusion of prostaglandins did not induce any change in blood flow. However, the thermocouple technique is not an ideal means of measuring blood flow, since a redistribution, e.g., from the iris to the ciliary processes, may have covered a net increase in the anterior uvea (STARR 1971 a). The vascular effects could be inhibited by polyphloretin phosphate, a nonspecific prostaglandin inhibitor (STARR 1971a). Topical application of PGE$_{1-2}$ and to some extent PGF$_{2\alpha}$ was reported to cause vasodilation and to increase the permeability of iridial blood vessels in rabbits as studied by fluorescein angiography (WHITELOCK and EAKINS 1973). The effects of PGE_{1-2} could be prevented by prior injection of polyphloretin phosphate subconjunctivally. Close injection of PGE_1 by iontophoresis to retinal blood vessels in pigs has been reported to induce vasodilation (POURNARAS et al. 1978). The estimated concentrations at the vessels were 0.7–5.5 μM. Prostaglandin synthetase inhibitors injected into the circulation reversibly inhibited vasodilation induced by hypercapnia, and partly also by hypoxia (POURNARAS et al. 1978). It was therefore suggested that prostaglandins play a role in hypercapnic vasodilation of the retina. In the baboon, indomethacin inhibits cerebral vasodilation during hypercapnia in a similar manner (PICKARD and MACKENZIE 1973). BILL (1979) found an approximately 20% reduction in retinal blood flow in conscious rabbits after indomethacin treatment, which fits the same pattern of prostaglandin involvement in the regulation of retinal blood flow. High doses (> 200 μg) of prostaglandins injected intravitreously in rabbits invariably caused pathological changes in retinal microcirculation (PEYMAN et al. 1975). The importance of these observations could be addressed by additional quantitative study.

2. Blood-Aqueous Barrier and Formation of Aqueous Humor

Injection of PGE_1 and PGE_2 into the anterior chamber of rabbits (BEITCH and EAKINS 1969), cats (EAKINS 1970), and monkeys (KELLY and STARR 1971) causes a disruption of the blood-aqueous barrier as judged from the increase in protein concentration of the aqueous humor. Prostaglandins $F_{1\alpha}$ and $F_{2\alpha}$ in high doses have been reported to be effective, at least in monkeys (KELLY and STARR 1971). In the very susceptible rabbit the discruption can be induced with as little as 5–10 ng PGE_1 or PGE_2 (BEITCH and EAKINS 1969). Topical administration of prostaglandins and arachidonic acid also cause a breakdown of the blood-aqueous barrier in rabbits (KASS et al. 1972; PODOS et al. 1973a; BENGTSSON et al. 1975). The effect of arachidonic acid could be prevented by prior treatment with indomethacin or aspirin (PODOS et al. 1973a; BENGTSSON et al. 1975). The effects of naturally occurring prostaglandins on the blood-aqueous barrier are summarized in Table 1.

In the rabbit it is evident that the disruption of the blood-aqueous barrier after prostaglandin treatment is localized to the ciliary and iridial processes (NEUFELD and SEARS 1973; COLE 1974; OHTSUKI et al. 1975; LATIES et al. 1976), but it is not clear whether this is based on a direct action on the epithelium (GREEN 1973) or primarily on the vasculature, leading to edema in the stroma and a subsequent breakdown of the epithelium (TAMURA 1974; OHTSUKI et al. 1975; PEDERSEN 1975a; PEDERSEN and TØNJUM 1975; LATIES et al. 1976). The latter is probable (NEUFELD and SEARS 1973). Electron microscopic studies with horseradish peroxidase as a tracer indicate that the critical disruption of the blood-aqueous barrier takes place at the intercellular tight junctions between the nonpigmented epithelial cells (Fig. 2) (VEGGE et al. 1975; PEDERSEN 1975a; MEYERS et al. 1975). However, the vigorous leakage of plasma proteins into the aqueous humor must also be based on a vascular component. Topical or intracameral administration of PGEs has also been reported to induce some leakage from the iridial vasculature, presumably by opening tight junctions between endothelial cells in the rabbit (PEDERSEN 1975b; PINTER et al. 1978) and the rat (SZALAY et al. 1976). Much of the tracer found in the iris

Table 1. Effects of naturally ocurring prostaglandins and prostacyclin on intraocular pressure (IOP), aqueous humor protein concentration, and pupil diameter as reported in various species. The values have been obtained from text as well as figures and tables in the respective papers and mostly represent the arithmetic mean

Species	Administration	Prostaglandin	Amount (µg)	Increase in IOP (mmHg)	Increase in aqueous protein (mg/100 ml)	Pupillary constriction (+/−)	Reference
Rabbit A	Topical	PGD_2	1–10	0–1	221–247	−	Kulkarni and Srinivasan 1982
A		PGE_1	5	15	1,500	−	Kass et al. 1972
U		PGE_1	10	16	ND	ND	Green and Kim 1975
A		PGE_1	50	40	ND	−	Kass et al. 1972
U		PGE_1	10	14	ND	ND	Green and Kim 1975
A		PGE_2	25–100	8–18	ND	ND	Bethel and Eakins 1972
A		$PGF_{2\alpha}$	200	12–14	ND	ND	Bethel and Eakins 1972
A		PGI_2	10–100	7–15	0[d]	−	Kulkarni and Srinivasan 1982
U	Intracameral	PGE_1	0.01	10	90	+	Waitzman and King 1967
		PGE_1	0.1–2.5	> 20	150–460	+	Waitzman and King 1967
		PGE_1	0.8	16	ND	−	Starr 1971b
		PGE_1	1	135%[a]	NS	+	Beitch and Eakins 1969
		PGE_1	10	38	ND	ND	Chiang and Thomas 1972a
		PGE_2	1	130%[a]	2,000	+	Beitch and Eakins 1969
		PGE_2	2.5	32	ND	+	Waitzman and King 1967
		PGE_2	1–10	31–38	ND	+	Chiang and Thomas 1972b
		$PGF_{1\alpha}$	1	20%[a]	ND	NS	Beitch and Eakins 1969
		$PGF_{2\alpha}$	1	90%[a]	ND	+	Beitch and Eakins 1969
		$PGF_{2\alpha}$	10	18	ND	ND	Chiang and Thomas 1972a
A	Intravitreal	PGD_2	1–10	4	16–216	−	Kulkarni and Srinivasan 1982
A		PGI_2	1–10	6	137–134[a]	−	Kulkarni and Srinivasan 1982
U	Intravenous	PGE_1	4	30	ND	−	Starr 1971b
		PGE_1	7.9	15	ND	ND	Chiang and Thomas 1972c
		PGE_1	7.9	10	ND	ND	Green and Kim 1975
		PGE_2	7.9	10	ND	NS	Chiang and Thomas 1972b
		PGE_2	7.9	17	ND	ND	Green and Kim 1975
		$PGF_{2\alpha}$	23.7	None	ND	ND	Chiang 1974

Species	Anesthesia	Route	Prostaglandin	Dose			±	Reference
Cat	P	Intracameral	PGE$_1$	1	12	>1,000	+	EAKINS 1970
			PGE$_2$	1	17	>1,000	+	EAKINS 1970
Dog	P	Intravenous	PGE$_1$	100[b]	2	ND	ND	NAKANO et al. 1973
			PGE$_2$	100[b]	1	ND	ND	NAKANO et al. 1973
			PGF$_{2\alpha}$	200[b]	5	ND	ND	NAKANO et al. 1973
Monkey	NS	Topical	PGE$_1$	100	None	–[c]	–	KELLY and STARR 1971
	KP		PGE$_2$	10	3	ND	+	CASEY 1974a, b
	T		PGE$_2$	100	None	–[c]	–	KELLY and STARR 1971
	NS		PGF$_{1\alpha}$	100	None	–[c]	–	KELLY and STARR 1971
	NS		PGF$_{2\alpha}$	100	None	–[c]	–	KELLY and STARR 1971
	NS	Intracameral	PGE$_1$	15	14	>1,200	–	KELLY and STARR 1971
	P		PDE$_2$	1	7	ND	+	CASEY 1974a, b
	PH		PGE$_2$	15	12	>800	–	KELLY and STARR 1971
	KP		PGF$_{1\alpha}$	15	6	>2,600	–	KELLY and STARR 1971
	T		PGF$_{2\alpha}$	15	6	ND	–	KELLY and STARR 1971
	P	Intravenous	PGE, PGF	300	None	ND	–	KELLY and STARR 1971
	PH							

ND, not determined; NS, not clearly specified; ±, constriction of the pupil in some but not all experiments

A, awake; U, urethane; P, pentobarbital; PH, phencyclidine; K, ketamine; T, thiamylal

[a] Percent increase above preinjection level. Preinjection pressures not given

[b] Calculated assuming weight of dogs 25 kg. Weights of dogs in Materials and Methods indicated to be 20–28 kg

[c] Indicates no flare

[d] Protein concentration increased bilaterally

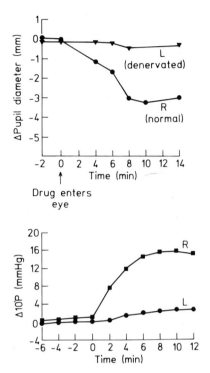

Fig. 2. Effect of sensory denervation on **a** pupil diameter and **b** intraocular pressure (*IOP*) responses to intracameral infusion of 1.25 µg PGE$_1$. Note the absent or weak response in the denervated eyes. Mean values of five and six experiments, respectively. *L*, left eye; *R*, right eye. (Butler and Hammond 1977)

stroma may originate from the ciliary processes (Ohtsuki et al. 1975; Vegge et al. 1975; Laties et al. 1976). The posterior chamber is the origin of the protein (Neufeld and Sears 1973).

In the cynomolgus monkey subconjunctival injection of 10–100 µg PGE$_1$ caused a breakdown of the blood-aqueous barrier in the anterior portion of the pars plicata, whereas alterations in the epithelium of the posterior portion and pars plana of the ciliary body were less marked (Okisaka 1976). In the cat it is not clear to what extent the ciliary epithelium is affected after treatment with prostaglandins, and clearly larger doses of prostaglandins have to be used to increase the protein concentration of the aqueous humor in this species (Eakins 1970). It is possible that part of the proteins after larger doses of prostaglandins enter the chamber system of the cat eye through a backflow from the circle of Hovius (van Alphen and Wilhelm 1978).

In the ciliary processes, as in many other tissues, the prostaglandins have been shown to stimulate the production of cAMP through an activation of adenylate cyclase (Waitzman and Woods 1971). Prostaglandins, especially of the E series, also increase the short-circuit current through the isolated rabbit iris-ciliary body preparate (Cole and Nagasubramanian 1972, 1973; Green 1973). This is thought to be due to an increased flux of Na$^+$ across the epithelium. However, the concentration (about 10 µg/ml) needed to obtain this effect is far above physiological levels, and there is no evidence that prostaglandins would increase secretion of aqueous humor.

3. Intraocular Pressure

Intracameral injection of E and F series of prostaglandins causes an increase in intraocular pressure (IOP) in the rabbit (WAITZMAN and KING 1967; BEITCH and EAKINS 1969; CHIANG and THOMAS 1972a, b), cat (EAKINS 1970), and monkey (KELLY and STARR 1971; CASEY 1974a). The cat seems to be the least susceptible, and small doses do not increase IOP (WAITZMAN and King 1967; Eakins 1970). Topical application of PGE$_{1-2}$ and PGF$_{2\alpha}$ in the rabbit (BETHEL and Eakins 1972; Kass et al. 1972; PODOS et al. 1973a, b; WHITELOCK and EAKINS 1973; GREEN and KIM 1975) is also effective, whereas the monkey eye responded less (KELLY and STARR 1971; CASEY 1974a). Arachidonic acid administered topically or subconjunctivally in rabbits and monkeys also increased IOP (PODOS et al. 1973a, b; CONQUET et al. 1975; KASS et al. 1975). Intravenous administration of prostaglandins has been reported to be effective in the rabbit (WAITZMAN and KING 1967; STARR 1971b; CHIANG and THOMAS 1972a, b, c; CHIANG 1974; GREEN and KIM 1975) and to some extent in the dog (NAKANO et al. 1973), but not in the monkey (KELLY and STARR 1971). It seems likely that after intravenous injection of prostaglandins the immediate increase in IOP is due to ocular vasodilation, whereas the more sustained increase is based on a disruption of the blood-aqueous barrier. Intravenous infusion of PGE$_{2\alpha}$ was reported to decrease IOP in rabbits and dogs (NAKANO et al. 1973; CHIANG 1974). A consensual response after intracameral or topical administration of E and F series of prostaglandins has been demonstrated in the fellow eye of rabbits (BEITCH and EAKINS 1969; CHIANG and THOMAS 1972a, b; KASS et al. 1972). The exact mechanism of this is not known, but it has been suggested that prostaglandins may reach the other eye through the circulation (CHIANG and THOMAS 1972a, b). However, since the prostaglandins are efficiently and rapidly inactivated by the lungs, the validity of this hypothesis remains uncertain. No consensual response was reported in the monkey (CASEY 1974a). The effect of naturally occurring prostaglandins on IOP is summarized in Table 1.

In the rabbit the initial hypertensive phase after intracameral administration of PGE$_1$ was shown to be followed by a prolonged hypotensive phase (STARR 1971b). The same has also been demonstrated in conscious rabbits after topical application of PGE$_2$ and PGF$_{2\alpha}$ (CAMRAS et al. 1977). A small dose (5 µg) of PGF$_{2\alpha}$ topically applied only induced the hypotensive phase of the response (CAMRAS et al. 1977). Thus the effect on IOP, at least in the rabbit, is biphasic, the increase in IOP but not the decrease being sensitive to blockade with polyphloretin phosphate (STARR 1971b).

Studies on the effects of prostaglandins on human eyes are naturally very sparse. Intravenous injection of PGE$_2$ and PGF$_{2\alpha}$ to interrupt middle-trimester pregnancies was reported not significantly to affect IOP (HILLIER and EMBREY 1972). In a subsequent study intravenous or intrauterine injection of PGF$_{2\alpha}$ used for the same purpose was reported to reduce IOP (ZAJACZ et al. 1976).

4. Outflow of Aqueous Humor

Although the prostaglandins increase IOP they also tend to increase gross facility of outflow of aqueous humor in all species studied (Waitzman and King 1967; Kass et al. 1972; Casey 1974a; Green and Kim 1975; Camras et al. 1977). Topical arachidonic acid also increased gross facility of outflow in rabbits (Podos et al. 1973a). Using the perilimbal suction cup technique to distinguish between gross facility, true facility, and pseudofacility, Masuda and Mishima (1973) demonstrated that most of the increase in gross facility after topical instillation of prostaglandins in rabbits was due to increased pseudofacility. An increased pseudofacility was also verified by Green and Padget (1979) in rabbits, and since the ultrafiltration component in aqueous humor formation in the hypertensive phase after prostaglandin treatment is increased, this is not unexpected. However, it has also been shown that gross facility is increased during the hypotensive phase at very low IOP values, both in living and dead rabbits (Camras et al. 1977). This increase in gross facility was suggested to be due to an increase in true facility. Neufeld et al. (1975) demonstrated that pharmacologic doses of cAMP infused into the anterior chamber of rabbits increase outflow facility. Prostaglandins stimulate the production of cAMP and perhaps this explains the apparent increase in true facility. However, it seems highly likely that secretion of aqueous humor is significantly reduced during the hypotensive phase, and measurement of outflow facility using manometic techniques in the rabbit eye tends to give an overestimation at very low IOP values. It is therefore not clear to what extent true facility is increased during the hypotensive phase.

It is evident from the foregoing that the increase in IOP is due to an abrupt increase in the rate of entry of aqueous humor, a plasmoid aqueous, mainly on the basis of a disruption of the blood-aqueous barrier (Sears 1960). This effect is naturally subject to tachyphylaxis. Subsequently, the decrease in formation of aqueous humor and possibly increase in true facility of outflow will reduce IOP to subnormal levels. While the initial increase in IOP is of short duration, usually 1–2 h, the decrease may be prolonged up to 20 h (Camras et al. 1977). This time course is compatible with the hypotony of acute cyclitis in the human and is undoubtedly related to the time required to repair the ciliary epithelia.

5. Iridial and Ciliary Smooth Muscles

Constriction of the pupil (Waitzman and King 1967; Beitch and Eakins 1969; Eakins 1970; Chiang and Thomas 1972b; Casey 1974b), as well as no response in pupil diameter (Starr 1971b; Kelly and Starr 1971; Kass et al. 1972), has been reported (see Table 1). Problems with differences among individual prostaglandins, amounts and possibly activity, as well as the route of administration, may at least partly explain these discrepancies, but a good explanation was also offered by van Alphen and Angel (1975). They found that both the sphincter muscle and the dilator muscle of the cat iris contracted to PGE_{1-2} and $PGF_{2\alpha}$ in vitro. Thus it is conceivable that different responses may be obtained, depending on the initial tone of the iridial smooth muscles, as well as on the amounts of prostaglandins used. Prostaglandins E_{1-2} and $F_{2\alpha}$ also strongly relaxes isolated preconstricted ciliary muscle strips from cats. This effect could be blocked by β-adrenergic antagonists

(VAN ALPHEN and ANGEL 1975). Free acids of prostaglandin precursors and the endoperoxide PGH_2 have also been shown to elicit comparatively strong responses in vitro in the cat sphincter muscle (CRAWFORD et al. 1978). The effect of PGH_2 may be based on a synthesis of TxA_2 in the preparate (CRAWFORD et al. 1978).

6. Miscellaneous Effects

In mice ptosis can be induced by intravenous injection of PGE_1. This seems to be based on an interference of prostaglandins with norepinephrine (HOLMES and HORTON 1968). In contrast to this, in the cat nictitating membrane prostaglandins have been reported to potentiate catecholamine-induced contraction (TÜRKER et al. 1969). Injection of PGE_1 or arachidonic acid into the third ventricle of the brain in rabbits has been reported to induce hyperthermia and increase IOP (KRUPIN et al. 1976). No miosis was elicited. The mechanism behind the effects remained unknown but aspirin treatment prevented the responses to arachidonic acid.

The information about the intraocular effects of prostacyclin and thromboxane so far is very sparse. Prostacyclin and its breakdown products 6-keto-PGE_1 and 6-keto-$PGF_{1\alpha}$ increased IOP in rabbits after intravitreal injection (KULKARNI and SRINIVASAN 1981). In addition, 6-keto-PGE_1, caused an increase in the aqueous humor protein concentration.

Intracameral injection of 5-HPETE or 5-HETE (500 ng) in rabbits has not been reported to have any effect on IOP, the blood-aqueous barrier, or leukocyte migration (BHATTACHERJEE et al. 1980, 1981). 12-Hydroxyeicosatetraenoic acid in a dose of up to 5 µg was also ineffective (BHATTACHERJEE et al. 1981). Administration of 25–400 ng 5,12-diHETE (leukotriene B_4) caused infiltration of otherwise cell-free aqueous humor by polymorphonuclear leukocytes in a dose-dependent manner, without affecting IOP (BHATTACHERJEE et al. 1980, 1981). In another study, intracameral injection of 12 µg 5-HETE, 4 µg 12-HETE, 0.7 µg 15-HETE, and 0.5 µg 15-HPETE in rabbits did not affect IOP, pupil size, or the blood-aqueous barrier, or cause leukocyte infiltration into the aqueous humor (STJERNSCHANTZ et al., to be published b), Leukotriene C_4 and D_4 in a dose of 10 µg were in a similar way ineffective, but leukotriene B_4 (0.9 µg) caused leukocyte infiltration into the anterior chamber (STJERNSCHANTZ et al., to be published b). Interestingly, it was recently shown that indomethacin treatment in rabbits with immunogenic uveitis increased the leukocyte infiltration into the aqueous humor (KULKARNI et al. 1981). It is possible that by blocking the cyclooxygenase pathway a facilitation of lipoxygenase pathway products with chemotactic properties takes place.

V. Interaction with the Autonomic and Sensory Nervous Systems in the Eye

Stimulation of adrenergic nerves has been shown to cause a release of prostaglandins in the periphery, e. g., in the spleen (GILMORE et al. 1968; DAVIES et al. 1968; HEDQUIST et al. 1971). The prostaglandins decrease release of norepinephrine from noradrenergic nerves (HEDQUIST 1969; 1973; HEDQUIST et al. 1971), thus forming a negative feedback system. Prostaglandins E_{1-2} but not $PGF_{2\alpha}$ were shown to inhibit the overflow of ^3H-norepinephrine during field stimulation of the rabbit iris, which indicates that a similar negative feedback system exists in the eye (NEUFELD and PAGE 1975). Also the ocular hyperemia after sympathetic ganglionectomy

(TREISTER and BÁRÁNY 1970) is probably caused by release of prostaglandins (NEU-FELD et al. 1973). The hyperemia was prevented by α-methyl-*p*-tyrosine administered before ganglionectomy to deplete norepinephrine stores, as well as by indomethacin, which blocks the prostaglandin synthesis. Norepinephrine released from degenerating adrenergic nerves triggers a prostaglandin synthesis and release in the innervated tissue, inducing hyperemia. A cofactor may be required.

Adrenergic agonists have been reported to antagonize prostaglandin effects at the postjunctional level (WAITZMAN 1970). Adrenergic antagonists do not inhibit prostaglandin responses in the eye except for the ciliary muscle, where β-antagonists prevent prostaglandin-induced relaxation in vitro (VAN ALPHEN and ANGEL 1975). Norepinephrine, an α-adrenergic agonist, and isoproterenol, a mixed β-adrenergic agonist, both antagonized the prostaglandin-induced miosis in cats and rabbits and increase in IOP in rabbits. Phenoxybenzamine, an α-adrenergic antagonist, blocked the antagonizing effect of norepinephrine on the pupil diameter, and in addition to some extent that of isoproterenol. Propranolol, a nonselective β-adrenergic antagonist, was less effective in blocking isoproterenol effects both in cats and rabbits (WAITZMAN 1969). Phenoxybenzamine also blocked the antagonizing effect of norepinephrine on IOP in rabbits, but propranolol was ineffective in blocking the effect of isoproterenol. Recently, it was reported that α-adrenergic agonists in rabbit eyes rendered supersensitive by sympathectomy cause a biphasic response in IOP, similar to that induced by prostaglandins, and hyperemia and aqueous flare (UNGER 1979). This effect could be prevented by phentolamine, an α-adrenergic antagonist, and by indomethacin, indicating that a synthesis and release of prostaglandins was somehow triggered through activation of α-adrenergic receptors. WAITZMAN et al. (1979) also reported an early increase in IOP in sympathectomized rabbits after topical norepinephrine that could be significantly reversed by indomethacin, implying an involvement of prostaglandins. Subsensitivity in the ocular response to topical norepinephrine was suppressed in rabbits pretreated with the cyclooxygenase inhibitor flurbiprofen. This observation supports the idea that cyclooxygenase products mediate the development of tolerance to catecholamines, perhaps by a postsynaptic inhibition of norepinephrine (DUFFIN et al. 1981). The prostaglandin feedback regulating the release of norepinephrine in the iris however, is not mediated at a postjunctional site (NEUFELD and PAGE 1975).

The prostaglandins have also been postulated to be involved in the maintenance of the iris sphincter tone (POSNER 1973). Prostaglandins E_{1-2} and $F_{2\alpha}$ and arachidonic acid in concentrations not affecting the sphincter tone potentiated the cholinergic effect of transmural stimulation of the bovine iris and the effect of exogenous acetylcholine (GUSTAFSSON et al. 1975, 1980). Prostaglandin synthetase inhibitors effectively reduced contraction responses to transmural stimulation, exogenous acetylcholine, and arachidonic acid (GUSTAFSSON et al. 1980). Thus it is possible that prostaglandins are involved in the modulation of cholinergic input to the eye, too, at the postganglionic postjunctional level.

BUTLER and HAMMOND (1977, 1980) found that the miotic and hypertensive effect of exogenous PGE_1 was greatly reduced by prior coagulation of the trigeminal nerve in rabbits (Fig. 2), as did JAMPOL et al. (1975) by denervation. This indicates that a considerable part at least of the immediate effect of exogenous PGE_1 and other prostaglandins is probably exerted through sensory nerves. Nonspecific depletion of sensory nerve endings with capsaicin has been reported to render the rat skin insensitive to many noxious compounds, e. g., formaldehyde, bradykinin, and prostaglandins (ARVIER et al. 1977). MANDAHL and BILL (1980, 1981) found that tetrodotoxin, which blocks sodium channels and thus nerve conduction, prevented the contraction of the iridial sphincter muscle to PGE_1 and PGE_2. The hypertensive effect of low doses of PGE_1 could also be blocked by tetrodotoxin, but high doses of PGE_1 or PGE_2 still induced a hypertensive response, probably because larger amounts of prostaglandin diffused to the target area, i. e., the ciliary processes. This implies that part of the breakdown of the blood-aqueous barrier caused by prostaglandins in the ciliary processes is independent of nerve conduction. Earlier evidence supporting a direct effect of endogenous prostaglandins on the blood vessels in the eye comes from the study by JAMPOL et al. (1975). They demonstrated that alcohol denervation of the eye did not prevent an increase in the aqueous humor protein concentration after paracentesis, whereas aspirin pretreatment markedly attenuated the response. Thus is seems evident that the miosis and perhaps the other elements of the irritative response occurring after intracameral injection of exogenous prostaglandins are mainly based on a neural mechanism, with the release of a substance or substances from sensory nerves in the processes of the ciliary body or in their immediate vicinity. Endogenous prostaglandins released in the ciliary body can in all likelihood act independently of sensory nerves, directly on the vasculature.

VI. Pathophysiological Considerations

The prostaglandins, PGI_2, thromboxane, and lipoxygenase products all are of interest from a pathophysiological point of view in the eye, although only the prostaglandins have been more thoroughly studied in this respect. The prostaglandins may be particularly important in injury reactions and inflammation of the eye. Some pathological conditions in the retina may also involve prostaglandins. The difficulties with extrapolation of data from animal models to the human eye should be stressed, however, since most of the studies reported in the text were performed in animals.

1. Immediate Response to Injury of the Eye

The eye of most mammalian species, including the human, typically responds to injury with hyperemia, disruption of the blood-aqueous barrier, increased IOP, and miosis. The rabbit eye is particularly sensitive. Such noxious stimuli comprise antidromic stimulation of the fifth cranial nerve, scratching of the cornea or the iris, local irritants such as nitrogen mustard and formaldehyde, alkali burns, paracentesis of the anterior chamber, and various kinds of irradiation, e. g., X-ray, laser, and infrared (MAGENDIE 1824; BERNARD 1858; WESSELY 1908; LARSSON 1930; DUKE-ELDER and DUKE-ELDER 1931; DAVSON and HUBER 1950; MAURICE 1954; PERKINS 1957; SEARS 1960, 1961; COLE 1961; DYSTER-AAS and KRAKAU 1964a; AMBACHE et al. 1965; NEUFELD et al. 1972; UNGER et al. 1974; PATERSON and PFISTER 1975; WORGUL et al. 1977; STJERNSCHANTZ et al. 1979). The immediate response to injury should be distinguished from the inflammatory response occurring later, involving in addition, for example, leukocyte infiltration and alterations connected to destruction and repair of the affected tissues. While direct stimulation of the trigeminal nerve or of its peripheral endings by irritants does not seem to elicit any immediate release of prostaglandins in the rabbit eye (COLE and UNGER 1973), direct trauma of the anterior uvea causes a release of substantial amounts of prostaglandins into the aqueous humor (AMBACHE et al. 1965; COLE and UNGER 1973; MILLER et al. 1973). PATERSON and PFISTER (1975) showed that alkali burns of the eye also cause a release of prostaglandins into the aqueous humor, and so does laser irradiation of the iris (UNGER et al. 1974, 1977).

JAMPOL et al. (1975) described the main mechanisms behind the acute reaction of the rabbit eye to injury. They found that in cases involving direct trauma of the anterior uvea, e. g., after paracentesis, a synthesis and release of prostaglandins account for most of the reaction. In cases involving noxious stimuli, e. g., topical application of nitrogen mustard, prostaglandins did not play any apparent role but the mechanism was based on an involvement of sensory nerves in an axon reflex with the release of one or many transmitters in the eye. Of course, situations falling between these two categories exist. For instance, laser irradiation of the iris induces an irritative response in the rabbit eye that involves both a release of prostaglandins and a direct stimulation of sensory nerves (UNGER et al. 1974, 1977; BUTLER et al. 1980b). It thus seems likely that, depending on the location of the laser burns, released prostaglandins could either diffuse to the ciliary processes and act independently of sensory nerves, or exert their effect mainly through sensory nerves on the basis of a neural mechanism. Recently, it was also shown that 3–12 h after the initial response to topical nitrogen mustard in rabbits, when a typical inflammatory response has been established, there is a release of prostaglandins and infiltra-

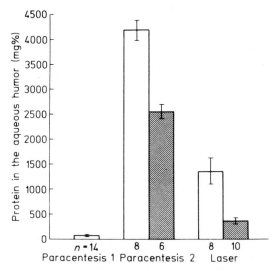

Fig. 3. Protein concentration in the aqueous humor of Dutch pigmented rabbit eyes in response to paracentesis and laser irradiation of the iris, after treatment with aspirin to block prostaglandin synthesis. Time interval between first and second paracentesis or laser irradiation and paracentesis 1–1.5 h. *Hatched columns* represent animals pretreated with aspirin; *empty columns*, control animals. Note the attenuated response in animals treated with aspirin. Mean ± SEM. (NEUFELD et al. 1972)

tion of polymorphonuclear leukocytes into the aqueous humor, as well as a secondary rise in IOP (CAMRAS and BITO 1980a).

NEUFELD et al. (1972) were the first to demonstrate that endogenous prostaglandins are involved in the disruption of the blood-aqueous barrier after certain stimuli. They showed that aspirin, a blocker of the cyclooxygenase step in the biosynthesis of prostaglandins, to a large extent prevented the disruption in rabbits after paracentesis or argon-laser irradiation (Fig. 3). Subsequently, works by PODOS et al. (1973a, b), BHATTACHERJEE and EAKINS (1974), and CONQUET et al. (1975) verified that the intraocular response to arachidonic acid could be prevented by cyclooxygenase inhibitors in rabbits, and numerous later studies have shown that cyclooxygenase inhibitors effectively attenuate ocular irritation associated with a release of prostaglandins. Unfortunately, the effect of systemic aspirin or indomethacin on the responses to anterior chamber paracentesis, subconjunctival arachidonic acid, or intravitreally injected *Shigella* endotoxin was very poor in monkeys (KASS et al. 1975). Either the primate eye may be less sensitive to cyclooxygenase inhibitors or some other agent released is more important in primates. However, ZIMMERMAN et al. (1975) reported that aspirin stabilized the blood-aqueous barrier in human eyes in connection with cataract surgery and penetrative keratoplasty, indicating that there is some effect of cyclooxygenase inhibitors in primate eyes too (MISHIMA and MASUDA 1977).

2. Inflammation of the Eye

Uveitis accomplished by intravitreal injection of bovine serum albumin or bacterial endotoxin has been shown to be accompanied by a release of prostaglandins in the rabbit (EAKINS et al. 1972a; BHATTACHERJEE 1975; YAMUCHI et al. 1979). EAKINS et al. (1972a) demonstrated that PGE_1 and some PGE_2 were released into the aqueous of rabbits suffering from bovine serum albumin uveitis. Since PGE_2 and $PGF_{2\alpha}$ are the only major endogenous prostaglandins in the iris, it was speculated that the PGE_1 activity was derived from polymorphonuclear leukocytes, which have been shown to release PGE_1 during phagocytosis (HIGGS and YOLTEN 1972). Rabbits with type III allergic reaction (Arthus' reaction) caused by serum-induced endophthalmitis or lens-induced uveitis also show a high content of PGE_{1-2} in the anterior uvea and the aqueous humor (RAHI et al. 1978). Isolated microsomes or homogenized iris-ciliary body tissue from rabbit eyes with anterior uveitis synthesized considerably more prostaglandins than normal tissue, indicating that the prostaglandin synthesis in inflamed eyes is increased (BHATTACHERJEE 1977). Treatment of rabbits with cyclooxygenase inhibitors attenuates the ocular inflammation remarkably (BHATTACHERJEE 1975; YAMUCHI et al. 1979). Prostaglandins apparently tend to accumulate in the intraocular fluids in chronic inflammation (BITO 1974), and from this observation it was reasoned that they may be causative and that the system postulated to remove them from the eye might be defective. It may be that there is no actual defect in a physiological mechanism but that the epithelia postulated to participate in removal are damaged or even necrotic from the inflammation.

In a preliminary communication, EAKINS et al. (1972b) reported that aqueous humor samples from untreated patients with acute anterior uveitis contained substantial amounts of E and F prostaglandin-like activity. The activities in the aqueous humor assayed as PGE_2 corresponded to 20–56 ng/ml, whereas control samples obtained from uninflamed eyes undergoing cataract surgery showed less than 2 ng/ml. MASUDA et al. (1973), using radioimmunoassay, demonstrated that both the PGE_1 and $PGF_{2\alpha}$ concentrations in the aqueous humor of the eye with glaucomatocyclitic crisis or with Behçet's disease were significantly greater than in a normal group. The values were lower than those reported by EAKINS et al. (1972 b) based on eyes with anterior uveitis. In glaucomatocyclitic crisis, oral indomethacin as well as subconjunctival polyphloretin phosphate effectively lowered IOP (MASUDA et al. 1975). In the first clinical study, PERKINS and MCFAUL (1965) indicated that indomethacin treatment had a favorable effect in cases of acute anterior uveitis. A beneficial effect of indomethacin in patients with uveitis and neuritis was also reported by TUOVINEN et al. (1966). Interestingly, before the use of glucocorticoids, aspirin was frequently used for the treatment of sympathetic ophthalmia and iritis (GIFFORD 1910). It is quite evident that at least certain kinds of uveitis both in animal models and in man involve an increased metabolism of prostaglandins. However, other components seem to be more important and, e. g., products of the lipoxygenase pathway could play an essential role in uveitis. This is further emphasized by the fact that cyclooxygenase inhibitors are only of limited value in the treatment of uveitis in man, in contrast to glucocorticoids, which block phospholipase A_2, thus depriving the cyclooxygenase as well as the lipoxygenase pathway of substrate.

3. Other Disorders in the Eye Possibly Involving Prostaglandins

Much speculation has arisen about the possible involvement of prostaglandins in diabetic retinopathy. Conflicting results have been reported concerning the plasma concentration of 6-keto-$PGF_{1\alpha}$, the end product of PGI_2, in diabetics with retinopathy as compared to healthy individuals (DOLLERY et al. 1979; DAVIS et al. 1980; BONNE et al. 1980). It is thought that PGI_2 may be important in preventing diabetic retinopathy because of its inhibiting effect on platelet aggregation, thus protecting the retina from microthrombi and vascular damage. A decrease in the vascular PGI_2 synthesis has been noted in diabetic animals as well as man (HARRISON et al. 1978, 1980; JOHNSON et al. 1979). So far, however, there is no clear evidence suggesting that prostaglandins, PGI_2, or thromboxane would be important in diabetic retinopathy. In amaurosis fugax, i. e., transient monocular blindness, aspirin treatment has been reported to be beneficial (HARRISON et al. 1971; MUNDALL et al. 1971, 1972), and an increased platelet aggregability may be a causative factor in this disorder (MUNDALL et al. 1972; BETTELHEIM et al. 1980). It is not clear whether the positive effect of aspirin is based on inhibition of the cyclooxygenase enzyme or, e. g., interference with platelet ADP, but it may be pertinent to note that the synthesis of TxA_2 is also inhibited by aspirin. As mentioned earlier, TxA_2 promotes platelet aggregation markedly.

Topical (MIYAKE 1977, 1978; MIYAKE et al. 1980) as well as oral (KLEIN et al. 1979) administration of indomethacin has been reported to prevent the development of aphakic cystoid macular edema (ACME) to some extent, implying an involvement of prostaglandins in this disorder. The beneficial effect of topical indomethacin was recently also verified by YANUZZI et al. (1981). MIYAKE et al.

(1978), in support of this hypothesis, have demonstrated that the prostaglandin concentration in the aqueous humor after cataract surgery is clearly elevated and that this may to a considerable extent be prevented by topical administration of indomethacin. According to BINKHORST et al. (1976), the incidence of ACME is clearly lower in extracapsular than in intracapsular cataract extractions because the remaining capsule is a barrier for diffusion of prostaglandins into the vitreous. Although ACME as determined by fluorescein angiography 4–8 weeks after cataract surgery seems to be very common (30%–50%) (IRVINE et al. 1971; HITCHINGS et al. 1975), the disorder in most cases heals spontaneously and only few of the patients get any permanent visual disability (GASS and NORTON 1969; JACOBSON and DELLAPORTA 1974). Therefore, at the present time it is not clear how beneficial indomethacin therapy is in ACME. Careful surgery is most important.

Prostaglandins E_{1-2} have also been reported to induce vascularization of the cornea in rabbits (BENEZRA 1978). It is interesting that PGE_1, being most powerful in this respect, has been shown to be released from polymorphonuclear leokocytes during phagocytosis in vitro (HIGGS and YOLTEN 1972). Using the hamster cheek pouch chamber technique, FROMER and KLINTHWORTH (1975a, b, 1976) presented evidence that leukocytes, particularly polymorphonuclear ones, are indeed necessary for the induction of blood vessel formation in the rat cornea in connection with various trauma. However, results contradicting this have subsequently been published (SHOLLEY et al. 1976; ELIASON 1978). Although it is not clear at the present time what the role of polymorphonuclear leukocytes is in corneal vascularization, the ability of prostaglandins to induce or enhance vascularization is interesting also with regard to neovascularization phenomena in diabetic retinopathy.

C. Histamine

I. General Background

Histamine (β-aminoethylimidazole) (Fig. 4) is formed from histidine after decarboxylation. Histamine is located primarily in mast cells and their circulating counterpart, the basophilic leukocytes. In addition, cells or the skin and enterochromaffin cells of the gastrointestinal tract contain histamine. There is also probably a neuronal pool of histamine in the central nervous system. Common effects of histamine comprise bronchoconstriction, contraction of intestinal smooth muscle, gastric secretion, contraction or relaxation of vascular smooth muscle, and stimulation of sensory nerve endings. It must be emphasized that marked species differences exist with regard to histamine sensitivity, the guinea pig being particularly sensitive. Most of the effects are mediated through H_1- and/or H_2-receptors. Effects exerted on vascular smooth muscle are mediated through H_1- as well as H_2-receptors. The effects on the vasculature are highly dependent on the vascular bed in question, as well as the species, and vasodilation or vasoconstriction may ensue, the overall effect being a decrease in peripheral resistance with a drop in blood pressure. A characteristic property of histamine is that it causes increased permeability of postcapillary venules, and therefore increased outflux of plasma proteins and edema. In the skin histamine is involved in the triple response. Several peptides and proteins release histamine, e. g., substance P, somatostatin, kinins, and components of the complement system.

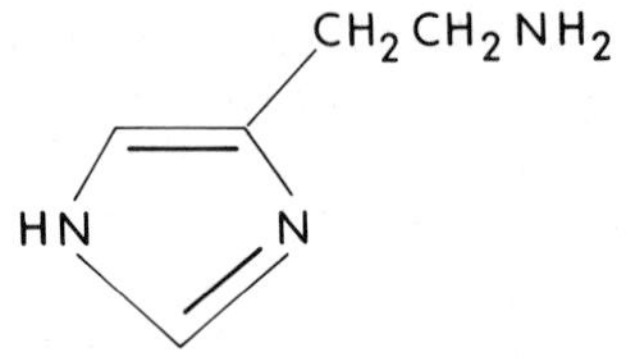

$$CH_2 CH_2 NH_2$$

a

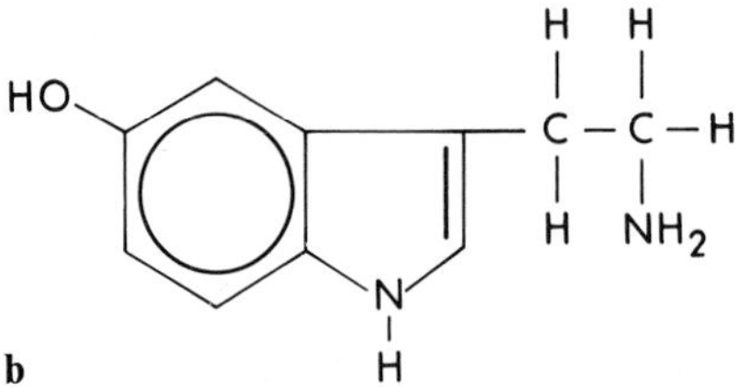

b

Fig. 4. Chemical structures of **a** histamine and **b** 5-hydroxytryptamine

II. Occurrence and Effects in the Eye

In the adult eye mast cells have been detected in the conjunctiva, the subconjunctival and episcleral tissues, at the limbus, and in the uvea of many species, including man (JORPES et al. 1937; HOLMGREN and STENBECK 1940; GÜNTHER 1956; LARSEN 1959; VANNAS 1959; LEVENE 1962; SMELSER and SILVER 1963; ALLAN-SMITH et al. 1978). In the anterior uvea, particularly in the iris, however, mast cells are sparsely distributed (LEVENE 1962; SMELSER and Silver 1963). The histamine content of ocular tissues in various species has been determined and is shown in Table 2. The uveal values are at least 10–100 times larger than those reported in the aqueous humor (LEVENE 1962). Human tears have been reported to contain about 10 ng histamine per milliliter. In vernal conjunctivitis this figure increased to about 40 ng/ml (ABELSON et al. 1977).

When administered topically or injected locally, histamine induces hyperemia and edema in the conjunctiva, as well as in the uvea (FRIEDENWALD and PIERCE 1930; RYCROFT 1934; BRÜCKNER 1946; PAYOT 1946; SCHLAEGEL 1949; SHEPARD 1949; VILSTROP 1952; COLE 1974; EAKINS and BHATTACHERJEE 1977). FRIEDEN-

Table 2. Histamine content of ocular tissues in various species. In most of the groups $n > 30$. Statistical variation not indicated in original article (LEVENE 1962)

Species	Choroid and retina (µg/g wet weight)	Anterior uvea (µg/g wet weight)	Eyelid (µg/g wet weight)
Rat	1.2	8.9	105.8
Guinea pig	3.7	3.4	14
Rabbit	2.4	1.4	11.2
Monkey	3.6	2.3	6.8

WALD and PIERCE (1930) demonstrated a substantial increase in IOP after intravitreal injection of histamine in several species, lasting for 10–90 min. COLE (1974) found that continuous perfusion with a total of 20 nmol (2.2 µg) histamine through the anterior chamber of the rabbit resulted in leakage of fluorescein as well as protein into the aqueous humor from the ciliary processes and their iridial extensions. However, EAKINS and BHATTACHERJEE (1977) did not find any increase in permeability of the blood-aqueous barrier after 50 µg (450 nmol) histamine intracamerally injected in rabbits. Intravenous injection of histamine in rabbits has not been reported to have any appreciable effect on the blood-aqueous barrier (CHIANG 1974). The effect on the pupil is constriction (RYCROFT 1934; SHEPARD 1949), although on a molar basis it is rather weak, at least in the rabbit (EAKINS and BHATTACHERJEE 1977).

Intracameral and intravitreal injections of histamine in cats and rats have been shown to induce increased permeability of venules in the iris and in the larger vessel layer of the choroid (ASHTON and CUNHA-VAZ 1966). In the ciliary processes leakage occurred in the capillaries, and the same was true for the choriocapillaries (ASHTON and CUNHA-VAZ 1966). Retinal as well as cerebral blood vessels were totally insensitive to histamine. The blood vessels in the conjunctiva showed a pattern of dilation and leakage similar to that in the iris (ASHTON and Cunha-Vaz 1966). Intravenous injection of histamine in the rat has also been demonstrated to cause increase in vessel diameter in the iris as studied with vital microscopy (CASTELHOLTZ 1967). Recently, the existence of H_2-receptors in the conjunctival blood vessels of human eyes was reported and vasodilation induced by dimethylaminopropylisothiourea, a selective H_2-receptor agonist, was effectively blocked by cimetidine, a H_2-receptor antagonist (ABELSON and UDELL 1981).

III. Pathophysiological Considerations

Since the anterior uvea contains relatively few mast cells, histamine is not thought to play a significant role in the acute injury response of the eye. Furthermore, supporting this theory, antihistaminic drugs (H_1-blockers) do not prevent the effects of fifth nerve injury in rats (MOSES and HOLEKAMP 1971), and in rabbits compound 48/80, depleting histamine, does not prevent the response (STJERNSCHANTZ and SEARS, unpublished results). In this respect the antridromic vasodilation and the accompanying permeability disturbance in the eye differ from the triple response in the skin, where mast cells and histamine are important (KIERNAN 1975; ARVIER et al. 1977; LEMBECK and HOLZER 1979). In the conjunctiva, however, histamine causes hyperemia, edema, and itching. In the rabbit conjunctiva, histamine-induced edema was amplified by prostaglandins (E_{1-2}) (EAKINS and BHATTACHERJEE 1977).

In chronic inflammation of the eye there is an increased number of mast cells in the affected tissue, but in the acute phase the number is decreased (ZOLLINGER 1949; GÜNTHER 1956; VANNAS 1959; LARSEN 1961). In the rat, limbal mast cells were reported to degranulate after injury and mast cells invade the cornea in connection with subsequent vascularization (SMITH 1961). Thyroidectomy and thyrotropin have been reported to increase the number of granules in ocular mast cells, whereas thyroxin, cortisone, and avitaminosis C have been reported to cause degranulation (LARSEN 1959).

The number of mast cells in the anterior uvea and sclera of patients with angle-closure glaucoma was found to decrease during acute attack and increase in the chronic congestive phase (GÜNTHER 1956; VANNAS 1959). An increased number of mast cells has also been found in inflammatory secondary glaucoma (VANNAS 1959). UNGER (1966) demonstrated an increased number of mast cells in specimens from Elliot's scleral trephining in two cases of primary glaucoma. In one case there was inflammatory reaction around a collector vein of Schlemm's canal with increased number of mast cells, and in the other case the trabecular meshwork contained an increased number of mast cells. However, it is not clear whether mast cells and histamine play any role at all in the development of acute glaucoma. They may merely reflect a secondary phenomenon of an already initiated process. From a pathological point of view, histamine is likely to be most important in allergic states of the surface of the eyeball.

D. 5-Hydroxytryptamine

I. General Background

5-Hydroxytryptamine (5-HT) or serotonin (Fig. 4) is synthesized from tryptophan through hydroxylation and subsequent decarboxylation. It is located primarily in the enterochromaffin system of the gastrointestinal tract in mammals. It also occurs in platelets and has been established as a neurotransmitter in the central nervous system. In rodents and cattle, mast cells also contain 5-HT. The main metabolite is 5-hydroxyindolacetic acid (5-HIAA). 5-Hydroxytryptamine exerts complex effects on the vascular tree, depending on the resting tone and the dose used, and vasodilation as well as vasoconstriction may result. The capillary permeability is not appreciably altered by 5-HT, except in the rat. Veins constrict to 5-HT.

II. Occurrence and Effects in the Eye

5-Hydroxytryptamine has been demonstrated in the vertebrate as well as invertebrate eye (LEVENE 1962; WELSH 1964; QUAY 1965a; ADOLPH and TUAN 1972; ADOLPH and EHINGER 1975; THOMAS and Redburn 1979; Floren and HANSSON 1980; EHINGER et al. 1981). A problem with quantitation of endogenous 5-HT in tissues is that in many species the platelets of the blood contain substantial amounts of 5-HT. Therefore, unless the blood is removed by perfusion, the 5-HT values measured represent overestimations. It is likely that most of the ocular 5-HT values reported in the literature grossly exaggerate the real 5-HT content. Recently, for example, it was shown that the 5-HT content of the rabbit retina was 24 ± 5 ng/ g tissue (EHINGER et al. 1981). If the blood was perfused away, the value decline to 4 ± 1 ng/g tissue, or even less, although the rabbit retina is poorly vascularized. In several mammalian species the 5-HT content of the nonperfused retina has been reported to be 4–100 ng/g wet weight of tissue (THOMAS and REDBURN 1979; FLOREN and HANSSON 1980; EHINGER et al. 1981). In the chicken retina, which is avascular, the concentration of 5-HT was reported to be 176 ± 12 ng/g wet weight (SUZUKI et al. 1977a).

The metabolism of 5-HT in the eye has been studied in several papers (e.g., BAKER 1966a, b; BAKER and QUAY 1969; CARDINALI and ROSNER 1971; SMITH 1973;

SMITH and BAKER 1974; SUZUKI et al. 1977 b; FLOREN and HANSSON 1980). The retina in lower vertebrates is unique in that it is the only other tissue besides the pineal containing hydroxyindole-*o*-methyltransferase activity (QUAY 1965 b). Thus the retina has the enzyme required for melatonin synthesis. The common embryologic origin of the pineal body and the retina may explain this. Experiments with ^3H-5-hydroxytryptophan injected intravitreously in rats have shown that the precursor, serotonin, or some of its metabolites can be traced in the hypothalmus, indicating a possible indolamine-containing nerve pathway from the eye to the hypothalmus (O'STEEN and VAUGHAN 1968). It is not known whether this pathway is associated with the retinohypothalmic pathway in the inferior accessory optic tract, which is involved in light-induced regulation of hydroxindole-*o*-methyltransferase activity in the pineal gland (MOORE et al. 1967). The influence of light on 5-HT synthesis and content in the rat retina was studied by O'STEEN (1970). The 5-HT content of the retina and the optic nerve was influenced by photoperiod fluctuations and the biogenic amine was suggested to be related to light-induced changes in neuroendocrine function.

Biochemical analyses indicates the presence of 5-HT and its metabolite 5-HIAA in the retina, but the histofluorescent demonstration of 5-HT has generally not been successful (HÄGGENDAHL and MALMFORS1 1965; EHINGER 1976; EHINGER et al. 1981). However, HAUSCHILD and LATIES (1973) reported spontaneously occurring indole-containing neurons in the chick retina. Both quantitative and morphological uptake studies show that retinal neurons of the goldfish, chick, pigeon, rabbit, cat, and cow accumulate 5-HT (EHINGER and FLOREN 1976, 1978; SUZUKI et al. 1978; FLOREN 1979; THOMAS and REDBURN 1979; OSBORN 1980), but no indolamine-accumulating neurons have been detected in Old World monkeys or the human (EHINGER and FLOREN 1979). A K^+ induced release of 5-HT from neurons of the bovine retina in a Ca^{++} dependent manner has also been shown (THOMAS and REDBURN 1979; OSBORNE 1980), and 5-HT has been demonstrated to alter responses in retinal ganglion cells (STRASCHILL 1968; AMES and POLLEN 1969). Thus some of the neurotransmitter criteria for 5-HT in the retina have been fulfilled, although the final localization of endogenous 5-HT still remains to be solved. A fact not supporting a neurotransmitter role of 5-HT is the relatively scarce amount of the amine found in the retina, e. g., as compared with the CNS (FLOREN and HANSON 1980). One has also to consider the possibility that a related indolamine rather than 5-HT is the transmitter. Indolamine-accumulating neurons that have been demonstrated in the retina have their perikarya in the innermost cell row of the inner nuclear layer among amacrine cells, sending processes to various parts of the inner plexiform layer (EHINGER and FLOREN 1976).

5-Hydroxytryptamine may also have a neurotransmitter role in the compound eye of the horse shoe crab (*Limulus*) (ADOLPH 1966; BEHRENS and WULF 1970; ADOLPH and TUAN 1972), and it has been suggested that it is involved in lateral inhibition. The amount of 5-HT in the eye of the horse shoe crab is considerably larger than that reported for the retina in vertebrates (1–23 µg/g wet weight [ADOLPH and TUAN 1972]).

Intravenous injection of 5-HT in dogs and rabbits has been reported to lower IOP (SCHUMACHER and CLASSEN 1962; CHIANG 1974). Intravenous injection of 5-HT in rats has been demonstrated to cause strong constriction of retinal vessels

(TAMMISTO 1965). Isolated bovine long posterior ciliary arteries also react with constriction to 5-HT in vitro (DALSKE 1974). However, these vessels do not have a normal resting tone, and may therefore react differently in vivo. 5-Hydroxytryptamine is unlikely to be involved in the acute vasomotor response to ocular injury (MOSES and HOLEKAMP 1971).

A single injection of a large dose of 5-HT systemically induces reversible cataract of short duration in rats (TILGNER and KUSCH 1969; DIETZE and TILGNER 1973). The lens opacity is located in the anterior subcapsular layer and usually lasts for 1–2 h. The mechanism of this phenomenon is not entirely clear, but it seems that the changed motility of the lids is an important factor. Closure of the lids prevents cataract formation (DIETZE et al. 1974), possibly by preventing evaporation through the cornea and an increase in the salt concentration of the aqueous humor. P-Chlorophenylalanine (PCP), which blocks the hydroxylation of tryptophan, in high doses causes an irreversible cataract in weanling rats, but no change was found in rhesus monkeys (GRALLA and RUBIN 1970). Although it is quite clear that 5-HT concentrations in animals treated with PCP are low, it is not clear whether the cataractogenic effect is due to lack of 5-HT or some other compound in indolamine metabolism.

E. Plasma Kinins

I. General Background

Bradykinin and kallidin are polypeptides that are referred to as plasma kinins. These agents contract as well as relax smooth muscle. They are split from precursor proteins in the α_2-globulin fraction of the plasma by proteolytic enzymes, preferentially kallikreins. The kallikreins are present in an inactive form as prekallikreins. Conversion of prekallikrein to kallikrein in plasma results in formation of bradykinin. Glandular and tissue kallikreins convert the precursors preferentially to kallidin. The half-life of kinins in plasma is extremely short, around 15 s. The amino acid sequence of bradykinin is shown in Table 3. Bradykinin has many powerful effects on vascular smooth muscle, causing relaxation of most resistance vessels but contraction of capacitance vessels, and big arteries. Like histamine, plasma kinins increase permeability of the microvasculature, probably in small venules rather than in capillaries. Bradykinin is also a very strong pain stimulator. Recently, bradykinin-like immunoreactivity was demonstrated in neurons of rat hypothalamus (CORREA et al. 1979).

II. Effects in the Eye

Introduction of bradykinin into the anterior chamber of rabbit eyes undergoing closed-circuit perfusion has been reported to induce miosis and a sharp rise in IOP, accompanied by an increased protein content of the effluent (COLE and UNGER 1974). The permeability of the vasculature in the ciliary processes has also been shown to be strongly increased (COLE 1974). There was no significant prostaglandin-like activity in the effluent, and indomethacin and atropine were both ineffective in preventing the responses (COLE and UNGER 1974). However, EAKINS et al.

Table 3. Amino acid sequences of some biologically active peptides of interest in the eye

Name	Amino acids		Sequence
	No.		
Bradykinin	9		Arg–Pro–Pro–Gly–Phe–Ser–Pro–Phe–Arg
Angiotensin II	8		Asp–Arg–Val–Tyr–Ile–His–Pro–Phe
Substance P	11		Arg–Pro–Lys–Pro–Gln–Gln–Phe–Phe–Gly–Leu–Met
Enkephalin			
Met–	5		Tyr–Gly–Gly–Phe–Met
Leu–	5		Tyr–Gly–Gly–Phe–Leu
Neurotensin	13		Glu–Leu–Tyr–Glu–Asn–Lys–Pro–Arg–Arg–Pro–Tyr–Ile–Leu
Somatostatin	14		Ala–Gly–Cys–Lys–Asn–Phe–Phe–Trp–Lys–Thr–Phe–Thr–Ser–Cys
Thyrotropin-releasing hormone (THR)	3		(pyro)Glu–His–Pro
Luteinizing-hormone-releasing hormone (LHRH)	10		(pyro)Glu–His–Trp–Ser–Tyr–Gly–Leu–Arg–Pro–Gly
Antidiuretic hormone (ADH)	9		Cys–Tyr–Phe–Gln–Asn–Cys–Pro–Arg–Gly[a]
Oxytocin	9		Cys–Tyr–Ile–Gln–Asn–Cys–Pro–Leu–Gly
α-Melanocyte-stimulating hormone	13		Ser–Tyr–Ser–Met–Glu–His–Phe–Arg–Trp–Gly–Lys–Pro–Val
Vasoactive intestinal polypeptide	28		His–Ser–Asp–Ala–Val–Phe–Thr–Asp–Asn–Tyr–Thr–Arg–Leu–Arg–Lys–Gln–Met–Ala–Val–Lys–Lys–Tyr–Leu–Asn–Ser–Ile–Leu–Asn
Glucagon	29		His–Ser–Gln–Gly–Thr–Phe–Thr–Ser–Asp–Tyr–Ser–Lys–Tyr–Leu–Asp–Ser–Arg–Arg–Ala–Gln–Asp–Phe–Val–Gln–Trp–Leu–Met–Asp–Thr
Gastrin	34		(pyro)Glu–Leu–Gly–Pro–Gln–Gly–His–Pro–Ser–Leu–Val–Ala–Asp–Pro–Ser–Lys–Lys–Gln–Gly–Pro–Trp–Leu–Glu–Glu–Glu–Glu–Glu–Ala–Tyr–Gly–Trp–Met–Asp–Phe
Cholecystokinin	39		Tyr–Ile–Gln–Gln–Ala–Arg–Lys–Ala–Pro–Ser–Gly–Arg–Val–Ser–Met–Ile–Lys–Asn–Leu–Gln–Ser–Leu–Asp–Pro–Ser–His–Arg–Ile–Ser–Asp–Arg–Asp–Tyr–Met–Gly–Trp–Met–Asp–Phe

[a] In swine ADH arginine in position 8 is replaced by lysine

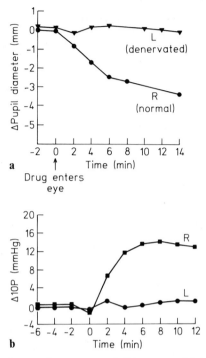

Fig. 5. Effect of sensory denervation on **a** pupil diameter and **b** intraocular pressure (*IOP*) responses to intracameral infusion of 25 ng bradykinin. Note the absent or very weak response in the denervated eyes. Mean values of eight and six experiments, respectively. *L*, left eye; *R*, right eye. (Butler and Hammond 1977)

(1976) found that both the miosis and the breakdown of the blood-aqueous barrier induced by bradykinin could to a considerable extent be prevented by prior treatment of the animals with inhibitors of prostaglandin synthesis. Butler and Hammond (1977, 1980) reported that the miotic and hypertensive effects of bradykinin in rabbits could be prevented by prior coagulation of the fifth cranial nerve (Fig. 5), implying that the effects are exerted through sensory nerves. This explains the rapid breakdown of the blood-aqueous barrier after injection of bradykinin into the anterior chamber, since the response is likely to be mediated by an axon reflex. Intravenous infusion of bradykinin in rabbits did not cause any disruption of the blood-aqueous barrier of increase in IOP (Chiang 1974). This may at least partly be attributed to the rapid inactivation of bradykinin in the blood.

F. The Renin-Angiotensin System

I. General Background

The main role of the renin-angiotensin system is to regulate blood pressure and volume homeostasis. Angiotensin I, a decapeptide, is split from the precursor angiotensinogen, and α-globulin in plasma, by renin or angiotensin-I-generating enzyme. Angiotensin I is activated to angiotensin II after removal of the terminal histidyl-leucine residues by angiotensin-converting enzyme (peptidyldipeptidase). The same enzyme (kininase II) also inactivates kinins, e. g., bradykinin. Angiotensin II exerts many physiological effects, the most important of which is vasoconstriction. It also releases aldosterone from the adrenal cortex. Angiotensin II is split to angiotensin III, a heptapeptide with a short half-life. Angiotensin III shares effects with angiotensin II. The amino acid sequence of angiotensin II is shown in Table 3. Angiotensin III is inactivated by various peptidases. Components of the renin-angiotensin system have also been demonstrated at extrarenal sites, e. g., in the brain.

II. Occurrence in the Eye

Angiotensin-I-generating enzyme activity has been investigated in primary and secondary aqueous humor of rabbits, dogs, and monkeys (IKEMOTO and YAMAMOTO 1978). Very little activity, if any, could be detected in the primary aqueous humor, but secondary aqueous contained enzyme activity. Since paracentesis causes an accumulation of plasma proteins in the aqueous humor, it was thought that the activity was due to plasma renin. This was further verified by the effect of nephrectomy (IKEMOTO and YAMAMOTO 1978). Angiotensin-converting enzyme, however, was recently reported in aqueous humor and tears from man and rabbit (VITA et al. 1981). The activity was around 5% of that in the serum. Tears contained more enzyme activity than the aqueous humor. Angiotensin – converting enzyme has been demonstrated in homogenates of the retina as well as in isolated retinal vessels (IGIĆ et al. 1977; WARD et al. 1979). The enzyme has also been demonstrated in the choroid and the ciliary body of human, bovine, pig, and rabbit eyes (IGIĆ and KOJOVIC 1980). Microvessels isolated from the pig retina showed the highest enzyme activity, approximately ten times that in the plasma. The angiotensin-converting enzyme has been detected in the eye, but its role is not at all clear.

G. Substance P

I. General Background

Substance P is an undecapeptide that was first discovered in tissue extracts from equine brain and gut (VON EULER and GADDUM 1931). The amino acid sequence of the peptide is shown in Table 3. Substance P is widely distributed in the nervous system and the intestinal tract of vertebrates (for a review see BURY and MASHFORD 1977; NICOLL et al. 1980). Substance P has also been found in other tissues, including the blood. Substantia nigra, the trigeminal nucleus, and the dorsal horn of the spinal cord contain large amounts of substance P. Substance P has been demonstrated in primary afferent nerve fibers, both in the central and peripheral portions. In addition, substance-P-positive nerve fibers have been detected in sympathetic ganglia (HÖKFELT et al. 1977a).

A substantial amount of evidence has accumulated suggesting that substance P may be involved in sensory neurotransmission or modulation of sensory input in C and possibly A delta fibers (NICOLL et al. 1980). These fibers relay information about noxious stimuli. Physiological experiments, as well as the morphological pattern of substance P within the nervous system, support this conclusion. Stimulation of sensory nerves does not only cause a release of substance P in the cephalad portion of the nerves but also in the periphery, as demonstrated in the superfused feline tooth pulp (OLGART et al. 1977) and in the anterior uvea of the rabbit (BILL et al. 1979). Thus substance P could very well be involved in an axon reflex mechanism. The mechanism of inactivation of substance P is not exactly known, but degradation by peptidases is a more likely alternative than uptake by neurons or other elements. Capsaicin, a derivative of homovanillic acid, causes depletion of substance P from sensory nerve terminals (JESSEL et al. 1978). However, capsaicin is not a selective depletor of substance P. Recently two analogs of substance P (D-Pro^2, D-Phe^7, D-Trp^9)-SP and (D-Pro^2, D-Trp^{7,9})-SP have been synthesized with some antagonizing effects (ENGBERG et al. 1981; FOLKERS et al. 1981; ROSELL et al. 1981).

II. Distribution in the Eye

Substance-P-like biological activity or immunoreactivity has been found particularly in the retina and in the iris and cornea. The retina, which is an extension of the diencephalon, has been shown to contain substance-P-like activity in the chick, pigeon, rat, guinea pig, rabbit, dog, cow, and monkey (DÜNER et al. 1954; HELD et al. 1966; WINDER and PATSALOS 1974; KANAZAWA and JESSEL 1976; REUBI and JESSEL 1978; ESKAY et al. 1980, 1981; STJERNSCHANTZ et al. 1982a; UNGER et al. 1981) (see Table 4). In the bullfrog and carp retina, immunoreactive substance P was shown to differ from synthetic substance P as determined by high-performance liquid chromatography (ESKAY et al. 1981). Immunohistochemical investigations indicate that substance P is localized to a distinct population of amacrine cells in the pigeon retina (KARTEN and BRECHA 1980). In other species the anterior uvea is also rich in substance-P-like immunoreactivity, and so is the cornea (see Table 4), although the absolute values per unit weight tissue in the cornea are lower due to the considerable connective tissue stroma. Substance-P-positive neurons have been verified immunohistochemically in the cornea, the iris, the ciliary body, and the trabecular meshwork (HÖKFELD et al. 1977b; MILLER et al., 1981; LATIES et al. 1981; TERVO et al. 1981; TÖRNQUIST et al. 1982; TERENGHI et al. 1982). Sensory denervation by coagulation of the epigasserian tract in the rabbit destroyed about 70% of the substance-P-like immunoreactivity in the anterior uvea (BUTLER et al. 1980a), indicating that most of the substances P in this tissue resides in sensory neurons of the fifth nerve. A beautiful separate localization of vasoactive intestinal polypeptide (anterior choroid) and substance P (iris) has been achieved in the guinea pig (TERENGHI et al. 1982). Normally, substance-P-like immunoreactivity of the aqueous humor in the rabbit corresponds to about 10 pg or less (BILL et al. 1979; STJERNSCHANTZ et al. 1982a), and no immunoreactivity identified as substance P has been found in the lens or the vitreous. However, the lens seems to be the only tissue that slowly accumulates ^{125}I-tyr^8-substance P or its metabolites after intracameral injection in rabbits (STJERNSCHANTZ and SEARS 1982). Substance-P-like immunoreactivity was recently also reported in the compound eye of the lobster (MANCILLAS et al. 1981). Each of the four optic neuropils contained substance-P-like immunoreactivity.

Table 4. Substance-P-like immunoreactivity (pmol/g wet weight) of ocular tissues in various species. Values have been converted to pmol/g tissue by using a molecular weight for substance P of 1,500. Mean ± SEM

Species	Cornea	Anterior uvea	Choroid	Retina	Reference
Pigeon		104 ±35		3 ±1	Reubi and Jessel 1978
Rat	5.2±0.3				Gamse et al. 1981
Rat				59 ±13	Kanazawa and Jessel 1976
Rat				43.3±7.1	Eskay et al. 1980
Guinea pig				46 ±9.1	Eskay et al. 1980
Rabbit		7.9±0.3			Camras and Bito 1980b
Rabbit	5.1±1.3	8.1±1.1	6.5±1.3	20.5±1.3	Stjernschantz et al. 1982a
Rabbit				25.3±4.8	Eskay et al. 1980
Cow				21.3±2	Eskay et al. 1980
Monkey				4.7±0.8	Eskay et al. 1980

Under in vivo conditions, exogenous substance P is rapidly inactivated in the anterior uvea, and only 0.02%–0.06% of the substance P injected into the anterior chamber of rabbit eyes could be recovered in biologically active form from the ciliary processes after a time period of 15–30 min (STJERNSCHANTZ and SEARS 1982). This was only 1%–3% of the corresponding amount of radioactive substance P that reached the ciliary processes after intracameral injection.

III. Effects in the Eye

The ocular functions of substance P are of definite interest with regard to retinal neurotransmission and nociception. The immediate response to injury is likely to be at least partly dependent on intact sensory innervation, and thus one or more agents released from sensory neurons must be crucial in the response. At first glance, substance P appears to be a good candidate for such a role.

1. Retina

The exact function of substance P in the retina is not known. Both in amphibian and carp retina increased spontaneous activity as well as enhancement of light-evoked excitation of ganglion cells can be achieved with exogenous substance P in vitro (DICK and MILLER 1980; GLICKMAN et al. 1980). The receptors for substance P are probably located in the membranes of the ganglion cells because the response of these cells to substance P occurs under synaptic blockade (GLICKMAN and ADOLPH 1982). This indicates that substance P or a closely related peptide may act as a neuromodulator or may be involved in neurotransmission directly in the retina. Visual deprivation in the rat was demonstrated to cause a decrease in the substance P content of various forebrain structures (PRADELLES et al. 1979).

2. Iridial Smooth Muscles

Studies in vivo as well as in vitro have shown that substance P has marked effects on the sphincter muscle of the iris (BILL et al. 1979; BUTLER and HAMMOND 1980;

COHEN et al. 1981; MANDAHL and BILL; NISHIYAMA et al. 1971a; SOLOWAY et al. 1981; STJERNSCHANTZ et al. 1981). In vivo the threshold concentration for constriction of the pupil seems to be around 1 ng/ml aqueous humor in the rabbit, corresponding to a molar concentration of about 10^{-9}. Quantitative studies in vitro determined the threshold concentration in whole rabbit to be $2 \times 10^{-10} M$ (SOLOWAY et al. 1981). The effect is direct on the smooth muscle (BUTLER and HAMMOND 1980; MANDAHL and BILL 1980, 1981). Substance P does not seem to have any appreciable effect on the dilator muscle (SOLOWAY et al. 1981). Recently, it was demonstrated that the contractile response to noncholinergic, nonadrenergic nerve stimulation of the rabbit iris sphincter could be antagonized by the substance P analog (D-Pro^2, D-Trp^{7,9})-SP, indicating that substance P or a closely related peptide is specifically involved in this response (LEANDER et al. 1981). The intense and sustained miosis in vivo has important consequences because it creates a pupillary block and increases IOP (AL-GHADYAN et al. 1979; Stjernschantz et al. 1981). It may be harmful during extracapsular cataract surgery.

3. Ocular Circulation and the Blood–Aqueous Barrier

Intracameral injection of substance P in the rabbit does not cause any significant increase in ocular blood flow (STJERNSCHANTZ 1981; STJERNSCHANTZ et al. 1982b). When administered from the adventitial side, substance P seems to be surprisingly ineffective vasodilator in the anterior uvea. Intraarterial infusion of large doses of substance P reduces peripheral resistance and induces ocular vasodilation at least momentarily (STJERNSCHANTZ et al. 1981). Although large doses of substance P cause vasodilation after intraarterial infusion, no disruption of the blood–aqueous barrier has been noticed (STJERNSCHANTZ et al. 1981). The effect on ocular capillary permeability of intraarterially infused substance P is also surprisingly weak, as studied with Evans' blue (STJERNSCHANTZ et al. 1982b). Injection of substance P into the anterior (BUTLER and HAMMOND 1980; STJERNSCHANTZ et al. 1981, to be published a) or posterior chamber (BUTLER and HAMMOND 1980) is also relatively ineffective in inducing a disruption of the blood–aqueous barrier in rabbits. Prior contradicting results have been presented (BILL et al. 1979; MANDAHL and BILL 1981; NISHIYAMA et al. 1981a). It is clear, however, that in doses that can easily cause intense miosis no disruption of the blood–aqueous occurs. It is therefore likely that the disruption of the blood–aqueous barrier that occurs during the irritative response of the rabbit eye is not caused by a release of substance P. The effect of substance P on the blood–aqueous barrier may be greater in eyes with increased blood flow (BILL et al. 1979; MANDAHL and BILL 1981), achieved by acute sympathectomy and/or by the use of pentobarbital as anesthetic (BILL and STJERNSCHANTZ 1980). Thus it is possible that substance P, together with some other agent causing vasodilation, e.g., ATP, may induce a breakdown of the barrier. Adenosine triphosphate has been shown to be released into the aqueous humor by antidromic stimulation of the trigeminal nerve in rabbits and to cause slight hyperemia after intravitreal injection (MAUL and SEARS 1979). Intracameral injection of high doses of ATP causes immediate disruption of the blood–aqueous barrier in rabbit eyes (STJERNSCHANTZ et al., to be published c).

Involvement of endogenous substance P in the disruption of the blood–aqueous barrier in rabbits after noxious stimuli has been claimed by CAMRAS and

Bito (1980 b) and Holmdahl et al. (1981). The first authors found that capsaicin-treated eyes did not react to topical nitrogen mustard with a typical increase in IOP and barrier breakdown. Holmdahl et al. (1981) showed that the aqueous flare response to infrared irradiation in rabbits could be attenuated by pretreating the eyes with a large dose of the substance P analog (D-Pro^2, D-Trp^{7,9})-SP. The response can also be blocked by indomethacin and β-adrenergic antagonists (Bengtsson et al. 1975; Bengtsson 1977). Furthermore, the data given in these reports are skimpy, especially with regard to the hyperemia response. Additionally, capsaicin, on irritant itself, is a nonspecific agent. It is likely that a peptide other than substance P is important in the mechanism leading to disruption of the blood–aqueous barrier in ocular irritation.

4. Intraocular Pressure

Intracameral injection of high doses (≥ 1 µg) of substance P induces a variable increase in IOP (Bill et al. 1979; Butler and Hammond 1980; Stjernschantz et al. 1981; Mandahl and Bill 1981). In the absence of a barrier disruption, the most likely explanation for this effect is a pupillary block and peripheral iridectomy prevents the response (Stjernschantz et al. 1981). In cases with barrier breakdown the increase in IOP is dependent both on this and the pupillary block. Low doses (≤ 10 ng) induce miosis but no appreciable increase in IOP (Nishiyama et al. 1981 a; Stjernschantz et al. 1981). Intraarterial infusion of substance P did not cause any increase in IOP (Stjernschantz et al. 1981).

5. Formation and Outflow of Aqueous Humor

Determination of outflow facility of aqueous humor in rabbit eyes after intracameral injection of substance P revealed a 50% decrease in gross facility (Stjernschantz et al. 1981). This seems to be due to a pupillary block with secondary bulging of the peripheral iris against the cornea to obstruct the iridocorneal angle. This also explains why the increase in IOP is so variable. It is conceivable that the anatomy of the chamber angle differs somewhat from eye to eye, thus making some eyes more and some less susceptible to the effect. No direct measurement of aqueous humor formation has been performed after administration of substance P. However, using the data for outflow facility (Stjernschantz et al. 1981), it can be calculated roughly that no major changes were likely to occur after intracameral injection of substance P with intact blood–aqueous barrier.

In conclusion, substance P is probably involved in the sustained and intense miosis in response to acute injury of the eye. The fact that PGE_1 and PGE_2, as well as bradykinin (Butler and Hammond 1977, 1980; Mandahl and Bill 1980, 1981) lose their miotic effect after sensory denervation of blockade of nerve conduction suggests rather strongly that a secondary agent, possibly substance P, is released from sensory nerves by these agents. At the present time, it has not been proved satisfactorily that substance P causes either ocular vasodilation or the breakdown of the blood–aqueous barrier after ocular irritation. A closely related peptide may be a more likely alternative. The increase in IOP frequently seen in the irritative response is largely a function of pupillary block induced by miosis (Al-Ghadyan et al. 1979; Stjernschantz et al. 1981), and partly related to the abrupt increase in entry of plasmoid aqueous (SEARS 1961) into the posterior chamber via a disrupted blood–aqueous barrier (NEUFELD and SEARS 1973). The effects of substance P in human eyes are not yet known.

H. Enkephalins

I. General Background

The enkephalins are pentapeptides with strong opioid properties, distributed mainly within the central nervous system. In contrast to the endorphins, which may have neurohormonal activity, the enkephalins are believed to function as neurotransmitters or modulators of synaptic transmission. The amino acid sequence of met- and leu-enkephalin are shown in Table 3. Enkephalin-positive and substance-P-positive nerve fibers coexist in many regions of the central nervous system, and it is now evident that there are opioid receptors not only in the central nervous system but also in primary afferent neurons (see NICOLL et al. 1980). An interesting interaction of enkephalin with substance P in the rat trigeminal nucleus has been demonstrated in that K^+ induced release of substance P is reduced by opiates and opioid peptides (JESSEL and IVERSEN 1976), an effect that can be blocked by naloxane, a specific antagonist of opioids. In vitro met-enkephalin has also been shown to inhibit the release of substance P from cultured neurons (MUDGE et al. 1979).

II. Occurrence and Effects in the Eye

Met- and leu-enkephalin have been demonstrated in the avian retina (BRECHA et al. 1979; HUMBERT et al. 1979; TÖRNQUIST et al. 1981). Immunohistochemical investigations indicate that leu-enkephalin is located in a selective population of amacrine cells (BRECHA et al. 1979). (D-Ala^2, Met^5)-enkephalinamide has been demonstrated to induce long-lasting inhibition of light-evoked responses and aspartate-activated spike activity in ganglion cells of the amphibian retina (DICK and MILLER 1980). (D-Ala^2, Met^5)-enkephalinamide has also been shown to inhibit the release of ^{3}H-GABA from goldfish amacrine cells and affect the firing pattern of ganglion cells (DJAMGOZ et al. 1981). Thus the output off the retina may be modulated by an opiate system. Visual deprivation was reported to decrease the content of met-enkephalin and substance P in various forebrain structures of the rat (PRADELLES et al. 1979). Intracameral injection of met-enkephalin in the rabbit has little effect on the pupil and inconsistent effects on IOP, the blood–aqueous barrier, or the ocular circulation (STJERNSCHANTZ et al., to be published d). No studies have been published on a possible interaction between the enkephalins and substance P in the eye.

Leu-enkephalin-positive immunoreactivity has also been demonstrated in the lobster eye (MANCILLAS et al. 1981). Interestingly, prominent enkephalin-like immunoreactivity was observed in the retinular cells, i.e., the primary photoreceptors of the compound eye (MANCILLAS et al. 1981).

J. Neurotensin

Neurotensin, a tridecapeptide, has been demonstrated in the central nervous system and in the gastrointestinal tract primarily (CARRAWAY and LEEMAN 1973; LEE-

MAN and CARRAWAY 1977; BISETTE et al. 1978). The amino acid sequence of neurotensin is shown in Table 3. Neurotensin exerts effects on the vasculature and glucose metabolism, as well as on the intestinal and uterine smooth muscles. The peptide has also been reported to induce hypothermia (NEMEROFF et al. 1977). The distribution of neurotensin within the central nervous system is somewhat reminiscent of that of the enkephalins, and neurotensin may also be involved in pain perception (SNYDER 1980).

Amacrine cells in the avian retina show positive immunoreactivity to neurotensin as demonstrated by immunohistochemistry (BRECHA et al. 1981; TÖRNQUIST et al. 1981). The effects of neurotensin on aqueous humor dynamics in the rabbit eye are modest (STJERNSCHANTZ et al., to be published d). However, uveal blood flow seems to be increased after intracameral as well as intraarterial injection of neurotensin (STJERNSCHANTZ et al. to be published d).

K. Hypothalamic Peptides Regulating the Adenohypophysis

The hypothalamic releasing or inhibiting factors regulate the release of glycoprotein hormones and growth hormone from the adenohypophysis.

I. Somatostatin

Somatostatin has been found in the nervous system and the gastrointestinal tract, including the pancreas (VALE et al. 1977). The peptide was first discovered for its ability to inhibit the release of growth hormone. Subsequent studies have revealed a wide variety of effects of somatostatin. The peptide seems to interfere with various peptide hormones in a complex way. Somatostatin may also have a modulating function on sensory input to the brain, and immunohistochemically the peptide has been localized to primary afferent neurons (HOKFELT et al. 1975, 1976). The amino acid sequence of somatostatin is shown in Table 3).

Somatostatin has been demonstrated in the goldfish, frog, bullfrog, chick, rat, guinea pig, rabbit, cow, and monkey retina (RORSTADT et al. 1979; SHAPIRO et al. 1979; ESKAY et al. 1980; LAKE and PATEL 1980; YAMADA et al. 1980) and has immunohistochemically been localized to amacrine cells as well as to ganglion cells in the frog, rat, and goldfish retina (MARSHAK et al. 1979). In the pigeon and chicken retina, somatostatin has immunohistochemically also been detected in amacrine cells (BRECHA et al. 1981; TÖRNQUIST et al. 1981). In the rat retina, horizontal cells, amacrine cells, and large neurons in the ganglionic cell layer seem to be specifically labeled with somatostatin-like immunoreactivity (KRISCH and LEONHARDT 1979). Rats suffering from hereditary degeneration of photoreceptor cells, as well as rats after transection of the optic nerve, show an increased amount of somatostatin-like immunoreactivity in the retina (RORSTAD et al. 1979). The function of somatostatin in the retina is not known, although an inhibitory effect on retinal neurons has been suggested (KRISCH and LEONHARDT 1979). Somatostatin has no major effect on aqueous humor dynamics or ocular blood flow as studied in the rabbit (STJERNSCHANTZ et al., to be published d).

II. Thyrotropin-Releasing Hormone

Thyrotropin-releasing hormone (TRH) is a tripeptide regulating the release of thyrotropin from the adenohypophysis. The amino acid of the peptide is shown in

Table 3. In the central nervous system neurons containing TRH have been demonstrated immunohistochemically, and TRH has been postulated to have a neurotransmitter or modulator role.

Thyrotropin-releasing-hormone-like immunoreactivity has been demonstrated in the retina of lower vertebrates, such as the frog, bullfrog, and eel (Jackson and Reichlin 1977; Eskay et al. 1980). In mammals, TRH-like immunoreactivity has also been demonstrated in the retina (Schaeffer et al. 1977; Martino et al. 1980), but it is not clear whether this is due to authentic TRH (Yongblood et al. 1979). It seems apparent that TRH is present in lower vertebrates in the inner retinal cells or ganglion cells (Eskay et al. 1980). Thyrotropin-releasing hormone could also be released by K^+ in a Ca^{++} dependent manner, and kainic acid, a neurotoxic agent, destroyed retinal TRH (Eskay et al. 1980). The function of TRH in the retina is not known.

III. Luteinizing-Hormone-Releasing Hormone

Luteinizing-hormone-releasing hormone (LHRH) is primarily located to neurons in the hypothalamus–it causes a release of luteinizing and follicle-stimulating hormones from adenohypophysis. It has also been found in other parts of the brain and in sympathetic ganglia (see Eiden and Brownstein 1981). The amino acid sequence of LHRH is shown in Table 3.

Recently, LHRH-positive nerve fibers were immunohistochemically found in the platyfish retina (Münz et al. 1981), near amacrine and bipolar cells. The LHRH-positive retinal fibers have been traced to nucleus olfactoretinalis via the optic nerve and tract. The function of LHRH in the retina is not known.

L. Peptide Hormones Secreted by the Neurohypophysis

I. General Background

Antidiuretic hormone (ADH) or vasopressin and oxytocin are nonapeptides secreted by the neurohypophysis. Both hormones are synthesized in the supraoptic and paraventricular nucleus of the hypothalamus, and then transported in the nerve fibers to the median eminence and pars nervosa of the hypophysis to be released into the blood. The main physiological role of ADH is reabsorption of water in the distal tubuli and collecting ducts of the kidney, while that of oxytocin is contraction of the uterine smooth muscle and the myoepithelium of the mammary gland. High doses of ADH also have vasopressor effects, whereas high doses of oxytocin seem to cause relaxation of vascular smooth muscle. The carrier proteins of ADH and oxytocin, the neurophysins, have also been demonstrated immunohistochemically in other parts of the central nervous system, indicating that the presence of these nonapeptides may not be restricted only to the hypothalamus and the hypophysis (Swanson 1977; Nilaver et al. 1980). The amino acid sequences of ADH and oxytocin are shown in Table 3.

II. Effects of Antidiuretic Hormone in the Eye

The literature on the ocular effects of ADH is somewhat confusing, although ADH has been much studied in ophthalmologic research. The contradiction may, however, largely be due to different preparations, doses, and routes of administration employed in different studies. Early studies indicated that vasopressin extracts could cause both mydriasis and miosis depending on the dose (SCHLAEPPI 1940). However, in a recent study with synthetic vasopressin and its analogs it was shown both in vitro and in vivo that the only consistent effect is contraction of the pupillary sphincter (HOROWITZ 1981). The efficiency was of about the same order of magnitude as that of substance P. The effect was positively correlated to the pressor property and not the antidiuretic property of vasopressin (HOROWITZ 1981).

SCHLAEPPI (1940) found a lowering effect on IOP of Pitressin, a vasopressin extract, both in man and rabbit after subconjunctival administration. Topical administration of 0.2–2 units ADH was also reported to induce a decrease in IOP in glaucomatous as well as normal human eyes (BECKER and CHRISTENSEN 1956; CONSTANT and BECKER 1956). It was assumed that this was due to a decrease in aqueous humor formation, and gross facility of outflow was shown to decrease (CONSTANT and BECKER 1956). The reduction in formation of aqueous humor could possibly have been secondary to local vasoconstriction. Such a vasoconstriction has been reported in the eye after administration of vasopressin (CONSTANT and BECKER 1956; WUDKA and LEOPOLD 1956). Intracameral infusion of 50–200 μ units ADH per milliliter in the rabbit caused an increase in gross facility of outflow (NAGASUBRAMANIAN 1974). The final concentration of ADH in the aqueous humor was far above the physiological level in these studies. Systemic administration of ADH, especially in anesthetized animals, tends to increase the blood pressure and possibly, secondarily to this, IOP (see review by KASS and SEARS 1977). A problem is encountered here, too, because the baroreceptor reflex is inhibited in anesthetized animals, thus tending to potentiate the pressor effect. Ethanol, a classic inhibitor of ADH secretion, lowers IOP, but it is not entirely clear whether this is based solely on a decrease in the plasma concentration of ADH (HOULE and GRANT 1967; LEYDHECKER et al. 1978).

In vitro ADH has been reported to increase the transepithelial short-circuit current in the rabbit iris-ciliary body preparation (COLE and NAGASUBRAMANIAN 1972, 1973). This was interpreted as due to increased flux of Na^+. 5 mM cAMP also tended to increase the short-circuit current, although with some variability (COLE and NAGASUBRAMANIAN 1972). BERGGREN (1970) did not find any evidence of a modulating effect of vasopressin on the active secretion of the rabbit ciliary epithelium in vitro. Ethanol loading in rabbits caused a decrease in IOP which could be counteracted by nicotine infusion, releasing ADH, and it was suggested that ADH in physiological concentrations would increase IOP by increasing the formation of aqueous humor (NAGASUBRAMANIAN 1977). Intraarterial infusion of ADH in anesthetized rabbits increased the blood pressure and decreased the blood flow through the anterior uvea, as measured by the thermocouple technique, and decreased IOP (NAGASUBRAMANIAN 1977). The decrease in IOP was explained on the basis of reduced blood flow through the anterior uvea from too high concentrations of intraarterially infused ADH. Intravenous administration of ADH in another study also performed in anesthetized rabbits lowered aqueous humor formation (NIEDERER et al. 1975). This was accompanied by a decrease in systemic blood pressure. However, the physiological concentrations of ADH were again clearly exceeded, and a local vasoconstriction in the eye possibly affecting aqueous humor formation cannot be excluded. DDAVP, a synthetic agonist with a much higher ratio of ADH to pressor activity than natural vasopressin, is useful to study secretory versus pressor mechanisms (HOROWITZ et al. 1983). While a pharmacologic dose of LVP (0.2 units) administered intravitreally produced a reduction in IOP, DDAVP had no effect on IOP. Vasopressin does not produce its ocular hypotensive effect by an action on an ADH-like receptor. This observation lends support to the contention that an effect on vascular smooth muscle, most plausibly mediated by a pressor receptor, explains any pharmacologic ocular hypotensive response to vasopressin. Could vasopressin act as a "first messenger" to stimulate adenylate cyclase in ciliary processes? Biochemical evidence stands against this hypothesis because vasopressin neither stimulates ciliary process adenylate cyclase nor affects cAMP phosphodiesterase activity or cAMP production in intact ciliary processes in vitro. Although ADH may influence IOP, the evidence for a homeostatic role of ADH either in the steady state regulation of IOP or in hypovolemic situations is lacking.

III. Effects of Oxytocin in the Eye

Information about the effect of oxytocin in the eye is very sparse. Systemic administration of synthetic oxytocin has not been reported to have any appreciable effect on the blood–aqueous barrier in rabbits (DYSTER-AAS and KRAKAU 1964b). Both in vivo and in vitro large doses of oxytocin contract the pupillary sphincter in the rabbit (HOROWITZ 1981).

M. Melanocyte-Stimulating Hormones

The melanocyte-stimulating hormones (MSHs) are secreted by the intermediate lobe of the hypophysis, and may play a role in regulating skin pigmentation in amphibia and fish. In man MSHs have not been detected in plasma, and it is likely that the effect of α-MSH is partly contained within ACTH, since the 13 amino acids of α-MSH are identical with the first 13 residues of ACTH. However, the effect on pigment dispersion of ACTH is only about 1/40 of that of αMSH. β-Melanocyte-stimulating hormone in most mammalian species is an octadecapeptide. α-Melanocyte-stimulating hormone has been demonstrated immunohistochemically also in extrahypophyseal sites of the brain (PELLETIER and DUBÉ 1977; DESY and PELLETIER 1978; DUBÉ et al. 1978; JACOBOWITZ and O'DONOHUE 1978; and others). The amino acid sequence of α-MSH is shown in Table 3.

I. Effects in the Eye

Subcutaneous injection of α-or β-MSH in pigmented rabbits causes a disruption of the blood-aqueous barrier and a transient increase in IOP (DYSTER-AAS and KRAKAU 1964b; DYSTER-AAS 1965; NEUFELD et al. 1972). The disruption of the barrier as well as the increase in IOP is slow in onset. There is no response in the pupil diameter. Pharmacologic experiments indicate that histamine, prostaglandins, and sensory nerves are unlikely to be involved in this response (DYSTER-AAS 1965; BENGTSSON et al. 1975). If anything, inhibitors of prostaglandin synthesis seem to enhance the response (NEUFELD et al. 1972; BENGTSSON et al. 1975). β-Adrenergic blockade is said to prevent the barrier disruption, while terbutalin, a β_2-adrenergic agonist, facilitates it (BENGTSSON 1977), and the effect has been suggested to involve an increase in cAMP as an important mechanism in the barrier disruption. Imidazole, one of the effects of which is that it activates the phosphodiesterase and thus presumably decrease cAMP levels, was reported to abolish the effect of α-MSH (BENGTSSON 1976). In connection with this it is interesting to note that both 5-ATP and 5-ADP have been demonstrated to cause hyperemia and a breakdown of the blood–aqueous barrier in rabbits after intravitreal injection (MAUL and SEARS 1979); 5-AMP was inactive in this respect. It should be pointed out that the possible role of cAMP in the breakdown of the blood–aqueous barrier is only hypothetical, and cAMP is involved in many physiological mechanisms as a second messenger. α-Melanocyte-stimulating hormone has also been shown to release ^3H-γ-aminobutyric acid from preloaded rabbit retinas in vitro (BAUER and EHINGER 1980). This may indicate a neurotransmitter or modulator role of α-MSH in the retina, particularly since the effect could be achieved with relatively low concentrations of the peptide. However, at the present time it is not known what the physiological or pathophysiological role of MSHs in the eye is, if any.

N. Vasoactive Intestinal Polypeptide

I. General Background

Vasoactive intestinal polypeptide (VIP) consists of 28 amino acids, and was originally found in the intestine (SAID and MUTT 1970). The amino acid sequence of VIP is shown in Table 3. Subsequently, the peptide has also been demonstrated in the central as well as peripheral nervous system, various parts of the gastrointestinal tract, the pancreas, the genitourinary tract, and the upper respiratory tract. Vasoactive intestinal polypeptide has also been found in autonomic ganglia. It has many potent effects causing, e.g., vasodilation, increased cardiac output, respiratory stimulation, and hyperglycemia.

II. Localization and Effects in the Eye

Immunoreactive VIP has been detected in a population of amacrine cells in the rat retina (LOREN et al. 1980). Processes of these cells reached both the inner and the outer half of the inner plexiform layer. Vasoactive-intestinal-polypeptide-positive nerve fibers have also been demonstrated in the lacrimal, tarsal, and harderian glands, as well as in the uvea of the cat (UDDMAN et al. 1980), but especially in the posterior uvea (TERENGHI et al. 1982). The nerve fibers are in close proximity to choroidal blood vessels but not to blood vessels of the anterior uvea. Extirpation of the pterygopalatine ganglion destroys the VIP-positive immunoreactivity (UDDMAN et al. 1980). UNGER et al. (1981) quantified the VIP-like immunoreactivity in the rabbit eye. Highest concentration (31 pmol/g wet weight) was found in the choroid. In the anterior uvea and the retina the concentration was about one-sixth of that in the choroid. Infusion of VIP intravenously or intraarterially in rabbits causes an increase in choroidal blood flow but not in the blood flow of the anterior uvea (NILSSON and BILL 1979). However, when VIP is administered from the adventitial side by intracameral injection it increases the blood flow of the anterior uvea too (NILSSON and BILL 1979). Both intraarterial and intravenous infusion of VIP in concentrations not appreciably affecting the blood pressure increase IOP in rabbits (NILSSON and BILL 1979). Large doses of VIP injected intracamerally in rabbits were reported to cause a breakdown of the blood–aqueous barrier (NISHIYAMA et al. 1981 b).

Stimulation of the facial intermediate nerve causes a marked increase in uveal, preferentially choroidal blood flow in rabbits (STJERNSCHANTZ and BILL 1979, 1980) and monkeys (NILSSON et al. 1980; LINDER 1981). These effects are resistant at least to muscarinic blockade. The blood flow to the eyelids and the harderian gland was also increased (STJERNSCHANTZ and BILL 1980). It is possible that the increase in blood flow is due to a release of VIP from stimulate nerve fibers. GLOSTER (1961) reported an increase in IOP in cats and rabbits during stimulation of the greater superficial petrosal nerve, and RUSKELL (1970) demonstrated a long-lasting decrease in IOP in monkeys after surgical interruption of the pterygopalatine ganglion. Ruskell also showed a cholinergic innervation of choroidal arteries, probably of facial nerve origin (RUSKELL 1971). It is possible that these results carried information about the effects of VIP-containing nerves in the eye. This is further supported by the fact that VIP and acetylcholine may coexist in the same neuron (HOKFELT et al. 1980).

It is not known at the present time whether VIP-positive nerve fibers may have any significant role in regulation of ocular blood flow or fluid dynamics. The specific location of VIP in the anterior choroid is intriguing because the choroid does not autoregulate its blood flow (ALM and BILL 1972, 1973).

O. Glucagon

Glucagon is a pancreatic peptide consisting of 29 amino acids. It is secreted by the α cells of Langerhans' islets and has opposite effects on glucose metabolism to those of insulin. There is also an intestinal form of glucagon. Glucagon-positive neurons have been deteced in the brain (see SNYDER 1980). The amino acid sequence of glucagon is shown in Table 3.

In the chicken retina, glucagon-positive cell bodies have recently been described in the innermost cell row of the inner nuclear cell layer (TÖRNQUIST et al. 1981). The cells have been suggested to be amacrine cells. The possible function of glucagon in the retina is not known.

P. Gastrin/Cholecystokinin

Gastrin and cholecystokinin are gastrointestinal polypeptides. The last five amino acid residues are the same in both peptides. There are many forms of gastrin. The main effect of gastrin is stimulation of gastric acid and pepsin secretion, whereas cholecystokinin (pancreozymin) is involved in the contraction of the gallbladder and secretion of the exocrine pancreas. Both peptides have also been demonstrated in the nervous system, and cholecystokinin has been demonstrated in primary afferent neurons (see SNYDER 1980; HOKFELT et al. 1980). The amino acid sequences of gastrin and cholecystokin are shown in Table 3.

Cholecystokinin-like immunoreactivity was recently demonstrated in the inner plexiform layer of the frog retina (OSBORNE et al. 1981). The somata of amacrine cells and their processes showed positive immunoreaction. The immunoreactivity was identified as cholecystokinin through combined chromatography and radioimmunoassay. Bovine and human retinas also showed quantitatively some cholecystokinin-like immunoreactivity (OSBORNE et al. 1981). Gastrin/cholecystokinin-like immunoreactivity was also demonstrated immunohistochemically in the inner plexiform layer of the rat retina (ERIKSEN and LARSSON 1981). The function of gastrin/cholecystokinin in the retina is not known.

Q. Summary

The occurrence and effects of autacoids and neuropeptides in the eye have been reviewed. Several ocular tissues, particularly the anterior uvea and the conjunctiva, have a marked capacity for prostaglandin synthesis. The prostaglandins may be involved in certain physiological processes, such as the maintenance of the iris sphincter tone and autoregulation of retinal blood flow. They play an important role in acute injury responses of the eye and perhaps in ocular inflammation. Very little is known about the effects of prostacyclin and thromboxane in the eye, although these compounds can be synthesized by ocular tissues. Some of the compounds in the lipoxygenase pathway of arachidonic acid metabolism, particularly leukotriene B_4, may play an important role in ocular inflammation due to their chemotactic properties. Histamine plays an important role in allergic states of the conjunctiva. 5-Hydroxytryptamine fulfills some of the criteria of a retinal neurotransmitter, but the histochemical localization in the retina of this indolamine has failed so far. Of the plasma kinins, bradykinin may play a role in the acute injury response of the eye. Of the renin–angiotensin system, the angiotensin-converting enzyme (kininase II) has been found in the anterior uvea, the choroid, the retina, the aqueous humor, and tears. However, it is not clear whether this system plays any important role in the eye.

Of the neuropeptides, substance P has been localized to sensory neurons conveying nociceptive impulses from the eye, and substance P is probably the cause of the miosis of the irritative response. It is not yet known what the effects of substance P in the human eye are. Substance P, the enkephalins, neurotensin, somatostatin, thyrotropin-releasing hormone (TRH), leuteinizing-hormone-releasing hormone (LHRH), vasoactive intestinal polypeptide (VIP), glucagon, and gastrin/cholecystokinin have all been demonstrated immunohistochemically in the retina, preferentially in amacrine cells. Each has been suggested to have a neurotransmitter or modulator function. It is not clear to what extent the immunohistochemical techniques employed can distinguish between individual neuropeptides and identical amino acid sequences in larger precursor proteins, and neither is it clear whether these peptides represent separate populations of amacrine cells. Antidiuretic hormone may influence aqueous humor dynamics and intraocular pressure to some extent, but there is no clear evidence of an important role for this peptide in the regulation of aqueous humor dynamics. The effects of oxytocin in the eye have been very little studied. The most prominent effect may be miosis when large doses are employed. The melanocyte-stimulating hormones have not been detected in the eye but exert effects both in the retina and in the anterior uvea. Finally, VIP has been localized to neurons in the eye originating in the pterygopalatine ganglion. These nerves innervate choroidal blood vessels as well as glandular tissue of the orbit, and may be involved in the regulation of choroidal and glandular tissue blood flow.

Acknowledgements. I would like to express my deep gratitude to Professor Marvin L. Sears for advice and criticism of the manuscript. I am also indebted to Mrs. Susan O'Hara for typing and library assistance. This work was supported in part by Fogarty International Research Fellowship I F05 TWO 2776-01 (Prof. Sears), and by USPHS grants EY-00237, EY-00785, the Connecticut Lions Eye Research Foundation Inc., and Research to Prevent Blindness Inc.

References

Abdel-Latif AA, Smith JP (1979) Distribution of arachidonic acid and other fatty acids in glycerolipids of the rabbit iris. Exp Eye Res 29:131–140

Abelson MB, Udell IJ (1981) H_2-receptors in the human ocular surface. Arch Ophthalmol 99:302–304

Abelson MB, Soter NA, Simon MA, Dohlman J, Allansmith MR (1977) Histamine in human tears. Am J Ophthalmol 83:417–418

Adolph AR (1966) Excitation and inhibition of electrical activity in the *Limulus* eye by neuropharmacological agents. In: Bernhard CG (ed) Funtional organization of the compound eye. Pergamon, New York, pp 465–482

Adolph A, Ehinger B (1975) Indolamines and the eccentric cells of the *Limulus* lateral eye. Cell Tiss Res 163:1–14

Adolph AR, Tuan FJ (1972) Serotonin and inhibition in *Limulus* lateral eye. J Gen Physiol 60:679–697

Al-Ghadyan A, Mead A, Sears M (1979) Increased pressure after paracentesis of the rabbit eye is completely accounted for by prostaglandin synthesis and release plus pupillary block. Invest Ophthalmol Vis Sci 18:361–365

Allansmith MR, Greiner JV, Baird RS (1978) Number of inflammatory cells in the normal conjunctiva. Am J Ophthalmol 86:250–259

Alm A, Bill A (1972) The oxygen supply to the retina. II. Effects of high intraocular pressure and of increased arterial carbon dioxide tension on uveal and retinal blood flow in cats. Acta Physiol Scand 84:306–319

Alm A, Bill A (1973) Ocular and optic nerve blood flow at normal and increased intraocular pressure in monkeys (*Macaca irus*): a study with radioactively labelled microspheres including flow determinations in brain and some other tissues. Exp Eye Res 15:15–29

Ambache N (1955) Irin, a smooth-muscle contracting substance present in rabbit iris. J Physiol (Lond) 129:65–66P

Ambache N (1956) Trigeminomimetic action of iris extracts in rabbits, J Physiol (Lond) 132:49–50P

Ambache N (1957) Properties of irin, a physiological constituent of the rabbit iris. J Physiol (Lond) 135:114–132

Ambache N (1959) Further studies on the preparation, purification and nature of irin. J Physiol (Lond) 146:255–294

Ambache N, Brummer HD (1968) A simple chemical procedure for distinguishing E from F prostaglandins, with application to tissue extracts. Br J Pharmacol Chemother 33:162–170

Ambache N, Kavanagh L, Whiting J (1965) Effect of mechanical stimulation on rabbits' eyes: release of active substances in anterior chamber perfusates. J Physiol (Lond) 176:378–408

Ambache N, Brummer HC, Rose JG, Whiting J (1966) Thin-layer chromatography of spasmogenic unsaturated hydroxy-acids from various tissues. J Physiol (Lond) 185:77–78

Ames A, Pollen DA (1969) Neurotransmission in central nervous tissue: a study of isolated rabbit retina. J Neurophysiol 32:424–442

Ängard E, Samuelsson B (1964) Smooth muscle stimulating lipids in sheep iris. The identification of prostaglandin $F_{2\alpha}$ prostaglandins and related factors 21. Biochem Pharmacol 13:281–283

Arvier PT, Chahl LA, Ladd RJ (1977) Modification by capsaicin and compound 48/80 of dye leakage induced by irritants in the rat. Br J Pharmacol 59:61–68

Ashton N, Cunha-Vaz JG (1965) Effect of histamine on the permeability of the ocular vessels. Arch Ophthalmol 73:211–223

Baker PC (1966a) Development of 5-hydroxytryptophan decarboxylase in the brain, eye, and whole embryo of *Xenopus laevis*. Neuroendocrinology 1:257–264

Baker PC (1966b) Monoamine oxidase in the eye, brain, and whole embryo of developing *Xenopus laevis*. Dev Biol 14:267–277

Baker PC, Quay WB (1969) 5-Hydroxytryptamine metabolism in early embryogenesis and the development of brain and retinal tissues, a review. Brain Res 12:273–295

Bauer B, Ehinger B (1980) Action of α-MSH on the release of neurotransmitters from the retina. Acta Phys Scand 180:105–107

Becker B (1960) The transport of organic anions by the rabbit eye. I. In vitro iodopyracet (Diodrast) accumulation by ciliary body-iris preparation. Am J Ophthalmol 50:862–867

Becker B, Christensen RE (1956) Beta-hypophamine (vasopressin), its effect upon intraocular pressure and aqueous flow in normal and glaucomatous eyes. Arch Ophthalmol 56:1–9

Behrens ME, Wulff VJ (1970) Neuropharmacological modification of response characteristics of sense cells in the *Limulus* lateral eye. Vision Res 10:679–689

Beitch BR, Eakins KE (1969) The effects of prostaglandins on the intraocular pressure of the rabbit. Br J Pharmacol 37:158–167

BenEzra D (1978) Neovasculogenic ability of prostaglandins, growth factors, and synthetic chemo-attractants. Am J Ophthalmol 86:455–461

Bengtsson E (1976) The effect of imidazole on the disruption of the blood-aqueous barrier in the rabbit eye. Invest Ophthalmol 15:315–320

Bengtsson E (1977) Interaction of adrenergic agents with α-melanocyte stimulating hormone and infrared irradiation of the iris in the rabbit eye. Invest Ophthalmol 16:209–217

Bengtsson E, Krakau CET, Öhman R (1975) The inhibiting effect of indomethacin on the disruption of the blood-aqueous barrier in the rabbit eye. With a technical note: Measurement of aqueous flare. Invest Ophthalmol 14:306–312

Berggren L (1970) Secretory activity in vitro of the rabbit eye ciliary processes incubated with corticosteroids, neurohypophyseal hormones and ascorbic acid. Acta Ophthalmol 48:284–292

Bernard C (1858) Leçons sur la physiologie et la pathologie du système nerveux, vol Z. Baillière, Paris, pp 96, 205

Bethel RA, Eakins KE (1972) The mechanism of the antagonism of experimentally induced ocular hypertension by polyphloretin phosphate. Exp Eye Res 13:83–91

Bettelheim H, Grabner G, Schuster H, Dudczak R, Lechner K, Niessner H, Valencak E (1980) Amaurosis Fugax Studien über Hämodynamik und Plättchenfunktion. Klin Monatsbl Augenheilkd 176:328–333

Bhattacherjee P (1974) Autoradiographic localization of intravitreally or intracamerally injected $[^3H]$-prostaglandins. Exp Eye Res 18:181–188

Bhattacherjee P (1975) Release of prostaglandin-like substances by *Shigella* endotoxin and its inhibition by non-steroidal anti-inflammatory compounds. Br J Pharmacol 54:489–494

Bhattacherjee P (1977) Stimulation of prostaglandin synthetase activity in inflamed ocular tissue of the rabbit. Exp Eye Res 24:215–216

Bhattacherjee P, Eakins KE (1974) Inhibition of prostaglandin synthetase systems in ocular tissues by indomethacin. Br J Pharmacol 50:227–230

Bhattacherjee P, Kulkarni PS, Eakins KE (1979) Metabolism of arachidonic acid in rabbit ocular tissues. Invest Ophthalmol Vis Sci 18:172–178

Bhattacherjee P, Hammond BR, Williams RN, Eakins KE (1980) Arachidonic acid lipoxygenase products in ocular tissues and their effect on leukocyte infiltration in vivo. Proc Int Soc Eye Res 1:32

Bhattacherjee P, Hammond B, Salmon JA, Stepney R, Eakins KE (1981) Chemotactic response to some arachidonic acid lipoxygenase products in the rabbit eye. Eur J Pharmacol 73:21–28

Bill A (1979) Effects of indomethacin on regional blood flow in conscious rabbits – a microsphere study. Acta Physiol Scand 105:437–442

Bill A, Stjernschantz J (1980) Cholinergic vasoconstrictor effects in the rabbit eye: vasomotor effects of pentobarbital anaesthesia. Acta Physiol Scand 108:419–424

Bill A, Stjernschantz J, Mandahl A, Brodin E, Nilsson G (1979) Substance P: release on trigeminal nerve stimulation, effects in the eye. Acta Physiol Scand 106:371–373

Binkhorst CD, Kats A, Tjan T, Loones LH (1976) Retinal accidents in pseudoaphakia. Intracapsular versus extracapsular surgery. Trans Am Acad Ophthalmol Otolaryngol 81:120–128

Bisette G, Manberg P, Nemeroff CB, Prange AJ Jr (1978) Mini-review. Neurotensin, a biologically active peptide. Life Sci 23:2173–2182

Bito LZ (1972a) Accumulation and apparent active transport of prostaglandins by some rabbit tissues in vitro. J Physiol (Lond) 221:371–387

Bito LZ (1972b) Comparative study of concentrative prostaglandin accumulation by various tissues of mammals and marine vertebrates and invertebrates. Comp Biochem Physiol 42A:65–82

Bito LZ (1973) Absorptive transport of prostaglandins from intraocular fluids to blood: a review of recent findings. Exp Eye Res 16:299–306

Bito LZ (1974) The effects of experimental uveitis ion anterior uveal prostaglandin transport and aqueous humor composition. Invest Ophthalmol 13:959–966

Bito LZ (1975) Saturable energy-dependent, transmembrane transport of prostaglandins against concentration gradients. Nature 256:134–136

Bito LZ, Salvador EV (1972) Intraocular fluid dynamics. III. The site and mechanism of prostaglandin transfer across the blood intraocular fluid barriers. Exp Eye Res 14:233–241

Bito LZ, Wallenstein MC (1977) Transport of prostaglandins across the blood-brain and blood-aqueous barriers and the physiological significance of these absorptive transport processes. Exp Eye Res [Suppl] 229–243

Bito LZ, Davson H, Hollingsworth J (1976) Facilitated transport of prostaglandins across the blood-cerebrospinal fluid and blood-brain barriers. J Physiol (London) 256:273–285

Bonne C, Lonchampt MO, Regnault F, Saint-Dizier D, Duhault J (1980) Plasma prostacyclin (PGI$_2$) in diabetic retinopathy. Proc Int Soc Eye Res 1:33

Borgeat P, Sirois P (1981) Leukotrienes: a major step in the understanding of immediate hypersensitivity reactions. J Med Chem 24:121–126

Brecha NC, Karten HJ, Laverack C (1979) Enkephalin-containing amacrine cells in the avian retina: immunohistochemical localization. Proc Natl Acad Sci USA 76:3010–3014

Brecha N, Karten HJ, Schenker C (1981) Neurotensin-like and somatostatin-like immunoreactivity within american cells of the retina. Neuroscience 6:1329–1340

Brückner R (1946) Über Histaminwirkung am Auge. Ophthalmologica 111:306–309

Bury RW, Mashford ML (1977) Substance P: its pharmacology and physiological roles. Aust J Exp Biol Med Sci 55:671–735

Butler JM, Hammond BR (1977) Effect of sensory denervation on the response of the rabbit eye to bradykinin and PGE$_1$. Trans Ophthalmol Soc UK 97:668–674

Butler JM, Hammond BR (1980) The effects of sensory denervation on the response of the rabbit eye to prostaglandin E$_1$, bradykinin and substance P. Br J Pharmacol 69:495–502

Butler JM, Powell D, Unger WG (1980a) Substance P levels in normal and sensorily denervated rabbit eyes. Exp Eye Res 30:311–313

Butler JM, Unger WG, Cole DF (1980b) Axon reflex in ocular injury: sensory mediation of the response of the rabbit eye to laser irradiation of the iris. Q J Exp Physiol 65:181–192

Camras CB, Bito LZ (1980a) The pathophysiological effects of nitrogen mustard on the rabbit eye. I. The biphasic intraocular pressure response and the role of prostaglandins. Exp Eye Res 30:41–52

Camras CB, Bito LZ (1980b) The pathophysiologic effects of nitrogen mustard on the rabbit eye. II. The inhibition of the initial hypertensive phase by capsaicin and the apparent role of substance P. Invest Ophthalmol Vis Sci 19:423–428

Camras CB, Bito LZ, Eakins KE (1977) Reduction of intraocular pressure by prostaglandins applied topically to the eyes of conscious rabbits. Invest Ophthalmol Vis Sci 16:1125–1134

Cardinali DP, Rosner JM (1971) Metabolism of serotonin by the rat retina in vitro. J Neurochem 18:1769–1770

Carraway R, Leeman SE (1973) The isolation of a new hypotensive peptide, neurotensin, from bovine hypothalami. J Biol Chem 248:6854–6861

Casey WJ (1974a) Prostaglandin E_2 and aqueous humor dynamics in the rhesus monkey eye. Prostaglandins 8:327–337

Casey WJ (1974b) The effect of prostaglandin E_2 on the rhesus monkey pupil. Prostaglandins 6:243–251

Castenholz A (1967) Beobachtungen und Analysen mikrozirkulatorischer Vorgänge am Rattenauge. II. Zur pharmakologischen Beeinflußbarkeit der Irisstrombahn, Albrecht von Graefes Arch Klin Exp Ophthalmol 172:326–345

Chiang TS (1974) Effects of intravenous infusions of histamine, 5-hydroxytryptamine, bradykinin and prostaglandins on intraocular pressure. Arch Int Pharmacodyn 207:131–138

Chiang TS, Thomas RP (1972a) Consensual ocular hypertensive response to prostaglandin. Invest Ophthalmol 11:169–176

Chiang TS, Thomas RP (1972b) Consensual ocular hypertensive response to prostaglandin E_2. Invest Ophthalmol 11:845–849

Chiang TS, Thomas RP (1972c) Ocular hypertension following intravenous infusion of prostaglandin E_1. Arch Ophthalmol 88:418–420

Christ EJ, van Dorp DA (1972) Comparative aspects of prostaglandin biosynthesis in animal tissues. Biochem Biophys Acta 270:537–545

Cohen S, Dusman E, Blumberg S, Teichberg VI (1981) In vitro contraction of the pupillary sphincter by substance P and its stable analogs. Invest Ophthalmol Vis Sci 20:717–721

Cole DF (1961) Prevention of experimental ocular hypertension with polyphloretin phosphate. Br J Ophthalmol 45:482–489

Cole DF (1974) The site of breakdown of the blood-aqueous barrier under the influence of vasodilator drugs. Exp Eye Res 19:591–607

Cole DF, Nagasubramanian S (1972) The effect of natural and synthetic vasopressins and other substances on active transport in ciliary epithelium of the rabbit. Exp Eye Res 13:45–57

Cole DF, Nagasubramanian S (1973) Substances affecting active transport across the ciliary epithelium and their possible role in determining intraocular pressure. Exp Eye Res 16:251–264

Cole DF, Unger WG (1973) Prostaglandins as mediators for the responses of the eye to trauma. Exp Eye Res 17:357–368

Cole DF, Unger WG (1974) Action of bradykinin on intraocular pressure and pupillary diameter. Ophthalmol Res 6:308–314

Conquet PH, Plazonnet B, LeDouarec JC (1975) Arachidonic acid-induced elevation of intraocular pressure and anti-inflammatory agents. Invest Ophthalmol 14:772–775

Constant MA, Becker B (1956) Experimental tonography. II. The effects of vasopressin, chlorpromazine and phentolamine methanesulfonate. Arch Ophthalmol 56:19–25

Correa FMA, Innis RB, Uhl GR, Snyder SH (1979) Bradykinin-like immunoreactive neuronal systems localized histochemically in rat brain. Proc Natl Acad Sci USA 76:1489–1493

Crawford CG, van Alphen GWHM, Cook HW, Lands WEM (1978) The effect of precursors, products, and product analogs of prostaglandin cyclooxygenase upon iris sphincter muscle. Life Sci 23:1255–1262

Dalske HF (1974) Pharmacological reactivity of isolated ciliary arteries. Invest Ophthalmol 13:389–392

Davies BN, Horton EW, Withrington PG (1968) The occurrence of prostaglandin E_2 in splenic venous blood of the dog following splenic nerve stimulation. Br J Pharmacol 32:127–135

Davis TME, Mitchell MD, Dornan TL, Turner RC (1980) Plasma 6-keto-$PGF_{1\alpha}$ concentrations and diabetic retinopathy. Lancet I:8164

Davson H, Huber A (1950) Experimental hypertensive uveitis in the rabbit. Ophthalmologica 120:118–124

Desy L, Pelletier G (1978) Immunohistochemical localization of alphamelanocyte stimulating hormone (α-MSH) in the human hypothalamus. Brain Res 154:377–381

Dhir SP, Garg SK, Sharma YR, Lath NK (1978) Prostaglandins in human tears. Am J Ophthalmol 87:403–404

DiBenedetto FE, Bito LZ (1980) Accumulation and apparent active transport of prostacyclin (PGI_2) and thromboxane B_2 (TxB_2) by the anterior uvea and prostaglandin $F_{2\alpha}$ ($PGF_{2\alpha}$) by the retina-choroid. Proct Int Soc Eye Res 1:19

Dick E, Miller R (1980) Opioids and substance P influence ganglion cells in amphibian retina. Invest Ophthalmol Vis Sci [Suppl] 19:132

Dietze U, Tilgner S (1973) Reversible Linsentrübungen bei Wistarratten nach einmaliger Applikation von Serotonin. Ophthalmologica 166:76–80

Dietze U, Tilgner S, Schröder K-D (1974) Einfluß des Lidschlusses auf die Ausbildung der reversiblen Serotonin Katarakt der Ratte. Ophthalmologica 168:230–237

Djamgoz MBA, Stell WK, Chin CA, Lam DMK (1981) An opiate system in the goldfish retina. Nature 292:620–623

Dollery CT, Friedman LA, Hensby CN, Kohner E, Lewis PJ, Porta M, Webster J (1979) Circulating prostacyclin may be reduced in diabetes. Lancet II:8156–8157

Dubé D, Lissitzky JC, Leulerc R, Pelletier G (1978) Localization of α-melanocyte stimulating hormone in rat brain and pituitary. Endocrinology 102:1283–1291

Duffin RM, Christensen RE, Bergamini MVW (1981) Suppression of adrenergic adaptation in the eye with a prostaglandin synthesis inhibitor. Invest Ophthalmol Vis Sci 21:756–759

Düner H, von Euler US, Pernow B (1954) Catecholamines and substance P in the mammalian eye. Acta Phys Scand 31:113–118

Duke-Elder PM, Duke-Elder WS (1931) The vascular responses of the eye. Proc R Soc Lond [Biol] 109:19–28

Dyster-Aas HK (1965) A comparison between the aqueous flare inducing effect of α-melanocyte stimulating hormone and a minimal trauma. Acta Ophthalmol 43:30–46

Dyster-Aas HK, Krakau CET (1964a) Aqueous flow determination in the rabbit by means of a minimal eye trauma. Invest Ophthalmol 3:127–134

Dyster-Aas HK, Krakau CET (1964b) Increased permeability of the blood-aqueous humor barrier in the rabbit's eye provoked by melanocyte-stimulating peptides. Endocrinology 74:255–265

Eakins KE (1970) Increased intraocular pressure produced by prostaglandins E_1 and E_2 in the cat eye. Exp Eye Res 10:87–92

Eakins KE (1977) Prostaglandin and non-prostaglandin mediated breakdown of the blood-aqueous barrier. Exp Eye Res [Suppl] 483–498

Eakins KE, Bhattacherjee P (1977) Histamine, prostaglandins and ocular inflammation. Exp Eye Res 24:299–305

Eakins KE, Whitelock RAF, Perkins ES, Bennett A, Unger WG (1972a) Release of prostaglandins in ocular inflammation in the rabbit. Nature 239:248–249

Eakins KE, Whitelock RAF, Bennett A, Martenet AC (1972b) Prostaglandin-like activity in ocular inflammation. Br Med J 19:452–453

Eakins KE, Atwal M, Bhattacherjee P (1974) Inactivation of prostaglandin E_1 by ocular tissues in vitro. Exp Eye Res 19:141–146

Eakins KE, Stier C, Bhattacherjee P, Greenbaum LM (1976) Actions and interactions of bradykinin, prostaglandins and nonsteroidal anti-inflammatory agents on the eye. Inflammation 1:117–125

Ehinger B (1973) Localization of the uptake of prostaglandin E_1 in the eye. Exp Eye Res 17:43–47

Ehinger B (1976) Biogenic amines as transmitters in the retina. In: Bonting SL (ed) Transmitters in the visual process. Pergamon, Oxford, pp 145–163

Ehinger B, Florén I (1976) Indolamine-accumulating neurons in the retina of rabbit, cat and goldfish. Cell Tiss Res 175:37–48

Ehinger B, Florén I (1978) Quantitation of the uptake of indolamines and dopamine in the rabbit retina. Exp Eye Res 26:1–11

Ehinger B, Florén I (1979) Absence of indolamine-accumulating neurons in the retina of humans and cynomolgus monkeys. Albrecht von Graefes Arch Klin Exp Ophthalmol 209:145–153

Ehinger B, Hansson C, Törnquist K (1981) 5-Hydroxytryptamine in the retina of some mammals. Exp Eye Res 33:663–672

Eiden LE, Brownstein MJ (1981) Extrahypothalamic distribution and functions of hypothalamic peptide hormones. Fed Proc 40:2553–2559

Eliason JA (1978) Leukocytes and experimental corneal vascularization. Invest Ophthalmol Vis Sci 17:1087–1095

Engberg G, Svensson TH, Rosell S, Folkers K (1981) A synthetic peptide as an antagonist of substance P. Nature 293:222–223

Eriksen EF, Larsson LI (1981) Neuropeptides in the retina: evidence for differential topographical localization. Peptides 2:153–157

Eskay RL, Long RT, Iuvone PM (1980) Evidence that TRH, somatostatin and substance P are present in neurosecretory elements of the vertebrate retina. Brain Res 196:554–559

Eskay RL, Furness JF, Long RT (1981) Substance P activity in the bullfrog retina: localization and identification in several vertebrate species. Science 212:1049–1051

Florén I (1979) Indolamine accumulating neurons in the retina of chicken and pigeon. A comparison with the dopaminergic neurons. Acta Ophthalmol 7:198–210

Florén I, Hansson HC (1980) Investigations into whether 5-hydroxytryptamine is a neurotransmitter in the retina of rabbit and chicken. Invest Ophthalmol Vis Sci 19:117–125

Flower RJ, Blackwell GJ (1979) Anti-inflammatory steroids induce biosynthesis of a phospholipase A_2 inhibitor which prevents prostaglandin generation. Nature 278:456–459

Folkers K, Horig J, Rosell S, Bjorkroth U (1981) Chemical design of antagonists of substance P. Acta Physiol Scand 111:505–506

Forbes M, Becker B (1960) The transport of organic anions by the rabbit eye. II. In vivo transport of iodopyracet (Diodrast). Am J Ophthalmol 50:867–873

Friedenwald JS, Pierce HF (1930) The pathogenesis of acute glaucoma. Arch Ophthalmol 3:574–582

Fromer CH, Klintworth GK (1975a) An evaluation of the role of leukocytes in the pathogenesis of experimentally induced corneal vascularization. I. Comparison of experimental models of corneal vascularization. Am J Pathol 79:537–554

Fromer CH, Klintworth GK (1975b) An evaluation of the role of leukocytes in the pathogenesis of experimentally induced corneal vascularization. II. Studies on the effect of leukocyte elimination on corneal vascularization. II. Studies on the effect of leukocyte elimination on corneal vascularization. Am J Pathol 81:531–544

Fromer CH, Klintworth GK (1976) An evaluation of the role of leukocytes in the pathogenesis of experimentally induced corneal vascularization. III. Studies related to the vasoproliferative capability of polymorphonuclear leukocytes and lymphocytes. Am J Pathol 82:157–170

Gamse R, Leeman SE, Holzer P, Lembeck F (1981) Differential effects of capsaicin on the content of somatostatin, substance P, and neurotensin in the nervous system of the rat. Naunyn Schmiedebergs Arch Pharmacol 317:140–148

Gass JD, Norton EWD (1969) Follow-up study of cystoid macular edema following cataract extraction. Trans Am Acad Opthalmol Otolaryngol 73:665–681

Gifford H (1910) On the treatment of sympathetic ophthalmia by large doses of salicylate of sodium, aspirin, or other salicylic compounds. Ophthalmoscope 8:257–258

Gilmore N, Vane JR, Wyllie JH (1968) Prostaglandin release by the spleen. Nature 218:1135–1140

Glickman RD, Adolph AR (1982) Acetylcholine and substance P: action via distinct receptors on carp retinal ganglion cells. Invest Ophthalmol Vis Sci 22:804–808

Glickman R, Adolph AR, Dowling JE (1980) Does substance P have a physiological role in the carp retina? Invest Ophthalmol Vis Sci 19 [Suppl] 281

Gloster J (1961) Influence of facial nerve on intraocular pressure. Br J Ophthalmol 45:259–278

Gralla EJ, Rubin L (1970) Ocular studies with para-chlorophenylalanine in rats and monkeys. Arch Ophthalmol 83:734–740

Green K (1973) Permeability properties of the ciliary epithelium in response to prostaglandins. Invest Ophthalmol 12:752–758

Green K, Kim K (1975) Pattern of ocular response to topical and systemic prostaglandin. Invest Ophthalmol 14:36–40

Green K, Padgett D (1979) Effect of various drugs on pseudofacility and aqueous humor formation in the rabbit eye. Exp Eye Res 28:239–246

Günther G (1956) Über das Vorkommen von Gewebsmastzellen am menschlichen Auge und seiner Adnexe bei pathologischen Zuständen. Ber Zusammenkunft Dtsch Ophthalmol Ges 59:278–281

Gustafsson L, Hedquist P, Lagercrantz H (1975) Potentiation by prostaglandns E_1, E_2, and $F_{2\alpha}$ of the contraction response to transmural stimulation in the bovine iris sphincter muscle. Acta Physiol Scand 95:26–33

Gustafsson L, Hedquist P, Lundgren G (1980) Pre- and post-junctional effects of prostaglandin E_2, prostaglandin synthetase inhibitors and atropine on cholinergic neurotransmission in guinea pig ileum and bovine iris. Acta Physiol Scand 110:401–411

Häggendal J, Malmfors T (1965) Identification and cellular localization of the catecholamines in the retina and the choroid of the rabbit. Acta Physiol Scand 64:58–66

Harrison HE, Reece AH, Johnson M (1978) Decreased vascular prostacyclin in experimental diabetes. Life Sci 23:351–356

Harrison HE, Reece AH, Johnson M (1980) Effect of insulin treatment on prostacyclin in experimental diabetes. Diabetologica 18:65–68

Harrison MJG, Marshall J, Meadows JC, Ross Russell RW (1971) Effect of aspirin in amaurosis fugax. Lancet II:743–744

Hauschild D, Laties AM (1973) An indolamine-containing cell in chick retina. Invest Ophthalmol 12:537–540

Hedquist P (1969) Modulating effect of prostaglandin E_2 on noradrenalin release from the isolated cat spleen. Acta Physiol Scand 75:511–512

Hedquist P (1973) Autonomic neurotransmission. In: Ramwell P (ed) Prostaglandins vol I. Plenum, New York pp 101–131

Hedquist P, Stjärne L, Wennmalm Å (1971) Facilitation of sympathetic neurotransmission in the cat spleen after inhibition of prostaglandin synthetase. Acta Physiol Scand 83:430–432

Held H, Heizmann A, Lembeck F, Schlote W (1966) Substanz P in der Retina. Naunyn Schmiedebergs Arch Exp Path Pharm 253:246–259

Higgs GA, Youlten LJF (1972) Prostaglandin production by rabbit peritoneal polymorphonuclear leukocytes in vitro. Br J Pharmacol 44:330P

Hillier K, Embrey MP (1972) High dose intravenous administration of PGE_2 and $PGF_{2\alpha}$ for the termination of mid-trimester pregnancies. J Obstet Gynaecol Br Comm 79:14–22

Hitchings RA, Chisholm IH, Bird AC (1975) Aphakic macular edema: incidence and pathogenesis. Invest Ophthalmol 14:68–72

Hökfelt T, Johansson O, Luft R, Arimura A (1975) Immunohistochemical evidence for the presence of somatostatin, a powerful inhibitory peptide, in some primary sensory neurons. Neurosci Lett 1:231–235

Hökfelt T, Elde R, Johansson O, Luft R, Nilsson G, Arimura A (1976) Immunohistochemical evidence for separate populations of somatostatin-containing and substance P-containing primary afferent neurons. Neuroscience 1:131–136

Hökfelt T, Elfvin L-G, Schultzberg M, Goldstein M, Nilsson G (1977a) On the occurrence of substance P-containing fibers in sympathetic ganglia: immunohistochemical evidence. Brain Res 132:29–41

Hökfelt T, Johansson O, Kellerth J-O, Ljungdahl Å, Nilsson G, Nygårds A, Pernow B (1977b) Immunohistochemical distribution of substance P. In: Von Euler US, Pernow B (eds) Substance P. Raven, New York, pp 117–145

Hökfelt T, Johansson O, Ljungdahl A, Lundberg JM, Schultzberg M (1980) Peptidergic neurons. Nature 284:515–521

Holmdahl G, Håkansson R, Leander S, Rosell S, Folkers K, Sundler F (1981) A substance P antagonist [D-Pro^2, D-Trp^{7,9}]-SP inhibits inflammatory responses in the rabbit eye. Science 214:1029–1032

Holmes SW, Horton EW (1968) Prostaglandins and the central nervous system, In: Ramwell PW, Shaw JE (eds) Prostaglandin symposium of the Worcester Foundation for Experimental Biology. Intersience, New York, pp 21–38

Holmgren H, Stenbeck A (1940) Frequency of mast cells in human eyes in different pathological conditions. Acta Ophthalmol 18:271–294

Horowitz JD (1981) The effects of neurohypophyseal peptides on the intraocular pressure and pupil of the rabbit. Dissertation, Yale University School of Medicine

Horowitz J, Gregory D, Sears M (to be published) Neurohypophyseal peptides and the eye: use of synthetic analogs in analyzing effects on pupil and intraocular pressure. Albrecht Von Graefes Arch Klin Exp Ophthalmol

Houle RE, Grant WM (1967) Alcohol, vasopressin and intraocular pressure. Invest Ophthalmol 6:145–154

Humbert J, Pradelles P, Cros C, Dray F (1979) Enkephalin-like products in embryonic chicken retina. Neurosci Lett 12:259–263

Igíc R, Kojović V (1980) Angiotensin I converting enzyme (kininase II) in ocular tissues. Exp Eye Res 30:299–303

Igie R, Robinson CJG, Erdös EG (1977) Angiotensin I converting enzyme activity in the choroid plexus and in the retina. In: Bucklye JP, Ferrario CM (eds) Central actions of angiotensin and related hormones. Pergamon, New York, pp 23–27

Ikemoto F, Yamamoto K (1978) Renin-angiotensin system in the aqueous humor of rabbits, dogs and monkeys. Exp Eye Res 27:723–725

Irvine AR, Bresky R, Crowder BB (1971) Macular edema after cataract extraction. Ann Ophthalmol 3:1234–1240

Jackson IMD, Reichlin S (1977) Thyrotropin releasing hormone: abundance in the skin of the frog, *Rana pipiens*. Science 198:414–415

Jacobowitz DM, O'Donohue TL (1978) Alpha-melanocyte stimulating hormone–immunohistochemical identification and mapping in neurons of rat brain. Proc Nat Acad Sci 75:6300–6304

Jacobson DR, Dellaporta A (1974) Natural history of cystoid macular edema after cataract extraction. Am J Ophthalmol 77:445–447

Jampol LM, Neufeld AH, Sears ML (1975) Pathways for the response of the eye to injury. Invest Ophthalmol 14:184–189

Jessel TM, Iversen LL (1976) Opiate analgesics inhibit substance P release from rat trigeminal nucleus. Nature 268:549–551

Jessel TM, Iversen LL, Cuello AC (1978) Capsaicin-induced depletion of substance P from primary sensory neurons. Brain Res 152:183–188

Johnson M, Harrison HE, Raftery AT, Elder JB (1979) Vascular prostacyclin may be reduced in diabetes in man. Lancet I:325–326

Jorpes E, Holmgren H, Wilander O (1937) Über das Vorkommen von Heparin in den Gefäßwänden und in den Augen. Z Mikrosk Anat Forsch 42:279–290

Kanazawa I, Jessel T (1976) Postmortem changes and regional distribution of substance P in the rat an mouse nervous system. Brain Res 117:362–367

Karten JH, Brecha N (1980) Localization of substance P immunoreactivity in amacrine cells of the retina. Nature 283:87–88

Kass MA, Holmberg NJ (1979) Prostaglandin and thromboxane synthesis by microsomes of rabbit ocular tissues. Invest Ophthalmol Vis Sci 18:166–171

Kass MA, Sears ML (1977) Review. Hormonal regulation of intraocular pressure. Surv Ophthalmol 22:153–176

Kass MA, Podos SM, Moses RA, Becker B (1972) Prostaglandin E_1 and aqueous humor dynamics. Invest Ophthalmol 11:1022–1027

Kass MA, Neufeld AH, Sears ML (1975) Systemic aspirin and indomethacin do not prevent the response of the monkey eye to trauma. Invest Ophthalmol 14:604–606

Kelly RGM, Starr MS (1971) Effects of prostaglandins and a prostaglandin antagonist on intraocular pressure and protin in the monkey eye. Can J Ophthal 6:205–211

Kiernan JA (1975) A pharmacological and histological investigation of the involvement of mast cells in cutaneous axon reflex vasodilatation. Q J Exp Physiol 60:123–130

Klein RM, Katzin HM, Yanuzzi LA (1979) The effect of indomethacin pretreatment of aphakic cystoid macular edema. Am J Ophthalmol 87:487–489

Krisch B, Leonhardt H (1979) Demonstration of somatostatin-like activity in retinal cells of the rat. Cell Tissue Res 204:127–140

Krupin T, Oestrich C, Podos SM, Becker B (1976) Increased intraocular pressure after third ventricle injections of prostaglandin E_1 and arachidonic acid. Am J Ophthalmol 81:346–350

Kuehl FA, Egan RW (1980) Prostaglandins, arachidonic acid and inflammation. Science 210:978–984

Kulkarni PS (1981) Synthesis of cyclo-oxygenase products by human anterior uvea from cyclic prostaglandin endoperoxide (PGH_2). Exp Eye Res 32:197–204

Kulkarni PS, Eakins KE (1977) The enzymatic conversion of prostaglandin endoperoxides to thromboxane-A_2-like activity in human iris microsomes. Prostaglandins 14:601–605

Kulkarni PS, Srinivasan BD (1981) Comparative effects of intravitreal cyclooxygenase products on intraocular inflammation. Invest Ophthalmol Vis Sci [Suppl] 32

Kulkarni PS, Eakins HMT, Saber WL, Eakins KE (1977) Microsomal preparations of normal bovine iris-ciliary body generate prostacyclin-like but not thromboxane-A_2-like activity. Prostaglandins 14:689–700

Kulkarni PS, Bhattacherjee P, Eakins KE, Srinivasan BD (1981) Anti-inflammatory effects of betamethasone phosphate, dexamethasone phosphate and indomethacin on rabbit ocular inflammation induced by bovine serum albumin. Curr Eye Res 1:43–47

Lake N, Patel YC (1980) Neurotoxic agents reduce retinal somatostatin. Brain Res 181:234–236

Larsen G (1959) The mast cells of the uveal tract of the eye and changes induced by hormones and avitaminosic-C. Am J Ophthalmol 47:509–519

Larsen G (1961) Experimental uveitis. Acta Ophthalmol 39:231–258

Larsson S (1930) Über den Augendruck und die vorderen intraokularen Gefäße. Norstedt, Stockholm

Laties AM, Neufeld AH, Vegge T, Sears ML (1976) Differential reactivity of rabbit iris and ciliary process to topically applied prostaglandin E_2 (Dinoprostone). Arch Ophthalmol 94:1966–1971

Laties AM, Stone RA, Brecha NC (1981) Substance P-like immunoreactive nerve fibers in the trabecular meshwork. Invest Ophthalmol Vis Sci 21:484–486

Leander S, Håkazson R, Rosell S, Folkers K, Sundler F, Törnquist K (1981) A specific substance P anatagonist blocks smooth muscle contractions induced by non-cholinergic, non-adrenergic nerve stimulation. Nature 294:467–469

Leeman SE, Carraway R (1977) Substance P and neurotensin. In: Gainer H (ed) Peptides in neurobiology. Plenum, New York, pp 99–144

Lembeck F, Holzer P (1979) Substance P as a neurogenic mediator of antidromic vasodilation and neurogenic plasma extravasation. Naunyn Schmiedebergs Arch Pharmacol 310:175¹83

Levene RZ (1962) Mast cells and amines in normal ocular tissue. Invest Ophthalmol 1:531–543

Leydhecker W, Krieglstein GK, Uhlich E (1978) Experimentelle Untersuchungen zur Wirkungsweise alkoholischer Getränke auf den Augeninnendruck. Klin Monatsbl Augenheilkd 172:75–79

Linder J (1981) Effects of facial nerve section and stimulation on cerebral and ocular blood flow in hemorrhagic hypotension. Acta Physiol Scand 112:185–193

Loren I, Törnquist K, Alumets J (1980) VIP (vasoactive intestinal polypeptide) – immunoreactive neurons in the retina of the rat. Cell Tissue Res 210:167–170

Magendie F (1824) De l'influence de la cinquième paire de nerfs sur la nutrition et les fonctions de l'oeil. J Physiol Exp Path 4:176–182, 302–315

Mancillas JR, McGinty JF, Selverston AI, Karten H, Bloom FE (1981) Immunocytochemical localization of enkephalin and substance P in retina and eyestalk neurones of lobster. Nature 293:576–578

Mandahl A, Bill A (1980) Effects of substance P, PGE_2 and capsaicin on the pupillae sphincter, modification by tetrodotoxin. Acta Physiol Scand 109:26

Mandahl A, Bill A (1981) Ocular responses to antidromic trigeminal stimulation, intracameral prostaglandin E_1 and E_2, capsaicin and substance P. Acta Physiol Scand 112:331–338

Marshak DW, Yamada T, Basinger SF, Walsh JH, Stell WK (1979) Characterization of immunoreactive somatostatin in retina. Invest Ophthalmol Vis Sci [Suppl] 85

Martino E, Nardi M, Vaudagna G, Simonetti S, Cilotti A, Pinchera A (1980) Presence of thyrotropin-releasing hormone in porcine and bovine retina. Experientia 36:622–623

Masuda K, Mishima S (1973) Effects of prostaglandins on inflow and outflow of the aqueous humor in rabbits. Jpn J Ophthalmol 17:300–309

Masuda K, Izawa Y, Mishima S (1973) Prostaglandins and uveitis: a preliminary report. Jpn J Ophthalmol 17:166–170

Masuda K, Izawa Y, Mishima S (1975) Prostaglandins and glaucomatocyclitic crisis. Jpn J Ophthalmol 19:368–375

Maul E, Sears ML (1979) ATP is released into the rabbit eye by antidromic stimulation of the trigeminal nerve. Invest Ophthalmol Vis Sci 18:256–262

Maurice DM (1954) Constriction of the pupil in the rabbit by antidromic stimulation of the trigeminal nerve. J Physiol [Lond] 123:45–46

Meyers RL, Shabo AL, Maxwell DS (1975) Effect of prostaglandin on the blood-aqueous barrier in the rabbit ciliary process. Prostaglandins 9:167–173

Miller A, Costa M, Furness JB, Chubb IW (1981) Substance P immunoreactive sensory nerves supply the rat iris and cornea. Neurosci Lett 23:243–249

Miller JD, Eakins KE, Atwal M (1973) The release of PGE_2-like activity into aqueous humor after paracentesis and its prevention by aspirin. Invest Ophthalmol 12:939–942

Mishima S, Masuda K (1977) Clinical implication of prostaglandins and synthesis inhibitors. Leopold IH, Burns RP (eds) Symposium on ocular therapy, vol 10. Wiley, New York, pp 1–19

Miyake K (1977) Prevention of cystoid macular edema after lens extraction by topical indomethacin. I. A preliminary report. Albrecht von Graefes Arch Klin Exp Ophthalmol 203:81–88

Miyake K (1978) Prevention of cystoid macular edema after lens extraction by topical indomethacin. II. A control study in bilateral extractions. Jpn J Ophthalmol 22:80–94

Miyake K, Sugiyama S, Norimatsu I (1978) Prevention of cystoid macular edema after lens extraction by topical indomethacin. III. Radioimmunoassay measurement of prostaglandins in the aqueous during and after lens extraction procedures. Albrecht von Graefes Arch Klin Exp Ophthalmol 209:83–88

Miyake K, Shizuko S, Hana M (1980) Long-term follow-up study on prevention of aphakic cystoid macular edema by topical indomethacin. Br J Ophthalmol 64:324–328

Moncada S, Flower RJ, Vane JR (1980) Prostaglandins, prostacyclin and thromboxane A_2. In: Goodman A, Gilman LS (eds) The pharmacological basis of therapeutics 6th edn. MacMillan, New York, pp 668–681

Moore RY, Heller A, Wurtman RJ, Axelrod J (1967) Visual pathway mediating pineal response to environmental light. Science 155:220–223

Moses R, Holekamp TLR (1971) Evidence against mediation of ocular lesion by exposure, histamine, or serotonin following fifth nerve injury in rats. Am J Ophthalmol 71:574–577

Mudge AW, Leeman SE, Fischbach GD (1979) Enkephalin inhibits release of substance P from sensory neurons in culture and decreases action potential duration. Proc Natl Acad Sci USA 76:526–530

Mundall J, von Kaulla KN, Austin JH (1971) Effect of aspirin in amaurosis fugax. Lancet I:92

Mundall J, Quintero P, von Kaulla KN, Harmon R, Austin J (1972) Transient monocular blindness and increased platelet aggregability treated with aspirin. Neurology 22:280–285

Münz H, Stumpf WE, Jennes L (1981) LHRH systems in the brain of platyfish. Brain Res 221:1–13

Nagasubramanian S (1974) The effect of vasopressin on the facility of aqueous humour outflow in the rabbit, Ophthalmol Res 6:301–307

Nagasubramanian S (1977) Role of pituitary vasopressin in the formation and dynamics of aqueous humour. Trans Ophthalmol Soc UK 97:686–701

Nakano J, Chang ACK, Fisher RG (1973) Effects of prostaglandins E_1, E_2, A_1, A_2, and $F_{2\alpha}$ on canine carotid arterial blood flow, cerebrospinal fluid pressure, and intraocular pressure. J Neurosurg 38:32–39

Nemeroff C, Bisette G, Prange A, Loosen P, Barlow T, Lipton M (1977) Neurotensin: central nervous system effects of a hypothalmic peptide. Brain Res 128:485–496

Neufeld AH, Page ED (1975) Regulation of adrenergic neuromuscular transmission in the rabbit iris. Exp Eye Res 20:549–561

Neufeld AH, Sears ML (1973) The site of action of prostaglandin E_2 on the disruption of the blood-aqueous barrier in the rabbit eye. Exp Eye Res 17:445–448

Neufeld AH, Jampol LM, Sears ML (1972) Aspirin prevents the disruption of the blood-aqueous barrier in the rabbit eye. Nature 238:158–159

Neufeld AH, Chavis RM, Sears ML (1973) Degeneration release of norepinephrine causes transient ocular hyperemia mediated by prostaglandins. Invest Ophthalmol 12:167–175

Neufeld AH, Dueker DK, Vegge T, Sears ML (1975) Adenosine 3′,5′-monophosphate increases the outflow of aqueous humour from the rabbit eye. Invest Ophthalmol 14:40–42

Nicoll RA, Schenker C, Leeman SE (1980) Substance P as a transmitter candidate. Ann Rev Neurosci 3:327–368

Niederer W, Richardson BP, Donatsch P (1975) Hormonal control of aqueous humour production. Exp Eye Res 20:329–340

Nilaver G, Zimmermann EA, Wilkins J, Michaels J, Hoffman D, Silverman A-J (1980) Magnocellular hypothalamic projections to the lower brain stem and spinal cord of the rat. Immunocytochemical evidence for predominance of the oxytocin neurophysin system compared to the vasopressin-neurophysin system. Neuroendocrinology 30:150–158

Nilsson S, Bill A (1979) Effect of the vasoactive intestinal polypeptide on the intraocular pressure (IOP) and regional blood flow. Acta Physiol Scand 108:51

Nilsson S, Linder J, Bill A (1980) Effects of facial nerve stimulation on ocular blood flow and the intraocular pressure (IOP) in the cynomolgus monkey. Acta Physiol Scand 109:26

Nishiyama A, Masuda K, Mochizuki M (1981 a) Ocular effects of substance P. Jpn J Ophthalmol 25:362–369

Nishiyama A, Masuda K, Mochizuki M (1981 b) Ocular effects of vasoactive intestinal polypeptide. Invest Ophthal Vis Sci 20 [Suppl]:64

Ohtsuki K, Minzuno K, Sears ML (1975) Disruption of the blood-aqueous barrier demonstrated by histofluorescence microscopy. Jpn J Ophthalmol 19:153–165

Okisaka S (1976) The effects of prostaglandin E_1 on the ciliary epithelium and the drainage angle of cynomologus monkeys: a light- and electron-microscopic study. Exp Eye Res 22:141–154

Olgart L, Gazelius B, Brodin E, Nilsson G (1977) Release of substance P-like immunoreactivity from the dental pulp. Acta Physiol Scand 101:510–512

Osborne NN (1980) In vitro experiments on the metabolism uptake and release of 5-hydroxytryptamine in bovine retina. Brain Res 184:283–297

Osborne NN, Nicholas DA, Cuello AC, Dockray GJ (1981) Localization of cholecystokinin immunoreactivity in amacrine cells of the retina. Neurosci Lett 26:31–35

O'Steen WK (1970) Retinal and optic nerve serotonin and retinal degeneration as influenced by photoperiod. Exp Neurol 27:194–205

O'Steen WK, Vaughan GM (1968) Radioactivity in the optic pathway and hypothalamus of the rat after intraocular injection of tritiated 5-hydroxytryptophan. Brain Res 8:209–212

Payot P (1946) Über die Beeinflussung der Histamin-Chemosis des Kaninchens durch Anästhetika. Ophthalmologica 112:25–38

Paterson CA, Pfister RR (1975) Prostaglandin-like activity in the aqueous humor following alkali burns. Invest Ophthalmol 14:177–183

Pedersen OØ (1975a) Electron microscopic studies on the blood-aqueous barrier of prostaglandin-treated rabbit eyes. I. Iridial and ciliary processes. Acta Ophthalmol 53:685–698

Pedersen OØ (1975b) Electron microscopic studies on the blood-aqueous barrier of prostaglandin-treated rabbit eyes. II. Iris. Acta Ophthalmol 53:699–709

Pedersen OØ, Tønjum AM (1975) In vitro studies on peroxidase movement in the epithelium of prostaglandin-treated rabbit ciliary bodies. Acta Ophthalmol 53:673–684

Pelletier G, Dubé D (1977) Electron microscopic immunohistochemical localization of α-MSH in the rat brain. Am J Anat 150:201–205

Perkins ES (1957) Influence of fifth cranial nerve on the intraocular pressure of the rabbit eye. Br J Ophthalmol 41:257–300

Perkins ES, McFaul PA (1965) Indomethacin in the treatment of uveitis: a double blind trial. Trans Ophthalmol Soc UK 85:53–58

Peyman GA, Bennett TO, Vlchek J (1975) Effects of intravitreal prostaglandins on retinal vasculature. An Ophthalmol 7:279–288

Pickard JD, Mackenzie ET (1973) Inhibition of prostaglandin synthesis and the response of baboon cerebral circulation to carbon dioxide. Nature 245:187–188

Pintér E, Takáts I, Trombitás K, Tigyi-Sebes A (1978) Effect of prostaglandin E_2 on the permeability of the iris vessels to horseradish peroxidase in the rabbit. Albrecht von Graefes Arch Klin Exp Ophthalmol 207:221–228

Podos SM, Becker B, Kass MA (1973a) Prostaglandin synthesis, inhibition and intraocular pressure. Invest Ophthalmol 12:426–433

Podos SM, Becker B, Kass MA (1973b) Indomethacin blocks arachidonic acid-induced elevation of intraocular pressure. Prostaglandins 3:7–15

Posner J (1973) Prostaglandin E_2 and the bovine sphincter pupillae. Br J Pharmacol 49:415–427

Pournaras C, Tsacopoulos M, Chapuis PH (1978) Studies on the role of prostaglandins in the regulation of retinal blood flow. Exp Eye Res 26:687–697

Pradelles P, Cros C, Humbert J, Dray F, Ben-Ari Y (1979) Visual deprivation decreases metenkephalin and substance P content of various forebrain structures. Brain Res 116:191–193

Quay WB (1965a) Indole derivatives of pineal and related neural and retinal tissues. Pharmacol Rev 17:321–345

Quay WB (1965b) Retinal and pineal hydroxyindole-o-methyl transferase activity in vertebrates. Life Sci 4:983–991

Rahi A, Bhattacherjee P, Misra R (1978) Release of prostaglandins in experimental immune complex endophthalmitis and phacoallergic uveitis. Br J Ophthalmol 62:105–109

Reubi JC, Jessel TM (1978) Distribution of substance P in the pigeon brain. J Neurochem 31:359–361

Rorstadt OP, Brownstein MJ, Martin JB (1979) Immunoreactive and biologically active somatostatin-like material in rat retina. Proc Natl Acad Sci USA 76:3019–3023

Rosell S, Olgart L, Gazelius B, Panopoulos P, Folkers K, Hörig J (1981) Inhibition of antidromic and substance P-induced vasodilation by a substance P antagonist. Acta Physiol Scand 111:381–382

Ruskell GL (1970) An ocular parasympathetic nerve pathway of facial nerve origin and its influence on intraocular pressure. Exp Eye Res 10:319–330

Ruskell GL (1971) Facial parasympathetic innervation of the choroidal blood vessels in monkeys. Exp Eye Res 12:166–172

Rycroft BW (1934) The relationship of histamine and the intraocular pressure. Br J Ophthalmol 18:149–156

Said SI, Mutt V (1970) Polypeptide with broad biologic activity: isolation from small intestine. Science 169:1217–1218

Sakata H, Yoshida H (1979) Cellular localization of prostaglandin E in the rabbit iris by indirect immunofluorescence method. Albrecht von Graefes Arch Klin Exp Ophthalmol 211:221–227

Schaeffer JM, Brownstein MJ, Axelrod J (1977) Thyrotropin-releasing hormone-like material in the rat retina: changes due to environmental lighting. Proc Nat Acad Sci USA 74:3579–3581

Schlaegel TF (1949) Histamine and uveal infiltration. Am J Ophthalmol 32:1331–1336

Schlaeppi V (1940) De l'influence des extraits post-hypophysaires sur la pupille et la tension intraoculaire. Ophthalmologica 100:321–344

Schumacher H, Classen HG (1962) Der Einfluß von 5-Hydroxytryptamin auf den Augeninnendruck. Albrecht von Graefes Arch Klin Exp Ophthalmol 164:538–542

Sears ML (1960) Miosis and intraocular pressure changes during manometry. Arch Ophthalmol 63:707–714

Sears ML (1961) The immediate reaction to ocular trauma. Ophthalmologica [Suppl] 142:558–561

Shapiro B, Kronheim S, Pimstone B (1979) The presence of immunoreactive somatostatin in rat retina. Horm Metabol Res 11:79–80

Shephard EM (1949) Histamine diphosphate used topically in the eye. West Va Med J 45:62–64

Sholley MM, Gimbrone MA, Cotran RS (1976) The relationship of leukocytic infiltration to neovascularization of the cornea. Anat Rec 184:528–529

Smelser GK, Silver S (1963) The distribution of mast cells in the normal eye. A method of study. Exp Eye Res 2:134–140

Smith MD (1973) 5-Hydroxytryptophan decarboxylase (5-HTPD) and monoamine oxidase (MAO) in the maturing mouse eye. Comp Gen Pharmacol 197:1231–1233

Smith MD, Baker PC (1974) The maturation of indolamine metabolism in the lateral eye of the mouse. Comp Biochem Physiol 49A:281–286

Smith RS (1961) The development of mast cells in the vascularized cornea. AMA Arch Ophthalmol 66:383–390

Snyder SH (1980) Brain peptides as neurotransmitters. Science 209:976–983

Soloway MR, Stjernschantz J, Sears ML (1981) The miotic effect of substance P on the isolated rabbit iris. Invest Ophthalmol Vis Sci 20:47–52

Starr MS (1971 a) Effects of prostaglandin on blood flow in the rabbit eye. Exp Eye Res 11:161–169

Starr MS (1971 b) Further studies on the effect of prostaglandin on intraocular pressure in the rabbit. Exp Eye Res 11:170–177

Stjernschantz J (1981) Neuropeptides in the eye, In: Sears ML (ed) Future directions in ophthalmic research. Yale University Press, New Haven, pp 327–358

Stjernschantz J, Bill A (1979) Effect of facial nerve stimulation on the blood flow of the eye and tongue. Acta Physiol Scand 105:44

Stjernschantz J, Bill A (1980) Vasomotor effects of facial nerve stimulation: noncholinergic vasodilation in the eye. Acta Physiol Scand 109:45–50

Stjernschantz J, Sears ML (1982) Identification of substance P in the anterior uvea and retina of the rabbit. Exp Eye Res 35:401–404

Stjernschantz J, Geijer C, Bill A (1979) Electrical stimulation of the fifth cranial nerve in rabbits: effects on ocular blood flow, extravascular albumin content and intraocular pressure. Exp Eye Res 28:229–238

Stjernschantz J, Sears M, Stjernschantz L (1981) Intraocular effects of substance P in the rabbit. Invest Ophthalmol Vis Sci 20:53–60

Stjernschantz J, Gregerson D, Bausher L, Sears M (1982a) Enzyme-linked immunosorbent assay of substance P. A study in the eye. J Neurochemistry 38:1323–1328

Stjernschantz J, Sears M, Mishima H (1982b) Role of substance P in the antidromic vasodilation, neurogenic plasma extravasation and disruption of the blood-aqueous barrier in the rabbit eye. Naunyn-Schmiedeberg's Arch Pharmacol 321:329–335

Stjernschantz J, Sherk T, Sears M (to be published b) Intraocular effects of lipoxygenase pathway products in arachidonic acid metabolism

Stjernschantz J, Sherk T, Sears M (to be published c) Effects of ATP and some of its derivatives in the rabbit eye

Stjernschantz J, Sherk T, Sears M (to be published d) Intraocular effects of somatostatin, neurotensin and enkephalins in the rabbit

Straschill M (1968) Actions of drugs on single neurons in the cat's retina. Vis Res 8:35–47

Suzuki O, Noguchi E, Miyakes S, Yagi K (1977a) Occurrence of 5-hydroxytryptamine in chick retina. Experientia 33:927–928

Suzuki O, Noguchi E, Yagi K (1977b) Monoamine oxidase in developing chick retina. Brain Res 135:305–313

Suzuki O, Noguchi E, Yagi K (1978) Uptake of 5-hydroxytryptamine by chick retina. J Neurochemistry 30:295–296

Swanson LW (1977) Immunohistochemical evidence for a neurophysin-containing autonomic pathway arising in the paraventricular nucleus of the hypothalamus. Brain Res 128:346–353

Szalay J, Goldberg R, Klug R (1976) The effect of prostaglandin on the iridial blood vessel permeability. Acta Ophthalmol 54:731–742

Tammisto T (1965) The effect of 5-hydroxytryptamine (serotonin) on retinal vessels of the rat. Acta Ophthalmol 43:430–433

Tamura T (1974) Effect of prostaglandins E_1 and E_2 on the ciliary body of albino rabbits: an electron microscopic study. Jpn J Ophthalmol 18:135–149

Terenghi G, Polak JM, Probert L, McGregor GP, Ferri GL, Blank MA, Unger WG, Zhang S, Cole DF, Bloom SR (1982) Mapping, quantitative distribution and origin of substance P and VIP containing nerves in the uvea of guinea pig eye. Histochemistry 75:399–417

Tervo K, Tervo T, Erankö L, Erankö O, Cuello AC (1980) Immunoreactivity for substance P in the gasserian ganglion, ophthalmic nerve and anterior segment of the rabbit eye. Histochem J 13:435–443

Thomas TN, Redburn DA (1979) 5-Hydroxytryptamine – a neurotransmitter of bovine retina. Exp Eye Res 28:55–61

Tilgner S, Kusch T (1969) Untersuchungen über reversible Linsentrübungen bei Ratten und Mäusen nach kombinierter Applikation von Phenelzin und Serotonin. Ophthalmologica 159:211–222

Törnquist K, Lorén I Håkanson R, Sundler F (1981) Peptide-containing neurons in the chicken retina. Exp Eye Res 33:55–64

Törnquist K, Mandahl A, Leander S, Lorén I, Håkanson R, Sundler F (1982) Substance P immunoreactive nerve fibers in the anterior segment of the rabbit eye: distribution ans possible physiological significance. Cell Tiss Res 222:467–477

Treister G, Bárány EH (1970) Degeneration mydriasis and hyperemia of the iris after superior cervical ganglionectomy in the rabbit. Invest Ophthalmol 9:873–887

Tuovinen E, Esilä R, Liesmaa M (1966) Experience of the use of indomethacin in inflammatory eye diseases. Acta Ophthalmol 44:585–589

Türker RK, Khairallah PA, Kayaalp SO, Kaymakcalan S (1969) Response of the nictitating membrane to prostaglandin E_1 and angiotensin. Eur J Pharmacol 5:173–179

Uddman R, Alumets J, Ehinger B, Håkanson R, Lorén I, Sundler F (1980) Vasoactive intestinal peptide nerves in ocular and orbital structures of the cat. Invest Ophthalmol Vis Sci 19:878–885

Unger H-H (1966) Mastzellen beim Glaukomanfall. Klin Monatsbl Augenheilkunde 148:355–368

Unger WG (1979) Prostaglandin mediated inflammatory changes induced by α-adrenoceptor stimulation in the sympathectomised rabbit eye. Albrecht von Graefes Arch Klin Exp Ophthalmol 211:289–300

Unger WG, Perkins ES, Bass MS (1974) The response of the rabbit eye to laser irradiation of the iris. Exp Eye Res 19:367–377

Unger WG, Cole DF, Bass MS (1977) Prostaglandin and neurogenically mediated ocular response to laser irradiation of the rabbit iris. Exp Eye Res 25:209–220

Unger WG, Butler JM, Cole DF, Bloom SR, McGregor GP (1981) Substance P, vasoactive intestinal polypeptide (VIP) and somatostatin levels in ocular tissue of normal and sensorily denervated rabbit eyes. Exp Eye Res 32:797–801

Vale W, Rivier C, Brown M (1977) Regulatory peptides of the hypothalamus. Annu Rev Physiol 39:473–527

Van Alphen GWHM, Angel MA (1975) Activity of prostaglandin E, F, A, and B on sphincter, dilator and ciliary muscle preparations of the cat eye. Prostaglandins 9:157–166

Van Alphen GWHM, Wilhelm P (1978) Effect of prostaglandins on the blood-aqueous barrier of the perfused cat eye. Invest Ophthalmol Vis Sci 17:60–63

Van Dorp DA, Jouvenaz GH, Struijk CB (1967) The biosynthesis of prostaglandin in the pig eye iris. Biochim Biophys Acta 137:396–399

Vannas S (1959) Mast cells in glaucomatous eyes. Acta Ophthalmol 37:330–339

Vegge T, Neufeld AH, Sears ML (1975) Morphology of the breakdown of the blood-aqueous barrier in the ciliary processes of the rabbit eye after prostaglandin E_2. Invest Ophthalmol 14:33–36

Vilstrop G (1952) Studies on the vascular capacity and tissue fluid content of the choroid and their variation under treatment with histamine. Acta Ophthalmol 30:173–180

Vita JB, Anderson JA, Hulem CD; Leopold IH (1981) Angiotensin-converting enzyme activity in ocular fluids. Invest Ophthalmol Vis Sci 20:255–257

Von Euler US, Gaddum JH (1931) An unidentified depressor substance in certain tissue extracts. J Physiol (Lond) 72:74–87

Waitzman MB (1969) Effects of prostaglandin and β-adrenergic drugs on ocular pressure and pupil size. Am J Physiol 217:1593–1598

Waitzman MB (1970) Possible new concepts relating prostaglandins to various ocular functions. Surv Ophthalmol 14:301–326

Waitzman MB, King CD (1967) Prostaglandin influences on intraocular pressure and pupil size. Am J Physiol 212:329–334

Waitzman MB, Woods WD (1971) Some characteristics of an adenyl cyclase preparation from rabbit ciliary process tissue. Exp Eye Res 12:99–111

Waitzman MB, Bailey WR, Kirby CG (1967) Chromatographic analysis of biologically active lipids from rabbit irides. Exp Eye Res 6:130–137

Waitzman MB, Woods WD, Cheek WV (1979) Effects of prostaglandins and norepinephrine on ocular pressure and pupil size in rabbits following bilateral cervical ganglionectomy. Invest Ophthalmol Vis Sci 18:52–60

Wallenstein MC, Bito LZ (1978) The effects of intravitreally injected prostaglandin E_1 on retinal function and their enhancement by a prostaglandin transport inhibitor. Invest Ophthal Vis Sci 17:795–799

Ward PE, Stewart TA, Hammon KJ, Reynolds RC, Igić R (1979) Angiotensin I converting enzyme (kininase II) in isolated retinal microvessels. Life Sci 24:1419–1424

Welsh JH (1964) The quantitative distribution of 5-hydroxytryptamine in the nervous system, eyes and other organs of some vertebrates. In: Richter D (ed) Comparative neurochemistry, proceedings of the fifth international neuro-chemical symposium. Pergamon New York, pp 355–366

Wessely K (1908) Experimentelle Untersuchungen über den Augendruck, sowie über qualitative und quantitative Beeinflussung des intraokularen Flüssigkeitwechsels. Arch F. Augenheilkd 60:97

Whitelock RAF, Eakins KE (1973) Vascular changes in the anterior uvea of the rabbit produced by prostaglandins. Arch Ophthalmol 89:495–499

Winder AF, Patsalos PN (1974) Substance P and retina neurotransmission. Biochem Soc Trans 4:1260–1261

Wolfe LS (1975) Possible roles of prostaglandins in the nervous system. Adv Neurochem 1:1–49

Worgul BV, Bito LZ, Merriam GR (1977) Intraocular inflammation produced by x-irradiation of the rabbit eye. Exp Eye Res 25:53–61

Wudka E, Leopold I (1956) Experimental studies of the choroidal vessels-IV. Pharmacologic observations. Arch Ophthalmol 55:857–885

Yamada T, Marshak D, Basinger S, Walsh J, Morley J, Stell W (1980) Somatostatin-like immunoreactivity in the retina. Proc Natl Acad Sci USA 77:1691–1695

Yamuchi H, Iso T, Iwao J, Iwata H (1979) The role of prostaglandins in experimental ocular inflammations. Agents Actions 9:280–283

Yanuzzi LA, Landau AM, Turtz AI (1981) Incidence of aphakic cystoid macular edema with the use of topical indomethacin. Ophthalmology 88:947–954

Youngblood WW, Humm J, Kizer JS (1979) TRH-like immunoreactivity in rat pancreas and eye, bovine and sheep pineals and human placenta: non-identity with synthetic pyroglu-*his*-pro-NH$_2$ (TRH). Brain Res 163:101–110

Zajacz M, Torok M, Mocsary P (1976) Effect on human eye of prostaglandin and a prostaglandin analogue used to induce abortion. IRCS Med Sci 4:316

Zimmerman TJ, Gravenstein N, Sugar A, Kaufman HE (1975) Aspirin stabilization of the blood-aqueous barrier in the human eye. Am J Ophthalmol 79:817–819

Zollinger R (1949) Über das Vorkommen von Gewebmastzellen in Iris und Ziliarkörper. Ophthalmologica 117:249–252

CHAPTER 8

Vitamin A

G. J. CHADER

A. Introduction

Vitamin A can be defined as that compound or series of β-carotene derivatives which are necessary for maintenance of vision, reproduction, and general epithelial cell growth and differentiation. It also appears to be involved in bone development, the immune response, mucopolysaccharide synthesis, and adrenocortical function. Deficiency interferes with rhodopsin regeneration (leading to night blindness) and with reproductive processes, lowers resistance to infection, leads to abnormal bone development, and induces keratinizing metaplasia of epithelial cells (xerophthalmia, keratomalacia). Retinoid deficiency has also been linked to an increased susceptibility to some types of epithelial cancer (SPORN and NEWTON 1979).

Strictly speaking, the term "vitamin A" refers only to the long-chain alcohol, retinol. In practice, however, vitamin A has been used in a much more general

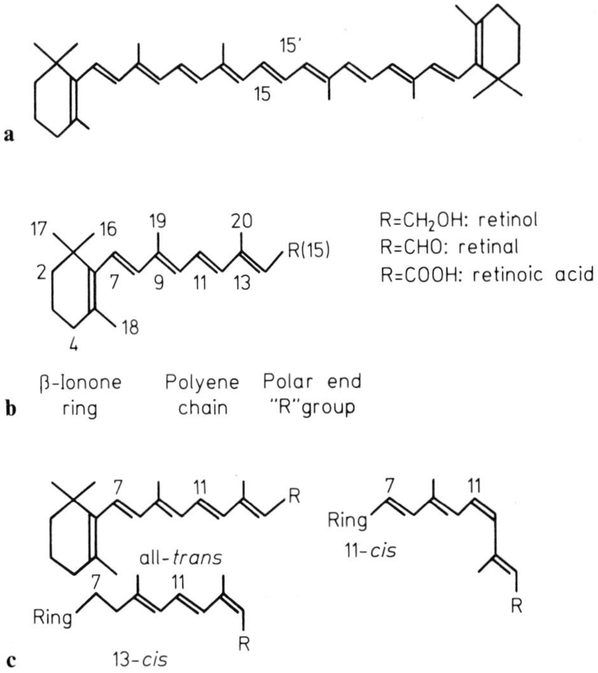

Fig. 1 a–c. Important retinoid structures. **a,** β-Carotene precursor; **b,** retinoids – chemical forms; **c,** retinoids – isomers

sense, encompassing all compounds which exhibit the pharmacological and physiological properties of the basic vitamin A alcohol moiety. It is now clear that the new term "retinoid" is more suitable as the generic name for the family of vitamin A compounds. This is especially true since the various retinoids are used in strikingly different manners in cellular processes. In this review, therefore, the term "retinoid" will be used in the parent or generic sense, while the names "retinol", "retinal", "retinoic acid", etc. will be reserved for the corresponding specific chemical structure (Fig. 1).

B. Retinoid Structure

Vitamin A was the first fat-soluble vitamin discovered. At the turn of the century, it was evident from nutrition studies that animals kept on grain meal alone failed to develop, but that supplementation of their diet with yellow vegetables such as corn allowed for normal growth (McCollum and Davis 1915; Steenbock 1919). McCollum and his coworkers further studied this "fat-soluble factor A," and along with other workers such as Drummond (1920) characterized the factor as a vitamin. It was not until 1931, however, that Karrer et al. (1931) were able to elucidate the chemical structure of vitamin A. Several years later, Holmes and Corbet (1937) crystallized the pure compound, and in the 1940s, Arens and van Dorp (1946a) and Isler and Huber (1947) achieved the first chemical synthesis of the vitamin. In the retina, the first work was performed by Kuhne in the middle of the nineteenth century. Direct evidence for the presence of vitamin A in the retina came only many years later, however, from the early work of Wald (1933), who found that a compound closely related to vitamin A ("retinene") could be extracted from dark-adapted retinas, while retinol was obtained after bleaching. Subsequent work, mainly by Morton (Morton and Goodwin 1944), identified retinene as the aldehyde form of vitamin A. It was ultimately shown that retinene (now called "retinal") formed the prosthetic unit of the rhodopsin moiety (Wald and Brown 1950) and was interconvertible with the alcohol (retinol) form.

Retinoids are derived from a basic five-carbon building block called isoprene (2-methyl-1,3-butadiene). Isoprenoids form a large family of compounds including various oils, resins, rubber, and more specifically, carotene, chlorophyll, steroids and steroid hormones, and the retinoid group. The immediate and most efficient natural precursor to the retinoids is β-carotene (Fig. 1). This isoprenoid hydrocarbon is composed of two symmetrical 20-carbon units, each consisting of a β-ionone ring and an unsaturated side chain. Oxidative cleavage at the 15–15′ position yields the retinoid skeleton and an oxygenated polar functional group at the end of the side chain. The polar end group is of importance in conferring vitamin A activity on the molecule, with the three main types of functional groups subserving different physiological functions in vivo. The hydroxyl function in retinol, for example, allows for transport of the retinoid, for normal reproductive processes, and for possible participation in intracellular glycosylation reactions. The aldehyde form, retinal, is specifically involved in vision, while the acid form may predominantly be involved in growth and differentiation in epithelial tissues but is ineffective in maintaining normal vision (DOWLING and WALD 1960) and reproduction. Variations can also occur in the ionone ring, as in vitamin A_2 or dehydroretinol, which has an extra double bond in the 3,4 position. Retinoids of this type produce "porphyropsins" when bound to pigment apoprotein and are common only in some fish and amphibia. They are not generally found in higher vertebrates. There are several isomeric forms of vitamin A which are also critical to specific biological processes. The all-*trans* configuration of the side chain is the most commonly found type and is the form transported in the blood (Fig. 1). The 11-*cis* isomer is important in the visual process and mainly found in the retina. The 13-*cis* form is found in small amounts in tissues and may be involved in some aspects of cellular differentiation and function.

Interest in synthetic retinoid analogs has been heightened by the possibility of their use in the chemoprevention of some types of cancer (SPORN and NEWTON 1979). Many retinoid analogs are now available which have increased potency and reduced toxicity to normal cells. These retinoids are potentially of great importance in treating ocular epithelial diseases; one retinoic acid preparation (tretinoin) has been used effectively in corneal wound healing (SMOLIN et al. 1979).

C. Retinoid Properties

Vitamin A has the empirical formula $C_{20}H_{30}O$, a molecular weight of 286.4, and is chemically a long-chain unsaturated alcohol. It forms yellowish prisms in petroleum ether with a melting point of 62–64 °C. See HUBBARD et al. (1971) for other retinoid melting points. It is distinctly nonsoluble in water but dissolves in alcohol, acetone, chloroform, ether, and several oils. Sesame oil is often the vehicle of choice for in vivo administration. Dimethylsulfoxide can also be used. Mainly due to its high degree of unsaturation, vitamin A is sensitive to oxidation (atmospheric O_2, oxidizing agents) and to metals (Co, Cu). It is unstable to light and heat and is particularly labile in ultraviolet (UV) light. It is more stable in basic solution than in acids, which tend to isomerize retinoids.

Dietary vitamin A is most often obtained in the diet as a "provitamin", i.e., a carotenoid precursor which is split in the gut to produce the actual retinoid moiety. The most common sources of the carotenoids are green leafy vegetables (e.g., lettuce, spinach) and the family of yellow vegetables (e.g., carrots, pumpkins). Fruits (peaches, apricots) also provide a carotenoid source. The retinoid moiety itself is also obtained through ingestion of animal tissues and products. Meats (liver, fat) are a good source of vitamin A. Fish and its liver and oils are well-known sources of dietary retinoids. Butter, cheese, and egg yolk are intermediate in retinoid content, while milk is relatively low in vitamin A value (except when fortified).

An international unit (IU) of vitamin A is defined as that biological activity exhibited by 300 ng of retinol; this corresponds to 344 ng of the more commonly used retinyl acetate derivative. One gram of pure retinol thus contains 3.33×10^6 IU. Vitamin A_2 has about 40% of the biopotency of retinol. The recommended daily allowances for vitamin A are 5000 IU for adults and about 2000–3500 IU for children. In serum, a concentration of 30–100 μg/100 ml is generally considered "normal." Levels of 10–20 μg/100 ml are considered "low," while below 10 μg/100 ml the level is "deficient." As defined in laboratory animal studies, deficiency symptoms include general growth retardation, night blindness (nyctalopia), bone damage, germinal epithelial atrophy, and keratinization of epithelial tissues (e.g., corneal xerosis and xerophthalmia). In man, the condition of keratomalacia, a generalized vitamin A and protein/calorie malnutrition syndrome, occurs in many underdeveloped countries. Overdoses of vitamin A ($> 10^5$ IU/day) are much less common and are mainly associated with vitamin fads and excessive liver consumption. Symptoms are general fatigue, irritability, and bone and joint pain, along with skin and epithelial cell changes due to conversion of normally keratinized cells to mucus-secreting types.

D. Retinoid Identification

Retinoids and their interactions with proteins have classically been identified and characterized by their absorptive properties (Fig. 2), although colorimetric and fluorescent methods have also been used. Many of these physicochemical methods have previously been described in detail (DRUJAN 1971; BRIDGES 1972; KNOWLES and DARTNALL 1977a). Biologically, an important index of vitamin A potency has been the growth rate of laboratory rats (BROWN and MORGAN 1948; ZILE et al. 1979). A sensitive radioimmunoassay for serum vitamin A has also been described (WESTFALL and WIRTZ 1980).

The most widely used physicochemical methods for identification and determination of vitamin A and other retinoids are:
1. Spectral methods which determine absorptive properties in the near UV range. This includes absorptive changes upon selective destruction of the vitamin with

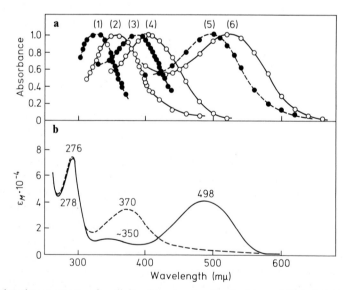

Fig. 2a. Absorbance spectra for digitonin extracts of retinoids and their interactions with visual proteins: (*1*) retinol; (*2*) 3-dehydroretinol; (*3*) retinal; (*4*) 3-dehydroretinal; (*5*)rhodopsin; (*6*) porphyropsin. (Adapted from WALD 1939). **b.** Absorbance spectra of bovine rhodopsin. Dark-adapted, *solid line*; light-bleached, *dashed line*. (Adapted from SHICHI et al. 1969)

UV irradiation (Bessey–Lowry procedure) and a distinctive shift in λ_{max} when vitamin A is dehydrated to anhydroretinol

2. Fluorescence based on the transient yellow–green fluorescent "glow" at 470 nm of retinol and its esters when excited at 325 nm
3. The Carr–Price colorimetric reaction, based on the formation of transient blue complexes when retinol or its esters are treated with Lewis acids
4. High-pressure liquid chromatography (HPLC) techniques.

I. Spectral Methods

The conjugated double-bond system of the retinoids yields an excellent diagnostic absorption spectrum in both pure solvent solution and in various biological fluids and tissues. Retinol, for example, exhibits a maximum at about 324–325 nm with $E_{1cm}^{1\%} = 1835$ (Fig. 2a). Peak maxima are sometimes affected by solvent (CAMA et al. 1951). Chemical changes in retinoid structure, as in dehydroretinol or retinal, lead to substantial spectral shifts (λ_{max} at about 351 and 373 respectively), although ester forms (acetate, palmitate) of retinol have maxima similar to the parent compound ($\lambda_{max} = 325$–328 nm). Stereoisomerism can also result in spectral shifts. Spectral properties of many of the important retinoids and their isomers have been summarized by HUBBARD et al. (1971).

In biological fluids and tissues, various substances can interfere in the spectral determination. This can be circumvented in several ways:

The multiple wavelength method of MORTON and STUBBS (1949), in which absorption is measured at several wavelengths and correction is made for non-vitamin-A components.

The difference spectrum at 326 nm before and after decomposition of vitamin A in the sample. This can be accomplished by strong acid or UV irradiation (BESSEY et al. 1946).

The EMBREE and SHANTZ (1940) method for conversion of vitamin A to anhydroretinol (BUDLOWSKI and BONDI 1957). This method is predicated on the characteristic absorption spectrum of anhydroretinol with λ_{max} of 358, 377, and 399 nm.

The interaction of retinoids with proteins alters the spectral properties of the retinoid, as well as having a new spectral contribution from the protein moiety (HUBBARD et al. 1971; KNOWLES and DARTNALL 1977a; also see Table VIII of KNOWLES and DARTNALL 1977b). The retinal–protein interaction in dark-adapted visual pigments from different species exhibits a wide range of absorption maxima ($\lambda_{max} = 345$–575 nm). Bovine rhodopsin, for example, has a λ_{max} of 498 nm (WALD and BROWN 1953; SHICHI et al. 1969), due primarily to the chemical interaction of 11-cis retinal and opsin to form a protonated Schiff base. In comparison, iodopsin from chicken retina exhibits a λ_{max} of 562 nm with the 11-cis retinal chromophore. The absorption band in the visible region of the dark-adapted retinal-protein moiety is abolished upon bleaching (or with denaturation) and is diagnostic of the interaction of retinal with a visual protein (Fig. 2b). Noncovalent interaction (e.g., hydrophobic bonding) can also result in retinoid spectral changes. When retinol interacts with the serum retinol-binding protein (RBP), it exhibits an absorption maximum at about 330 nm, a value similar to that seen with retinol in benzene solution. Binding of retinol to the cellular retinol-binding protein (CRBP), however, shifts the peak to 343–348 nm and induces other changes in band shape (Ross et al. 1978).

II. Fluorescence Methods

If excited by UV light in the range of its absorption maximum ($\lambda_{max} = 330$ nm), retinol emits a transient bright green fluorescence. The uncorrected emission maximum is between 470 and 490 nm. Several other retinoids, such as retinoic acid (excitation max = 340 nm; emission max = 480 nm), also fluoresce (THOMPSON 1969). Thus both detection and quantification of many retinoids can be accomplished (VON PLANTA et al. 1962) using assay techniques outlined by KAHAN (1971). The method is suited for vitamin A determination in serum and other biological fluids and tissues (KAHAN 1971; HANSEN and WARWICK 1968) and appears to be well correlated with spectrophotometric and colorimetric determinations. A simple and effective fluorimetric determination specifically for serum vitamin A has been described by FUTTERMAN et al. (1975) and is based on the enhancement of retinol fluorescence when the ligand is bound to the serum RBP.

Fluorescence measurements are also useful in characterizing vitamin-A-binding proteins. The purified serum RBP–retinol complex exhibits excitation and emission maxima at 332 and 463 nm respectively, with the relative fluorescence intensity considerably higher than exhibited by retinol alone in solvent solution (GOODMAN 1969). Binding to RBP thus changes both the retinol fluorescence intensity and the λ_{max} (blue shift of about 15–20 nm). Ross et al. (1978) and ONG and CHYTIL (1978) have studied the binding of retinol to purified CRBP, but observed no marked change in the spectrum from that exhibited by pure retinol in ethanolic solution. SAARI et al. (1978) reported a slight blue shift of retinol bound to purified CRBP of bovine retina ($\lambda_{max} = 470$ nm). Fluorescence of retinoic acid bound to purified bovine retina CRABP has been reported to be similar to the retinol–CRBP spectrum, with excitation and emission maxima at 350 and 465 nm respectively (SAARI et al. 1978). Fluorescence of vitamin A can also be determined in tissue extracts in vitro and in tissue samples in situ. A transient whitish-green fluorescence has been observed in oil droplets isolated from frog pigment epithelium (BIDGES 1975). Fluorescence determination coupled with sucrose gradient ultracentrifugation has been used in the characterization of cellular receptor proteins in the cytosol of chick and bovine retina (WIGGERT et al. 1977a). POPPER (1944) has used the fluorescent properties of retinol to visualize the tissue distribution of the retinoid in situ by fluorescence microscopy. He and others have been able to pinpoint areas of retinol storage as in retina (GREENBERG and POPPER 1941). Such compartmentalization has been correlated with vitamin A nutrition (OLSON 1968).

III. Colorimetric Methods

The simplest and most rapid technique used for the detection and quantification of vitamin A has been the Carr–Price reaction. (CARR and PRICE 1926). The assay is based on the reaction of the retinoid with antimony trichloride in an anhydrous solvent producing a transient blue-colored complex with an absorption maximum at 620 nm. The specificity of the technique is not absolute and the experimental conditions (e.g., moisture, temperature) must be rigidly controlled to obtain reliable results. A somewhat similar method using trifluoroacetic acid has also been described (NEELD and PEARSON 1963).

IV. High-Pressure Liquid Chromatography

Separation of retinoids has generally been effected by chromatography techniques, including thin-layer chromatography (FUNG et al. 1978) and column chromatography (e.g., alumina). These methods are useful for simple separation and preliminary identification of retinoids (e.g., R_f values), but are less adequate when complex mixtures of retinoids must be separated, identified, and quantified. High-pressure liquid chromatography (HPLC) appears to be able rapidly to effect all three of these parameters. Utilizing either normal phase or reverse phase methods, retinoids can be quickly separated – based on differences in functional groups (alcohol/aldehyde/acid), isomers, esters, and chemical and natural product derivatives (ROTMANS and KROPF 1975; PAANAKKER and GROENENDIJK 1979; BRIDGES et al. 1980; BHAT et al. 1980).

The HPLC technique is very sensitive and can rapidly separate and tentatively identify virtually the entire range of retinoids, ranging in polarity from the highly hydrophobic fatty acid esters to the free aldehydes and alcohols. This is particularly useful in examining the movement of retinoids between retina and pigmented epithelium and the fluxes in retinoid chemical types and isomeric forms in these tissues. In other tissues (e.g., epithelial), retinoids also undergo rapid conversion to more polar metabolites such as retinoic acid; minute amounts of these compounds can be separated and identified by HPLC (FROLIK et al. 1978; ROBERTS and FROLIK 1979).

E. Retinoid Metabolism

The best-defined and understood series of reactions involving retinoids are in the visual process in the retina–pigmented epithelium functional unit (WALD and HUBBARD 1960). These will be addressed in the sections on retinoid uptake and action (Sects. F and G). Demonstration of such retinoid chemical transformations and identification of retinal (retinene) as the actual functional chromophore in the visual process indicated, however, that other retinoid forms might act as active metabolites in tissues known to be responsive to vitamin A. This is especially true in light of the diverse functions of the vitamin in reproduction, bone formation, and general growth and differentiation of epithelial tissues. The chemical synthesis of retinoic acid and the discovery that it could substitute for retinol in all vitamin-A-dependent processes except vision and reproduction (ARENS and VAN DORP 1946b) greatly stimulated the investigation of vitamin A metabolism.

Many tissues can convert retinol to retinoic acid through the aldehyde, retinal (Fig. 3). FUTTERMAN (1962) was one of the first to demonstrate the general nature of retinal oxidation to retinoic acid. The acid then appears to be the key intermediate for studying both active form metabolism of the vitamin and catabolism to inactive excretion products. Retinoic acid is found in only small amounts in tissues and itself is quickly metabolized. Oxidation at the 4-position of the ionone ring may constitute a primary step in elimination of the retinoid from tissues (Frolik et al. 1979; Roberts and Frolik 1979). Retinoid isomers (13-*cis*-retinoids) have been reported, e.g., the 13-*cis*-oxo metabolite (Frolik et al. 1980), indicating the probability of *trans* to *cis* isomeric conversion, in some cases in vivo. Oxidative decarboxylation of retinoic acid can also occur (Roberts and deLuca 1967). An interesting epoxidation reaction takes place in the intestinal mucosa of the rat, resulting in the formation of 5,6-epoxy-retinoic acid (McCormick et al. 1978), which isomerizes to the 5,8-oxide upon treatment with dilute HCl (McCormick and Napoli 1982). Chen and Heller (1977) and DeLuca (1977) have reported the presence of a "retinol-like" metabolite of retinoic acid (metabolite "X") in pigmented epithelium and other tissues. It is as yet unknown whether the epoxy compound and the retinol-like metabolite are involved in vitamin A activation or in its catabolism.

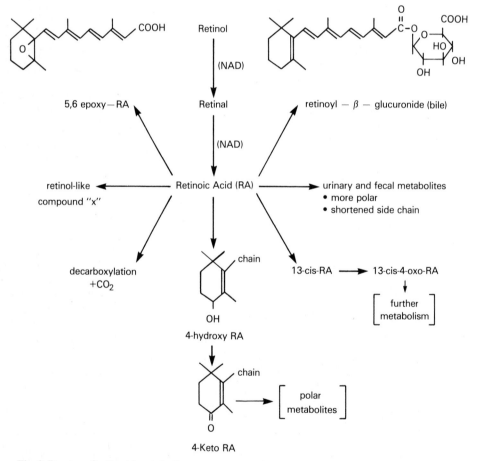

Fig. 3. Routes of retinoid metabolism

Excretory products of vitamin A are well known. Olson and co-workers (DU-NAGIN et al. 1965) and ZILE et al. (1980) have demonstrated the excretion of a gluc-uronide metabolite in rat bile. Using radiolabeled retinol and retinoic acid, ROBERTS and DeLUCA (1967) showed the excretion of several radiolabeled metab-olites in feces and urine, as well as bile; they further demonstrated that portions of the side chain could be cleaved, with C-15 and C-14 appearing as expired CO_2. Many of these metabolites have been summarized by RIETZ et al. (1974) and by DeLUCA (1979). Use of the sensitive technique of HPLC should give a clearer view of the cellular aspects of retinoid activation and catabolism in the future.

F. Retinoid Uptake

After ingestion or formation in the gut (Fig. 4), vitamin A is esterified and trans-ported to the liver in the chylomicra (GOODMAN 1979). In the liver, it is stored main-

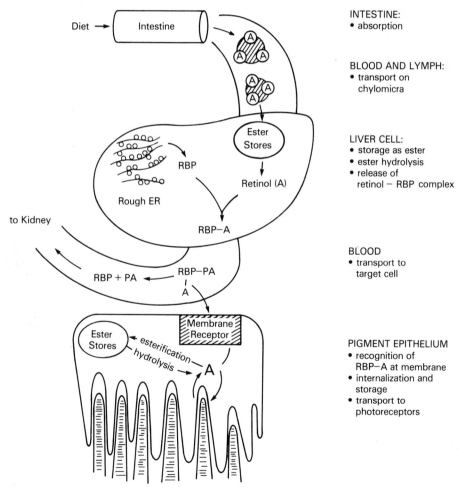

Fig. 4. Vitamin A transport to target pigmented epithelium cell. *RBP*, retinol. binding pro-tein; *PA*, prealbumin; *ER*, endoplasmic reticulum

ly as the retinyl ester. Upon demand, retinol is released from the liver in a 1:1 molar complex with RBP. This complex, in turn, is also usually bound to another protein, the plasma prealbumin PA. Target tissues, such as the pigmented epithelium, have plasma membrane receptors which tightly bind the retinol–RBP complex and effect the translocation of the retinoid into the cell (HELLER 1975; MARAINI 1979). Autoradiography studies using ^{125}I-labeled RBP have confirmed the presence of membrane receptors for the retinol–^{125}I-RBP complex on the pigmented epithelial cell surface (BOK and HELLER 1976). As might be expected from the polarity of the pigmented epithelial cell in vivo, the receptors are only found on the plasma membrane surrounding the basal and lateral surfaces of the cell. It appears that only the retinol moiety is taken up into the cell; the RBP remains in the plasma to be processed elsewhere in the body (e.g., in the kidney). Similar membrane receptors have been described in intestinal mucosal cells (RASK and PETERSON 1976). Uptake into epithelial cells of the cornea is somewhat different, since the cornea is avascular. A recent study by RASK et al. (1980) demonstrates that vitamin A (complexed with RBP) is delivered by a diffusional process from the episcleral blood vessels at the limbus.

Within the target cell, retinol is bound to a specific soluble CRBP. Cellular retinol-binding protein is a low-molecular-weight (2-S) binding protein of high specificity for retinol, and is found in high concentration in retina and pigmented epithelium (WIGGERT et al. 1977a), cornea (WIGGERT et al. 1977b), and cultured retinoblastoma cells (WIGGERT et al. 1977c). A separate and distinct receptor is present for retinoic acid, i.e., the cellular retinoic acid binding protein (CRABP), in many tissues (SANI 1974; ONG and CHYTIL 1975), including most ocular tissues (WIGGERT et al. 1978a). Both the CRBP and CRABP have been isolated and purified from bovine retina (SAARI et al. 1978; LIOU et al. 1981). Another separate soluble binding protein for 11-*cis* retinal (STUBBS et al. 1979) has been identified. In the retinas of some species, a 7-S binding protein for retinol is present (WIGGERT et al. 1978b) that appears to be compartmentalized in the subretinal space (LAI et al. 1982). Differences in 7-S binding are seen in light and dark, possibly due to differential loading of the 7-S protein under the two conditions (WIGGERT et al. 1979; LAI et al. 1982). This has led to the postulate that the 7-S interphotoreceptor retinol-binding protein could act as a transport vehicle between and within tissues (CHADER 1982; CHADER et al. 1983).

G. Retinoid Action

I. The Visual Process

Retinoid interconversions and interactions with proteins are best understood in the retina–pigmented epithelium unit. The visual cycle, driven by alternating sequences of light and dark, results in movement of retinoid between the retina and pigmented epithelium and cyclic chemical and conformational changes in retinoid forms. In most species, the pigmented epithelium is the main site of retinoid storage (WALD 1935); from there it moves to the retinal photoreceptor upon demand. In the pigmented epithelium it is primarily in the ester form, stored in oil droplets in many species (BRIDGES 1975, 1976). Figure 5 summarizes many of the steps in-

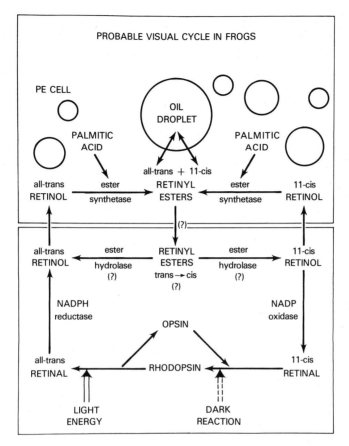

Fig. 5. Retinoid movement and interconversions in pigmented epithelium (*PE*) and retina of the frog. (Adapted from BRIDGES 1976)

volved in the flow of retinoids between pigmented epithelium and retina and the chemical transformations involved in the visual process. During bleaching, the rhodopsin chromophore, 11-*cis*-retinal, is isomerized in the photoreceptor to the all-*trans* configuration, is split from the opsin moiety, and can be reduced to the alcohol (WALD and HUBBARD 1949; FUTTERMAN et al. 1970). The retinol can then diffuse or be transported back to the pigmented epithelium, where it is reesterified and stored (DOWLING 1960; BERMAN et al. 1980a). Proportions of retinoids in the various chemical forms (alcohol, aldehyde, ester, etc.) have been calculated during light- and dark-adaptation by several investigators, including ZIMMERMAN (1974), BRIDGES (1975, 1976), and BERMAN and her co-workers (BERMAN et al. 1979, 1980b).

After photon capture by rhodopsin, a series of short-lived intermediates can be detected, each with special spectral characteristics (Fig. 6). Recent interest in rhodopsin chemistry has centered around defining the first changes in the retinal moiety after bleaching. In the dark-adapted photoreceptor outer segment, retinal

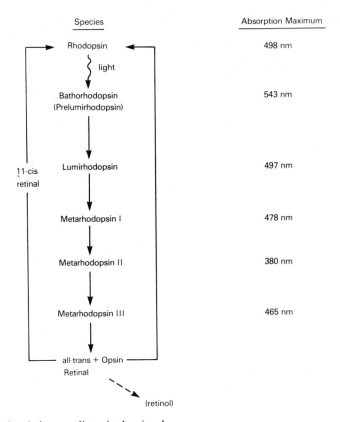

Fig. 6. Rhodopsin intermediates in the visual process

is bound through a Schiff base linkage (C=N) to a lysine residue of the opsin (WANG et al. 1980). Most probably the Schiff base is protonated, but is protected from hydrolysis by negative groups of the protein (HONIG and EBRY 1974). Studies on deuterium effects on the kinetics of bathorhodopsin formation at low temperatures have led Rentzepis and his colleagues (PETERS et al. 1977) to postulate that proton translocation may be the primary event in the visual process. The locus of the proton translocation is not known, however.

It has also been proposed that the conversion of 11-*cis*-retinal in rhodopsin to a strained all-*trans* retinal via a "bicycle-pedal" isomerization may be the initial result of photon capture (WARSHEL 1976). HONIG et. al. (1979) have also provided strong evidence that photon capture results in isomerization of the 11-*cis* chromophore to an all-*trans* configuration, and that this change is a likely candidate for triggering the cascade of rhodopsin intermediates that have been observed between the initial photic stimulation and the splitting of the retinal from the opsin (Fig. 6). Low-temperature spectroscopy has allowed for identification of each of these intermediates by their distinctive spectra, which are probably generated in the main by protein effects on the delocalization of π electrons of the chromophore (DOUKAS et al. 1978). These reactions have been thoroughly reviewed previously (EBREY and

HONIG 1975; OSTROY 1977). Evidence from resonance Raman spectroscopy indicates that isomerization of the 11-*cis* retinal to a distorted form of the all-*trans* isomer takes place within picoseconds of photic stimulation (HAYWARD et al. 1981). The speed of this reaction is consistent with the hypothesis that such a change may consitute the initial step in the visual process. Whether this reaction does initiate the cascade sequence or not, the techniques of picosecond absorption spectroscopy and Raman spectroscopy should be extremely useful in delineating these reactions over the next few years.

II. Glycoprotein Biosynthesis

Evidence from several laboratories indicates that retinoids may be involved in cellular glycoprotein biosynthesis (WOLF and DELUCA 1969; PETERSON et al. 1976). Vitamin A deficiency causes a dramatic decrease in the incorporation of radiolabeled mannose into rat liver glycoprotein, whereas vitamin A repletion leads to a marked stimulation of mannose incorporation (DELUCA 1977). Vitamin A deficiency also leads to a specific decrease in the synthesis of rat serum α-macroglobulin, a decrease that can be directly attributed to a defect in glycosylation (WOLF et al. 1979). DELUCA (DELUCA et al. 1979 b) and others have also suggested that the well-known effect of retinoids on cell adhesion in tissue culture may be due to regulation of glycosylation of cell membrane glycoproteins. The striking effects of retinoids on the morphology and biochemistry of cultured cells have been reviewed by LOTAN (1980).

Such data have led to the general postulate that vitamin A may act in mammalian membranes as dolichol does in lower animal species, i.e., as a lipid intermediate in protein glycosylation. In such a scheme, the lipid (dolichol or retinol) would first be phosphorylated (e.g., retinol-*P*). This activated species would then interact with a sugar moiety (e.g., retinyl-*P*-mannose) and ultimately donate the sugar group to a nascent glycoprotein. It has been proposed that retinyl-*P* could act as a sugar carrier across biological membranes through an enzymatic *trans* to *cis* isomerization reaction (DELUCA et al. 1979 a, b). Although the synthesis of retinyl-*P* has been demonstrated, as well as the presence of small amounts of retinyl-*P*-mannose in liver microsomes, the physiological importance of such reactions in vivo has yet to be firmly established. The role of retinoic acid is also questionable in such a process, although a "retinol-like" metabolite of retinoic acid (CHEN and HELLER 1977; DELUCA 1977; DELUCA et al. 1979 a) could, at least theoretically, act as a lipid carrier.

III. Hormone-like Action

It has long been considered that vitamin A has "hormone-like" characteristics (WOLF and DELUCA 1970; MORTON 1974). There are, for example, specific target tissues for retinoids, a specific serum transport protein (RBP), and specific intracellular carrier proteins. This is all very similar to the situation seen in vivo and in vitro for the steroid hormones.

Nuclear uptake of ^3H-retinoic acid in cultured retinoblastoma cells has been observed biochemically (Wiggert et al. 1977c) and by autoradiography (Chader et al. 1981). In a similar vein, Takase et al. (1979) have found that purified CRBP facilitates the binding of ^3H-retinol to isolated nuclei from livers of vitamin-A-deficient rats. The specific action of retinoids in the nucleus is still unknown, but effects on synthesis of DNA (Zile et al. 1977, 1979) and of RNA (Kaufman et al. 1972; Blalock and Gifford 1977; Tsai and Chytil 1978) have been reported. Differences between retinol and retinoic acid are apparent but have yet to be better defined. In cultured retinoblastoma cells, for example, it is only retinoic acid, not retinol, that is quickly taken up by nuclei. This general area has been recently reviewed in detail (Chytil and Ong 1978; Chader et al. 1981; Chader 1982).

References

Arens J, VanDorp D (1946a) Synthesis of some compounds possessing vitamin A activity. Nature 157:190–191

Arens J, VanDorp D (1946b) Activity of vitamin-A-acid in the rat. Nature 158:622–623

Berman E, Segal N, Feeney L (1979) Subcellular distribution of free and esterified forms of vitamin A in the pigment epithelium of the retina and in liver. Biochim Biophys Acta 572:167–177

Berman E, Horowitz J, Segal N, Fisher S, Feeney-Burns L (1980a) Enzymatic esterification of vitamin A in the pigment epithelium of bovine retina. Biochim Biophys Acta 630:36–46

Berman E, Segal N, Schneider A, Feeney L (1980b) An hypothesis for a vitamin A cycle in the pigment epithelium of bovine retina. Neurochem Res 1:113–122

Bessey O. Lowry O, Brock M, Lopez J (1946) The determination of vitamin A and carotene in small quantities of blood serum. J Biol Chem 166:177–188

Bhat P, DeLuca L, Wind M (1980) Reverse phase high-pressure liquid chromatographic separation of retinoids, including retinylphosphate and mannosylretinylphosphate. Anal Biochem 102:243–248

Blalock J, Gifford G (1977) Retinoic acid (vitamin A acid) induces transcriptional control of interferon production. Proc Natl Acad Sci USA 74:5382–5386

Bok D, Heller J (1976) Transport of retinol from the blood to the retina: an autoradiographic study of the pigment epithelial cell surface receptor for plasma retinol-binding protein. Exp Eye Res 22:395–402

Bridges CD (1972) The rhodopsin-porphyropsin visual system. In: Dartnall HJA (ed) Photochemistry of vision, pt1. Springer, Berlin Heidelberg New York, pp 417–480 (Handbook of sensory physiology, vol 7)

Bridges CD (1975) Storage, distribution and utilization of vitamin A in the eyes of adult amphibians and their tadpoles. Vision Res 15:1311–1323

Bridges CD (1976) Vitamin A and the role of the pigment epithelium during bleaching and regeneration of rhodopsin in the frog eye. Exp Eye Res 22:435–455

Bridges CD, Fong S-L, Alvarez R (1980) Separation by programmed-gradient high-pressure liquid chromatography of vitamin A isomers, their esters, aldehydes, oximes and vitamin A_2: presence of retinyl ester in dark-adapted goldfish pigment epithelium. Vision Res 20:355–360

Brown E, Morgan A (1948) The effect of vitamin A deficiency upon nitrogen metabolism of the rat. J Nutr 35:425–438

Budlowski P, Bondi A (1957) Determination of vitamin by conversion to anhydrovitamin A. Analyst 82:751–760

Cama H, Collins F, Morton R (1951) Studies in vitamin A. Spectroscopic properties of all-trans-vitamin A and vitamin A acetate. Analysis of liver oils. Biochem J 50:48–59

Carr F, Price E (1926) Colour reactions attributed to vitamin A. Biochem J 20:497–501

Chader G (1982) Retinoids in ocular tissues: binding proteins, transport and mechanism of action: In: McDevitt D (ed) Cell biology of the eye. Academic, New York, pp 377–433

Chader G, Wiggert B, Russell P, Tanaka M (1981) Retinoid binding proteins of retina and retinoblastoma cells in culture. Ann NY Acad Sci 359–115–133

Chader G, Wiggert B, Lai Y-L, Fletcher R (1983) Interphotoreceptor retinol-binding protein: a possible role in retinoid transport to the retina. In: Osborne N, Chader G (eds) Progress in retinal research, vol 2. Pergamon, Oxford

Chen C-C, Heller J (1977) Uptake of retinol and retinoic acid from serum retinol-binding protein by retinal pigment epithelial cells. J Biol Chem 252:5216–5221

Chytil F, Ong D (1978) Cellular vitamin A binding proteins. Vitam Horm 36:1–32

DeLuca H (1979) Retinoic acid metabolism. Fed Proc 38:2519–2523

DeLuca L (1977) The direct involvement of vitamin A in glycosyl transfer reactions of mammalian membranes. Vitam Horm 34:1–57

DeLuca L, Adamo S, Bhat P, Sasak W, Silverman-Jones C, Akalovsky I, Frot-Coutaz J, Fletcher T, Chader G (1979a) Recent developments in studies on biological functions of vitamin A in normal and transformed tissues. Pure Appl Chem 51:581–591

DeLuca L, Bhat P, Sasak W, Adamo S (1979b) Biosynthesis of phosphoryl and glycosyl phosphoryl derivatives of vitamin A in biological membranes. Fed Proc 38:2535–2539

Doukas A, Aton B, Callender R, Ebry T (1978) Resonance Raman studies of bovine metarhodopsin I and metarhodopsin II. Biochemistry 17:2430–2439

Dowling J (1960) Chemistry of visual adaptation in the rat. Nature 188:114–118

Dowling J, Wald G (1960) The biological function of vitamin A acid. Proc Natl Acad Sci USA 46:587–592

Drujan B (1971) Determination of vitamin A. Methods Enzymol 18:565–573

Drummon J (1920) Researches on the fat-soluble accessory substance III. Technique for carrying out feeding tests for vitamin A (fat-soluble A). Biochem J 14:661–664

Dunagin P, Meadows E, Olson J (1965) Retinoyl β-glucuronic acid: a major metabolite of vitamin A in rat bile. Science 148:86–87

Ebrey T, Honig B (1975) Molecular aspects of photoreceptor function. Q Rev Biophys 8:129–184

Embree N, Shantz E (1940) Cyclization of vitamin A_2. J Biol Chem 132:619–626

Frolik C, Tavela T, Newton D, Sporn M (1978) In vitro metabolism and biological activity of all-*trans*-retinoic acid and its metabolites in hamster trachea. J Biol Chem 253:7319–7324

Frolik C, Roberts A, Tavela T, Roller P, Newton D, Sporn M (1979) Isolation and identification of 4-hydroxy- and 4-keto-retinoic acid. In vitro metabolites of all-*trans*-retinoic acid in hamster trachea and liver. Biochemistry 18:2092–2097

Frolik C, Roller P, Roberts A, Sporn M (1980) In vitro and in vivo metabolism of all-*trans*- and 13-*cis*-retinoic acid in hamsters. J Biol Chem 255:8057–8062

Futterman S (1962) Enzymatic oxidation of vitamin A aldehyde to vitamin A acid. J Biol Chem 237:677–680

Futterman S, Hendrickson A, Bishop P, Rollins M, Vacano E (1970) Metabolism of glucose and reduction of retinaldehyde in retinal photoreceptors. J Neurochem 17:149–156

Futterman S, Swanson D, Kalina R (1975) A new rapid fluorimetric determination of retinol in serum. Invest Ophtalmol 14:125–130

Fung Y, Rahwan R, Sams R (1978) Separation of vitamin A compounds by thin layer chromatography. J Chromatog 147:528–531

Goodman DeW (1969) Retinol transport in human plasma. In: DeLuca H, Suttie J (eds) The fat-soluble vitamins. University of Wisconsin Press, Madison pp 203–211

Goodman DeW (1979) Vitamin A and retinoids: recent advances. Fed Proc 38:2501–2503

Greenberg R, Popper H (1941) Demonstration of vitamin A in the retina by fluorescence microscopy. Am J Physiol 134:114–118

Hansen L, Warwick W (1968) A fluorometric micromethod for serum vitamin A. Am J Clin Pathol 50:525–529

Hayward G, Carlsen W, Siegman A, Stryer L (1981) Retinal chromophore of rhodopsin photoisomerizes within pico-seconds. Science 211:942–944

Heller J (1975) Interaction of plasma retinol-binding protein with its receptor. Specific binding of bovine and human retinol-binding protein to pigment epithelium cells from
bovine eyes. J Biol Chem 250:3613–3619

Holmes H, Corbet R (1937) The isolation of crystalline vitamin A. J Am Chem Soc 59:2042–
2047

Honig B, Ebrey T (1974) The structure and spectra of the chromophore of the visual pigments. Ann Rev Biophys Bioeng 3:151–177

Honig B, Ebrey T, Callender R, Dinur U, Ottolenghi M (1979) Photoisomerization, energy
storage and charge separation: a model for light energy transduction in visual pigments
and bacteriorhodopsin. Proc Natl Acad Sci USA 76:2503–2506

Hubbard R, Brown D, Bownds D (1971) Methodology of vitamin A and visual pigments.
Methods Enzymol 18:615–653

Isler O, Huber W (1947) Ronco A, Kufler M: Synthese des Vitamins A. Helv Chim Acta
30:1911–1927

Kahan J (1971) The fluorescence properties of vitamin A. Methods Enzymol 18:574–591

Karrer P, Morf R, Schopp K (1931) Zur Kenntnis des Vitamins-A aus Fischtränen II. Helv
Chim Acta 14:1431–1436

Kaufman D, Baker M, Smith J, Henderson W, Harris C, Sporn M, Saffiotti U (1972) RNA
metabolism in tracheal epithelium: alteration in hamsters deficient in vitamin A. Science
177:1105–1108

Knowles A, Dartnall J (1977a) The characterization of visual pigments by adsorption spectroscopy. In: Davson H (ed) The eye, vol 2B. Academic, New York, pp 53–101

Knowles A, Dartnall H (1977b) Structure of the visual pigment molecule: In: Davson D (ed)
The eye, vol 2B. Academic, New York pp 103–174

Lai Y, Wiggert B, Liu Y, Chader G (1982) Interphotoreceptor retinol-binding proteins: possible transport vehicles between compartments of the retina. Nature 298:848–849

Liou G, Fong SL, Bridges CD (1981) Companson of cytosol retinol binding proteins from
bovine retina, dog liver and rat liver. J Biol Chem 256:3153–3155

Lotan R (1980) Effects of vitamin A and its analogs (retinoids) on normal and neoplastic
cells. Biochim Biophys Acta 605:33–91

Mariani G (1979) Binding proteins for retinol in retina and pigment epithelium. In: Zadunaisky J, Davson H (eds) Current topics in eye research. Acadmic, New York, pp 143–174

McCollum E, Davis M (1915) The nature of the dietary deficiences of rice. J Biol Chem
23:181–190

McCormick A, Napoli J (1982) Identification of 5,6-epoxyretinoic acid as an endogenous
retinol metabolite. J Biol Chem 257:1730–1735

McCormick A, Napoli J, DeLuca H (1978) High-pressure liquid chromatographic resolution of vitamin A compounds. Anal Biochem 86:25–33

Morton R (1974) The vitamin concept. Vitam Horm 32:155–166

Morton R, Goodwin R (1944) Preparation of retinene *in vitro*. Nature 153:405–406

Morton R, Stubbs A (1949) Photoelectric spectrophotometry applied to the analysis of mixtures and vitamin A oils. Analyst 71:348–356

Napoli J, McCormick A, Schnoes H, DeLuca H (1978) Identification of 5,8-oxyretinoic acid
isolated from small intestine of vitamin A-deficient rats dosed with retinoic acid. Proc
Natl Acad Sci USA 75:2603–2605

Neeld J, Pearson W (1963) Macro- and micromethods for the determination of serum vitamin A using trifluoroacetic acid. J Nutr 79:454–462

Olson J (1968) Some aspects of vitamin A metabolism. Vitam Horm 26:1–63

Ong D, Chytil F (1975) Retinoic acid-binding protein in rat tissues. Partial purification and
comparison to rat tissue retinol-binding protein. J Biol Chem 250:6113–6117

Ong D, Chytil F (1978) Cellular retinol-binding protein from rat liver. Purification and
characterization. J Biol Chem 253:828–832

Ostroy S (1977) Rhodopsin and the visual process. Biochim Biophys Acta 463:91–125

Paanakker J, Groenendijk G (1979) Separation of geometric isomers of retinyl ester, retinal
and retinol pertaining to the visual cycle. J Chromatogr 168:125–132

Peters K, Applebury M, Rentzepis P (1977) Primary photochemical event in vision: proton translocation. Proc Natl Acad Sci USA 74:3119–3123

Peterson P, Rask L, Helting T, Ostberg L, Fernstend Y (1976) Formation and properties of retinylphosphate galactose. J Biol Chem 251:4986–4995

Popper H (1944) Distribution of vitamin A in tissue visualized by fluorescence microscopy. Physiol Rev 24:205–224

Rask L, Peterson P (1976) In vitro uptake of vitamin A from the plasma retinol-binding protein to mucosal epithelial cells from the monkey's small intestine. J Biol Chem 251:6360–6366

Rask L, Geijor C, Bill A, Peterson P (1980) Vitamin A supply of the cornea. Exp Eye Res 31:201–211

Rietz P, Wiss O, Weber F (1974) Metabolism of vitamin A and the determination of vitamin A status. Vitam Horm 32:237–249

Roberts A, DeLuca H (1967) Pathways of retinol and retinoic acid metabolism in the rat. Biochem J 102:600–611

Roberts A, Frolik C (1979) Recent advances in the in vivo and in vitro metabolism of retinoic acid. Fed Proc 38:2524–2527

Ross A, Takahashi Y, Goodman DeW (1978) The binding protein for retinol from rat testes cytosol. Isolation and partial characterization. J Biol Chem 253:6591–6598

Rotmans J, Kropf A (1975) The analysis or retinal isomers by high speed liquid chromatography. Vision Res 15:1301–1302

Saari J, Futterman S, Bredberg L (1978) Cellular retinol- and retinoic acid-binding proteins of bovine retina. Purification and properties. J Biol Chem 253:6432–6436

Sani B (1974) Retinoic acid: a binding protein in chick embryo metatarsal skin. Biochem Biophys Res Comm 61:1276–1282

Shichi H, Lewis M, Irreverre F, Stone A (1969) Biochemistry of visual pigments. I. Purification and properties of bovine rhodopsin. J Biol Chem 224:529–536

Smolin G, Okumoto M, Friedlander M (1979) Tretinoin and corneal epithelial wound healing. Arch Ophthalmol 97:545–546

Sporn M, Newton D (1979) Chemoprevention of cancer with retinoids. Fed Proc 38:2528–2534

Steenbock H (1919) White corn vs yellow corn and a probable relationship between the fat soluble vitamins and yellow plant pigments. Science 50:352–354

Stubbs G, Saari J, Futterman S (1979) 11-*cis*-Retinal binding protein from bovine retina. Isolation and partial characterization. J Biol Chem 254:8529–8533

Takase S, Ong D, Chytil F (1979) Cellular retinol-binding protein allows specific interaction of retinol with the nucleus in vitro. Proc Natl Acad Sci USA 76:2204–2208

Thompson A (1969) Fluorescence spectra of some retinyl polyenes. J Chem Phys 51:4106–4116

Tsai C, Chytil F (1978) Effect of vitamin A deficiency on RNA synthesis in isolated rat liver nuclei. Life Sci 23:1461–1472

VonPlanta C, Schwieter U, Chopard-dit-Jean L, Ruegg R, Kofler M, Isler O (1962) Synthesen in der Vitamin-A_2-Reihe. Helv Chem Acta 45:548–554

Wald G (1933) Vitamin A in the retina. Nature 132:316–317

Wald G (1935) Carotenoids and the visual cycle. J Gen Physiol 19:351–371

Wald G (1939) The porphyropsin visual system. J Gen Physiol 22:775–794

Wald G, Brown P (1950) The synthesis of rhodopsin from retinene. Proc Natl Acad Sci USA 36:84–92

Wald G, Brown P (1953) The molar extinction of rhodopsin. J Gen Physiol 37:189–200

Wald G, Hubbard R (1949) The reduction of retinene to vitamin A in vitro. J Gen Physiol 32:289–290

Wald G, Hubbard R (1960) Enzymic aspects of the visual processes. In: Boyer P, Lardy H, Myrback K (eds) The enzymes, vol 3. Academic, New York, pp 369–386

Wang J, McDowell J, Hargrave P (1980) Site of attachment of 11-*cis*-retinal in bovine rhodopsin. Biochemistry 19:5111–5117

Warshel A (1976) Bicycle-pedal model for the first step in the vision process. Nature 260:678–683

Westfall S, Wirtz G (1980) Vitamin A antibodies: application to radioimmunoassay. Experientia 36:1351–1352

Wiggert B, Bergsma D, Lewis M, Chader G (1977a) Vitamin A receptors: retinol binding in neural retina and pigment epithelium. J Neurochem 29:947–954

Wiggert B, Bergsma D, Helmsen R, Alligood J, Lewis M, Chader G (1977b) Retinol receptors in corneal epithelium, stroma and endothelium. Biochim Biophys Acta 491:104–113

Wiggert B, Russell P, Lewis M, Chader G (1977c) Differential binding to soluble nuclear receptors and effects on cell viability of retinol and retinoic acid in cultured retinoblastoma cells. Biochem Biophys Res Comm 79:218–225

Wiggert B, Bergsma D, Helmsen R, Chader G (1978a) Vitamin A receptors: retinoic acid binding in ocular tissues. Biochem J 169:87–94

Wiggert B, Mizukawa A, Kuwabara T, Chader G (1978b) Vitamin A receptors: multiple species in retina and brain and possible compartmentalization in retinal photoreceptors. J Neurochem 30:653–659

Wiggert B, Derr J, Fitzpatrick M, Chader G (1979) Vitamin A receptors of the retina. Differential binding in light and dark. Biochim Biophys Acta 582:115–121

Wolf G, DeLuca L (1969) Recent studies on some metabolic functions of vitamin A. In: DeLuca H, Suttie J (eds) The fat-soluble vitamins. University of Wisconsin Press, Madison, pp 257–265

Wolf G, DeLuca L (1970) Recent studies on some metabolic functions of vitamin A. In: DeLuca H, Suttie J (eds) The fat-soluble vitamins. University of Wisconsin Press, Madison, pp 257–265

Wolf G, Kiorpes T, Masushige S, Schreiber J, Smith M, Anderson R (1979) Recent evidence for the participation of vitamin A in glycoprotein synthesis. Fed Proc 38:2540–2543

Zile M, Bunge E, DeLuca H (1977) Effect of vitamin A deficiency on intestinal cell proliferation in the rat. J Nutr 107:552–560

Zile M, Bunge E, DeLuca H (1979) On the physiological basis of vitamin A-stimulated growth. J Nutr 109:1787–1796

Zile M, Schnoes H, DeLuca H (1980) Characterization of retinoyl β-glucuronide as a minor metabolite of retinoic acid in bile. Proc Natl Acad Sci USA 77:3230–3233

Zimmerman W (1974) The distribution and proportions of vitamin A compounds during the visual cycle in the rat. Vision Res 14:795–802

CHAPTER 9

Anti-Infective Agents

I. H. LEOPOLD

A. Introduction

In the 50-year period since Fleming made his monumental discovery of penicillin, a vast array of anti-infective agents have been developed to combat the plethora of infectious microorganisms plaguing mankind. While once the ophthalmologist had only penicillin to resort to when faced with ocular infection, his choice now includes myriads of antibiotics. This variety of anti-infective agents has brought tremendous benefits, but it has also brought the need for greater knowledge on the part of the physician. He must be aware of newly introduced antimicrobial agents and reevaluate older drugs for new uses in the light of the development of tolerance and toxic side effects.

B. Accurate Diagnosis and Drug Choice

The selection of the correct anti-infective agent requires accurate diagnosis, but it also demands an understanding of the anti-infective agents themselves and their effects. Tables 1 and 2 summarize the drugs of choice for specific microorganisms.

I. Mechanisms of Action

Antibiotics can be either bactericidal (killing bacteria) or bacteriostatic (inhibiting multiplication of the microorganism). Bactericidal agents include the penicillins, the cephalosporins, and aminoglycosides such as gentamicin, tobramycin, amikacin, neomycin, kanamycin, and streptomycin. Other bactericides are vancomycin, bacitracin, polymycin B, and colistin. The sulfonamides, trimethoprim, the tetracyclines, chloramphenicol, erythromycin, clindamycin, and lincomysin are all bacteriostatic agents.

Successful antimicrobial agents perform by destroying the structural parts of microorganisms or by interfering in their biosynthetic functions. Agents such as chloramphenicol, the tetracyclines, erythromycin, lincomycin, kanamycin, neomycin, streptomycin, and gentamicin impair protein synthesis, affecting ribosomal subunits. Vancomycin and bacitracin, the penicillins, and the cephalosporins alter the synthesis of the mucopolypeptide layer of the bacterial cell wall. Agents such as the polymyxins, colistin, amphotericin, and nystatin function by altering the permeability of the bacterial cell membrane, allowing the cell contents to leak out. Rifampin exerts its antimicrobial effect by selectively inhibiting bacterial DNA-de-

Table 1. Drugs of choice for specific infections. (Adapted from Leopold 1978)

Infecting organism	First choice	Alternative
Gram-positive cocci		
Staphylococcus aureus[a] Non-penicillinase-producing	Penicillin G	A cephalosporin; clindamycin; vancomycin
Penicillinase-producing	A penicillinase-resistant penicillin	A cephalosporin; clindamycin; vancomycin
Streptococcus pyogenes	Penicillin G	An erythromycin
Streptococcus, viridans group[a]	Penicillin G	Chloramphenicol, an erythromycin, a cephalosporin, vancomycin
Streptococcus, enterococcus group (endocarditis or other severe infection)[a]	Ampicillin or penicillin G with streptomycin	Vancomycin with or without streptomycin, kanomycin or gentamicin; tetracycline
Streptococcus, anaeerobic	Penicillin G	Clindamycin; a tetracycline; an erythromycin; chloramphenicol
Streptococcus pneumoniae (pneumococcus)[a]	Penicillin G	An erythromycin; a cephalosporin; chloramphenicol; vancomycin
Gram-negative cocci		
Neisseria gonorrhoeae[a]	Penicillin G	Ampicillin; amoxicillin; a tetracycline; an erythromycin
Neisseria meningitidis	Penicillin G	Chloramphenicol; trimethoprim; sulfamethoxazole
Gram-positive bacilli		
Bacillus anthracis (anthrax)	Penicillin G	An erythromycin; tetracycline chloramphenicol; clindamycin; tetracycline
Clostridium perfringens (welchii)	Penicillin G	
Clostridium tetani	Penicillin G	Tetracycline; a cephalosporin
Corynebacterium diphtheriae	An erythromycin	Penicillin G
Listeria monocytogenes	Ampicillin with or without streptomycin	An erythromycin; tetracycline; chloramphenicol
Enteric gram-negative bacilli		
Bacteroides[a]	Penicillin G	Clindamycin; an erythromycin; tetracycline
	Clindamycin	Chloramphenicol; carbenicillin or ticarcillin; tetracycline
Enterobacter[a]	Gentamicin or tobramycin	Carbenicillin or ticarcillin; kanamycin; amikacin; chloramphenicol; tetracycline

Table 1 (continued)

Infecting organism	First choice	Alternative
Escherichia coli[a]	Gentamicin or tobramycin	Ampicillin; carbenicillin or ticarcillin; a cephalosporin; kanamycin; amikacin; tetracycline; trimethoprim-sulfamethoxazole; chloramphenicol
Klebsiella pneumoniae[a]	Gentamicin or tobramycin	A cephalosporin; kanamycin; amikacin; tetracycline; trimethoprim-sulfamethoxazole; chloramphenicol
Proteus mirabilis[a]	Ampicillin	Gentamicin or tobramycin; carbenicillin or ticarcillin; a cephalosporin; kanamycin; amikacin; trimethoprim-sulfamethoxazole, chloramphenicol
Other *Proteus*[a]	Gentamicin or tobramycin	Carbenicillin or ticarcillin; kanamycin; amikacin; tetracycline; trimethoprim-sulfamethoxazole; chloramphenicol
Salmonella typhi[a]	Chloramphenicol	Ampicillin; amoxicillin; trimethoprim-sulfamethoxazole
Serratia[a]	Gentamicin or tobramycin	Carbenicillin or ticarcillin kanamycin; amikacin; trimethoprim-sulfamethoxazole; chloramphenicol
Other gram-negative bacilli		
Acinetobacter (*Mima, Herellea*)[a]	Gentamicin or tobramycin	Kanamycin; amikacin; chloramphenicol; minocycline
Hemophilus influenzae[a]	Chloramphenicol	Ampicillin; tetracycline
Other infections	Ampicillin or amoxicillin	Tetracycline; trimethoprim-sulfamethoxazole; a sulfonamide; streptomycin
Legionnaires' disease, agent of	An erythromycin	Tetracycline
Leptotrichia buccalis (Vincent's infection)	Penicillin G	Tetracycline; an erythromycin
Pasteurella multocida	Penicillin G	Tetracycline
Pseudomonas aeruginosa[a] (urinary tract infection)	Carbenicillin or ticarcillin	Gentamicin or tobramycin; amikacin; a polymyxin
Acid-fast bacilli		
Mycobacterium tuberculosis	Isoniazid with ethambutol, with or without rifampin	Streptomycin; *p*-aminosalicyclic acid; kanamycin
Atypical mycobacteria	Isoniazid with rifampin, with or without ethambutol	Streptomycin; kanamycin; erythromycin; *p*-aminosalicyclic acid
Mycobacterium leprae (leprosy)	Dapsone with or without rifampin	Acedapsone; rifampin; clofazimine

Table 1 (continued)

Infecting organism	First choice	Alternative
Actinomycetes		
Actinomyces israelii[a] (actinomycosis)	Penicillin G	Tetracycline
Nocardia[a]	Trisulfapyrimidines	Trimethoprim-sulfamethoxazole; trisulfapyrimidines with minocycline or ampicillin or erythromycin
Chlamydiae		
Chlamydia psittaci (psittacosis; ornithosis)	Tetracycline	Chloramphenicol
Chlamydia trachomatis (trachoma; inclusion conjunctivitis)	Tetracycline (topical plus oral)	A sulfonamide (topical plus oral)
	An erythromycin (topical plus oral)	Tetracycline (topical plus, in adults, oral); a sulfonamide (topical plus oral)
(pneumonia)	An erythromycin	A sulfonamide
(urethritis)	Tetracycline	A sulfonamide
(lymphogranuloma venereum)	Tetracycline	Chloramphenicol; a sulfonamide
Fungi		
Aspergillus	Amphotericin B	No dependable alternative
Blastomyces dermatitidis	Amphotericin B	Hydroxystilbamidine
Candida albicans	Amphotericin B	Flucytosine; nystatin (oral or topical); miconazole (topical); clotrimazole (topical)
Coccidioides immitis	Amphotericin B	Miconazole
Cryptococcus neoformans	Amphotericin B with or without flucytosine	No dependable alternative
Histoplasma capsulatum	Amphotericin B	
Mucor	Amphotericin B	
Sporothrix schenckii	An iodide	Amphotericin B
Mycoplasma		
Mycoplasma pneumoniae	An erythromycin or a tetracycline	
Pneumocystis carinii	Trimethoprim-sulfamethoxazole	Pentamidine
Rickettsia [Rocky Mountain spotted fever; endemic typhus (murine); tick bite fever; typhus; rickettsial pox; scrub typhus; Q fever]	Tetracycline	Chloramphenicol

Table 1 (continued)

Infecting organism	First choice	Alternative
Spirochetes		
Leptospira	Penicillin G	Tetracycline
Treponema pallidum (syphilis)	Penicillin G_1	Tetracycline; an erythromycin
Treponema pertenue (yaws)	Penicillin G	Tetracycline
Parasites		
Toxoplasma	Pyrimethamine (Daraprim) Sulfonamides	Clindamycin
Worms		
Onchocerca	Diethylcarbamazine (Hetrazan)	

[a] Because resistance may be a problem, susceptibility tests should be performed

Table 2. Trade names of most commonly used antibiotics

Antibiotic	Trade name
Ampicillin	Amcil
	Omnipen
	Penbritin
	Polycillin
	Drincipen
Carbenicillin	Geopen
	Pyopen
Cephalothin	Keflin
Cephaloridine	Loridine
Cefazolin	Ancif
	Kefzol
Chloramphenicol	Chloromycetin
Colistin (Sodium)	Coly-Mycin M
Gentamicin	Garamycin
Methicillin	Staphcillin
Nofcillin	Unipen
Cloxacillin	Orbenin, Tegopen
Dicloxacillin	Dyapen
	Pathocil
	Veracillin
Oxacillin	Prostaphlin
Potassium penicillin G (intraocular)	
Buffered potassium penicillin G (intraocular)	
Penicillin G (Repository)	Crepatcillin
	Depopenicillin
	Lentopen
Tobramycin	Nebcin
Vancomycin	Vancocin

pendent RNA polymerase. The sulfonamides act through inhibition of microbial synthesis of folic acid by competing with their structural analog, p-aminobenzoic acid (PABA), for transport into the bacterial cell and subsequently inhibiting the enzymatic incorporation of PABA into a precursor of folic acid.

II. Penetration and Absorption

After the anti-infective agent has been chosen, correct dosage must be determined for the individual. Dosage is established through consideration of the penetration of the agent itself, as well as the age and health of the particular individual

Dosage schedules for other parts of the body may not be adequate for ocular infection. Since penetration varies, new agents must be tested for their absorption into the ocular chambers and tissues. Often massive doses must be administered systemically in order to assure adequate drug levels in ocular tissue. Therefore, various routes of administration should be investigated.

Most drugs penetrate into the infected tissues from the bloodstream by passive diffusion. The rate of penetration into the eye is proportional to the concentration of free drug in the plasma or extraocular fluid.

1. Protein and Tissue Binding

Drugs which are bound to protein, such as aminoglycosides (gentamicin), the tetracyclines, and clindamycin, are less likely to penetrate than those which are free or loosely bound, like penicillin or the cephalosporins. Some binding seems to take place in all ocular tissue, but it is particularly pronounced in the pigmented tissue. In vitro experiments have shown that melanin acts as an inhibitor of antibiotic activity (BARZA et al. 1976), presumably due to its binding ability. Less binding takes place in albino tissue than in highly pigmented tissue (BARZA et al. 1979). Though antibiotic activity is probably reduced by pigment, in some situations it could possibly enhance effectiveness by providing a mechanism for keeping an antibiotic in the tissue for a longer period of time (BLOOME et al. 1970).

2. The Blood–Aqueous Barrier

Permeability of the blood–aqueous barrier is a factor in determining the ability of an antibiotic to penetrate the site of infection. In the normal eye, concentrations of antibiotics are much lower than in the serum or plasma. However, when the eye is inflamed the blood–aqueous barrier becomes more permeable, allowing increased amounts of antibiotics from the bloodstream to enter the eye (LEOPOLD and LA MOTTE 1945; LEOPOLD and SCHEIE 1943). When the infection and inflammation begin to subside and the blood–aqueous barrier regains its original integrity, viable microorganisms may still persist within the eye. Therefore, drug dosage should not be reduced as the patient improves, until it can be assured that fluids and tissue are free from pathogenic microorganisms.

3. Physicochemical Influences

Any antibiotic applied topically to the eye will either penetrate into the ocular tissue or be washed away with the tear flow. The conjunctiva can take up appreciable amounts of some drugs, such as sulfacetamide, from the tears and discharge them into the eye over a long period of time (RIDLEY 1958; SALAZAR and PATIL 1975). However, there is considerable evidence that drug penetration into the aqueous humor across the conjunctiva and limbal sclera is negligible compared with that across the cornea (DOANE et al. 1978; MAURICE 1951). The limbal vasculature probably carries away most of the drug that penetrates the conjunctiva before it enters the anterior chamber.

The amount of drug entering the cornea will be determined by the drug contact time with the cornea, the permeability of the corneal epithelium, the tear flow, and the characteristics of the drug itself. Lipophilic substances, such as chloramphenicol and some of the tetracyclines, penetrate the epithelium much more readily than nonlipophilic substances. Polar compounds readily transverse the corneal stroma and then pass into the anterior chamber through the corneal endothelium The latter may offer hindrance to some drugs. According to the time it takes to cross the endothelial barrier, antibiotics may reach their peak in the anterior aqueous in 10–20 min, or it may take as long as a few hours. The cornea may act as a reservoir for the drug, gradually releasing it into the anterior chamber. Drug levels within the anterior chamber will depend on outflow facility, as well as on the amount taken up by the iris and ciliary body tissue.

4. Aqueous and Uveoscleral Outflow

After the drug passes into the aqueous humor it bathes the lens, iris, and anterior chamber and flows with the aqueous through the filtration angle of the root of the iris, through the trabecular meshwork, and out of the eye via Schlemm's canal. Approximately 1.5% of the volume of the anterior chamber is lost each minute in both man and rabbit. Drugs may also be absorbed into the tissues of the anterior uvea and the blood circulating through them or into the lens. This loss varies greatly for different substances (MAURICE 1980).

A small, questionable significant portion of the drug in humans flows out with the aqueous along the uveoscleral pathway (BILL and PHILLIPS 1971), from the anterior chamber into the anterior uvea, and from there into the suprachoroid and out of the eye, perhaps through perivascular spaces.

III. Limiting Factors

1. Age

Usual doses need to be reduced for the very young and the very old. Premature infants and newborns have imperfectly developed capacities for excreting drugs. The gray baby syndrome is an example of the effects of chloramphenicol on infants who are unable to metabolize this agent. In the elderly patient, renal elimination of drugs frequently diminishes. Even in the absence of overt renal disease, dosage schedules should be reduced in the aged, particularly with toxic antibiotics such as aminoglycosides.

2. Renal Disease

Certain drugs which depend on renal function for excretion, such as aminogly-cosides, polymyxins, vancomycin, and flucytosine, should be used carefully in patients with renal disease. Due to reduced elimination, these drugs can build up to toxic levels in the plasma and tissue. Tetracyclines, which have an antianabolic action, increase the kidney's workload and may lead to decreased renal function. Careful dosage modification programs have been worked out for kanamycin and gentamicin according to the degree of renal impairment encountered (MAWER 1976; DETTLI 1976). For these drugs it is better to lengthen the dose interval rather than reduce the dose. Blood assays are a valuable tool for verifying the correctness of the schedule (BARZA and LAUERMAN 1978).

The foregoing considerations apply to drugs administered systemically, rather than those applied topically or periocularly. However, when large doses are administered by periocular injection, the patient's renal function should be assessed.

3. Liver Disease

In patients with hepatic dysfunction, dosage reduction is required for antibiotics excreted largely by the liver, such as erythromycin, chloramphenicol, lincomycin, clindamycin, rifampin, and isoniazid. Drugs excreted in high concentrations in the bile may also be influenced by infection in the biliary tract, hepatic disease, or biliary obstruction. If the ophthalmologist limits his administration to periocular injection or topical therapy, these systemic factors are definitely not as important, but would still have to be considered in a patient who was treated for a long period of time with large doses by the periocular route.

4. Enzymes

Drug metabolism may be altered by various enzymatic factors which are genetically inherited. Acute hemolysis may result in patients with glucose-6-phosphate dehydrogenase deficiency taking sulfonamides or chloramphenicol.

5. Pregnancy

Some antibiotics can cross the placenta and affect the unborn child. They can also be transmitted through the nursing mother's milk to her baby. Tetracyclines taken during pregnancy cause injury to developing teeth, particularly during the second and third trimesters. This drug may cause fatty necrosis of the liver in pregnant women. Pancreatitis and associated renal damage has also been reported with the use of tetracyclines during pregnancy.

PHILIPSON (1977) has observed that it is more difficult to maintain satisfactory concentrations of ampicillin in pregnant than in nonpregnant women. This might possibly hold true for other penicillins as well.

6. Ocular Damage and Disease

Ocular damage and disease may impede or enhance drug penetration and dosage. In experiments comparing topical penetration of gentamicin to corneas burned with lye and those with pyocyaneus ulcers, it was found that higher drug levels were found in the eyes with lye-buned corneas, although the epithelial barrier was breached in both cases (BAUM et al. 1974). Perhaps only the endothelial barrier was damaged by lye. Obstruction to drug penetration can be caused by various disease conditions, such as dense keratinization of the conjunctiva and cornea, or dense scaling seen in advanced cases of pemphigoid or Stevens–Johnson syndrome. Conjunctival flap, in addition to providing further epithelial covering, adds vascularization that can provide a route of removal for medication. Old chemical burns and scars, particularly those causing vascularization, provide an obstruction to drug penetration (FOULKS 1980).

IV. Routes of Administration

There are many choices in regard to the route of ocular anti-infective administration. Thought should be given to the site of infection within the eye, penetration of the antibiotic, toxic effects, and the health profile of the patient being treated. Though clinically the most common methods of ocular antibiotic administration are topical, subconjunctival, and systemic, experimental studies continue to explore alternative methods. Table 3 summarizes various routes of administration

Table 3. Experimental studies of methods of administration of antibiotics and chemotherapeutic agents for ocular purposes. (Adapted from LEOPOLD 1971)

Method of administration	Reference
Topical	
Drops (solutions, emulsions, suspensions; detergents added)	BELLOWS and GUTMAN (1943)
	LEOPOLD and SCHEIE (1943)
	SWAN (1944)
	LEOPOLD (1945)
	LEOPOLD (1945)
Ointments (compound bases)	RICHTER (1957)
Cotton pledget	VON SALLMANN (1945)
	STRUBLE and BELLOWS (1944)
	STRUBLE and BELLOWS (1946)
Powder	
Sulfonamide	CAMERON (1949)
Penicillin crystals	JULES and YOUNG (1945)
	AINSLIE (1946)
Iontophoresis	
Sulfonamide	BELLOWS and CHINN (1941)
	BOYD (1942)
	VON SALLMANN (1943, 1944)
Penicillin	VON SALLMANN and MEYER (1944)
	WRIGHT and STUART HARRIS (1945)
	LEOPOLD et al. (1947)
Streptomycin	LEOPOLD and NICHOLS (1946)
Bacitracin	LOCKE (1949)
Neomycin	WITZEL et al. (1956)
Tetracycline	DE ROETTH (1949)
Polymyxin	BELLOWS et al. (1950)
Spray (penicillin)	MELODIA and BOVO (1953)
Lamellae	MUNOZ (1955)

Table 3 (continued)

Method of administration	Reference
Ocusert	
Injection	
Subconjunctival injection	
Penicillin	Struble and Bellows (1944)
	Leopold (1945 b)
	Struble and Bellows (1946)
Streptomycin	Leopold et al. (1947)
	Sorsby et al. (1952)
Polymyxin	Ainslie and Smith (1952)
	Ainslie and Cairns (1960)
Oxytetracycline	Cannon et al. (1952)
Chloramphenicol	Sorsby et al. (1953)
Sub-Tenon	Swan et al. (1956)
Retrobulbar	
Penicillin	Sorsby and Ungar (1946)
Streptomycin	Leopold et al. (1947)
Chlortetracycline	Michiels (1953)
Intracameral – anterior chamber	
Penicillin	Dunnington and von Sallmann (1944)
	Leopold (1945)
	Mann (1946)
	Saubermann (1957)
Streptomycin	Leopold et al. (1947)
	Grignolo (1948)
Chloramphenicol	Capalbi and Centanni (1949)
	Leopold et al. (1950)
Intracameral – vitreous	
Penicillin	Rycroft (1945)
	von Sallmann (1945)
	Leopold (1945 a)
	Mann (1946)
	Weizenblatt (1946)
Streptomycin	Leopold et al. (1947)
Chloramphenicol	Leopold et al. (1950)
	Capalbi and Centanni (1949)
Oral	
Sulfonamide	Bellows and Chinn (1939)
	Scheie and Souders (1941)
	Davson (1949)
Chloramphenicol	Leopold and Nichols (1946)
	Abraham and Burnett (1955)
Intramuscular and intravenous	
Penicillin	Struble and Bellows (1944)
	Rycroft (1945)
	Leopold (1945 b)
	von Sallmann (1947)
	Saubermann (1953)
Streptomycin	Leopold and Nichols (1946)
	Langham (1951)

and the experimental studies supporting these methods. Tables 4–7 present common drug dosages used for various routes chosen.

Penetration studies with antibiotics can provide guidelines for selecting systemic dosage schedules for ophthalmic infections (Table 8). Drugs rated as demonstrating fair penetration can be expected to provide therapeutic concentrations against many organisms in the inflamed eye.

Table 4. Dosage for systemic therapy in intraocular infection. (LEOPOLD 1972b)

Agent	Dosage
Agents effective against gram-positive and gram-negative organisms	
Ampicillin (Penbritin)	2-g priming dose orally, i.m., or i.v., and 1 g every 6 h
Carbenicillin (Pyopen)	5–7 g i.v. every 4 h (see Agents effective against gram-positive infections)
	1-g priming dose i.m., and 0.5 g every 8 h
Cephalothin (Keflin)	2 g i.m. every 4 h
Cephalexin (Keflex)	2-g priming dose orally, and 1 g every 8 h
Cephaloridine (Loridine)	2-g priming dose i.m., and 1 g every 8 h
Chloramphenicol (Chloromycetin)	3-g priming dose orally, i.m., or i.v., and 1 g every 8 h
Gentamicin (Garamycin)	1 mg/kg i.m. every 8 h
Kantamycin (Kantrex)	0.5 g i.m. every 8 h
Sulfadiazine (Cremodiazine)	2-g priming dose orally or i.v., and 1 g every 6 h
Tetracycline	1-g priming dose orally, i.m., or i.v., and 0.15 g every 8 h
Agents effective against gram-positive infections	
Erythromycin (Erythrocin)	
propionate (Ilosone)	1-g priming dose orally, and 0.5 g every 6 h
succinate	100 mg i.v. every 4 h
lactobionate	250–500 mg i.v. every 4 h
Lincomycin (Lincocin)	2-g priming dose orally, and 1 g every 6 h
	1 g i.m. initially, and 600 mg every 8 h
	600 mg i.v. every 8 h
Methicillin (Staphcillin) (for penicillinase-producing bacteria)	4 g i.m. every 6 h
Oxacillin (sodium oxacillin) (Prostaphlin) (for penicillinase-producing bacteria)	2 g i.m. or i.v. every 6 h
Penicillin G (aqueous) (for non-penicillinase-producing bacteria)	20 million units daily, interrupted or continuous i.v. infusion
Novobiocin (Albamycin)	0.5 g orally every 6 h, and 0.5 mg i.m. or i.v. every 12 h
Vancomycin (Vancocin)	2-g priming dose i.v., and 1 g i.v. every 12 h
Agent effective against fungi	
Amphotericin B (Fungizone)	0.25–1.5 mg/kg i.v.

Table 5. Dosage for subconjunctival therapy in intraocular infections. (LEO-POLD 1972 b)

Agent	Dosage
Bacitracin	10,000 units
with polymyxin B	10 mg (1 mg = 10,000 units)
or colistin (Coly-Mycin)	15 mg
Cephalothin (Keflin)	50 mg
Cephaloridine (Loridine)	25–50 mg
Chloramphenicol (Chloromycetin)	1.25 mg
0.7 ml 15% suspension of micronized material, sodium succinate	100 mg
Erythromycin (lactobionate) (Ery-throcin)	2.5 mg up to 50 mg
or novobiocin with polymyxin B	10 mg (1 mg = 10,000 units)
Gentamicin (Garamycin)	1.25–2.5 mg
Kanamycin (Kantrex)	10–20 mg
Lincomycin (Lincocin)	50–75 mg
Neomycin	100–500 mg
Penicillin G	500,000 to 1 million units
or methicillin (Staphcillin)	150 mg
with streptomycin	50 mg
Tetracycline	2.5–5 mg

Table 6. Solutions for intracameral injection or irrigation. (LEOPOLD 1972 b)

Agent	Dosage
Bacitracin	500–1,000 units
Chloramphenicol (Chlormycetin)	1–2 mg
Colistin (Coly-Mycin)	0.1 mg
Erythrocycin (Erythrocin)	1–2 mg
Methicillin (Staphcillin)	1 mg
Neomycin	2.5 mg
Penicillin G	1–4 M units
Polymyxin B	0.1 mg
Streptomycin	0.5–5 mg
Tetracycline	2.5–5 mg

    Recently there has been a renewed interest in intravitreal antibiotic administration, which was begun in the 1940s (VON SALLMANN 1944; LEOPOLD 1945 b; MANN 1946; PEYMAN et al. 1974 a; ZACHARY and FORSTER 1976). Antibiotics placed in the vitreous can leave the eye directly across the retinal surface or by passing through the anterior hyaloid membrane into the posterior chamber and out of the eye with aqueous drainage. The rate of disappearance of antibiotics placed in the vitreous has been studied (MAURICE 1976; KLEINBERG et al. 1979), as has the toxicity of various concentrations of antibiotics (PEYMAN et al. 1974 b; FORSTER et al. 1976 a).

    In a review of the routes of antibiotic therapy for corneal infections, PETTIT (1976) noted that high therapeutic levels of most antibiotics can be delivered to the

Table 7. Intravitreal antibiotic injection. (LEOPOLD 1978)

Antibiotic	Intravitreal dosage (mg)
Aminoglycosides	
Gentamicin	0.4
Tobramycin	0.5
Amikacin	0.4
Kanamycin	0.5
Penicillins	
Methicillin	2
Oxacillin	0.5
Ampicillin	5
Carbenicillin	2
Miscellaneous	
Cephaloridine	0.25
Erythromycin	0.5
Lincomycin	1.5
Clindamycin	1
Vancomycin	1
Chloramphenicol	2
Amphotericin B	0.005–0.01

Table 8. Intraocular penetration of systemically administered antibiotics. (Adapted from LEOPOLD 1971)

Antibiotics	Investigators
Good	
Ampicillin	KUROSE and LEOPOLD (1965)
	RECORDS and ELLIS (1967)
Chloramphenicol	LEOPOLD et al. (1950)
	LANGHAM (1951)
	SORSBY et al. (1953)
	SAUBERMANN (1953)
Cephaloridine	MIZAKAWA et al. (1965)
	RILEY et al. (1968)
Cephalexin	BOYLE et al. (1970)
Dicloxacillin	RECORDS (1968 b)
Linocmycin	COLES et al. (1971)
	BOYLE et al. (1971)
	MERCER et al. (1978)
	KLEINBERG et al. (1979)
Cephalothin	MIZAKAWA et al. (1965)
	RECORDS (1968 a)
Fair	
Penicillin	LEOPOLD (1945 b)
	VON SALLMANN (1944)
	STRUBLE and BELLOWS (1946)
	BLEEKER and MAAS (1958)
	SORSBY and UNGAR (1946, 1948)
	SAUBERMANN (1953)

Table 8 (continued)

Antibiotics	Investigators
Methicillin	GREEN and LEOPOLD (1965)
	RECORDS and ELLIS (1967)
Neomycin	VOGEL et al. (1951)
	SORSBY and UNGAR (1958)
Vancomycin	PRYOR et al. (1962a)
Gentamicin	LITWACK et al. (1969)
	FURGIUELE (1970)
Colistin	PRYOR et al. (1962b)
	ROSS et al. (1959)
Polymyxin	AINSLIE and SMITH (1952)
Oleandomycin	McCOY and LEOPOLD (1959)
Erythromycin	HALLETT and LEOPOLD (1957)
Cefoxitin	AXELROD and KOCHMAN (1980a)
Cefamandole	AXELROD and KOCHMAN (1980b)
Poor	
Amphotericin	MONTANA and SERY (1958)
	GREEN et al. (1965)
Oxacillin	RECORDS (1967)
	RECORDS and ELLIS (1967)
Novobiocin	SERY et al. (1957)
Streptomycin	LEOPOLD and NICHOLS (1946)
	BELLOWS and FARMER (1947)
	GRIGNOLO (1948)
Tetracyclines	DEROETTH (1949)
	CANNON and LEOPOLD (1952)
Ristocetin	FURGIUELE et al. (1960)

site of the corneal ulcer by a variety of different techniques. These include classic iontophoresis, corneal bathing with an eyecup, and gel foam pledgets, as well as the newer hydrophilic inserts. He recommended using one or a combination of the following three techniques for delivering antibiotics to the ulcer:

1. Frequent administration of antibiotic drops (every 15–20 min)
2. Continuous lavage of the cornea with antibiotic solutions
3. Subconjunctival injections of antibiotics.

1. Topically Applied Antibiotic Drops

Since commercially available ophthalmic antibiotic preparations are available in fairly low concentrations (Tables 9–10), it has become a common practice among physicians frequently treating bacterial corneal ulcers to formulate their own concentrated antibiotic drops for topical use (THEODORE 1972; JONES 1973). Concentrated antibiotic solutions may be prepared for this purpose by diluting commercially available parenteral antibiotic preparations with tear substitutes or a bal-

Table 9. Commercially available topical ophthalmic antibiotic and chemotherapeutic preparations

---

Chloramphenicol
    Solution 0.5%   Ointment 1%
        Chloroptic (Allergan)   (Allergan)
        Econochlor (Alcon)   (Alcon)
        Ophthochlor (Parke-Davis)   (Parke-Davis)

Erythromycin
    Ilotycin   Ointment 0.5%
                                  (Dista)

Gentamicin
    Solution 3 mg/ml   Ointment 3 mg/g
                                  Garamycin (Schering)
                                  Genoptic (Allergan)

Neomycin   Ointment 5 mg/g
                                  Myciguent (Upjohn)

Bacitracin   Ointment 500 units/35 g
                                  Baciguent (Upjohn)

Sodium sulfacetamide
    Solution 10%–30%   Ointment 10%
        Bleph-10 (Allergan)   Cetamide (Alcon)
        Bleph-30 (Allergan)   Sulamyd (Schering)
        Isopto Cetamide 15% (Alcon)
        Sulamyd 10% (Schering)
        Sulamyd 30% (Schering)
        Sodium sulfacetamide 10%–30% (Barnes-
           Hind)
        Sodium sulfacetamide 10% (Cooper)

Sodium sulfadiazine   Ointment 5% generic

Sulfisoxazole diolomine
    Solution 4% (Barnes-Hind)   Ointment 4%
                                  Gantrisin (Roche)

---

anced salt solution (JONES 1973). Suggested concentrations of commonly used antibiotics in the treatment of corneal ulcers are included in Table 11.

    Allergic reactions and local irritation secondary to the intensively applied anti-
biotic drops may occur, but generally these changes are not severe enough to ne-
cessitate discontinuance of treatment prior to resolution of the ulcer. Since hyperemia and edema of the conjunctiva and diffuse superficial punctate keratitis
may be caused by both the infection and the treatment, clinical judgment of what
is happening to the ulcer itself is critical in evaluating the therapeutic response.

2. Continuous Corneal Lavage with Antibiotic Solutions

To reduce the demands of frequent instillation of eye drops, other methods of delivering a constant level of antibiotic solution to the cornea have been developed.
The drug can flow through a small plastic catheter traversing the lid (HESSBURG

Table 10. Commercially available topical ophthalmic preparations containing mixtures of antibiotics

	Ophthalmic ointment	Ophthalmic solution
Polymyxin B + neomycin		
Mycitracin (Upjohn)	Polymyxin B 5,000 units, neomycin 3.5 mg	
Polyspectrin (Allergan)		Polymyxin B 5,000 units, neomycin 3.5 mg
Statrol (Alcon)	Polymyxin B 6,000 units, neomycin 3.5 mg	Polymyxin B 16,250 units, neomycin 3.5 mg
Polymyxin B + neomycin + bacitracin		
Neo-Polycin (Dow)	Neomycin 3.5 mg, polymyxin B 10,000 units, bacitracin zinc 500 units	
Neosporin (Burroughs Wellcome)	Neomycin 3.5 mg, polymyxin B 5,000 units, bacitracin zinc 400 units	
Polycidin (Smith, Miller, and Patch)		
Polyspectrin, SOP (Allergan)		
Polymyxin B + neomycin + gramicidin		
Neosporin (Burroughs Wellcome)		Polymyxin B 5,000 units, neomycin 1.75 mg, gramicidin 0.025 mg
Neo-Polycin (Dow)		
Polymyxin B + bacitracin		
Polysporin (Burroughs Wellcome)	Polymyxin B 10,000 units, bacitracin zinc 500 units	
Polymyxin B + chloramphenicol		
Chloromyxin (Parke Davis)	Chloramphenicol 10 mg, polymyxin B 5,000 units	
Polymyxin B + oxytetracycline		
Terramycin (Pfizer)	Oxytetracycline 5 mg, polymyxin B 10 000 units	

Table 11. Concentrations of antibiotic solutions that may be prepared for topical use in corneal ulcers [a]

Bacitracin	10,000 units/ml
Carbenicillin	100 mg/ml
Cephaloridine	50 mg/ml
Cephalothin	50 mg/ml
Chloramphenicol	5 mg/ml
Colistin	5–10 mg/ml
Erythromycin	50 mg/ml
Gentamicin	15 mg/ml
Lincomycin	50–150 mg/ml
Methicillin	50–100 mg/ml
Neomycin	50–100 mg/ml
Penicillin G	100,000–200,000 units/ml
Polymyxin B	5–10 mg/ml
Streptomycin	50–100 mg/ml
Vancomycin	50 mg/ml

[a] Topical use of the penicillins should be avoided if equally good alternate antibiotics are available

1969), or via a cannulated contact lens, such as the Mediflow lens (JONES 1973). Antibiotic solutions used for constant bathing of the cornea with these techniques are given in low dilutions of 0.05%–0.1% in Ringer's solution at the rate of 6–8 drops/min. Not only do these techniques deliver a constant level of antibiotic to the ulcer, but the continuous irrigation also cleanses the ulcer surface.

3. Subconjunctival Injections of Antibiotics

Subconjunctival antibiotic injections should be used as part of the initial therapy in all severe corneal ulcers, and should be repeated every 12–24 h as follows:

Topical anesthetic (0.5% proparacaine or tetracaine) 5 drops
Lidocaine (2%) 0.5 ml subconjunctivally and 0.2–1.0 ml antibiotic solution (Table 12) subconjunctivally in anesthetized area.
Rotate sites of injection on bulbar conjunctiva and avoid tearing vessels.

Pain following injection may occur even though a small amount of lidocaine is injected subconjunctivally prior to injection of the antibiotic. Also, signs of inflammation, already present in the eye with an ulcerated cornea, may be expected to increase, and oozing from the injection site frequently occurs. Because the use of concentrated antibiotic drops and the subconjunctival injections of antibiotics are not officially approved by the manufacturer or the Food and Drug Administration (FDA), it is wise to have the patient sign an informed consent when antibiotics are to be used in this manner. This procedure is justified by the clinical situation and by accepted community practices. The ability to deliver therapeutic levels of antibiotics to the anterior segment of the eye by subconjunctival injections is supported by extensive animal data and is consistent with clinical experience in treating bacterial ulcers of the cornea (PETTIT 1976; BARZA et al. 1973; GOLDEN and COPPEL 1970; GOLDMAN et al. 1973; LITWACH et al. 1969; PATERSON 1973; PRYOR et al. 1962a; RECORDS and ELLIS 1967; RECORDS 1969). The recommended antibiotic

Table 12. Subconjunctival antibiotic dosages for treatment of corneal ulcers

Ampicillin	50–250 mg
Bacitracin	10,000 units
Carbenicillin	100 mg
Cephaloridine	100 mg
Cephalothin	100 mg
Chloramphenicol, sodium succinate suspension	50–100 mg
Colistin	15–30 mg
Erythromycin (lactobionate or gluceptate)	50–100 mg
Gentamicin	10–20 mg
Kanamycin	10–20 mg
Lancomycin	50–150 mg
Methicillin	100–200 mg
Neomycin	100–500 mg
Penicillin G	300,000 to 1 million units
Polymyxin B	10 mg
Streptomycin	50–100 mg
Vancomycin	25 mg

dosages for subconjunctival use as previously published in the ophthalmic literature are tabulated in Table 12 (ALLEN 1971; JONES 1973; THEODORE 1972; LEOPOLD
1971, 1972a, 1978).

V. Use of Antibiotics in Combination

The simultaneous use of multiple antibiotics in a shotgun fashion should be
avoided because of the problems of drug toxicity and sensitizations, microbial
superinfections, and antagonisms between certain agents. However, there are a
limited number of reasons whereby the simultaneous administration of more than
one chemotherapeutic agent is warranted (JAWETZ 1975; RAHAL 1978):

1. Prevention of emergence of resistance to one or both drugs
2. Treatment of polymicrobic infections for which one antibiotic is not sufficient
3. Initial treatment of vision-threatening infections prior to isolation of the causative agent
4. Synergism between two antimicrobials against a specific infecting agent.

1. Prevention of Emergence of Drug-Resistant Mutants

In a few chronic infections in which large numbers of organisms are present, the
continued use of a single drug is likely to lead to the emergence of resistant mutants. This development can be prevented by the simultaneous administration of
a second drug that attacks a different locus in the microbial cell and is able to suppress of kill any mutants resistant to the first drug. The best example of this therapeutic approach is the administration of isoniazid and ethambutol in the treatment of tuberculosis.

2. Treatment of Mixed Infections

Certain types of polymicrobic infections can be treated satisfactorily with a single
drug. On the other hand, other polymicrobic infections are due to a mixed flora
– including enteric gram-negative bacilli, *Bacteroides* species, various gram-positive cocci, and *Clostridia*. These organisms have a wide spectrum of antimicrobial
susceptibilities, and combination therapy with clindamycin plus gentamicin or ampicillin plus chloramphenicol is logically employed. This treatment is suggested not
for synergistic action against individual bacterial species but for coverage of the
multiplicity of organisms involved.

3. Initial Treatment of Vision-Threatening Infections

In critically ill patients with severe infections, such as in an immunosuppressed
patient with ocular infection of unknown etiology, several antimicrobial drugs are
employed simultaneously to provide adequate initial tratment for the most likely
etiologic agents while the results of cultures are awaited. In the treatment of a vitreous abscess prior to surgery and definitive bacteriologic diagnosis, a combination
of penicillin and chloramphenicol may be employed to cover the spectrum or organisms implicated in this infection – *Streptococci*, *Bacteroides*, and other anaerobes, and Enterobacteriaceae. Treatment of unknown sepsis in neutropenic

patients receiving antineoplastic chemotherapy involves the use of combinations of drugs aimed at *Pseudomonas aeruginosa* and other causes of severe infections. Such combinations include carbenicillin and gentamicin, carbenicillin and amikacin, and cephalothin with gentamicin (KLASTERSKY et al. 1976; SCHIMPFF et al. 1976). An aminoglycoside effective against *Pseudomonas aeruginosa* is an essential element in any such program. The selection of the aminoglycoside for initial empirical therapy will depend on local epidemiologic considerations and on whether one of those agents (gentamicin, tobramycin, or amikacin) has been used previously.

4. Antibiotic Synergism and Antagonism

Combinations of antibiotics are very effective against a specific infecting organism if they provide an additive or synergistic effect. However, sometimes combining antibiotics produces an indifferent or even antagonistic effect. Caution must be used in injecting two or more antibiotics together intravenously, as some combinations are incompatible when administered in the same containers. Table 13 gives guidelines for usage of combined antibiotics, and Table 14 summarizes intravenous incompatibilities.

Table 13. Guidelines on synergetic and antagonistic antimicrobial combinations. (LEOPOLD 1978)

Combinations	Antimicrobials	Interaction	Organism
Two bactericidal agents	Penicillin and streptomycin	Synergistic	Streptococci
	Most	Additive or indifferent	Most
Two bacteriostatic agents	Most	Additive or indifferent	Most
	Trimethoprim and sulfamethoxazole	Synergistic	Many
	Erythromycin and lincomycin	Antagonistic	Few gram-positive
	Erythromycin and chloramphenicol	Antagonistic	Few gram-negative
	Lincomycin and chloramphenicol	Antagonistic	Few gram-negative
One bactericidal plus one bacterio-static	Penicillin and tetracycline	Antagonistic	Pneumococci
	Most	Additive or indifferent	Most
	Polymyxin and sulfonamides	Synergistic	*Proteus*
	Erythromycin and streptomycin	Synergistic	Streptococci

Table 14. Intravenous incompatibilities. (Leopold 1978)

Drug	Incompatible with
Tetracycline	Amphotericin B Corticosteroids Cephalothin Chloramphenicol Polymyxin B Penicillin G
Polymyxin B	Cephalothin Chloramphenicol Tetracycline
Penicillin G	Vancomycin Phenylephrine Tetracycline Amphotericin B
Vancomycin	Chloramphenicol Methicillin; penicillin G Hydrocortisone
Methicillin	Kanamycin Vancomycin tetracycline

a) Antagonism

Antibiotic antagonism occurs when the combined effect of two or more antimicrobial drugs is smaller than the sum of the effects of the individual drugs. In in vitro studies, antagonism

Is commonly observed when a inhibitory concentration of a bacteriostatic drug interacts with a minimal bactericidal concentration of a penicillin or another inhibitor of cell wall synthesis or an aminoglycoside

Is usually not observed when high concentrations of either the bactericidal or bacteriostatic drugs are used

Is generally manifested by a reduction of the number of viable bacteria to the level produced by the bacteriostatic drug alone.

Transposed to the in vivo situation, antagonism may not show its effect in the presence of adequate levels of antibody and numbers of leukocytes. However, in the immunosuppressed or granulocytopenic host, antibiotic antagonism can be a source of therapeutic failure.

The mechanism of antibiotic antagonism varies with the specific pair of antibiotics involved. The inhibition of the bacterial multiplication needed to allow the bactericidal action of penicillin and other drugs that interfere with cell wall synthesis probably accounts for the antagonistic effect of bacteriostatic drugs such as tetracycline. Chloramphenicol can antagonize the bactericidal action of gentamicin in vitro, either by blocking the small amount of protein synthesis needed for the bactericidal effect of an amminoglycoside or by binding to the ribosome, which in some way blocks aminoglycoside uptake elsewhere on the ribosome complex.

In experimental infections, antagonism can be observed when a bacteriostatic drug (chloramphenicol) and a bactericidal drug (penicillin) are administered simultaneously. This antagonism, however, is not observed when the bactericidal drug is administered first, or when multiple doses of both drugs are given (WALLACE et al. 1967). Similarly, in experimental *Proteus mirabilis* meningitis, chloramphenicol can interfere with the bactericidal action of gentamicin (STRAUSBAUGH and SANDE 1978). Such antagonism, however, is not important when the effects of the bacteriostatic drug (in the presence of normal host defenses) are sufficient to effect cure. Because of very specific timing and dose relationships, antimicrobial antagonism is not commonly observed clinically. The most convincing evidence for clinically important antagonism is in the combined use of two specific antibiotics (chlortetracycline and penicillin) in the treatment of meningitis due to a specific microorganism, *Streptococcus pneumoniae* (LEPPER and DOWLING 1951). There are very few other clinical examples of antimicrobial antagonism that have been well documented.

b) Synergism

Antibiotic synergism occurs when the combined antimicrobial effect of two or more drugs is more than the sum of the effect of the individual drugs. Several different mechanisms of antimicrobial synergism are known.

Enhancement by One Drug of the Entry of a Second Drug into Microbial Cells. The synergistic action of penicillin and an aminoglycoside has been most extensively studied with enterococci, both in vitro (MOELLERING et al. 1971) and in vivo. Penicillin alone inhibits growth of enterococci but is not bactericidal. Aminoglycosides alone cannot enter enterococci because of a permeability barrier. Penicillin-induced changes in the enterococcus cell wall, however, enable the aminoglycosides to enter so that bactericidal action takes place (unless the enterococcal strain has an R-factor-mediated resistance to the aminoglycoside) (KROGSTAD et al. 1978).

About 50% of enterococcal isolates at some hospitals are resistant to high levels of streptomycin (over 2,000 µg/ml); these strains are not susceptible to penicillin-streptomycin combination (MOELLERING et al. 1971). Many strains of enterococci are similarly resistant to kanamycin and amikacin, and consequently are immune to combined therapy with penicillin. Enterococcal isolates resistant to penicillin–gentamicin synergism have not yet appeared, which makes this drug pair the synergistic combination of choice for treatment of enterococcal infections. Synergism between vancomycin and aminoglycosides against enterococci has also been demonstrated (MANDELL et al. 1970), but cephalosporins do not show synergistic activity with aminoglycosides in the treatment of enterococcal infections.

Inhibition by One Drug of a Microbial Enzyme that Inactivates the Second Drug. Organisms that produce β-lactamase (penicillinase) are usually highly resistant to penicillin. If, however, β-lactamase is exposed to a substrate that has a high binding affinity, but is not hydrolyzable (methicillin or cloxacillin), then the enzyme may be so tightly bound as to render it unavailable for destruction of a readily cleavable penicillin, such as ampicillin. In this way, a penicillinase-susceptible penicillin may be protected from enzymatic hydrolysis and enabled to exert its antibacterial effect. Though in general this approach has had little practical application, the isolation of very potent inhibitors of microbial β-lactamases, such as clavulanic acid, may provide an effective means of maintaining the efficacy of otherwise hydrolyzable penicillins against *Staphylococcus aureus* and a variety of resistant gram-negative bacilli (READING and COLE 1977).

Inhibition of Successive Steps in a Metabolic Sequence. Sulfonamides act as competitive inhibitors of PABA, which many bacteria require as a precursor in the biosynthesis of folic acid. The conversion of folic acid to its coenzyme form, which is involved in purine synthesis, requires enzymatic reduction of dihydrofolate to tetrahydrofolate. This latter enzymatic step is inhibited by trimethoprim. Thus the combination of a sulfonamide and trimethoprim blocks two sequential steps in the pathway of purine and nucleic acid synthesis, resulting in more effective suppression of microbial growth than is achieved by either drug used alone. This combination has been effective in the treatment of urinary tract infections due to enteric gram-negative bacilli, typhoid fever due to chloramphenicol-resistant organism, and pneumocystosis.

VI. Adverse Drug Interactions

When several unrelated drugs are administered simultaneously, interactions can occur that alter the anticipated responses of one or more of the drugs administered. Such interactions may be an unexpected response or an increase or decrease in the usual reaction. They may involve several antimicrobial agents or an antimicrobial agent and one or more drugs of an unrelated class (Table 15) (ABRAMOWICZ 1977).

A variety of mechanisms may account for observed drug interactions:
1. Accelerated or decreased metabolism of one agent produced by the induction of microsomal enzymes by administration of a second agent
2. Decreased absorption of one drug due to the presence of a second drug in the gastrointestinal tract when oral administration is employed
3. Increased circulating levels of one drug in its active form due to its displacement from plasma proteins or secondary tissue receptor sites
4. Decreased renal excretion of one drug produced by the administration of a second drug.

Some interactions occur only with high drug dosage, while others are the result of inherited differences in drug metabolism. If drugs must be administered together, the smallest number of drugs is the safest, and drug dosage must be altered accordingly.

In vitro incompatibilities may also occur on mixing several drugs or on adding certain drugs to specific diluents. Some antibiotics form a precipitate when they come in contact with each other, e.g., when erythromycin lactobionate is mixed in the same solution with another antibiotic. One drug may also inactivate another; gentamicin acitivity is lost when mixed with carbenicillin or ampicillin in normal saline solution (NOONE and PATTISON 1971).

Individually, microbial agents are capable of causing adverse side effects, some of which are life-threatening; these effects include hypersensitivity to penicillin,

Table 15. In vivo drug interactions involving antimicrobials. (Adapted from SWARTZ 1980)

Antimicrobial agent	Second drug	Possible adverse effect
Aminoglycosides	Cephhalosporins	Increased nephrotoxicity
	Curare-like drugs	Neuromuscular blockade
	Digoxin	Possible decreases digoxin effect with neomycin
	Ethacrynic acid; furosemide	Increased ototoxicity
	Polymyxins	Increased nephrotoxicity
p-Aminosalicylic acid (PAS)	Probenecid	Increased PAS toxicity
Amphotericin B	Curare-like drugs	Increased neuromuscular blockade
	Digitalis glycosides	Increased digitalis toxicity
Ampicillin	Allopurinol	Increased frequency of rashes from ampicillin
	Oral anticoagulants	Increased prothrombin time
Cephalosporins	Aminoglycosides	Increased nephrotoxicity
	Ethacrynic acid	Increased nephrotoxicity
	Furosemide	Increased nephrotoxicity
Chloramphenicol	Oral anticoagulants	Increased anticoagulant effect
	Oral hypoglycemic agents	Increased sulfonylurea hypoglycemia
	Phenytoin	Increased phenytoin toxicity
Polymyxins	Aminoglycosides	Increased nephrotoxicity
	Curare-like drugs	Increased neuromuscular blockade
Sulfonamides	Oral anticoagulants	Increased anticoagulant effect
	Oral hypoglycemic drugs	Increased sulfonylurea hypoglycemia
Tetracyclines	Oral antacids	Decreased effect of tetracycline
	Barbiturates	Decreased doxycycline effect
	Oral anticoagulants	Increased anticoagulant effect
	Phenytoin	Decreased doxycycline effect

blood dyscrasias from chloramphenicol and the sulfonamides, and superinfections, particularly those induced by the tetracyclines. Toxic features of each antibiotic must therefore be known. In addition, dosage, duration of administration, age of patient, state of the kidney and liver, and known sensitivities to antibiotics should be considered. In patients with impaired liver or kidney function, careful monitoring of drug blood concentrations and electrolyte balance studies should be done. All drugs should be administered with caution to pregnant women and newborns.

Allergic reactions are most frequently caused by penicillin and sulfonamides, and they are more frequent with parenteral than with oral administration. Since allergy to one penicillin usually means allergy to the others, cephalosporins are usually used in patients allergic to penicillin (though instances of cross-hypersensitivity have been reported).

Gastrointestinal disturbances are more frequent with oral than with parenteral administration, and are most common with the tetracyclines. This side effect may be due to irritation of the gastrointestinal tract by antimicrobial drugs or their metabolites, or it may result from superinfection. Superinfections are most common

Table 16. Direct drug toxicity

Kidney
    Aminoglycosides
    Polymyxins
    Cephaloridine
    Amphotericin B
    Tetracycline
    Carbenicillin
    Rifampin
Hematopoietic system
    Chloramphenicol
    Sulfonamides
    Penicillin
    Cephalosporins
    Rifampin
Nervous system
    Ototoxicity – vestibular > auditory
        Streptomycin
        Gentamicin
        Minocycline
    Ototoxicity – auditory > vestibular
        Neomycin
        Kanamycin
        Amikacin
        Tobramycin
    Neuromuscular blockade
        Aminoglycoside – reversed by neostigmine and calcium gluconate
        Colistin
        Polymyxin B } – reversed by calcium gluconate but not by neostimine
    Seizures
        Penicillin
        Cephalosporins
    Peripheral neuropathy
        Isoniazid
    Papilledema
        Tetracycline
        Nalidixic acid
    Optic neuritis
        Ethambutal
        Chloramphenicol
Liver
    Isoniazid
    Rifampin
    P-Amino salycilic acid
    Tetracycline
    Oxacillin
Gastrointestinal tract
    Direct irritation
    Bacterial overgrowth
        Erythromycin
        Tetracyclines
        Neomycin
        Chloramphenicol
        Clindamycin – pseudomembranous colitis

---

with broad-spectrum drugs, such as the tetracyclines. Stomatitis and glossitis are fairly common side effects, often resulting from superinfection by *Candida* species.

Most antimicrobial drugs and their metabolites are excreted primarily in the urine, with some excretion by the biliary tract. During the first 24 h of therapy, most patients with impaired kidney function can tolerate the usual doses of antimicrobial drugs that are excreted mainly by kidneys. Subsequent doses, however, should be reduced to minimize the risk of renal insufficiency with increased drug concentration in blood and tissues. If the patient is dehydrated, maintenance doses of all agents excreted by the kidneys should be reduced. Some of the antimicrobials excreted mainly by the kidneys are themselves capable of causing renal imbalance. These include amphotericin B, bacitracin, neomycin, kanamycin, polymyxins, vancomycin, cephaloridine and the sulfonamides.

Tetracycline has caused severe liver damage in pregnant women, bone lesions, and staining and deformity of teeth in children up to the age of 8 years and in the newborn when given to pregnant women in about the 4th month of gestation. Pseudotumor cerebri can occur in infants under 6 months of age. Except for tetracycline, congenital defects have not been described convincingly with any antimicrobial agent.

Table 16 is a summary of the various internal systems which can be effected by drug toxicity. More detailed considerations of anti-infective toxicities will be described in Sect. D under individual drug headings.

C. Postoperative Intraocular Infections (Endophthalmitis)

Various regimes (Tables 17–19) have been suggested for management of intraocular infections. They all stress the necessity for prompt cultures of the contents of the ocular chambers and introduction of therapy. Once the aqueous and vitreous humors have been obtained for culture, antibiotics may be given topically, systemically, subconjunctivally, and directly into the anterior and vitreous chambers according to the following pharmacological principles:

1. Antibiotic should be selected on the basis of:
   a) Smear
   b) Culture
   c) Sensitivity
   (LEOPOLD and APT 1960; LEOPOLD 1952, 1971, 1978; FORSTER 1978; BAUM 1978; ALLEN and MANGIARACINE 1973).
2. Route of administration should be selected to provide effective concentration of proper antibiotic at site of infection.
3. Treatment should be started early (LEOPOLD 1952; LEOPOLD and APT 1960).
4. The topical and systemic toxic potential of the antibiotics, alone and in combination should be known (LEOPOLD and APT 1960; LEOPOLD 1952, 1971).
5. Topical therapy is superior to systemic for conjunctival and corneal infections (LEOPOLD et al. 1944).
6. Lipid-soluble antibiotics penetrate the cornea better than water-soluble antibiotics (SWAN and WHITE 1942; LEOPOLD et al. 1950; LANGHAM 1951).

Table 17. Therapeutic regimen for endophthalmitis. (Adapted from BAUM and PEYMAN 1977)[a]

---

1. Periocular injection[b]
   a) Gentamicin 40 mg (1 ml)
      and
   b) Cefazolin 100 mg (0.75 ml)

2. Systemic administration
   a) Gentamicin 4 mg/kg i.m. daily in three divided doses
      and
   b) Cefazolin 1.0 g i.v. every 4 h
      and
   c) Probenecid 0.5 g orally four times a day

After 12 h of the above therapy, repeat the retrobulbar injections of gentamicin and cefazolin and give:

3. Retrobulbar injection of dexamethasone phosphate 4 mg (1 ml) or prednisolone succinate 25 mg (1 ml)

4. Prednisone 60 mg orally

---

[a] The retrobulbar injections are then given daily for 4–7 days, each drug in a separate syringe. Systemic antibiotic and corticosteroid therapy is continued for 7–14 days. Modify antibiotic therapy if necessary on the basis of clinical condition and results of culture and sensitivity report of anterior chamber and vitreous tap. Do not switch therapy if clinical state is improving but culture studies indicate a change of antibiotic

[b] Injections are made with a disposable tuberculin syringe, 25 gauge, $^5/_8$-in. needle

7. Penetration into cornea and anterior segment is increased by employing means to prolong contact time:
   a) Increasing frequency of drop instillation. (Wash out preceding drop by instillation intervals of less then 5 min.) (BAUM et al. 1974; DAVIS et al. 1977)
   b) Cotton packs (LEOPOLD 1971)
   c) Corneal baths (LEOPOLD 1971)
   d) Detergent (surface-tension-lowering agent in vehicle) (SWAN and WHITE 1942; LEOPOLD 1945a)
   e) Iontophoresis
   f) Presoaked (soft) contact lens (PRAUS and KREJCI 1977)
   g) Ointments, powders, viscous vehicles (ADLER et al. 1971)
   h) Denuded corneal epithelium (LEOPOLD and LaMOTTE 1945)
   i) Periocular injection (OAKLEY et al. 1976; SAUBERMANN 1957; LEOPOLD 1947, 1971)
   j) Adding vasoconstrictor to periocular injection, if no contraindications are present (SORSBY and UNGAR 1946)
8. Most systemically administered antibiotics penetrate better across the blood–aqueous barrier of the inflamed eye than the normal eye (LEOPOLD 1945b; BARZA and BAUM 1973).
9. It is difficult to produce adequate concentrations of antibiotics in the vitreous humor by all indirect methods (ABEL et al. 1974; BARZA and BAUM 1973; BAR-

Table 18. Therapeutic regimen for endophthalmitis. (Adapted from FORSTER et al. 1980)

1) Intraocular
   a) Gentamicin (Garamycin) 0.1 mg (100 µg) and
   b) Cephaloridine (Loridine) 0.25 mg (250 µg) or
      Cefazolin 2.25 mg (presently being evaluated but needs further clinical experience
      before recommendation)

2) Subconjunctival
   a) Gentamicin 40 mg and
   b) Cephaloridine or cefazolin 100 mg and
   c) Triamcinolone diacetate (Aristocort) 40 mg[a]

3) Topical
   a) Gentamicin 9 mg/ml and
   b) Cephaloridine or cefazolin 50 mg/ml and
   c) Prednisolone acetate 1%

4) Systemic
   a) Cefazolin (Ancef or Kefzol) 1,000 mg every 6–8 h or
   b) Gentamicin (Garamycin) 80 mg every 6–8 h.

[a] Subconjunctival corticosteroids should be deferred for 48–72 h to await culture growth
and confirmation if a fungal organism is suspected

Table 19. Suggested choice of antibiotic for intraocular infection pending results of micro-
biologicol analyses

	1st choice	2nd choice	3rd choice
Topical	Bacitracin	Chloromycetin +	Vancomycin
	Gentamicin	cephaloridine	Neomycin, polymyxin bacitracin
Subconjunctival	Gentamicin	Tobramycin +	Gentamicin
	Methicillin	cephaloridine	Vancomycin
Intravenous	Gentamicin + methicillin + penicillin G	Gentamicin + cephalothin	Gentamicin Vancomycin

ZA et al. 1973, 1977, 1978; GOLDEN and COPPEL 1970; LEOPOLD 1945b). Intravitreal injection produces greater levels than periocular, which is better than
parenteral (LEOPOLD 1945b; PEYMAN 1977; SORSBY and UNGAR 1946).

10. Clinical course is a better guide to therapeutic course than in vitro sensitivity
    tests (LEOPOLD 1971).

11. Nonspecific anti-inflammatory therapy can be helpful when judiciously em-
    ployed (LEOPOLD 1971).

12. Parenteral injection will augment levels provided by other methods, e.g.,
    periocular routes (GOLDEN and COPPEL 1970).

13. All intracameral injections inflict ocular trauma, but reasonably tolerated doses have been determined for available antibiotics based on ophthalmoscopic examinations, electrophysiological tests, histological analyses, and clinical trial (Peymann 1977; Forster 1974).
14. Probenecid orally administered decreases renal excretion of penicillins and cephalosporins, as well as transport out of eye (Forbes and Becker 1960; Barza et al. 1973).

During this time the use of cycloplegics is usually advisable.

I. Incidence

Since intraocular infections can result in visual loss, infection following elective intraocular surgery is particularly dreaded. The incidence of intraocular infection after surgery varies, but is most frequent after cataract extraction, the most commonly performed intraocular surgical procedure. It is estimated that 1,100 cases of postoperative endophthalmitis will develop each year, with an incidence of 2–3 per 1,000, as a result of all types of intraocular surgery (Allansmith et al. 1970) (Table 20).

Even in preantiseptic days, postoperative infection of the eye was relatively infrequent, occurring in less than 3% of cases, the rate for general surgery being much higher. This definite difference in incidence between general and ocular surgery is just as apparent today, when postoperative ocular infection may be expected to occur in less than 0.3% of cases, as against 1.3%–10% in various fields of general surgery.

A survey of reported intraocular infections following intraocular surgery over seven decades reveals some interesting information, including some concerning the organisms responsible for postoperative cataract infection and their declining occurrence (Leopold 1971). (However, it must be realized that these records are not 100% accurate. It is not always possible to be certain of a diagnosis of endophthalmitis, particularly in those eyes that recover, and microbiological studies have been negative.) The greatest decline in frequency of endophthalmitis occurred before the

Table 20. Preparation of antibiotics for periocular injection. (Adapted from Bohigian 1981)

	Available vials	Diluent added to vial	Resulting concentrate
Ampicillin	1,000 mg	5.0 ml	0.5 ml = 100 mg
Carbenicillin	1,000 mg	5.0 ml	0.5 ml = 100 mg
Cephalothin	1,000 mg	5.0 ml	0.5 ml = 100 mg
Chloramphenicol	1,000 mg	5.0 ml	0.5 ml = 100 mg
Methicillin	1,000 mg	5.0 ml	0.5 ml = 100 mg
Cefazolin	500 mg	2.5 ml	0.5 ml = 100 mg
Neomycin	500 mg	1.0 ml	0.5 ml = 250 mg
Vancomycin	500 mg	5.0 ml	0.25 ml = 25 mg
Penicillin G	5 Munits	2.5 ml	0.5 ml = 1 Munit
Gentamicin	80 mg/2 ml	–	0.5 ml = 20 mg
Colestimethate (Sodium)	150 mg	2.0 ml	0.3 ml = 25 mg
Bacitracin	50,000 units	5.0 ml	0.5 ml = 5,000 units

advent of antibiotics, possibly being attributable to improved aseptic technique. The significant drop in incidence of infection between 1920 and 1940 probably reflects the introduction of antiseptic practices in surgery.

II. Results of Therapy

Unfortunately, the outcome of clinically diagnosed postoperative endophthalmitis is far from satisfactory. Of 145 eyes with intraocular infections reported in 14 papers, 87 were either removed or totally blind, and only 58 had visual acuity of counting fingers or above, representing a loss of over 60% (LEOPOLD 1971). In other words, in the period during which antibiotics have been available, in approximately two-thirds of all eyes with intraocular infections, the infection could not be controlled. Even though the range and choice of antibiotics have improved tremendously in the last decades, in the 1960s 57% of the eyes contracting endophthalmitis were lost. Except for the series collected by Freeman and Gay, outstanding for its high rate of recovery, there has been little improvement in the number of eyes saved after postoperative endophthalmitis over the decades.

III. Contributory Factors

Many studies relevant to the attempt to further reduce the occurrence of endophthalmitis after elective surgery have been reported. These shed light on various aspects of the problem, including:
1. Source of infection in the surgical environment
2. Ophthalmic operative area
3. Influence of host tissue
4. Organisms responsible for infection.

1. Sources of Infection in the Surgical Environment

Exogenous sources of intraocular infection are diverse and numerous. Bacteria or fungi can be introduced into the globe by contaminated surgical instruments or irrigating fluid. Medications instilled during or after surgery may not be sterile (AYLIFFE et al. 1966) . Foreign material, such as cotton fibers, talc powder, or starch granules may harbor the spores of some fungi species. Microorganisms may be present on the skin in the operative field or in the cul-de-sac, and can be transferred into the eye (LEOPOLD and APT 1960). Contamination may come from the surgeon's breath or gloves, and from the air in the operating room. Another more remote cause of postoperative infection is bacteremia from a distant focus.

Though most postoperative infections appear immediately after surgery, intraocular infections may not be manifested until weeks or years after operations are performed. Trephine procedures are more prone to postoperative infection than iridencleisis, but complications have been recorded subsequent to all types of filtering procedures. Fungal infections following cataract extraction surgery are often not evidenced for weeks or months afterwards. The emergence of postoperative intraocular viral infections has not been observed.

2. Ophthalmic Operative Area

In spite of excellent aseptic techniques for preparation of the ophthalmic operative area, there have still been demonstrations of contamination of the operating field

(MAUMENEE and MICHLER 1951; MCMEEL and WAPNER 1965). *Staphylococcus aureus* was found after preoperative skin preparation in one or more sites of 85% (17 of 20) of the ocular surgical cases studied by MCMEEL and WAPNER. Not one case was completely free of contamination. Similarly, after studying cultures of the skin and conjunctiva after preparation of the area for cataract extraction, MAUMENEE and MICHLER concluded that tissues cannot be sterilized in all cases. This was substantiated by studies undertaken at the Mt. Sinai Hospital (LEOPOLD 1971) determining the microbial flora of 245 postoperative eyes following cataract surgery. Microorganisms were present in 79% (194 of 245) of the cases and no growth could be cultured in 21% (51 of 245). None of these eyes developed ocular infection, although many of them harbored pathogenic bacteria.

Infections are observed after sterile preoperative cultures, yet have been absent when highly pathogenic bacterial species have appeared in postoperative cultures (DUNNINGTON and LOCATCHER-KHORAZO 1945; CALLAHAN 1953; LEOPOLD and APT 1960). Although there have been direct correlations of postoperative infection with preoperative cultures (ALLEN and MANGIARACINE 1973), the preoperative eye culture itself does not provide adequate information in predicting the development of postoperative infection.

3. Influence of Host Tissue

The tissues of the host vary in their ability to withstand infecting agents. Mutilated and necrotic tissue, poor blood supply, weak immunologic responses, the presence of foreign bodies (sutures, cotton fibers, etc.) all increase the chances of infection. Some sites in the eye seem to be more susceptible to infection than others, as can be seen in the following studies. Fifteen out of 25 patients developed intraocular infection after intraocular surgery following erroneous instillation of a contaminated solution. Extraocular operations (including 16 strabismus operations) performed when contaminated solution was used resulted in no postoperative infections (AYLIFFE et al. 1966). In another study, rabbit aqueous was injected with a strain of nonhemolytic coagulase negative *Staphylococcus aureus*, producing only transitory hyperemia of the eyes. When a similar inoculum was injected into the lens or vitreous, a purulent infection resulted (MAUMENEE and MICHLER 1951; MAYLATH and LEOPOLD 1955).

4. Organisms Responsible for Intraocular Infection

The organisms most usually responsible for causing intraocular infection have proved to be *Staphylococcus aureus*, resistant or nonresistant *Proteus*, *Pseudomonas aeruginosa*, *Bacillus subtilis*, enterococci, *Streptococcus*, and pneumococcus. These organisms can vary in virulence, numbers, and resistance to therapeutic onslaught. The increased recognition of *Staphylococcus epidermidis* as causative agent in endophthalmitis is supported by the work of VALENTON and co-workers (1973). Other organisms which have been found to cause intraocular infection include *Haemophilus influenza*, *Yersinia pestus*, *Pasteurella septica* (GALLOWAY and ROBINSON 1973), and *Escherichia coli* (BRISTOW et al. 1971; BHARGAVA and CHOPDAR 1971). *Neisseria meningitidis* has also been reported (JENSEN and NAIDOFF 1973). *Clostridium perfringens* may cause intraocular infections following penetrating wounds of the eye, but these organisms are only rarely responsible for postoperative infection. Postoperative fungus endophthalmitis is becoming an increasing problem, but still remains quite rare. *Volutella* (FOSTER et al. 1958), *Neurospora sitophila* (THEODORE et al. 1962), *Candida* (WALINDER and KOCH 1971; GREENE and WIERNIK 1972), *Fusarium*, and *Aspergillus* have all been reported as causative agents in postoperative endophthalmitis.

IV. Antibiotic Prophylaxis

The continued appearance of intraocular infection after attention to asepsis in elective surgery and the frequent failure of therapy bring up the question to what extent antibiotics can justifiably be used to prevent possible infection in intraocular surgery?

There are several reports of successful prophylactic antibiotic techniques for ophthalmic surgery. The success of these prior approaches and the awareness of the inability completely to sterilize the operative field in ophthalmology justifies further evaluation of this method. Topical preoperative prophylaxis has been advocated by DUNNINGTON and LOCATCHER-KHORAZO (1945), HUGHES and OWENS (1947), ALLEN and MANGIARACINE (1964), and others. There have been advocates of systemically administered drugs for prophylaxis (NEVEU and ELLIOTT 1959), but the majority of proponents of prophylaxis for intraocular surgery have used a subconjunctival approach. These include PEARLMAN (1956), CHALKLEY and SHOCK (1967), CASSADY (1967) and KOLKER et al. (1967) . Various antibiotics have been used for this purpose, singly and in combinations, usually being injected at the end of the surgical procedure. Although several reports indicate that with such therapy the incidence of intraocular infection was reduced almost to zero, others indicate little change in the incidence of infection. Several of these note that the onset of the bacterial infection was not prevented but simply delayed for weeks, thus masking the correct diagnosis and falsely suggesting the presence of fungal endophthalmitis (ARONSTAM 1964; CHALKLEY and SHOCK 1967).

Meticulous attention to operating room detail may reduce the incidence of such infections to a very low figure, but obviously does not eliminate it. For the past several years, McPherson (MCPHERSON et al. 1968) has used prophylactic subconjunctival antibiotics given at the beginning of an operation in an attempt to prevent the occurrence of operative infection. He points out that using antibiotics presurgically may enable the ophthalmologist to operate in a field protected by antibacterial levels of antibiotic in the aqueous throughout the course of the average intraocular operation. McPherson administered ampicillin (31 mg in 0.25 ml sterile water) subconjunctivally to patients who are not sensitive to penicillin, and cephaloridine (50 mg in 0.25 ml sterile water) to those with a history of penicillin sensitivity. Approximately 2,000 intraocular procedures have been carried out with no evidence of local or systemic hypersensitivity reaction, and no patient has developed endophthalmitis.

There are several dangers of prophylactic antibiotic use, however. Subconjunctival injections prior to operation may balloon the conjunctiva, providing a little less room for the surgical field. Prophylactic antibiotics may lead to the alteration of the local conjunctival flora and permit the development of pathogens which flourish only because competitive organisms have been inhibited. This method may also allow resistant pathogens to grow successfully, increasing their chances of invasion. Hypersensitivity reactions or systemic toxic effects can occur, and superinfections may develop.

CHALKLEY and SHOCK (1971) studied the use of antibiotic solutions of neomycin and polymyxin for irrigation of the anterior chamber at the close of surgery. They abandoned the randomized study after trying the method in 43 eyes. Although no infection occurred, the irritation was greater than they felt justified in inflicting for protective purposes. It is possible that the drug concentration they used may be reduced in subsequent studies and be less damaging. Perhaps the use of a single antibiotic in solution, such as gentamicin (Garamycin), might afford protection similar to the combination of neomycin and polymyxin, with some reduction in irritation.

V. Use of Steroids

If no improvement in intraocular infection is noted with in 24 h, other antibiotics must be selected and ACTH or corticosteroid therapy may be initiated. Usually ACTH or corticosteroid therapy is withheld until after the first 24 h of antibacterial therapy because these anti-inflammatory agents may mask the influence of the antibiotic. They certainly will not be helpful, however, unless the proper antibiotic to control the specific pathologic organism can be found.

The most to be gained by using steroids is the reduction of the inflammatory reaction. Even where useful vision has been lost because of the extensive inflammatory damage resulting from the infection, an infectious process has been halted. Steroids have been recommended to reduce this damage by allowing time for specific medication to become effective.

Experimental studies have demonstrated that steroids do not usually interfere with the effectiveness of a specific antibiotic (MAYLATH and LEOPOLD 1955). However, there is no clinical proof that the eventual result is better when steroids are used in combination with an effective antibiotic than when the antibiotic is used alone (FREEMAN and GAY 1967; KLASTERSKY et al. 1971).

VI. Vitrectomy

Vitrectomy, though still experimental, is another approach to controlling intraocular infection. With increased refinement and technical experience, the therapeutic incision into the vitreous and drainage of the bulk of infectious organisms and associated inflammatory debris could convert the vitreous cavity into a permeable chamber, allowing greater mobility of instilled antibiotics. COTTINGHAM and FORSTER (1976) have demonstrated that rabbit eyes with endophthalmitis caused by *Staphylococcus aureus* and *Staphylococcus epidermidis* treated by vitrectomy and intraocular gentamicin (24–31 h or 40–49 h after inoculation) had a significantly greater number of negative cultures 1 week later than when treated with intraocular antibiotics alone.

In clinical studies, PEYMAN and co-workers (1980) have demonstrated that pars plana vitrectomy with intravitreal antibiotics is an effective treatment of culture-proved endophthalmitis. Of 20 eyes, 17 (85%) were saved with some degree of useful vision; 3 eyes were lost. Best results occurred when treatment was begun during the first 36 h after onset of symptoms.

Nonspecific supportive therapy must also be considered for each patient, as well as agents that may heighten blood and ocular levels, such as probenecid, which favorably affect penicillin concentrations. Obviously attention must be paid to asepsis, to early diagnosis, to bacteriologic cultures, to antibiotic prophylaxis, and to vigorous prompt active therapy. Perhaps the next step to take in improving the odds against intraocular infection is to improve the patient's local and systemic resistance to infection or to employ techniques such as vitrectomy drainage.

D. Antibiotics

I. Penicillin Derivatives

Penicillins are naturally occurring or synthetic derivatives of 6-aminopenicillanic acid. They fall into three groups: acid-resistant penicillins, penicillinase-resistant penicillins, and broad-spectrum penicillins. At the present time, acid-resistant penicillins (phenethecillin, propicillin, and phenbenicillin) are of little value to the ophthalmologist because they are given orally and do not provide the high blood level concentrations favorable to ocular penetration.

Of the penicillinase-resistant penicillins (methicillin, oxacillin, cloxacillin, diphenicillin, nafcillin), methicillin has been the most extensively studied for ophthalmologic use. It has been found to penetrate poorly into the normal eye, but will penetrate through the disrupted blood–aqueous barrier in the inflamed eye (GREEN and LEOPOLD 1965).

Since all the semisynthetic penicillins are bound to protein in the serum, not all the antibiotics in the serum are free to cross the blood–aqueous barrier. Methicillin

Table 21. Undesirable side effects of individual penicillins

Common
    Rashes – most common with ampicillin
    Allergic reactions – rashes, anaphylaxis, serum sickness
    Diarrhea – most common with ampicillin

Less frequent
    Drug fever
    Hemolytic anemia – with high doses parenterally
    Central nervous system effects
        Convulsions – with high parenteral doses
        Muscle jerkings
    Hyperkalemia – with large doses of penicillin G rapidly delivered
    Blood dyscrasias
        Agranulocytopenia – with semisynthetic penicillin
        Platelet dysfunction – with carbenicillin
    Gastrointestinal disturbance
        Pseudomembranous colitis – ampicillin

and ampicillin have been found to be the least serum-bound of the newer penicillins (RECORDS and ELLIS 1967).

Side effects for the general class of penicillins are included in Table 21. The well-known allergic reaction to penicillin, occurring in approximately 5%–10% of the population of the United States (ZIMMERMAN 1958), is the most serious side effect.

1. Ampicillin

Ampicillin (Penbriten), α-aminobenzyl penicillin, was the first available semisynthetic penicillin effective against a wide variety of gram-negative bacteria. It is active against strains of *Escherichia coli*, *Shigella*, and *Salmonella*, as well as *Hemophilus influenzae*. It is not effective against many strains of *Pseudomonas*, nor is it very effective against non-penicillinase-producing staphylococci or gram-negative bacteria such as *Proteus* bacilli. Absorption studies (KUROSE and LEOPOLD 1965; RECORDS and ELLIS 1967) show that ampicillin penetrates adequately into the normal eye (both human and experimental animal) and passes readily into the inflamed eye. Since no parenteral preparation is available, it is administered orally.

2. Amoxicillin

Amoxicillin is a new semisynthetic penicillin that is similar in structure and spectrum of activity to ampicillin. It is distinguished from ampicillin by more complete absorption from the gastrointestinal tract and lack of interference with absorption by meals. Gastrointestinal side effects are less frequent with amoxicillin than with ampicillin. Following oral administration, drug levels in the blood are approximately twice those achieved by a similar oral dose of ampicillin, and are equivalent to those achieved by comparable doses of intramuscular ampicillin. Pharmacokinetic parameters of intramuscular amoxicillin, including peak serum levels and time of peaking, are nearly identical to those for oral administration (SPYKER et al. 1977). Approximately 20% of the amoxicillin is bound to serum protein.

The recommended adult dose of amoxicillin is 500 mg to 1.0 g at 8-h intervals. An approximate comparable daily dose (50 mg/kg) given by single lavage produced peak levels of 0.8 μg/ml in aqueous humor of normal rabbit eyes 2 h after administration (FAIGENBAUM et al. 1976). The ocular penetration ratio (aqueous humor/serum) of oral amoxicillin in the noninflamed rabbit eye was comparable to that of other penicillins (FAIGENBAUM et al. 1976).

The principal indications of amoxicillin in ocular infections are mild forms of suspected *Hemophilus* infections, such as nonsuppurative, preseptal cellulitis and conjunctivitis.

3. Carbenicillin

Another semisynthetic penicillin, carbenicillin, is an α-carboxybenzylpenicillin having a wide antimicrobial range of activity against gram-positive and gram-negative pathogens. This antibacterial spectrum is similar to that of ampicillin, except that carbenicillin extends the spectrum to include most strains of *Pseudomonas aeruginosa*, indole-positive *Proteus*, and some strains of *Enterobacter* not susceptible to ampicillin. Carbenicillin is bactericidal, unstable to staphylococcal penicillinase, and not highly bound to serum protein.

Carbenicillin appears to be virtually nontoxic and has no local irritant effects (ACRED et al. 1967), though potential to cause hypersensitivity reactions such as drug fever and eosinophilia has been reported. Carbenicillin appears to be well tolerated when administered intramuscularly or intravenously, but it is not absorbed following oral administration and passes with difficulty into the cerebrospinal fluid. Due to its low toxicity, it is possible to prescribe large doses of carbenicillin for prolonged time periods.

Investigators indicate that superinfection is enhanced following therapy with carbenicillin (MARKS and EICKOFF 1970). This may be due, in part, to the effects of a complex therapeutic regimen, e.g., steroids, immunosuppressive and cytotoxic agents.

Synergistic combination of carbenicillin and gentamicin has been suggested to overcome strains of *Pseudomonas* emerging with an increase in resistance to carbenicillin (HOFFMAN and BULLOCK 1958). Antagonism of the antimicrobial activity of gentamicin by the antibiotic carbenicillin has been reported in patients and in laboratory animals (MCLOUGHLIN and REEVES 1971). It was concluded that treatment by both antimicrobial agents together may, in certain circumstances, be less effective than with gentamicin or carbenicillin alone.

Results of investigations on the intraocular penetration of carbenicillin following subconjunctival injection in patients scheduled for elective ocular surgery show that carbenicillin penetrates the human noninflamed eye. Aqueous humor levels achieved with a subconjunctival dose of 250 mg (0.5 ml) could be therapeutically effective against susceptible pathogens (BOYLE et al. 1972).

4. Ticarcillin

Ticarcillin is the disodium salt of carboxythienylacetamidopenicillanic acid, similar in structure and antimicrobial activity to carbenicillin. The distinctive features of ticarcillin are the greater in vitro activity (two to four times that of carbenicillin) against the majority of isolates of *Pseudomonas*, and the broader activity against indole-positive and indole-negative *Proteus*, *Escherichia coli*, and *Enterobacter* (SUTHERLAND et al. 1971).

Like carbenicillin, ticarcillin is less active than penicillin against streptococci and penicillin-sensitive staphylococci and is not active against penicillinase-producing staphylococci. With the exception of *Bacteroides fragilis*, the majority of non-spore-forming anaerobic bacteria are inhibited by 10 µg/ml or less of ticarcillin (ROY et al. 1977). The in vitro synergism of ticarcillin with gentamicin and other aminoglycosides is similar to that of carbenicillin.

Intravenous administration of ticarcillin produces higher and more prolonged levels of the drug in the blood than are achieved by a comparable dose of carbenicillin, due in part to the lower renal excretion and slower hepatic conversion to penicillanic acid. Approximately 45% of the drug concentration is bound to serum protein (SUTHERLAND et al. 1971). The recommended adult daily dose of ticarcillin is 200–300 mg/kg in three divided doses. Intravenous administration of 1 g produces speak serum levels of 100 µg/ml within 15 min (SUTHERLAND et al. 1971). As with other penicillins, serum levels can be increased and prolonged by the concomitant administration of probenecid. Adverse reactions to ticarcillin are similar to those reported for carbenicillin. On the basis of the smaller dose requirement, certain dose-related side effects of carbenicillin should occur less frequently with ticarcillin. These include sodium retention, hypokalemia related to sodium excretion, and platelet aggregation defects with bleeding (BROWN et al. 1974).

II. Probenecid

Carinamide and probenecid (Benemid) are examples of drugs developed for the specific purpose of depressing the tubular secretion of penicillin in an effort to prolong the antibiotic in the body (BEYER et al. 1951). The action of probenecid is chiefly the inhibition of transport or organic acids across epithelial barriers. Through this action, probenecid inhibits the tubular secretion of many drugs and drug metabolites, thereby raising the concentrations of these drugs in the plasma. The transport of drugs such as penicillin G across the blood–aqueous and the blood–brain barriers may also be affected (SPECTOR and LORENZO 1974). Penicillin and other organic acids are rapidly secreted from the ocular and cerebrospinal fluid by an active process. Probenecid inhibits this process and thus elevates the concentration of penicillin in the aqueous and vitreous humor, as well as in the cerebrospinal fluid.

III. Cephalosporins

The cephalosporins are semisynthetic, bactericidal, antibacterial agents similar in structure, mechanism of action, and pharmacology to the penicillins. These have groups added to 7-aminocephalosporanic acid as compared to the basic 6-aminopenicillanic acid of the penicillins. Both interfere with the terminal step in cell wall synthesis by inactivating a transpeptidase, thereby preventing cross-linkage of peptidoglycan chains. The cephalosporins are active in vitro against streptococci (with the exception of enterococci), staphylococci (including penicillinase-producing strains), and the majority of isolates of *Escherichia coli*, *Klebsiella*, and indole-negative *Proteus*. The susceptibility of non-spore-forming anaerobes is variable. The cephalosporins are not active against *Pseudomonas* and indole-positive *Proteus*. Cephalosporin therapy is not effective in *Hemophilus influenzae* infections. As with penicillins, the cephalosporins are hydrolyzed into microbiologically inactive products by β-lactamases.

While once there were only three cephalosporins (parenteral cephalothin, cephaloridine and oral cephalexin), now there are more than 33. In addition, a further major criterion of classification has been added, β-lactamase-sensitive versus β-lactamase-resistant.

The group of enzymes known as β-lactamases can open β-lactam bonds of nuclei of some of the penicillins and cephalosporins, thus rendering the antibiotics inactive. Originally, *Staphylococcus aureus*, a gram-positive organism, presented the most clinical problems due to β-lactamases; however, in recent years, gram-negative organisms have been causing more difficulties. As a group, cephalosporins are much less susceptible than penicillin to staphylococcal β-lactamases, but many cephalosporins may be hydrolyzed by β-lactamases produced by gram-negative organisms, ranging from total susceptibility to complete resistance (although β-lactamase resistance does not automatically confer high antibacterial activity).

Parenteral cephalosporins susceptible to β-lactamases:

Cephalothin   Ceftezole
Cephapirin   Ceforanide
Cephacetrile   Cefazedone
Cephaloridine   Cefotiam
Cefazolin

Oral cephalosporins susceptible to β-lactamases:

Cephadrine   Cephaloglycin
Cefadroxil   Cefatrizine
Cephalexin   Cefaclor.

Another approach to combating β-lactamase has been to find compounds that inhibit the antibiotic-destroying enzyme itself and which, although not antibiotics themselves, can be added to antibiotic therapy. Clavulanic acid was the first compound studied in this regard. It has weak antibacterial action, but is a potent and progressive inhibitor of many β-lactamases. For example, a β-lactamase-producing *Staphylococcus aureus*, requiring 500 µg/ml of ampicillin to inhibit its growth, needs only 0.8 µg/ml of ampicillin plus 1 µg/ml of clavulanic acid for similar growth inhibition. It also enhances activity against ampicillin-resistant *Hemophilus influenzae* and penicillin-resistant gonococci. Another similar compound, CP-45, 899 from Pfizer, has been found to be slightly less potent as a β-lactamase inhibitor, but apparently is more stable in solution.

Whether this will mean an increase in the use of such agents as benzypenicillin and ampicillin, which in some areas may be losing their clinical usefulness, is not yet known. Though there are still a number of unanswered questions, with the advances in β-lactam research that are being made, a cephalosporin resistant to β-lactamase attack may prove to be better as a single agent than a combination of antibiotic and inhibitor (JOHNSON et al. 1979). Two new β-lactam antibiotics, mezlocillin and azlocillin, appear to be helpful in the treatment of serious infections by sensitive pathogens and, so far, the adverse effects of these agents have not been significant (ELLIS et al. 1979).

Adverse reactions to cephalosporins are generally related to the route of administration: pain on intramuscular injection, phlebitis with intravenous administration, and gastrointestinal disturbances with oral preparations (MOELLERING and SWARTZ 1976).

The newer cephalosporin derivatives vary with respect to the kinds of adverse reaction that they may produce. Allergic reactions occur in approximately 5% of cases and include anaphylaxis, serum sickness, urticarial and morbilliform rashes, fever, neutropenia, and thrombocytopenia (MOELLERING and SWARTZ 1976). Therapy with cephalosporins may lead to the development of a positive direct Coombs' reaction and, more rarely, a hemolytic anemia. Dose-related nephrotoxicity has limited the use of cephaloridine as a parenteral compound.

A frequent and pertinent clinical question is the risk of reactions to cephalosporins in patients who are allergic to penicillins. Studies suggest that specific as well as cross-reacting antibodies to the various semisynthetic penicillins and cephalosporins are formed, and that the intensity of the cross-reaction varies with the compound employed (KUWAHARA et al. 1971). Available data suggest that the risk of allergic reactions to cephalosporins among patients with a history of penicillin allergy is in the range of 5%–16%, with a mean rate of approximately 8% (PETZ 1971). The frequency of true cross-reactions is unknown, since penicillin-allergic patients also have an increased rate of reactivity to unrelated drugs (SMITH et al. 1966). On the basis of these considerations, cephalosporin therapy should be avoided in patients with a past history of anaphylaxis or immediate hypersensitivity reaction to any of the penicillins. It seems reasonable, however, to prescribe cephalosporins for patients with a history of less severe reactions, particularly in light of the limited number of safe alternate systemic agents effective against streptococci and staphylococci (AMERICAN MEDICAL ASSOCIATION 1977; MOELLERING and SWARTZ 1976; SMITH et al. 1966).

In contrast to the newer penicillins, none of the new semisynthetic cephalosporin derivatives differ markedly in antibacterial spectrum or pharmacology from the prototype compound, cephalothin. Recent reviews have enumerated the distinctive features of these compounds (WASHINGTON 1976; MOELLERING and SWARTZ 1976; O'CALLAGHAN 1975), though knowledge of the ocular pharmacokinetics of the new oral and parenteral cephalosporins is incomplete. Intravenous cephalothin (1 g) and cephaloridine (1 g) produced mean peak concentrations of 0.55 and 28.4 μg/ml respectively in secondary aqueous humor of human eyes undergoing surgery (RECORDS 1968 a, 1969).

There may be a clinical place for the newer cephalosporins. The more recently developed cephalosporins possess high activity against enterobacteria and at least some activity against *Pseudomonas aeruginosa*.

Cefotaxime (HR 756, Hoechst-Roussel) has a broad spectrum of activity, which includes all the enterobacteria, *Hemophilus*, *Neisseria*, *Acinetobacter*, and most pseudomonads, anaerobes, staphylococci (not methicillin-resistant), and streptococci (not *Streptococcus faecalis*). There is doubt about its value against *Bacteroides*. Cefotaxime, like cefuroxime, is stable against β-lactamases (but not against enzymes of *Bacteroides fragilis* and *Proteus vulgaris*). Blood levels reach 40–300 mg/l following 2 g i.v. dose, with a half-life of 1–1.6 h.

Moxalactam (LY 127, 935, Lilly; 6059-S, Shinogi) is an oxa-β-lactam (oxacephalosporin) with the 7-methoxy group of the "cephamycins." Its activity is similar to that of cefotaxime, though it is less active against gram-positive organisms and more active against *Bacteroides fragilis*. It is highly resistant to β-lactamases and provides similar blood levels to those of cefotaxime.

Cefoperazone (T 1551, Toyama; CP-52, 640-2, Pfizer) is less active than the two cephalosporins above, but it is more active against *Pseudomonas aeruginosa*. Its β-lactamase stability is not yet clearly defined, but it can be hydrolyzed.

Cefsulodin (SCE-129, Takeda; CGP 7174/E, Ciba-Geigy; 46 811 Abbott) is active against many, but not all, *Pseudomonas aeruginosa* variants, including carbenicillin-resistant strains, but is not very active against other gram-negative organisms. It is fairly resistant to β-lactamases but can be hydrolyzed by some enzymes. A 2 g i.v. dose provides blood levels of 16–70 mg/l.

Other new cephalosporins have been reported. Ceftizoxime (FK 749, FR 13,749, Fujisawa) and ceftazidime (GR 20,263, Glaxo) apparently resemble cefotaxime, but YM 09330 (Yamanouchi), another cephamycin, seems less active. SM 1652 (Sumitomo) is, like cefsulodin, antipseudomonal, but is more active than cefsulodin against the enterobacteria. Ceforanide (BLS 786, Bristol) and cefazaflur (Smith, Kline and French) seem less active than the others. It cannot be disputed that several of these new cephalosporins have very promising antibacterial activity, but it is less clear what their clinical ophthalmologic role should be. There may well be roles for some of them against such organisms as *Pseudomonas* and aminogly-coside-resistant enterobacteria.

IV. Aminoglycosides

The aminoglycosides, having a greater spectrum of activity than cephalosporins, are useful agents for treatment of serious infections due to *Pseudomonas, Entero-bacter, Klebsiella, Serratia, Escherichia*, and other gram-negative aerobic or-ganisms. The aminoglycoside group consists of a large number of strucurally re-lated, polycationic compounds derived from different species of *Streptomyces*. All inhibit protein synthesis and are bactericidal through binding of the aminogly-coside to the 30-S subunit of the bacterial ribosome, with consequent misreading of the genetic code. The spectra of action of the aminoglycosides differ. This may be attributable to differences in drug penetration, abilities of the ribosome to bind the drug, and capacities of the bacteria to alter the drugs chemically (PRATT 1977). All the aminoglycosides are poorly absorbed from the gastrointestinal tract and must be administered parenterally. The aminoglosides are not metabolized to a sig-nificant degree and are excreted unchanged by glomerular filtration. All have pro-duced nephrotoxicity, ototoxicity, neuromuscular toxicity, hypersensitivity reactions, and superinfection. The introduction of gentamicin in 1969 greatly ex-panded the therapeutic capabilities against aerobic gram-negative organisms, par-ticularly *Pseudomonas*.

1. Streptomycin and Dihydrostreptomycin

These antibiotics serve most widely in the treatment of tuberculosis, tularemia, and gram-negative bacterial infections due to sensitive strains, and are particularly ef-fective against *Hemophilus influenzae, Klebsiella pneumoniae* infections, and some strains of *Proteus vulgaris*. Occasional strains of *Pseudomonas aeruginosa* are no-minally sensitive to the streptomycin drugs.

Absorption through the gastrointestinal tract is poor, and streptomycin and di-hydrostreptomycin are usually injected intramuscularly. LEOPOLD and NICHOLS (1946) found that systemic streptomycin in rabbits penetrated significantly into the extraocular muscles, conjunctiva, sclera, and aqueous humor, but less adequately into the chorioretinal tissue and vitreous body. An appreciable increase in the con-centration of the drug appeared in the secondary aqueous humor.

The most important side effect of these drugs is a neurotoxicity affecting the eighth cranial nerve. Streptomycin, however, is essentially toxic to the vestibular function, causing impairment which is promptly recognized, but for which the patient is able to compensate. Dihydrostreptomycin exerts a toxicity on the audi-tory system, and the development of deafness is often progressive after the cessa-tion of therapy. Irreversible loss of hearing is a potential consequence, even from small doses (1–5 g); it may occur within a few weeks, or a period up to 6 months may pass before any symptoms are manifest. Since streptomycin is basically as ef-fective as dihydrostreptomycin and is not as toxic, it is preferable to the latter.

2. Gentamicin

At least three-fourths of the strains of *Pseudomonas, Klebsiella, Aerobacter,* and *Escherichia coli* and most of the strains of staphylococci are sensitive to reasonable concentrations of gentamicin; many *Proteus* strains are also inhibited.

Gentamicin is relatively insoluble in lipids and approximately 25%–30% protein bound. Topically applied gentamicin, 0.3% solution or ointment, may produce aqueous humor levels as high as 1.6 µg/ml in rabbit eyes whose corneas have been mechanically abraded or chemically burned (Furgiuele 1967). Subconjunctival injections of 0.5 ml 0.3% gentamicin solution or of intravenous dosages of 1 mg/kg produce levels of approximately 0.8 µg/ml in the experimental rabbit eye (Furgiuele 1967). In the human eye, subconjunctival injection of 10 mg gentamicin in 0.25 ml produced aqueous humor levels ranging from 2 to 7 µg/ml at 1 h and from 1 to 9 µg/ml at 2½ h (Furgiuele 1970).

The most serious adverse effects of gentamicin are ototoxicity, renal damage, and ataxia. In a recent study by Libert and co-workers (1979), it was found that subconjunctival injections of gentamicin induced a lysosomal storage process within the conjunctival fibroblast in rats, rabbits, and humans. Under electron microscopoy the accumulated substance was shown to be composed of a granular material and pleomorphic lamellar structures, corresponding to the presence of complex lipids. In the animal studies, the proximal convoluted tubles of the kidneys developed lesions. Although human kidneys were not examined following subconjunctival injections, there is the possibility that a treated patient might also develop kidney lesions. There have been reports in the literature of therapeutic accidents with low parenteral doses (Hewitt 1974; Wilfert et al. 1971).

3. Tobramycin

Tobramycin is a member of a broad-spectrum antibiotic complex, nebramycin, similar in structure to gentamicin. It is highly soluble in water and stable for extended periods at extremes of pH (1–11) and temperature (5 °C–37 °C) (Neu 1976). Tobramycin and gentamicin bind permanently to the 30-S ribosome subunit to cause depletion of the ribosome pool. Like gentamicin, tobramycin is active against staphylococci (including penicillinase-producing strains) but not streptococci. Tobramycin is more active than gentamicin on a weight basis (two- to fourfold) against *Pseudomonas aeruginosa (*Neu 1976). The comparative sensitivity of *Klebsiella, Enterobacter, Serratia,* and *Proteus* to tobramycin and gentamicin is variable.

Bacterial resistance to tobramycin and other aminoglycosides is achieved by inactivation of the antibiotics by enzymes present in the periplasmic space of bacteria (Neu 1976). These enzymes vary in prevalence among *Pseudomonas* and the Enterobacteriaceae. There is variation among hospitals and other institutions in the percentage of gentamicin-resistant strains of *Pseudomonas* that are sensitive to tobramycin; strains resistant to both gentamicin and tobramycin have also appeared (Neu 1976). In contrast to *Pseudomonas*, most strains of *Klebsiella, Enterobacter, Escherichia coli,* and *Serratia* that are resistant to gentamicin are resistant to tobramycin. Although in vitro synergism of tobramycin and carbenicillin against *Pseudomonas* has been demonstrated, the clinical significance has not been determined.

Synergistic effects have also been produced to tobramycin and ticarcillin against *Pseudomonas aeruginosa, Escherichia coli,* and *Enterobacter* infections in mice (COMBER et al. 1977).

The human pharmacokinetics of tobramycin are similar to those of gentamicin. The recommended daily dose in an adult with normal renal function is 3–5 mg/kg, either by intramuscular injection or by slow intravenous infusion. Peak serum levels of 6.5 µg/ml can be achieved by a single intramuscular dose of 1.5 mg/kg (NEU 1976). The drug is not bound to serum protein. The serum half-life following intramuscular injection is approximately 2 h. Adverse reactions to tobramycin are similar in type and frequency to those to gentamicin. Renal toxicity of some degree occurs in approximately 1.5%–4.4% of patients receiving these drugs (NEU 1976). Severe nephrotoxicity is rare. Tobramycin therapy should be monitored by serum levels of creatinine. The efficacy of tobramycin in treating a variety of infections has been established by extensive clinical reports (FINLAND and NEU 1976).

The ocular pharmacokinetics of intramuscular and intravenous tobramycin have not been thoroughly defined. Subconjunctival injection of 5 and 10 mg of tobramycin produced mean peak concentrations of 5.5 and 6.7 µg/ml respectively in normal rabbit eyes without toxicity (UWAYDAH and FARIS 1976). Although tobramycin may ultimately replace gentamicin as the systemic agent for documented *Pseudomonas aeruginosa* infections, its use in ocular infections should currently be reserved for infections caused by gentamicin-resistant strains of *Pseudomonas aeruginosa* or the Enterobacteriaceae. Recently, DAVIS and co-workers (1979) have shown that the topical route of administration was consistently more effective than either subconjunctival or intramuscular routes. Subconjunctival injection of antibiotic did not enhance the effectiveness of topical therapy in either guinea pigs or rabbits. Intramuscular tobramycin was more effective than saline in guinea pigs with keratitis but not in rabbits with keratitis.

4. Neomycin

Neomycin is a powerful bactericidal antibiotic with a wide spectrum. Among its advantages are the fact that resistance is not readily developed by organisms and it is not inactivated by exudates or enzymes. The drug has limited application for systemic use, however, because of its oto- and nephrotoxicity. It has been extensively and advantageously employed in ophthalmology by means of local administration and subconjunctival injection. Occasional hypersensitivity to the local application of neomycin on the conjunctiva or skin about the eye has been seen.

Penetration of neomycin into the rabbit eye by local, subconjunctival, and intraocular instillation was evaluated by VOGEL et al. (1951). Studies by SORSBY and UNGAR (1958) disclosed that subconjunctival neomycin was effective against strains of penicillin-resistant staphylococci and *Pseudomonas aeruginosa*, and ineffective against intraocular infections with *Bacteroides proteus*, although control of the latter could be obtained by prophylactic application of the drug. Subconjunctival doses of 500 mg were tolerated and elevated concentrations produced in the cornea and aqueous humor for 16 h. The authors suggested subconjunctival neomycin (500 mg/ml), to which is added epinephrine (0.25 ml diluted 1:1,000), as a standard method for the treatment of intraocular infections.

Neomycin is poorly absorbed from the gastrointestinal tract. Intramuscular injection actuates a high plasma concentration but, because of renal impairment and irreversible damage to the eighth cranial nerve, is used only in critical situations. If the drug is given parenterally, the established average is 8 mg/kg/day in four doses and should not exceed 14 mg/kg/day or 1 g in 10 days.

Neomycin is employed widely in many ophthalmic preparations. At the onset it was felt that if the excessive and indiscriminate use of these preparations occurred, more reactions and increased bacterial resistance would result. This development would be unfortunate, because neomycin is of considerable value to the ophthalmologist at the present time. However, when hypersensitivity has occurred, it has not been of great significance, and the agent has been very useful in ophthalmic practice over several decades.

5. Kanamycin

Kanamycin (Kantrex) is a bactericidal antibiotic which is closely related to neomycin and, to a lesser extent, streptomycin. Its antibacterial spectrum is identical to that of neomycin, and a cross-resistance exists between the drugs. This drug also appears to be effective against some strains of tubercle bacilli which are resistant to streptomycin, isoniazid, and p-aminosalicyclic acid, but resistance to kanamycin may be acquired during treatment.

Kanamycin, like neomycin, is negligibly absorbed from the gastrointestinal tract, and systemic treatment must therefore be implented by the intramuscular route. Another similarity exists in the fact that parenteral use should be avoided except in the case of staphylococcal or other infections which cannot be effectively treated with less toxic antibiotics.

Studies concerning ocular penetrability were performed in rabbits by Furgiuele et al. (1960). They found the drug to enter the normal eye satisfactorily when given subconjunctivally, but inadequately when given by intramuscular injection. Penetration via the intramuscular route is increased by the presence of ocular inflammation. A 2.5% solution administered topically or 10 mg given subconjunctivally was well tolerated by the normal rabbit eye. For patients, the authors recommended large systemic doses to ensure intraocular penetration.

6. Amikacin

Amikacin is a semisynthetic aminoglycoside similar in structure to kanamycin. It is readily soluble in water and stable for 24 months at room temperature. Amikacin is resistant to many of the bacterial R-factor-mediated enzymes that inactivate kanamycin, gentamicin, and tobramycin; consequently, a large percentage of gram-negative bacteria resistant to these aminoglycosides are sensitive to amikacin (Price et al. 1974; Finland et al. 1976). It should be noted, however, that nonenzymatic mechanisms can confer resistance on amikacin and the other aminoglycosides. Organisms resistant to amikacin are generally resistant to kanamycin, gentamicin, and tobramycin. Amikacin has no advantage over these aminoglycosides for infections caused by organisms sensitive to this group. It possesses in vitro activity beyond that of streptomycin, kanamycin, and rifampin against isolates of the *Mycobacterium fortuitum* complex (Sanders et al. 1977).

The pharmacokinetics and toxicity of amikacin are similar to those of kanamycin. Cochlear toxicity is more common than vestibular toxicity. Amikacin should not be administered concurrently with other nephrotoxic or ototoxic antimicrobials such as polymyxin B, colistin, vancomycin, or other aminoglycosides. The recommended daily dose in an adult with normal renal function is 15 mg/kg, either by intramuscular injection or by slow intravenous infusion. Peak serum concentrations of 21 µg/ml are produced 1 h following intramuscular injection of 500 mg amikacin in normal adults. The effectiveness of amikacin in diverse gram-negative infections has been widely reported (FINLAND et al. 1976; SANDERS et al. 1977).

The ocular pharmacokinetics of amikacin have not been adequately investigated. As for other infections, amikacin should be reserved for ocular infections caused by susceptible strains of *Pseudomonas aeruginosa* or other gram-negative organisms known to be resistant to kanamycin, gentamicin, or tobramycin.

7. Spectinomycin

Spectinomycin is different from the other aminoglycosides in structure and mechanism of action. The interaction of spectinomycin and the 30-S ribosomal subunit is reversible (ANDERSON et al. 1967) and requires a single protein for drug susceptibility (BOLLEN et al. 1969). Although spectinomycin has broad in vitro activity against gram-positive and gram-negative aerobic organisms, the drug was released by the FDA in 1971 exclusively for the treatment of acute, uncomplicated gonococcal urethritis and proctitis in the male and gonococcal cervicitis and proctitis in the female. Use of this drug should be considered in patients with a history of penicillin allergy and infections due to suspected or proved penicillinase-producing strains of *Neisseria gonorrhoeae*.

8. Others

Two other aminoglycosides, sisomicin and netilmicin, are currently under investigation and may offer therapeutic advantages over their prototypes. Netilmicin is active against a wide variety of bacteria including many strains that are resistant to gentamicin, tobramycin, and amikacin (JAHRE et al., 1979; MEYERS et al. 1981).

V. Erythromycin

Since its isolation in 1952, erythromycin has withstood the test of time and has shown no serious toxicity. Gastrointestinal distress sometimes follows oral administration of the antibiotic. The estolate preparation occasionally produce some jaundice, but the stearate and ethylsuccinate preparations are satisfactory alternatives. Intramuscular administration of erythromycin is best avoided due to pain and insolubility.

In its earlier years of use, as an alternative for penicillin in penicillin-resistant infections, restricted use was advocated. However, since widespread staphylococcal resistance has not proved to be a significant problem, it will probably be used more extensively in the future. It has been noted, though, that drug withdrawal rapidly leads to a reemergence of sensitive strains.

Erythromycin has traditionally been used for patients with allergies to penicillin, in the treatment of streptococcal infections, and for prophylactic treatment of rheumatic fever. Additionally, erythromycin has activity against *Hemophilus influenzae* and is effective against *Mycoplasma pneumoniae*. It is useful in clostridial infections in penicillin-allergic patients. Among the sexually transmitted diseases, syphilis is usually treated with penicillin G, although erythromycin 2 g/day for 10–20 days is being used. *Chlamydia* and mycoplasmas are increasingly involved as agents of sexually transmitted disease and are highly sensitive to erythromycin.

Intravenous or intramuscular forms of the drug, especially in normally tolerated doses, show marked penetrability across the blood–aqueous barrier (NAIB et al. 1955). It also enters the aqueous humor in adequate concentrations when administered topically or subconjunctivally (QUERENGESSER and ORMSBY 1955).

VI. Lincomycin

Lincomycin was named after Lincoln, Nebraska, where the soil it was isolated from was obtained. It is a bactericidal agent against a wide range of gram-positive organisms, but is ineffective against most gram-negative bacteria. A dose of 500 mg will result in plasma levels of about 2–5 ng/kg lasting for about 6 h following oral administration, longer after intramuscular (JACKSON et al. 1965).

Lincomycin's antibacterial activity is through inhibition of protein synthesis at the 50-S ribosome. The antibiotic spectrum covers gram-positive cocci and gram-positive anaerobes. An in vitro concentration of less than 0.5 µg/ml will inhibit *Bacillus anthracis* and the following species of *Streptococcus; pneumoniae pyogenes*, and *viridans* (KLEINBERG et al. 1979). A concentration of less than 2 µg/ml of lincomycin hydrochloride is active against *Corynebacterium diptheriae, Clostridium tetani*, and *Clostridium perfringens*. Its use in penicillin-sensitive individuals, based on its spectrum of activity in vitro, suggests a potential use for the treatment of ocular infections.

Therapeutic levels of lincomycin hydrochloride have been found after intramuscular injection of 600 mg (BOYLE et al. 1971; COLES et al. 1971) and after five topical instillations every 5 min (NAKATSUE 1961; IMAI 1969). Penetration studies of topical 1% lincomycin hydrochloride indicate that peak concentrations occur within 45 min after the last instillation. Removal of the epithelial barrier allowed a greater penetration of lincomycin than when the epithelial barrier was intact, which is somewhat different from the data for clindamycin showing the epithelium acting as a reservoir (MERCER et al. 1978).

Lincomycin injected into the vitreous humor penetrates to some degree into the aqueous humor of the anterior chamber (KLEINBERG et al. 1979; MAURICE 1976). MAURICE has shown that water-soluble antibiotics injected into the vitreous body diffuse rapidly through the vitreous and may leave the compartment by two known ways. They diffuse anteriorly to the aqueous humor or are removed by active transport through the retina-choroid.

Experiments by KLEINBERG et al. (1979) have yielded a first-order disappearance rate from the vitreous chamber, and their findings were virtually identical with those reported for clindamycin hydrochloride by MAURICE. It appears that the mechanisms for vitreal elimination of the two antibiotics are identical, both being predominantly cleared by way of the retina-choroid. These findings are consistent with the similarity of their chemical structures. Although there is substantial loss of drugs through the retina-choroid, intravitreous injection does produce steady therapeutic levels of lincomycin in the anterior chamber.

VII. Clindamycin

Clindamycin is a 7-chloro analog of the antibiotic lincomycin hydrochloride. Although its spectrum of activity is similar to that of lincomycin, the chlorination has increased its effectiveness (HEMAN-ACKAH 1975). It is active against gram-positive cocci and gram-positive and gram-negative anaerobic pathogens except clostridian species (TABBARA and O'CONNOR 1975). The effectiveness of clindamycin phosphate in the treatment of experimental toxoplasmic retinochoroiditis in rabbits has been demonstrated (TABBARA and O'CONNOR 1975). O'CONNOR has suggested that clindamycin 300 mg every 6 h, coupled with sulfadiazine 1 g four times daily, may be useful for therapy of toxoplasmosis (O'CONNOR 1980a).

Intraocular penetration studies have been performed with the use of oral clindamycin palmitate (TOKUDA et al. 1973; MIKUNI et al. 1973) and with subconjunctival intramuscular injection of clindamycin phosphate (TABBAR and O'CONNOR 1975; MERCER et al. 1978). Substantial tissue penetration and bioactivity of clindamycin occur in cornea, aqueous humor, iris, and ciliary body following topical administration. Very little is absorbed by other ocular tissue or into the serum after this means of application.

Comparison of topically applied clindamycin hydrochloride and clindamycin phosphate was made feasible with a gas chromatographic method of analysis (DEVLIN et al. 1978). Results indicate that clindamycin phosphate undergoes hydrolysis in the eye, liberating the biologically active clindamycin. However, topical clindamycin hydrochloride produced higher levels than those achievable with the phosphate ester in the uvea, aqueous humor, and cornea, presumably due to clindamycin hydrochloride's higher lipid solubility.

VIII. Oleandomycin

The antibacterial spectrum of oleandomycin is similar to that of erythromycin. Erythromycin, though, is effective at a lower concentration and consequently is preferable for infections by organisms sensitive to both agents. However, a strain of staphylococci will occasionally be resistant to erythromycin and not to oleandomycin. A new form of the drug, currently marketed as triacetyloleandomycin (Cyclamen, TAO), is claimed to be more rapidly and completely absorbed from the gastrointestinal tract and to produce more elevated blood levels.

Oleandomycin enters the eye when given in massive doses orally or intravenously. A single administration of 1 g successfully penetrates the aqueous humor of rabbits (McCOY and LEOPOLD 1959). DUMAS et al. (1958) have reported the phosphate form of the drug to penetrate the animal eye when applied locally, intravenously, and subconjunctivally. Subconjunctival injections were poorly tolerated, even in dosages as low as 2.5 mg/ml, and are therefore not recommended.

IX. Carbomycin

Carbomycin has an antibacterial spectrum resembling that of erythromycin. Organisms gain resistance slowly, in the same way that they respond to penicillin.

Both erythromycin and oleandomycin are more active and potent than carbomycin, but there is almost complete cross-resistance among the three agents. The absorption and excretion pattern is similar to that of erythromycin.

Carbomycin has been used topically in the form of the hydrochloride ointment to facilitate penetration into the aqueous humor (HALLIDAY and ORMSBY 1955). It has been shown to cross the blood–aqueous barrier after oral, intravenous, or subconjunctival administration (HAUSLER and ORMSBY, unpublished data).

X. Spiramycin

Spiramycin has a narrow antibacterial spectrum, resembling penicillin, erythromycin, and novobiocin in range of activity. JONES and FINLAND (1957) consider it less active than erythromycin or oleandomycin. The drug penetrates the eye when used locally, subconjunctivally, and orally, but requires the use of large doses (FURGIUELE et al. 1958).

Spiramycin has been reported to be effective against toxoplasmosis in animals (BOQACZ 1954; GARIN and EYLES 1958). Investigations of patients with posterior uveitis, due possibly to toxoplasmosis, were conducted at the Wills Eye Hospital. The results in cases treated by alternative means were not as satisfactory as those treated with pyrimethamine and sulfonamides (FAJARDO et al. 1962).

XI. Novobiocin

Novobiocin (Cathomycin, Albamycin) is another narrow-spectrum antibiotic which is most active against some strains of *Bacteroides proteus* and *Streptococcus faecalis*; staphylococci rapidly develop resistance to novobiocin. The drug is given orally and is usually well tolerated. Side effects that have been reported include skin eruption, leukopenia, and yellowish discoloration of the plasma due to a drug degradation product.

Novobiocin penetrates the ocular tissues poorly when given systemically unless the dosage is large. Intravenous administration in animals produces detectable levels following doses of 0.1 g/kg body wt (SERY et al. 1957), and effective concentrations are obtained after subconjunctival doses of 12.5 mg.

XII. Ristocetin

Ristocetin (Spontin) has an antibacterial spectrum similar to that of erythromycin and novobiocin. However, it is bactericidal rather than bacteriostatic. Staphylococci develop resistance to ristocetin very slowly, and no cross-resistance with other antibiotics has been demonstrated. The drug must be given intravenously for the treatment of systemic infections. It is not absorbed from the gastrointestinal tract and intramuscular injection causes extreme irritation.

The ocular penetration was evaluated in rabbits by FURGIUELE et al. (1960). No evidence of penetration in normal or inflamed eyes was demonstrated after intravenous doses of 50–100 mg/kg body wt. Subconjunctival injection of 10 mg did produce irritation, but no penetration of drug into the eye.

XIII. Vancomycin

Vancomycin is highly active against gram-positive cocci. It is a glycopeptide soluble in water to concentrations of over 100 mg/ml. Resistance to the agent develops very slowly, and no cross-resistance has yet been demonstrated. It should be reserved for serious staphylococcal infections or other organisms resistant to the more commonly used antibiotics.

Vancomycin is not absorbed from the gastrointestinal tract, is irritating intramuscularly, and is therefore administered by the intravenous route. The plasma concentration is maintained for 12 h and two daily doses are sufficient. The drug diffuses well into the ocular tissues and appears in the ocular and spinal fluid when inflamed membranes have induced increased permeability (PRYOR et al. 1962 b).

Hypersensitivity reactions do occur. Phlebitis and pain at the site of intravenous injection may be common. Chills, fever, and shock-like state (red neck syndrome) happen rarely during the course of intravenous therapy. A drop in blood pressure may occur if vancomycin is given rapidly. Auditory impairment is frequent but not usually permanent. Ototoxicity is not common if concentrations in the plasma are kept below 30 µg/ml. However, this toxicity and renal damage are more common if vancomycin is administered concomitantly with other nephrotoxic and ototoxic agents.

XIV. Bacitracin

Bacitracin is a bactericidal antibiotic derived from a strain of *Bacillus subtilis*, and has the same general spectrum as penicillin, with which it exhibits a pronounced synergism. Resistance to this antibiotic is rare, and its potency is not diminished by blood, pus, or necrotic tissue.

Bacitracin is most frequently utilized in the topical therapy of infections caused by *Staphylococcus aureus* and other gram-positive bacteria, especially if the bacteria are resistant to other antibiotics. While parenteral application of the drug can induce kidney (tubular) damage, the condition is usually reversible. Systemic therapy has been limited to serious penicillin-resistant staphylococcal infections, including meningitis and endocarditis. The intramuscular dosage is 10,000–20,000 units three or four times daily.

The drug is not absorbed from the gastrointestinal tract. When administered intramuscularly, bacitracin appears in tissues and pleural and ascitic fluid, but diffuses negligibly into the cerebrospinal fluid. It is excreted slowly, primarily by glomerular filtration.

Bacitracin penetrates the ocular tissues by the subconjunctival route and can be topically instilled into the anterior chamber of the eye. For intraocular infections, it is most effective in combination with drugs such as streptomycin or polymyxin B, which act against the gram-negative group of bacteria. It is perhaps the most effective topical antibiotic available for treating staphylococcal blepharoconjunctivitis (BAUM 1980).

XV. Polymyxin B

The polymyxins are cationic detergents, basic polypeptides, which form water-soluble salts. Polymyxin B is the least toxic and the one currently available for clinical use. It is not absorbed from the gastrointestinal tract, and is therefore given parenterally for systemic infections. The intramuscular dose should not exceed 2.5 mg/

kg body wt./day for patients with normal kidney function. The plasma concentration decreases rapidly, but detectable blood levels persist for 12 h – an indication that the drug should be given at 8- or 12-h intervals. There is no appreciable diffusion into the cerebrospinal fluid.

The factors which limit the use of polymyxin by the parenteral route in general medicine are nephrotoxicity and central nervous system side effects. The ophthalmologist gains the advantage of a potent antibiotic and avoids toxic complications by utilizing the subconjunctival and topical routes. AINSLIE and SMITH (1952) have demonstrated that polymyxin E can satisfactorily penetrate the eye from subconjunctival sites. Polymyxin B also enters the ocular tissues in this fashion and can also be used in solution for intracameral injection or irrigation. A 2% aqueous solution has a pH of approximately 5.7.

XVI. Soframycin

AINSLIE and HENDERSON (1958) found soframycin particularly suitable for subconjunctival antibiotic therapy: the drug was highly soluble in water, did not cause undue tissue irritation, and gained therapeutic concentrations in the aqueous humor (in rabbits). AINSLIE and CAIRNS (1960) reported satisfactory results for the subconjunctival treatment of corneal infections (both clinical and experimentally produced) induced by *Staphylococcus aureus*, pneumococcus, *Escherichia coli*, and *Pseudomonas aeruginosa*. In the clinical study, a subconjunctival dose of 500 mg was generally employed.

XVII. Colistin

Colistin (Coly-Mycin) is an antibiotic which has been isolated from the bacterium *Aerobacillus colistinus*. It is a polypeptide that is similar to but not identical with the polymyxins in chemical composition and spectrum of activity. In vitro, a potent bacteriostatic and bacteriocidal action is exerted on a wide variety of gram-negative bacteria (*Aerobacter aerogenes*, *Pseudomonas aeruginosa*, *Salmonella*, *Shigella*), but there is a lesser effect against *Proteus*, fungi, and gram-positive bacteria (staphylococci, streptococci). Resistance to colistin has not readily occurred in vitro, and no cross-resistance to the present broad spectrum is known.

The activity of colistin is approximately equal to that of polymyxin B but, as opposed to polymyxin, the clinical and laboratory experience to date have shown virtually no nephrotoxicity after recommended systemic doses. ROSS et al. (1960) found slight azotemia, but only in very young infants, and observed no other side effects.

Two forms of colistin are available: colistin sulfate (Coly-Mycin S), a nonabsorbable form which has been used for bowel sterilization and topical medication, and colistin methanesulfonate (Coly-Mycin M), the absorbable form which is employed parenterally, subconjunctivally, and topically. One milligram of pure colistin base has been assigned a potency of 30,000 units. No corneal or conjunctival irritation follows instillation of 0.12% drops. Subconjunctival injection of 10 mg colistin sodium methanesulfonate is not very irritating (PRYOR et al. 1962b).

SCHWARTZ and co-workers (1960) document a study in which colistin was shown to penetrate the subretinal fluid of 7 of 18 patients given an intramuscular dose of 33 mg pure base. GORDON and McLEAN (1960) successfully treated a *Pseudomonas* infection of the cornea with colistin eyedrops (500,000 units in 7.5 ml sterile water) and two instramuscular injections (500,000 units). Subconjunctival injections (50,000–100,000 units in water) and solutions for intracameral irrigation (100,000 units/ml) were estimated by the authors to be effective for the treatment of intraocular infections caused by *Pseudomonas aeruginosa*. LUND (1969) treated 165 patients with 0.12% colistin sulfate drops with only one adverse reaction, a local allergy.

In man, single therapeutic doses of intramuscular colistin sodium methanesulfonate provide high blood levels for 8–12 h. The dosage for systemic infections is 2 mg colistin base/kg body wt./day, although as much as 7.5 mg/kg body wt./day has been administered in critical situations without nephrotoxicity.

XVIII. Sulfonamides

By virtue of their ability to prevent bacterial utilization of PABA, all the sulfonamides are essentially bacteriostatic and act against a variety of gram-positive and gram-negative bacteria. Except in the case of meningococci, the appropriate antibiotic is superior to a sulfonamide drug for any given infection. The sulfonamides invariably act more slowly and less effectively than antibiotics, and their effect is curtailed by the presence of purulent material and bacterial products. sulfacetamide solution (10%–30%) has been useful for topical ocular therapy; although SCHNEIERSON (1958) found only a small percentage of isolated staphylococcal strains to be sensitive to sulfonamides in vitro. Systemic sulfonamides caused some undesirable reactions, e.g., hematuria, anuria, crystalluria, agranulocytosis, hemolytic anemia, rashes, transitory myopia, and allergies.

The long-acting sulfonamides sulfamethoxypyridazine (Kynex, Midicel) and sulfadimethoxine (Madribon) have been introduced. Adequate blood levels of free drug are maintained with one or two daily doses, and the total requirement is less than that of the short-acting sulfonamides because of the reduced rate of renal excretion. Another sulfonamide, sulfaethylthiadiazole, referred to also as sulfaethiodole (Sul-Spanison liquid, Sul-Spantab tablets), is conveniently available in a sustained release form given every 12 h.

Intraocular penetration of topically applied sulfonamides seems directly related to their solubility and protein binding (GALLARDO and THOMPSON 1942). Most commonly used sulfonamides readily penetrate the ocular tissues and fluids. CRABB et al. (1957) noted therapeutic levels of sulfisoxazole (Gantrisin) in the aqueous humor of rabbits following topical and subconjunctival administration or injection. Since the blood–aqueous and blood–cerebrospinal fluid barriers are analogous, the study of the diffusion of sulfonamides into the cerebrospinal fluid of normal adults should give an indication of drug penetration across the blood–aqueous barrier. The accessibility of a group of these drugs to the cerebrospinal fluid was ranked in the following descending order: sulfamethazine, sulfadiazine, triple sulfapyrimadine mixture, sulfamerazine, sulfamethoxypyridazine, sulfioxazole, and sulfaethylthiadiazole. The intraocular penetration of sodium sulfadiazine is increased by iontophoresis and by loss or damage to corneal epithelium.

All sulfonamides have the same range of therapeutic action and are characterized by a mutual cross-resistance. The only advantages of the long-acting sulfonamides over those whose effective duration is more limited are their convenience of administration and lower cost. A major disadvantage of the former is that the occurrence of a sensitization reaction may be prolonged by the free sulfonamide, which persists in the blood for a period of days.

XIX. Trimethoprim-Sulfamethoxazole

Trimethoprim-sulfamethoxazole (Co-trimoxazole, Proloprim, Trimpex, Septra, Bactrim) is a synergistic combination available as an oral preparation consisting of trimethoprim 80 mg and sulfamethoxazole 400 mg. The half-life of sulfamethoxazole is similar to that of trimethoprim, and usually a dosage of two tablets every 12 h is employed. Excretion is primarily through the kidneys.

This fixed ratio combination is effective in vitro against a wide variety of gram-positive and gram-negative organisms including staphylococci, streptococci, *Escherichia coli*, *Hemophilus influenzae*, *Proteus mirabilis*, and *Salmonella* and *Shigella* species. The combination also has limited antiprotozoal and antifungal activity. Although this mixture is used primarily for urinary infections, it has been helpful against typhoid resistance to chloramphenicol, uncomplicated gonorrhea, septicemias, brucellosis, and subacute bacterial endocarditis.

Trimethoprim inhibits bacterial folate production. Some bacteria, e.g., *Pseudomonas*, *Neisseria*, and anaerobes, have intrinsic resistance to it, while others may acquire resistance through plasmid-borne R factors. Trimethoprim may protect sulfamethoxazole from resistance by organisms, but the reverse does not seem to occur. London has already seen an epidemic of plasmid-borne trimethoprim resistance. Diagnostic laboratories should test both trimethoprim and sulfamethoxazole individually as well as in combination (ANONYMOUS 1980).

XX. Chloramphenicol

Chloramphenicol is an antibacterial and antirickettsial agent isolated from *Streptomyces* species, acting by rapidly but reversibly inhibiting bacterial ribosomal protein synthesis. It is lipid-soluble and largely water-insoluble. Water solubility is improved by the addition of a succinate group. The succinate and palmitate preparations are hydrolyzed to free chloramphenicol by the body.

Chloramphenicol is inactive against viruses, fungi, yeasts, protozoa and almost all strains of *Pseudomonas*, but is effective against coliforms, *Mycoplasma*, *Rickettsia*, *Schistosoma*, anaerobes, *Neisseria*, *Staphylococcus*, *Streptococcus*, and ampicillin-resistant *Hemophilus influenzae* type B, for which it is the drug of choice in invasive infections. It is also the drug of choice for *Salmonella typhosa* (except in Mexico and Asia, where resistance to chloramphenicol appears to be common).

Bacterial resistance to chloramphenicol develops slowly. When it occurs, it is usually due to inactivating enzymes (as in *Escherichia coli* and *Staphylococcus aureus*). Resistance may also be acquired during treatment by the transfer of genetic information from resistant organisms to chloramphenicol-sensitive bacteria. During conjugation, a resistance factor (the R factor) is passed from the resistant to the previously sensitive strain, thus conferring resistance on this strain. Rarely, resistance may be due to a permeability barrier.

Chloramphenicol is administered orally and intravenously but not intramuscularly (probably due to delayed hydrolysis). It is rapidly distributed throughout the body with high concentrations in liver, kidney, saliva, and eye.

1. Penetration and Absorption

Chloramphenicol has a high ether–water partition coefficient, resulting in high intraocular penetrations following various routes of administration. Subconjunctival injection of 10 mg chloramphenicol succinate per kilogram produces high levels in the aqueous humor (BROUGHTON and GOLDMAN 1973).

Oral administration of chloramphenicol at the level of 3 g per initial dose will produce comparable levels to those following intravenous or intramuscular administration. Parenteral administration therefore appears to be indicated only if the patient cannot or should not take the drug by mouth.

Intravenously administered chloramphenicol penetrates well into the aqueous humor of experimental rabbit eyes. One hour after intravenous injection of 50 mg chloramphenicol per kilogram, serum concentration reached 12 µg/ml, and the aqueous humor concentration was 6 µg/ml. None could be detected in the vitreous after 1 h. Chloramphenicol obviously penetrates the eye more readily than penicillin, streptomycin, chlortetracycline, and oxytetracycline (FURGIUELE et al. 1960; LEOPOLD et al. 1950; LEOPOLD 1951, 1952).

Increased levels are obtained in the eye when the blood–aqueous barrier has been altered by surgery or paracentesis (LEOPOLD et al. 1950).

Blood levels of chloramphenicol in excess of 15 µg/ml are readily attained in man after oral administration of 3–5 g/day in divided dose given every 4 h. The drug is rapidly absorbed after oral administration, with a peak serum level at 2 h, and a half-life of 2 h with normal renal and hepatic function. It is 60% protein-bound. Probenecid seems to have no effect on the concentration of the active drug; generally, however, there is some evidence that intraperitoneal injection of probenecid 30 min prior to subconjunctival chloramphenicol injection increases the chloramphenicol aqueous humor concentration. Perhaps the probenecid may block the active transport of antibiotic out of the eye (BROUGHTON and GOLDMAN 1973).

2. Toxicity and Side Effects

Dose reduction is not required for patients with renal failure. However, in hepatic failure conjugation may be decreased, with a corresponding increase in the risk of toxicity (usually depression of erythropoietic function) from higher concentrations of the metabolically active drug.

Until neonatal pharmacokinetics are better understood, chloramphenicol should not be used for neonatal infections without careful monitoring of blood levels. In the newborn, active chloramphenicol is excreted in the urine in a similar proportion to that in adults (5%–10% of total dose). Due to the immaturity of the enzyme system, conjugation is much delayed and the newborn has a reduced ability to metabolize many lipid-soluble drugs, including chloramphenicol. This can lead to higher active drug levels and possible accumulation with increased risk of toxicity. Newborns of low birth weight who began chloramphenicol treatment in the first 2 days of life have been found to develop a change in feeding pattern, regurgitation, abdominal distension, hypotonia, hypothermia, and a characteristic gray color. This gray baby syndrome is associated with a 40% fatality rate within 24–48 h, and occurs with doses greater than 75 mg/kg/day (blood levels greater than 50 µg/mg). If the drug is discontinued, symptoms may be reversed in 24–36-üh. For full-term neonates within the 1st week of life (and in premature infants within the first 4 weeks) the recommended intravenous dose is 25 mg/kg/day in two divided doses. Because of the rapid maturation of hepatic and renal function, this can be increased to 50 mg/kg/day (in two doses) between 1 and 4 weeks for full-term infants, and 50–100 mg/kg/day (in four divided doses) beyond that.

The most serious side effects of chloramphenicol are from interaction with the hematopoietic system, consisting of reversible, dose-related reactions and irreversible, idiopathic reactions. Of 830 cases of drug-induced agranulocytosis reported to the Council of Drugs, 56 were attributed to chloramphenicol, 92 were attributed to sulfonamides, and 370 to phenothiazines (HUGULEY 1966).

Dose-related anemia (with normal bone marrow), sometimes with leukopenia or thrombocytopenia, can be minimized by maintaining blood concentration at less than 25 µg/ml (within the therapeutic range). Complete recovery usually occurs with in less than 12 days of stopping the drug. One theory postulates that this reaction results from inhibition of phenylalanine incorporation into protein of early erythroid and granulocyte cells. The administration of phenylalanine to reverse this toxicity is being studied. The second major hematologic reaction that may occur with chloramphenicol therapy is aplastic anemia, which can be fatal. This probably occurs in one out of every 40,000 therapeutic courses of the drug; it is unrelated to dose, duration of treatment, or route of administration, and usually begins weeks to months after treatment has ended.

At least three cases of persistent bone marrow hypoplasia have been reported following the use of chloramphenicol eye drops (CARPENTER 1975; ROSENTHAL and BLACKMAN 1965; ABRAMS et al. 1980). The reports of marrow hypoplasia following the use of chloramphenicol eye drops and ointment suggest that systemic effects result either from absorption through conjunctival membranes, or from drainage down the lacrimal duct with eventual gastrointestinal tract absorption. It is remarkable that so small an amount of chloramphenicol could be responsible for so devastating a complication, but the lack of dose relationship has been pointed out (CONE and ABELSON 1952). This would support the hypothesis that there is an individual, possibly genetic predisposition to this toxicity (YUNIS 1973). In all of the topical cases, there were many months of constant use prior to the onset of the bone marrow hypoplasia. In the case following the use of ointment there was a 3-month lag after cessation of the long-term ointment use. It has been claimed that the longer the interval between the last dose of chloramphenicol and the first sign of hematologic abnormality, the greater the mortality. The precise mechanism of chloramphenicol-induced aplastic anemia remains undefined. The reversible erythroid suppression variety is likely to be a result of mitochondrial injury, while aplastic anemia appears to be related to an impairment of DNA synthesis.

There are a number of other reversible dose-related effects. Diarrhea, vomiting, and severe glossitis, which may be due to bacterial or fungal superinfection, may occur with doses of 6–12 g/day for more than 1 week. Central nervous system disturbances include paresthesias, blurring of vision, retrobulbar and peripheral neuritis, and acute encephalopathy.

The prolonged use of chloramphenicol has been suggested to cause optic atrophy in children. Thirteen of 98 cystic fibrosis patients who have received long-term chloramphenicol therapy of almost 5 years developed visual disturbances. Visual loss was sudden, bilateral, and associated with an ophthalmoscopic picture of optic neuritis. According to HARLEY and co-workers (1970), the condition was dose-related, depending on the amount and duration of chloramphenicol therapy. Vision improved on withdrawal of the drug in most of the patients. The pathology in three patients who had suffered visual disturbance, including bilateral optic atrophy, revealed loss of retinal ganglion cells, gliosis of the nerve fiber layer, and involvement of the papillomacular bundle (HARLEY et al. 1970).

Allergic reactions may also occur, and include rash, fever, and hemorrhage into skin or intestinal mucosa.

Chloramphenicol may inhibit the humoral immune response, which may be related to bone marrow suppression. This has been reported in adults on 2–4 g/day. It was suggested that there is an inhibition of the growth of rapidly dividing β-lymphocytes following antigenic stimulation; however, no clinical significance has been attributed to this reaction so far (MEISSNER and SMITH 1979).

XXI. Tetracyclines

Tetracyclines are bacteriostatic agents acting by inhibition of microbial ribosomal protein synthesis. They are broad spectrum antibiotics against gram-positive and gram-negative bacteria such as *Escherichia coli*, *Aerobacter*, *Klebsiella*, and *Bacillus subtilis*, as well as other organisms such as rickettsiae, actinomycetes, and protozoa. *Pseudomonas*, *Proteus*, and many strains of *Staphylococcus* are resistant to the tetracyclines.

Members of the tetracycline group, extracted from *Streptomyces* species or produced synthetically, include the following compounds:

Chlortetracycline (Aureomycin)   Tetracycline (Anchromycin,
Oxytetracycline (Terramycin)   Panmycin, Tetracyn)
Robitet   Methacycline (Rondomycin)
Demeclocycline (Declomycin)   Tetracycline phosphate complex (Tetrex)
Minocycline (Minocin, Bectrin)
Tetracycline buffered with sodium hexametaphosphate (SK-tetracycline)
Tetracycline buffered with potassium methaphosphate (Sumycin)

1. Penetration and Absorption

When administered in doses sufficient to provide adequate serum levels, tetracyclines diffuse into most fluids and tissues. They will diffuse into the spinal fluid and into the ocular fluid if the systemic dose is sufficiently high. Tetracycline passes through the placenta and is present in the milk of lactating women. When applied as a corneal bath, it does not penetrate the intact normal cornea. However, if the epithelium is removed, penetration is facilitated (DOUVAS et al. 1951).

When given intravenously in rabbits in a dose of 30 mg/kg, only 3 µg oxytetra-cycline could be found 1½ h later. Chlortetracycline did not penetrate as well (DOUVAS et al. 1951).

CANNON and associates (1952) found that topically administered oxytetra-cycline solution and ointment failed to penetrate the normal cornea into the aqueous humor in a significant amount. Subconjunctival injections of 50 mg pro-duce transient levels of oxytetracycline in the aqueous humor, but none in the vit-reous humor. Intravenously administered oxytetracycline produced detectable levels in the cornea, sclera, aqueous, iris, and rectus muscle of the rabbit eye 30 min after the injection of 50 mg/kg body wt., but no detectable amounts could be found 2 and 6 h after the intravenous injection (CANNON et al. 1952).

Topical tetracycline has been used prophylactically in the eyes of newborn chil-dren, and it has been suggested as a substitute for Credé's prophylaxis. External infections due to susceptible organisms respond well to topical tetracyclines.

It has been shown by ROBSON and SCOTT (1943b) and CANNON and LEOPOLD (1952) that oxytetracycline may be highly successful against a variety of organisms producing experimental corneal infection, particularly following local therapy. This is particularly true if the therapy is instituted early in the course of the infec-tion. Acute trachoma may be arrested by topical tetracycline. Three to four weeks of therapy is recommended, usually in ointment form.

The rates of absorption, achievemant of peak blood concentrations, and dura-tion of action vary among the tetracyclines. These drugs are bound to plasma pro-teins, but the chemical nature of a tetracycline is more important than the degree of protein binding in determining the duration of its serum half-life. Peak serum levels are generally attained within 2–4 h of oral administration. Average serum half-lifes following repeated doses are 5.5 h for chlortetracycline, 8.5 h for tetra-cycline, 9.5 h for oxytetracycline, 12 h for demeclocycline, 15 h for methacycline, 15–17 h for doxycycline, and 17–19 h for minocycline. The longer half-life of the newer tetracyclines permits administration of smaller doses at longer intervals.

2. Fluorescence

Tetracycline has been used experimentally to study the formation of cortical bone, and urinary calculi, and clinically to detect new growths. The tetracyclines fluoresce bright yellow when exposed to ultraviolet radiation of 360 nm. After a single dose of 3–4 g, fluorescence may be detected within 24 h in all tissues except the brain. The drug remains visible in bone and neoplastic tissue for several weeks. The fact that oxytetracycline concentrates in rapidly growing neoplastic tissue has been used as a way of detecting the presence of such tissue (NEWELL et al. 1963). Intraocular neoplasms do not selectively concentrate enough oxytetracycline to be diagnostically helpful. It may be related to the inability of tetracycline to penetrate into the eye as compared with other tissue. HAVENER (1978) has pointed out that although melanomas will not selectively fluoresce within the eye, such tissue will fluoresce when it has extended extraocularly into the orbital tissue. Approximately 1 g/day for an adult for 3 days is required to bring about such fluorescent detection of the neoplasm, and it has to be stopped for at least 12 h prior to surgery to permit the high concentrations of the drug to leave normal structures.

3. Toxicity and Side Effects

About 10% of people taking large doses will develop gastrointestinal disturbances. Nausea and diarrhea are not uncommon complications. Other undesirable reactions include dryness of the mouth, hoarseness, stomatitis, glossitis, black hairy tongue, pharyngitis, dysphagia, proctitis, and inflammatory lesions of the vulvovaginal and perianal regions. Thrombophlebitis has occurred at sites of intravenous injection. Most of these effects are related to suppression of normal enteric flora with overgrowth of other organisms. Superinfections, including severe staphylococcal enterocolitis and infection with *Candida albicans*, have occurred during oral and rarely intravenous or intramuscular administration.

Hypersensitivity reactions do occur, with rare anaphylactic shock. Cross-sensitization among the tetracyclines is common. Photosensitivity reactions have been noted, particularly after demeclocycline. Minocycline has not produced such reactions to date.

Tetracyclines differ in their excretion. Doxycycline and minocycline are excreted much less by the kidney than the other tetracyclines and may not accumulate in patients with renal insufficiency. This is because these two analogs are very soluble in fat, which may interfere with their renal clearance.

Reaction products of tetracyclines can produce Fanconi's syndrome by damaging the proximal renal tubules. This usually clears after withdrawal of tetracycline. In all reported cases of this syndrome the patient has ingested outdated capsules. Outdated tetracyclines have been known to cause renal tubular acidosis, a syndrome of potassium depletion secondary to nephropathy and an illness simulating systemic lupus erythematosus. It is important, therefore, that the patient only use tetracyclines that are within the expiration date.

Fatty degeneration of the liver has been reported with tetracyclines used during pregnancy. The drug is attracted to embryonic and growing osseous tissue, where it may form a tetracycline calcium-phosphate complex due to its chelating property. The danger of adverse effects of fetus and child is greatest from mild-pregnancy to 3 years of age. Changes have been reported in deciduous and permanent teeth, including dysgenesis, staining, and increased tendency to caries. Discoloration may be progressive, and varies from yellowish-brown to dark gray. There may also be discolorization of nails when exposed to ultraviolet light.

In infants and children, tetracyclines given in therapeutic doses can cause pseutotumor cerebri. Tense bulging of the fontanelles has been observed with increased intracranial pressure in infants. Papilledema and meningeal irritation have been observed in adults. There are no abnormalities of the spinal fluid, and the diagnosis, chiefly one of exclusion, may require careful neurological appraisal. Withdrawal of the antibiotic leads to reversal of the condition. Tetracyclines may have an effect on the blood function, e.g., coagulation, and may potentiate the effects of dicoumaral-type anticoagulants.

XXII. Pyrimethamine

Pyrimethamine, or 2,4-diamino-5 (*p*-chlorophenyl)-6-ethylpyrimine (Daraprim), is a potent folic acid antagonist and an effective antiparasitic agent which has been used clinically in the treatment of malaria and toxoplasmosis. Inhibition of the growth of the parasite is probably due to deprivation of folic acid (HITCHINGS 1952). Pyrimethamine can kill proliferating *Toxoplasma* organisms both in vivo and in vitro, but seems to be without effect unless the cells are actively dividing. It is essential for pyrimethamine to penetrate into the cell in order to attack the *Toxoplasma* organisms, which are intracellular; otherwise fresh cysts will be formed, which will be a potential source of recurrence (EYLES and COLEMAN 1953; RYAN et al. 1954; BEVERLY and FRY 1957; BEVERLY 1958; COOK and JACOBS 1956).

1. Value

There is clinical evidence that pyrimethamine is of considerable value in toxoplasmosis, particularly when given systemically in association with sulfonamides (KAYHOE et al. 1957). Remarkably effective synergism between sulfadiazine and pyrimethamine has been demonstrated in studies of mice infected with toxoplasmosis (EYLES 1956).

However, conflicting opinions exist as to the effect of pyrimethamine for the treatment of the disease in the human eye. Perhaps this is due to the persistence of resistant strains, or to slow-growing parasites, or to the inability of the drug to penetrate within the cells to attack the intracellular parasites (HOGAN 1958; FAJARDO et al. 1962; ACERS 1964; PERKINS et al. 1956). PERKINS and his co-workers treated alternate patients in a series of 164 individuals with uveitis with 25 mg pyrimethamine per day or a placebo. Of the patients with positive dye tests treated with pyrimethamine, 76% improved within a month. However, the study of ACERS (1964) cast doubt on the clinical value of pyrimethamine and sulfonamides. He could find no significant difference in the response of therapy between the treated group (pyrimethamine + triple sulfonamides + prednisone) and the control group (prednisone and placebo). JACOBS and his co-workers were able to show in experimental toxoplasmosis in rabbits that the dosage of pyrimethamine and sulfadiazine was important and that dosage must be continued for a long period of time at an adequate level in order to be successful and to reduce recurrences (JACOBS et al. 1964).

2. Toxicity

When pyrimethamine is used for malaria prophylaxis at a dosage of 25 mg/week, no significant toxic symptoms are reported, but when it is used in larger daily doses for ocular disease, hematologic depression is the outstanding undesirable effect. Although general bone marrow depression is seen, which produces a decrease in red cells, white cells, and platelets, thrombocytopenia has been the most severe manifestation of pyrimethamine toxicity. When platelet suppression begins in a patient receiving pyrimethamine, the platelet count usually declines 3–9 days after the drug is discontinued (KAUFMAN and GISLER 1960). Normal levels are regained in 1–2 weeks.

Other toxic manifestations of pyrimethamine include convulsions, which have been described in monkeys and in accidentally poisoned children (GRISHAM 1962). It is also capable of producing teratogenic effects (SAND 1963). Hematologic complications of pyrimethamine may be treated with folinic acid [citrovorum factor (Leucovorin), formyl tetrahydroperoylglutamic acid] administered intramuscularly in amounts of 3–9 mg/day. Folinic acid should be administered whenever the platelet count drops below 200,000. If only mild cellular depression is observed, it is not necessary to stop the pyrimethamine. Folinic acid (3 mg/day) is usually used prophylactically along with pyrimethamine in order to prevent and ameliorate the bone marrow depression. Since the *Toxoplasma* organism cannot use folinic acid, it does not inhibit the effect of pyrimethamine on *Toxoplasma*. It does not impair the effectiveness of pyrimethamine in experimental studies (FRANKEL and HITCHINGS 1957). HARRIS (1956) has demonstrated that vitamin B12 can accentuate folinic acid efficiency and should not be used during pyrimethamine therapy. Multivitamin preparations containing folinic acid or PABA will protect *Toxoplasma* organisms against pyrimethamine, and should therefore not be used during the course of therapy.

3. Penetration and Dosage

Measurement of pyrimethamine in the eye reveal that the drug may concentrate in the retina 12 h after intramuscular injection of 2.5 ml labeled pyrimethamine per kilogram body wt. in monkeys. The pyrimethamine concentrations were 1.02 µg/ml in the retina and 0.03 µg/ml in the aqueous; none could be detected in the vitreous. It requires about 0.25 µg/ml to destroy most *Toxoplasma* organisms in tissue culture, and the organisms have to be exposed to this concentration for about 4 days. Subconjunctival injections of pyrimethamine produced detectable levels in the aqueous humor, but not in the vitreous. There is insufficient evidence that periocular injections would produce adequate levels in the retina to be effective against toxoplasmic retinitis (CHOI 1958; KAUFMAN and CALDWELL 1959).

Today dosage programs for the use of pyrimethamine and sulfonamides in toxoplasmic uveitis (ocular toxoplasmosis) employ 75 mg daily for 2 days orally, followed by 25 mg daily for 6 weeks, and sulfadiazine or trisulfapyrimidines 2 g immediately followed by 1.5 g four times daily for 6 weeks. Folinic acid 3 mg twice a week is also employed. Leukocyte and platelet counts have to be monitored at least weekly. Clindamycin 300 mg ever 6 h along with sulfadiazine 1 g four times daily may be tried, but does not have FDA approval as yet. Periocular clindamycin may prove effective but has not had adequate clinical trial (O'CONNOR 1974, 1980 b).

XXIII. Drugs Used in the Treatment of Fungal Infections

Mycoses fall into three principal classes: (a) those due to dermatophytes, affecting only the skin, hair, and nails; (b) local and usually superficial infections caused by *Candida albicans;* and (c) systemic infections, which may also be caused by *Candida* species, of which other examples are aspergillosis, coccidioidomycosis, cryptococcosis, and histoplasmosis (MEDOFF and KOBAYASHI 1980). The drugs available for their treatment are discussed below.

1. Griseofulvin, Nystatin, and Amphotericin B

Griseofulvin was discovered and characterized nearly 40 years ago, but had to be rediscovered and survive a period when it was unjustly suspected of toxicity. It is unique in being deposited in keratin as this is laid down, and is therefore concentrated and persists in precisely the area attacked by dermatophytes. It now provides the standard treatment for dermatomycoses.

Nystatin was the first of the polyenes to be discovered, a group of antibiotics acting on a wide range of fungi, particularly *Candida* species. It has an exceedingly low solubility (so low, indeed, that its therapeutic effect is surprising), and is used in the form of a suspension for application to mucous and other surfaces attacked by *Candida albicans*. These areas include the mouth and alimentary tract; bronchial lesions can be treated by inhalation, vaginal by pessary or cream, and skin by various forms of application. Other polyenes also used for some of these purposes are candicidin, and natamycin (Pimaricin).

Amphotericin B is a later-discovered polyene active against all fungi causing systemic infections, and can be solubilized to permit intravenous injection.

a) Ocular Penetration

Montana and Sery found no detectable penetration of the eye by amphotericin B, whether given topically, subconjunctivally, or intravenously (MONTANA and SERY 1958). GREEN et al. (1965) also believed the blood–eye barrier to be highly resistant to the passage of amphotericin B. However, they did show that in the inflamed eye penetration improved.

b) Ocular Tolerance

Topical application of ointments containing amphotericin B 5 mg/g (0.5%) is safely tolerated, but a concentration of 50 mg/g (5%) causes corneal edema and iritis (FOSTER et al. 1958). The anterior chambers of experimental animal eyes appear to tolerate single injections of 25 µg in 0.05 ml of distilled water, causing a temporary iritis and floating anterior lens opacity. Concentrations of 5–10 µg placed in the center of the vitreous were well tolerated by the rabbit eye (AXELROD et al. 1973). Such a dose can be successful against experimental *Candida* endophthalmitis (AXELROD and PEYMAN 1973).

Clinically, amphotericin B topically applied has been successful in the management of fungal corneal ulcers. Hourly instillations of amphotericin B solution 1 mg/ml (0.1%) resulted in improvement in five patients with keratitis from various fungi, e.g., *Aspergillus versicolor*, *Penicillinum*, *Fusidium terricola*, *Gibberella fujikuroi*, *Curvularia lunate*, and a corn smut (ANDERSON et al. 1959).

Although intravenous administration of amphotericin has been successful in controlling experimental intraocular histoplasmosis resulting from introductions of organisms into the anterior chamber, the results in presumed ocular histoplasmosis are not clear cut (SETHIE and SCHWARZ 1966; FALLS and GILES 1960).

Amphotericin may be the most toxic of all antibiotics in clinical use: the individual dose, given at 2-day intervals, should not exceed 1 mg/kg, or the total dose 3 g. Even so, vomiting, fever, thrombophlebitis, hypokalemia, and a raised blood urea are common effects, and some degree of permanent renal damage results from a full course. Thus although success has often been achieved with this drug in treating systemic mycoses, it has for long been hoped that some other better-tolerated treatment might be found.

Amphotericin is generally effective in treating ocular mycoses (GRIFFIN et al. 1973; ELLIOTT et al. 1979; LARSEN et al. 1978; JONES 1975), but it has potentially serious adverse effects which can complicate the already difficult course of an illness in debilitated and immune-suppressed patients.

2. 5-Fluorocytosine

5-Fluorocytosine is a synthetic compounds which interferes in a well-ascertained way with the metabolism of yeast-like fungi. It is absorbed when given orally, and large doses, which appear to be quite safe, produce high concentrations not only in the blood but also in cerebrospinal fluid. There are now fairly numerous reports of its successful use in some cases of cryptococcal meningitis and of systemic candidiasis.

The most promising recent development has been combined treatment with fluorocytosine and amphotericin B. One effect of this combination is that amphotericin B increases the permeability of the fungal cell, thus permitting a higher concentration of fluorocytosine to be attained within it. There is evidence that it also permits a lower dose of the more toxic drug to be given, and that the development of resistance to its partner is discouraged. A synergic action has been demonstrated in several experimental mycoses in mice. Favorable clinical reports are those of UTZ et al. (1975) on the treatment of cryptococcosis and of ELLARD et al. (1976) on success in cases of *Candida* endophthalmitis, *Candida* septicemia, and *Torulopsis* endocarditis. Failure with fluorocytosine treatment is sometimes accompanied by a large increase in resistance of the infecting organism.

There is some evidence of synergistic action of amphotericin and fluorocytosine in some *Candida* infections (JONES 1975; RABINOVICH et al. 1974). Some isolates of *Candida* species are known to be resistant to fluorocytosine (JONES et al. 1974; FISHMAN et al. 1972).

3. Imidazoles

Clotrimazole, introduced some years ago as a systemic antifungal agent, had serious side effects, and is now used mainly for the local treatment of candidiasis. Miconazole which in addition to a wide antifungal spectrum has some action an gram-positive bacteria, can be administered not only locally for infections due to yeasts and dermatophytes, but also both orally and parenterally, and is well tolerated (SAWYER et al. 1975). Miconazole is an imidazole with a broad spectrum of activity against gram-positive cocci and most fungal diseases, including candidiasis, aspergillosis, histoplasmosis, and infections with *Torulopsis*. In low doses it is fungistatic, and therefore treatment may need to be prolonged to ensure adequate eradication of the fungus. At very high doses it is fungicidal. It penetrates well into most infected tissues, including vitreous humor (SYMOENS 1977), but penetration into normal spinal fluid is poor. Minor side effects include pruritus, rash, chills, phlebitis, and gastrointestinal symptoms, but no major adverse reactions have been reported to date. A transitory increase in blood lipids may occur because of the lipids present in the parenteral form of the drug.

Success with miconazole has been claimed in the treatment of various deep-seated mycoses. An impressive report is that by DERESENSKI et al. (1977) on the treatment of meningitis due to *Coccidioides immitis*. These authors administered miconazole intrathecally by several routes, including the intraventricular. It does not seem possible yet to assess the relative merits of this drug and amphotericin B, but certainly miconazole has an advantage in lower toxicity. Econazole is another imidazole which has also been successfully used locally in infections due to yeasts and dermatophytes. It has also been investigated in deep-seated mycoses (HEEL et al. 1978).

Pimaricin is a polyene antifungal produced by *Streptomyces natalensis*, and has poor ocular penetration properties. A 5% suspension applied topically every 2 h for 2 weeks was well tolerated in the human eye (NEWMARK et al. 1970). Intravitreal injection of 50 µg was toxic to experimental rabbit eyes, though 25 µg could be tolerated. However, this suppressed experimental *Aspergillus* infection in only 40% of the rabbits studied (ELLISON 1976). *Fusarium solani* keratitis does respond to topical therapy (JONES et al. 1972).

XXIV. Diethylcarbamazine in the Treatment of Onchocerciasis

Onchocerciasis is a major ocular disease, and along with trachoma, cataract, and xerophthalmia is one of the great blinding diseases of the tropics. Relatively simple and effective means are available to prevent or treat trachoma, cataract, and xerophthalmia. However, the prevention of ocular onchocerciasis is far from satisfactory (ANONYMOUS 1978). The treatment under study consists of diethylcarbamazine citrate (DEC) (Hetrazan), a microfilaricide, plus suramin, a macrofilaricide. Other agents employed include levamisole, mebendazole, and corticosteroids.

It is generally accepted (BUCK 1974) that ocular disease in onchocerciasis is caused by microfilariae of *Onchocerca volvulus* in the ocular tissues. However, it is not clear how much disease is caused by presence of living microfilariae and how much by their death and dissolution (ANDERSON and FUGLSANG 1977). Host reactions to microfilariae vary not only between different individuals, but also within the same individual at different stages of the infection (BRYCESON 1976; BARTLETT et al. 1978). Variations might therefore be expected in response to the administration of macro- and microfilaricidal drugs.

Diethylcarbamazine citrate is the most effective microfilaricide available for treating ocular or other forms of onchocerciasis. It is therefore potentially of great public health importance in the prevention of blindness from onchocerciasis and for treating certain other filarial diseases, but it is a very difficult drug to handle in cases of severe ocular onchocerciasis (ANDERSON et al. 1976). It has low toxicity for animals and man, but serious adverse systemic reactions can occur when it is given orally by ordinary therapeutic schedules to heavily parasitized patients. These reactions include itching, papular and exfoliative skin eruptions, arthralgia, vertigo, collapse (FUGLSANG and ANDERSON 1974; BRYCESON et al. 1977), and even death (OOMEN 1969; ANDERSON et al. 1976).

Ocular adverse reactions occur also with systemic administration of the drug. These comprise acute exacerbations of ocular inflammation with watering, photophobia, bulbar and circumcorneal hyperemia, the formation of minute globular infiltrates at or near the limbus, and snowflake or fluffy punctate corneal opacities (ANDERSON et al. 1976). Twice-daily administration of 1–1.5 mg β-methasone may diminish but not prevent these ocular reactions. There is evidence that a 10- to 14-day oral course of DEC followed by a weekly maintenance dose may improve vision in onchocercal sclerosing keratitis or iritis, but it seems not to benefit the other ocular lesions, and may even worsen the visual deficit from retinal or optic nerve disease (ANDERSON et al. 1976).

The topical administration of 3% DEC drops four times daily, without steroid therapy, to patients with ocular onchocerciasis can lead to severe adverse ocular reactions, including severe itching, redness, swelling of lids and conjunctiva, or severe iritis with hypopyon (ANDERSON and FUGLSANG 1973).

A single topical administration of 5% DEC to the rabbit eye rapidly gives a level of 10 µg/ml at 3 h (LAZAR et al. 1968). The more severe adverse reactions seen clinically with 3% DEC eye drops may thus relate to repeated high peak levels in the ocular tissues. Weaker solutions would be expected to give lower peak levels, but the duration of an effective drug level would be shortened. To maintain an effective tissue drug level without peak levels giving adverse reactions in heavily parasitized eyes, it might suffice to use very frequent applications of weaker solutions of DEC with the addition of agents to prolong the contact time. But the frequency of application required might well be prohibitive. The levels of drug that are respectively beneficial or damaging, the margin between these, and the rate of rise and fall of tissue drug levels following topical administration will determine whether beneficial therapy or prophylaxis could be achieved with DEC eye drops, or whether continuous controlled delivery of the drug would be needed to achieve that goal (JONES et al. 1978 a).

Diethylcarbamazine was given as eye drops in varying concentrations in half-log dilution series from 1% to 0.0001% to patients with ocular onchocerciasis. Migration of microfilariae into the cornea, followed by their straightening and disintegration, was observed with delivery rates as low as 0.1 µg/h. Dose related adverse inflammatory reactions, including the development of globular limbal infiltrates with itching and redness, were seen with delivery rates as low as 0.6 µg/h, but substantial inflammatory reactions, including severe vasculitis, were seen only with delivery rates of or above 1.0 µg/h. This suggests that it should be possible to achieve beneficial clearing of the microfilarial load, without adverse reactions, by continuous nonpulsed delivery of the drug. Technology exists for such delivery, either directly into the eye or systemically by a transdermal system that could give 3–7 days' treatment from each application. The observations reported suggest that after preliminary clearing of the microfilarial load by carefully controlled delivery of DEC, it may be possible to maintain therapy by less strictly controlled delivery in DEC-medicated salt, or to use treatment with suramin, without incurring substantial adverse reactions, such as a deterioration in vision in cases in which the optic nerve is already compromised. Continuous nonpulsed DEC delivery systems could have a place in the management of onchocercal sclerosing keratitis. The unique opportunities for using the ocular model to define the requirements for beneficial nondamaging therapy with DEC should be explored in further field trials (JONES et al. 1978 a).

Recently JONES et al. (1978 b) applied increasing concentrations of levamisole and of mebendazole to one eye in groups of four patients with ocular onchocerciasis in northern Cameroon. No effects resulted from up to 3.0% mebendazole suspensions, but 3.0% levamisole solutions rapidly caused entry of microfilariae, straightening out and subsequent opacification of previously curled-up living microfilariae, the rapid formation of typical limbar globular infiltrates, and the subsequent formation of fluffy opacities around the microfilariae. These changes are typical of all other drugs they studied that have a microfilaricidal action on *Onchocerca volvulus* – DEC, suramin, and metrifonate. The efficacy of 3% levamisole approximated to that of 0.03% DEC. This is in keeping with published observations on the filaricidal activity of these two compounds. It is suggested that this system of drug testing should be considered for systematic use in the search for more effective and safer drugs for onchocerciasis.

ANDERSON and FUGLSANG (1978) observed 54 heavily infected patients with ocular onchocerciasis, who were treated with an initial 2-week course of DEC in which the dose was increased slowly from 25 mg on the 1st day to 150–200 mg twice daily on days 8–14. *β*-methasone 1.5 mg was given twice daily 2 days before DEC administration and during the days of increasing DEC dosage, after which it was tailed off. This course was followed by three to five weekly injections of suramin. It was found to be possible to rid these heavily infected patients of most of their microfilariae during the initial course without intolerable side effects. The subsequent suramin course was in general well accepted except in one case, where there was a serious aggravation of anterior uveitis. Three patients developed retinal pigment atrophy, optic atrophy occurred in three others, and both showed retinal and optic atrophy.

References

Abel R Jr, Boyle GL, Furman M, Leopold IH (1974) Intraocular penetration of cefazolin sodium in rabbits. Am J Ophthalmol 78:779

Abraham RK, Burnett HH (1955) Tetracycline and chloramphenicol studies on rabbit and human eyes. Arch Ophthalmol 54:641

Abramowicz M (ed) (1977) Adverse interactions of drugs. Med Lett Drugs Ther 19:5

Abrams SM, Degnan PJ, Viciguerra V (1980) Marrow aplasia following topical application of chloramphenicol eye ointment. Arch Intern Med 140:576

Acers TE (1964) Toxoplastic retinochoroiditis, a double-blind therapeutic study. Arch Ophthalmol 71:58

Acred P, Brown DM, Knudsen ET, Rolinson GN, Sutherland R (1967) New semi-synthetic penicillin active against *Pseudomonas pyocyanea*. Nature 215:25

Adler CA, Maurice DM, Paterson ME (1971) The effect of viscosity of the vehicle on the penetration of fluorescein into the human eye. Exp Eye Res 11:34

Ainslie D (1946) Use of solid penicillin in case of endophthalmitis following lens extraction. Br J Ophthalmol 30:208

Ainslie D, Cairns JE (1960) Subconjunctival administration of soframycin in the treatment of corneal infections. Br J Ophthalmol 44:25

Ainslie D, Henderson WG (1958) Soframycin. Its penetration into the eye and its effect upon experimentally produced *Staph. aureus* and *Ps. pyocyanea* corneal infections. Br J Ophthalmol 42:513

Ainslie D, Smith C (1952) Polymyxin E. Penetration into the eye and therapeutic value in experimental infections due to *Ps. pyocyanea*. Br J Ophthalmol 36:353

Allansmith M, Skaggs C, Kimura S (1970) Anterior chamber paracentesis. Arch Ophthalmol 84:745

Allen HF (1971) Current status of prevention, diagnosis and management of bacterial corneal ulcers. Ann Ophthalmol 3:235

Allen HF, Mangiaracine AB (1964) Bacterial endophthalmitis after cataract extraction, a study of 22 infections in 20,000 operations. Arch Ophthalmol 72:454

Allen HF, Mangiaracine AB (1973) Bacterial endophthalmitis after cataract extraction II, incidence in 36,000 consecutive operations with special reference to pre-operative topical antibiotics. Trans Am Acad Ophthalmol Oto 77:581

American Medical Association (1977) AMA Drug Evaluations. Publishing Services Group, Littleton, MA

Anderson B, Roberts S, Gonzalez C, Chick E (1959) Mycotic ulcerative keratitis. Arch Ophthalmol 62:169

Anderson J, Fuglsang H (1973) Topical diethylcarbamazine in ocular onchocerciasis. Trans R Soc Trop Med Hyg 67:710

Anderson J, Fuglsang H (1977) Ocular onchocerciasis. Tropical Diseases Bulletin 74:257

Anderson J, Fuglsang H (1978) Further studies on the treatment of ocular onchocerciasis with diethylcarbamazine and suramin. Br J Ophthalmol 62:450

Anderson J, Fuglsang H, Marshall TF de C (1976) Effects of diethylcarbamazine on ocular onchocerciasis. Tropenmed Parasitol 22:279

Anderson P, Davies J, Davies BD (1967) Effect of spectinomycin on polypeptide synthesis in extracts of *Escherichia coli*. J Mol Biol 29:203

Anonymous (1978) Onchocerciasis – out of the oublitte. Br J Ophthalmol 62:427 (editorial)

Anonymous (1980) Bacterial resistance to trimethoprim. Br Med J 281:571 (editorial)

Aronstam RH (1964) Pitfalls of prophylaxis: alteration of post-operative infection by penicillin-streptomycin. Am J Ophthalmol 57:312

Axelrod AJ, Peyman GA (1973) Intravitreal amphotericin B treatment of experimental fungal endophthalmitis. Am J Ophthalmol 76:584

Axelrod AJ, Peyman GA, Apple DJ (1973) Toxicity of intravitreal injection of amphotericin B. Am J Ophthalmol 76:598

Axelrod JL, Kochman RS (1980a) Cefoxitin levels in human aqueous humor. Am J Ophthalmol 90:388

Axelrod JL, Kochman RS (1980b) Cefaclor levels in human aqueous humor. Arch Ophthalmol 98:740

Ayliffe GAJ, Barry DR, Lowbury EJL, Roper Hall MJ, Walker WM (1966) Post-operative infection with *Pseudomonas aeruginosa* in an eye hospital. Lancet I:1113

Bartlett A, Turk J, Ngu J, Mackenzie CD, Fuglsang H, Anderson J (1978) Variation in delayed hypersensitivity in onchocerciasis. Trans R Soc Trop Med Hyg 72:372

Barza M, Baum J (1973) Penetration of ocular compartments by penicillin. Analysis of factors affecting concentration and half life. Surv Ophthalmol 18:71

Barza M, Lauermann M (1978) Why monitor serum levels of gentamicin. Clin Pharmacokinet 3:202

Barza M, Baum J, Birkby AB, Weinstein L (1973) Intraocular penetration of carbenicillin in the rabbit. Am J Ophthalmol 75:307

Barza MM, Baum J, Kane A (1976) Inhibition of antibiotic activity in vitro by synthetic melanin. Antimicrob Agents Chemother 10:569

Barza M, Kane A, Baum JL (1977) Regional differences in the ocular concentration of gentamicin after subconjunctival or retrobulbar injection of rabbit. Am J Ophthalmol 83:407

Barza M, Kane A, Baum JL (1978) Intraocular penetration of gentamicin after subconjunctival and retrobulbar injection. Am J Ophthalmol 85:541

Barza M, Kane A, Baum J (1979) Marked differences between pigmented and albino rabbits in the concentration of clindamycin in iris and choroid retina. J Infect Dis 139:203

Baum JE (1978) The treatment of bacterial endophthalmitis. Ophthalmology 85:350

Baum JL (1980) Antibiotic use in ophthalmology. In: Duane TD (ed) Clinical ophthalmology, vol 4. Chap 6. Harper and Row, New York

Baum JL, Peyman GA (1977) Antibiotic administration in the treatment of bacterial endophthalmitis. Viewpoints Surv Ophthalmol 21:332

Baum JL, Barza M, Shushan D, Weinstein L (1974) Concentration of gentamicin in experimental corneal ulcers. Arch Ophthalmol 92:315

Bellows JG, Chinn H (1939) Distribution of sulfanilamide in eye. JAMA 112:2023

Bellows JG, Chinn H (1941) Penetration of sulfathiazole in eye. Arch Ophthalmol 25:294

Bellows JG, Farmer CJ (1947) Streptomycin in ophthalmology. Am J Ophthalmol 30:1215

Bellows JG, Gutmann M (1943) Application of wetting agents in ophthalmology, with particular reference to sulfonamide compounds. Arch Ophthalmol 30:352

Bellows JG, Richardson VM, Farmer CJ (1950) Aureomycin in ophthalmology. Am J Ophthalmol 33:273

Beverley JK (1958) A rational approach to the treatment of toxoplasmic uveitis. Trans Ophthalmol Soc UK 78:109

Beverley JK, Fry BA (1957) Sulphadimidine, pyrimethamine and dapsone in the treatment of toxoplasmosis in mice. Br J Pharmacol Chemother 12:189

Beyer KH, Russo HF, Tillson EK, Miller AG, Veruey WF, Gass SR (1951) Benemid, its renal affinity and its elimination. Am J Physiol 166:625

Bhargava SK, Chopdar A (1971) Gas gangrene panophthalmitis. Br J Ophthalmol 55:136

Bill A, Phillips CI (1971) Uveoscleral drainage of aqueous humor in human eyes. Exp Eye Res 12:275

Bleeker GM, Maas EH (1958) Penetration of penethamate, a penicillin ester, into the tissues of the eye. Arch Ophthalmol 60:1013

Bloome M, Golden B, McKee A (1970) Antibiotic concentration in ocular tissues of penicillin G and dehydrostreptomycin. Arch Ophthalmol 83:78

Bogacz J (1954) Comparative effect of various synthetic agents and various antibiotics including spiramycin on toxoplasma. Bull Soc Pathol Exot Filiales 47:903

Bohigian GM (1981) Postoperative infection: endophthalmitis. In: Waltman SR, Krupin T (eds) Complications in ophthalmic surgery. Lippincott, Philadelphia, Chap 2

Bollen A, Davies J, Ozaki M, Mizushima S (1969) Ribosomal protein conferring sensitivity to the antibiotics spectinomycin in *Escherichia coli*. Science 165:85

Boyd JL (1942) Sodium sulfathiazole iontophoresis. Arch Ophthalmol 28:205

Boyle GL, Hein HF, Leopold TH (1970) Intraocular penetration of cephalexin in man. Am J Ophthalmol 69:868

Boyle GL, Lichtig ML, Leopold IH (1971) Lincomycin levels in human ocular fluids and serum following subconjunctival injection. Am J Ophthalmol 71:1303

Boyle GL, Gwon AE, Zinn KM, Leopold IH (1972) Intraocular penetration of carbenicillin after subconjunctival injection in man. Am J Ophthalmol 73:754

Bristow JH, Kassar B, Sevel D (1971) Gas gangrene panophthalmitis treated with hyperbaric oxygen. Br J Ophthalmol 55:139

Broughton W, Goldman JN (1973) The intraocular penetration of chloramphenicol succinate in rabbits. Ann Ophthalmol 5:71

Brown CH III, Natelson EA, Bradshaw MW, Williams TW Jr, Alfrey CP Jr (1974) The hemostatic defect produced by carbenicillin. N Engl J Med 291:265

Bryceson ADM (1976) What happens when microfilariae die? Trans R Soc Trop Med Hyg 70:397

Bryceson ADM, Warrell DA, Pope HM (1977) Dangerous reactions to treatment of onchocerciasis with diethylcarbamazine. Br Med J 1:742

Buck AA (ed) (1974) Onchocerciasis. World Health Organization, Geneva

Callahan A (1953) Effect of sulfonamides and antibiotics on panophthalmitis complicating cataract extraction. Arch Ophthalmol 49:212

Cameron EH (1949) Treatment of hypopyon ulcer of cornea. Br J Ophthalmol 33:368

Cannon EJ, Leopold IH (1952) Effectiveness of Terramycin and other antibiotics against experimental bacterial keratitis. Arch Opthalmol 47:426

Cannon EJ, Nichols AC, Leopold IH (1952) Studies on intraocular penetration and toxicity of Terramycin. Arch Ophthalmol 47:344

Capalbi S, Centanni L (1949) Il chloroamfenicolo in oculistica; prime recerche cliniche e sperimentali. Arch Ottal 53:408

Carpenter G (1975) Chloramphenicol eye drops and marrow aplasia. Lancet 2:326

Cassady JR (1967) Prophylactic subconjunctival antibiotics following cataract extraction. Am J Ophthalmol 64:1081

Chalkley THF, Shoch D (1967) An evaluation of prophylactic subconjunctival antibiotic injection in cataract surgery. Am J Ophthalmol 64:1084

Chalkley THF, Shoch D (1971) Porphylactic intraocular antibiotics in cataract surgery. 105th annual meeting, American Ophthalmological Society, 25 May 1971

Choi SC (1958) Penetration of pyrimethamine (Daraprim) into ocular tissues of rabbits. Arch Ophthalmol 60:603

Coles RS, Boyle GL, Leopold IH, Schneierson SS (1971) Lincomycin levels in rabbit ocular fluids and serum. Am J Ophthalmol 72:464

Comber KR, Basker MJ, Osborne CD, Sutherland R (1977) Synergy between ticarcillin and tobramycin against Pseudomonas aeruginosa and Enterobacteriaceae in vitro and in vivo. Antimicrob Agents Chemother 11:956

Cone TE Jr, Abelson SM (1952) Aplastic anemia following two days of chloramphenicol therapy. J Pediatr 41:349

Cook MK, Jacobs L (1956) The effect of pyrimethamine and sulfadiazine on toxoplasmic in tissue culture. Am J Trop Med 5:376

Cottingham AJ, Forster RK (1976) Vitrectomy in endophthalmitis. Arch Ophthalmol 94:2078

Crabb AM, Fielding IL, Ormsby HL (1957) Bacillus Proteus endophthalmitis. Am J Ophthalmol 43:86

Davis SD, Sarff LD, Hyndiuk RA (1977) Antibiotic therapy of experimental Pseudomonas keratitis in guinea pigs. Arch Ophthalmol 95:1638

Davis SD, Sarff LD, Hyndiuk RA (1979) Comparison of therapeutic routes in experimental keratitis. Am J Ophthalmol 87:710

Davson H (1949) Penetration of some sulphonamides into intra-ocular fluids of cat and rabbit. J Physiol 110:416

Deresenski SC, Lilly RB, Levine HB, Galgiani JM, Stevens DA (1977) Treatment of fungal meningitis with miconazole. Arch Intern Med 137:1180

de Roetth A (1949) Penetration of Aureomycin into the eye. Arch Ophthalmol 42:365

Dettli L (1976) Drug dosage in renal disease. Clinical Pharmacokinetics 1:126

Devlin JL, Mercer KB, Dea FJ, Leopold IH (1978) Intraocular penetration of topical clindamycin in rabbits. Arch Ophthalmol 96:1650

Doane MG, Jensen AD, Dohlman CH (1978) Penetration routes of topically applied eye medications. Am J Ophthalmol 85:383

Douvas MG, Featherstone RM, Braley AE (1951) Role of Terramycin in ophthalmology. Arch Ophthalmol 46:57

Duke BOL, Vincelette J, Moore PJ (1973) Microfilariae in the cerebrospinal fluid, and neurological complications, during treatment of onchocericiasis with diethylcarbamazine. Tropenmed Parasitol 27:123

Dumas J, Fielding IL, Ormsby HL (1958) Oleandomycin. Am J Ophthalmol 46:10

Dunnington JH, Locatcher-Khorazo D (1945) Value of cultures before operation for cataract. Archives of Ophthalmol 34:215

Dunnington J, von Sallmann L (1944) Penicillin therapy in ophthalmology. Arch Ophthalmol 32:353

Ellard T, Beskow D, Norrby R, Wahlen T, Alestig K (1976) Combined treatment with amphotericin B and flucytosine in severe fungal infections. J Antimicrob Chemother 2:239

Elliott JH, O'Day DM, Gutow GS, Podgorski SF, Abrabawi P (1979) Mycotic endophthalmitis in drug abusers. Am J Ophthalmol 88:66

Ellis CJ, Geddesham, Davey PG, Wiser, Andrews JM, Grimley RP (1979) Mezlocillin and azlocillin: an evaluation of two new β-lactam antibiotics. J Antimicrob Chemother 5:517

Ellison AC (1976) Intravitreal effects of pimaricin in experimental fungal endophthalmitis. Am J Ophthalmol 81:157

Eyles DE (1956) Newer knowledge of the chemotherapy of toxoplasmosis. Ann NY Acad Sci 64:252

Eyles DE, Coleman N (1953) Synergistic effect of sulfadiazine and Daraprim against experimental toxoplasmosis in the mouse. Antibiot Chemother 3:483

Faigenbaum SJ, Boyle GC, Prywes AS, Abel R Jr, Leopold IH (1976) Intraocular penetration of amoxicillin. Am J Ophthalmol 82:598

Fajardo RV, Furgiuele FP, Leopold IH (1962) Treatment of toxoplasmosis uveitis. Arch Ophthalmol 67:712

Falls H, Giles C (1960) The use of amphotericin B in selected cases of chorioretinitis. Am J Ophthalmol 49:1288

Finland M, Neu HC (1976) Tobramycin. J Infect Dis 134 [Suppl]:1–234

Finland M, Brumfitt W, Kass EH (1976) Advances in aminoglycoside therapy: amikacin. J Infect Dis 134 [Suppl]:242

Fishman LS, Griffin JR, Sapico FL, Hecht R (1972) Hematogenous *Candida* endophthalmitis, a complication in candidemia. N Engl J Med 286:675

Forbes M, Becker B (1960) The transport of organic anions by the rabbit eye. II. In vivo transport of iodopyrocet (Diodrast). Am J Ophthalmol 50:867

Forster RK (1974) Endophthalmitis. Diagnostic cultures and visual results. Arch Ophthalmol 92:387

Forster RK (1978) Etiology and diagnosis of bacterial postoperative endophthalmitis. Ophthalmology 85:320

Forster RK, Zachary IG, Cottingham AJ Jr (1976a) Diagnosis and treatment of endophthalmitis. In: Leopold IH, Burns RP (eds) Symposium on ocular therapy, vol 9. Wiley, New York chap 5, p 51

Forster RK, Zachary IG, Cottingham AJ Jr, Norton EWD (1976b) Further observations on the diagnosis, cause and treatment of endophthalmitis. Am J Ophthalmol 81:52

Forster RK, Abbott RL, Gelender H (1980) Management of infectious endophthalmitis. Ophthalmology 87:313

Foster JB, Almeda E, Littman ML et al (1958) Some intraocular and conjunctival effects of amphotericin B in man and in the rabbit. Arch Ophthalmol 60:55

Foulks GN (1980) Effect of pathological conditions on drug penetration into the anterior segment. Int Ophthalmol Clin 20:51

Frankel JK, Hitchings GH (1957) Relative reversal by vitamin (para-amino-benzoic-folic and folinic acids) on the effects of sulfadiazine and pyrimethamine on *Toxoplasma* – the mouse and man. Antibiot Chemother 7:630

Freeman MI, Gay AJ (1967) Systemic steroid therapy in post-cataract endophthalmitis. In: Becker B, Drews R (eds) Current concepts on opthalmology. Mosby, St. Louis, chap 12

Fuglsang H, Anderson J (1974) Collapse during treatment of onchocerciasis with diethylcarbamazine. Trans R Soc Trop Med Hyg 68:72

Furgiuele FP (1967) Ocular penetration and intolerance of gentamicin. Am J Ophthalmol 64:421

Furgiuele FP (1970) Penetration of gentamicin into the aqueous humor of human eyes. Am J Ophthalmol 69:481

Furgiuele FP, Sery TW, Leopold IH (1958) The ocular penetration and tolerance of a new antibiotic: spiramycin. Antibiotics annual, 1958–1959. Medical Encyclopedia, New York, p 204

Furgiuele FP, Sery TW, Leopold IH (1960) Newer antibiotics: their intraocular penetration. Am J Ophthalmol 50:614

Gallardo E, Thompson R (1942) Sulfonamide content of aqueous humor following conjunctival application of drug powders. Am J Ophthalmol 25:1210

Galloway NR, Robinson GE (1973) Panophthalmitis due to *Pasteurella septica*. Br J Ophthalmol 57:153

Garin JP, Eyles DE (1958) Treatment of experimental toxoplasmosis in the mouse with spiramycin. Presse Med 66:957. [Abstract in JAMA 168:835]

Golden B, Coppel SP (1970) Ocular tissue absorption of gentamicin. Arch Ophthalmol 84:792

Goldman JN, Broughton W, Javed H, Lauderdale V (1973) Ampicillin, erythromycin and chloramphenicol penetration into rabbit aqueous humor. Ann Ophthalmol 5:147

Gordon DM, McLean JM (1960) Colistin in *Pseudomonas* infection. Am J Ophthalmol 50:33

Green WR, Leopold IH (1965) Penetration of methicillin. Am J Ophthalmol 60:800

Green WR, Bennett JE, Goos RD (1965) Ocular penetration of amphotericin B. Arch Ophthalmol 73:769

Greene WH, Wiernik PH (1972) *Candida* endophthalmitis. Successful treatment in a patient with acute leukemia. Am J Ophthalmol 74:1100

Griffin JR, Pettit TH, Fishman LS, Foos RY (1973) Blood-borne *Candida* and endophthalmitis, a clinical and pathologic study of 21 cases. Arch Ophthalmol 89:450

Grignolo A (1948) Primi risultati spermimentali e clinici sull'impiego della streptomicina nelle infezioni tubercolari dell'occhio

Grisham RSC (1962) Central nervous toxicity of pyrimethamine (Daraprim) in man. Am J Ophthalmol 54:1119

Hallett JW, Leopold IH (1957) Clinical trial of erythromycin ophthalmic ointment. Am J Ophthalmol 44:519

Halliday JA, Ormsby HL (1955) Carbomycin in ocular infection. Am J Ophthalmol 39:51

Harley RD, Huang NN, Macri CH, Green WR (1970) Optic neuritis and optic atrophy following chloramphenicol in cystic fibrosis patients. Trans Am Acad Ophthalmol Otolaryngol 74:1011

Harris JW (1956) Aggravation of clinical manifestations of folic acid deficiency by small doses of vitamin B12. Am J Med 21:461

Havener WH (1978) Ocular pharmacology, 4th edn. Mosby, St. Louis, p 176

Heel RC, Brogden RN, Speight TM, Avery GS (1978) Econazole, a review of its anti-fungal activity in therapeutic efficacy. Drugs 16:177

Heman-Ackah SM (1975) Microbial kinetics of drug action against gram-positive and gram-negative organisms. II. Effect of clindamycin on *Staphylococcus aureus* and *Escherichia coli*. J Pharm Sci 64:1612

Hessburg PC (1969) Management of *Pseudomonas* keratitis. Surv Ophthalmol 14:43

Hewitt WL (1974) Gentamicin toxicity in perspective. Postgrad Med J 50 [Suppl 7]:55

Hitchings GH (1952) Daraprim as an antagonist of folic and folinic acid. Trans R Soc Trop Med Hyg 46:467

Hoffman TA, Bullock WE (1970) Carbenicillin therapy of *Pseudomonas* and other gram-negative bacillary infections. Ann Intern Med 73:165

Hogan MJ (1958) Ocular toxoplasmosis. Am J Ophthalmol 46:467

Hughes WF, Owens WC (1947) Post-operative complications of cataract extractions. Arch Ophthalmol 38:577

Huguley CMJ, Lea JW, Butts JA (1966) Adverse hematologic reactions to drugs. In: Brown EB, Moore CV (eds) Progress in hematology, vol 5. Grune and Stratton, New York

Imai M (1969) Penetration of lincomycin into the tissues of rabbit eyes. Jpn Clin Ophthalmol 23:1175

Jackson H, Cooper J, Mellinger WJ, Olsen AR (1965) Group AB hemolytic streptococcal pharyngitis results in treatment with lincomycin. JAMA 194:1189

Jacobs L, Melton ML, Kaufman HE (1964) Treatment of experimental ocular toxoplasmosis. Arch Ophthalmol 71:111

Jahre JS, Fu KP, Neu HC (1979) Clinical evaluation of netilmicin therapy in serious infections. Am J Med 66:67

Jawetz E (1975) Combined actions of antimicrobial drugs. In: Gillete JR, Mitchell JR (eds) Concepts in biochemical pharmacology. Springer, Berlin Heidelberg New York, p 343 (Handbook of experimental pharmacology, vol 28, pt 3)

Jensen AD, Naidoff MA (1973) Bilateral meningococcal endophthalmitis. Arch Ophthalmol 90:396

Johnson M, Harrison HE, Raftery AT, Elder JB (1979) Vascular prostacyclin may be reduced in diabetes in man. Lancet I:325

Jones BR (1975) Principles in the management of oculomycosis. Am J Ophthalmol 79:719

Jones BR, Robertson DM, Riley FC, Hermans PE (1974) Endogenous *Candida* oculomycosis. Arch Ophthalmol 91:33

Jones BR, Anderson J, Fuglsang H (1978 a) Effects of various concentrations of diethylcarbamazine citrate applied as eye drops in ocular onchocerciasis, and the possibilities of improved therapy from continuous non-pulsed delivery. Br J Ophthalmol 62:428

Jones BR, Anderson J, Fuglsang H (1978 b) Evaluation of microfilaricidal effects in the cornea from topically applied drugs in ocular onchocerciasis: trials with levamisole and mebendazole. Br J Ophthalmol 62:440

Jones D, Foster RK, Rebell C (1972) *Fusarium solani* keratitis treated with natamycin (Pimaricin). Arch Ophthalmol 88:147

Jones DB (1973) Early diagnosis and therapy of bacterial corneal ulcers. Int Ophthalmol Clin 13(4):1

Jones WF Jr, Finland M (1957) Antibiotic combinations. Tetracycline, erythromycin, oleandomycin and spiramycin, and combinations of tetracycline with each of the other three agents – comparisons of activity in vitro and antibacterial action of blood after oral administration. N Engl J Med 247:481

Jules F, Young MY (1945) Treatment of septic ulcer of cornea by local applications of penicillin. Br J Ophthalmol 29:312

Kaufman HE, Caldwell LA (1959) Pharmacological studies of pyrimethamine (Daraprim) in man. Arch Ophthalmol 61:885

Kaufman HE, Gisler PH (1960) Hematologic toxicity of pyrimethamine in man. Arch Ophthalmol 64:140

Kayhoe DE, Jacobs L, Beye HK, McCullough NB (1957) Acquired toxoplasmosis: observations on two parasitologically proved cases treated with pyrimethamine and triple sulfonamides. N Engl J Med 257:1247

Klastersky J, Cappel R, Debrusscher L (1971) Effectiveness of betamethasone in management of severe infections. N Engl J Med 284:1248

Klastersky J, Hensgens C, Meunier-Carpentier F (1976) Comparative effectiveness of combinations of amikacin with penicillin G and amikacin with carbenicillin in gram-negative speticemia; double-blind clinical trial. J Infect Dis 134:S433

Kleinberg J, Dea FJ, Anderson JA, Leopold IH (1979) Intraocular penetration of topically applied lincomycin hydrochloride in rabbits. Arch Ophthalmol 97: 933

Kolker AE, Freeman MI, Pettit TH (1967) Prophylactic antibiotics and post-operative endophthalmitis. Am J Ophthalmol 63:434

Krogstad DJ, Korfhagen TR, Moellering RC Jr, Wennerstein C, Swartz MN (1978) Plasmid-mediated resistance to antibiotic synergism in enterococci. J Clin Invest 61:1645

Kurose Y, Leopold IH (1965) Intraocular penetration of ampicillin-1: animal experiment. Arch Ophthalmol 73:361

Kuwahara S, Mime S, Nishida M (1971) Immunogenicity of cefazolin. In: Antimicrobial agents and chemotherapy 1970. American Society for Microbiology, Bethesda, p 374

Langham M (1951) Factors affecting penetration of antibiotics into aqueous humour. Br J Ophthalmol 35:614

Larsen PA, Lindstrom RL, Doughman DJ (1978) *Torulopsis glabrata* endophthalmitis after keratoplasty with an organ cultured cornea. Arch Ophthalmol 96:1019

Lazar M, Lieberman TW, Furman M, Leopold IH (1968) Ocular penetration of Hetrazan in rabbits. Am J Ophthalmol 66:215

Leopold IH (1945 a) Local toxic effect of detergents on ocular structures. AMA Arch Ophthalmol 34:99

Leopold IH (1945 b) Intravitreal penetration of penicillin and penicillin therapy of infections of the vitreous. Arch Ophthalmol 33:211

Leopold IH (1951) Clinical trial with chloramphenicol in ocular infections. Arch Ophthalmol 45:44

Leopold IH (1952) Surgery of ocular trauma. Arch Ophthalmol 48:738

Leopold IH (1971) Management of intraocular infection. Doyle memorial lecture. Trans Ophthalmol Soc UK 16:577

Leopold IH (1972a) Discussion in Burns and Oden's paper 1972. Antibiotic prophylaxis in cataract surgery. Trans Am Ophthalmol Soc 70:43

Leopold IH (1972b) Problems in the use of antibiotics. In: Leopold IH (ed) Symposium on ocular therapy, vol 5. Mosby, St. Louis, chap 13, pp 113

Leopold IH (1978) Secondary ocular infections. Aust J Ophthalmol 6:101

Leopold IH, Apt L (1960) Postoperative intraocular infections. Am J Ophthalmol 50:1225

Leopold IH, LaMotte WO (1945) Penetration of penicillin in rabbit eyes with normal, inflamed and abraded cornea. Arch Ophthalmol 33:43

Leopold IH, Nichols A (1946) Intraocular penetration of streptomycin following systemic and local administration. AMA Arch Ophthalmol 35:33, 1946

Leopold IH,, Scheie HG (1943) Studies with microcrystalline sulfathiazole. Arch Ophthalmol 29:811

Leopold IH, Holmes LF, LaMotte WO Jr (1944) Local versus systemic penicillin therapy of rabbit corneal ulcers. Arch Ophthalmol 32:193

Leopold IH, Wiley M, Dennis R (1947) Vitreous infections and streptomycin. Am J Ophthalmol 30:1345

Leopold IH, Nichols AC, Vogel AW (1950) Penetration of chloramphenicol U.S.P. (Chloromycetin) into the eye. Arch Ophthalmol 44:22

Lepper MH, Dowling HF (1951) Treatment of pneumococcic meningitis with penicillin compared with penicillin plus Aureomycin: studies including observations on an apparent antagonism between penicillin and Aureomycin. Arch Intern Med 88:489

Libert J, Ketelbant-Balasse PE, Van Hoff F, Aubert-Tulkens G, Tulkens P (1979) Cellular toxicity of gentamicin. Am J Ophthalmol 87:405–411

Litwack KD, Pettit T, Johnson BL Jr (1969) Penetration of gentamicin, administered intramuscularly and subconjunctivally into aqueous humor. Arch Ophthalmol 82:687

Locke JC (1949) Experimental studies with antibiotics; bacitracin, streptomycin, penicillin, and antibiotic mixtures in intraocular infections with penicillin-resistant staphylococci. Am J Ophthalmol 32 (pt 2):135

Lund MH (1969) Colistin sulfate ophthalmic in the treatment of ocular infections. Arch Ophthalmol 81:4

Mandell GL, Lindsey E, Hook EW (1970) Synergism of vancomycin and streptomycin for enterococci. Am J Med Sci 259:346

Mann I (1946) Intra-ocular use of penicillin. Br J Ophthalmol 30:134

Marks ML, Eickoff TC (1970) Carbenicillin: a clinical and laboratory evaluation. Ann Intern Med 73:179

Maumenee AE, Michler RC (1951) Sterility of the operative field after ocular surgery. Trans Pac Coast Oto-Ophthalmol Soc Annu Meeting 32:172

Maurice DM (1951) The permeability of sodium ions of the living rabbit's cornea. J Physiol 112:367

Maurice D (1976) Injection of drugs into the vitreous body. In: Leopold IH, Burns RP (eds) Symposium on ocular therapy, vol 9. Wiley, New York, chap 6, pp 59

Maurice D (1980) Factors influencing the penetration of topically applied drugs. Int Ophthalmol Clin 20 (3):21

Mawer GE (1976) Computer assisted prescribing of drugs. Clin Pharmacokinet 1:67

Maylath Fr, Leopold IH (1955) Study of experimental intraocular infection: I. The recoverability of organisms inoculated into ocular tissues and fluids; II. The influence of antibiotics and cortisone alone and combined on intraocular growth of these organisms. Am J Ophthalmol 40:86

McCoy G, Leopold IH (1959) Penetration of oleandomycin. Am J Ophthalmol 48:666

McLoughlin JE, Reeves DS (1971) Clinical and laboratory evidence for inactivation of gentamicin by carbenicillin. Lancet I:261

McMeel JW, Wapner JM (1965) Infections and retinal surgery. I. Bacteriologic contamination during scleral buckling surgery. Arch Ophthalmol 74:42

McPherson SD Jr, Presley GD, Crawford JR (1968) Aqueous humor assays of subconjunctival antibiotics. Am J Ophthalmol 66:430

Medoff G, Kobayashi GS (1980) Strategies in the treatment of systemic fungal infections. N Engl J Med 302:145

Meissner HC, Smith AL (1979) The current status of chloramphenicol. Pediatrics 64:348

Melodia C, Bovo I (1953) L'aerosol nella teratia oculare. Ann Ottalm 79:105

Mercer KB, DeOlden JE, Leopold IH (1978) Intraocular penetration of topical clindamycin in rabbits. Arch Ophthalmol 96:880

Meyers B, Hirschman SZ, Strougo LG, Wormser GP (1981) Clinical study of netilmicin therapy. Mt Sinai J Med (NY) 48:42

Michiels J (1953) Les antibiotiques autres que la penicilline en ophthalmologie. Ann Oculist (Paris) 186:617

Mikuni M, Oshi M, Imai M, et al. (1973) Ophthalmic use of clindamycin palmitate. Jpn J Antibiot 26:409

Mizakawa T, Azuma I, Kawaguchi S (1965) Intra-ocular distribution of cephalothin and cephaloridine. J Antibiot (Tokyo) 18:525

Moellering RC Jr, Swartz MN (1976) The newer cephalosporins. N Engl J Med 294:24

Moellering RC Jr, Wennersten C, Medrek T, et al. (1971) Prevalence of high-level resistance to aminoglycosides in clinical isolates of enterococci. Antimicrob Agents Chemother 10:335

Montana JA, Sery TW (1958) Effect of fungistatic agents in corneal infections with *Candida albicans*. Arch Ophthalmol 60:1

Munoz L (1955) Gelatinoides de fluoresceina. Arch Soc Oftal Hispano-Am 15:1246

Naib K, Hallett JW, Leopold IH (1955) Observations on the ocular effects of erythromycin. Am J Ophthalmol 39:395

Nakatsue T (1961) Intraocular penetration of antibiotics into rabbit eye with experimental uveitis. Nippon Ganga Gakkai Zasshi 75:1244

Neu HC (1976) Tobramycin: a overview. J Infect Dis 134 [Suppl]:1

Neveu M, Elliott AJ (1959) Prophylaxis and treatment of endophthalmitis. Am J Ophthalmol 48:368

Newell FW, Goren SB, Brizel HE, Harper PV (1963) The use of iodine-125 as a diagnostic agent in ophthalmology. Trans Am Acad Ophthalmol Otolaryngol 67:177

Newmark E, Ellison AC, Kaufman HE (1970) Pimaricin therapy of cephalosporin and *Fusarium* keratitis. Am J Ophthalmol 69:458

Noone P, Pattison JR (1971) Therapeutic implications of interaction of gentamicin and penicillins. Lancet II:575

Oakley DE, Weeks RD, Ellis PP (1976) Corneal distribution of subconjunctival antibiotics. Am J Ophthalmol 81:307

O'Callaghan CH (1975) Classification of cephalosporins by their antibacterial activity and pharmacokinetic properties. Antimicrob Agents Chemother 1:1

O'Connor GR (1974) Manifestations and management of ocular toxoplasmosis. Bull NY Acad Med 50:192

O'Connor GR (1980a) Chemotherapy of toxoplasmosis and toxocariasis. In Sriniausan BD (ed) Ocular therapeutics. Masson, New York, pp 51

O'Connor GR (1980b) Ocular toxoplasmosis. Symposium, management of intraocular inflammation, University of Southern California, 2 Oct 1980

Oomen AP (1969) Fatalities after treatment of onchocerciasis with diethylcarbamazine. Trans R Soc Trop Med Hyg 63:548

Paterson CA (1973) Intraocular penetration of ^{14}C-labeled penicillin after sub-Tenon's or subconjunctival injection. Ann Ophthalmol 5:171

Pearlman MD (1956) Prophylactic subconjunctival penicillin and streptomycin after cataract extraction. Arch Ophthalmol 55:516

Perkins ES, Smith CH, Schofield PB (1956) Treatment of uveitis with pyrimethamine (Daraprim). Br J Ophthalmol 40:577

Pettit TH (1976) Management of bacterial croneal ulcers. In: Leopold IH, Burns R (eds) Symposium on ocular therapy, vol 8. Wiley, New York, pp 57

Petz LD (1971) Immunologic reactions of humans to cephalosporins. Postgrad Med J 47 [Suppl 2]:64

Peyman GA (1977) Antibiotic administration in the treatment of bacterial endophthalmitis. II. Intravitreal injections. Surv Ophthalmol 21:332

Peyman GA, May DR, Ericson ES, Apple D (1974a) Intraocular injection of gentamicin. Arch Ophthalmol 91:487

Peyman GA, Vastine DW, Crouch ER, Herbst RW (1974b) Clinical use of intravitreal antibiotics to treat bacterial endophthalmitis. Trans Am Acad Ophthalmol Otolaryngol 78:862

Peyman GA, Raichand M, Bennett TO (1980) Management of endophthalmitis with pars plana vitrectomy. Br J Ophthalmol 64:472

Philipson A (1977) Pharmacokinetics of ampicillin during pregnancy. J Infect Dis 136:370

Pratt WB (1977) Bactericidal inhibitors of protein synthesis (the aminoglycosides). Chemotherapy of infection. Oxford University Press, New York, chap 3, p 85

Praus R, Krejci L (1977) Release from hydrophilic gel contact and intraocular penetration. Ophthalmol Res 9:213

Price KE, Pursiano TA, Defuria MD (1974) Activity of BBK-8 (amikacin) against clinical isolates resistant to one or more aminogylcoside antibiotics. Antimicrob Agents Chemother 5:143

Pryor JG, Apt L, Leopold IH (1962a) Intraocular penetration of vancomycin. Arch Ophthalmol 67:608

Pryor JG, Apt L, Leopold IH (1962b) Intraocular penetration of colistin. Arch Ophthalmol 67:612

Querengesser EI, Ormsby HL (1955) Ocular penetration of erythromycin. Can Med Assoc J 72:200

Rabinovich S, Shaw BD, Bryan T, Donta ST (1974) The effect of 5-fluorocytosine and amphotericin B on *Candida albicans* infection in mice. J Infect Dis 130:28

Rahal JJ (1978) Antibiotic combinations: the clinical relevance of synergy and antagonism. Medicine (Baltimore) 57:179

Reading C, Cole M (1977) Clavulanic acid: a beta-lactamase-inhibiting beta-lactam from *Streptomyces clavuligerus*. Antimicrob Agents Chemother 11:852

Records RE (1967) Human intraocular penetration of sodium oxacillin. Arch Ophthalmol 77:693

Records RE (1968a) Intraocular penetration of cephalothin II. Human studies. Am J Ophthalmol 66:441

Records RE (1968b) Intraocular penetration of dicloxacillin in experimental animals. Invest Ophthalmol 7:663

Records RE (1969) Intraocular penetration of cephaloridine. Arch Ophthalmol 81:331

Records RE, Ellis PP (1967) The intraocular penetration of ampicillin, methicillin and oxacillin. Am J Ophthalmol 64:135

Richter G (1957) Die Rolle der Salbengrundlagen bei der lokalen Antibiotikatherapie am Auge, dargestellt am Beispiel des Chloramphenicols. Klin Monatsbl Augenheilkd 131:215

Ridley AF (1958) Use of topical antibiotics in ophthalmology. Trans Ophthalmol Soc UK 78:335

Riley FC, Boyle GL, Leopold IH (1968) Intraocular penetration of cephaloridine in humans. Am J Ophthalmol 66:1042

Robson JM, Scott GI (1943a) Production and treatment of experimental pneumococcal hypopyon ulcers in the rabbit. Br J Exp Pathol 24:50

Robson JM, Scott GI (1943b) Local chemotherapy in experimental lesions of the eye produced by *Staphylococcus aureus*. Lancet 1:100, 1943

Rosenthal RL, Blackman A (1965) Bone marrow hypoplasia following use of chloramphenicol eye drops. JAMA 191:136

Ross S, Puig JR, Zaremba EA (1960) Colistin: some preliminary laboratory and clinical observations in specific gastroenteritis in infants and children. In: Antibiot annual 1959–1960. Antibiotics, New York

Roy I, Back V, Thadepalli H (1977) In vitro activity of ticarcillin anaerobic bacteria compared with that of carbenicillin and penicillin. Antimicrob Agents Chemother 11:258

Ryan RW, Hart WM, Culligan JJ, Gunkel RD, Jacobs L, Cook MK (1954) Diagnosis and treatment of toxoplasmic uveitis. Trans Am Acad Ophthalmol 58:867

Rycroft BW (1945) Penicillin control of deep intraocular infection. Br J Ophthalmol 29:57

Salazar M, Patil PN (1975) An explanation for the long duration of mydriatic effect of atropine in the eye. Invest Ophthalmol 15:671

Sand BJ (1963) Teratogenesis from Daraprim. Am J Ophthalmol 56:1011

Sanders WE Jr, Hartwig EC, Schneider NJ, Cacciatore R, Valdez H (1977) Susceptibility of organisms in the *Mycobacterium fortuitum* complex to antituberculous and other antimicrobial agents. Antimicrob Agents Chemother 12:295

Saubermann G (1953) Experimental results with antibiotics for clinical use. Trans Ophthalmol Soc UK 73:181

Saubermann G (1957) Broad spectrum antibiotics in intraocular infection. Ophthalmologica 133:249

Sawyer PR, Brogden RN, Pinder RM, Speight RM, Avery GS (1975) Miconazole, a review of its anti-fungal activity and therapeutic efficacy. Drugs 9:406

Scheie HG, Souders BF (1941) Penetration of sulfanilamide and its derivatives into aqueous humor of eye. Arch Ophthalmol 25:1025

Schimpff SC, Landesman S, Hahn DM et al. (1976) Ticarcillin in combination with cephalothin or gentamicin as empiric antibiotic therapy in granulocytopenic cancer patients. Antimicrob Agents Chemother 10:837

Schneierson SS (1958) Survey of current bacterial susceptibility to anti-microbial agents. Comparison with previous survey. J Mt Sinai Hosp 25:52

Schwartz BS, Warren MR, Barkley FA, Landis L (1960) Microbiological and pharmacological studies of colistin sulfate and sodium colistin methanesulfonate. Antibiot Annual 1959–1960, p 41

Sery TW, Paul SD, Leopold IH (1957) Novobiocin, a new antibiotic. AMA Arch Ophthalmol 57:100

Sethie KK, Schwarz S (1966) Amphotericin B in ocular histoplasmosis of rabbits. Arch Ophthalmol 75:818

Smith JW, Johnson JE, Cluff LD (1966) Studies on the epidemiology of adverse drug reactions. II. An evaluation of penicillin allergy. N Engl J Med 274:998

Sorsby A, Ungar J (1946) Pure penicillin in ophthalmology. Br Med J 2:723

Sorsby A, Ungar J (1948) Intravitreal injection of penicillin: study on the levels of concentration reached and therapeutic efficacy. Br J Ophthalmol 32:857

Sorsby A, Ungar J (1958) Neomycin in ophthalmology. Ann R Coll Surg Engl 22:107

Sorsby A, Ungar J, Bailey NL (1952) Streptomycin in opthalmology. Br Med J 1:119

Sorsby A, Ungar J, Crick RP (1953) Aureomycin, chloramphenicol, and Terramycin in ophthalmology. Br Med J 2:301

Spector R, Lorenzo AV (1974) The effects of salicylate and probenecid in the cerebrospinal fluid transport of penicillin, aminosalicylic acid and iodide. J Pharmacol Exp Ther 188:55

Spyker DA, Rugloski RJ, Vann RL, O'Brien WM (1977) Pharmacokinetics of amoxicillin: dose dependence after intravenous, oral and intramuscular administration. Antimicrob Agents Chemother 11:132

Strausbaugh LJ, Sande MA (1978) Factors influencing the therapy of experimental *Proteus mirabilis* meningitis in rabbits. J Infect Dis 137:251

Struble GC, Bellows JG (1944) Studies on the distribution of penicillin in the eye and its clinical application. JAMA 125:685

Struble GC, Bellows JG (1946) Contact eye cup for corneal baths with solutions of penicillin. Arch Ophthalmol 35:173

Sutherland R, Burnett J, Rolinson GN (1971) A-carboxy-3-thienylmethylpenicillin (BRL 2288): a new semisynthetic penicillin: in vitro evaluation. In: Antimicrobial agents and chemotherapy – 1970. American Society of Microbiology, Bethesda, p 390

Swan KC (1944) Reactivity of ocular tissues to wetting agents. Am J Ophthalmol 27:1118

Swan KD, White NG (1942) Corneal permeability: I. Factors affecting penetration of drugs into the cornea. Am J Ophthalmol 25:1043

Swan KC, Crisman HR, Bailey PF (1956) Subepithelial versus subcapsular injections of drugs. Arch Ophthalmol 56:26

Swartz MN (1980) In: Federman, Rubinstein (eds)

Symoens J (1977) Clinical and experimental evidence on miconazole for the treatment of systemic mycosis – a review. Proc R Soc Med 70 [Suppl]:4–8

Tabbara KF, O'Connor GR (1975) Ocular tissue absorption of clindamycin phosphate. Arch Ophthalmol 93:1180

Theodore FH (1972) Points in treatment of bacterial corneal ulcers. In: Leopold IH (ed) Symposium on Ocular therapy, vol 5. Mosby, St. Louis, pp 48

Theodore FH, Littman ML, Almeda E (1962) Endophthalmitis following cataract extraction due to *Neurospora sitophila*, a so-called non-pathogenic fungus. Am J Ophthalmol 53:35

Tokuda H, Hiroshi H, Kayaba T (1973) The use of clindamycin palmitate in ophthalmology. Jpn J Antibiot 26:404–404

Utz JP, Garriques IL, Sande MA et al. (1975) Therapy of *Cryptococcus* with a combination of flucytosine and amphotericin B. J Infect Dis 132:368

Uwaydah MM, Faris BM (1976) Penetration of tobramycin sulfate in the aqueous humor of the rabbit. Arch Ophthalmol 94:1173

Valenton MJ, Brubaker RF, Allen HF (1973) *Staphylococcus epidermidis albus* in endophthalmitis. Arch Ophthalmol 89:94

Vogel AW, Leopold IH, Nichols A (1951) Neomycin. Ocular-tissue tolerance and penetration when locally applied in the rabbit eye. Am J Ophthalmol 34:1357

von Sallmann L (1943) Penicillin and sulfadiazine in treatment of experimental intraocular infection with pneumococcus. Arch Ophthalmol 30:426

von Sallmann L (1944) Simultaneous local application of penicillin and sulfacetamide. Arch Ophthalmol 32:190

von Sallmann L (1945) Penetration of penicillin into the eye; further studies. Arch Ophthalmol 34:195

von Sallmann L (1947) Controversial points in ocular penicillin therapy. Trans Ophthalmol UK 45:570

von Sallmann L, Meyer K (1944) Penetration of penicillin into the eye. Arch Ophthalmol 31:1

Walinder P, Koch E (1971) Endogenous fungus endophthalmitis. Acta Ophthalmol 49:50

Wallace JF, Smith RH, Garcia M et al. (1967) Studies on the pathogenesis of meningitis: VI. Antagonism between penicillin and chloramphenicol in experimental pneumococcal meningitis. J Lab Clin Med 70:408

Washington JA II (1976) The in vitro spectrum of the cephalosporins. Mayo Clin Proc 51:237

Weizenblatt S (1946) Penicillin in treatment of acute endophthalmitis. Arch Ophthalmol 36:736

Wilfert JN, Burke JP, Bloomer HA, Smith CB (1971) Renal insufficiency associated with gentamicin therapy. J Infect Dis 124:148

Witzel SH, Fielding IZ, Ormsby HL (1956) Ocular penetration of antibiotics by iontophoresis. Am J Ophthalmol 42:89

Wright RE, Stuart-Harris CH (1945) Penetration of penicillin into eye. Br J Ophthalmol 29:428

Yunis A (1973) Chloramphenicol induced bone marrow suppression. Semin Hematol 10:225

Zachary IG, Forster RK (1976) Experimental intravitreal gentamicin. Am J Ophthalmol 82:604

Zimmermann MC (1958) The prophylaxis and treatment of penicillin reactions with penicillinase. Clin Med 5:305

Anti-Inflammatory Agents
Steroids as Anti-Inflammatory Agents

J. R. POLANSKY and R. N. WEINREB

A. Introduction

Corticosteroids have provided an effective means of controlling many ocular inflammatory conditions for over 30 years. Although information concerning the use of these drugs continues to expand rapidly, the pharmacologic action of steroids in ocular tissues has not been clearly defined. Interpretations of clinical and experimental studies with steroids are often limited by our lack of knowledge concerning the basic pharmacology of these hormones in the eye. In order to develop improved therapeutic approaches, it is essential the devise quantitative studies of drug efficacy (and side effects) relevant to specific ocular conditions. Recent advances in endocrinology and immunology provide some useful insights which may help to explain the observed steroid effects and provide new methods to employ these agents in the treatment of ophthalmic disorders.

In this chapter, we will first examine some of the early investigations which led to the introduction of steroids as ocular anti-inflammatory agents. More recent aspects of ophthalmic steroid hormone therapy will then be examined, using selected data from both clinical and basic science research. A particular emphasis will be given to: (a) factors which may influence the activity of different ophthalmic steroid preparations; (b) various routes of administration; (c) therapeutic approaches; and (d) complications. Finally, current concepts concerning the mechanisms by which steroids alter cellular and molecular processes will be reviewed.

It is hoped that this presentation will serve to improve the understanding of the pharmacology of steroids as anti-inflammatory agents, and will aid in the future experimental and clinical use of steroid hormones in the eye.

B. Historical Development

I. Cortisone

Since the early descriptions of the "suprarenal capsules" (one of the earliest names for the adrenal glands), the function of these structures has provided one of the most challenging and controversial areas in scientific research. In 1716, the Academie de Sciences de Bordeaux offered a prize for anyone who could produce a satisfactory answer to the question, *„Quel est l'usage des glands surrénales?"* Montesquieu, who served as judge for the competition, decided that none of the proposed theories for the function of the adrenals was acceptable, and the prize money was unclaimed (GAUNT 1975).

In 1855, ADDISON described a clinical syndrome of "general languor and debility" (among other features) leading to a morbid state, which he postulated was associated with a diseased condition of the "supra-renal capsules." A year later, BROWN-SEQUARD (1856) provided support for the "vital" role of the adrenal glands by showing that adrenalectomy resulted in death in a variety of animals. The role of the adrenals in sustaining life, however, was not universally accepted at this time. In fact, many physiologists challenged Brown-Sequard's findings, probably because of the difficulty in removing all of the adrenal tissue in rats. Further, considerable confusion developed over the function of the adrenals because of the growing list of physiological processes which could be attributed to these glands (GAUNT 1975), and there were a number of fiercely debated controversies. Some of the early investigators in this field postulated that the adrenal glands were involved in the regulation of glucose metabolism; some postulated that these glands were involved in the maintenance of fluid and electrolyte balance; others held on to the belief that the adrenals were a center for the detoxification of lethal humors circulating in the blood.

Although the confusion surrounding the possible physiological effects of the adrenal glands had not been resolved, detailed chemical evaluation of the adrenal cortex began after 1930. Reports by HARTMAN and BROWNELL (1930) and SWINGLE and PFIFFNER (1930, 1931) that extracts of the adrenal cortex and active biological properties stimulated the search for cortin, the hypothetical major hormone of this gland. Use of lipid extracts, in particular, provided sufficiently high activity for chemical fractionation of adrenal products. The most concerted studies were conducted in the laboratories headed by KENDALL, REICHSTEIN, WINTERSTEINER, and PFIFFNER. Numerous analytical products of the adrenal hormone. In addition, investigators searching for cortin were confused by the diverse biological effects which could apparently be attributed to the adrenal hormones, as in the earlier studies of adrenal function (see INGLE 1950). By 1936, however, it appeared that many of the problems in adrenal research were resolved when Reichstein's laboratory (DE FREMERY et al. 1937) isolated corticosterone, which they considered to be the major adrenal hormone. Soon after this, STEIGER and REICHSTEIN (1937) demonstrated that corticosterone probably had a structure based on the steroid ring by performing the partial synthesis of the similar steroid, deoxycorticosterone.

Some of the excitement in adrenal chemistry waned following these reports, and a number of laboratories decided to pursue other areas of research. Nevertheless, KENDALL and INGLE continued their studies of the adrenal hormones, because their quantitative measurements suggested that corticosterone was not the physiologically active adrenal hormone (see KENDALL 1971). Instead, "compound E" (known today as cortisone) appeared to be the most likely candidate, but the methods available were not sufficient to obtain enough of this hormone to evaluate this proposal. Impetus to the synthesis of cortisone was provided by the war effort. Rumors circulated that German scientists were preparing extracts of the adrenal glands which would permit their pilots to fly at remarkably high altitudes. Because preliminary evidence suggested that compound E had some effect on oxygen consumption and might increase the ability to withstand stress, the National Research Council assembled a group of scientists to produce this compound. As the war came to a close, however, these scientists had failed to obtain enough cortisone for testing. In 1946, SARETT described a method to achieve a partial synthesis of cortisone, and by 1948 KENDALL had finally obtained enough cortisone for medical use. KENDALL presented his findings with high expectations at a conference at the newly established Sloan-Kettering Institute in New York, but his paper received only minor attention and generated little clinical interest. It appeared that no one wished to be involved in the testing of this drug, which most physicians believed would have little medical value (KENDALL 1971).

KENDALL returned disillusioned to the Mayo Clinic. On a chance meeting in the hallway, PHILLIP HENCH, Director of the Rheumatic Disease Section at the Mayo Clinic, learned from KENDALL that cortisone had been isolated. Eight years before, HENCH and KENDALL had discussed the possibility that an adrenal product might be the missing factor "X" which was responsible for the improvement observed in rheumatic disease patients who became pregnant or developed jaundice. HENCH requested enough of this compound to administer to one patient with rheumatoid arthritis who had failed to respond to the accepted therapeutic manipulations. Although only enough cortisone was available for a limited therapeutic trial, the patient responded rapidly and dramatically (HENCH et al. 1949). News of the general success of cortisone in rheumatoid arthritis and certain other conditions (HENCH et al. 1950) created a great interest in other possible therapeutic uses for adrenal hormones, and steroid therapy was soon evaluated in ophthalmology as well as many other fields of medicine. KENDALL, HENCH, and REICHSTEIN were awarded the Nobel Prize in Medicine in 1950 for their studies of cortisone.

II. Use of Steroids in Ophthalmology

After the demonstration that both cortisone and ACTH were beneficial in rheumatoid arthritis, these agents were employed for the treatment of ocular disease. Using these drugs, it was possible to intervene in the pathogenesis of many ocular inflammatory lesions which were resistant to the other means of therapy that were available. For example, OLSON et al. (1951) reported that patients with acute iridocyclitis responded dramatically to steroid therapy within 24 h, with relief of pain and photophobia, a marked decrease in anterior chamber flare and cells, and the resolution of fibrin deposition. The patients who responded to steroids in this study had previously failed to respond to cycloplegics, foreign protein therapy, salicylates, local heat, and antibiotics. After the initial clinical success of systemic steroid therapy, the possibility of a direct effect of steroids on ophthalmic tissues was also explored. Importantly, topical cortisone proved useful in the treatment of diseases of the anterior segment (e.g., OLSON et al. 1950; WOODS 1950; GORDON and McCLEAN 1950). These observations provided the first clinical evidence that steroids could exert anti-inflammatory effects at the tissue level. The clinical value of topical therapy was important because the side effects associated with the systemic administration of cortisone and ACTH were avoided.

The eye soon became an ideal setting for the investigation of both the clinical and experimental effects of steroid therapy. Early experimental studies of JONES and MEYER (1950) demonstrated that steroids could inhibit corneal neovascularization, and ASHTON and COOKE (1951) reported that steroids could interfere with cellular wound healing. WOODS and WOOD (1950, 1952, 1958) using experimental models of ocular tuberculosis and allergy, examined the ability of steroids to inhibit inflammatory processes in the eye. The studies of ocular tuberculosis, in particular, called attention to the danger that steroid therapy might disseminate an infectious process. In most cases of systemic infection, it was readily apparent that steroid therapy was contraindicated. However, in the eye, the desire to preserve the delicate structure of ocular tissues often required that steroid therapy be considered even in the presence of active infections. The decision to use steroids became increasingly more difficult because of the growing list of ocular and systemic side effects which were reported with steroid therapy (Hogan et al. 1955).

The clinical usefulness of cortisone raised the possibility that still more potent and possibily more specific steroid compounds could be produced. This was desirable in both ophthalmology and other fields of medicine. By 1952, hydrocortisone (cortisol) had become available in addition to cortisone (Fig. 1); this compound differs from cortisone in that the 11-position of the steroid molecule is a hydroxyl rather than a keto group. Although cortisone was generally ineffective when applied to the skin in dermatologic disorders, this compound was effective in systemic and ocular testing. Hydrocortisone did appear to be slightly more effective than cortisone for some ophthalmic disorders (McDonald et al. 1953).

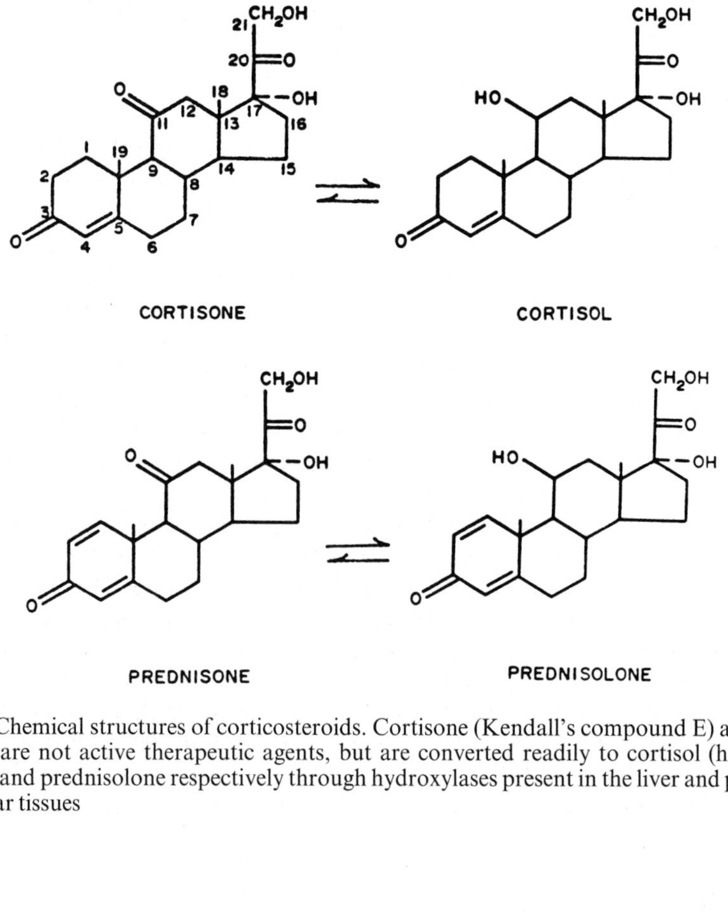

CORTISONE   CORTISOL

PREDNISONE   PREDNISOLONE

Fig. 1. Chemical structures of corticosteroids. Cortisone (Kendall's compound E) and prednisone are not active therapeutic agents, but are converted readily to cortisol (hydrocortisone) and prednisolone respectively through hydroxylases present in the liver and probably in ocular tissues

Attempts to increase the therapeutic effectiveness of hydrocortisone by altering chemical groups of the steroid molecule resulted in failure, and most new changes and substitutions in the steroid ring reduced or eliminated steroid activity. Clinically inactive compounds resulted when oxygen groups in the 3- or 11-positions were removed, when the carbon side chain beginning at the 17-position was eliminated, or when the double bond at the 4-position was removed from cortisone. The first lead to the development of potentially more active synthetic steroids came with the testing of 9α-fluorocortisol, a by-product of the synthesis of cortisone (FRIED and SABO 1954). This compound demonstrated considerably more anti-inflammatory activity than hydrocortisone, but was not useful as a systemic anti-inflammatory agent because it also markedly increased the mineralocorticoid activity (and was associated with unacceptable fluid retention and electrolyte disturbances). 9α-Fluorocortisol was briefly evaluated as a topical ophthalmic steroid, but prednisone and prednisolone (Fig. 1) soon became available and were popularized for use in the eye (KING and WEIMER 1955; GORDON 1956). Prednisone and prednisolone were more active than the cortisone derivatives when compared after topical or systemic administration. In addition, these compounds differed from 9α-fluorocortisol in that they showed a decrease rather than an increase in mineralocorticoid side effects compared to cortisone and hydrocortisone. Although prednisone and prednisolone appeared equal to each other as anti-inflammatory agents when applied locally in the eye, prednisolone derivatives were chosen for therapeutic formulations. The rationale for this choice was probably influenced by the superiority of topical prednisolone to topical prednisone in dermatologic disorders, and perhaps by reports which suggested that 11-hydroxyl compounds were more effective than corresponding 11-keto compounds (i.e., hydrocortisone compared to cortisone) in certain ophthalmic conditions, such as sclerosing keratitis (HOGAN ET AL. 1955).

Knowledge gained from the studies of prednisolone and 9α-fluorocortisol pointed the way to the synthesis of new and more active anti-inflammatory steroid compounds. One of the most important compounds produced with this information was dexamethasone (Fig. 2). Dexamethasone combined the $\Delta\ddot{a}^1$ group (double bond between carbons 1 and 2) of the former compound and the 9α-fluoro group of the latter compound. A 16α-methyl group was also added because this group had been shown further to diminish the enhanced mineralocorticoid activity produced by the 9α-fluoro substitution. Other synthetic steroids with increased anti-inflammatory activity were also produced and tested in the eye. These included β-methasone (nearly identical to dexamethasone, but with the methyl group at the 16-position in the β-rather than α-configuration), triamcinolone acetonide, 6α-methylprednisolone, and fluocinolone acetonide (see Fig. 2).

The introduction of dexamethasone and some of the other synthetic steroids generated enthusiasm that an improved and perhaps more specific ocular anti-inflammatory therapy would be achieved (NIELSEN 1959; GORDON 1959). However, the increased anti-inflammatory potency of these agents appeared to be inextricably associated with an increased incidence of deleterious side effects. In fact, topical β-methasone and dexamethasone appeared to be particularly prone to raise the intraocular pressure (IOP). Possibly for this reason, these steroids became the standard drugs employed in the topical testing protocols (BECKER 1965; ARMALY

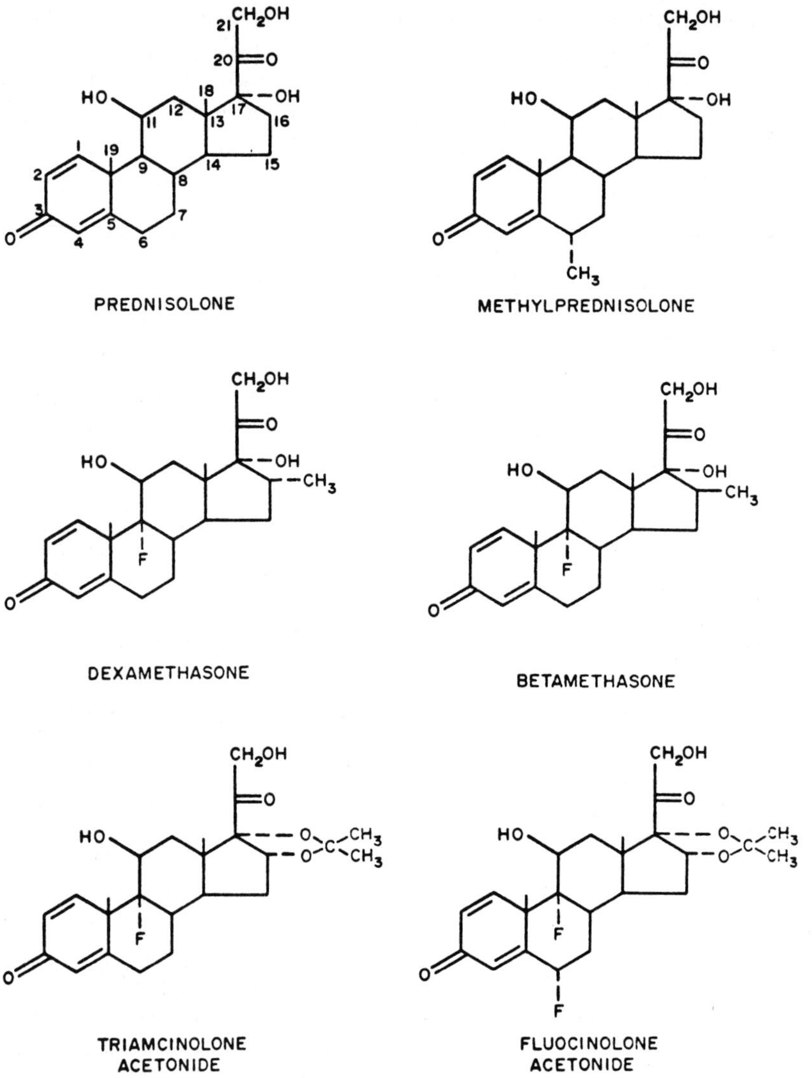

Fig. 2. Chemical structures of potent synthetic steroids

1965). Methylprednisolone and triamcinolone acetonide (which were less active than dexamethasone in systemic testing) were employed for injectable ophthalmic preparations. Fluocinolone acetonide and other compounds which had increased anti-inflammatory potency compared to dexamethasone were not introduced into clinical ophthalmologic practice because of the fears that even greater side effects would be observed and because no separation between beneficial and detrimental steroid effects was anticipated.

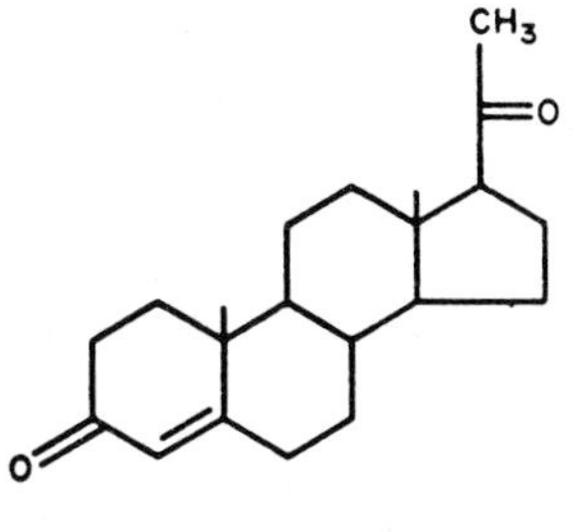

PROGESTERONE

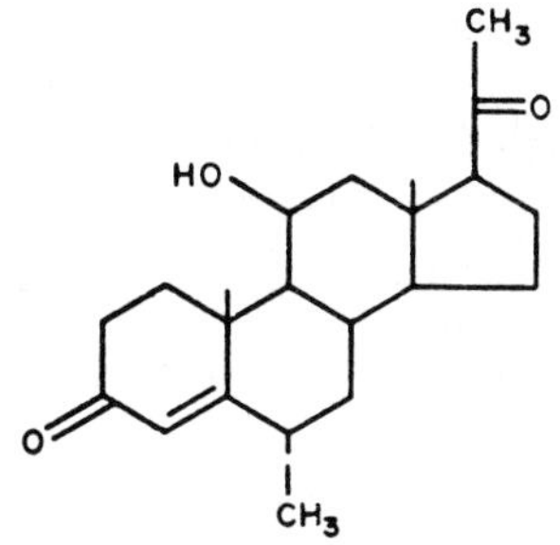

MEDRYSONE

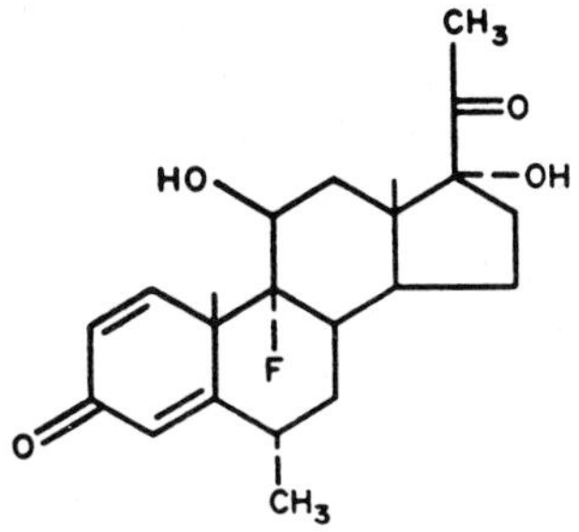

FLUOROMETHOLONE

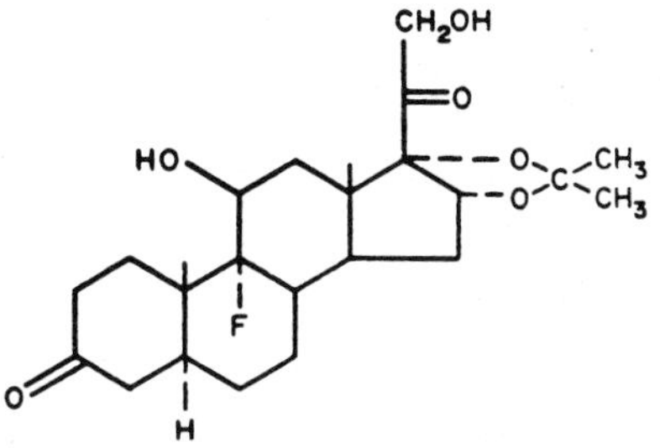

TETRAHYDROTRIAMCINOLONE ACETONIDE

Fig. 3. Chemical structures of some of the newer ophthalmic steroids, medrysone and fluorometholone, compared to progesterone and tetrahydrotriamcinolone acetonide

Attempts were subsequently focused on the sythesis of ophthalmic steroids which resembled progesterone. Prior studies suggested that progesterone was a steroid that might lower IOP (Posthumus 1952). Progesterone itself has no anti-inflammatory effect, and "necessary" chemical groups were added to produce steroids with reasonable anti-inflammatory potency. Medrysone and fluorometholone (Fig. 3) were two of the newer steroids produced by this method, both of which have been introduced into ophthalmic practice. There is evidence that these compounds do show a partial split in activity compared to other steroids, i.e., they can provide effective topical anti-inflammatory activity with a relative decrease in their propensity to raise IOP. However, as discussed in later sections, it is likely that this is due to the particular pharmacokinetics of these steroids, rather than being related to a progesterone-like activity. Tetrahydrotriamcinolone acetonide (Fig. 3) was also thought to achieve a split in activity; the rationale in this case was that this steroid might not penetrate the cornea. Subsequent evaluation showed this supposition to be in error, and tetrahydrotriamcinolone acetonide has not found a place in ophthalmic practice.

C. Steroid Therapy

I. Activity of Steroid Compounds

1. Potency

Estimates for the relative dosages of steroids have been primarily developed by observing the therapeutic efficacy after oral administration. Table 1 (Williams et al. 1980) presents the accepted values for the relative potencies of systemic steroids based on these clinical and experimental estimates. Of the steroids employed in systemic therapy, dexamethasone has the highest estimated potency, approximately 30- to 40-fold greater than hydrocortisone. Systemic prednisolone, methylprednisolone, and triamcinolone are approximately four- to fivefold more active than hydrocortisone. Orally administered cortisone and prednisone have potencies which closely approximate hydrocortisone and prednisolone (respectively), probably due to the rapid conversion of the inactive keto compounds to the active 11-hydroxyl derivatives by the liver. Table 1 also provides estimates of the mineralocorticoid effects of the different systemic steroids. Systemic cortisone and hydrocortisone are both associated with significant mineralocorticoid activity in the doses required to achieve a therapeutic effect in many clinical settings. Use of prednisone or prednisolone is associated with a fourfold decrease in mineralocorticoid potency relative to the cortisone compounds. When this effect is combined with the fourfold increase in glucocorticoid potency, the result is a markedly diminished tendency to fluid retention and electrolyte disturbances when these compounds are employed in therapy. Other synthetic steroids (as indicated in Table 1) show even less mineralocorticoid activity, but the mineralocorticoid side effects of prednisone are usually not clinically significant.

The estimates of the glucocorticoid potency are used to calculate comparable doses when a change in therapeutic regimen is desired for the different systemic steroids. On this basis, doses of 20 mg hydrocortisone, 25 mg cortisone, 5 mg prednisone or prednisolone, 4 mg methylprednisolone or triamcinolone, and 0.75 mg dexamethasone are calculated to be equivalent. It is always assumed that the amound of drug administered may then have to be adjusted further to achieve the desired therapeutic effect in individual patients.

As shown in Table 1, steroids are classified as short-acting, intermediate-acting, or long-acting compounds, based originally on the estimated duration of hypothalamic–pituitary suppression (see Dluhy et al. 1975). Recently, the importance of this method of distinguishing steroid drugs received renewed attention. Evidence from both clinical and experimental studies suggests that the duration of drug action can have important consequences for the clinical effectiveness of steroid therapy. For example, it has been observed that the use of long-acting systemic steroids, such as dexamethasone, is associated with an increased incidence of systemic complications, and that major cushingoid changes can develop even with very low doses of these agents (see discussions by Meikle and Tyler 1977; Tyrrell and Baxter 1981). It is possible that individual differences exist in the rate at which steroids are eliminated (Kozower et al. 1974; Meikle et al. 1976). Use of long-acting steroids in a patient with slowed elimination may cause a higher incidence of complications. Even when evaluated in patients with apparently normal

Table 1. Systemic glucocorticoid preparations (WILLIAMS et al. 1980)

Commonly used name[a]	Estimated potency relative to cortisol	
	Glucocorticoid	Mineralocorticoid
Short-acting		
Hydrocortisone	1	1
Cortisone	0.8	0.8
Intermediate-acting		
Prednisone	4	0.25
Prednisolone	4	0.25
Methylpredniso-lone	5	±
Triamcinolone	5	±
Long-acting		
Paramethasone	10	±
β-Methasone	25	±
Dexamethasone	30–40	±

[a] Short-acting preparations have a biological half-life of less than 12 h; long-acting, greater than 48 h; and intermediate, between 12 and 36 h. Triamcinolone has the longest half-life of the intermediate-acting preparations

steroid metabolisms, it is clear that the duration of drug action can have a major influence on the magnitude of the steroid response. MEIKLE and TYLER (1977), for example, have provided compelling evidence that the potency of hydrocortisone, prednisone, and dexamethasone varies considerably, depending upon the amount of time since the therapeutic dose. They compared the potency of oral steroids by measuring the suppression of endogenous corticosterone 8 h and 14 h after oral administration. Using hydrocortisone as a standard, prednisone was three times as potent after 8 h, and was 5.2 times as potent after 14 h. Dexamethasone was 52 times as potent as hydrocortisone 8 h after the steroid dose, but was 154 times as potent as hydrocortisone 8 h after the steroid dose, but was 154 times as potent when evaluated 14 h later. These studies emphasize the role of pharmacokinetics in determining drug effects, and suggest that the rate of drug clearance and/or persistence in ocular tissues will be important factors in determining ophthalmic therapeutic responses (see NAGATAKI and MISHIMA 1980; SHELL 1982 a).

To obtain quantitative information concerning the potencies of different ophthalmic steroids, it is possible to compare the ability of different anti-inflammatory steroids to bind to glucocorticoid receptors. The anti-inflammatory as well as many other tissue effects of steroids appear to be mediated through these glucocorticoid receptors, which are specialized cytoplasmic proteins. In general, the affinity of a given steroid for these glucocorticoid receptors should be a primary determinant of the potency of a steroid to induce a glucocorticoid response in target cells. Steroids that do not bind a glucocorticoid receptors do not produce glucocor-

Table 2. Relative binding of different steroid compounds to human glucocorticoid receptors. Data for human fetal lung receptor (Ballard et al. 1975)

Steroid	Glucocorticoid-receptor binding[a]
Cortisol	1
9α-Fluorocortisol	3.5
Prednisolone	2.1
Dexamethasone	7.1
Fluocinolone acetonide	11.4

[a] Binding affinities expressed relative to cortisol

ticoid effects. Most biological metabolites of active steroids show very low glucocorticoid binding and are not capable of producing a glucocorticoid response in target cells. For example, tetrahydrocortisol, the major product of hydrocortisone metabolism, does not bind to these receptors and is inactive. Cortisone and prednisone have a very low affinity for glucocorticoid receptors and only produce a clinical effect after they are converted to their respective 11-hydroxyl compounds (cortisol and prednisolone), which bind with significantly higher affinities.

Table 2 presents some of the early measurements comparing the receptor binding of different anti-inflammatory steroids in human tissues (Ballard et al. 1975). The order of binding affinities for glucocorticoid receptors is dexamethasone > ↔ prednisolone > cortisol. 9α-Fluorocortisol, the first synthetic steroid with enhanced anti-inflammatory activity, has a binding affinity 3.5 times greater than cortisol, while prednisolone has an affinity 2.1 times greater. Dexamethasone and flurcinolone acetonide show an affinity 7.1 and 11.4 times greater, respectively. There have been a number of detailed structure/activity studies of therapeutic steroids (e.g., Rousseau and Baxter 1979; Bloom et al. 1980), but many of these prior investigations employed rat hepatoma cells, and also did not evaluate ophthalmic steroids directly.

The receptor-binding characteristics of ophthalmic steroids can be studied using cultured human cell lines. The use of human cells may be important because responses to anti-inflammatory steroids in animal tissues do not always provide clinically relevant information (C. Schlaegel, Upjohn Pharmaceuticals, personal communication). Figure 4a shows the results of a representative experiment in which the ability of fluorometholone, medrysone, and tetrahydrotriamcinolone acetonide to bind glucocorticoid receptors was tested in a competitive binding assay. Of these, fluorometholone clearly shows the highest binding affinity for the glucocorticoid receptor, with an affinity comparable to dexamethasone (see Fig. 4b). It is therefore expected to be a potent steroid, capable of inducing a therapeutic response at relatively low drug concentrations. Medrysone and tetrahydrotriamcinolone show a tenfold lower affinity than fluorometholone, and considerably higher concentrations of these two compounds would be required at the target tissue to elicit a steroid response. Fluorometholone was originally developed as a

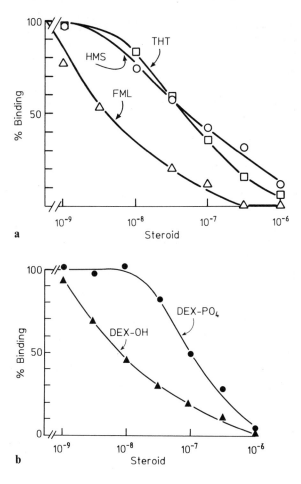

Fig. 4a, b. Potency of ophthalmic steroids evaluated in glucocorticoid-receptor-binding assays. Suspensions of $2–5 \times 10^6$ human skin fibroblasts were incubated with $5\,nM\ ^3H$-dexamethasone and varying concentrations of unlabeled steroid in a competitive binding assay for 60 min at 37 °C, using Dulbecco's modified Eagle's medium in a 10% CO_2 incubator. Cells were washed extensively at 0 °C, counted using liquid scintillation spectroscopy, and expressed as the percentage of control binding ($5\,nM\ ^3H$-dexamethasone alone). *FML*, fluorometholone; *HMS*, medrysone; *THT*, tetrahydrotriamcinolone actonide; *DEX-OH*, dexamethasone 21-alcohol; *DEX-PO$_4$*, dexamethasone 21-phosphate. (POLANSKY et al., to be published)

potent topical anti-inflammatory agent for dermatologic disorders and has 25–50 times the potency of hydrocortisone.

Fluorometholone has been shown to be effective in ocular inflammation (e.g., FAIRBAIRN and THORSON 1971; KUPFERMAN and LEIBOWITZ 1975). Receptor data support the idea that it should provide potent anti-inflammatory activity when delivered to the site of inflammation. The receptor binding of tetrahydrotriamcinolone and medrysone suggests that these agents are relatively weaker glucocorticoids and possess an inherent anti-inflammatory potency similar to hydrocortisone.

Dexamethasone alcohol and dexamethasone phosphate have been compared using the glucocorticoid receptor assay. Prior studies on experimental keratitis (LEIBOWITZ and KUPFERMAN 1980a) suggested that there might be a difference in the anti-inflammatory potencies of these compounds. As shown in Fig. 4b, dexamethasone alcohol is approximately 15 times more potent than dexamethasone phosphate in its ability to compete for glucocorticoid receptors. This finding may help to explain why some investigators have reported a relatively decreased topical anti-inflammatory effect with phosphate derivatives (LEIBOWITZ and KUPFERMAN 1980a; HARTER et al. 1970). However, the relatively potent effect of dexamethasone phosphate on the IOP suggests that ocular tissues may have phosphatases that can convert the less active phosphate derivative to the fully active alcohol derivative.

Knowledge of the differential binding of steroids to the glucocorticoid receptor may provide a more rational approach to the therapeutics use of these agents. This line of inquiry may be particular value for steroid therapy in the eye, since potency estimates may be influenced by the drug formulation, the route of administration, and the experimental for clinical system evaluated. The data compiled by NELSON (1970) demonstrate that available estimates for the potency of steroids of ophthalmic interest vary over a rather wide range. With receptor-binding data as a starting point, it may be possible to evaluate the contribution of other factors which regulate steroid potency. Using values for the relative binding to the receptor as a measure of the underlying steroid activity, it will be possible to analyze the factors which might account for observed differences in steroid efficacy. These factors include absorption and/or distribution of the steroid, the tissue half-life and clearance, and metabolism and cellular interactions which may modify the biological response.

2. Absorption and Distribution

When steroids are administered systemically, an equilibrium is established between the hormone which is bound by plasma proteins and that which remains in its free, unbound form. The amount of hormone in the free form determines the degree of steroid effect (BALLARD 1979), since only the unbound hormone appears to enter the cell and interact with the glucocorticoid receptor. As shown in Fig. 5, most of the cortisol (hydrocortisone) in the plasma is bound to corticosteroid-binding globulin (CBG). Over the physiological range of 5–25 µg cortisol per 100 ml plasma, the unbound hormone represents approximately 8% of the total (0.4–1.6 µg/100 ml). Administration of hydrocortisone in excess of 25 µg/100 ml results in a saturation of CBG binding. At this point, albumin becomes the major plasma protein which binds the steroids, because it has a binding capacity considerably greater than CBG. Approximately 50% of the additional hydrocortisone in the plasma binds to albumin, leaving 50% free to interact with target tissues. Importantly, many synthetic steroids show a decreased binding affinity to CBG (BALLARD 1979), and this may be a significant factor contributing to the increased potency of these compounds relative to hydrocortisone. It is also believed that the free ste-

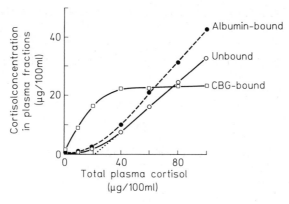

Fig. 5. Distribution of cortisol in plasma. (BALLARD 1979)

roid level determines the amount that is transferred from the circulation to systemic and ocular tissues, where the drugs exert their effects.

The penetration of steroids after topical application to the eye has been an active area of investigation. Early studies reported that topical steroids penetrated the cornea and entered the aqueous (GREEN et al. 1955a, b), but the methods employed in the early studies have come under criticism, and probably overestimated the amount of hormone that reached the aqueous humor (KROMAN and LEOPOLD 1961). Following this, measurement of radioactively labeled steroids became the accepted method of evaluating penetration of steroid into ocular tissues (see SCHWARTZ 1966a), although there were some initial difficulties in the use of this technique. For example, Cox et al. (1972) could not detect labeled dexamethasone phosphate in the aqueous humor after topical application. Later, KRUPIN et al. (1974) showed that this steroid could be found in both the cornea and aqueous humor, confirming an earlier report by SHORT et al. (1966), but the steroid employed had to be labeled with a sufficiently high specific activity.

Because there was evidence that some ophthalmic steroids penetrated the cornea more effectively than others, it was proposed that absorption would be a major determinant in pedicting the IOP response of a given steroid. Most recent evidence, however, suggests that this concept is not as useful as originally believed. For example, it was proposed that tetrahydrotriamcinolone acetonide did not penetrate the cornea as well as triamcinolone acetonide, and this might explain the lower propensity of the former to raise IOP. When SUGAR et al. (1972) investigated this question, they found that tetrahydrotriamcinolone acetonide penetrated the cornea as well as or better than triamcinolone acetonide. A more likely explanation for the decreased IOP effect observed with tetrahydrotriamcinolone acetonide is that its potency is five- to tenfold lower than that of triamcinolone acetonide, as determined by glucocorticoid receptor binding (ZLOCK and POLANSKY, unpublished observations). Another proposal was that topical fluorometholone did not penetrate the cornea as well as other steroids. HULL et al. (1974), however, showed that fluorometholone penetrated the cornea as well as or better than steroids which

Table 3. Corneal permeability (mean ± SEM) of tritiated labeled steroids with epithelium intact and absent (data obtained from Hull et al. 1974)

Steroid	Epithelium intact (nmol/cm^2/h)	Epithelium absent (nmol/cm^2/h)
Dexamethasone phosphate	7.1 ± 0.6 [a]	32.4 ± 1.8 [b]
Prednisolone phosphate	12.1 ± 0.5	37.7 ± 2.6 [b]
Prednisolone acetate	14.3 ± 1.1	11.5 ± 1.2
Fluorometholone	15.4 ± 2.2	14.4 ± 3.3

[a] Significantly different from the other three steroids at a p value of <0.05
[b] Significantly different from the corneal permeability of the same drug with the epithelium intact at a p value of <0.001

have a greater effect on IOP. In this study (Table 3), fluorometholone showed a slightly higher permeability than prednisolone acetate and prednisolone phosphate. All these steroids penetrated better than dexamethasone phosphate when the epithelium was intact. These permeabilities are in the opposite order to that expected if absorption were the major determinant of steroid effects on IOP. Other studies of fluorometholone have suggested that it may involve special ocular pharmacokinetics (see Yamauchi et al. 1975), and this may partly explain the reduced tissue levels of fluorometholone observed after topical administration reported by Leibowitz and Kupfermann (1975), Kupferman and Leibowitz (1975).

Another interesting observation has been that an increased steroid permeability can be observed after injury or removal of the corneal epithelium (Leopold et al. 1955, Hull et al. 1974; Leibowitz and Kupferman 1980a; see Tables 3 and 4). The water-soluble steroids with highly charged phosphate groups (dexamethasone phosphate and prednisolone phosphate) show the largest increases in corneal permeability after removal of the epithelium. The steroids which are less water-soluble, such as prednisolone acetate and fluorometholone, show only small changes after the epithelium is removed. Although it might be logical to assume that the increased corneal permeability would result in a proportionate increase in steroid effect, this does not appear to be the case. In fact, the studies of Leibowitz and Kupferman (1980a) emphasize that steroid bioavailability measurements did not correlate with anti-inflammatory efficacy when different steroid derivates were compared in their experimental keratitis model. As shown in Table 4, phosphate derivatives achieve the highest bioavailability measured, but the anti-inflammatory effectiveness is the lowest. Dexamethasone acetate achieves the lowest corneal bioavailability, but produces the highest anti-inflammatory effectiveness with the epithelium intact or absent. The alcohol derivative demonstrates values between those obtained with the other two compounds, both for bioavailability and anti-inflammatory effect. The major increase in corneal bioavailability shown by the alcohol and phosphate derivatives after removal of the epithelium is not accompanied by a corresponding increase in anti-inflammatory effect. These data emphasize that changes in steroid permeability and bioavailability must be interpreted cautiously, and an effort must be made to develop appropriate models of therapeutic effectiveness for different ocular inflammatory conditions. This is especially

Table 4. Experimental anti-inflammatory effects and corneal bioavailability of various topical dexamethasone derivations (21-substitutions) (LEIBOWITZ and KUPFERMAN 1980a)

Corticosteroid	Anti-inflammatory effect (%)	Corneal bioavailability (µg min/g)
Epithelium intact		
Dexamethasone acetate 0.1%	55	111
Dexamethasone alcohol 0.1%	40	543
Dexamethasone sodium phosphate 0.1%	19	1,068
Epithelium absent		
Dexamethasone acetate 0.1%	60	118
Dexamethasone alcohol 0.1%	42	1,316
Dexamethasone phosphate 0.1%	22	4,642

true when comparing different steroid derivatives. Further, it would be desirable to evaluate the bioavailability of the different ophthalmic steroids directly in appropriate models of inflammation, and to measure potential changes in drug permeability and changes in drug binding in these system.

3. Metabolism

Metabolism was assumed to be the major determinant of the potency of systemic steroids before the role of glucocorticoid receptors and the influence of steroid binding to plasma proteins was appreciated. A number of investigators have reported that the more active steroids appear to be more resistant to degradation (see GLENN et al. 1957; FLORINI and BUYSKE 1959). Thereafter it was also recognized that enzymes present in tissues could activate certain steroids. For example, cortisone and prednisone are converted into cortisol and prednisolone, respectively, after oral administration. Figures 6 and 7 illustrate these two different aspects of steroid metabolism.

The conversion of prednisone into prednisolone after an oral dose accounts for the therapeutic efficacy of prednisone therapy. As shown in Fig. 6, during the first 30 min following a 10-mg oral dose of prednisone, prednisolone becomes the major steroid found in the circulation, and there is very little prednisone (prednisolone/prednisone > 10). The levels of prednisolone reach a peak within 1–2 h and then decline over the next 8 h due to metabolism, excretion, and redistribution. The small amount of prednisone present in the circulation is not involved in the effects of steroid therapy, and much of this steroid is derived by a conversion back to this steroid from prednisolone.

Figure 7 presents the major pathways for the metabolic degradation and deactivation of steroid hormones. Pathways (1) and (2) involve the "A" ring of the steroid molecule. The enzymes responsible for this step, including conjugation to glucuronides (and other products which favor excretion by the kidney) are located primarily in the liver. The existence of pathways (3), (4), and (5), as well as side chain cleavage, are found in many peripheral tissues and also in the liver. The presence of cortoic acids, previously unnoticed steroid degradation products, has been de-

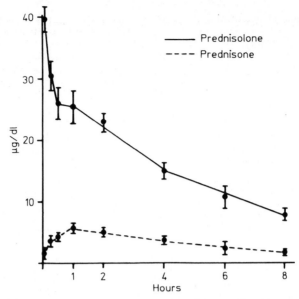

Fig. 6. Plasma concentrations of prednisolone and prednisone after 10-mg oral dose of prednisone. (MEIKLE et al. 1975)

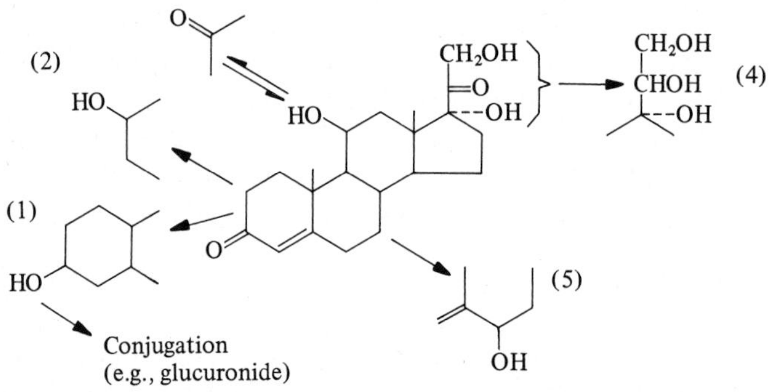

Fig. 7. Major metabolic fates of cortisol: (*1*) reduction of the 4–5 double bond, hydroxylation of the 3-keto group, with subsequent conjugation at the hydroxyl position; (*2*) hydroxylation at the 2-position; (*3*) conversion of the 11-hydroxyl to an 11-keto group; (*4*) reduction of carbonyl group at C-20 to isomeric alcohols; and (*5*) hydroxylation at the 6-position. (COPE 1972)

scribed recently (MONDER and BRADLOW 1980). It is of particular interest that the specific structure of the groups associated with many of the more potent synthetic steroids appears to inhibit certain degradative pathways. For example, hydrocortisone elimination from the circulation is achieved primarily through "A" ring changes [pathways (1) and (2)]. Prednisolone (which has an extra double bond in the "A" ring) is excreted either unchanged or with the side chain at (4) degraded, while both pathways (3) and (5) also contribute to this process (see COPE 1972). Dexamethasone and triamcinolone are more resistant to degradation than prednisolone, and are excreted primarily unchanged with only a partial alteration through pathway (5), because other degradative pathways are blocked (VERMEULEN 1959; FLORINI et al. 1961). More details of specific structure/activity changes are provided by WOLFF (1979). In addition, it is of interest that progesterone (which lacks a 21-hydroxyl group) is removed more rapidly from the circulation than steroids with a hydroxyl group at the 21-position. This finding might be relevant to the metabolism of other steroids, such as fluorometholone and medrysone, which also lack a 21-hydroxyl group. Studies of degradative pathways in the individual ocular tissues may provide explanations for some of the anti-inflammatory and tissue effects of steroids applied to the eye.

Few studies of steroid metabolism have been conducted in the eye, but there is evidence to suggest that ocular tissues may be particularly active in the metabolism of steroids. Metabolic conversions may have an important role in determining the success and/or failure of a particular therapeutic modality. For example, as previously mentioned, direct steroid effects were first observed in ocular tissues with topical cortisone due to the ability of tissues to convert cortisone to hydrocortisone, the active 11-hydroxyl derivative. The fact that cortisone and prednisone appeared to be fully active when tested clinically indicates the presence of an active 11-β-hydroxylase system in the cornea and perhaps other ocular tissues. The lack of a similar hydroxylase activity in the skin is notable, and steroids requiring a similar conversion are inactive in dermatologic disorders (MAIBACH and STOUGHTON 1975). Phosphatase activity in the cornea can convert a less active phosphate derivative to a more active alcohol form (SUGAR et al. 1972). Ocular tissues also appear to possess degradative enzymes. SOUTHREN et al. (1976) have demonstrated that the iris-ciliary body and cornea show high levels of "A" ring reductase activity. As mentioned above, "A" ring reduction (primarily by the liver) accounts for the inactivation of circulating steroids such as cortisol. Prednisolone is considerably more protected from "A" ring reductions than hydrocortisone, and other synthetic steroids, such as dexamethasone, are even more resistant to these degradative pathways. GARZON et al. (1976) and GALLEGOS et al. (1976) have shown that the cornea has other degradative enzyme systems capable of attack at the 20-keto and 6-β-positions of progesterone, and possibly also for 16-keto steroids. YAMAUCHI et al. (1975) showed that fluorometholone is rapidly converted to an unknown metabolite after passage through the cornea, while dexamethasone appears more resistant to degradation.

Enzyme systems capable of metabolizing steroids in ocular tissues may have important therapeutic implications. The biological activity of steroid metabolites must also be determined. The use of ophthalmic steroids will become increasingly rational when this information can be correlated with data about steroid potency, absorption, and distribution.

II. Routes of Administration

1. Topical

Topical therapy provides a simple and direct method of steroid application to external ocular structures. This route is effective for the treatment of many external ocular inflammatory diseases, as well as for inflammation of the anterior segment.

A major advantages of topical steroids is that a much lower total dose is administered compared with oral steroid therapy, markedly diminishing the chances of systemic complications.

A variety of steroid preparations are formulated for topical application to the eye (see PODOS et al. 1971; LEIBOWITZ and KUPFERMAN 1980a). However, relatively little quantitative information is available concerning the advantages or disadvantages of the different preparations. Table 5 provides a summary of the corticosteroid eye drops and ointments currently available in the United States. These preparations are listed according to the steroid bases (different steroid compounds), their derivatives (alterations at the 21-position), and examples of the commercial names by which the drugs are marketed. As shown in Table 5, topical steroids are formulated at different drug concentrations, which vary according to the type of steroid employed. The concentrations available for each drug appear to be formulated in accordance with the estimates of the systemic steroid potency listed in Table 1. For eye drops, the maximum concentration of hydrocortisone is two and a half times that of prednisolone, which in turn is ten times that of dexamethasone. A similar pattern is also observed for ointments: hydrocortisone is formuated at two and five times the concentration of prednisolone, which is five times that of dexamethasone. The concentrations chosen for the different topical steroids also correlate well with relative affinities of the various steroids for the glucocorticoid receptor; i.e., the steroids with the highest affinities require the lowest drug concentrations to produce a therapeutic effect, those with the lowest require the highest concentrations. Dexamethasone and fluorometholone show a greater affinity for the glucocorticoid receptor than prednisolone, and prednisolone appears to have a greater affinity than hydrocortisone and medrysone. When topical steroids are administered directly to the site of inflammation (e.g., in external ocular diseases), the relative degree of binding to the glucocorticoid receptor is likely to be a major determinant of therapeutic efficacy. In cases where topical steroids must pass through other tissues to reach their site of action (e.g., in intraocular inflammation or steroid glaucoma), drug absorption, distribution, and metabolism may play a proportionately greater role.

Although the different ophthalmic steroids have been formulated to provide a beneficial therapeutic effect, it is possible that one compound may be preferable to another, depending upon the clinical setting. For example, dexamethasone is generlly resistant to degradation and is likely to have a relatively long half-life in tissues. If this is confirmed in ocular tissues, topical dexamethasone may be preferable to shorter-acting steroids when maximal suppression of intraocular inflammation is desired. For similar reasons, however, topical dexamethasone is likely to have a proportionately greater effect on IOP (and may also be more likely to produce other steroid-induced complications) than other topical steroids. Fluorometholone, on the other hand, appears to have a relatively rapid rate of degradation and a reduced tissue half-life, providing a different therapeutic option. Since fluorometholone shows a high affinity for the glucocorticoid receptor as well as a high degree of topical anti-inflammatory action, this steroid appears to be an effective agent for the treatment of external ocular disease. An increased susceptibility of fluorometholone to degradation or increased rate of removal in ocular tissues may account for the lesser propensity of this drug to elevate the IOP (and per-

Table 5. Topical steroids

Steroid base	Derivative	Commercial preparation	
Eye drops			
Hydrocortisone	Acetate	2.5%	(Optef) (Hydrocortisone Ophthal-
	Alcohol	0.2%	mic)
Prednisolone	Acetate	1%	(Econopred Plus, Pred Forte)
		0.125%	(Econopred, Pred Mild)
	Phosphate	1.0%	(Inflamase Forte)
		0.125%	(Inflamase)
Dexamethasone	Alcohol	0.1%	(Maxidex)
	Phosphate	0.1%	(Decadron Phosphate)
Fluorometholone	Alcohol	0.1%	(Fluorometholone)
Medrysone	Alcohol	1%	(Medrysone)
Ointments			
Hydrocortisone	Acetate	1.5%	(Hydrocortisone)
		0.5%	(Acetate Ophthalmic)
Prednisolone	Phosphate	0.25%	(Hydeltrasol Ophthalmic)
Dexamethasone	Phosphate	0.05%	(Decadron Phosphate Ophthalmic, Maxidex Ophthalmic)

haps to result in other steroid complications), because a relatively smaller amount of the drug reaches the desired target tissues in the eye. For this reason, fluorometholone may be less effective than other potent steroids in the treatment of intraocular inflammation, unless it is administered more frequently.

When selecting a topical steroid preparation, one must consider practical as well as theoretical factors. The advantages of water-soluble steroids (phosphate derivatives of prednisolone and dexamethasone) have recently been reviewed by APT et al. (1979). Phosphate derivatives provide a clear solution (compared to acetate and alcohol derivatives, which are less water-soluble and are in suspension), are associated with enhanced patient compliance, and allow a more reproducible dose to be administered. Aside from these considerations, other factors may influence the choice among the different steroid derivatives. LEIBOWITZ et al. (1978) and LEIBOWITZ and KUPFERMAN (1980a) have shown that the phosphate derivatives are not as effective as the other steroid derivatives in experimental keratitis, confirming earlier studies by HARTER et al. (1970) in experimental uveitis.

The presence of the phosphate group diminishes glucocorticoid receptor binding of a steroid when evaluated in whole cells (Fig. 4b). Together these date suggest that phosphate derivatives in some cases may be less effective than alcohol or acetate compounds when a maximal therapeutic effect is desired and when compliance is controlled. Given sufficient time in ocular tissues, the phosphate group will probably be removed by phosphatases in ocular tissues, producing a fully active alcohol compound. However, the rate of this process in different ocular sites is unknown.

Table 6. Experimental anti-inflammatory activity of topical steroids (LEIBOWITZ and KUPFERMAN 1980a)

Corneal epithelium intact	Decrease (%)	Corneal epithelium absent	Decrease (%)
Prednisolone acetate 1%	51	Prednisolone acetate 1%	53
Dexamethasone alcohol 0.1%	40	Prednisolone sodium phosphate 1%	47
Fluorometholone alcohol 0.1%	31	Dexamethasone alcohol 0.1%	42
Prednisolone sodium phosphate 1.0%	28	Fluorometholone alcohol 0.1%	37
Dexamethasone sodium phosphate 0.1%	19	Dexamethasone sodium phosphate 0.1%	22
Dexamethasone sodium phosphate 0.05% (ointment)	13		

LEIBOWITZ and KUPFERMAN (1980a) have recently summarized man of their experimental findings using a clove-oil-induced keratitis model to evaluate quantitatively the anti-inflammatory effects of different topical steroid preparations. On the basis of comparative anti-inflammatory effects (see Table 6), these investigators reported that prednisolone acetate 1% is the most potent of the commercially available steroids. Therefore, these investigators suggest that prednisolone acetate formulations (e.g., Econopred Plus, Pred Forte; KUPFERMAN and LEIBOWITZ 1976) provide the most appropriate anti-inflammatory therapy for acute inflammatory keratitis. The data also show fluorometholone alcohol and dexamethasone alcohol to be effective anti-inflammatory agents in the keratitis model, while dexamethasone phosphate is the least effective agent. Since dexamethasone derivatives are more potent than corresponding prednisolone derivatives, it should be possible to achieve a greater anti-inflammatory effect with 1% dexamethasone acetate, if this formulation were commercially available. However, an unacceptable increase in complications might accompany the use of such a concentrated dexamethasone preparation.

One practical method for increasing the effectiveness of topical steroid preparations is to increase frequency of application. When a maximal effect is desired (e.g., in impending central corneal involvement by inflammatory keratitis), a useful clinical approach is to administer topical steroids hourly, or even more frequently. Table 7 shows that hourly administration of prednisolone acetate suppresses corneal inflammation approximately five times better than when the drug is administered every 4 h in the clove oil keratitis model. A maximal anti-inflammatory effect is achieved when the drops are administered every 5 min, but such a regimen is not clinically practical. As an alternative method, LEIBOWITZ and KUPFERMAN (1980a) suggest the application of five consecutive doses at 1-min intervals, on an hourly basis. When intensive steroid therapy is not required, application of steroids every 4 h, daily or even weekly, may be adequate in certain inflammatory conditions (see Sect. c). Less frequent administration of steroid drops (as well as short-term regimens) would be expected to produce fewer ocular and systemic side effects. The employment of more dilute steroid formulations (e.g., 0.125% prednisolone) represents another potential means of reducing complications. Similarly, rel-

Table 7. Anti-inflammatory topical effect of different dosage schedules for administration of prednisolone acetate 1% (LEIBOWITZ and KUPFERMAN 1980a)

Treatment regimen	Total no. doses delivered	Decrease in corneal inflammation (%)
1 drop every 4 h	6	11
1 drop every 2 h	10	30
1 drop every hour	18	51
1 drop every 30 min	34	61
1 drop every 15 min	66	68
1 drop each min for 5 min every hour	90	72

atively weak steroids (such as medrysone) may be appropriate for mild external inflammatory conditions, and the dilution of dexamethasone to a concentration of 0.001% has been proposed as another method of reducing side effects such as elevated IOP (KAUFMAN 1975; PAVAN-LANGSTON and ABELSON 1978). Dilute dexamethasone is not commercially available but can be individually prepared.

Anti-inflammatory therapy with steroid ointments may be particularly useful when prolonged contact in desirable and hard to achieve (e.g., during sleep). Theoretically, the increased contact time of the ointment with the cornea delivers a greater amount of steroid to ocular tissues. Although the available ointment formulations may not produce an increased anti-inflammatory effect (see SCHLAEGEL and O'CONNOR 1977; LEIBOWITZ and KUPFERMAN 1980a), other methods of topical steroid application based on prolonged contact time with the cornea are being developed to increase drug levels. For example, use of high-viscosity gels reportedly results in very high levels of steroid in both the aqueous and cornea (SCHOEN-WALD and BALTROVIK 1979). The anti-inflammatory efficacy of this method of steroid delivery requires further investigation, and the possibility that the high levels of steroids delivered by this method will predispose to a high incidence of steroid-induced complications must also be evaluated.

One other method of topical steroid administration which offers considerable promise is the use of continuous drug delivery systems. These systems allow a controlled steady-state release of drug (SHELL and BAKER 1974; SHELL 1982b; PAVAN-LANGSTON 1976; LAMBERTS 1980), and achieve a therapeutic effect while delivering a much lower total dose of steroid than conventional eye drops and ointments. The effectiveness of constant rate delivery systems using hydrocortisone inserts has been reported in a number of experimental studies (DOHLMAN et al. 1972; LERMAN et al. 1973; KELLER et al. 1976). A clinical study by ALLANSMITH et al. (1975) reported the efficacy of hydrocortisone ocular inserts when tested in a variety of inflammatory conditions. The rationale for controlled release systems is to avoid the transient overdoses and underdoses that accompany other methods of local steroid administration (SHELL 1982b). Further development of controlled release systems may help to define and expand the clinical value of this method of topical steroid therapy. There are many opportunities for improving both the theoretical understanding and technical capabilities by which topical steroidal agents are delivered.

2. Periocular

A number of ocular inflammatory conditions have been reported to respond favorably to periocular steroid injections with a therapeutic effect above that achieved by other methods of drug administration (ARONSON et al. 1970; SCHLAEGEL 1970; NOZIK 1972; SMITH and NOZIK 1982). NOZIK has emphasized that the effectiveness of periocular injections is critically dependent upon the proper technique and placement of the drug. Specific sites are advocated for periocular steroids in particular ocular diseases: (a) subconjunctival injection in the treatment of corneal diseases; (b) anterior subTenon's injection for iritis or iridocyclitis; (c) posterior subTenon's injection for equatorial and mid-zone posterior uveitis; and (d) retrobulbar injection for inflammation of the macula, optic nerve, or disc. It is generally agreed that the type of injection and the precise anatomic location for the steroid must be individualized for the particular clinical setting, and that the periocular steroid should be placed in a position to maximize the concentration of the drug at the desired site of action.

Table 8 presents some currently available injectable corticosteroid preparations. Aside from hydrocortisone, the corticosteroid preparations listed in this table are potent anti-inflammatory agents. The formulation of the steroid preparations probably plays an important role in determining the rate at which drug is released from the depot, and therefore the duration of steroid effects. Water-soluble preparations are characteristically short-acting because they diffuse from the depot more rapidly, even when steroids which are thought to be relatively long-acting by other methods of drug delivery (such as dexamethasone) are employed. Less soluble steroid preparations have a longer duration of action, although the duration of action of any of the periocular steroids may vary depending upon the anatomic location of the depot injection and distribution into surrounding tissues.

One problem with periocular steroids is that repeated injections may be required, particularly when short-acting preparations are employed. These injections often result in patient discomfort and additional inflammatory insults at the injection site. Also, there is a risk of inadvertent intraocular injection, and there

Table 8. Injectable corticosteroid preparations (HERSCHLER 1976)

Water-soluble, short-acting compounds
    Dexamethasone sodium phosphate (Decadron)
    Hydrocortisone sodium succinate (Solu-Cortef)

Suspensions of moderately soluble compounds in polyethylene glycol
    Triamcinolone diacetate (Aristocort)
    Methylprednisolone acetate (Depo-Medrol)

Suspensions of poorly soluble compounds
    Triamcinolone acetonide (Kenalog)
    Triamcinolone hexacetonide (Aristopan)

Mixtures of soluble and moderately soluble compounds
    β-Methasone sodium phosphate and β-methasone acetate (Celestone)

---

may be a greater chance of adrenal suppression with periocular injections than with the topical route (SCHLAEGEL 1970). Since less soluble preparations are designed to release active steroid over a sustained interval, their use may limit the need for repeated injections. Unfortunately, there are reports that injections of long-acting steroid preparations may increase the risk of serious ocular complications. Moderately soluble repository corticosteroids were initially reported to raise IOP and induce steroid glaucoma (KALINA 1969). With sparingly soluble preparations, such as triamcinolone acetonide, the duration of steroid action may be even longer and the chance of ocular complications even greater (HERSCHLER 1976). HERSCHLER proposes that triamcinolone acetonide may produce effects for months after an injection, and use of this agent can result in a glaucoma that is particularly severe and difficult to control. Surgical excision of the steroid may be indicated, and may be the only way to relieve uncontrolled IOP. SMITH and NOZIK (1982) believe that Depo-Medrol preparations may likewise show steroid effects for a longer duration than is generally appreciated, and that the commercially available preparations can also produce unwanted inflammatory reactions at the site of injection.

The major advantage of injectable corticosteroid preparations is that the drug can be placed near the site of active inflammation, and this may allow the quick delivery of an effective amount of steroid to the desired ocular site for a sustained period of time. HYNDIUK and REAGAN (1968) examined tissue localization of ^3H-methylprednisolone acetate (Depo-Medrol) in monkeys 2 and 9 days after subconjunctival injection. Steroids were concentrated in the posterior uvea-retina following subTenon's injection, and these levels remained high for at least 9 days. Similarly, retrobulbar injections resulted in high steroid levels in the posterior uvea-retina, as well as in the optic nerve and vitreous (HYNDIUK 1969; LEVINE and ARONSON 1970). These studies emphasize that the periocular route provides a means to deliver steroids to intraocular tissues, some of which are difficult to reach by other methods. Although the precise pathway by which the periocular steroid reaches different anatomic sites in the eye has not been clearly established, a direct absorption of the injected steroid through ocular tissues is most probable. Control experiments in these studies have shown that the same steroid dose administered did not result in appreciable drug levels in comparable ocular tissues. These experiments, however, do not prove the superiority of the periocular route over the systemic route; and it would be most useful to examine whether sufficiently high steroid levels could be achieved in ocular tissues if maximal systemic therapy were given.

The evaluation of subconjunctival steroids in experimental animals may not provide information that can be compared with the effectiveness of steroids administered by this route in patients. In the rabbit, the amount of subconjunctival steroid required to produce an anti-inflammatory effect is often well in excess of that employed in patients. Also, the fact that rabbits are much smaller than humans may explain why investigators have observed systemic effects (and occasionally toxic effects) of steroids after periocular injections in these animals (ROSENTHAL et al. 1976; SMOLIN et al. 1977). Thus it is possible that some of the anti-inflammatory effects of periocular steroids in these animals could involve steroid suppression of systemic immunity, and some of the other effects could involve an alteration of overall metabolism.

Among the new possibilities that can be considered in these studies is the placement of controlled release steroid devices at strategic periocular sites. With these limitations in mind, it is particularly important to study the time course of steroid release from periocular injections to help resolve some of the controversies concerning this route of drug delivery. In this connection reference should be made to the sections on local injection (see Chap. 2).

3. Systemic

Systemic therapy offers certain advantages. Oral steroid regimens are easily self-administered, and this route provides a relatively simply means of delivering steroids to many ocular tissues which cannot be reached by topical therapy. The tissue levels of steroids may not be as high with systemic therapy as those achieved through depot steroid injections, but for some disorders steroid levels may be adequate to produce the desired therapeutic result. It is important to realize that certain ocular sites, such as the cornea, may not be readily accessible to systemic therapy, but this can prove advantageous, e.g., in active viral epithelialitis accompanied by uveitis.

High-dose (60–100 mg prednisone per day) short-term (less than 2 weeks) administration of systemic steroids provides a potentially valuable tool for the treatment of inflammatory and immunologically mediated ophthalmic disease. A direct effect on the systemic immune response can also be achieved. Oral steroid therapy may be particularly useful in treating the ophthalmic complications of general connective tissue disorders, such as sarcoid.

It is often possible to avoid many of the complications of high-dose steroid therapy by administering steroids for a short time. Long-term systemic steroids can be dangerous, even with moderate anti-inflammatory doses. In this regard, Kaufman (1975) cautions that chronic steroid administration should not be used as therapy for low-grade ocular inflammatory processes, even though such a regimen may be necessary to suppress ocular symptoms completely. Long-term systemic steroids can result in the retardation of growth in children and in the progression of osteoporosis in older patients, among other complications. Epstein (1977) has suggested that cytotoxic agents may be preferable to steroids for certain conditions, especially when high-dose, prolonged steroid therapy would otherwise be employed. Of course, the lowest effective dose should be employed in order to reduce glucocorticoid side effects (Kimura 1977).

Prednisone is the steroid most often chosen for oral therapy. This drug is rapidly converted to prednisolone by the liver in most patients, although an improved therapeutic response is expected with prednisolone if the liver function has been impaired and is incapable of sufficient conversion of the prednisone to prednisolone. Use of prednisone or prednisolone appears to be relatively safer than longer-acting steroids such as dexamethasone, which may be more likely to suppress the hypothalamic–pituitary–adrenal (HPA) axis and produce cushingoid changes. Current evidence indicates that effective blood levels of steroid persist for 8 h after a 15-mg dose of prednisolone, but higher doses of steroid may be required to influence less sensitive tissues and to achieve the desired anti-inflammatory effects.

Since approximately 100 mg of prednisone achieves nearly complete glucocorticoid receptor saturation (BAXTER and TYRELL 1981), the exceedingly large prednisone doses (up to 1,000 mg) which have been used in acute renal transplant rejection or in shock may not actually add to the therapeutic response. In renal transplant recipients (VINCENTI et al. 1980), considerably less steroid is just as effective in preventing rejection as were the earlier extra high dose protocols. Importantly, the decrease in steroid dosages in this study was associated with a significant increase in patient survival.

Alternate-day steroid regimens have been employed in an attempt to reduce complications such as suppression of the HPA axis and the deleterious effects of steroids on growth, osteoporosis, and immunosuppression (HARTER et al. 1963; HARTER 1974; FAUCI 1978; TYRRELL and BAXTER 1981). It is not known whether or not alternate-day therapy will lessen the undesirable effects of steroids on ocular tissues.

Alternate-day steroid regimens are not useful for all medical conditions. The patient must be carefully observed to assure that there is no flare-up of the disease process or rebound upon steroid withdrawal. FAUCI (1978) has emphasized that alternate-day therapy is usually not effective for the suppression of an ongoing inflammatory response of serious proportions, and this mode of therapy should be instituted only after the inflammatory process has ben brought under control. Steroid effects on some inflammatory cells may require a relatively continuous presence of hormone, which alternate-day therapy will not provide. For example, neutrophil responses rapidly return to normal on the "off" day of alternate-day steroid regimens (PARILLO and FAUCI 1979). In the eye, neutrophils are regarded as extremely destructive inflammatory cells involved in many rapidly progressive lesions; alternate-day therapy is not likely to be useful in attempting to control such inflammatory processes. On the other hand, when the pathogenic mechanism primarily involves the monocyte-macrophage system, alternate-day therapy may prove useful. In studies of this cell type, DALE et al. (1974) report that steroid effects persist on the off day of alternate day therapy. The macrophage is known to play a central role in many immune processes (MOLLER 1980; MARCHALONIS 1980), and a steroid effect on this cell type is one mechanism by which alternate-day therapy can prevent the renewal of inflammatory reactions.

Alternate-day steroid therapy has received mixed reviews when evaluated for the treatment of ocular inflammatory conditions. O'CONNOR has major reservations about its use for cases where inflammatory processes threaten vital structures, such as the macula; in his experience, such regimens provide poor overall results, with increased symptoms on the off day of therapy (SCHLAEGEL and O'CONNOR 1977). In the same review, SCHLAEGEL reports good results with alternate-day steroids in his patients. There is general agreement, however, that alternate-day therapy should not be employed for the initial treatment of ocular inflammation, and this is especially true in cases where inflammation may cause irreversible damage to essential ocular structures. In this case, a short course of high-dose systemic therapy, possibly with combined topical or periocular steroids, may be considered for initial control. Alternate-day therapy should be considered only when it is necessary to continue systemic steroid therapy for extended periods.

4. Intravitreal

The injection of steroids into the vitreous cavity has received substantial attention (Machemer et al. 1979; Tano et al. 1980a, b, c, 1981). The intravitreal route has been employed in an attempt to prevent the serious consequences of fibroblastic proliferation and contraction band (strand) formation in endophthalmitis, perforating injuries of the eye, and vitreous surgery. In earlier studies, Graham and Peyman (1974) employed a combination of intravitreal dexamethasone and gentamicin in experimental endophthalmitis, and showed that the steroid could provide a useful means of reducing inflammation if administered early.

Machemer's experiments provide further evidence that intravitreal steroids may be useful in reducing unwanted cellular proliferations. He suggests that intravitreal administration allows a sufficiently high concentration of steroids to be delivered to the desired location and produce a therapeutic effect. Triamcinolone acetonide appears to remain in the eye longer than dexamethasone following these injections, and thus may be preferred for this method of drug delivery. As shown in Fig. 8, the choice of triamcinolone acetonide is supported by the effectiveness of this steroid in reducing the incidence of retinal detachments after experimental injection of cultured fibroblasts into the vitreous cavity (Tano et al. 1980c).

It is entirely possible that complications of intravitreal steroids will be seen in humans which were not observed when McCuen et al. (1981) examined this in Machemer's experimental systems. In patients, it is possible that triamcinolone acetonide will be associated with steroid glaucoma and steroid cataract, neither of which are readily detected in animal studies. Also, the sustained release of intravitreal triamcinolone acetonide may increase the incidence of systemic steroid side effects. Nevertheless, such considerations are often outweighed by the consequences of serious inflammatory conditions in which irreversible destruction of ocular tissues is imminent. Experimental data suggesting intravitreal steroids may limit some of the devastating pathological processes that affect this part of the eye argue for continued evaluation of the intravitreal administration of steroids, as well as other drugs.

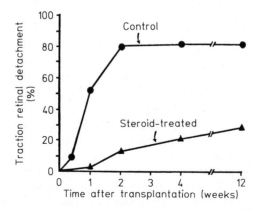

Fig. 8. Number of developing traction retinal detachments after intravitreal injection, with and without triamcinolone injections. (Adapted from Tano et al. 1980b)

III. Therapeutic Approaches

1. Specific Clinical Problems and Controversies

LEVINE and LEOPOLD (1973) have listed ocular conditions responsive to corticosteroids (Table 9). Degenerative conditions do not have a major inflammatory or immunologic component (e.g., involutional cataracts or macular degeneration) and are unresponsive to steroids. In other cases, an overlying inflammatory component appears to be steroid-responsive, while the underlying disease process is steroid-resistant (e.g., reticulum cell sarcoma or optic neuritis). Some ocular diseases with prominent inflammatory components characteristically show improvement after steroid therapy, while others display little or no response. For example, the use of steroids (either topical or systemic) for the treatment of Terrien's marginal corneal disease has been disappointing, despite the increasing awareness that recurrent, disabling, episodic inflammation can be a dominant feature in this disease (AUSTIN and BROWN 1981). Similarly, steroids do not have an impressive effect on the course of Mooren's ulcer or Fuchs' heterochromic iridocyclitis. In the latter disorder, as in certain instances of serous cyclitis, underlying flare may persist despite steroid therapy.

Table 9. Ocular conditions reported to respond to corticosteroids (LEVINE and LEOPOLD 1973)

Allergic blepharitis and conjunctivitis
Vernal conjunctivitis
Contact dermatitis of the conjunctiva and eyelid
Immune graft reaction
Irritant conjunctivitis
Optic neuritis
Progressive thyroid exophthalmos
Phlyctenular conjunctivitis and keratitis
Pseudotumor of the orbit
Temporal arteritis
Marginal corneal ulcers
Viral ocular diseases
Herpes simplex (diskiform stage)
Herpes zoster
Adenovirus
Superficial punctate keratitis
Posterior uveitis
Juvenile xanthogranuloma
Sympathetic opthalmia
Chemical burn of the cornea and conjunctiva
Scleritis and episcleritis
Acne rosacea keratitis
Ocular pemphigus
Iritis, iridocyclitis
Mucocutaneous conjunctival lesions
Interstitial keratitis
Retinal vasculitis
Infiltrative corneal disease

The use of steroids may be detrimental to the ultimate visual outcome in bacterial, fungal, and some viral infections of the eye (e.g., the epithelial stage of herpes simplex), especially if the offending agent has not been neutralized with appropriate specific therapy. However, steroids may be used in conjunction with effective antimicrobial therapy to reduce severe structural damage, e.g., loss of central vision, optic nerve or macular involvement in toxoplasmic retinochoroiditis). In some cases, one route of administration may be more advisable than another. For example, local steroids may be indicated in herpes zoster (see JONES 1974) of the eye to prevent destruction by inflammatory lesions and for keratitis, while systemic steroids represent a potential hazard in this disorder due to dissemination of the virus (KAUFMAN 1966), and have been reserved only for certain complications of herpes zoster (e.g., progressive proptosis with third nerve palsy or the onset of optic neuritis) (MARSH 1980). On the other hand, systemic steroids may be indicated to achieve adequate therapeutic levels in the uvea of an eye with the keratouvitis of herpes simplex in order to avoid high corneal concentrations that might exacerbate viral epithelialitis.

a) Ocular Allergy

Ocular inflammation due to allergy often responds rapidly to topical steroids. For mild allergic conditions, however, other therapeutic modalities which are associated with fewer complications are usually sufficient, and may be preferred to steroids (FRIEDLAENDER, to be published). Cold compresses and antihistamine/vasoconstrictor eye drops are useful adjunctive therapies to relieve the itching and redness in mild allergic conjunctivitis (such as that caused by pollens or dander). In more severe forms of allergic conjunctivitis (such as vernal and atopic keratoconjunctivitis), these measures may not be sufficient. Topical steroids often achieve symptomatic improvement in these patients, but frequent, long-term steroid administration may be required to achieve apparent suppression of the disease process. The recent introduction of disodium cromoglycate (Cromolyn) may decrease the need for long-term steroid therapy in many of these cases. Cromolyn may function to reduce steroid requirements by preventing the release of histamine and other vasoactive mediators from mast cells. Steroids are generally prescribed to patients with allergic conjunctivitis who do not adequately respond to more conservative regimens, or in cases where it is necessary to suppress the inflammatory response before subsequent control with nonsteroidal therapy. It is safest to use the lowest dose and frequency of steroids necessary to control the patient's symptoms. Steroids with relatively low potency, such as medrysone, may also be useful to achieve a therapeutic effect in these patients and decrease the chance of complications.

For certain allergic diseases, specific antimicrobial therapy may also decrease the steroid requirements, possibly by eliminating or effectively blocking the antigenic stimuli. Phlyctenular keratoconjunctivitis, for example, is thought to be a delayed hypersensitivity reaction to foreign protein (e.g., from tubercle bacillus or staphylococcus organisms). Although a brief course of steroids often, but not always, leads to resolution of this condition, chronic steroid administration is occasionally necessary (OSTLER and LANIER 1974). In some of these cases, systemic tetracycline brings rapid relief of symptoms and an apparent arrest of the nontuberculous form of this disease (ZAIDMAN and BROWN 1981).

b) Keratitis

The use of steroids for the treatment of keratitis is particularly controversial because of the possibility that these drugs suppress the host immune response, and result in the dissemination of infectious agents and a more destructive lesion (THYGESEN et al. 1960). On the other hand, maximum steroid therapy in central stromal keratitis may be essential to avert permanent corneal scarring and irreversible structural changes which can predispose to repeated infection (ARONSON and MOORE 1969; ARONSON and ELIOT 1972). It is particularly dangerous to use steroids without the proper neutralization of the infectious agents, but steroids are occasionally employed to "buy time" when severe corneal destruction appears imminent (see discussion, LEOPOLD 1970).

The use of steroids to treat herpes simplex is particularly cotroversial (OSTLER 1978; PAVAN-LANGSTON and ABELSON 1978; COSTER 1980). On the basis of his extensive clinical experience, THYGESEN (THYGESEN et al. 1960; THYGESEN 1977) asserts that steroids should not be used for this disorder, and that much of the morbidity and the progressive nature of this disease are directly due to the administration of steroids in this condition. Among the complications of steroid therapy in herpes simplex cited by THYGESEN are increased stromal involvement, superinfection with bacteria and fungi, and corneal perforation. Although these are potentially serious complications, it is generally agreed that there is a place for steroid therapy in both stromal disease and in keratouveitis. Furthermore, the use of steroids after keratoplasty helps a favorable recovery in herpetic patients. Guidelines for the rational use of steroids in herpetic disease have been summarized (PA-VAN-LANGSTON 1978):

1. Use a concomitant prophylactic antiviral agent.
2. Use steroids only in the presence of an intact corneal epitheliums.
3. Taper steroid regimens to avoid rebound effects.
4. Look for the possibility of superinfection.
5. Use the lowest dose of steroids that will control the inflammation (by dilution of commercially available preparations).

Steroid therapy for bacterial infections of the cornea has also been a source of controversy. In experimental bacterial keratitis, LEIBOWITZ and KUPFERMAN (1980 b) observed that the number of viable organisms was unchanged when antibiotic-treated and antibiotic/corticosteroid-treated groups were compared. On the other hand, STERN et al. (1980) observed in their keratitis model that steroid treatment resulted in an increase in the number of viable pseudomonas organisms when the antibiotic therapy was marginally effective against the infectious agents. Because of the potential dangers of steroid therapy in the presence of pathogenic agents (such as is often the case in infectious keratitis), the risks and benefits must be considered carefully for individual patients before a therapeutic decision is made. Corticosteroids probably have a place in the treatment of bacterial keratitis when there is central or paracentral corneal involvement, but effective antibiotic therapy prior to the initiation of steroids is advisable.

c) Uveitis

The optimal use of steroids in the different inflammatory disorders of the uveal tract requires further clarification. There are many problems in defining appropriate parameters for an objective assessment of the therapeutic response. Appropriate experimental models are lacking. There are multiple causes for uveitis, and in many instances the underlying pathophysiological mechanisms are poorly understood (SCHLAEGEL 1977; SCHLAEGEL and O'CONNOR 1977). The initial stimulus for inflammation often occurs long before the initiation of treatment. Although the inflammatory processes in many forms of uveitis are self-limiting, steroids can be effective in reducing major inflammatory symptoms, relieving pain, preventing synechiae, and alleviating the secondary glaucoma and elevated IOP that may accompany anterior segment inflammation. There have been a number of reviews concerned with the clinical use of steroids in uveitis (e.g., COLES 1966; SCHLAEGEL 1970), and some practical guidelines have been reviewed recently (GANLEY 1980; SMITH and NOZIK 1982).

Most of the useful information has been gained by the qualitative assessment of therapy, but attempts to quantitate the efficacy of steroids in patients with uveitis may help to define improved therapeutic approaches. For example, DUNNE and TRAVERS (1979) have recently conducted a controlled double-blind clinical trial in which quantitative criteria were developed to evaluate the effectiveness of different anti-inflammatory steroids in uveitis. In this study, clobetasone butyrate (a relatively new therapeutic steroid) appeared to be equivalent to β-methasone phosphate in reducing the clinical symptoms and was superior to β-methasone in improving the ocular signs of uveitis. Another approach to obtaining quantitative information about steroid therapy in uveitis is to define relevant biochemical parameters of the disease process. In this regard, WEINREB and KIMURA (1979) have suggested that measurement of serum angiotensin-converting enzyme in sarcoid uveitis may provide a marker for the response to systemic or topical steroids.

Steroids have also been used to treat postoperative uveitis (e.g., following cataract surgery). Although there was originally some question whether such therapy could interfere with surgical wound healing, complications with contemporary surgical techniques (such as wound leak) do not appear to occur with increased frequency (CORBOY 1976). There are also reports suggesting that preoperative steroids can help to diminish active postoperative inflammation following lensectomy/vitrectomy (DIAMOND and KAPLAN 1978; KAPLAN et al. 1979) and after filtering surgery (CHANDLER and GRANT 1979b). In addition, PEYMAN et al. (to be published) have recently demonstrated that the use of steroids in intravitreal infusion fluid reduces postvitrectomy intravitreal albumin.

Considerable caution should be exercised in the administration of steroids for uveitis unless it is absolutely necessary. KAUFMAN (1975) warns against the use of long-term systemic steroids in low-grade uveitis. For severe uveal inflammation, on the other hand, high-dose topical steroids and/or periocular injections near the site of inflammation may be required to prevent irreversible damage. Again, however, steroid therapy should not be continued indefinitely. Cytotoxic drugs may be useful as adjunctive therapy (KIMURA 1977), and these agents appear to produce fewer side effects than long-term systemic steroids (EPSTEIN 1977). Cytotoxic agents may be particularly beneficial for sympathetic ophthalmia, Behçet's syndrome, and rheumatoid sclerouveitis (GODFREY et al. 1974; O'CONNOR 1980; JAMPOL et al. 1978). In other cases, however, cytotoxic agents do not appear to be effective in replacing anti-inflammatory steroids (e.g., chronic cyclitis, Vogt–Koyanagi–Harada syndrome, sarcoid).

d) Optic Neuritis

Although systemic corticosteroids appear to provide symptomatic relief in cases of optic neuritis, a number of studies suggest that the visual outcome is not altered (LUBOW and ADAMS 1972; GOULD et al. 1977; BIRD 1977; PERKIN and ROSE 1979). In these studies it is difficult to evaluate the efficacy of steroid therapy because of the following factors:
1.) There may be differences in the patient populations, especially with regard to age, sex, and clinical findings.
2.) The disease course may be dependent on the patient's location and environment.
3.) The clinically observed disease may have different causes.
4.) Steroid treatment is instituted at different times in the disease course and different dosage levels are employed.

The present evidence indicates that use of steroids in optic neuritis results in a shorter recovery time and relief of pain for many patients. Short-term, high-dose steroid therapy involves some risk, as mentioned, but complications of such therapeutic regimens are usually few if the patient is appropriately monitored. Since steroid therapy does not appear to worsen the disease course, steroids may be useful in cases of painful optic neuritis in which analgesics do not provide relief. Also, in patients who maintain a slowly progressive course of optic neuritis, it is not unreasonable to attempt a steroid trial, although the sporadic nature of the disease makes it difficult to interpret either the immediate benefits of such therapy or the long-term effect on visual outcome.

There have been reports that ACTH therapy could be more useful than systemic steroids in this disorder (WRAY 1977). It is possible that an unknown hormone effect of ACTH (independent of known anti-inflammatory or immunosuppressive effects of steroids) could account for this reported efficacy. The rationale for such regimens is based on opinions that ACTH therapy is also superior to oral steroids in dermatomyositis and multiple sclerosis (see WILLIAMS et al. 1980). On the other hand, the difficulty of defining the response in these conditions and the possibility that inadequate doses of systemic steroids were employed (MEYERS et al. 1980; TYRRELL and BAXTER 1981) provides considerable room for skepticism. Also, there are many other problems with ACTH therapy, and it is generally not recommended for clinical use (TYRRELL and BAXTER 1981). More compelling evidence is necessary to demonstrate that ACTH therapy has a therapeutic effect in optic neuritis beyond that achieved by maximal systemic steroid therapy.

Optic neuritis, therefore, remains one of the most difficult disorders in which to evaluate the efficacy of steroid therapy or to specify an appropriate therapeutic regimen.

2. Current Assessment

It is clear that the clinical effects of steroid therapy depend upon the nature of the disease process and the host response. Ocular inflammatory and immunologic responses are complex and involve many cellular actions and interactions. The results of steroid therapy will be determined by the differential steroid sensitivity of the various cell types which participate in the disease process. The timing and duration of steroid administration may also have important therapeutic consequences for a particular disease, depending upon (among other factors) whether the inflammatory stimulus is continous or intermittent.

The action of steroids through high-affinity glucocorticoid receptors suggests that some anti-inflammatory actions may occur at low drug concentrations. Also, there is likely to be a time lag of between 30 min and 3 h before steroid receptor-mediated changes in specific protein synthesis will produce a therapeutic response. In some cases the cellular response to steroids may last for a considerable amount of time (depending upon the half-life of the macromolecular products involved), possibly explaining why a single dose of steroid produces anti-inflammatory effects in some conditions long after the drug is no longer present in the tissue. Receptor-mediated actions of steroids may also explain why some patients with herpes keratitis show a steroid dependency with only 1 drop of 0.005% dexamethasone every 3–7 days, and why a daily drop of 0.1% dexamethasone can be used to prevent corneal graft rejection. A dilemma confronts the therapist in the use of steroids in ocular inflammatory disease. Some investigators feel that the possibility of serious structural alterations demands the use of maximal steroid therapy (Aronson et al. 1970). Others believe that steroids should not be used because the disease process will be exacerbated by steroids (Thygeson 1977; also see Havener 1976). Controversies in the use of steroids persist because it is difficult to evaluate the therapeutic response.

It may be possible to use a low concentration of steroid to produce the desired clinical effects (Kaufman 1968). The dose–response curve for individual steroid effects would be most useful. In some cases, dilute steroids can be employed to achieve the desired anti-inflammatory effect and to decrease the chance of developing side effects. It is also possible that new routes of steroid administration (e.g., intravitreal), new methods of drug delivery (e.g., continuous release device), or the use of steroids which differ in their potency or metabolism may allow a separation of therapeutic effects from those side effects. Selective adjunctive anti-inflammatory therapy used along with steroids may further decrease the dose requirements for steroids, and may occasionally produce a synergistic effect. The development of improved antimicrobial agents and the use of substances which may enhance host resistance (such as interferon or vitamin A) offer new therapeutic avenues which may replace steroid therapy or augment its effectiveness.

IV. Complications

Two prominent ocular side effects of steroid therapy are the development of elevated (IOP) and posterior subcapsular cataracts (PSCs). The possibility of steroid glaucoma is a major concern, expecially when suppression of ocular inflammation requires long-term corticosteroid administration. Steroid-induced cataract has been a particularly difficult problem to investigate, and quantitative information is not readily obtained in this disorder. Most retrospective studies have shown that lower steroid doses are generally associated with a decreased incidence of PSCs, but there are also a number or reports that demonstrate a considerable variability in the development of this condition. At the present time it is not possible to define an absolutely safe therapeutic regimen, and the factors which may influence individual susceptibility to steroid-induced cataracts require further investigation.

1. Glaucoma

Soon after corticosteroids were introduced, a report appeared suggesting that steroid therapy might increase IOP (McLean 1950). The first case of "cortisone glaucoma" was reported by Francois (1954); local steroids had been applied for 3 years in a patient with vernal conjunctivitis. When this patient was examined, significant visual field loss and markedly elevated IOP were observed, without signs of active inflammation. The IOP returned to normal soon after steroids were discontinued in one eye, while the other eye required surgery. Other investigators who examined the question of steroid glaucoma, however, reported little or no change in the IOP when they attempted to study the effects of prolonged steroids on the eye. The problem of steroid glaucoma after topical administration of steroid became generally appreciated with the reports of Goldmann (1962) and Valerio et al. (1962). Also, Bernstein and Schwartz (1962) and Bernstein et al. (1963) demonstrated that systemic steroids could have a significant effect on IOP, confirming earlier case reports.

Interest in the IOP response to topical steroids increased dramatically following reports by Armaly (1963a, b) and Becker and co-workers (Becker and Mills 1963a, Becker and Hahn 1964) in which the ocular steroid-sensitivity of different populations was examined. The use of dexamethasone phosphate 0.1% or β-methasone phosphate 0.1%, administered three to four times a day for 3–6 weeks, produced a surprisingly high incidence of elevated IOP in the general population. Between 30% and 40% of the control group showed IOPs that exceeded 20 mmHg by Becker's criteria (and a change of more than 6 mmHg by Armaly's criteria). Also, the fact that approximately 6% of the patients in the population showed IOPs that exceeded 31 mmHg under the standard testing protocols (and 80%–90% of those with glaucoma showed this response) further emphasized the danger that steroid therapy might produce clinically significant elevations in IOP. These studies argued strongly against the indiscriminate use of topical steroids. This point was again emphasized by the case reports of Burde and Becker (1970), in which steroid glaucoma and permanent visual field defects were found in two young patients in which steroids were employed to relieve minor ocular irritation associated with the wearing of contact lenses. Chandler and Grant (1979a) point out that it is important to take a careful history in making the diagnosis of open-angle glaucoma, because a number of patients self-prescribe corticosteroid drops and may actually have a steroid glaucoma. In some cases, patients have employed topical steroids to relieve the burning due to epinephrine treatment (Becker and Mills 1963b), making the glaucoma more difficult to control. In spite of the problems associated with the inappropriate use of steroids, steroid therapy should not be abandoned when required in patients with glaucoma or in patients who are high steroid responders. It is often possible to compensate for the IOP effects of steroids in these patients by increased antihypertensive therapy (e.g., SCHWARTZ 1966c; ARMALY 1967). The use of dilute steroid preparations or some of the newer steroid agents may also provide the necessary anti-inflammatory activity with a lesser effect on IOP.

BECKER and HAHN (1964) and ARMALY (1965) examined the pharmacogenetic basis of the IOP response to topical steroid testing by comparing IOP response in patients with primary open-angle glaucoma, their relatives, and volunteer controls who were selected to exclude a family history of glaucoma or a positive water-provocative tonogram (Po/C > 100). On the basis of the distributions of IOP response in the different populations, these investigations suggest that three separate populations of steroid responders could be distinguished. According to Becker's criteria, homozygous poor responders had IOP responses of less than 20 mmHg, heterozygous intermediate responders had IOP responses between 20 and 31 mmHg, and homozygous high responders had IOP responses exceeding 31 mmHg. BECKER and HAHN (1964) and BECKER (1965) proposed that the high responders were homozygous for the glaucoma gene, and that the inheritance was recessive. Although ARMALY stressed the change in IOP after steroid therapy rather than absolute pressure levels, he also extrapolated a similar distribution of steroid responsiveness in the different groups. In contrast to BECKER, he suggested the high-responder gene was associated with but not identical to the glaucoma gene.

The precise genetic relationship between the IOP response to steroids and primary open-angle glaucoma has not been resolved, and several have questioned the finding of distinct populations of steroid responders (e.g., FRANCOIS et al. 1966; SCHWARTZ 1966b). When SCHWARTZ et al. (1973a, b) evaluated the inheritance patterns of steroid responsiveness in twins, they concluded that the data did not support the mendelian recessive pattern that was proposed. To explain this apparently contradictory study, PALMBERG et al. (1975) suggested that concordance results (65%) presented by SCHWARTZ et al. were actually in agreement with the genetic hypothesis, because the reproducibility of the steroid response in the populations evaluated would predict a similar result (73%). Other objections notwithstanding, KOLKER and HETHERINGTON (1976) asserted that the classification of steroid responsiveness may help in the selection of patients for the study of the pathogenesis of glaucoma, as well as in distinguishing some cases of primary open-angle glaucoma from some secondary glaucomas. Studies of the effect of topical steroids do emphasize the importance of determining a family history of glaucoma before the institution of steroid therapy.

One of the most important questions raised by the studies of topical steroid testing is whether the high-responder group would later show an incidence of glaucomatous change, with further increases in IOP and visual field loss. KITAZAWA and HORIE (1981) have recently reported the results of a 10-year follow-up study conducted on a group of 35 high responders (change in IOP exceeding 16 mmHg after 4 weeks of β-methasone phosphate 0.1% four times a day). A sustained rise in pressure exceeding 21 mmHg developed in 5 of the 22 previously normotensive patients in this group, and 2 of these patients demonstrated glaucomatous field changes. Of the 13 ocular hypertensives in the original group, 7 had a further rise in pressure associated with glaucomatous field changes. If the results obtained in this study are proved to be applicable to other patient populations, this will imply that development of primary open-angle glaucoma is somehow linked to the high-pressure response to steroids. Perhaps a compromised meshwork is more susceptible to the effect of topical steroid. In other studies (BAYER and NEUNER 1967; NEUNER and DARDENNE 1968) it has been shown that patients with Cushing's syndrome have a high incidence of elevated IOP compared to the general population. The case study of a patient with an adrenal adenoma presented by HAAS and NOOTEN (1974) also emphasizes that endogenous circulating steroids can contribute to the development of elevated IOP in some individuals. Interestingly, the older steroid-responsive relatives of the propositors showed no evidence of glaucoma. SCHWARTZ (1981 b) studied the possibility that increased concentrations of steroids in patients with glaucoma might help to explain the elevated IOP in glaucoma as an alternative to the increased ocular steroid sensitivity hypothesis in these patients. It is conceivable that both humoral and cellular responsiveness play a role.

In the search for a genetic marker for glaucoma the proposal has been made that primary open-angle glaucoma is associated with a generalized cellular defect in steroid sensitivity. The genetic hypothesis for steroid sensitivity, as well as inherited traits and disease associations (e.g., phenylthiocarbamide testing and diabetes mellitus, see KOLKER and HETHERINGTON 1976), suggested that there might be a cellular basis for the increased steroid sensitivity. Initial studies of the ability of steroids to inhibit phytohemagglutinin stimulation in lymphocytes (BIGGER et al. 1972, 1975) and the evaluation of the sensitivity of the hypothalamic–pituitary axis by dexamethasone suppression testing (BECKER et al. 1973) supported the concept of a generalized cellular hypersensitivity to steroids in glaucoma patients. Previously, an evaluation of the response of eosinophils to systemic steroids by AR-MALY (1967) did not show a correlation with the ocular steroid response. Further investigations of the lymphocyte sensitivity to steroids did not produce consistent results, and many failed to support the original observations (FOON et al. 1977; BEN EZRA et al. 1976; SOWELL et al. 1977). Likewise, a recent study by McCARTY et al. (1981), using concanavalin A stimulation of lymphocytes to assay for steroid effects, revealed no more cellular sensitivity in the glaucoma patients than in controls. In studies performed on cultured skin fibroblasts from patients with primary open-angle glaucoma and matched controls, POLANSKY et al. (to be published) again found no differences in steroid sensitivity, either at the receptor level or when cellular responsiveness to cortisol was measured. Overall, most studies argue against the presence of a generalized cellular sensitivity to steroids in patients with glaucoma.

a) Dose–Response Relationships

ARMALLY (1965) originally demonstrated that the ocular response to dexamethasone phosphate in high steroid responders decreased significantly when the steroid was diluted from 0.1% to 0.05%, with a further decrease observed using a 0.01% dilution. The IOP responses obtained by ARMALY are shown in Fig. 9a, in which the date are expressed to show the average rise in IOP. One particularly important control in this study was the demonstration that a rechallenge using 0.1% dexamethasone phosphate after all dilutions had been tested produced an increase in

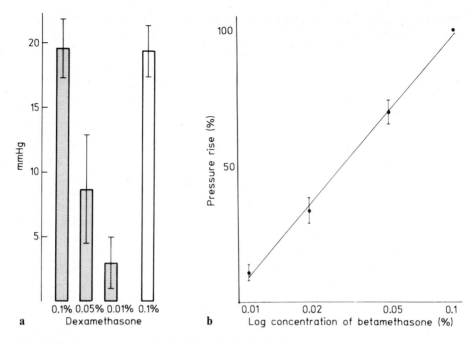

Fig. 9a, b. Dose-response relationships obtained after topical testing with dilutions of (**a**) dexamethasone phosphate (adapted from ARMALY 1965) and (**b**) β-methasone phosphate (KITAZAWA 1976), when evaluated in known high steroid responders

IOP equivalent to that seen initially. This result indicated that the IOP response remained unchanged after repeated steroid challenge and that high responders could be used to evaluate the dose–response effect of potent steroids on the IOP. In support of this concept, KITAZAWA (1976) used regression analysis (Fig. 9 b) to show that the β-methasone phosphate dose–response relationship could be described as a linear relationship in high responders.

The ability to obtain quantitative information concerning the IOP response also enabled the examination of possible differences between the different ophthalmic steroid preparations. Of the topical steroids, the newer steroids (such as fluorometholone, medrysone, and tetrahydrotriamcinolone acetonide were of particular interest, because it was proposed that they might not raise IOP as much as other compounds. Among the initial studies performed, CANTRILL et al. (1975) reported that the commercially available concentrations of fluorometholone 0.1% and medrysone 1% had significantly less effect on the average IOP response than dexamethasone 0.1% and even dexmethasone phosphate 0.005%. Fluorometholone and medrysone showed approximately 36% and 5% of the effect of 0.1% dexamethasone phosphate on IOP, respectively. It is of interest that in this study prednisolone 1% appeared to raise the IOP significantly less than dexamethasone 0.1%, but this result requires further confirmation. KITAZAWA (1976) also measured IOP changes after topical administration of β-methasone and the newer steroids, using a number of different drug dilutions (Table 10). Importantly, KI-

Table 10. Increase in intraocular pressure after topical administration of various corticosteroids (KITAZAWA 1976)

	No. of eyes		
	5 mm Hg	6–15 mm Hg	16 mm Hg
β-methasone			
0.1%	0	0	24
0.05%	3	10	11
0.02%	7	12	5
0.01%	20	4	0
Medrysone			
1.0%	18	6	0
Tetrahydrotriamcinolone			
1.25%	10	5	9
0.25%	24	0	0
0.05%	24	0	0
Fluorometholone			
0.1%	10	12	2
0.05%	17	7	0
0.01%	24	0	0

TAZAWA reported the steroid response for individual patients instead of the average values for IOP changes (Table 10). This study confirmed that the commercially available preparations of fluorometholone and medrysone have a reduced propensity to raise IOP relative to β-methasone. However, it was also clear that some patients showed a major rise in IOP while using fluorometholone 0.1%. In this study, about 7% of the high responders tested showed a rise in IOP > 16 mmHg using this concentration of fluorometholone (also see STEWART and KIMBROUGH 1979).

Rather than study the IOP response to topical steroids in high responders, MINDEL et al. (1980) investigated the activity of different steroid compounds in non-selected populations of hospitalized patients, under conditions where compliance could be assured (see Fig. 10). Although the differences in the IOP response were less than that seen in high responders, his study likewise confirmed that fluorometholone and medrysone show a reduced propensity to raise the IOP compared with dexamethasone phosphate.

Overall, these data support the concept that fluorometholone has a reduced propensity to raise IOP, although we have shown that it has a potency equal to dexamethasone in receptor-binding assays and provides effective topical anti-inflammatory activity for a variety of ocular conditions. It is possible that fluorometholone is more susceptible to degradation than dexamethasone. A shorter half-life in ocular tissues could cause a lower effective concentration of fluorometholone to reach the trabecular meshwork. A similar effect may be true for medrysone. Medrysone is a substantially weaker steroid than fluorometholone, and has a binding affinity comparable to tetrahydrotriamcinolone acetonide. However, use of tetrahydrotriamcinolone acetonide 1.25% results in a rather large num-

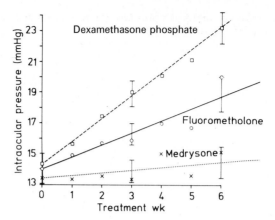

Fig. 10. Comparison of effects of dexamethasone phosphate, fluorometholone, and medrysone on intraocular pressure in nonselected hospitalized patients. (Mindel et al. 1980)

ber of patients being classified in the high-responder category, while medrysone 1% shows even less of an IOP effect than fluorometholone 0.1%.

The evaluation of the pharmacokinetics and metabolism of the different ophthalmic steroids may help to explain why certain steroids appear to show a beneficial split between their glucocorticoid receptor potency and their ability to raise IOP.

b) Temporal Aspects

The temporal responses to steroids have important clinical implications. It has been generally believed that sustained and significant elevations of IOP are not found prior to 2 or 3 weeks of steroid therapy. This may not be the case. For example, in one of the patients studied by Armaly (1965), the data demonstrate an elevated IOP response that occurred within the 1st week of steroid treatment (Fig. 11). It is possible that frequent administration of potent steroids may result in significant elevations of IOP which are often not detected. For example, when attention was given to this possibility, major elevations in the IOP were observed 2–5 days following administration of topical steroid drops or ointments in at least five patients (Weinreb, unpublished observations). Increases in IOP may continue with increased duration of steroid administration (Armaly 1965). In the study by Mindel et al. (1980) (Fig. 10), the increase in IOP appeared linear over a 6-week period when tested in an unselected population of patients. Although it is likely that the IOP response will stabilize in some patients, this has not been investigated adequately. In any case, the studies that have been performed show that elevations in IOP are maintained for the duration of steroid treatment. The rate at which IOP falls after cessation of topical or systemic corticosteroids varies considerably from patient to patient (Spaeth et al. 1977; Chandler and Grant 1979a). In some patients the increased pressure is sustained (for a considerable amount of time); in unusual cases, the pressure increase is irreversible after steroids are withdrawn, and may require pharmacologic or surgical intervention.

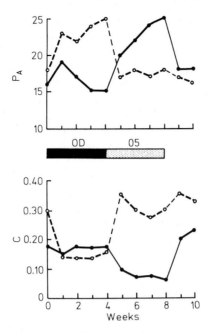

Fig. 11. Intraocular pressure response (P_A) and outflow facility (C) measurements in a patient receiving topical dexamethasone phosphate. (ARMALY 1965)

Generally speaking, prolonged use of steroids may produce a rise in IOP regardless of the route employed, and prior topical testing for steroid sensitivity may not always predict the response for injectable steroids (HERSCHLER 1976). The primary determinant for the steroid effect on IOP of repository steroids may be the rate at which the drug is released from the depot site, with the longer-acting steroid preparations demonstrating a greater chance of producing sustained elevations of IOP ad steroid glaucoma. HERSCHLER suggests that an initial depot injection of a water-soluble steroid preparation with a brief duration of activity is a rational means of testing this complication. In the case of systemic steroids, GODEL et al. (1972 a, b) have reported that the IOP response of a given individual correlates reasonably well with the response to topical steroids, but their interesting observations require further study.

Whereas the IOP response and decreased outflow facility after prolonged topical steroid administration have been widely accepted, there have been conflicting assessments of the rapid effect (i.e., within hours) of glucocorticoids on IOP. LINNER (1959) reported that elevation of ocular tension could be observed 2½–6 h after topical administration of 0.3% prednisolone in healthy volunteers without glaucoma. KIMURA and MAEKAWA (1976) subsequently reported a significant rise in IOP 5–9 h after 20 mg hydrocortisone was administered orally to subjects with primary open-angle glaucoma. In contrast, SPAETH (1969) found no rapid increase in IOP after oral dexamethasone. In other studies, investigators noted a potential relationship between the diurnal curves of ocular pressure and plasma cortisol (e.g., Boyd et al. 1962; Smith et al. 1962). The parallelism between IOP and plasma cortisol found in earlier studies was elegantly confirmed by Weitzman et al. (1975). However, these authors concluded that these were temporally related and not a causally related phenomenon, after evaluating the IOP response to dexamethasone in one patient with pigmentary glaucoma. More recently, Weinreb et al. (1979) investigated the possibility of a rapid steroid effect on IOP in four patients with primary open-angle glaucoma. Oral dexamethasone (3 mg) or placebo was administered in a double-blind fashion after a period of hospitalization. All patients demonstrated a clear rise in IOP in both eyes within 3–6 h of the steroid dose. When compared to the control days the effects of steroids in this study were statistically significant ($P < 0.01$). A typical response for one patient is shown in Fig. 12. The oral steroid was readily absorbed (as shown by the rise in plasma-free steroid levels,) and the downward trend in IOP was reversed within a rather short time course. This study supports the concept that a rapid effect of steroids on IOP may be significant, and that comparisons between the IOP response of normal controls and glaucoma patients could provide useful information. It is possible that

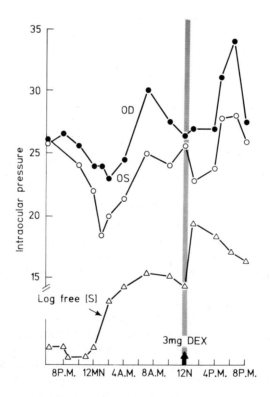

Fig. 12. Intraocular pressure (*IOP*) response in one of the four hospitalized primary open-angle glaucoma patients evaluated by Weinreb et al. (1978). 3 mg oral dexamethasone (*DEX*) or placebo was given at 12 noon (double-blind). Plasma-free steroid hormones (*S*) were measured using a whole-cell receptor-binding assay (for convenience, the data are expressed as the logarithm of the dexamethasone equivalents)

an IOP response to endogenous steroids may contribute to the elevations in IOP and diurnal changes observed in patients with primary open-angle glaucoma.

It is thus possible that the effect of steroids on IOP may involve two different types of response. First, a rapid and perhaps transient increase in IOP is noted within hours after a topical or systemic dose of glucocorticoid. This could involve an increase in aqueous inflow as suggested by LINNER (1959). Such a response may be of considerable importance if levels of endogenous glucocorticoids contribute to the regulation of diurnal variations of IOP. A second type of IOP response is observed after a period of several days or weeks of steroid administration and is sustained for the duration of steroid therapy. In the case of prolonged administration of topical steroids, the effect on IOP predominantly involves a decreased outflow facility. The effect of long-term systemic steroids is less clear, with significant effects on both inflow and outflow reported. By considering the actions of steroids on separate target tissues in the aqueous inflow and outflow pathways, it may be possible to understand these apparently different mechanisms. The continued evaluation of the temporal and dose–response relationships is necessary if we are to understand steroid-induced effects on IOP, and may lead to a better knowledge of the endogenous control of IOP.

c) Biochemical Studies

Although the pressure elevations after prolonged topical steroid administration involve a decrease in outflow facility, the biochemical mechanism has not been characterized. Functional steroid receptors have been demonstrated in both cultured human trabecular meshwork cells (WEINREB et al. 1981) and human trabeculectomy specimens (HERNANDEZ et al. 1981). It is therefore conceivable that a glucocorticoid-induced alteration in outflow facility could be mediated by a direct steroid action on the cells of the meshwork. One recent proposal has been that active corticosteroids inhibit the production of important prostaglandin products by trabecular cells, and that this may be related to the decrease in outflow facility (WEINREB et al. 1983).

Many different biochemical changes could be induced by the action of steroids on meshwork cells, but one important possibility that has been considered is an effect on glycosaminoglycan (formerly called mucopolysaccharide) production or metabolism. Particular interest was generated in hyaluronic acid and other glycosaminoglycans because studies by BÁRÁNY and SCOTCHBROOK (1954) suggested that removal of these substances by hyaluronidase increased outflow facility. FRANCOIS and VICTORIA-TRONCOSO (1977) have proposed that steroid glaucoma results from a direct effect on the lysosomes of cells at the filtration angle, with a buildup of undegraded mucopolysaccharides in the outflow pathway. KNEPPER (1978) has reported that alterations in glycosaminoglycans occur after dexamethasone administration to rabbits. Cultured human trabecular cells have relatively high levels of endogenous hyaluronidase (ZUMBRUN et al. 1981). Primate trabecular cells in tissue culture have been shown to produce hyaluronic acid (SCHACHTSCHABEL et al. 1977), and cultured human trabecular cells have been shown to produce hyaluronic acid and fibronectin (POLANSKY et al. 1978; ALVARADO and POLANSKY 1979). It is also possible that steroids might induce alterations in the outflow pathway by an unknown effect on the structural or functional properties of trabecular cells. One proposal has been that steroids prevent normal trabecular cell phagocytosis, the physiological mechanism for the meshwork's "self-cleaning filter" (Bill 1975). Although trabecular cells appear to be the most likely site at which steroid-mediated changes in outflow facility are modulated, it is also possible that steroid-induced alterations in the composition of aqueous humor or in other tissues (e.g., the ciliary muscle), could secondarily produce changes in the structure or function of the trabecular meshwork.

Structural alterations in the trabecular meshwork of patients with steroid glaucoma have been examined. These studies are difficult to interpret because limited numbers of steroid glaucoma specimens are available and appropriate control specimens have not been defined. Increased amounts of connective tissue in the juxtacanalicular tissue have been emphasized as one possible change due to steroids (see Rohen et al. 1973; Kayes and Becker 1964; Sano and Miyata 1971). Also, Alcian blue hyaluronidase-sensitive material has been reported in the cytoplasmic granules of trabecular endothelial cells in rabbits with steroid-induced ocular hypertension (Ticho et al. 1979). Questions which must be addressed to these reports include:

1. Do these changes represent primary pathogenic changes or are they secondary to other cellular processes or to the effects of elevated IOP?
2. Are the reported changes age-related rather than a result of the glaucomatous process?
3. Are the earliest changes functional or biochemical rather than anatomic?

2. Cataract

Black et al. (1960) first demonstrated an association between steroid therapy and the development of posterior subcapsular cataracts (PSCs). In patients receiving relatively high doses of systemic steroids (exceeding the equivalent of 15 mg prednisone) for over 2 years, there was a greater than 30% chance that these patients would eventually show PSC changes. Although objections have been raised concerning the possible role of the underlying disease state in some of these studies, Spaeth and von Sallmann (1966) have argued strongly that the control groups analyzed did not show higher incidence of PSCs than the normal population. On the basis of the initial, studies of Ogelsby et al. (1961), Giles et al. (1962), and Crews (1963), it has been proposed that a dose of less than 10 mg prednisone per day orally for less than a year is rarely associated with development of PSCs. Nevertheless, Skalka and Prchal (1980) have recently suggested that the concept of a safe dose of systemic steroids should be abandoned. Instead, they indicate that individual susceptibility may be more important than the dosage or duration of steroid therapy.

Systemic debility could have contributed to the development of cataractous changes in their study because the control group had an unusually high incidence (almost 15%) of PSC changes. Other evidence indicates that certain disease states may contribute to the development of cataract formation (e.g., see the report of a very high incidence of PSCs in diabetics receiving topical steroids, Yablonski et al. 1978), and the possibility of circulating metabolic factors should be considered in the assessment of individual variability in the development of steroid cataracts.

Steroid PSCs may be reversible, especially in younger patients (FORMAN et al. 1977; ROOKLIN et al. 1979). They may also be progressive despite discontinuance of steroid therapy. The development of PSCs may indicate a need to taper steroid levels even if chronic therapy is required, although the problem of steroid cataracts must be balanced with the need to suppress the underlying disease process. Even though most PSCs require a considerable amount of time to develop, LOREDO et al. (1972) have reported that children may develop cataracts in a 3–10-month period. A short course of topical or systemic steroid therapy will probably not result in the development of PSCs. Some data concerning steroid-induced cataracts after postkeratoplasty topical steroid therapy have been presented by DONSHIK et al. (1981). The data concerning injectable steroid preparations are particularly difficult to interpret, and often they are used in the presence of underlying inflammatory conditions which can cause changes similar to steroid cataracts. PHILLPOTTS (1969) has emphasized that only the lowest doses of methylprednisolone can be placed in the anterior chamber at the time of surgery without resulting in cataracts, which develop over approximately $2\frac{1}{2}$ months. Insufficient quantitative data are available to evaluate whether the injectable steroids themselves are more likely to predispose to PSCs than steroids administered by other routes. Also, it is possible that one injectable steroid could have a greater cataractogenic effect than others, but this has not been proved. HYNDIUK (1969) has shown that the lens concentrates methylprednisolone considerably more than other tissues, but comparisons among various steroid preparations have not been conducted.

Overall, the quantitative data concerning PSCs are much more difficult to obtain than those concerning steroid effects on IOP. The relatively rapid time course and the reversibility of the IOP response have been used to obtain a considerable amount of information relevant to the development of steroid glaucoma. By contrast, the development of PSCs occurs over a long period, and the process is not reversible in most cases. Thus clinical testing for steroid cataracts cannot be readily performed except when patients are receiving steroids for other indications. It will be useful to analyze the effects of different steroid preparations independently in future studies, in addition to employing the usual conversion of the steroids to prednisone (or prednisolone) equivalents. As with steroid glaucoma, no definitive animal models for PSCs have been developed, and the experimental models of steroid cataract are equivocal (KUCK 1977).

Although there are difficulties with the experimental animal systems, an understanding of the biochemistry of steroid hormone action on the lens may prove useful in understanding human disease. Specific glucocorticoid receptors have been identified in lens epithelium (SOUTHREN et al. 1977), and the enzymatic degradation of cortisol by the lens tissues has been reported (ONO et al. 1971; SOUTHREN et al. 1976). In an attempt to understand steroid-induced changes that could lead to cataract, some investigators have found evidence for altered lens transport mechanisms (BECKER and COTLIER 1965), while others have reported changes in phospholipid metabolism after high doses of steroids in experimental animals (TAMADA et al. 1980). The available studies of steroid action on the lens do not clarify the relationship of steroids to the development of posterior subcapsular cataracts.

It is likely that some of the questions concerning the role of steroids in the development of PSCs will be resolved when the factors that contribute to individual susceptibility to this disorder are better defined. Aside from specific disease associations and the age of the patient, it is possible that individual differences in the absorption or concentration of steroids or metabolism of steroid by the lens may contribute to the differences in patient susceptibility (see Sect. 2.2).

3. Other Ocular Effects

Steroid-induced changes are likely to occur in most ocular tissues because of the presence there of glucocorticoid receptors. Physiological evidence for changes in ocular tissues induced by steroids includes effects on corneal thickness and metabolism, changes in the composition of the aqueous humor, an increase in the relative viscosity and mucopolysaccharide content of the vitreous, alterations in the intermediary metabolism of the retina, and vasoconstrictive effects in the conjunctiva and other tissues (SCHWARTZ 1966a). Clinically recognized ocular complications of steroid therapy include retardation in wound-healing processes and the possibility of progressive corneal ulceration (see BROWN et al. 1970; DONSHIK et al. 1978), steroid uveitis (KRUPIN et al. 1970), possible alteration of muscular function related to the development of mydriasis or ptosis (ARMALY 1964; SPAETH 1980; BEARD 1981), toxic effects on the retina (ZIMMERMANN et al. 1973), and damage due to inadvertent intraocular injections (ELLIS 1978; ZINN 1981), while some complications may involve the toxic effect of the vehicle in which the steroid is prepared. Other steroid side effects may involve the interaction of the steroid with other hormones, and may be influenced by regulatory factors in the cellular environment at the time of drug administration. The presence of active infection or the use of other drugs may also influence the development of complications during steroid therapy. It is important to define the mechanisms involved in the different complications of steroid administration in order to understand where it may be possible to limit the clinically significant side effects.

The effects of steroids on corneal wound healing appear to be complex, with differential effects on the various cell types involved in the healing process and different effects for various types of incision (DOHLMAN 1966). It is possible that delaying steroid administration after surgery, or employing less potent steroid formulations and/or less frequent steroid administration, may reduce some of the effects of steroids on corneal wounds (see LORENZETTI 1970). The rapidly destructive corneal ulcers that are associated with steroid therapy presumably involve the uncontrolled release of collagenase; however, a direct interaction of the steroid with the collagenase enzyme, as originally proposed, does not appear to be a promising line of inquiry. It is possible that steroids could exert a direct effect on collagenase by regulating its synthesis or the production of factors which control the activation of this enzyme. Apparently, collagenase activity in the cornea has a critical dependence upon the interaction of epithelial and stromal cells (JOHNSON-WINT 1980). Inflammatory products of lymphocytes and neutrophils may also influence the expression of corneal collagenase (NEWSOME and GROSS 1979). Steroid-induced corneal ulcerations may, of course, result from an alteration in the cellular relationships in the repair process (DONSHIK et al. 1978). Reports of a beneficial effect from progestational steroids in these ulcers may provide new clues to the regulation of corneal collagenase(s) (NEWSOME and GROSS 1977).

There are a number of other complications associated with steroid therapy in which the formulation of the drug may play an important role. In this regard, Newsome et al. (1971) have proposed that the vehicle and not the steroid may be responsible for the mydriasis associated with topical steroid therapy that has been described previously by Armaly (1964). This proposal requires further examination in which different ophthalmic steroids and drug vehicles are compared. It is possible that the drug vehicle may also contribute to the complications associated with inadvertent intraocular steroid injections (Schlaeger and Wilson 1974; Ellis 1978; Byers 1979; Whiteman et al. 1980; Zinn 1981), but a direct effect of the high concentration of steroid has not been totally ruled out. The question of whether steroid-induced changes in the electroretinogram are due to the vehicle or the steroid itself has not been adequately clarified, nor has the clinical importance of this alteration (Zimmerman et al. 1973).

With the development of new methods to deliver drugs to previously inaccessible ocular tissues, it is possible that previously unrecognized complications or advantages of steroid therapy may appear. For each steroid complication, it is important to distinguish receptor-mediated effects of the drugs from other nonspecific steroid effects, some of which may be related to toxicity of the drug vehicle.

4. Systemic Complications

The major metabolic, structural, and functional changes which occur after prolonged use of high-dose systemic steroids have been described as "iatrogenic Cushing's syndrome." Typical features include weight gain with redistribution of fat to the truncal area, moon face, plethora, "buffalo hump," thin skin, easy bruising, osteoporosis, and striae, as well as an increased incidence of infections, psychiatric problems, myopathy and muscle weakness, decreased carbohydrate tolerance, negative nitrogen balance, renal calculi, etc. (Tyrrell and Baxter 1981; Williams et al. 1980). Some of these pathological changes are due to the direct action of steroid hormones on the target tissues. Others may involve the action of other hormones, such as insulin or epinephrine, whose tissue effects are altered by steroid therapy. In either case, it is likely that the steroid hormones exert their influence on tissues by acting directly at the cellular level by binding to cytoplasmic glucocorticoid receptors (present in most tissues of the body) that affect protein synthesis (Baxter and Rousseau 1979). Use of synthetic steroids does not reduce the tendency for the development of cushingoid side effects, although the undesirable mineralocorticoid effects (such as hypokalemia, fluid retention, edema, and hypertension) are markedly less with synthetic steroids than with hydrocortisone or ACTH. An additional problem encountered with ACTH therapy is the production of adrenal androgens, and use of ACTH in females is associated with hirsutism and the development of virilizing features.

Many complications of steroid therapy require weeks or even months to appear. Therefore, short-term therapeutic regimens provide a margin of safety, even if high doses are employed. For example, steroid effects on growth and osteoporosis, which are major concerns in long-term steroid therapy, need not be considered in short-term (high-dose) regimens. Other complications, such as myopathy, skin changes, and cushingoid appearance, likewise require some time to develop. Short-term therapy can be associated with rapid alterations in carbohydrate metabolism, mood changes (usually mood elevation and/or sleeplessness), and suppression of inflammatory and immunologic responses. Hyperosmotic nonketotic coma has been described in apparently healthy individuals receiving short courses of steroids, probably as a result of a latent partial insulin deficiency (Nozik, personal communication). Although such cases are probably extremely rare, it is possible to have patients check their urine for glucose with a dipstick during the course of oral steroid therapy. In any case, patients receiving steroid should be instructed to consult their physicians if any signs of diabetes (e.g., polyuria or polydipsia) occur.

Certain conditions which may be of concern with the use of systemic steroids deserve special consideration. Steroids are contraindicated in most cases of sys-temic infection, except in very unusual circumstances. If active tuberculosis is pres-ent, however, steroids can be used if appropriate antitubercular therapy is em-ployed concomitantly. Reactivation of inactive tuberculosis does not appear with increased frequency in patients receiving chronic steroid therapy (Tyrrell and Baxter 1981) and antitubercular therapy is not indicated unless active disease is present. Steroid therapy alters carbohydrate metabolism, and the insulin dose must be increased appropriately in patients with diabetes mellitus. In rare cases a patient with circulating insulin antibodies may actually show a decrease in insulin require-ment with immunosuppressive doses of steroids.

The presence of peptic ulcer disease is also a matter of concern. It has been clearly established that steroids can induce ulcers in experimental animals, but the evidence in humans is less clear. A controversial evaluation of the literature by Conn and Blitzer (1976) proposes that there is no association between steroid therapy and ulcer formation, but analysis of the data presented in this paper reveals an increasing incidence of ulcers in patients treated with high doses of steroids (Baxter and Tyrrell 1981) and those with cirrhosis and renal disease (which may be associated with a decreased steroid clearance rate). Current recommendations suggest that steroids may be used along with appropriate ulcer therapy and careful medical monitoring (Williams et al. 1980).

Psychological disturbances are another concern with steroid therapy. Mood changes and sleep disturbances can occur even with short courses of steroid. The appearance of major psychological symptomatology does not appear to be directly related to prior psychiatric illness (Tyrrell and Baxter 1981), and a psychiatric history does not contraindicate the use of steroids when required; it seems reason-able, however, to inquire whether there is a history of psychological disorders and to contact the patient's psychiatrist at the time steroid therapy is initiated. Another aspect of the withdrawal of steroids is that some patients demonstrate major symp-toms similar to those of adrenal insufficiency when steroids are discontinued; this is known as the "steroid-withdrawal snydrome" (Amatruda et al. 1965; Dixon and Christy 1965). The physician must guard against administering steroids in the long term because of the psychological component in this syndrome, but it is pos-sible that the change in steroid level may also be accompanied by true physiological alterations. The use of systemic steroids in pregnancy is to be avoided if at all pos-sible, especially during the first trimester (Tyrrell and Baxter 1981). Experimen-tal animal systems show a high incidence of abortion, placental insufficiency, cleft palate, etc. with steroid administration. Fortunately, problems associated with ste-roid therapy during pregnancy in humans have not been as frequent as expected

(SCHATZ et al. 1975; COPE 1977). Surgery in patients who are receiving high-dose systemic steroid therapy, especially abdominal surgery, appears to be particularly troublesome, with poor wound healing and an increased incidence of infection and electrolyte imbalance as potential risks.

Suppression of the hypothalamic–pituitary–adrenal (HPA) axis can result in a relative adrenal insufficiency and, occasionally, addisonian crisis after withdrawal of steroid therapy. Usually, a gradual tapering of the steroid dose is employed, although it is possible that a switch to alternate-day therapy may be useful (WILLIAMS et al. 1980). Patients who are appropriately tapered to maintenance steroid doses of 5 mg prednisone may continue to show a diminished adrenal response to stressful stimuli until the axis has fully recovered (BYNNY 1976). This could be important, because significantly more steroids may be required in the case of major accidents, surgery, and infections. Less acute situations, such as dental extractions and upper respiratory infections, may also require additional steroids. A variety of different tests are available to assess the HPA axis, including the metyrapone, ACTH, and insulin tolerance tests (see TYRRELL and BAXTER 1981), but if there is no time to perform a test the patient should receive sufficiently high steroid therapy for surgery or major stress. The most rigorous one is the insulin tolerance test, which gives a reasonable but not absolute assurance that the patient can withstand stress. Even with normal results of the test, the possibility of some degree of adrenal insufficiency remains a concern for the severe stress accompanying surgery.

The degree of adrenal suppression has been correlated with the dose, duration, and time of day at which specific steroids are administered (NICHOLS et al. 1965; LIVANOU et al. 1967; STRECK and LOCKWOOD 1979), although individual variability does exist. If steroids are administered for 7–10 days in relatively high doses (greater than 60 mg of prednisone), a certain amount of adrenal insufficiency may be expected. The axis usually recovers quickly, and the return of adrenal function is essentially inevitable even with major suppression of the HPA axis, given sufficient time. Patients who have received long-term high-dose therapy may show major adrenal suppression and need careful follow-up for up to a year before the HPA axis is fully recovered. In cases of adrenal the use of ACTH to "prime" the adrenal cortex is not generally recommended insufficiency secondary to steroid administration. The effectiveness of this therapy may be limited by a suppression of endogenous ACTH production which might delay full recovery (see TYRRELL and BAXTER 1981).

D. Cellular and Molecular Mechanisms

I. The Immune System

Immunologic and inflammatory reactions defined in nonocular tissues are also likely to participate in the pathogenesis of ocular disease (LEOPOLD 1974; SILVERSTEIN 1974; KAUFMAN 1974; O'CONNOR 1975, 1981 a, b; DAVIES and BONNEY 1981). The expression of immune responses involves interaction of several interdependent cell populations. Some of these are presented schematically in Fig. 13. An awareness of the immune cell interactions in both cell-mediated and antibody-mediated pathways is necessary in order to understand the actions of steroids and nonsteroi-

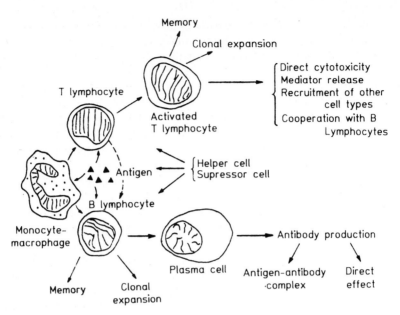

Fig. 13. Cellular interactions involved in the development of T and B lymphocyte activation. The macrophage is a central cell type in both cell-mediated and antibody-mediated immune pathways. (FAUCI 1979)

dal agents. The interaction of different cells is required for the expression of immune responses (for example, see the numerous relationships the monocyte-machrophage demonstrates with T lymphocytes and B lymphocytes, as well as with helper cells and suppressor cells). Thus a drug effect on a cell type not directly involved in tissue injury may be an important consequence. Furthermore, a steroid effect on a sensitive cell type (such as the macrophage or T lymphocyte) can have a subsequent effect through these cellular interactions on the immune response of a more steroid-resistant cell type (for example, lymphocyte or plasma cell). Steroid effects on immune cell interaction may also be modulated by preventing entry of the cell into an inflammatory locus. Glucocorticoids also suppress the production of specific inflammatory mediators. These cellular and molecular mechanisms are reviewed in the following section.

1. Leukocyte Kinetics and Function

Glucocorticoids alter the kinetics of circulating immune cells by altering the entry as well as disappearance of leukocytes from the circulation and other compartments such as the thymus, lymphocyte glands, and bone marrow; steroids also decrease the ability of certain leukocyte populations to accumulate at the site of inflammation, and influence specialized functional properties of cells involved in effector immune responses (see review by FAUCI 1979). Qualitatively different steroid effects are observed in certain steroid-sensitive species (such as the rat, mouse, and rabbit) as compared to those in more resistant species (such as man, monkey, and guinea pig) (CLAMAN 1975). The differences between the qualitative sensitivity and resistance to steroids can ultimately be understood on the basis of quantitative differences at the cellular level (see FAHEY et al. 1981).

With increased adrenocorticosteroid activity and administration of extracts of the adrenal cortex (SELYE 1936, 1946; INGLE 1938; DOUGHTERTY and WHITE 1944), profound decrease in lymphoid cells and tissues have been observed in steroid-sensitive species. Administration of even moderate doses of steroids in sensitive animals results in involution of thymus tissue and extensive lymphocyte cell death. These dramatic effects on rat and mouse lymphocytes are dependent upon the binding of steroid hormones to specific glucocorticoid receptors and the subsequent regulation of specific protein synthesis (MUNCK and YOUNG 1975; MUNCK et al. 1979). Steroid effects in human leukocytes also appear to be mediated through similar receptor mechanisms (BAXTER and HARRIS 1975; FAUCI 1979; FAHEY et al. 1981), but the changes observed are considerably less dramatic and lymphocyte cell death is usually not prominent (except possibly in the treatment of leukemia [LIPPMANN 1979]).

In man, it is likely that the effects of steroid therapy are the result of more subtle changes (such as alterations in the distribution of circulating leukocytes and inhibition of the ability of certain immune effector cells to accumulate at inflammatory sites [FAUCI 1979]). In addition, steroid-induced alterations in leukocyte kinetics may affect the movement of these cells to an from lymphoid compartments, such as in the thymus and lymph nodes, and thereby suppress important cellular interactions required for the development of immune responses. In support of this concept, HARRIS and BAXTER (1979) have discussed changes in the distribution of immune cells in the thymus with steroid therapy.

Table 11 summarizes some of the alterations in leukocyte kinetics and function with appear to be particularly applicable to the human systems, primarily derived from reviews by FAUCI (1979) and PARRILLO and FAUCI (1979), and with some additional data from FAHEY et al. (1981). One important aspect of steroid effects on human immune cells is that the various leukocyte populations show different degrees of sensitivity to steroid therapy.

When the effects of systemic steroids on lymphocyte populations are examined, T lymphocytes (which are the major cell type in the recirculating lymphocyte pool) appear considerably more sensitive to steroid-induced changes than B lymphocytes. The relative resistance of B lymphocytes and plasma cells probably accounts for the inability of even high doses of steroids to inhibit production of specific antibodies. If steroids are administered experimentally with the antigenic challenge, antibody production can be inhibited, probably as a result of steroid effects on other cell types, such as the macrophage. All T lymphocyte functions are not equally sensitive to steroids when assessed by standard immunologic tests. For example, responses to antigens are reportedly suppressed more readily than responses to nonspecific mitogens, such as phytohemagglutinin (BALOW et al. 1975; VISCHER 1972). It has also been observed that the autologous mixed leukocyte reaction is suppressed more readily than the allogenic mixed leukocyte reaction; this has led investigators to speculate that the steroids normally present in the circulation may serve to suppress autoimmune reactions (ILFELD et al. 1977). According to PARILLO and FAUCI (1979), the production of lymphokines (antibody-mediated cellular immunity) is generally unaffected by steroid therapy. However, CRABTREE et al.

Table 11. Steroid-induced alterations in leukocyte kinetics and function

Observations	Current evidence	Comment
Lymphocytes		
Circulating lympho-cytopenia	Redistribution into other lymphoid compartments; no lymphocytolysis of resting cells in humans and other steroid-resistant species; possibly some lymphocytolysis of activated lymphocytes	Recirculating pool most affected, T lymphocytes affected to a greater degree than non-T lymphocytes
Suppression of delayed hypersensitivity	Effect of lymphokines on monocyte-macrophages inhibited	This effect may be due to a direct steroid effect on the macrophages, since lymphokine production was not affected. Other studies indicate some steroid effect on specific lymphocyte products
Suppression of lymphocyte proliferation	Responses to antigens more readily affected than responses to mitogens (such as phytohemagglutinin); production of cell growth factor affected at relatively low steroid concentrations	Emphasizes steroid inhibition of specific lymphocyte responses; effect of steroids on T cell proliferative factor may explain inhibition of phytohemagglutinin response
Suppression of mixed leukocyte reactions	Physiological concentrations of steroids suppress autologous mixed leukocyte reaction, higher concentrations suppress allogenic mixed leukocyte reaction	Consistent with potential physiological role of steroids to prevent T cell autoimmune reactions to self-antigens
Suppression of T-lymphocyte-mediated cytotoxicity	Only demonstrated with high in vitro concentrations	Antibody-dependent cell-mediated immunity not decreased
Antibody production by B cells relatively unaffected	Minor effect on immunoglobulin levels (increased catabolism and decreased synthesis) during active antibody production, but no significant effect on polyclonal immunoglobulin production	Experimentally induced reductions in antibody occur only if steroid administered concurrently with antigenic challenge
Monocyte-macrophage		
Circulating mono-cytopenia	Redistribution of cells and inhibition of release from bone marrow	Subsets of monocytes may be affected

Table 11 (continued)

Observations	Current evidence	Comment
Inhibition of accumulation at inflammatory loci	Macrophage response to lymphokines blocked; decreased monocyte plasminogen activator may contribute to reduced ability to enter inflammatory loci	Possible role of monocytopenia; however, monocyte-macrophage accumulation blocked after circulating monocyte levels return to normal during alternate-day therapy
Decreased functional activity	Monocyte-macrophage functions appear relatively sensitive to steroids, but conflicting information exists regarding steroid effects on bactericidal activity and lysosomal enzymes	Variable steroid effects on phagocytosis in animal models; recent studies do demonstrate a decrease in Fc receptor sites; decreased removal of antibody-coated target cells observed after chronic steroid administration
Decreased granuloma formulation	May be related to above phenomena	Steroid inhibition of macrophage development not adequately assessed in humans
Neutrophil Circulating neutrophilia	Accelerated release from bone marrow; reduced adherence to blood vessels	Could involve direct steroid effects on properties of the neutrophil, endothelial cells, or possibly the induction of a soluble factor
Inhibition of accumulation at inflammatory loci	Reduced adherence to vascular endothelium: steroids do not inhibit chemotaxis at doses that can be readily attained or sustained in vivo	Probable major mechanism for steroid suppression of neutrophil effects
Functional activities relatively steroid-resistant	May have an effect on release of lysosomal products, but no effect on phagocytic or bactericidal ability at usually attainable concentrations	Concept of lysosomal stabilization probably not functional in vivo; steroid lysis and stabilization of membranes at suprapharmacologic doses possibly due to nonspecific detergent effects
Eosinophils Circulating eosinopenia	Probably secondary to redistribution	Eosinopenia initially used to evaluate the structural activity and dose-responses of different steroids
Decreased migration into immediate hypersensitivity sites	Preliminary evaluations in dermatology only	Steroid effects on this cell type in relation to allergic and parasitic phenomena need further investigation

(1979) have recently demonstrated that moderate doses of dexamethasone can suppress the production of T cell proliferative factors, and that this effect may help to explain steroid inhibition of mitogenic responses by lymphocytes. It is worth noting that the steroid sensitivity of lymphoid cells appears to depend upon the developmental stage of these cells during the immune process. Baxter and Harris (1975) propose that some cells have a decreased sensitivity to steroids as they become more committed in their immune development. Another possible change in steroid sensitivity has been reported with the activation of human lymphocytes by Galili et al. (1980); the T lymphocytes stimulated in mixed lymphocyte cultures appeared more sensitive to steroid-mediated cell lysis than other lymphocytes (although the hormone concentrations employed in this study suggest a nonspecific effect).

When the monocyte-macrophage system is considered, most evidence points to this cell type as being quite sensitive to steroids, with major effects observed in both cell kinetics and function. Steroid effects on the macrophage may be relatively long-lived compared to effects on other leukocytes. In support of this concept, Dale et al. (1974) reported that macrophage accumulations at inflammatory loci remained depressed on the off day of alternate-day therapy, while neutrophil accumulation had already returned to normal. Interestingly, the effect on macrophage accumulation persisted even after circulating monocytes no longer showed a change in their kinetics. This suggests that steroids may have a specific effect on the macrophage, inducing changes in the structure and function of this cell type which differ from the effect on the monocyte. Alternatively, there may be subpopulations of monocytes which have a differential response to steroids, but these possibilities have not been investigated adequately. Some evidence demonstrates that steroids may exert specific effects on certain macrophage populations, i.e., effector macrophages appear particularly sensitive to steroids when tested in models for delayed hypersensitivity reactions (Rosenthal and Balow 1980). Claman (1975) has suggested that steroids may influence the cell surface of the effector macrophage, accounting for the decreased ability of lymphokines to recruit these cells for type IV immune reactions (see Fig. 14). Certain macrophage functions, such as those involved in phagocytosis and antigen processing, are reportedly resistant to steroids (Fauci 1979; Parrillo and Fauci 1979). Recent evidence does suggest, however, that the Fc-receptors involved in monocyte-macrophage functions are relatively sensitive to steroids, through an effect on the production of Fc-receptor-augmenting factor (Fahey et al. 1981). A number of other macrophage functions may also respond to relatively low steroid concentrations, including the ability to secrete plasminogen activator (Vassalli et al. 1976; Werb 1978) and neutral proteases (Werb et al. 1978) and the ability to express bactericidal activity (see Fahey et al. 1981).

Steroid effects on neutrophils have also received substantial attention, but investigation of the mechanisms of these effects is often confused by the original concept of "lysosomal stabilization" proposed by Weissmann and Thomas (1963). More recent considerations of the lysosomal stabilization theory have been unfavorable, and the supposedly direct interactions of the steroids with cell membranes are observed only at extremely high drug concentrations (between 10^{-4} and 10^{-5} M), and are probably due to a nonspecific detergent-like action of the steroids (e.g.,, see

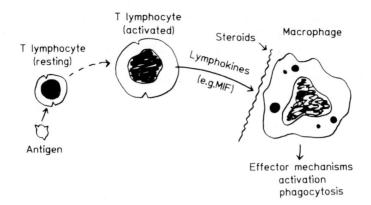

Fig. 14. Proposal that steroid hormones block the effect of lymphokines on the macrophage, possibly by an alteration of macrophage cell membrane. *MIF*, macrophage migration inhibitory factor (CLAMAN 1975)

THOMPSON 1979 b; FAHEY et al. 1981). Further, lysosomal stabilization was proposed before the current knowledge of glucocorticoid hormone action was achieved, and the stabilization does not show the appropriate specificity for anti-inflammatory steroids. Also, a lysis as well as stabilization can be observed (BRIGGS and BROTHERTON 1970). FAUCI (1979) proposes that the most important of steroids on neutrophils is achieved indirectly by inhibiting the access of this cell type to the inflammatory locus, rather than a direct action of steroids on neutrophil function. The inhibition of neutrophil accumulation at the site of inflammation appears relatively sensitive to steroids, since moderate doses of steroids influence this process. The mechanism for the decreased access of to neutrophils to sites of inflammation is unknown, but recent evidence suggests that steroids induce a soluble factor which may contribute to this effect (MACGREGOR 1976). Although the alteration of neutrophil kinetics is undoubtedly important in explaining some steroid effects on these cells, it is not possible to rule out a direct effect on an important neutrophil function at the present time. It has been proposed that steroid therapy may selectively inhibit the release of certain lysosomes (see DAVIES et al. 1981); but if this is confirmed, it will probably not involve a direct interaction of the steroid to stabilize lysosomal membranes.

HILLS et al. (1948) and FORSHAM et al. (1948) demonstrated that adrenal stimulation in man also resulted in a decrease in circulating eosinophils. Since this time, eosinopenia has proven to be a useful quantitative indicator of the systemic potency of a given steroid regimen. However, the possible importance of steroid effects on eosinophils in inflammatory processes has not been assessed adequately, although it is likely that steroid administration decrease the number of eosinophils at immediate hypersensitivity sites (PARRILLO and FAUCI 1979). Further investigation is needed to define steroid effects on eosinophils and other cell types, such as basophils, mast cells, and tissue cells, which participate in a variety of specialized immune and inflammatory processes.

The differential sensitivity of immune cells may underlie the effectiveness of steroids in ocular anti-inflammatory therapy. If steroid-sensitive cells are a major part of the active disease process, a major therapeutic effect is expected. Conversely, a minimal therapeutic effect is expected when the cells involved in the pathogenic process are relatively steroid-resistant. Sarcoid and other granulomatous diseases of the eye, in which T cells and macrophages appear to have a prominent role, usually respond well to steroid hormone therapy. As mentioned, T lymphocytes and macrophages are thought to be particularly responsive to anti-inflammatory steroids. Some of the problems reported with the use of steroids in the presence of active infections (e.g., tuberculosis, parasitic infections, herpes simplex may be due to the relative sensitivity of the immune cells responsible for the host defense to steroids, possibly the effector macrophage and/or the T cell. On the other hand, steroids do not markedly alter the disease course in Fuchs' syndrome, in which B cells and mature antibody-forming cells are prominent. As mentioned, B cells and plasma cells are generally thought to be less responsive to steroids than other leukocytes. Also in Fuchs' syndrome, steroids may produce a transient amelioration of symptoms, with the cells involved in the underlying pathogenic process remaining unaffected. This effect probably involves the suppression of inflammatory mediators released from local cells or from more steroid responsive immune cells. It is possible that the symptomatic relief obtained with steroid therapy in optic neuritis may be similarly explained.

The sensitivity of certain immune cells to steroids and the resistance of others may partially explain the rebound destruction of corneal tissues which can occur if steroids are withdrawn rapidly in cases of herpes simplex. Viral infections of the eye, such as herpes simplex, involve complex immune mechanisms (including both antibody-mediated and cell-mediated reactions in stromal disease: MEYERS and PETTIT 1974; METCALF and KAUFMAN 1976; NAGY et al. 1980; NESBURN 1981) that may participate in both host defense and tissue destruction. As mentioned earlier, moderate doses of steroids block the migration of leukocytes into the site of injury and also prevent the recruitment and, perhaps, function of destructive macrophages. During the time that these effector cells are blocked, the production of antibodies and/or lymphokines can continue, since these processes are generally steroid-resistant. The buildup of the antibodies and lymphokines may then provide a strong signal for an aggressive immune response if steroid therapy is withdrawn too rapidly. Other explanations of the rebound syndrome are possible.

2. Vascular and Inflammatory Effects

Some of the anti-inflammatory actions of steroids may be mediated by vascular effects and/or by a regulation of inflammatory mediators at the site of injury. MENKIN (1940) was the first to demonstrate that adrenal extracts prevented the increase in vascular permeability usually observed following injection of inflammatory products. However, he attributed these observations to a general physiological effect of steroids on vascular permeability, rather than an anti-inflammatory effect. With the availability of cortisone and ACTH, a number of investigators began to study steroid anti-inflammatory effects (see INGLE 1950). WOODS and WOOD (1950) examined steroid-induced inhibition of ocular inflammatory reactions in conjunctivitis and iritis following foreign protein injection into the anterior chamber of the eye, and EBERT and BARCLAY (1952) observed steroid inhibition of the allergic response in the rabbit ear chamber.

Direct vasoconstrictive effects of steroids on arterioles and venules were described by ASHTON and COOK (1952). ZWEIFACH et al. (1953) showed that vasoconstrictive actions of steroids were modulated by the arteriolar response to epinephrine or norepinephrine. Although substantial attention has been given to the interaction of steroid hormones and catecholamines on blood vessels, it is quite possible that this effect is distinct from the ability of steroids to protect vascular integrity during inflammation (see, e.g., KAZUO and TSURUFUJI 1981).

ALLISON et al. (1955) suggested that the action of cortisone on inflammation might be due to a protective effect on vascular endothelial cells and leukocytes, to account for the decreased leukocyte adherence and decreased migration into the inflamed area. WEISSMANN and THOMAS (1963) suggested that steroids might prevent inflammatory responses by directly stabilizing lysosomal membranes.

It has become apparent that some therapeutic actions of steroids might be due to a direct or indirect interaction with these vasoactive mediators. SCHAYER (1963) proposed that glucocorticoid-induced vasoconstriction may physiologically antagonize histamine-induced vasodilation. Other studies have investigated the role of glucocorticoids in antagonizing the kinin system of vasoactive peptides (CLINE and MELMON 1966; SUDDICK 1966), and later TSURUFUJI et al. (1979, 1980) reported that dexamethasone in some systems can block the inflammatory effects of bradykinin.

Of particular interest has been the concept that corticosteroids might inhibit prostaglandin production or release from tissues and thereby suppress inflammatory responses (see KANTROWITZ et al. 1975; LEWIS and PIPER 1975; FLOMAN and ZOR 1977; DAVIES et a. 1981). Prostaglandin release from damaged tissues has been proposed as a major mechanism for the production of the cardinal signs of inflammation after injury in the eye and other tissues (see Chaps. 7 and 10b), and the anti-inflammatory action of aspirin-like drugs probably involves prostaglandin pathways by inhibition of fatty acid cyclooxygenase, the key enzyme which acts on arachidonic acid for prostaglandin synthesis. It was appreciated that other putative inflammatory mediators could be derived from arachidonic acid. These other inflammatory mediators are derived by the action of lipoxygenases rather than cyclooxygenases. Normally the amount of arachidonic acid available is the rate-limiting step in the production of prostaglandins and other inflammatory mediators. The release of arachidonic acid is controlled to a large extent by phospholipase A_2 on phospholipids in cell membranes (Table 12). A considerable amount of evidence has accumulated over the last 5 years (see FLOWER 1981) to indicate that corticosteroids exert some of their anti-inflammatory effects by an inhibition of phospholipase A_2 activity. Recently, it has been reported that corticosteroids induce the biosynthesis of an inhibitor of phospholipase A_2 (FLOWER and BLACKWELL 1979; CARNUCCIO et al. 1980), and that the inhibitor can mimic the anti-inflammatory effects of steroids. Although this mechanism of steroid action may only be part of the story, it provides an exciting experimental lead to understanding the anti-inflammatory effects of steroids, by themselves and in relation to the actions of nonsteroidal anti-inflammatory agents.

Table 12. Some putative proinflammatory mediators generated from arachidonic acid and their interrelationships. (FLOWER 1981)

Prostaglandins	Hydroxyacids	Leukotrienes
Fever Erythema Edema Hyperalgesia	Leukocyte chemotaxis	Leukocyte chemotaxis, bronchospasm (increases in vascular permeability?)

Membrane phospholipids

|

(Phospholipase A$_2$)

|
↓

Prostaglandins ← (cyclooxygenase) — arachidonic acid — (lipoxygenases) → hydroxyacids, leukotrines

3. Ocular Immune Mechanisms

Direct observation is often possible in studies of steroid effects on immunologic and inflammatory processes in the eye. The interpretation of the therapeutic response is complicated by the fact that each ocular tissue represents an individual setting for the expression of immune responses (O'CONNOR 1981 a, b; FRIEDLAEN-DER 1979, 1981). Few data are available. Inflammatory responses in the eye may be altered by many stimuli, including neuronal mechanisms, individual reactions to irritation, injury, and surgery, as well as the host response to infectious agents. The eyelids, conjunctiva, cornea, uveal tract, etc. all have distinctive anatomic structures and possess unique cellular and biochemical environments that can influence ocular responses to inflammatory stimuli. In attempting to rationalize and quantify the therapeutic use of steroids in ocular tissues, it will therefore be useful to define individual steroid effects on specific cell types, both local cells and circulating leukocytes. By understanding direct steroid effects on these cells in the context of their hormonal environment, it may be possible to develop improved models for steroid therapy in the eye.

II. The Glucocorticoid Receptor

It has become apparent that most of the effects of glucocorticoid hormones are mediated by specialized steroid receptor proteins (BAXTER and ROUSSEAU 1979; MUNCK et al. 1979). These glucocorticoid receptors are present in virtually all cells, and this ubiquity probably contributes to the many different physiological and pharmacologic effects observed after corticosteroid hormone administration. There are also other classes of steroid hormone receptors for mineralocorticoids, estrogens, androgens, and progestins. These receptors have a more restricted distribution (McLEOD and BAXTER 1980) and are probably not involved in the therapeutic effects of anti-inflammatory steroids.

1. The Target Cell

A target cell is defined as a cell which responds to the actions of a given drug or hormone. Most cells are likely to be target cells for corticosteroid hormones because of the widespread distribution of glucocorticoid receptors. A steroid target cell uses its glucocorticoid receptors as highly specialized receivers to distinguish glucocorticoid hormonal signals from background noise produced by other hormones and molecules which impinge upon the cell (BAXTER and FUNDER 1979). Once received, the signal is relayed in a manner which allows for a specialized response. Figure 15 presents in diagrammatic form some of the basic steps in the action of steroid hormones (glucocorticoids) on an idealized target cell.

Circulating glucocorticoids are partially bound to plasma corticosteroid-binding globulin and albumin and partially free or unbound. Free steroid hormone concentrations are not readily measured in tissues, but will have an important influence on the steroid response because only the free hormone is able to influence cell function (BALLARD 1979). The unbound hormone passes through the cell membrane, which does not limit steroid penetration but may in some systems provide for specialized transport (BALLARD 1979).

Once inside the cell, the steroid binds in a reversible manner to the glucocorticoid receptor proteins present in the cytoplasm. There is evidence that the binding of an active hormone to the glucocorticoid receptor results in a conformational

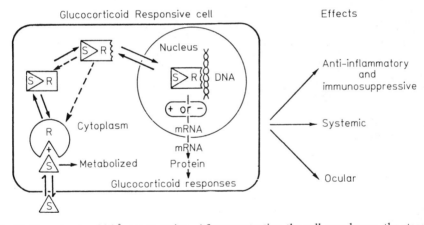

Fig. 15. Steps in steroid hormone action. After penetrating the cell membrane, the steroid (*S*) combines with the receptor (*R*), altering its conformation. S · R then binds chromatin and stimulates (or represses) the synthesis of specific mRNA species. Consequently, the changes in mRNAs result in alterations in the synthesis of specific proteins that mediate steroid hormone responses. (Adapted from BAXTER and HARRIS 1975) Steroid-induced alterations in protein synthesis appear to be individualized for different target cells. This permits steroids to modulate many specialized cellular responses in a wide range of differentiated tissues. Although the specialized responses to steroids (and possible interactions with other hormones) in specific target cells need considerably more investigation, it is likely that the in vivo effects of steroids will involve similar receptor-mediated mechanisms. The immunosuppressive and anti-inflammatory, as well as the systemic and ocular, effects of steroids are likely to involve a direct glucocorticoid effect on protein synthesis, but may also involve the interaction of other hormones in the expression of the steroid response

change in the receptor necessary for the subsequent expression of the steroid effect (ROUSSEAU and BAXTER 1979; SHERMAN 1979). Inactive glucocorticoids do not bind effectively to the receptor and do not induce the appropriate conformational change, while antagonists may induce a different conformational change in the receptor, which blocks further steps in glucocorticoid action. Recent kinetic studies of steroid antagonists suggest that these steroids have a very rapid "off-rate," and the antagonist-receptor complex may not be stable enough to allow transduction of the hormone signal (NGUYEN and BAXTER, personal communication).

When agonists bind to receptors, an activation step occurs wich leads to translocation of the steroid-receptor complex into the nucleus (HIGGINS et al. 1979). The step of nuclear tanslocation of the steroid-receptor complex is necessary for the subsequent regulation of gene transcription. Nuclear translocation is usually completed within 30–40 min following dexamethasone addition, and more rapidly (within 10 min) following hydrocortisone addition to target cells (MUNCK et al. 1979). The molecular mechanisms by which the steroid-receptor complex interacts with nuclear receptor sites and then alters chromatin structure and/or function are under active investigation in many laboratories; hormone regulation of eukaryotic gene expression provides challenges which are at the frontier of molecular biological research. In any case, the major result of the interaction of the steroid–receptor complex with chromatin is to modulate the levels of specific mRNA species: these may be influenced in either a positive or negative direction. Once the mRNA is transcribed from the appropriate part of the DNA code (and has been processed), it leaves the nucleus and enters the cytoplasm, where it serves as a template for the synthesis of specific proteins. Only certain mRNA species are regulated by steroid hormones. Thus only a limited number of proteins synthesized are affected. In fact, when the "domain" of the cellular response to glucocorticoids was evaluated by two-dimensional gel electrophoresis (O'FARRELL and IVARIE 1979), the steroid-induced changes in protein synthesis was restricted to less than 1% of the polypeptide products. The regulation of specific protein synthesis and the onset of the steroid response can be relatively rapid (e.g., within 1–2 h), but there is usually a perceptible time lag in which inhibitors of protein synthesis will prevent the appearance of the steroid effect (PETERKOFSKY and TOMKINS 1967; THOMPSON 1979 a).

The regulated production of specific proteins through the mechanism outlined above provides a means by which steroids can control a large number of individual physiological effects in diverse target tissues. Evidence from model cell systems has demonstrated that steroids can induce diverse changes and can influence the synthesis of important cytoplasmic proteins, including enzymes, result in alterations in cell surface proteins and cell transport mechanisms, and regulate the synthesis and secretion of extracellular protein products, including other hormones and local mediators of inflammation (see reviews by BAXTER and ROUSSEAU 1979; FAHEY et al. 1981). The specific gene products which are modulated by steroids are dependent upon the differentiated properties of the target cells; clearly, the ability of individual cell types to respond differently to the steroid hormone stimulus is at the foundation of the many different regulatory effects observed after steroid administration. The regulation of protein synthesis as outlined above provides the general mechanism by which steroids exert their effects on the different target cells. However, there are some cases which may appear to involve other steroid hormone

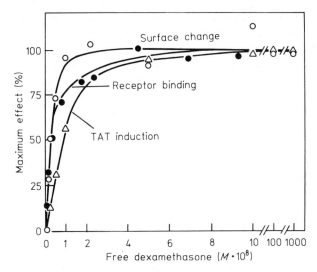

Fig. 16. Correlation between glucocorticoid-receptor binding, induction of tyrosine amino-transferase (*TAT*), and change in cell surface adhesion in rat hepatoma cells. Replotted from data compiled by ROUSSEAU (1974)

mechanisms, e.g., when a very rapid steroid response is required for the regulation of ACTH secretion (BAXTER and TYRRELL 1981).

Figure 16 illustrates the binding of dexamethasone to glucocorticoid receptors in rat hepatoma cells, one of the original cell systems used to investigate steroid hormone action (SAMUELS and TOMPKINS 1970). Figure 16 (from ROUSSEAU 1974) shows that a close correlation exists between receptor binding, the induction of a change in the adhesive properties of the cell surface, and the induction of a specific enzyme, tyrosine aminotransferase, after addition of dexamethasone to the cells. Receptor binding and cellular response are proportionately related over a wide range of hormone concentrations. Hormone binding as well as the observed cellular responses are saturable at relatively low drug concentrations.

For many biological responses involving the glucocorticoid receptor, the levels of steroid required are considerably lower than the concentrations employed in ophthalmic steroid preparations. In Fig. 16, maximal receptor binding of dexamethasone is achieved at 500 nM, which is equivalent to a 0.00002% solution. Even if only 1% of the steroid applied to the eye is absorbed, and even on the assumption that not all of the steroid will be in the unbound form when it reaches the target tissue, it is clear from a consideration of these data that new methods of steroid drug delivery are indicated to achieve the desired therapeutic effects with much less steroid than has commonly been employed.

2. Cellular Sensitivity and Modulation of Steroid Responses

The sensitivity of different target cells in the immune system and in ocular tissues to corticosteroid represents another important variable to consider in evaluating the effects of anti-inflammatory therapy. Also, variations in the cellular sensitivity to steroids could play a role in the development of side effects, such as glaucoma and cataract. The specific factors which regulate the cellular sensitivity to steroids in ocular tissues are unknown, but there are several levels at which the modulation of steroid sensitivity could occur: alterations in receptor-binding characteristics, the activation and translocation of the steroid-receptor complex to the nucleus, interaction of the complex with chromatin, transmission of the hormonal signal into mRNA and protein products, or subsequent steps in the expression of a differentiated response (as recently reviewed by HARRIS and BAXTER 1979). Evidence supporting modifications of cellular sensitivity at each of these steps has been primarily derived from genetic selection of steroid-resistant lymphoma cells in vitro. However, it is unlikely that similar selection pressures are relevant to the use of steroids in anti-inflammatory therapy in vivo. There is some evidence that steroid selection of resistant populations may play a role in determining the therapeutic response when steroids are employed in therapy for leukemia (LIPPMAN 1979). In the case of leukemia, differences in the number of glucocorticoid receptors have been useful in predicting the sensitivity of transformed cells to steroid, but this has not been the case for normal cell types. For example, although T cells and monocytes are more steroid-sensitive than B cells, this finding is not explained by differences in the characteristics or receptor binding (LIPPMAN 1979; HARRIS and BAXTER 1979). Also, major increases in glucocorticoid receptors accompany mitogen stimulation of lymphocytes, but this increase did not predict the sensitivity of the cells to steroid inhibition (MUNCK et al. 1979).

Recently, SCHWARTZ (1981a) has a reviewed mechanisms by which cellular sensitivity to hormones is regulated. One of the important possibilities raised by this review is whether the cellular sensitivity to glucocorticoids could be regulated by the homologous hormone. BLOOM et al. (1980) showed this to be unlikely for at least one glucocorticoid-responsive system. Prior exposure of rat hepatoma cells to dexamethasone resulted in no change in the number, affinity, or nuclear translocation of glucocorticoid receptors. Also, the ability of the cells to respond to steroids in the production of a specific protein product (tyrosine aminotransferase) was not diminished by the dexamethasone exposure. This response to glucocorticoid hormones contrasts with the finding that a "down-regulation" of the receptors occurs after addition of the homologous hormone for insulin (other polypeptides) and catecholamine receptors. Glucocorticoid receptors are also different from a variety of membrane receptors which show evidence for an "uncoupling" of receptors from effector pathways, an important mechanism by which decreased cellular sensitivity to repeated catecholamine stimulation occurs.

Hormones other than steroids can markedly alter the response to steroids at the cellular level. A full glucocorticoid effect may not be observed unless the target cell is exposed to the appropriate hormonal environment. For example, in cultured rat pituitary cells, thyroid hormone is necessary for the full induction of synthesis of growth hormone by glucocorticoids (MARTIAL et al. 1979). In isolated hepatocytes, cAMP or glucagon is required for induction of tyrosine aminotransferase (GRANNER 1979). Some of the interactions of glucocorticoids with other hormones are termed "permissive." One particularly interesting modulation of the glucocorticoid response was illustrated by JOHNSON et al. (1979). A variety of environmental conditions and, particularly, addition of cAMP to cultured GHl cells results in a reversal of steroid effects on specific gene synthesis. These investigators reported

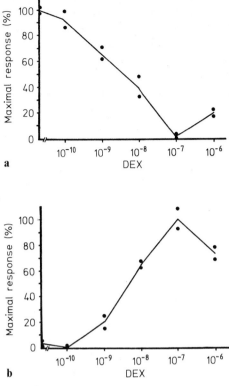

Fig. 17a, b. Effect of 36-h exposure to dexamethasone (*DEX*), as measured by ^3H-thymidine uptake (6-h labeling) in cultured human skin fibroblasts. Dexamethasone was added at differing doses to (**a**) cells in the logarithmic phase of growth and (**b**) cells at very high density, close to confluency

that dexamethasone repressed rather than stimulated specific gene products in the presence of cAMP.

These observations may be applicable to the effects of steroids on growing fibroblasts (ZUMBRUN and POLANSKY, unpublished data). As shown in Fig. 17, dexamethasone could either inhibit (Fig. 17a) or stimulate (Fig. 17b) the incorporation of ^3H-thymidine (used as a measure of cell growth). These opposite effects were induced at comparable hormone concentrations, but the cell cultures differed in their degree of confluency. Inhibition of cell division was characteristically observed during the active phase of cell proliferation when the cells were at low densitiy. Stimulation was observed during the late log phase of growth, as the cell cultures were at high density near confluency. It is possible that intracellular cAMP or other factors which increase at high cell density may help to explain these observations. Although the mechanisms involved in this dramatic modulation of dexamethasone effects require considerably more study, this example illustrates the more general finding that changes in the cellular environment can determine the response observed after steroid administration.

Thus the therapeutic response to steroids may be changed by altering the local cellular environment, for example, by using agents such as antimetabolites or inhibitors of prostaglandin pathways, or by employing other agents which can affect cells. Also, changes in steroid responsiveness with cell density may help to explain why early proliferation of cells in corneal wounds is particularly sensitive to steroids, and only slight effects of steroids are observed later.

As indicated earlier, a generalized cellular defect in steroid responsiveness is probably not present in glaucoma (POLANSKY et al., to be published; McCARTY et al. 1981), but an altered cellular environment might explain increased sensitivity to steroids in patients with primary open-angle glaucoma. For example, the disparate reports of the steroid sensitivity of peripheral blood lymphocytes in glaucoma might be due to a modulation of steroid responses to circulating factors, such as epinephrine in certain patient populations studied. It is also reasonable to consider that circulating or local factors could play a prominent role in altering the sensitivity of ocular cells to steroids in patients with primary open-angle glaucoma. A search for these factors could prove profitable.

3. Permissive Effects and Hormonal Interactions

INGLE (1952) succinctly stated the hypothesis that many of the metabolic effects of steroids were permissive, and could be attributed to the role of steroids as general tissues hormones. His studies of the effects of adrenal hormones on a variety of tissues suggested that steroids "support the capacity of tissues to attain maximal rates of metabolic processes." As reviewed more recently by GRANNER (1979), some of the actions of steroids on metabolism have been shown to involve the action and interaction of many different hormones. GRANNER suggests that the permissive action of glucocorticoid hormones on metabolic processes can best be understood by considering the role of steroids as biological "amplifiers" in specific target tissues. At first this may appear to be a new mechanism for steroid hormone action, but most evidence suggests that the permissive effects of steroids involve the induction of specific protein products, similar to the direct action of steroids on target cells discussed previously. However, in the case of permissive actions, the steroid-induced protein products act as obligate or enhancing factor to amplify the effects of other hormones. An example is provided by the amplification of epinephrine effects by steroids; steroids enhance the effects of epinephrine on vascular reactivity, cardiovascular function, glucose uptake in lymphocytes, and gluconeogenesis in the liver. Steroids also appear to amplify the effects of a wide range of other hormones, e.g., insulin-induced gluconeogenesis in the liver and thyroid-simulating hormone effects on the thyroid gland.

GRANNER suggests that many of the interactions of steroids with other hormones occur at the level of the "second messenger" in target cells, possibly involving the effects of intracellular cAMP and/or intracellular calcium. In this regard, there is considerable evidence that cAMP is a major pathway through which catecholamines, polypeptide hormones, and prostaglandins exert some of their regulatory effects on target cells. Additionally, the studies of BOURNE et al. (1974) have emphasized that hormones which influence the cAMP levels in cells of the immune system can be important regulators of the immune responses. Therefore, glucocorticoid effects on specialized immune cells may involve the coordinate regulatory effects of cAMP, and this may be particularly important to consider in ocular inflammation, in which changes in the neural and hormonal environment may produce second-messenger changes in cells. For example, glucocorticoid-induced contraction of vascular beds in the eye and steroid-induced enhancement of norepinephrine action in this process also suggest that the permissive effects of steroids may be relevant to ocular tissues. A variety of local potent regulatory hormones (autacoids) are released as cells respond to injury. The presence of these factors may modulate the steroid effect. The exogenous administration of cytoxic or adjunctive therapeutic regimens in the eye could also have an important influence on the steroid response.

4. Glucocorticoid Receptors in Ocular Tissues

Few investigations of glucocorticoid receptors or glucocorticoid induction of specific protein products have been conducted in ocular tissues, although there is some evidence available. MOSCONA and PIDDINGTON (1966) investigated the glucocorticoid hormone induction of glutamine synthetase, a specific protein that is produced in developing chick retina. This system has been of continuing interest, and steroid-receptor-binding studies in this tissue have been reported by CHADER et al. (1972) and PIPERBERG (1978). WEINSTEIN et al. (1977) reported the presence of specific glucocorticoid-receptor binding in homogenates of rabbit iris-ciliary body and adjoining corneoscleral meshwork, and SOUTHREN et al. (1977) demonstrated glucocorticoid-receptor binding in bovine lens epithelium. Using autoradiography, these investigators have described the nuclear translocation of glucocorticoid receptors in the rabbit outflow pathway and in human trabecular meshwork specimens (TCHERNITCHIN et al. 1980; HERNANDEZ et al. 1981). SOUTHREN et al. (1979; 1982 a) investigated the use of rabbit iris-ciliary body preparations to evaluate glucocorticoid receptors following steroid administration, and McCARTY and SCHWARTZ (1980) have employed a similar system to measure the levels of circulating glucocorticoid hormones. In another recent publication, WENK et al. (1982) have presented evidence from which they conclude that the steroid receptors in the lens epithelium (and perhaps other ocular tissues) have different binding properties from those reported in systemic tissues. However, considerably more study of steroid receptors in the eye (including binding studies using whole cells at 37 °C under physiological conditions) will be necessary before the possible importance of this suggestion can be properly evaluated.

Glucocorticoid hormone receptors in human ocular tissues are being studied using cell culture techniques. Cell culture provides a means of obtaining populations of a single cell type in sufficient quantities to perform quantitative hormone-binding studies and to evaluate the molecular mechanisms of steroid hormone action on these cells. Cultured human trabecular cells are of particular interest because of the role of this cell in the maintenance of the aqueous humor outflow pathway.

Figure 18 a shows a differentiated monolayer of human trabecular cells at the fourth passage, grown according to techniques described previously (POLANSKY et

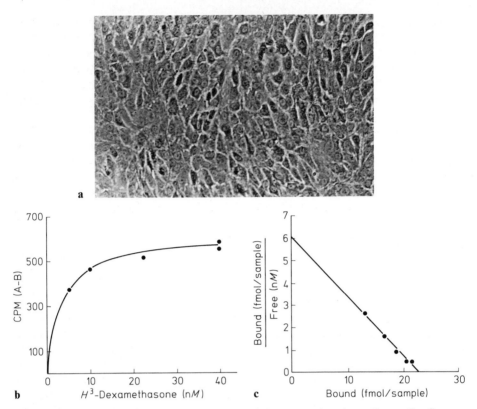

Fig. 18a–c. Glucocorticoid receptors in cultured human trabecular cells. **a**, Confluent fourth-passage monolayer; **b**, specific cell binding as a function of dexamethasone concentration; **c**, SCATCHARD plot of data; the intercept corresponds to 24 fmol/sample or 62,000 dexamethasone molecules bound per trabecular cell (WEINREB et al. 1981). *CPM*, counts per minute ^3H-dexamethasone; (A–B) represents specific binding

al. 1979; ALVARADO et al., to be published). Quantitative evaluation of the affinity and number of receptor sites for glucocorticoid hormones (defined by specific ^3H-dexamethasone binding) was performed on these cells using increasing concentrations of labeled steroids (WEINREB et al. 1978, 1981). A saturation of binding was apparent for the 10–40 nM range of dexamethasone (Fig. 18 b); Scatchard analysis (Fig. 18 c) showed one class of high-affinity receptor sites with the dissociation constant (K_d) of 5 nM and 60,000 binding sites per cell. A concise explanation of the derivation of binding parameters and Scatchard analysis is provided by BAXTER and FUNDER (1979). In other experiments, incubation of human trabecular cells with 40 nM dexamethasone for 60 min revealed that 62% of the specific binding was in the nuclear fraction and 38% was in the cytoplasmic fraction, indicating the presence of functional nuclear translocation of glucocorticoid receptors in the cells. Preliminary studies of the affinity of different compounds for the glucocorticoid receptors have shown that the order of binding affinity agrees with that normally seen in steroid-responsive systems, i.e., dexamethasone > cortisol > progesterone.

Future studies with these cells will allow a comparison of the different ophthalmic steroids (as well as other hormones), and this may provide additional information concerning the ability of these steroids to influence IOP. Also, the action of glucocorticoid agonists, partial agonists, and antagonists can be evaluated directly using these target cells. With regard to the action of other hormones, it is of particular interest that human trabecular cells have β-adrenergic receptors and respond to PGE_1, epinephrine, norepinephrine, and isoproterenol, but not to phenylephrine, with increases in intracellular cAMP (POLANSKY et al. 1980). In view of the preceeding discussion of hormonal interrelationships, it is possible that the effects of steroids on the trabecular cell type may involve interactions with other hormones, particularly those which regulate the generation of intraocular cAMP. There is evidence that drugs working via a cyclic AMP mechanism can affect outflow resistance (NEUFELD et al. 1975; Neufeld 1978) as well as aqueous humor formation (GREGORY et al. 1981; CAPRIOLI and SEARS 1983; SEARS and MEAD 1983). It is also possible that an interaction of steroids with local hormonal mediators (autacoids) may be relevant to the IOP response to glucocorticoids (WEINREB et al. 1983; HARRIS and SCHWARTZ 1983). Use of the cultured human trabecular cell or other ocular cells as target cells may make it possible to analyze these potentially important hormonal interrelationships.

5. Implications

The molecular basis for most clinically important steroid hormone effects in target tissues has not been examined adequately; however, certain salient features of the molecular biology of steroid hormone actions deserve emphasis in relation to ocular pharmacology:

1. Most physiological and pharmacologic effects of anti-inflammatory steroids are likely to be mediated through glucocorticoid receptors and the subsequent regulation of specific protein synthesis.

2. Action of steroid hormones through these receptors can account for a wide range of diverse effects on target cells, including alteration of cellular enzymes and cell surface structures, secretion of extracellular products, and the regulation of local mediators of inflammation.

3. It may be possible to achieve therapeutic effects by employing low steroid concentrations to separate therapeutic from side effects.

4. A steroid-induced response may persist for a considerable amount of time (hours to days) after the drug is no longer present in target tissues, depending upon the half-life of the macromolecular products regulated by the steroid. This may partially explain the need for reduced steroid administration to control some ocular disease processes.

5. The glucocorticoid receptor shows a differential binding affinity for various steroid hormone compounds (for example, dexamethasone > prednisolone > hydrocortisone).

6. The relative potency of steroids to elicit therapeutic responses (as well as side effects) is in general agreement with the receptor-binding activities of the steroid. Where an apparent split in activity is observed (for example, with fluorometholone), then the role of metabolism and absorption/distribution must be considered.

7. The similarity of glucocorticoid receptors in different tissues of the body may explain the difficulty in separating beneficial from detrimental effects of ste-

roid therapy. These effects include steroid actions on ocular and systemic tissues, as well as the anti-inflammatory and immunosuppressive actions of these agents. However, mineralocorticoid effects (e.g., potassium balance) of steroid hormones are mediated through separate mineralocorticoid receptors, which show different binding characteristics.

8. It may be possible to achieve some selectivitiy in the therapeutic use of steroids by:
   a) Employing methods to control the delivery of drug to the target tissue
   b) Choosing drugs which may be distributed or metabolized selectively in specific ocular tissues
   c) Understanding the timing of therapy in relation to pathogenic processes (and side effects) in ocular tissues
   d) Understanding the dose of steroids which is necessary to elicit an effect on target cells
   e) Evaluating the role of external influences and adjunctive therapy which may alter the effects of steroid hormones on their target cells.

9. Other drugs or hormones that interact with steroids to produce effects on target cells may be particularly important for modulation of immune responses or regulation of IOP.

10. Further evaluation of the ocular pharmacology of steroid hormones and the effects of steroid therapy in different ocular inflammatory conditions may lead to improved approaches to steroid therapy in the eye.

Acknowledgments. This work was supported by grants EY02477 (Dr. POLANSKY), EY03833 (Dr. WEINREB), EY01785 (Dr. BAXTER), and EY02162 (Departmental Core Grant). We would like to thank Dr. JOHN BAXTER and Dr. RICHARD O'CONNOR for consultation in their areas of expertise. We appreciate the advice of Dr. JORGE ALVARADO and Dr. STEVEN KRAMER, as well as the many other investigators who discussed their clinical experience with us. We are grateful to Patti Watson for editing the manuscript. That Man May See Inc. graciously provided their facilities for the work on this review.

References

Addison T (1855) On the constitutional and local effects of disease of the suprarenal capsules. Highley, London

Allansmith MR, Lee JR, McClellan BH, Dohlman CH (1975) Evaluation of a sustained release hydrocortisone ocular insert in humans. Trans Am Acad Ophthalmol Otolaryn 79:OP128–OP136

Allison F, Smith MR, Wood WB (1955) Studies on the pathogenesis of acute inflammation. I. The inflammatory reaction to thermal injury as observed in the rabbit ear chamber. J Exp Med 102:655–668

Alvarado J, Polansky JR (1979) Biological activity of cultured human trabecular cells. Invest Ophthalmol Vis Sci [ARVO Suppl] 18:241

Alvarado J, Wood I, Polansky JR (1982) Human trabecular cells II. Ultrastructural characteristics of cultured trabecular cells. Invest Ophthalmol Vis Sci 23:464–478

Amatruda TT, Hurst MM, D'Esopo DN (1965) Certain endocrine and metabolic facets of the steroid withdrawal syndrome. J Clin Endocrinol Metabol 25:1207–1217

Apt L, Henrick A, Silverman LM (1979) Patient compliance with use of topical ophthalmic corticosteroid suspensions. Am J Ophthalmol 87:210–214

Armaly MF (1963a) Effect of corticosteroids on intraocular pressure and fluid dynamics. 1. The effect of dexamethasone in the normal eye. Arch Ophthalmol 70:98–105

Armaly MF (1963b) Effect of corticosteroids on intraocular pressure and fluid dynamics. 2. The effect of dexamethasone in the glaucomatous eye. Arch Ophthalmol 70:492–499

Armaly MF (1964) Effect of corticosteroids on intraocular pressure and fluid dynamics. Arch Ophthalmol 71:636–644

Armaly MF (1965) Statistical attributes of the steroid hypertensive response in the clinically normal eye. Invest Ophthalmol 4:187–197

Armaly MF (1967) Steroids and glaucoma. In: Sampson CLM, Bahn GC, Schoel RE, Allen JH (eds) Symposium on glaucoma. Mosby, St. Louis, p 74

Aronson SB, Elliott JH (1972) Ocular inflammation. Mosby, St. Louis

Aronson SB, Moore TE (1969) Corticosteroid therapy in central stromal keratitis. Am J Ophthalmol 67:8733–896

Aronson SB, Moore TE, Williams FC, Goodner EK (1970) Corticosteroids in infectious ocular disease. In: Kaufman HE (ed) Symposium on ocular anti-inflammatory therapy. Thomas, Springfield, p 15

Ashton N, Cook C (1951) Effect of cortisone on healing of corneal wounds. Br J Ophthalmol 35:708–717

Ashton N, Cook C (1952) In vivo observations of the effects of cortisone upon the blood vessels in rabbit ear chambers. Br J Exper Path 33:445–450

Austin P, Brown SI (1981) Inflammatory Terrien's disease. Am J Ophthalmol 92:189–192

Ballard PL (1979) Delivery and transport of glucocorticoids to target cells. In: Baxter JD, Rousseau GG (eds) Glucocorticoid hormone action. Springer, Berlin Heidelberg New York, p 25

Ballard PL, Carter JP, Graham BS, Baxter JD (1975) A radioreceptor assay for evaluation of the plasma glucocorticoid activity of natural and synthetic steroids in man. J Clin Endocrinal Metab 41:290–304

Balow JE, Hurley DL, Fauci AS (1975) Immunosuppressive effects of glucocorticoids: differential effects of acute versus chronic administration on cell mediated immunity. J Immunol 114:1072–1076

Bárány EH, Scotchbrook S (1954) Influence of testicular hyaluronidase on the resistance to flow through the angle of the anterior chamber. Acta Physiol Scand 30:240–248

Baxter JD, Funder JW (1979) Hormone receptors. N Engl J Med 301:1149–1161

Baxter JD, Harris AW (1975) Mechanism of glucocorticoid action: general features, with reference to steroid-mediated immunosuppression. Transplant Proc 7:55–62

Baxter JD, Rousseau GG (1979) Glucocorticoid hormone action: an overview. In: Baxter JD, Rousseau GG (eds) Glucocorticoid hormone action. Springer, Berlin Heidelberg New York, p 1

Baxter JD, Tyrrell JB (1981) The adrenal cortex. In: Felig P, Baxter JD, Bioadus AE, Frohman LA (eds) Endocrinology and metabolism. McGraw-Hill, New York, p 385

Bayer JM, Neuner HP (1967) Cushing Syndrom und erhöhter Augeninnendruck. Deutsch Med Wochenschr 92:1791–1799

Beard C (1981) Ptosis. Mosby, St. Louis, p 61

Becker B (1965) Intraocular pressure response to topical corticosteroids. Invest Ophthalmol 4:198–205

Becker B, Cotlier E (1965) Topical corticosteroids and galactose cataracts. Invest Ophthalmol 4:806–814

Becker B, Hahn KA (1964) Topical corticosteroids and heredity in primary open-angle glaucoma. Am J Ophthalmol 57:543–551

Becker B, Mills DW (1963a) Corticosteroids and intraocular pressure. Arch Ophthalmol 70:500–507

Becker B, Mills DW (1963b) Elevated intraocular pressure following corticosteroid eye-drops. JAMA 185:170–172

Becker B, Podos SM, Asseff CF, Cooper DG (1973) Plasma cortisol suppression in glaucoma. Am J Ophthalmol 75:73–76

Ben Ezra D, Ticho U, Sachs U (1976) Lymphocyte sensitivity to glucocorticoids. Am J Ophthalmol 82:866–870

Bernstein HN, Schwartz B (1962) Effects of long-term systemic steroids on ocular pressure and tonographic values. Arch Ophthalmol 68:742–753

Bernstein HN, Mills DW, Becker B (1963) Steroid-induced elevation of intraocular pressure. Arch Ophthalmol 70:15–18

Bigger JF, Palmberg PF, Becker B (1972) Increased cellular sensitivity to glucocorticoids in primary open-angle glaucoma. Invest Ophthalmol 11:832–837

Bigger JF, Palmberg PF, Zink HA (1975) In vitro corticosteroid response. Correlation with primary open-angle glaucoma and ocular corticosteroid sensitivity. Am J Ophthalmol 79:92–97

Bill A (1975) the drainage of aqueous humor. Invest Ophthalmol 14:1–3

Bird AC (1977) Is there a place for corticosteroids in the treatment of optic neuritis? In: Brockhurst RJ, Boruchoff SA, Hutchinson B, Lessell S (eds) Controversies in ophthalmology. Saunders, Philadelphia, pp 822–829

Black RL, Oglesby RB, von Sallmann L, Bunim JJ (1960) Posterior subcapsular cataracts induced by corticosteroids in patients with rheumatoid arthritis. JAMA 174:150–171

Bloom E, Matulich DT, Lan N, Higgins SJ, Simons SS, Baxter JD (1980) Nuclear binding of glucocorticoid receptors: relations between cytosol binding, activation and the biological response. J Steroid Biochem 12:175–184

Bourne HR, Lichtenstein LM, Melmon KL, Henney CS, Weinstein Y, Shearer GM (1974) Receptors for vasoactive hormones and mediators of inflammation regulate many leukocyte functions. Science 184:19–28

Boyd TAS, Hassard DTR, Patrick A, McLeod LE (1962) The relation of diurnal variation of plasma corticoid levels and intraocular pressure in glaucoma. Trans Can Ophthalmol Soc 24:119–134

Briggs MH, Brotherton J (1970) Steroid biochemistry and pharmacology. In: Briggs MH, Brotherton J (eds) Steroid biochemistry and pharmacology. Academic, London, p 176

Brown SI, Weller CA, Vidrich AM (1970) Effect of corticosteroid on corneal collagenase of rabbits. Am J Ophthalmol 70:744–747

Brown-Sequard CE (1856) Recherches expérimentales sur la physiologie et la pathologie des capsules surrénales. Compt Rend 43:422–425

Burde RM, Becker B (1970) Corticosteroid induced glaucoma and cataracts in contact lens wearers. JAMA 213:2075–2077

Byers B (1979) Blindness secondary to steroid injection into the nasal turbinates. Arch Ophthalmol 97:79–80 Bynny RL (1976) Withdrawal from glucocorticoid therapy. N Engl J Med 295:30–32

Cantrill HL, Palmberg PF, Zink HA, Waltman SR, Podos SM, Becker B (1975) Comparison of in vitro potency of corticosteroids with ability to raise intraocular pressure. Am J Ophthalmol 79:1012–1017

Caprioli J, Sears M (1983) Forskolin lowers intraocular pressure in rabbits, monkeys and man. Lancet I:958–960

Carnuccio R, DiRosa M, Persico P (1980) Hydrocortisone-induced inhibition of prostaglandin biosynthesis in rat leukocytes. Br J Pharmacol 68:14–16

Chader GJ, Meltzer R, Silver J (1972) A soluble receptor for corticoids in the neural retina of the chick embryo. Biochem Biophys Res Comm 46:2026–2033

Chandler PA, Grant WM (1979a) Corticosteroid glaucoma. In: Chandler PA, Grant WM (eds) Glaucoma. Lea and Febriger, Philadelphia, p 276

Chandler PA, Grant WM (1979b) Filtering operations. In: Chandler PA, Grant WM (eds) Glaucoma. Lea and Febriger, Philadelphia, p 287

Claman HN (1975) How corticosteroids work. J Allergy Clin Immunol 55:145–151

Cline MJ, Melmon KL (1966) Plasma kinins and cortisone: a possible explanation of the anti-inflammatory actin of cortisol. Science 153:1135–1138

Coles RS (1966) Steroid therapy in uveitis. In: Schwartz B (ed) Corticosteroids and the eye. Little, Brown, Boston, p 869

Conn HO, Blitzer B (1976) Nonassociation of adrenocorticosteroid therapy and the peptic ulcer. N Eng J Med 294:473–479

Cope CL (1972) Metabolic breakdown. In: Cope CL (ed) Adrenal steroids and disease, 2nd edn. Lippincott, Philadelphia, p 80

Cope CL (1977) Adrenal steroids and disease. Pitman Medical, London

Corboy JM (1976) Corticosteroid therapy for the reduction of postoperative inflammation after cataract extraction. Am J Ophthalmol 82:923–927

Coster DJ (1980) Herpes simplex. In: Fraunfelder FT, Roy FH (eds) Current ocular therapy. Saunders, Philadelphia, p 60

Cox WV, Kupferman A, Leibowitz HH (1972) Topically applied steroids in corneal disease. Arch Ophthalmol 88::308–313

Crabtree GR, Gillis S, Smith KA (1979) Glucocorticoids and immune responses. Arthritis Rheum 22:1246–1256

Crews SJ (1963) Posterior subcapsular lens opacities in patients on long-term corticosteroid therapy. Br J Med 5346:1644–1647

Dale DC, Fauci AS, Wolff SM (1974) Alternate day prednisone. Leukocyte kinetics and susceptibility to infections. N Engl Med 291:1154–1158

Davies P, Bonney RJ (1981) Some basic mechanisms in inflammatory responses. In: Suran A, Gery I, Nussenblatt RB (eds) Immunology of the eye: workshop III. Information Retrieval Inc, Washington DC, p 273

Davies P, Bonney R, Humes J, Kuehl F (1981) The mechanism of action of antiinflammatory drugs at the cellular level. In: Suran A, Gery I, Nussenblatt RB (eds) Immunology of the eye: workshop III. Information Retrieval Inc, Washington DC, p 411

DeFremery P, Laquer E, Reichstein Q, Spanhoff RW, Uyldert IE (1937) Corticosterone, a crystallized compound with the biological activity of the adrenal corticol hormone. Nature 139:26

Diamond JG, Kaplan HJ (1978) Lensectomy and vitrectomy for complicated cataract secondary to uveitis. Arch Ophthalmol 96:1798–1804

Dixon RB, Christy NP (1965) On the various forms of corticosteroid withdrawal syndrome. Am J Med 68:224–230

Dluhy RG, Newmark SR, Lauler DP, Thorn GW (1975) Pharmacology and chemistry of adrenal glucocorticoids. In: Azarnoff D (ed) Steroid therapy. Saunders, Philadelphia, p 1

Dohlman CH (1966) Corticosteroids in corneal surgery. In: Schwartz B (ed) Corticosteroids and the eye. Little, Brown, Boston, p 845

Dohlman CH, Pavan-Langston D, Rose J (1972) A new ocular insert device for continuous constant-rate delivery to the eye. Ann Ophthalmol 4:823–832

Donshik PC, Berman MB, Dohlman CH, Gage J, Rose J (1978) Effect of topical corticosteroids on ulceration in alkali-burned corneas. Arch Ophthalmol 96:2117–2120

Donshik PC, Cavanaugh HD, Boruchoff SA, Dohlman CH (1981) Posterior subcapsular cataracts induced by topical corticosteroids following keratoplasty for keratoconus. Ann Ophthalmol 13:29–32

Dougherty TF, White A (1944) Influence of hormones on lymphoid tissue structure and function. The role of the pituitary adrenotrophic hormone in the regulation of the lymphocytes and other cellular elements of the blood. Endocrinology 35:1–14

Dunne JA, Travers JP (1979) Double-blind clinical trial of topical steroids in anterior uveitis. Br J Ophthalmol 63:762–767

Ebert RH, Barclay WR (1952) Changes in connective tissue reaction induced by cortisone. Ann Intern Med 37:506–518

Ellis PP (1978) Occlusion of the central retinal artery after retrobulbar corticosteroid injection. Am J Ophthalmol 85:352–356

Epstein WV (1977) A rheumatologist's perspective on the use of immunosuppressants. In: Brockhurst RJ, Boruchoff SA, Hutchenson B, Lessell S (eds) Controversies in ophthalmology. Saunders, Philadelphia, p 758

Fahey JV, Guyre PM, Munck A (1981) Mechanisms of antiinflammatory actions of glucocorticoids. Adv Inflamm Res 2:21–51

Fairbairn WD, Thorson JC (1971) Fluorometholone, Arch Ophthalmol 86:138–141

Fauci AS (1978) Alternate-day corticosteroid therapy. Am J Med 64:729–731

Fauci AS (1979) Immunosuppressive and anti-inflammatory effects of glucocorticoids. In: Baxter JD, Rousseau GG (eds) Glucocorticoid hormone action. Springer, Berlin Heidelberg New York, p 449

Floman N, Zor U (1977) Mechanism of steroid action in ocular inflammation: inhibition of prostaglandin production. Invest Ophthalmol 16:69–73

Florini JR, Buyske DA (1959) A comparison of the rate of metabolism and biological activity of 16 *OH*-hydrocortisone derivatives. Arch Biochem 79:8–12

Florini JR, Smith LL, Buyske DA (1961) Metabolic fate of a synthetic corticosteroid (triamcinolone) in the dog. J Biol Chem 236:1038–1042

Flower R (1981) Glucocorticoids, phospholipase A_2 and inflammation trends. Pharmacol Sci 2:186–189

Flower RJ, Blackwell GJ (1979) Anti-inflammatory steroids induce biosynthesis of a phospholipase A_2 inhibitor which prevents prostaglandin generation. Nature 278:456–459

Foon KA, Yuen K, Ballintine EJ, Rosensteich DL (1977) Analysis of the systemic corticosteroid sensitivity of patients with primary open angle glaucoma. Am J Ophthalmol 83:167–173

Forman AR, Loreto JA, Tina LV (1977) Reversibility of corticosteroid-associated cataracts in children with the nephrotic syndrome. Am J Ophthalmol 84:75–78

Forsham PH, Thorn GW, Runty FTG, Hills AG (1948) Clinical studies with pituitary adrenocorticotropin. J Clin Endocrinol 8:15–66

Francois J (1954) Cortisone et tension oculaire. Am Oculistique 187:805–816

Francois J, Victoria-Troncoso V (1977) Corticosteroid glaucoma. Ophthalmologia (Basel) 174:195–209

Francois J, Heintz-Debree C, Tripathi RC (1966) The cortisone test and the heredity of primary open-angle glaucoma. Am J Ophthalmol 62:844–852

Fried J, Sabo EF (1954) 9α-Fluoro derivatives cortisone and hydrocortisone. J Am Chem Soc 76:1455–1456

Friedlaender MH (1979) Allergy and immunology of the eye. Harper and Row, New York, p 1

Friedlaender MH (1981) Models of ocular inflammation. In: Suran A, Gery I, Nussenblatt RB (eds) Immunology of the eye: workshop III. Information Retrieval Inc, Washington DC, p 231

Friedlaender MH (to be published) Steroid therapy. Int Ophthalmol Clin

Galili N, Galili J, Klein E, Rosenthal L, Nordenskjold B (1980) Human T lymphocytes become glucocorticoid-sensitive upon immune activation, Cell. Immun. 50:440–444

Gallegos AJ, Delgado-Partida P, Garzon P (1976) The presence of 6-steroid hydroxylase in human cornea. J Steroid Biochem 7:135–137

Ganley JP (1980) Uveitis. In: Fraunfelder FT, Roy FH (eds) Current ocular therapy. Saunders, Philadelphia, p 485

Garzon P, Delgado-Partida P, Gallegos AJ (1976) Progesterone metabolism by human cornea. J Steroid Biochem 7:377–379

Gaunt R (1975) History of the adrenal cortex. In: Greep RO, Astwood EB (eds) Handbook of physiology vol 7, endocrinology. American Physiology Society, Washington DC, p 12

Giles CL, Mason GL, Duff IF, McLean JA (1962) The association of cataract formation and systemic corticosteroid therapy. JAMA 182:719–722

Glenn EM, Stafford RO, Lyster SC, Bowmann BJ (1957) Relation between biological activity of hydrocortisone analogues and their rates of inactivation by rat liver enzyme systems. Endocrinology 61:128–142

Godel V, Feiler-Ofry V, Stein R (1972a) Systemic steroids and ocular fluid dynamics. I. Analysis of the sample as a whole. Influence of dosage and duration of therapy. Acta Ophthalmol 50:655–662

Godel V, Feiler-Ofry V, Stein R (1972b) Systemic steroids and ocular fluid dynamics. II. Systemic versus topical steroids. Acta Ophthalmol 50:664–676

Godfrey WA, Epstein WV, O'Connor GR, Kimura SJ, Hogan MJ, Nozik RA (1974) The use of chlorambucil in intractable idiopathic uveitis. Am J Ophthalmol 78:415–429

Goldmann H (1962) Cortisone glaucoma. Arch Ophthalmol 68:621–626

Gordon DM (1956) Prednisone and prednisolone in ocular disease. Am J Ophthalmol 41:593–600

Gordon DM (1959) Dexamethasone in ophthalmology. Am J Ophthalmol 48:656–660

Gordon DM, McLean JM (1950) Effects of pituitary adrenocorticotropic hormone (ACTH) therapy in ophthalmologic conditions. JAMA 142:1271–1276

Gould ES, Bird AC, Leaver PK, McDonald WI (1977) Treatment of optic neuritis by retrobulbar injection of triamcinolone. Br Med J 6075:1495–1497

Graham RO, Peyman GA (1974) Intravitreal injection of dexamethasone. Arch Ophthalmol 92:149–154

Granner DK (1979) The role of glucocorticoid hormones as biological amplifiers. In: Baxter JD, Rouseau GG (eds) Glucocorticoid hormone action. Springer, Berlin Heidelberg New York, p 593

Green H, Kroman HS, Leopold IH (1955a) Corticosteroids in the aqueous humor of the rabbit. Arch Ophthalmol 54:853–857

Green H, Sawyer IL, Leopold IH (1955b) Investigation of corticosteriods in the aqueous humor of normal rabbit eyes. Am J Ophthalmol 30:871–873

Gregory D, Sears M, Bausher L, Mishima H, Mead A (1981) Intraocular pressure and aqueous flow are decreased by cholera toxin. Invest Ophthalmol Vis Sci 20:371–381

Haas JS, Nooten RH (1974) Glaucoma secondary to benign adrenal adenoma. Am J Ophthalmol 78:497–500

Harris AW, Baxter JD (1979) Variations in cellular sensitivity to glucocorticoids: observations and mechanisms. In: Baxter JD, Rousseau GG (eds) Glucocorticoid hormone action. Springer, Berlin Heidelberg New York, p 423

Harris MA, Schwartz B (1983) Dexamethasone-induced stimulation of beta-adrenergic sensitive adenylate cyclase in ciliary process epithelium. ARVO Abstracts, Suppl 24:5

Harter JG (1974) Alternate day therapy. In: Thorn GW (ed) Steroid therapy. Medcom, Kalamazoo, p 42

Harter JG, Reddy WJ, Thorn GW (1963) Studies on an intermittent corticosteroid dosage regimen. N Engl J Med 269:591–596

Harter JG, Borgmann AR, Leaders FE (1970) Steroid potency and the determination of potency, effectiveness and toxicity of anti-inflammatory drugs for use in the eye. In: Kaufmann HE (ed) Symposium on ocular anti-inflammatory therapy. Thomas, Springfield, p 234

Hartman FA, Brownell KA (1930) The hormone of the adrenal cortex. Science 72:76

Havener WH (1976) Corticosteroid misuse. In: Leopold IH, Burns RP (eds) Symposium on ocular therapy. Wiley, New York, p 25

Hench PS, Kendall EC, Slocumb CH, Polley HF (1949) The effect of a hormone of the adrenal cortex (17-hydroxy-11-dehydrocorticosterone: compound E) and of pituitary adrenocorticotrophic hormone on rheumatoid arthritis. Proc Staff Meetings Mayo Clinic 24:181–197

Hench PS, Kendall EC, Slocumb CH, Polley HF (1950) Effects of cortisone acetate and pituitary ACTH on rheumatoid arthritis, rheumatic fever and certain other conditions. Arch Intern Med 85:845–560

Hernandez MR, Wenk EJ, Weinstein BI, Ritch R, Dunn MW, Southren AL (1981) Glucocorticoid target cells in human trabeculectomy specimens. Invest Ophthalmol Vis Sci [ARVO Suppl] 20:23

Herschler J (1976) Increased intraocular pressure induced by repository corticosteroids. Am J Ophthalmol 82:90–93

Higgins SJ, Baxter JD, Rousseau GG (1979) Nuclear binding of glucocorticoid receptors. In: Baxter JD, Rousseau GG (eds) Glucocorticoid hormone action. Springer, Berlin Heidelberg New York, p 135

Hills AG, Forsham PH, Finch CA (1948) Changes in circulating leukocytes induced by the administration of pituitary adrenocorticotrophic hormone (ACTH) in man. Blood 3:755–768

Hogan MJ, Thygesen P, Kimura SJ (1955) Uses and abuses of adrenal steroids and corticotropin. Arch Ophthalmol 53:165–176

Hull DS, Hine JE, Edelhauser HF, Hyndiuk RA (1974) Permeability of the isolated rabbit cornea to corticosteroids. Invest Ophthalmol 13:457–459

Hyndiuk RA (1969) Radioactive depot-corticosteroid penetration into monkey ocular tissue. II. Subconjunctival administration. Arch Ophthalmol 82:259–262

Hyndiuk RA, Reagan MG (1968) Radioactive depot-cortisol penetration into monkey ocular tissue. I. Retrobulbar and systemic administration. Arch Ophthalmol 80:499–503

Ilfeld DN, Krakauer RS, Blaese RM (1977) Suppression of the autologous mixed lymphocyte reaction by physiologic concentrations of hydrocortisone. J Immunol 119:428–434

Ingle DJ (1938) Atrophy of the thymus in normal and hypophysectomized rats following administration of cortin. Proc Soc Exp Biol Med 38:443–444

Ingle DJ (1950) The biologic properties of cortisone: a review. J Clin Endocrinol Metab 10:1312–1354

Ingle DJ (1952) The role of the adrenal cortex in homeostasis. J Endocrinol 8:23–37

Jampol LM, West C, Goldberg MF (1978) Therapy of scleritis with cytotoxic agents. Am J Ophthalmol 86:266–271

Johnson LK, Baxter JD, Rousseau GG (1979) Mechanisms of glucocorticoid receptor function. In: Baxter JD, Rousseau GG (eds) Glucocorticoid hormone action. Springer, Berlin Heidelberg New York, p 305

Johnson-Wint B (1980) Regulation of stromal cell collagenase production in adult rabbit cornea: in vitro stimulation and inhibition by epithelial cell products. Proc Natl Acad Sci USA 77:5331–5335

Jones DB (1974) Herpes zoster ophthalmicus. In: Golden B (ed) Ocular inflammatory disease. Thomas, Springfield, p 198

Jones IS, Meyer K (1950) Inhibition of vascularization of the rabbit cornea by local application of cortisone. Proc Soc Expt Biol Med 74:102–104

Kalina RE (1969) Increased intraocular pressure following subconjunctival corticosteroid administration. Arch Ophthalmol 18:788–790

Kantrowitz F, Robinson DR, McGuire MB, Levine L (1975) Corticosteroids inhibit prostaglandin production by rheumatoid synovia. Nature 258:737–739

Kaplan HJ, Diamond JG, Brown SA (1979) Vitrectomy in experimental uveitis II. Method in eyes with protein-induced uveitis. Arch Ophthalmol 97:336–339

Kaufman HE (1966) Use of corticosteroids in corneal disease and external diseases of the eye. In: Schwartz B (ed) Corticosteroids and the eye. Little, Brown, Boston, p 827

Kaufman HE (1968) Topical corticosteroids: dose response relationships. In: Leopold IH (ed) Symposium on ocular therapy. Mosby, St. Louis, p 106

Kaufman HE (1974) Summary. In: Golden B (ed) Ocular inflammatory disease. Thomas, Springfield, p 321

Kaufman HE (1975) Practical considerations in the selection of anti-inflammatory agents. Trans Am Ophthalmol Otolaryn 79:OP89–OP94

Kayes J, Becker B (1969) The human trabecular meshwork in corticosteroid induced glaucoma. Trans Am Ophthalmol Soc 67:339–354

Kazuo S, Tsurufuji S (1981) Mechanism of anti-inflammatory action of glucocorticoids: reevaluation of vascular constriction hypothesis. Br J Pharmacol 73:605–608

Keller N, Longwell AM, Birss SA (1976) Intermittent vs continuous steroid administration. Arch Ophthalmol 94:644–652

Kendall E (1971) Cortisone. Scribner, New York

Kimura SJ (1977) The use of corticosteroids and immunosuppressive drugs in uveitis. In: Brockhurst RJ, Boruchoff SA, Hutchinson B, Lessell S (eds) Controversies in ophthalmology. Saunders, Philadelphia, p 762

Kimura R, Maekawa N (1976) Effect of orally administered hydrocortisone on the ocular tension in primary open angle glaucoma subjects. Acta Ophthalmol 54:430–436

King JH, Weimer JR (1955) Prednisone (Meticorten) and prednisolone (Meticortelone) in opthalmology: experimental and clinical studies. Arch Ophthalmol 54:46–54

Kitazawa Y (1976) Increased intraocular pressure induced by corticosteroids. Am J Ophthalmol 82:492–495

Kitazawa Y, Horie T (1981) The prognosis of corticosteroid-responsive individuals. Arch Ophthalmol 99:819–823

Knepper PA, Breen M, Weinstein HG, Black LT 1978) Intraocular pressure and glycosaminoglycan distribution in the rabbit eye: effect of age and dexamethasone. Exp Eye Res 27:567–575

Kolker AE, Hetherington J (1976) Primary open-angle glaucoma. In: Kolker AE, Hetherington J (eds) Becker-Shaffer's diagnosis and therapy of the glaucomas. Mosby, St. Louis, p 219

Kozower M, Veatch L, Kaplan MM (1974) Decreased clearance of prednisolone, a factor in the development of corticosteroid side effects. J Clin Endocrinol Metab 38:407–412

Kroman HS, Leopold IH (1961) Studies upon methyl- and fluro-substituted prednisolones in the aqueous humor of the rabbit. Am J Ophthalmol 52:77–81

Krupin T, Waltman SR, Becker B (1974) Ocular penetration in rabbits of topically applied dexamethasone. Arch Ophthalmol 92:312–314

Kuck JFR (1977) Drugs influencing the lens. In: Dikstein S (ed) Drugs and ocular tissues. Karger, New York, p 433

Kupferman A, Leibowitz HM (1975) Therapeutic effectiveness of fluorometholone in inflammatory keratitis. Arch Ophthalmol 93:1011–1014

Kupferman A, Leibowitz HM (1976) Biological equivalence of ophthalmic prednisolone acetate suspensions. Am J Ophthalmol 82:109–112

Lamberts DW (1980) Solid delivery devices. Int Ophthalmol Clin 20(3):63–77

Leibowitz HM, Kupferman A (1975) Penetration of fluorometholone into the cornea and aqueous humor. Arch Ophthalmol 93:425–427

Leibowitz HM, Kupferman A (1980 a) Antiinflammatory medications. Int Ophthalmol Clin 20:117–134

Leibowitz HM, Kupferman A (1980 b) Topically administered corticosteroids: effect on antibiotic-treated bacterial keratitis. Arch Ophthalmol 98:1287–1290

Leibowitz HM, Kupferman A, Steward RH, Kimbrough RL (1978) Evaluation of dexamethasone acetate as a topical ophthalmic formulation. Am J Ophthalmol 86:418–423

Leopold IH (1970) Summation. In: Kaufman EH (ed) Symposium on ocular anti-inflammatory therapy. Thomas, Springfield, p 245

Leopold IH (1974) Consideration of antiinflammatory drugs in ophthalmology. In: Leopold IH, Burns RP (eds) Symposium on ocular therapy. Wiley, New York, p 41.

Leopold IH, Kroman HS, Green H (1955) Intraocular penetration of prednisone and prednisolone. Tr Am Ophthalmol Otolaryn 59:771–777

Lerman S, Davis P, Jackson WB (1973) Prolonged release hydrocortisone therapy. Can J Ophthalmol 8:114–118

Levine ND, Aronson SB (1970) Orbital infusion of steroids in the rabbit. Arch Ophthalmol 83:599–607

Levine SB, Leopold IH (1973) Advances in ocular corticosteroid therapy. Med Clin North Am 57:62–77

Lewis GP, Piper PJ (1975) Inhibition of release of prostaglandins as an explanation of some of the actions of anti-inflammatory corticosteroids. Nature 254:308–311

Linner E (1959) Adrenocorticosteroids and aqueous humor dynamics. Doc Ophthalmol 13:210–222

Lippman ME (1979) Glucocorticoid receptors and effects in human lymphoid and leukemic cells. In: Baxter JD, Rousseau GG (eds) Glucocorticoid hormone action. Springer, Berlin Heidelberg New York, p 377

Livanou T, Ferriman D, James VHT (1967) Recovery of the hypothalamo-pituitary-adrenal function after corticoid steroid therapy. Lancet II:856–859

Loredo A, Rodriguez R, Murillo L (1972) Letter to the editor. N Eng J Med 286:160

Lorenzetti DWC (1970) Therapeutic and toxic dose-response effects of corticosteroids. In: Kaufman HE (ed) Symposium on ocular anti-inflammatory therapy. Thomas, Springfield, p 205

Lubow M, Adams L (1972) The changing management of acute optic neuritis. In: Smith JL (ed) Neuroophthalmology. Mosby, St. Louis

McDonald PR, Leopold IH, Vogel AW, Mulberger RD (1953) Hydrocortisone (compound F) in ophthalmology. Arch Ophthalmol 49:400–412

MacGregor RR (1976) The effect of anti-inflammatory agents and inflammation on granulocyte adherence. Evidence for regulation by plasma factors. Am J Med 61:597–607

Machemer R, Sugita G, Tano Y (1979) Treatment of intraocular proliferation with intraviteal steroids. Trans Am Ophthalmol Soc 77:172–179

Maibach HI, Stoughton RB (1975) Topical corticosteroids. In: Azarnoff DL (ed) Steroid therapy. Saunders, Philadelphia, p 174

Marchalonis JJ (1980) Cell interactions in immune responses. In: Fudenberg HH, Stites DP, Caldwell JL, Wells JV (eds) Basic and clinical immunology. Lange, Los Altos, p 115

Marsh RJ (1980) Herpes zoster. In: Fraunfelder FT, Roy FH (eds) Current ocular therapy. Saunders, Philadelphia, p 62

Martial JA, Seeburg PH, Matulich DT, Goodman HM, Baxter JD (1979) Regulation of growth hormone messenger RNA. In: Baxter JD, Rousseau GG (eds) Glucocorticoid hormone action. Springer, Berlin Heidelberg New York, p 279

McCarty G, Schwartz B (1980) Receptor-assessed plasma glucocorticoid activity in glaucoma. Invest Ophthalmol Vis Sci [ARVO Suppl] 19:125

McCarty G, Schwartz B, Miller K (1981) Absence of lymphocyte glucocorticoid hypersensitivity in primary open angle glaucoma. Arch Ophthalmol 99:1258–1260

McCuen II BW, Bessler M, Tano Y, Chandler D, Machemer R (1981) The lack of toxicity of intravitreally administered triamcinolone acetonide. Am J Ophthalmol 92:785–788

McDonald PR, Leopold IH, Vogel AW, Mulberger RD (1953) Hydrocortisone (compound F) in ophthalmology. Arch Ophthalmol 49:400–412

McLean JM (1950) In discussion of Woods AC (77). Clinical and experimental observation on the use of ACTH and cortisone in ocular inflammatory disease. Trans Am Ophthalmol Soc 48:259

McLeod KM, Baxter JD (1980) Molecular basis for hormone action. In: Bandy PK, Rosenberg LE (eds) Duncan's diseases of metabolism. Saunders, Philadelphia, p 104

Meikle AW, Tyler FH (1977) Potency and duration of action of glucocorticoids. Am J Med 63:200–207

Meikle AW, Weed JA, Tyler FH (1975) Kinetics and interconversion of prednisolone and prednisone studied with new radioimmunoassays. J Clin Endocrinol Metab 4:717–721

Meikle AW, Clark DH, Tyler FH (1976) Cushing syndrome from low doses of dexamethasone. JAMA 235:1592–1593

Menkin V (1940) Effect of adrenal cortex extract on capillary permeability. Am J Physiol 129:691–697

Metcalf JF, Kaufman HE (1976) Herpetic stromal keratitis – evidence for cell-mediated immunopathogenesis. Am J Ophthalmol 82:827–834

Meyers FH, Jawetz E, Goldfien A (1980) The adrenocorticol steroids. In: Meyers FH, Jawetz E, Goldfien A (eds) Review of medical pharmacology. Lange, Los Altos, p 353

Meyers RL, Pettit TH (1974) Chemotaxis of polymorphonuclear leukocytes in corneal inflammation: tissue injury in herpes simplex virus infection. Invest Ophthalmol 13:187–197

Mindel JS, Tavitan HO, Smith H, Walker EC (1980) Comparative ocular pressure elevation by medrysone, fluorometholone and dexamethasone phosphate. Arch Ophthalmol 97:1577–1578

Moller G (1980) Role of macrophages in the immune response. Immunol Rev 40:1

Monder C, Bradlow L (1980) Cortoic acids: explorations at the frontier of corticosteroid metabolism. Recent Prog Horm Res 36:345–400

Moscona AA, Piddington R (1966) Stimulation by hydrocortisone of premature changes in the developmental pattern of glutamine synthetase in embryonic retina. Biochem Biophys Acta 121:409–411

Munck A, Young DA (1975) Corticosteroids and lymphoid tissue. In: Geiger SR (ed) Handbook of physiology, vol VI. American Physiological Society, Washington DC, p 231

Munck A, Crabtree GR, Smith KA (1979) Glucocorticoid receptors and actions in rat thymocytes and immunologically stimulated human peripheral lymphocytes. In: Baxter JD, Rousseau GG (eds) Glucocorticoid hormone action. Springer, Berlin Heidelberg New York, p 341

Nagataki S, Mishima S (1980) Pharmacokinetics of instilled drugs in the human eye. Int Clin Ophthalmol 20:33–49

Nagy RM, McFall RC, Sery TW (1980) Cell-mediated immunity in herpes corneal stromal disease. Invest Ophthalmol Vis Sci 19:271–277

Nelson EL (1970) Ophthalmic steroids. In: Kaufman HE (ed) Symposium on ocular anti-inflammatory therapy. Thomas, Springfield, p 217

Nesburn AB (1981) Immunological aspects of ocular herpes simplex disease. In: Suran A, Gery I, Nussenblatt RB (eds) Immunology of the eye: workshop III. Information Retrieval, Washington DC, p 21

Neufeld AH (1978) Influences of cyclic nucleotides on outflow facility in the vervet monkey. Exp Eye Res 27:387–397

Neufeld AH, Dueker DK, Vegge T, Sears ML (1975) Adenosine 3′,5′-monophosphate increases the outflow of aqueous humor from the rabbit eye. Invest Ophthalmol 14:40–42

Neuner HP, Dardenne V (1968) Augenveränderungen bei Cushing Syndrom. Klin Monatsbl Augenheilkd 152:570–574

Newsome DA, Gross J (1977) Prevention by medroxyprogesterone of perforation in alkaliburned rabbit cornea: inhibition of collagenolytic activity. Invest Ophthalmol 16:21–31

Newsome DA, Gross J (1979) Regulation of corneal collagenase production: stimulation by serially passaged stromal cells by blood monocular cells. Cell 16:895–900

Newsome DA, Wong VG, Cameron TP, Anderson RA (1971) "Steroid-induced" mydriasis and ptosis. Invest Ophthalmol 10:424–429

Nichols T, Nugent CA, Tyler FH (1965) Diurnal variation in suppression of adrenal function by glucocorticoids. J Clin Endocrin Metab 25:343–349

Nielsen RH (1959) The use of dexamethasone in ophthalmologic steroid therapy. Arch Ophthalmol 62:438–444

Nozik RA (1972) Periocular injection of steroids. Trans Am Ophthalmol Otolaryngol 76:695–705

O'Connor GR (1975) Basic mechanisms responsible for the initiation and perpetuation of anterior segment inflammation. Trans Am Ophthalmol Otolaryngol 79:OP56–OP61

O'Connor GR (1980) Corticosteroids and immunosuppressives reviewed. In: Srinivasan (ed) Ocular therapeutics. Masson, New York, p 69

O'Connor GR (1981 a) The inflammatory response. In: Suran A, Gery I, Nussenblatt RB (eds) Immunology of the eye: workshop III. Information Retrieval, Washington DC, p 225

O'Connor GR (1981 b) Workshop on inflammation, infection, and allergy: general summary. In: Suran A, Gery I, Nussenblatt RB (eds) Immunology of the eye: workshop III. Information Retrieval, Washington DC, p 519

O'Farrell PH, Ivarie RD (1979) The glucocorticoid domain of response: measurement of pleiotropic cellular responses by two-dimensional gel electrophoresis. In: Baxter JD, Rousseau GG (eds) Glucocorticoid hormone action. Springer, Berlin Heidelberg New York, p 189

Oglesby RB, Black RL, von Sallmann T, Bunim JJ (1961) Cataracts in rheumatoid arthritis patients treated with corticosteroids. Arch Ophthalmol 66:519–523

Olson JA, Steffensen EH, Margulis RR, Smith RW, Whitney EL (1950) Effect of ACTH on certain inflammatory diseases of the eye. JAMA 142:1276–1278

Olson JA, Steffenson EH, Smith RW, Margulis RR, Whitney EL (1951) Use of adrenocorticotropic hormone and cortisone in ocular disease. Arch Ophthalmol 45:274–300

Ono S, Hirano H, Obara K (1971) Degradation of the side chain of cortisol by lens homogenate. Tohoku J Exp Med 104:171–175

Ostler HB (1978) Glucocorticoid therapy in ocular herpes simplex. I. Limitations. Surv Ophthalmol 23:35–43

Ostler HB, Lanier JD (1974) Phlyctenular keratoconjunctivitis with special reference to the staphylococcal type. Trans Pac Coast Otoophthalmol Soc Ann Mtg 55:237–252

Palmberg PF, Mandell L, Wilensky JT, Podos SM, Becker B (1975) The reproducibility of the intraocular pressure response to dexamethasone. Am J Ophthalmol 80:844–856

Parrillo JE, Fauci AS (1979) Mechanisms of glucocorticoid action on immune processes. Ann Rev Pharmacol Toxicol 19:179–201

Pavan-Langston D (1976) New drug delivery systems. In: Leopold IH, Burns RP (eds) Symposium on ocular therapy. Wiley, New York, p 17

Pavan-Langston D, Abelson MB (1978) Glucocorticoid therapy in ocular herpes simplex. II. Advantages. Surv Ophthalmol 23:35–48

Perkin GD, Rose FC (1979) Treatment. In: Perkin GD, Rose FC (eds) Optic neuritis and its differential diagnosis. Oxford University Press, Oxford, p 172

Peterkofsky B, Tomkins GM (1967) Effect of inhibitors of nucleic acid synthesis on steroid-mediated induction of tyrosine aminotransferase in hepatoma cell cultures. J Mol Biol 30:49–61

Phillpotts JS (1969) Intra-ocular medication with special reference to depomedrone. Trans Ophthalmol Soc UK 138:729–735

Piperberg JB (1978) Binding of steroids to the cytoplasmic receptor of the embryonic chick retina: kinetics and structural considerations. Arch Biochem Biophys 191:367–374

Podos SM, Krupin T, Asseff C, Becker B (1971) Topically administered corticosteroid preparations. Arch Ophthalmol 86:251–254

Polansky JR, Gospodarowicz D, Weinreb RN, Alvarado JJ (1978) Human trabecular meshwork cell culture and glycosaminoglycan synthesis. Invest Ophthalmol Vis Sci [ARVO Suppl] 17:207

Polansky JR, Weinreb RN, Baxter JD, Alvarado JJ (1979) Human trabecular cells. I. Establishment in tissue culture. Invest Ophthalmol 18:1043–1049

Polansky JR, Weinreb RN, Alvarado JJ (1980) Studies on human trabecular cells propagated in vitro. Vision Res 21:155

Polansky JR, Palmberg PF, Nakanistu M, Coit D, Matulich DI, Lan NC, Hajek S, Becker B, Baxter JD (to be published) Cellular sensitivity to glucocorticoids in patients with primary open-angle glaucoma: steroid receptors and biological responsiveness of cultured skin fibroblasts. Invest Ophthalmol Vis Sci

Posthumus RG (1952) The use and the possibilities of progesterone in the treatment of glaucoma. Ophthalmologica 124:2

Raichaind M, Peyman G, Schwartz H, Roe C (1982) Anti-inflammatory action of dexamethasone in vitrectomy infusion fluid. Ophthalmic Surg 13:493–498

Rocklin RE (1980) Mediators of cellular immunity. In: Fudenberg HH, Stites DP, Caldwell JL, Wells JV (eds) Basic and clinical immunology. Lange, Los Altos, p 144

Rohen JW, Linner E, Witmer R (1973) Electron microscopic studies on the trabecular meshwork in two cases of corticosteroid-glaucoma. Exp Eye Res 17:19–31

Rooklin AR, Lampert SI, Jaeger EA, McGeady SJ, Mansmann HC (1979) Posterior subcapsular cataracts in steroid-requiring asthmatic children. Allergy Clin Immunol 63:383–386

Rosenthal AR, Balow JE (1980) Mechanisms of glucocorticosteroid suppression of cell-mediated immunity. Immunol Rev 40:701

Rosenthal AR, Appelton B, Zimmerman R, Hopkins JL (1976) Intraocular copper foreign bodies: use of dexamethasone to suppress inflammation. Arch Ophthalmol 94:1571–1576

Rousseau GG (1974) Interaction of steroids with hepatoma cells: molecular mechanisms of glucocorticoid hormone action. J Steroid Biochem 6:75–89

Rousseau GG, Baxter JD (1979) Glucocorticoid receptors. In: Baxter JD, Rousseau GG (eds) Glucocorticoid hormone action. Springer, Berlin Heidelberg New York, p 49

Samuels H, Tompkins GM (1970) Relation of steroid structure to enzyme induction in hepatoma tisue culture cells. J Mol Biol 52:57–74

Sano T, Miyata Y (1971) Autopsy findings in a case of steroid glaucoma. Jpn J Clin Ophthalmol 25:153–160

Sarett LH (1946) Partial synthesis of 4-pregne-17 beta, 20 beta, 21-triol-3, 11-dione and 4-pregne-17 beta-21 diol-3, 11-30-trione monoacetate. J Biol Chem 162:601–631

Schachtschabel B, Bigalke B, Rohen JW (1977) Production of glycosaminoglycans by cell cultures of the trabecular meshwork of the primate eye. Exp Eye Res 24:71–80

Schatz M, Patterson R, Zeit S, O'Rourke J, Melam H (1975) Corticosteroid therapy for the pregnant asthmatic patient. JAMA 233:804–807

Schayer RW (1963) Induced synthesis of histamine, microcirculatory regulation and the mechanism of action of the adrenal glucocorticoid hormones. Progr Allergy 7:187–212

Schlaegel TF (1970) Depot corticosteroids by the cul-de-sac route. In: Kaufman HE (ed) Symposium on ocular anti-inflammatory therapy. Thomas, Springfield, p 117

Schlaegel TF (1977) Complications of uveitis. Int Ophthalmic Clin 17:65–85

Schlaegel TF, O'Connor GR (1977) Nonspecific treatment. Int Ophthalmol Clin 17:43–62

Schlaegel TF, Wilson FM (1974) Accidental intraocular injection of depot corticosteroids. Trans Am Acad Ophthalmol Otolaryngol 78:847

Schoenwald RD, Boltralik JJ (1979) A bioavailability comparison in rabbits of two steroids formulated as high-viscosity gels and reference aqueous preparations. Invest Ophthalmol 18:61–66

Schwartz B (1966a) Physiological effects of corticosteroids on the eye. In: Schwartz B (ed) Corticosteroids and the eye. Little, Brown, Boston, p 753

Schwartz B (1966b) The response of ocular pressure to corticosteroids. In: Schwartz B (ed) Corticosteroids and the eye. Little, Brown, Boston, p 929

Schwartz B (1966c) Use of corticosteroids in the management of patients with glaucoma. In: Schwartz B (ed) Corticosteroids and the eye. Little, Brown, Boston, p 1017

Schwartz B (1981a) Ocular glucocorticoid therapy: a review of mechanisms of receptor and cellular action. In: Suran A, Gery I, Nussenblat RB (eds) Immunology of the eye: workshop III. Information Retrieval, Washington DC, p 425

Schwartz B (1981b) Increased plasma cortisol levels in ocular hypertension. Arch Ophthalmol 99:1791–1794

Schwartz JT, Rueling FH, Feinleib M, Garrison RJ, Collie DJ (1973a) Twin study on ocular pressure after topical dexamethasone. 1. Frequency distribution of pressure response. Arch Ophthalmol 76:126–136

Schwartz JT, Rueling FH, Feinleib M, Garrison RJ, Collie DJ (1973b) Twin study on ocular pressure following topically applied dexamethasone. 2. Inheritance of variation in pressure response. Arch Ophthalmol 90:281–286

Sears ML, Mead A (1983) A major pathway for the regulation of intraocular pressure. Internatl Ophthalmol 6:201–212

Selye H (1936) Thymus and adrenals in the response of the organism to injuries and intoxications. Br J Exp Pathol 17:234–248

Selye H (1946) The general adaptation syndrome and the diseases of adaptation. J Clin Endocrin 6:117–230

Shell JW (1982a) Pharmacokinetics of topically applied ophthalmic drugs. Surv Ophthalmol 6:207–218

Shell JW (1982b) Ocular drug delivery systems – a review. Cutan Ocular Toxicol 1:49–63

Shell JW, Baker RW (1974) Diffusional systems for controlled release of drugs to the eye. Ann Ophthalmol 6:1037–1045

Sherman MR (1979) Allosteric and competitive steroid-receptor interactions. In: Baxter JD,, Rousseau GG (eds) Glucocorticoid hormone action. Springer, Berlin heidelberg New York, p 123

Short C, Keates RH, Donovan EF, Wyman M, Murdick PW (1966) Ocular penetration studies. Arch Ophthalmol 75:689–692

Silverstein AM (1974) Mechanisms of ocular immunologic disease. In: Golden B (ed) Ocular inflammatory disease. Thomas, Springfield, p 3

Skalka HW, Prchal JT (1980) Effect of corticosteroids on cataract formation. Arch Ophthalmol 98:1773–1777

Smith JL, Stempfel RS, Campbell HS, Hudnell AB, Richman DW (1962) Diurnal variation of plasma 17-hydroxycorticoids and intraocular pressure in glaucoma. Am J Ophthalmol 54:411–418

Smith R, Nozik RA (1982) Uveitis: a clinical approach to diagnosis and management. Williams and Wilkins, Baltimore, p 1

Smolin G, Hall JM, Okumoto M, Ohno S (1977) High doses of subconjunctival corticosteroid and antibody-forming cells in the eye and draining lymph nodes. Arch Ophthalmol 95:1631–1633

Southren AL, Altman K, Vittek J, Boniuk V, Gordon GG (1976) Steroid metabolism in ocular tissues of the rabbit. Invest Ophthalmol 15:222–228

Southren AL, Gordon GG, Yeh HS, Dunn MW, Weinstein BI (1977) Receptors for glucocorticoids in the lens epithelium of the calf. Science 200:1177–1178

Southren AL, Gordon CG, Yeh HS, Dunn MW, Weinstein BI (1979) Nuclear translocation of the cytoplasmic glucocorticoid receptor in the iris-ciliary body of the rabbit. Invest Ophthalmol Vis Sci 18:517–521

Southren AL, Ochoa Dominguez M, Gordon GG, Dunn MW, Weinstein BI (1982a) Nuclear translocation of the glucocorticoid receptor in the rabbit iris-ciliary body following topical administration of various anti-inflammatory steroids. Invest Ophthal Vis Sci [Suppl] 56:93

Sowell JG, Levene RZ, Bloom J, Bernstein M (1977) Primary open angle glaucome and sensitivity to corticosteroids in vitro. Am J Ophthalmol 84:715–720

Spaeth GL (1969) General medications, glaucoma and disturbances of intraocular pressure. Med Clin North Am 53(5):1109–1121

Spaeth GL (1980) The effect of autonomic agents on the pupil and the intraocular pressure of eyes treated with dexamethasone. Br J Ophthalmol 64:426–429

Spaeth GL, von Sallmann L (1966) Corticosteroids and cataracts. In: Schwartz B (ed) Corticosteroids and the eye. Little, Brown, Boston, p 915

Spaeth GL, Rodrigues MM, Weinreb S (1977) Steroid induced glaucoma. Trans Am Ophthalmol Soc 75:353–381

Steck WF, Lockwood DH (1979) Pituitary adrenal recovery following short-term suppression with corticosteroids. Am J Med 66:910–914

Steiger M, Reichstein Q (1937) Desoxy-corticosterone (21-oxy-progesterone) aus Delta 5-3-oxy-atiokohlensäure. Helv Chim Acta 20:1164–1179

Stern GA, Okumoto MA, Friedlaender M, Smolin G (1980) The effect of combined gentamicin-corticosteroid treatment on gentamicin-resistant pseudomonas keratitis. Ann Ophthalmol 12:9

Stewart RH, Kimbrough RL (1979) Intraocular pressure response to topically administered fluorometholone. Arch Ophthalmol 97:2139–2140

Suddick RP (1966) Glucocorticoid-kinin antagonism in the rat. Am J Physiol 211:844–850

Sugar J, Burde RM, Sugar A, Waltman SR, Kripalani KJ, Weliky I, Becker B (1972) Tetrahydrotriamcinolone and triamcinolone I. Ocular penetration. Invest Ophthalmol 11:890–893

Swingle WW, Pfiffner JJ (1930) An aqueous extract of the suprarenal cortex which maintains the life of bilaterally adrenalectomized cats. Science 71:321–322

Swingle WW, Pfiffner JJ (1931) Studies on the adrenal cortex. I. The effect of lipid fraction upon the life span of adrenalectomized-cats. Am J Physiol 96:153–163

Tamada Y, Miyashita H, Ono S (1980) Studies on the phospholipid metabolism of rabbit lens with special reference to long-term topical administration of steroid. Jpn J Ophthalmol 24:289–296

Tano Y, Chandler D, Machemer R (1980a) Treatment of intraocular proliferation with intravitreal injection of triamcinolone acetonide. Am J Ophthalmol 90:810–816

Tano Y, Sugita G, Abrams G, Machemer R (1980b) Inhibition of intraocular proliferations with intravitreal corticosteroids. Am J Ophthalmol 89:131–136

Tano Y, Chandler BS, Machemer R (1980c) Treatment of intraocular proliferation with intravitreal injection of triamcinolone acetonide. Am J Ophthalmol 90:810–816

Tano Y, Chandler DB, McCuen BW, Machemer R (1981) Glucocorticosteroid inhibition of intraocular proliferation after injury. Am J Ophthalmol 91:184–189

Tchernitchin A, Wend EJ, Hernandez M, Weinstein B, Dunn MW, Gordon G, Southren AL (1980) Glucocorticoid localization by radioautography in the rabbit eye following systemic administration of ^3H-dexamethasone. Invest Ophthalmol Vis Sci 19:1231–1235

Thompson EB (1979a) Glucocorticoid induction of tryosine aminotransferase in cultured cells. In: Baxter JD, Rousseau GG (eds) Glucocorticoid hormone action. Springer, Berlin Heidelberg New York, p 203

Thompson EB (1979b) Glucocorticoids and lysosomes. In: Baxter JD, Rousseau GG (eds) Glucocorticoid hormone action. Springer, Berlin Heidelberg New York, p 575

Thygesen P (1977) The unfavorable role of corticosteroids in herpetic keratitis. In: Brockhurst RJ, Boruchoff SA, Hutchinson B, Lessell S (eds) Controversies in ophthalmology. Saunders, Philadelphia, p 450

Thygesen P, Hogan MJ, Kimura SJ (1960) The unfavorable effect of topical steroid therapy on herpetic keratitis. Trans Am Ophthalmol Soc 58:245–262

Ticho V, Vilahav M, Berkowitz S, Yoffe B (1979) Ocular changes in rabbits with corticosteroid-induced ocular hypertension. Br J Ophthalmol 63:646–650

Tsurufuji S, Sugio K, Takemasa F (1979) The role of glucocorticoid receptor and gene expression in the anti-inflammatory action of dexamethasone. Nature 280:408–410

Tsurufuji S, Sugio K, Takemasa F, Yoshizawa S (1980) Blockade by antiglucocorticoids, actionomycin D and cycloheximide of anti-inflammatory action of dexamethasone against bradykinin. J Pharmacol Exp Ther 212:225–231

Tyrrell JB, Baxter JD (1981) Glucocorticoid therapy. In: Felig P, Baxter JD, Broadus AE, Frohman LA (eds Endocrinology and metabolism. McGraw-Hill, New York, p 599

Valerio M, Carones AV, DePoli A (1962) Il quadro clinico del glaucoma da cortisonoterapia locale. Gior Ital Oftal 15:143–150

Vassalli J, Hamilton J, Reich E (1976) Macrophage plasminogen activator modulation of enzyme production by anti-inflammatory steroids, mitotic inhibitors and cyclic nucleotides. Cell 8:271–281

Vermeulen A (1959) The metabolism of 4–14 C prednisolone. J Endocrinol 18:278–291

Vincenti F, Amend W, Feduska NJ, Duca RM, Salvatierra Jr O (1980) Improved outcome following renal transplantation with reduction in the immunosuppression therapy for rejection episodes. Am J Med 69:107–112

Vischer TL (1972) Effect of hydrocortisone on the reactivity of thymus and spleen cells of mice to in vitro stimulation. Immunology 233:777–784

Weinreb RN, Kimura SJ (1979) Uveitis associated with sarcoidosis and angiotensin converting enzyme. Trans Am Ophthalmol Soc 77:280–293

Weinreb RN, O'Donnell JT, Alvarado JJ, Baxter JD, Polansky JR (1978) Specific nuclear steroid binding in cultured human trabecular cells. Invest Ophthalmol Vis Sci [ARVO Suppl] 17:204

Weinreb RN, Polansky JR, Kramer SG, Baxter JD (1979) Acute intraocular pressure response to steroids in glaucoma. Invest Ophthalmol Vis Sci [ARVO Suppl] 18:41

Weinreb RN, Bloom E, Baxter JD, Alvarado J, Lan N, O'Donnell J, Polansky JR (1981) Detection of glucocorticoid receptors in cultured human trabecular cells. Invest Ophthalmol 21:403–407

Weinreb RN, Mitchell M, Polansky JP (in press) Prostaglandin synthesis by human trabecular cells: inhibitory effect of dexamethasone. Invest Ophthalmol Vis Sci [ARVO Suppl]

Weinstein BI, Altman K, Gordon G, Dunn M, Southren AL (1977) Specific glucocorticoid receptor in the iris-ciliary body of the rabbit. Invest Ophthalmol Vis Sci 16:973–976

Weissmann G, Thomas L (1963) Studies on lysosomes. II. The effect of cortisone on the release of acid hydrolases from a large granule fraction of rabbit liver induced by an excess of vitamin A. J Clin Invest 42:661–669

Weitzman ED, Henkind P, Leitman M, Hellman L (1975) Correlative 24-hour relationships between intraocular pressure and plasma cortisol in normal subjects and patients with glaucoma. Br J Ophthalmol 59:566–572

Wenk EJ, Rosario-Hernandez M, Weinstein BI, Gordon GG, Dunn MW, Southren AL (1982) Glucocorticoid receptor binding in bovine lens. Invest Ophthalmol Vis Sci 22:599–605

Werb Z (1978) Biochemical actions of glucocorticoids on macrophages in culture. Specific inhibition of elastase, collagenase, and plasminogen activator secretion and effects on other metabolic functions. J Exp Med 147:1695–1712

Werb Z, Foley R, Munck A (1978) Glucocorticoid receptors and glucocorticoid-sensitive secretion of neutral proteinase in a macrophage line. J Immunol 121:115–121

Whiteman DW, Rosen DA, Pinkerton RMH (1980) Retinal and choroidal microvascular embolism after intranasal corticosteroid injection. Am J Ophthalmol 89:851–853

Williams GH, Dluhy RG, Thorn GW (1980) Diseases of the adrenal cortex. In: Isselbacher KJ, Adams RD, Braunwald E, Petersdorf RG, Wilson JD (eds) Harrison's principles of internal medicine, 9th edn, McGraw-Hill New York, p 1734

Wolff ME (1979) Structure-activitiy relationships in glucocorticoids. In: Baxter JD, Rousseau GG (eds) Glucocorticoid hormone action. Springer, Berlin Heidelberg New York, p 97

Woods AC (1950) Clinical and experimental observation on the use of ACTH and cortisone in ocular inflammatory disease. Am J Ophthalmol 333:1325–1349

Woods AC, Wood RM (1950) Action of ACTH and cortisone on experimental ocular inflammation. Bull Johns Hopkins Hosp 87:482–504

Woods AC, Wood RM (1952) Studies in experimental ocular tuberculosis, Arch Ophthalmol 47:477–512

Woods AC, Wood RM (1958) Studies in experimental ocular tuberculosis. Arch Ophthalmol 59:559–578

Wray S (1977) ACTH and oral corticosteroids in the treatment of acute optic neuritis. In: Brockhurst RT, Boruchoff SA, Hutchinson B, Lessell S (ed) Controversies in ophthalmology. Saunders, Philadelphia, pp 830–838

Yablonski ME, Burde RM, Kolker AE, Becker B (1978) Cataracts induced by topical dexamethasone in diabetics. Arch Ophthalmol 96:474–476

Yamauchi H, Kito H, Uda K (1975) Studies on intraocular penetration and metabolism of fluorometholone in rabbits: a comparison between dexamethasone and prednisolone acetate. Jpn J Ophthalmol 19:339–347

Zaidman GW, Brown SI (1981) Phlyctenular keratoconjunctivitis. Am J Ophthalmol 92:178–182

Zimmerman TJ, Dawson WW, Fitzgerald CR (1973) Part I: Electroretinographic changes in normal eyes during administration of prednisone. Ann Ophthalmol 5:757–765

Zinn K (1981) Iatrogenic intraocular injection of depot corticosteroid and its surgical removal using the pars plana approach. Ophthalmology 88:13–17

Zumbrun FA, Weinreb RN, Alvarado JA, Polansky JR (1981) Endogenous hyaluronidase and degradation of hyaluronic acid by human trabecular cells. Invest Ophthalmol Vis Sci [ARVO Suppl] 20:23

Zweifach BW, Shorr E, Black MM (1953) The influence of the adrenal cortex on behaviour of terminal vascular bed. Ann NY Acad Sci 56:626–633

Anti-Inflammatory Agents:
Nonsteroidal Anti-Inflammatory Drugs

K. MASUDA

A. Introduction

Nonsteroidal anti-inflammatory compounds (NSAIDS) have been used since 1763, when EDWARD STONE described the therapeutic properties of an extract of willow bark upon ague. Although almost four centuries have passed since the first medical use of aspirin and more than four decades since its use for ocular conditions (GIFFORD 1947; for review see SEARS 1974; LEOPOLD and MURRAY 1979), the mechanism of the anti-inflammatory action of NSAIDS has yet to be clarified. The strong influence of these drugs on the phenomena of fever, pain, and inflammation, taken together with the known undesirable side effects of steroids, has made them of prime interest in ophthalmic therapeutics (LEOPOLD and MURRAY 1979).

B. Mechanism of Action of Nonsteroidal Anti-Inflammatory Drugs

Among substances liberated locally in tissues during inflammation are histamine, 5-hydroxytryptamine (5-HT), bradykinin, chemotactic factors, the slow reactive substance of anaphylaxis (SRS-A) [now known to be LTC_4 and LTD_4 (see Fig. 1)], the rabbit aorta-contracting substance [mainly thromboxane A_2 (TXA_2)], and PGEs and PGF_αs. Attempts to identify these substances, singly or in combination, as mediators of inflammation have been made by using specific antagonists. In some instances success has resulted. Antagonists of histamine, 5-HT, and bradykinin, however, may exert little or no anti-inflammatory effect. Further, potent anti-inflammatory drugs may have little antagonistic action against histamine, 5-HT, or the kinins. This discrepancy shows that these substances individually are unlikely to be able to initiate or sustain inflammation.

Prostaglandins have been proposed as mediators of ocular inflammation (VANE 1976). They are certainly synthesized and released into the eye when it is exposed to irritative stimuli such as physical injury, iris stroke, paracentesis (UNGER et al. 1975; MASUDA et al. 1977), chemical trauma, laser irradiation, trigeminal stimulation, or surgery (HUANG et al. 1971; Miyake 1978). The eye responds to irritative stimuli with miosis, vasodilation in the conjunctiva and iris, rise of protein concentration in aqueous humor, and an abrupt transient rise in intraocular pressure (IOP). That part of the response manifested by hyperemia and disruption of the blood–ocular barrier can partially be prevented by prior treatment with NSAIDS (NEUFELD et al. 1972; PODOS et al. 1973; MISHIMA and MASUDA 1979). In the rabbit, at least, the miotic part of the response is separate and related to the release of substance P (Soloway et al. 1981; Stjernschantz et al. 1981; see Chap. 7). These immediate reactions to trauma are at least quantitatively different from the responses, cellular and reparative, that characterize inflammatory responses.

An outline of the metabolism of arachidonic acid illustrates how prostaglandins are synthesized and released into the eye and at what point NSAIDS could act in an inflammatory response. The metabolites of arachidonic acid, the precursor of prostaglandins, are shown in Fig. 1. From arachidonic acid released from the cell membrane by the enzyme phospholipase A_2, the cyclic endoperoxides PGG_2 and PGH_2 are generated by a cyclooxygenase. They are unstable in aqueous solution, with a half-life of about 5 min, and the enzyme-complex-containing isomerase generates PGD_2, PGE_2, and $PGF_{2\alpha}$ from PGH_2. Prostaglandin E_2 has several of the properties of an inflammatory mediator. Thromboxane A_2 (previously rabbit aorta-contracting substance) is generated from PGG_2 or PGH_2. Of very great importance is a second pathway catalyzed by a lipoxygenase, by which are generated the leukotrienes (Fig. 1) (Borgeat and Samuelsson 1979 a, b; Goetzl and Sun 1979; Goetzl etal. 1980). The leukotrienes are eicosanoids, derived from 20-carbon unsaturated fatty acids. The action of a 5-lipoxygenase generates a monohydroxyeicosatetraenoic acid (5-HPETE). 5-HPETE, via an unstable intermediate, leukotriene A_4 (LTA_4), is converted into dihydroxyeicosatetraenoic acid, leukotriene B_4 (LTB_4), or into C_4, D_4, and E_4 (see Fig. 1). Leukotriene B_4 is chemotactic for leukocytes, while the others may cause vasoconstriction followed by capillary leakage and edema (Bhattacherjee et al. 1980, 1981). Nonsteroidal anti-inflammatory drugs do not inhibit the lipoxygenase but do inhibit the cyclooxygenase to prevent formation of prostaglandins and TXA_2 (Vane 1976). These two separate pathways and the effects of their interaction are of great importance for the development of inflammation, and therefore for the development of compounds that might prevent or ameliorate inflammation. (Further details are given in Chap. 7.) Current nonsteroidal anti-inflammatory drugs only inhibit the effects mediated by the cyclooxygenase pathway. Specific inhibitors of the lipoxygenase pathway have not yet been made available, although recently it was found that (7E,9E,11Z,14Z)-trans-5,6-methano 7,9,11,14-eicosatetraenoic acid (5,6-methanoleukotriene A_4) was a potent and specific inhibitor of 5-lipooxygenase. Of additional interest was the finding that the endogenous compounds LTA_4, 5-HETE, and 5,12-diHETE are inhibitory at micromolar concentrations (Arai et al. 1983). Both the cyclooxygenase pathway and the lipoxygenase pathway are inhibited by steroids because the latter induce an inhibitor of phospholipase A_2 (Flower and Blackwell 1979). Anti-inflammatory glucocorticoids induce a protein which inhibits phospholipase A_2. This protein, which has been named variously macrocortin (Flower and Blackwell 1979) and lipomodulin (Hirata and Axelrod, personal communication), may be an important regulatory one in many cell events whose functions depend on arachidonic acid or its metabolites.

The theory that NSAIDS act as anti-inflammatory drugs by inhibiting prostaglandin synthesis has been questioned (Ham et al. 1972; Lee 1974). Some potent inhibitors of prostaglandin synthesis in vitro are only poor anti-inflammatory drugs in vivo. This descrepancy, however, was explained by Brune (1977), showing that only acidic NSAIDS (pKa values of about 4) bind to plasma proteins and are highly concentrated in inflamed tissue. Capillary damage and extravasation of

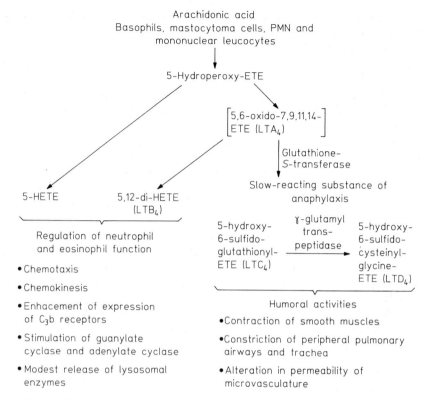

Fig. 1. Metabolites of arachidonic acid. LTA_4, leukotriene A_4 (etc.); PMN, polymorphonuclear

plasma protein take place in inflammation. Intensive absorption of the acids NSAIDS in the stomach and back diffusion in the renal tubules causes high concentration of the drugs in the serum and consequent high concentration of the drugs in the extracellular space at the inflammatory site. pH values in the extracellular spaces that are low in comparison to the intraocular ones force acidic NSAIDS into cell membranes and into the intracellular space. Thus only acidic NSAIDS can concentrate in inflamed tissues in the stomach or kidney, an event which might account for the high incidence of side effects in these organs. Different tissues respond differently and show individual sensitivities to NSAIDS (FLOWER and VANE 1972; BATTACHERJEE and EAKINS 1974a) because the rate-limiting factors and other conditions for the biosynthesis of prostaglandins vary. For example, comparisons of microsomal fractions show that the strength of indomethacin required to inhibit prostaglandin synthesis in the eye is 400 times that required for the spleen. Furthermore, in the eye, the strength of indomethacin required to inhibit prostaglandin synthesis is much higher in the conjunctiva than in the iris-ciliary body (BHATTACHERJEE and EAKINS 1974a, b).

These features, as well as routes of delivery, metabolism, and excretion of the drugs must be considered in understanding their relative order of potency when they are used for ocular conditions. There are very few data for the use of NSAIDS in the eye. Further details are given for each drug category.

C. Salicylates

Aspirin (acetylsalicylic acid) was first used in ophthalmology in 1899 (GIFFORD 1947), for the treatment of patients with uveitis. Experimental confirmation of the efficacy of this drug was made in an animal model of uveitis (WOODS 1961): 5% salicylate ameliorated ocular inflammation.

After VANE (1971) showed that aspirin-like drugs prevented prostaglandin synthesis, studies in ocular tissues began to appear. The first study of the effect of the synthesis and release of endogenous prostaglandins showed that aspirin helped to prevent disruption of the blood–aqueous barrier in the rabbit eye (NEUFELD et al. 1972; MILLER et al. 1973). When 600 mg aspirin was administered per rectum, the concentration of the drug in serum 1 h later was 46 ± 5 mg% (mean $\pm$ SEM) and 38 ± 5 mg% in aqueous humor (NEUFELD et al. 1972), and according to another report (MILLER et al. 1973), 13 ± 2 mg% in serum and 5.5 ± 1.9 mg% in aqueous humor. In the anterior uvea, the concentration was 25 mg% (MILLER et al. 1973). Although the values differ, it is clear that aspirin can penetrate into the eye. Pretreatment with aspirin incompletely but largely prevents the disruption of the blood–aqueous barrier. This effect could be correlated well with PGE_2-like activity in aqueous humor (MILLER et al. 1973). Topical administration of arachidonic acid provoked a significant increase of IOP in the rabbit eye (PODOS et al. 1973). Aspirin (600 mg per rectum) completely prevented the elevation of IOP. Pretreatment with aspirin stabilized lysosomal enzymes (acid phosphatase and β-glucuronidase) after paracentesis and prevented their release (HAYASAKA et al. 1981). As expected, aspirin had no effect on the rise in IOP after instillation of 5 µg of PGE_1 or PGE_2 (PODOS et al. 1973). Although all unsaturated fatty acids have an ocular irritative effect, these results indicate that aspirin probably blocked the biosynthesis of PGs from arachidonic acid. Aspirin also stabilized rat retinal lysosomes both in the absence and presence of 1.5 µg retinol per milligram (DEWAR et al. 1975). Pretreatment of rabbits with aspirin reduced the inflammatory response caused by cyclo-cryotherapy (CHAVIS et al. 1976).

As a consequence of these and other studies done in animals, it was suggested by SEARS et al. (1973), PERKINS (1975), PODOS and SUGAR, and MISHIMA and MASUDA (1977) that compounds inhibiting prostaglandin synthesis and release might be of value in treating or preventing inflammation in humans. The results have not been as dramatic as logic would have predicted; however, the nonsteroidal compounds tested have only had inhibitory effects on the products of the cyclooxygenase pathway. The role of the leukotrienes has only begun to be evaluated.

Experiments done in subhuman primates where the blood–aqueous barrier is less susceptible to trauma than in the rabbit have given less consistent results. Systemic aspirin in varying doses from 600 to 1800 mg per rectum failed to prevent the response to irritative stimuli in the rhesus monkey eye (KASS et al. 1975). In humans five doses of 10 grains of aspirin were given orally at 4-h intervals before surgery to patients who were about to undergo either cataract extraction or combined cataract extraction and penetrating keratoplasty. These patients did show a significantly low protein content in the secondary aqueous humor compared to the controls (ZIMMERMAN et al. 1975). The rise in pressure in other patients after penetrating keratoplasty was not prevented (ZIMMERMAN et al. 1976). The mechanism of the latter is probably different. The miotic response to irritation in humans may be lessened (MISHIMA and MASUDA 1977; see also Sect. D).

Aspirin had little activity in inhibiting prostaglandin biosynthesis (BHATTACHERJEE and EAKINS 1974a) in in vitro experiments done with microsomal fractions from the conjunctiva or iris-ciliary body of rabbit eyes. The discrepancy between the in vivo and the in vitro experiments has not been explained yet. Either only a modest inhibition is required or the effect of aspirin may be differently mediated.

The systemic side effects of aspirin have been well documented (SEARS 1974; ABRISHAMI and THOMAS 1977). Ocular side effects following orally administered aspirin include retinal hemorrhages (MORTADA and ABBOUND 1973) and rebleeding in traumatic hyphema due to diminished platelet aggregation (CRAWFORD et al. 1975).

D. Indomethacin

Indomethacin 1-(p-chlorobenzolyl)-5-methoxy-2 methylindole-3 acetic acid is a synthetic drug introduced in 1962. It has been widely used for its anti-inflammatory, antipyretic, and analgesic properties. However, the mode of action of this drug had not been clarified until VANE (1971) reported that indomethacin was the potent inhibitor of prostaglandin biosynthesis.

Prostaglandin synthetase systems in different tissues and organs have different sensitivities to the inhibitory drugs (FLOWER and VANE 1972; BHATTACHERJEE and EAKINS 1974a, b). BHATTACHERJEE and EAKINS (1974a, b) reported prostaglandin biosynthesis activities in various tissues of rabbits and various inhibitory activities of indomethacin on prostaglandin formation, as shown in Tables 1 and 2. The conjunctiva and anterior uvea required 200 and 400 times more indomethacin, respectively, than did the spleen. In the in vitro system (BHATTACHERJEE and EAKINS 1974 a), the nonacidic NSAID indoxole was the most potent inhibitor of prostaglandin biosynthesis, followed by pirprofen and indomethacin, in descending order. Indomethacin, phenylbutazone, and oxyphenbutazone were approximately equiactive on the anterior uvea, although indomethacin was twice as active as phenylbutazone and four times as active as oxyphenbutazone in the conjunctiva.

In the in vivo system (PODOS and BECKER 1976), indomethacin was more active than indoxole in inhibiting the IOP rise by arachidonic acid administration. The potency of the various NSAIDS to inhibit IOP rise introduced by arachidonic acid application is not exclusively dependent on prostaglandin synthesis and release.

The effectiveness of penetration of systemic indomethacin into the eye has been questioned because of the system for outward transport of organic acids in the ciliary epithelium (MOCHIZUKI 1980). After topical administration, indomethacin was found to penetrate readily into the eye (HANNA and SHARP 1972). 0.1% and 0.5% indomethacin administered topically suppressed the postsurgical inflammation in the human eye (MISHIMA and MASUDA 1977, 1979; MIYAKE 1978; MIYAKE et al.

Table 1. Prostaglandin (PG) biosynthesis from added substrate by various tissues in vitro (Bhattacherjee and Eakins 1974a)

	PG-like activity (ng/mg protein)[a]		
	Zero time	20 min	Increase in activity[c]
Spleen	18.9 ± 3.3 (9)	56 ± 10.5 (9)	38 ± 10 (9)
Kidney (medulla)	69 ± 12 (7)	648 ± 10 (7)	578.5 ± 96 (7)
Anterior uvea[b]	60 ± 5 (15)	179 ± 14 (15)	117 ± 11 (15)
Conjunctiva	39 ± 7 (5)	244 ± 34 (5)	205 ± 28 (5)
Cornea	15 ± 6 (5)	30.5 ± 5 (5)	15 ± 1 (5)
Retina	18 ± 3 (6)	32 ± 5 (6)	14 ± 2 (6)

[a] ng prostaglandin-like activity assayed as PGE_2 generated by microsomes in incubation fluid containing 10 µg/ml arachidonic acid. Numbers in parentheses refer to the number of separate microsomal fractions from pooled tissue samples used for each determination. Results expressed as mean $\pm$ SEM

[b] Iris and ciliary body

[c] Calculated from individual differences between zero-time and 20-min samples

Table 2. Comparison of the inhibitory activity of indomethacin on prostaglandin formation from added arachidonic acid by microsomal fractions of different rabbit tissues (Bhattacherjee and Eakins 1974a)

Tissue	Indomethacin ID_{50}	Comparative ID_{50} (spleen = 1)
Spleen	0.045	1
Kidney (medulla)	0.55	12
Conjunctiva	8.4	187
Anterior uvea	18.5	410
Retina	50.0	1,111

1978). In experimental uveitis induced by bovine serum albumin, topical indomethacin decreased the iris hyperemia, but increased leukocyte migration into the eye (Kulkarni et al. 1981).

The effect of indomethacin to inhibit prostaglandin biosynthesis, thereby preventing signs of ocular irritation, has been summarized (Sears et al. 1973; Eakins 1974; Perkins 1975; Mishima et al. 1977) (see also Chap. 7). Pretreatment of humans or rabbits with either indomethacin or aspirin prevents the IOP rebounding after ocular compression (Zimmerman et al. 1975). Pretreatment with indomethacin prevents the intense inflammatory reaction seen after injection of α-chymotrypsin into the posterior chamber of rabbits (Sears and Sears 1974). Pretreatment with systemic indomethacin or topically administered indomethacin reduces the miosis induced by intraocular surgery in humans or rabbits (Kramer et al. 1976; Sawa and Masuda 1976; Mochizuki et al. 1977). If the inhibition of miosis proves effective, pretreatment with indomethacin becomes a useful adjunct for cataract aspiration procedures. A good deal of interest in preventing any domino effect caused by ocular irritation and the biosynthesis of prostaglandins has surfaced because of the importance of cystoid macular edema, a condition developing after cataract surgery and surmised to be a prostaglandin effect.

Approximately 40%–50% of patients undergoing cataract extraction develop macular edema demonstrable by fluorescein angiography at some time in the postoperative period (KATZ 1981), within days to 4–6 months after surgery. The actual incidence of reduced visual acuity is much lower, and thought to be even further reduced by a technically satisfactory operation. In this latter regard, as well as others, a recent trend has been to prefer extracapsular cataract extraction to the intracapsular procedure. Therapy and/or pretreatment of this condition with indomethacin has been based on the concept first enunciated that disruption of the blood–aqueous barrier, induced by prostaglandin synthesis and release, may play a role (SEARS et al. 1973). In 1974 it was proposed that prostaglandins produced by the iris were causative (TENNANT 1974). The surgical observation (MIAMI STUDY GROUP 1979) that extracapsular cataract extraction was associated with a lower incidence of cystoid macular edema than intracapsular extraction suggested that diffusion of prostaglandins from the iris posteriorly to the macula might be limited by the remaining posterior capsule. Whatever the anatomic origin of the prostaglandins and the role of the mechanics of cataract extraction, numerous reports have appeared dealing with therapy versus prophylaxis of cystoid macular edema utilizing indomethacin. These have recently been reviewed (KATZ 1981). The results generally tend to support the supposition, based on the physiology of prostaglandin synthesis and release, that once cystoid macular is established, blockade of prostaglandin synthesis and release is to no avail (YANNUZZI et al. 1977). Prophylaxis, however, may be of value (MIYAKE 1977). Conflicting results and marginally satisfactory statistics suggest that other factors, especially the mechanics of surgical preparation of the patient and the surgery itself, or other pathways may be involved. Indeed, the presence of inflammatory cells (MARTIN et al. 1977) suggests that chemotactic factors may be involved and, in this regard, either prophylaxis with steroid to block *both* cyclooxygenase and lipooxygenase pathways or specific inhibition or antagonism of the leukotrienes may be required.

Reported ocular side effects (BURNS 1968) of long-term use of indomethacin are macular degeneration, retinal degeneration, corneal deposits, ocular rebleeding and vitreous hemorrhage (PALIMERIS et al. 1972), but these have been appropriately disputed (CARR and SIEGEL 1973). Side effects after topical administration of the drug have not been reported.

E. Pyrazolon Derivatives

Oxyphenbutazone, the parahydroxy derivative of phenylbutazolidine, has been used as an anti-inflammatory, antipyretic, and analgesic drug. Oxyphenbutazone systemically administered penetrates into the eye (WILLIAMSON et al. 1976). A dose of 100 mg given four times daily for 4 days before cataract surgery resulted in concentrations in serum of 5–19 mg%, ten times the level found in aqueous humor and other tissues. Topical administration of the drug as a 10% ointment four times daily for 4 days before surgery showed much less drug in aqueous humor. In animals, adequate drug penetration was shown in aqueous humor by either systemic or topical routes (THOMAS and HANNA 1973).

In clinical studies of the use of oxyphenbutazone, a trial of the efficacy of the drug was favorable in episcleritis (WATSON et al. 1973), scleritis (WATSON et al. 1968), foreign bodies in the cornea (DYSTER-AAS 1973), anterior uveitis (FOWLER and WILKINSON 1973), and postsurgical inflammation (ARNAUD 1971). As might be expected, no beneficial effects of the drug were reported on dendritic keratitis (NORRU 1973) or marginal corneal ulcers (McGILL et al. 1971).

F. Propionic Acid Derivatives

Flurbiprofen (FP), 2-(2-fluoro-4-biphenylyl) propionic acid, is a potent anti-inflammatory agent. One of its first uses was as an antivascularizing agent, reported by COOPER et al. (1980). Flurbiprofen was 12.5 times as potent as indomethacin in inhibiting biosynthesis of PGE_2 from arachidonic acid in bovine seminal vesicular microsomes (NOZU 1978). Like indomethacin, FP exerts its inhibitory effect on prostaglandin biosynthesis by competition (CROOK et al. 1976). The K_i values were estimated to be 0.12 μM for FP and 3.18 μM for indomethacin (NOZU 1978).Penetration of FP (ISHI et al., to be published) after its topical administration to the rabbit eye is shown in Fig. 2. ^{14}C-Flurbiprofen could be detected in the cornea, aqueous humor, iris, and ciliary body. The highest concentration was measured 20 min after the administration. The concentration decreased rapidly thereafter for 3 h. It decreased exponentially after 3 h, the disappearance rate being 0.17 h^{-1} in the cornea, 0.23 h^{-1} in the aqueous humor, 0.22 h^{-1} in the iris, and 0.23 h^{-1} in the

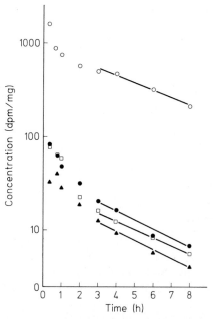

Fig. 2. Time course study of flurbiprofen in the anterior parts of the rabbit eye. ^{14}C-Flurbiprofen (0.1%, pH 6.9) was instilled into the eye of the albino rabbit. *Empty circles*, cornea; *solid circles*, aqueous humor; *squares*, iris; *triangles*, ciliary body. The number of experiments was four to six (mean ± SD). (ISHII et al., to be published)

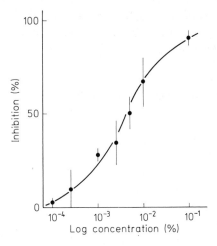

Fig. 3. The effects of topical flurbiprofen on the rise in intraocular pressure induced by arachidonic acid administration. The intraocular pressure was measured 1 h after arachidonic acid. The number of experiments was four to six for each dose (mean $\pm$ SD). (ISHII et al., to be published)

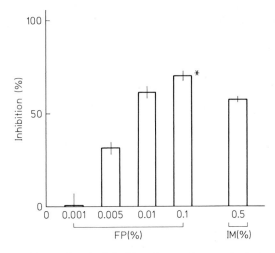

Fig. 4. The inhibitory effects of topical flurbiprofen on the protein leakage from disruption of the blood–aqueous barrier after paracentesis. *FP*, flurbiprofen; *IM*, indomethacin (0.5%). *Asterisk* denotes significant difference between 0.1% flurbiprofen and 0.5% indomethacin ($p < 0.05$). (ISHII et al., to be published)

ciliary body. Disappearance rate of indomethacin from aqueous humor was calculated from Hanna's report (HANNA and SHARP 1972), being 0.34 h^{-1} in aqueous suspension and 0.49 h^{-1} in oil solution.

Effects of FP on the rise in IOP after arachidonic acid administration were examined (GEISER et al. 1981) and are shown in Fig. 3. The rise in protein content in aqueous humor after paracentesis was significantly suppressed by prior treatment with FP (Fig. 4).

A dose of 50 µl 0.1% FP was applied topically to rabbit eyes three times a day for 3 months. Electroretinography was carried out and analyzed. No abnormalities were found in the electroretinogram. No FP effects on corneal wound healing were found.

The compound was well absorbed into rabbit ocular tissues and was highly concentrated in the rabbit cornea. In aphakic eyes, more drug penetrated to the vitreous and choroid-retina area than in normal rabbit eyes, although corneal concentration were still high. No ocular metabolism of FP could be detected, and the ocular route of application did not lead to any changes in blood elimination rates or metabolism when compared with intravenously injected drug. Currently, no NSAID is available for topical ocular use, and the development of such a drug is desirable for treatment of ocular inflammations (SUKAMOTO 1976), especially when long-term treatment is indicated (ANDERSON et al. 1982).

G. Anthranilic Acid Derivatives

Ever since amaurosis fugax was treated successfully with aspirin, the potential effect of the prostaglandins and their metabolites has been considered in dealing with vascular diseases of various sorts. The fenamates are known to prevent aggregation of platelets and propagation of thrombi. In one study of migraine, a therapeutic trial of flufenamic acid was done and it was reported that marked alleviation of headaches occurred (RABEY et al. 1977).

References

Abrishami MA, Thomas J (1977) Aspirin intolerance – a review. Ann Allergy 39:28
Anderson JA, Chen CC, Vita JB, Shackleton M (1982) Disposition of topical flurbiprofen in normal and aphakic rabbit eyes. Arch Ophthalmol 100:642–645
Arai Y, Shimoji K, Konno M, Konishi Y, Okuyama S, Iguchi S, Hayashi M, Miyamoto T, Toda M (1983) Synthesis and 5-lipoxygenase inhibitory activities of eicosanoid compounds. J Med Chem 26:72–78
Arnaud B (1971) The prevention of postoperative inflammation in ocular surgery by the use of Tandearil. Arch Ophthalmol (Paris) 31:349
Bhattacherjee P, Eakins KE (1974a) Inhibition of the prostaglandin synthetase systems in ocular tissues by indomethacin. Br J Pharmacol 50:227–230
Bhattacherjee P, Eakins KE (1974b) A comparison of the inhibitory activity of compounds on ocular prostaglandin biosynthesis. Invest Ophthalmol 13:967
Bhattacherjee P, Hammond BR, Williams RN, Eakins KE (1980) Arachidonic acid lipoxygenase products in ocular tissues and their effect on leukocyte infiltration in vivo. Proc Int Soc Eye 1:32
Bhattacherjee P, Hammond BR, Salmon JA, Stepney R, Eakins KE (1981) Chemotactic response to some arachidonic acid lipoxygenase products in the rabbit eye. Eur J Pharmacol 73:21–28
Borgeat P, Samuelsson B (1979a) Metabolism of arachidonic acid in polymorphonuclear leukocytes: structure analysis of novel hydroxylated compounds. J Biol Chem 254:7865–7869
Borgeat P, Samuelsson B (1979b) Arachidonic acid metabolism in polymorphonuclear leukocytes: unstable intermediate in formation of dihydroxy acids. Proc Natl Acad Sci USA 76:3213–3217

Brune K (1977) The importance of pharmacokinetics for the action of nonsteroid anti-inflammatory drugs. In: Ritshel WA (ed) Clinical pharmacokinetics, proceedings of an international sysmposium at Salzgitter-Rinzelheim (Germany). Fischer, Stuttgart, p 96

Burns CA (1968) Indomethacin, reduced retinal sensitivity, and corneal deposit. Am J Ophthalmol 66:825

Carr RE, Siegel IM (1973) Retinal function in patients treated with indomethacin. Am J Ophthalmol 75:302

Chavis RM, Uygantas CM, Uygantas A (1976) Experimental inhibition of prostaglandin-like inflammation after cryotherapy. Am J Ophthalmol 82:310

Cooper CA, Bergamini MVW, Leopold IH (1980) Use of flurbiprofen to inhibit corneal neovascularization. Arch Ophthalmol 98:1102–1105

Crawford JS, Lewandowski RL, Chan W (1975) The effect of aspirin on rebleeding in traumatic hyphema. Am J Ophthalmol 80:543–545

Crook D, Collins AJ, Rose AJ (1976) A comparison of the effects of flurbiprofen on prostaglandin synthetase from human rheumatoid synovium and enzymatically active animal tissues. J Pharm Pharmacol 28:535

Dewar AJ, Gillian B, Readin HW (1975) The effect of retinol and acetylsalicylic acid on the release of lysosomal enzymes from rat retina in vitro. Exp Eye Res 20:63

Dyster-Aas K (1973) Oxyphenbutazone eye ointment in the treatment of foreign bodies in the cornea. Acta Ophthalmol 51:791

Eakins KE (1974) Prostaglandins and prostaglandin synthetase inhibitors: actions in ocular disease: In: Robinson HJ, Vane JR (eds) Prostaglandin synthetase inhibitors. Raven, New York, p 343

Flower RJ, Blackwell GJ (1979) Anti-inflammatory steroids induce biosynthesis of a phospholipase A_2 inhibitor which prevents prostaglandin production. Nature 278:456

Flower RJ, Vane JR (1972) Inhibition of prostaglandin synthetase in brain explains the antipyretic activity of paracetamol (4-acetamido-phenol). Nature 238:104

Fowler PD, Wildinson P (1973) Treatment of anterior uveitis, comparison of oral oxyphenbutazone and topical steroids. BrJ Ophthalmol 57:892

Gieser DK, Hodapp E, Goldberg I, Kass MA, Becker B (1981) Flurbiprofen and intraocular pressure. Ann Ophthalmol 13:831–833

Gifford SR (1947) A handbook of ocular therapeutics. Lea and Febinger, Philadelphia, p 92

Goetzl EJ, Sun FF (1979) Generation of unique mono-hydroxy-eicosatetraenoic acids from arachidonic acid by human neutrophils. J Exp Med 150:406

Goetzl EJ, Hill HR, Gorman RR (1980) Unique aspects of the modulation of human neutrophil function by 12-L-hydroperoxy-5,8,10,14-eicosatetraenoic acid. Prostaglandins 19:71

Ham EA, Cirillo VJ, Zanetti M, Shen TY, Kuehl FA (1972) Studies on the mode of action of non-steroidal anti-inflammatory agents. In: Ramwell PW, Pharriss BB (eds) Prostaglandins in cellular biology. Plenum, New York, p 345

Hanna C, Sharp JD (1972) Ocular absorption of indomethacin by rabbit. Arch Ophthalmol 88:196–198

Hayasaka S, Masuda K, Sears ML (1981) Nonsteroid anti-inflammatory drugs stabilize the blood-aqueous barrier and lysosomal enzymes in the rabbit eye. Jpn J Ophthalmol 25:210–216

Huang K, Peyman GA, McGetrick J, Janevicius R (1977) Indomethacin inhibition of prostaglandin-mediated inflammation following intraocular surgery. Invest Ophthalmol 16:760–762

Ishii H, Sakai Y, Masuda K, Matsumura Y, Masuda K, Takase M (to be published) Nonsteroid anti-inflammatory drugs: basic studies on flurbiprofen eye drop. Jpn J Ophthalmol 25

Kass MA, Neufeld AH, Sears ML (1975) Systemic aspirin and indomethacin do not prevent the response of the monkey eye to trauma. Invest Ophthalmol 14:604–606

Katz I (1981) Indomethacin. Ophthalmology 88:455–458

Kramer SG, Oyakawa RT, Drake M (1976) Enhancement of pupillary dilation during intraocular surgery by prostaglandin inhibition. Association for research in vision and ophthalmology meeting, 25–29 April 1976, Sarasota

Kulkarni PS, Bhattacherjee P, Eakins, KE, Srinivasan BD (1981) Anti-inflammatory effects of betamethasone phosphate, dexamethasone phosphate and indomethacin on rabbit ocular inflammation induced by bovine serum albumin. Curr Eye Res 1:43

Lee RE (1974) The influence of psychotropic drugs on prostaglandin biosynthesis. Prostaglandins 5:63

Leopold IH, Murray D (1979) Noncorticosteroidal anti-inflammatory agents in ophthalmology. Ophthalmology 86:142–155

Martin NF, Green WR, Martin LW (1977) Retinal phlebitis in the Irvine-Gass syndrome. Am J Ophthalmol 83:377–386

Masuda K, Izawa Y, Mishima S (1977) Breakdown of the blood-aqueous barrier and prostaglandins. Bibl Anat 16:99

McGill JI, Easty DL, Levuy I, Holt-Wilson AD, Shilling J (1971) The etiology and treatment of marginal corneal ulcers. Trans Ophthalmol Soc UK 91:501

Miami Study Group (1979) Cystoid macular edema in aphakic and pseudophakic eyes. Am J Ophthalmol 88:45–48

Miller JD, Eakins KE, Atwal M (1973) The release of PGE_2-like activity into aqueous humor after paracentesis and its prevention by aspirin. Invest Ophthalmol 12:939

Mishima S, Masuda K (1977) Clinical implication of prostaglandins and synthesis inhibitors. In: Burns RP, Leopold IH (eds) Symposium on ocular therapy, vol 10. Wiley, New York, pp 1–19

Mishima S, Masuda K (1979) Prostaglandins and the eye: a review on clinical implications. Metab Pediatr Ophthalmol 3:179

Mishima S, Masuda K, Tamura T (1977) The drugs influencing the intraocular pressure. In: Dikstein S (ed) Drugs and ocular tissues. Karger, Basel, p 128

Miyake K (1977) Prevention of cystoid macular edema after lens extraction by topical indomethacin: a preliminary report. Albrecht von Graefes Arch Klin Exp Ophthalmol 203:81–88

Miyake K (1978) Prophylaxis of aphakic cystoid macular edema using topical indomethacin. Am Intra-Ocular Implant Soc J 4:174

Miyake K, Sugiyama S, Norimatsu I, Ozawa T (1978) Prevention of macular cystoid macular edema after lens extraction by topical indomethacin (III) radio-immunoassay measurement of prostaglandins in the aqueous during and after lens extraction procedure. Albrecht von Graefes Arch Ophthalmol 209:83

Mochizuki M (1980) Transport of indomethacin in the anterior uvea of the albino rabbit. Jpn J Ophthalmol 24:363

Mochizuki M, Sawa M, Masuda K (1977) Topical indomethacin in intracapsular extraction of senile cataract. Jpn J Ophthalmol 21:215

Mortada A, Abboud I (1973) Retinal haemorrhages after prolonged use of salicylates. Brit J Ophthalmol 57:199–200

Neufeld AH, Jampol LM, Sears ML (1972) Aspirin prevents the disruption of the blood-aqueous barrier in the rabbit eye. Nature 238:158–159

Norru MS (1973) Oxyphenbutazone (Tandearil R) as an adjuvant in treatment of dendritic keratitis, double blind trial using fluorescein-rose Bengal vital staining. Acta Ophthalmol 51:591

Nozu K (1978) Flurbiprofen: highly potent inhibitor of prostaglandin synthesis. Biochimica Biophysica Acta 529:493

Palimeris G, Koliopoulos J, Velissaropoulos P (1972) Ocular side effects of indomethacin. Ophthalmologica 164:339

Perkins ES (1975) Prostaglandins and the eye. Adv Ophthalmol 29:2

Podos SM, Becker B (1976) Comparison of ocular prostaglandin synthesis inhibitors. Invest Ophthalmol 15:841–844

Podos SM, Sugar A (1980) The use of nonsteroidal anti-inflammatory drugs in ocular conditions. In: Srinivasan BD (ed) Ocular therapeutics. Masson, New York, Chap 9, pp 73–81

Podos SM, Becker B, Kass MA (1973) Indomethacin blocks arachidonic acid-induced elevation of intraocular pressure. Prostaglandins 3:7–15

Rabey JM, et al. (1977) Ophthalmoplegic migraine: amelioration by flufenamic acid, a prostaglandin inhibitor. Ophthalmologica 175:158

Sawa M, Masuda K (1976) Topical indomethacin in soft cataract aspiration. Jpn J Ophthalmol 20:514

Sears ML (1974) The use of aspirin and aspirin-like drugs in ophthalmology. In: Leopold IH (ed) Symposium on ocular therapy, vol 7. Mosby, St. Louis, Chap 10, pp 104–115

Sears ML, Neufeld AH, Jampol LM (1973) Prostaglandins. Invest Ophthalmol 12:161–164

Sears D, Sears M (1974) Blood-aqueous barrier and alpha chymotrypsin glaucoma in rabbits. Am J Ophthalmol 77:378–383

Soloway HR, Stjernschantz J, Sears ML (1981) The miotic effect of substance P on the isolated rabbit iris. Invest Ophthalmol Vis Sci 20:47–52

Stjernschantz J, Sears M, Stjernschantz L (1981) Intraocular effects of substance P in the rabbit. Invest Ophthalmol Vis Sci 20:53–60

Stone E (1763) An account of the success of the bark of the willow in the cure of agues. Philos Trans R Soc Lond 53:195

Sukamoto H (1976) Clinical use of flurbiprofen as a postoperative anti-inflammatory agent. Folia Ophthalmol Jpn 27:87

Tennant JL (1978) Prostaglandins in ophthalmology. In: Emery JM (ed) Current concepts in cataract surgery. Selected proceedings of the fifth biennial cataract congress. Mosby, St. Louis, pp 360–362

Thomas AH, Hanna C (1973) Oxyphenbutazone in ocular inflammation. Arch Ophthalmol 89:340–341

Unger WG, Cole DF, Hammond B (1975) Disruption of the blood-aqueous barrier following paracentesis in the rabbit. Exp Eye Res 20:255–270

Vane JR (1971) Inhibition of prostaglandin-synthesis as a mechanism of action for aspirin-like drugs. Nature [New Biol] 231:232

Vane JR (1976) The mode of action of aspirin and similar compounds. J Allergy Clin Immun 58:691

Watson PG, Hayreh SS, Awdry PN (1968) Episcleritis and scleritis. Br J Ophthalmol 52:348–349

Watson PG, MacKay DAR, Clement RS, Wilkinson P (1973) Treatment of episcleritis, a double blind trial comparing betamethasone 0.1 percent, oxyphenbutazone 10 percent and placebo eye ointments. Br J Ophthal 57:866–870

Williamson J, Sim AK, Chawla JC, Tham HM, Forrester JV, Mammo NV (1976) Estimation of oxyphenbutazone concentrations in human serum and aqueous humor. Eye Ear Nose Throat Mon 55:176

Woods AC (1961) Endogenous inflammation of the uveal tract. Williams and Wilkins, Baltimore, p 458

Yannuzzzi LA, Klein RM, Wallyn RH, Cohen N, Katz I (1977) Ineffectiveness of indomethacin in the treatment of chronic cystoid macular edema. Am J Ophthalmol 84:517–519

Zimmerman TJ, Gravenstein N, Sugar A, Kaufman HE (1975) Aspirin stabilization of the blood-aqueous barrier in the human eye. Am J Ophthalmol 79:817–819

Zimmermann TJ, Binder P, Abel RA, Kaufman H (1976) Aspirin and the intraocular pressure rise following aphakic penetrating keratoplasty: a negative report. Ann Ophthalmol 8:611–613

CHAPTER 11

Chemotherapy of Ocular Viral Infections and Tumors

P. H. FISCHER and W. H. PRUSOFF

A. Introduction

This review will focus on drugs useful in the chemotherapy of ocular viral infections. Three drugs now approved for the treatment of herpes simplex virus (HSV) keratitis, iododeoxyuridine (IdUrd), adenine arabinoside (ara-A), and trifluorothymidine (CF₃dUrd), will be discussed. In addition, several agents now under development, acycloguanosine (acyclovir), ethyldeoxyuridine (EtdUrd), bromovinyldeoxyuridine (BVdUrd), 1-(2-deoxy-2-fluoro-β-D-arabinosyl)-5-iodo-cytosine (FIAC), 5-iodo-5′-amino-2′,5′-dideoxyuridine (AIdUrd), and the phosphonates will be reviewed. Each of these compounds was chosen for a particular reason. Acyclovir is a highly unusual acyclic guanosine derivative and is a most promising antiviral agent. Bromovinyldeoxyuridine, EtdUrd, and FIAC represent new pyrimidine derivatives which possess higher degrees of antiviral selectivity than the two thymidine analogs now available (CF₃dUrd, IdUrd). 5-Iodo-5′-amino-2′,5′-dideoxyuridine is a novel amino nucleoside that is activated only in herpes-infected cells. The phosphonates, in contrast, are not nucleosides, neither are they metabolized, and they represent inhibitors of the virally induced DNA polymerases. Such highly specific chemotherapy is not available for the treatment of ocular tumors and this topic will be only briefly discussed.

The high degree of selectivity which has now been achieved in viral chemotherapy depends on the exploitation of virus-specified enzymes. The substrate and inhibitor specificity of these enzymes is sufficiently different from that of their host cell counterparts for preferential drug activation or inhibition to be achieved. Thus the HSV-specified thymidine kinase, but not the host cell enzyme, can phosphorylate acyclovir (FYFE et al. 1978) and AIdUrd (CHEN and PRUSOFF 1979). Similarly, the herpesvirus-encoded DNA polymerase is preferentially inhibited by the triphosphates of acyclovir (FURMAN et al. 1979) and ara-A (MÜLLER et al. 1977b) and the phosphonates (MAO and ROBISHAW 1975; RENO et al. 1978). Thus it is clear that antiviral drug design can now be based on the qualitative as well as the quantitative exploitation of virally associated enzymatic activities. As our understanding of the many virally induced enzymes (KIT 1979) increases, the development of new, highly selective antiviral agents can be expected to continue.

Virally induced enzymes that are unique to the virus-infected cell and are also necessary for viral replication are good targets for selective chemotherapy. The

The research emanating from our laboratories was supported by U.S. Public Health Service Grant CA-05262 from the National cancer Institute (WHP) and Al-19043 (PHF)

RNA transcriptases, RNA replicases, and the reverse transcriptases are examples (see KIT 1979). Certain other virally induced enzymes, although catalyzing reactions which normally occur in uninfected cells, are sufficiently different from their host cell couterparts for chemotherapeutic attack to be possible. As was mentioned, the DNA polymerase (KEIR and GOLD 1963) and the thymidine kinase (KIT and DUBBS 1963) induced by herpesviruses are in this group. The deoxycytidine deaminase (CHAN 1977), deoxyribonuclease (KEIR and GOLD 1963), and ribonucleotide diphosphate reductase (COHEN 1972) activities induced by herpes infections are also possible targets.

Since the antiherpes activity of so many nucleoside analogs is dependent on the HSV thymidine kinase (DECLERCQ et al. 1977), this enzyme requires further discussion. It differs from the host cell enzyme in molecular weight, substrate specificity, electrophoretic mobility, isoelectric point, and immunologic properties (see KIT 1979, for a review). The herpes enzyme has an unusually broad substrate specificity, catalyzing the phosphorylation of 2'-deoxythymidine (dThd) and 2'-deoxycytidine (dCyd) (JAMIESON et al. 1974; JAMIESON and SUBAK-SHARPE 1974) and interacting with a variety of nucleoside analogs (CHENG 1976, 1977; CHENG et al. 1976). CHEN and PRUSOFF (1978) extended the activity of this enzyme to include thymidine monophosphate kinase activity. The critical nature of this enzyme in the biochemistry of many antiviral agents will be stressed.

Many aspects of antiviral chemotherapy have been recently reviewed (PRUSOFF and WARD 1976; KAUFMAN 1977; SIDWELL and WITKOWSKI 1979; MÜLLER 1979, 1980; DECLERCQ 1979; DECLERCQ and TORRENCE 1978; PRUSOFF and FISCHER 1979; CHANG and SNYDMAN 1979; SMITH et al. 1980; HERRMANN and HERRMANN 1979; KAUFMAN 1980, RENIS 1980; HIRSCH and SWARTZ 1980; PAVAN-LANGSTON 1979; 1980; BECKER and Hadar 1980; HELGSTRAND and OBERG 1980; FISCHER and PRUSOFF 1982). These and other reviews dealing with specific agents will be cited as a further guide to the primary literature.

The chemotherapy of ocular tumors, as is the case in other malignancies, is limited by the lack of highly selective agents. However, several protocols which may improve therapy are now being evaluated (see KITCHIN and ELLSWORTH 1980 for a review). One study is designed to prevent death in children with advanced unilateral retinoblastoma. Cyclophosphamide and vincristine, both active as single agents, are being employed. Other trials involving patients with metastatic neuroblastoma are also under way. BISHOP and MADSON (1975) and ROSENBAUM et al. (1980) have recently reviewed retinoblastoma. The treatment of orbital rhabdomyosarcoma has been discussed by ABRAMSON (1979). Current therapy involves radiation in combination with vincristine, cyclophosphamide, and actinomycin D.

B. Clinically Available Antiviral Agents

I. 5-Iodo-2'-deoxyuridine (Idoxuridine)

1. Synthesis

PRUSOFF (1959) synthesized IdUrd as part of an anticancer program (WELCH and PRUSOFF 1960).It is an analog of thymidine (Fig. 1) in which the methyl group is replaced by an iodine atom. Although the substitution is nearly isosteric, the induc-

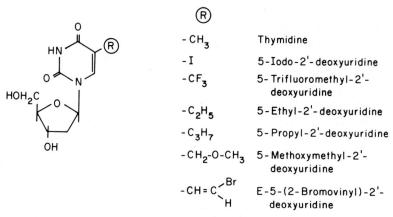

	®ᴿ	
	- CH₃	Thymidine
	- I	5-Iodo-2'-deoxyuridine
	- CF₃	5- Trifluoromethyl-2'-deoxyuridine
	- C₂H₅	5-Ethyl-2'-deoxyuridine
	- C₃H₇	5-Propyl-2'-deoxyuridine
	- CH₂-O-CH₃	5-Methoxymethyl-2'-deoxyuridine
	- CH = C⟨Br/H	E-5-(2-Bromovinyl)-2'-deoxyuridine

Fig. 1. Structures of various analogs of thymidine

tive effect of the halogen reduced the pKa from 9.8 for dThd to 8.2 for IdUrd (BERENS and SHUGAR 1963). The physicochemical properties and biological actions of IdUrd have been thoroughly reviewed (PRUSOFF 1967; GOZ and PRUSOFF 1970; SUGAR and KAUFMAN 1973; PRUSOF and GOZ 1975; LANGEN 1975; PRUSOFF et al. 1979 a; FISCHER and PRUSOFF 1982).

2. Antiviral Activity

HERRMANN (1961) first described the inhibitory effects of IdUrd on the replication of HSV and vaccinia virus. Although a wide variety of viruses are inhibited by the drug (PRUSOFF and GOZ 1975), its activity is restricted to those viruses in which DNA is synthesized during the replicative cycle. This is consistent with the fact that IdUrd is an analog of dThd.

The efficacy of IdUrd in experimental herpes keratitis was first demonstrated by KAUFMAN et al. (1962a) and confirmed by PERKINS et al. (1962). Subsequently, considerable in vivo evaluation of IdUrd against a number of viruses was done (SCHABEL and MONTGOMERY 1972; PRUSOFF and GOZ 1975). The reports of activity in experimental keratitis were of particular importance, since IdUrd was then shown to be effective in herpes simplex infections of the corneal epithelium in man (KAUFMAN 1962; KAUFMAN et al. 1962 b). For the first time an antiviral agent had been proved clinically efficacious in an established virus infection. 5-Iodo-2'-deoxyuridine has been widely used in herpes keratitis and its clinical utility well reviewed (KAUFMAN 1965; VERBOV 1979). The use of IdUrd in other viral diseases, including herpetic whitlow, genital herpes, cutaneous herpes, herpes zoster, and vaccinia whitlow, has been described (JUEL-JENSEN 1973, 1974). The systemic use of IdUrd in herpes encephalitis is limited by the associated myelosuppression (CALABRESSI et al. 1961; BOSTON INTERHOSPITAL VIRUS STUDY GROUP 1975).

3. Effects on Normal Cells

5-Iodo-2'-deoxyuridine resembles dThd so closely that few differences in the metabolism of these two compounds are evident in normal cells. The presence of dThd

(MATHIAS and FISCHER 1962), or the deletion of cellular thymidine kinase (KIT et al. 1963), confers resistance against the cytotoxic effects of IdUrd. These data are consistent with the idea that IdUrd is an analog of dThd, but do not distinguish between the various possible sites of action.

Recently, however, KAUFMAN and DAVIDSON (1979) presented evidence which strongly indicates that the cytotoxicity of IdUrd is dependent on its anabolism to the 5'-triphosphate and its subsequent incorporation into DNA. They isolated IdUrd-resistant cells which accumulate 5-iodo-2'-deoxyuridylate (IdUMP) but do not convert it to the triphosphate. The thymidine monophosphate kinase of these cells has an altered substrate specificity and a markedly reduced capacity to phosphorylate IdUMP. These results indicate that IdUrd and IdUMP are not per se cytotoxic, and that further metabolic activation, presumably to the triphosphate, is required. The relationship between the incorporation of halogenated deoxyuridines into DNA and their biological effects has been extensively studied and recently reviewed (GOZ 1978). PRUSOFF and GOZ (1973a, b, 1975) have described the metabolic handling and biochemical effects of IdUrd in detail.

4. Mechanism of Action

The antiviral selectivity of IdUrd is apparently dependent on the induction of viral thymidine kinase activity. Although IdUrd is phosphorylated by the host cell enzyme as efficiently as by the HSV thymidine kinase, the marked enhancement of activity present in virally infected cells leads to an accumulation of toxic metabolites. This increase in the anabolism of IdUrd in virally infected cells as compared to uninfected cells accounts for the selective antiherpes effects of IdUrd (PRUSOFF and GOZ 1973a, b, 1975). Extensive analyses of the metabolic handling of IdUrd and dThd have revealed no critical differences between normal and virus-infected cells. The pathways affected and the biochemical effects exerted have been reviewed in detail by PRUSOFF and GOZ (1975).

Among the enzymes involved in DNA biosynthesis, several are inhibited by IdUrd or one of its phosphorylated derivatives. Thymidine kinase, thymidylate kinase, and DNA polymerase are competitively inhibited and utilize the appropriate metabolite as an alternate substrate. In addition, the regulatory enzymes thymidine kinase, deoxycytidylate deaminase, and ribonucleoside diphosphate reductase are inhibited by 5-iodo-2'-deoxyuridine-5'-triphosphate. None of these effects, however, accounted for the antiviral activity of IdUrd. Thus PRUSOFF et al. (1965) proposed that incorporation of the analog into viral DNA was the key biochemical event.

Several lines of evidence support this suggestion. The replacement of thymidine by IdUrd in SV40 DNA correlated with a loss of infectivity of the viral DNA (BUETTNER and WERCHAU 1973). Similarly, a parallelism between the incorporation of IdUrd into viral DNA and the inhibition of HSV replication was shown (FISCHER et al. 1980). The earlier work of KAPLAN and BEN-PORAT (1966) on pseudorabies virus also focused on the importance of the incorporation of IdUrd into viral DNA. Their data suggested that fraudulent viral proteins were synthesized from DNA in which dThd was replaced by IdUrd. Thus encapsidation of the viral DNA was inhibited. KAN-MITCHELL and PRUSOFF (1979) showed that IdUrd inhibited the synthesis of the late but not early proteins in adenovirus-2-infected cells.

This is quite important, since only the late proteins are translated from RNA that had been transcribed from progeny DNA, the DNA that had been synthesized in the presence of IdUrd. The drug did not, however, induce changes in the physiological or immunologic characteristics of the adenovirus capsid proteins (WIGAND and KLEIN 1974). MAASS and HAAS (1966) found a reduction in the formation of SV40 antigens when IdUrd was present during viral replication.

The time course of IdUrd action and the reversal of its effects by dThd also implicate the incorporation of IdUrd into viral DNA as the critical event. Thus the absorption of herpesviruses to cells or the release of mature virus particles from infected cells is not inhibited by IdUrd (SMITH 1963; SMITH and DUKES 1964). Exposure of HSV-infected cells to IdUrd for only the first 2 h after infection does not inhibit virus replication. The antiviral activity of IdUrd can be reversed by dThd if the infected cells are exposed to IdUrd from 2 to 4 h after infection. In contrast, the effects caused by commencing IdUrd treatment 4 h after infection are not sensitive to dThd reversal (ROIZMAN et al. 1963).

The molecular mechanism by which the incorporation of IdUrd into DNA is translated into an antiviral effect is not known. Extensive investigations have been performed and a wide variety of biochemical effects reported. Recent reviews of the subject have examined a number of possibilities (PRUSOFF and GOZ 1975; GOZ 1978; PRUSOFF et al. 1979 a, b). Recently, OTTO et al. (1982) found a marked effect on viral proteins produced either when HSV was grown in the presence of IdUrd, or when HSV substituted with IdUrd in the DNA was grown in the absence of IdUrd.

II. 9-β-D-Arabinofuranosyladenine (Adenine, Arabinoside, Vidarabine)

1. Synthesis

9-β-D-Arabinofuranosyladenine (ara-A) was synthesized by LEE et al. (1960), and was isolated in 1967 from *Streptomyces antibioticus* (Parke Davis).

9-β-D-Arabinofuranosyladenine and 2'-deoxyadenosine are structural analogs, as shown in Fig. 2. There is an extensive literature on the biological effects of ara-A, and a number of reviews have been cited to provide a detailed guide to the primary literature (CH'IEN et al. 1973; CASS 1979; COHEN 1966, 1976; LEPAGE 1975; MÜLLER

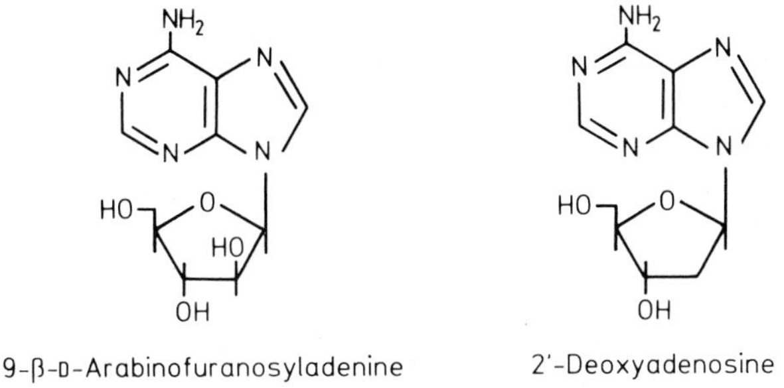

9-β-D-Arabinofuranosyladenine   2'-Deoxyadenosine

Fig. 2. Structures of 9-β-D-Arabinofuranosyladenine (Vidarabine) and 2'-deoxyadenosine

1980; North and Cohen 1979; Whitely et al. 1980 b). In addition, a monograph on the antiviral actions of ara-A is available (Pavan-Langston et al. 1975).

2. Antiviral Activity

Early reports described the activity of ara-A against several DNA viruses, including HSV and vaccinia virus (DeRudder and Privat-DeGarilhe 1965) and varicella-zoster virus and cytomegalovirus (Miller et al. 1969). The work has been extended to include other DNA viruses and the RNA tumor viruses. Shannon (1975) and Connor et al. (1975) have reviewed the in vitro antiviral effects of ara-A in detail.

9-β-D-Arabinofuranosyladenine is effective in experimental herpes keratitis (Schabel 1968) and herpes encephalitis (Sloan et al. 1973). Pavan-Langston and Dohlman (1972) demonstrated the clinical efficacy of ara-A in viral keratoconjunctivitis. Subsequently, a controlled study was conducted to evaluate ara-A versus IdUrd in HSV keratitis (Pavan-Langston and Buchanan 1976). The mean time to healing and the proportion of treatment failures were both slightly less in the ara-A-treated group. Abel et al. (1975) treated deep HSV eye infections with intravenously administered ara-A and demonstrated significant improvement. 9-β-D-Arabinofuranosyladenine also appears promising in the treatment of herpes zoster infections in immunosuppressed patients (Whitley et al. 1976). Importantly, successful therapy of biopsy-proved herpes simplex encephalitis in humans has been reported (Whitley et al. 1977, 1980 b). A beneficial effect in neonatal HSV infections is also evident (Whitley et al. 1980 a).

3. Effects on Normal Cells

9-β-D-Arabinofuranosyladenine inhibits DNA synthesis and is toxic to mammalian cells (Brink and LePage 1964; Doering et al. 1966; Müller et al. 1975). Cytotoxicity is apparently dependent on the metabolic activation of ara-A to its 5′-triphosphate (ara-ATP) (LePage 1975; Cohen 1976). Several biochemical effects of ara-ATP, including inhibition of DNA polymerase (York and LePage 1966; Furth and Cohen 1967, 1968) and ribonucleotide reductase (York and LePage 1966; Moore and Cohen 1967) and its incorporation into DNA (Waqar et al. 1971; Plunkett et al. 1974), may contribute to the cytotoxicity of ara-A. The K_i's for inhibition of DNA polymerase α and β by ara-ATP are 7.4 μM and 5.6 μM respectively (Müller et al. 1975), whereas the reduction of ribonucleotides seems considerably less sensitive (Moore and Cohen 1967).

The catabolism of ara-A to arabinofuranosylhypoxanthine by adenosine deaminase is the major pathway of detoxification. Potent inhibitors of deamination, such as the tight-binding compound deoxycoformycin (Cha 1975; Agarwal et al. 1977), potentiate the lethality of ara-A (Plunkett and Cohen 1975; Cass and Ah-Yeung 1976).

In clinical studies of herpes zoster in which ara-A was given systemically, the therapeutic index of the drug was found to be satisfactory (Whitley et al. 1976). In rodents the toxicity of ara-A is low, and quite large doses (75 g/kg) are required to reach the acute LD_{50} (Kurtz 1975). 9-β-D-Arabinofuranosyladenine did not reduce the healing time in experimental corneal wounds, and was found to produce fewer changes in the regenerating epithelium than did IdUrd (LANGSTON et al. 1974). A detailed review of the pharmacokinetics, disposition, toxicity and human pharmacology of ara-A recently appeared (WHITLEY et al. 1980 b).

4. Mechanism of Action

9-β-D-Arabinofuranosyladenine inhibits the replication of herpesviruses at concentrations that are not toxic to the host cells. This selectivity, as well as the antiviral action of ara-A, is apparently related to a preferential inhibition of viral DNA synthesis. Such inhibition of HSV DNA synthesis by ara-A was demonstrated in the absence (SHIPMAN et al. 1976) or presence (SCHWARTZ et al. 1976) of an adenosine deaminase inhibitor.

The preferential marked inhibition of the viral DNA polymerase by ara-ATP relative to cellular DNA polymerases may be the critical biochemical event producing the antiviral actions of ara-A. MÜLLER et al. (1977 b) have reported that ara-ATP inhibits the HSV DNA polymerase more potently than either the α or β DNA polymerases derived from uninfected cells. The K_i/K_m ratios (WEBB 1963) of ara-ATP for the various enzymes were used for comparison, but the differential binding ratio of ara-ATP to 2'-deoxyadenosine-5'-triphosphate (dATP) for HSV DNA polymerase relative to cellular DNA polymerase was not confirmed by OSTRANDER and CHENG (1980). In a study using a crude preparation this differential sensitivity was not detected (BENNETT et al. 1975).

In addition, it has been reported that ara-A produces chain termination more frequently in HSV DNA than in cellular DNA (MÜLLER et al. 1977 a). However, more recent studies by PELLING et al. (1981) show that ara-A is incorporated in internucleotide linkage in the DNA of both HSV and host cell. Other potential sites of inhibition include a direct effect of ara-A, at the nucleoside level, on S-adenosylhomocysteine hydrolase. The results of such inhibition would be a failure to methylate mRNA (HERSHFIELD 1979).

III. 5-Trifluoromethyl-2'-deoxyuridine (Trifluorothymidine, Viroptic, Trifluridine)

1. Synthesis

HEIDELBERGER et al. (1964) synthesized the trifluoro derivative of deoxyuridine as a dThd analog (Fig. 1). Although CF$_3$dUrd is stable under acidic conditions, the 5-carboxy derivative is generated under mildly alkaline conditions (HEIDELBERGER et al. 1964). Extensive reviews of the pharmacology and biochemistry of CF$_3$dUrd and other fluorinated pyrimidines are available (HEIDELBERGER 1975 a, b; HEIDELBERGER and KING 1969).

2. Antiviral Activity

5-Trifluoromethyl-2'-deoxyuridine functions as a dThd analog and potently inhibits the replication of DNA viruses, including HSV, vaccinia virus, and adenovirus. The replication of vaccinia virus, for example, is inhibited by CF$_3$dUrd at $10^{-7} M$ in HeLa cells (UMEDA and HEIDELBERGER 1969).

KAUFMAN and HEIDELBERGER (1964) first demonstrated the efficacy of CF$_3$dUrd in the treatment of herpes keratitis in rabbits. Interestingly, a strain of

HSV that was resistant to IdUrd in vivo and in vitro was sensitive to CF_3dUrd in vivo. It appears that CF_3dUrd is superior to IdUrd and ara-A for this disease (SUGAR et al. 1973; PAVAN-LANGSTON 1979). ITOI et al. (1975) have reported that topical administration of IdUrd, but not of CF_3dUrd, was teratogenic in pregnant rabbits; CF_3dUrd has also been shown to be effective in experimental herpes keratitis (CLOUGH and PARKHURST 1977).

For the treatment of superfical HSV infections of the eye in humans, CF_3dUrd appears to be the best available drug (for reviews see HEIDELBERGER and KING 1979; KAUFMAN 1980). Importantly, recent studies indicate that patients who have failed to respond to IdUrd or ara-A are effectively treated with CF_3-dUrd (McGILL et al. 1974; JONES et al. 1975). A number of clinical studies have documented that CF_3dUrd is efficacious in superficial herpes keratitis and that the drug compares favorably with ara-A (McKINNON et al. 1975; COSTER et al. 1976; TRAVERS and PATTERSON 1978) and IdUrd (WELLINGS et al. 1972; LAIBSON et al. 1977; PAVAN-LANGSTON and FOSTER 1977).

O'BRIEN and EDELHAUSER (1977) have shown that CF_3dUrd effectively penetrates the cornea and that some conversion to the 5-carboxy derivative occurs. 5-Trifluoromethyl-2′-deoxyuridine does not, however, inhibit the healing of corneal wounds (FOSTER and PAVAN-LANGSTON 1977).

3. Effects on Normal Cells

The anabolism of CF_3dUrd is similar to that of IdUrd and dThd. It is phosphorylated to the 5′-monophosphate by thymidine kinase (BRESNICK and WILLIAMS 1967) and, after metabolism to the triphosphate, is incorporated into DNA (FUJIWARA et al. 1970). In contrast to the case with IdUrd, inhibition of thymidylate synthetase by 5-trifluoromethyl-2′-deoxyuridylate (CF_3dUMP) (REYES and HEIDELBERGER 1965) rather than its incorporation into DNA appears to account for the cytotoxicity of CF_3dUrd (UMEDA and HEIDELBERGER 1968). Thus, in addition to its antiviral effects, CF_3dUrd is active against cancer (HEIDELBERGER and ANDERSON 1964) and is toxic upon systemic administration.

4. Mechanism of Action

Studies detailing the mechanisms by which CF_3dUrd exerts its antiviral effects have been reviewed (HEIDELBERGER 1975a, b; HEIDELBERGER and KING 1979). These workers have suggested that, although the metabolism of CF_3dUrd in virally infected cells and host cells is similar, toxicity is mediated through different mechanisms. Thus TONE and HEIDELBERGER (1973) presented data suggesting that preferential incorporation of CF_3dUrd into viral DNA accounts for its selective antiviral activity. In the case of vaccinia virus, the critical difference is at the level of the DNA polymerase. Although 5-trifluoromethyl-2′-deoxyuridine-5′-triphosphate inhibited both the cellular and viral DNA polymerases, the analog was more effectively utilized as an alternate substrate by the viral enzyme (TONE and HEIDELBERGER 1973).

The importance of the incorporation event is supported by other studies. PARKHURST et al. (1976) found that CF_3dUrd inhibited virus replication most effectively if it was added within 2 h of infection. In addition, dThd reverses the antiviral effect only if it is added before the synthesis of progeny DNA (UMEDA and HEIDELBERGER 1969). Morphologically defective virions, containing fragmented DNA, are produced in the presence of CF_3dUrd (FUJIWARA and HEIDELBERGER 1970). In vaccinia-virus-infected cells, CF_3dUrd leads to the synthesis of an altered late mRNA (OKI and HEIDELBERGER 1971) that has about 30% fewer sequences than the normal transcript (DEXTER et al. 1973). The mechanism of action of CF_3dUrd in HSV-infected cells remains to be elucidated.

C. Newer Agents Under Development

I. 9-(2-Hydroxyethoxymethyl)guanine (Acyclovir, Acycloguanosine)

1. Synthesis

Acyclovir is an acyclic analog of deoxyguanosine (Fig. 3). It and other acyclic nucleoside derivatives were synthesized by SCHAEFFER et al. (1978) as a result of their finding that the intact cyclic carbohydrate moiety was not necessary for binding to enzymes. In particular, it had been shown that adenosine deaminase could be inhibited by acyclic adenine derivatives (SCHAEFFER et al. 1971). Another procedure for the synthesis of acyclovir has been recently reported (BARRIO et al. 1980).

2. Antiviral Activity

a) In Vitro

The selective antiherpes action of acyclovir was first described by ELION et al. (1977). The compound, at a concentration of $0.1 \mu M$, inhibited by 50% the replication of HSV-1 in Vero cells. In contrast, a 3000-fold greater concentration was required to inhibit the growth of uninfected Vero cells. Acyclovir is highly effective against a large number of HSV-1 and HSV-2 strains in vitro (COLLINS and BAUER 1979; CRUMPACKER et al. 1979; CENTIFANTO and KAUFMAN 1979). The replication of varicella-zoster virus (SCHAEFFER et al. 1978; CRUMPACKER et al. 1979; BIRON and ELION 1980), Epstein-Barr virus (COLBY et al 1980; DATTA et al. 1980), and,

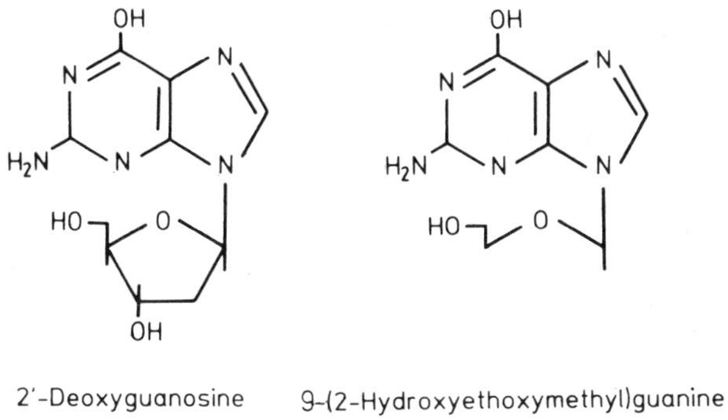

2'-Deoxyguanosine   9-(2-Hydroxyethoxymethyl)guanine

Fig. 3. Structures of 9-(2-hydroxyethoxymethyl)guanine (acyclovir, acycloguanosine) and 2'-deoxyguanosine

to a much lesser extent, cytomegalovirus (SCHAEFFER et al. 1978; CRUMPACKER et al. 1979) are inhibited by this agent. It is not active against vaccinia virus, adenovirus type 5, or a large number of RNA viruses (SCHAEFFER et al. 1978).

b) In Vivo

A high degree of antiherpes selectivity in vivo was initially demonstrated by SCHAEFFER et al. (1978). These investigators showed that acyclovir had good antiviral activity against herpes encephalitis in mice, herpes keratitis in rabbits, and cutaneous herpes infections in guinea pigs. Very little, if any, toxicity was associated with the drug therapy.

The in vivo antiherpes activity of acyclovir has been confirmed and extended by many other investigators. In general, acyclovir appears to be a safe, highly efficacious drug. The effectiveness of acyclovir in the treatment of experimental herpes virus keratitis in rabbits is well established (PAVAN-LANGSTON et al. 1978; KAUFMAN et al. 1978; FALCON and JONES 1979; SHIOTA et al. 1979; BAUER et al. 1979). Efficacy has been established in the cutaneous herpes infections in guinea pigs (PARK et al. 1980b) and mice (KLEIN et al. 1979a), herpes encephalitis in mice (PARK et al. 1979b), and ear infections in mice (FIELD et al. 1979).

Two recent double-blind clinical studies have documented the efficacy of acyclovir in the treatment of HSV-induced corneal dendritic ulcers. Acyclovir was equally (COSTER et al. 1980) or more effective than IdUrd (COLLUM et al. 1980).

An important observation has been the ability of acyclovir to prevent the establishment of latent HSV infections in ganglia. Using a mouse model in which HSV-1 (strain SC-16) is inoculated subcutaneously in the pinna, FIELD et al. (1979) showed that systemically administered acyclovir reduced the frequency of latent infections in the dorsal root ganglia. In HSV-1 (strain S)-induced skin infections in hairless mice, acyclovir effectively inhibited the establishment of ganglionic infections when applied topically (KLEIN et al. 1979a). A delay in the initiation or a shortening of the duration of therapy reduced this effect. Similarly, PAVAN-LANGSTON et al. (1979) have shown that systemically administered acyclovir reduced the incidence of trigeminal ganglionic latent HSV-1 infections after acute ocular infections in mice. The recurrence of HSV-1 skin lesions in mice was reported to be reduced by subcutaneous acyclovir treatment (BLYTH et al. 1980). The ganglionic infections resulting from oral (mouse lip) inoculation with HSV-1 (PARK et al. 1979a) or HSV-2 (PARK et al. 1980a) can also be reduced with acyclovir therapy.

Acyclovir was reported apparently to eliminate established latent ganglionic infections (PAVAN-LANGSTON et al. 1979). Three weeks after ocular infection of mice with HSV-1, 15 days of acyclovir treatment reduced the persistence of HSV-1 in the trigeminal ganglion from 100% to 12%. The duration of therapy appeared critical: if treatment was continued for only 5 days, virus persisted in all of the animals. FIELD et al. (1979), however, did not find acyclovir effective against latent infections established after inoculation of the mouse pinna. Similarly, negative findings regarding effects on established viral infections were reported by BLYTH et al. (1980) and by TROUSDALE et al. (1980).

Although HSV-1 strains resistant to acyclovir in vitro can be readily obtained, it appears that the in vivo pathogenicity of some of these strains is reduced (FIELD and DARBY 1980; KLEIN et al. 1980). This attenuation might be related to a loss of thymidine kinase activity in these strains (FIELD and DARBY 1980; FIELD and Wildy 1978). This is supported by the isolation of an acyclovir-resistant HSV-1 strain which induces a thymidine kinase with an altered substrate specificity, but which retains pathogenicity (DARBY et al. 1981). K. O. SMITH et al. (1980) have also isolated a HSV-1 mutant resistant to acyclovir which retains its virulence in rabbit corneas. It is proposed that certain drug-resistant, latency-negative HSV mutants may provide a good approach to the development of an attenuated vaccine (KLEIN et al 1980).

3. Effects on Normal Cells

Since acyclovir is phosphorylated and activated to a quite limited extent in normal cells, it is associated with very little toxicity (ELION et al. 1977). This lack of toxicity has been documented in many of the vitro antiviral studies, and extended to a number of cell types. The replication of granulocyte progenitor cells, which is frequently inhibited by antimetabolites, was found to be relatively insensitive to the effects of acyclovir (MCGUFFIN et al. 1980). Mitogen-stimulated in vitro lymphocyte blastogenic responses were not inhibited by acyclovir at 20 µg/ml (STEELE et al. 1980).

In a study of the disposition of acyclovir in humans, DEMIRANDA et al. (1979) found no indication of toxicity. Plasma concentrations decreased biphasically and the half-life in the slow disposition phase ranged from 2.2 to 5 h. The drug, as well as a metabolite, 9-carboxy-methoxymethylguanine, was excreted in the urine. The lack of toxicity, kinetic profile, and metabolism of acyclovir make it a promising antiviral agent suitable for systemic administration (SELBY et al. 1979).

4. Mechanism of Action

The biochemical bases of the highly selective antiviral effects of acyclovir were elucidated by ELION et al. (1977), FURMAN et al. (1979), and DERSE et al. (1981). Two features contribute to the drug's selectivity: (a) preferential phosphorylation by the herpesvirus-specified thymidine kinase; and (b) selective inhibition of, and/or substrate for, the viral DNA polymerase by the triphosphate of acyclovir. These investigators analyzed the extracts of HSV-1-infected and uninfected Vero cells for the presence of the mono-, di-, and triphosphates of acyclovir. These metabolites were present in high concentrations in the virally infected cells, but not in the control cells. In addition, cells infected with a thymidine kinase deficient mutant of HSV-1 did not accumulate phosphorylated derivatives of acyclovir. The probable site of action of acyclovir, inhibition of the viral DNA polymerase, was also reported in this study. The 5'-triphosphate of acyclovir was found to be a competitive inhibitor of the HSV-1 DNA polymerase with respect to 2'-deoxyguanosine-5'-triphosphate, (dGTP) ($K_i = 0.08$ µM). In contrast, the K_i was 2.1 µM for the host cell (HeLa S-3) α-DNA polymerase. This unusual drug thus acts as a thymidine analog at the phosphorylation step by the viral thymidine kinase, but as a deoxyguanosine analog as an inhibitor of, and/or substrate for, the viral DNA polymerase.

Rigorous evidence that the thymidine kinase from HSV-1-infected cells does indeed catalyze the phosphorylation of acyclovir was provided by FYFE et al. (1978). The 5'-monophosphate of acyclovir is converted to the diphosphate by quanosine monophosphate kinase (MILLER and MILLER 1980). Nucleoside diphosphokinase presumably catalyzes the formation of the triphosphate.

Several reports characterizing the nature and specificity of acyclovir triphosphate inhibition of DNA polymerases have appeared. The acyclic triphosphate is a better substrate and inhibitor of the HSV-1 enzyme than the α polymerase of the host cell (Furman et al. 1979). St. Clair et al. (1980) showed that the DNA polymerases induced by HSV-2 and human cytomegalovirus were more sensitive than the enzymes from vaccinia virus and Friend leukemia virus to inhibition by acyclovir triphosphate. The Epstein-Barr virus DNA polymerase is also quite sensitive to inhibition by the acyclic triphosphate (Datta et al. 1980).

Further evidence in support of an action by acyclovir at the level of DNA polymerase has been provided in studies utilizing cells biochemically transformed by HSV-1. The work of Furman et al. (1980) indicates that the growth of cells biochemically transformed by HSV-1 thymidine kinase is inhibited by acyclovir. DNA synthesis was also reduced and small, chain-terminated products were generated. It appears that cells transformed by HSV-1 are more sensitive to acyclovir than HSV-2-transformed cells (Nishiyama and Rapp 1979). It is interesting that, although the K_i for acyclovir triphosphate inhibition of the vaccinia virus enzyme (3.7 μM) is considerably higher than that for the HSV-1 enzyme (0.08 μM) (St. Clair et al. 1980), it is still low enough to inhibit viral replication if the metabolite can be generated. Thus vaccinia and pseudorabies viruses are normally refractory to the effects of acyclovir, but when the viruses replicate in HSV-1-transformed cells, inhibition is evident Darby et al. 1980). These data underscore the importance of the activation reaction and highlight the critical nature of DNA polymerase as a site of action.

Examination of HSV-1 mutants that are resistant to acyclovir has revealed two distinct loci of resistance (Coen and Schaeffer 1980; Schnipper and Crumpacker 1980; Crumpacker et al. 1980). Consistent with the studies on drug activation and the mechanism of action, these investigations show that either reduced levels of thymidine kinase activity or an altered polymerase can confer resistance. A recent report by Darby et al. (1981) indicates that resistance can also develop in HSV-1 mutants that induce a thymidine kinase with an altered substrate specificity.

II. 5-Ethyl-2′-deoxyuridine (Aedurid)

1. Synthesis

The synthesis of 5-ethyl-2′deoxyuridine (EtdUrd) was described by Gauri and Malorny (1967) and by Swierkowski and Shugar (1969) (Fig. 1).

2. Antiviral Activity

5-Ethyl-2′-deoxyuridine inhibits the replication of herpesvirus (Gauri and Malorny 1967; DeClercq and Shugar 1975; Cheng et al. 1976) and vaccinia virus (DeClercq and Shugar 1975) in cell culture. This nucleoside is effective in the treatment of herpetic keratitis in rabbits (Gauri and Malorny 1967; Gauri 1968), in therapy of deep ocular herpes infection in rabbits (Martenet 1975), and in reduction of mortality associated with herpes simplex encephalitis in mice (Davis et al. 1978, 1979). Topical application of EtdUrd was not significantly effective against HSV-1 cutaneous infections in athymic nude mice (Descamps et al. 1979). This compound does not appear to be immunosuppressive (Gauri et al. 1969).

GUARI and ELZE (1977) and ELZE (1979) have reported that EtdUrd is effective in the therapy of herpes keratitis in humans. This compound is used clinically in West Germany for the topical treatment of herpetic keratitis.

3. Effects on Normal Cells

5-Ethyl-2'-deoxyuridine is not very cytotoxic, even when it is incorporated into the DNA of mouse (SILAGI et al. 1977) and human (SINGH et al. 1974; SWIERKOWSKI et al. 1973) cells. Chromosome damage was not apparent after such incorporation (SWIERKOWSKI et al. 1973; SINGH et al. 1974) and the analog was not mutagenic (PIETRZYKOWSKA and SHUGAR 1966; SWIERKOWSKI and SHUGAR 1969).

4. Mechanism of Action

The basis of the antiviral activity of EtdUrd has not been worked out, but its selectivity may be due to higher levels of thymidine kinase activity in the virally infected cells. Induction of the viral enzyme appears to be necessary for the antiviral activity of EtdUrd (CHENG et al. 1976; DECLERCQ et al. 1977). HeLa cells which are thymidine kinase deficient are not inhibited by EtdUrd at 25 μM, whereas 1 μM of the compound inhibits HSV-1-transformed variants of these cells (CHENG et al. 1976). These data suggest an important activation role for the viral thymidine kinase. The monophosphate of EtdUrd has been reported to inhibit thymidylate synthetase isolated from *Escherichia coli* (WALTER and GAURI 1975).

III. E-5-(2-Bromovinyl)-2'-deoxyuridine

A series of novel deoxyuridine derivatives with halogenated vinyl substituents at the 5-position have been synthesized (JONES et al. 1979; DECLERCQ et al. 1979a). Of these, the bromovinyl compound Fig. 1) appears to be the most potent inhibitor of HSV replication (DECLERCQ et al. 1979a, 1980b). E-5-(2-Bromovinyl)-2'-deoxyuridine (BVdUrd) is highly selective against a large number of HSV-1 and HSV-2 strains, but HSV-1 is considerably more sensitive (DECLERCQ et al. 1980c). Thymidine kinase deficient mutants of HSV-1 are resistant to BVdUrd, suggesting that this enzyme is necessary for the preferential activation of BVdUrd (DECLERCQ et al. 1980c). E-5-(2-Bromovinyl)-2'-deoxyuridine and E-5-(2-iodovinyl)-2'-deoxyuridine (IVdUrd) are preferentially phosphorylated by this enzyme (CHENG et al. 1981b; DESCAMPS and DECLERCQ 1981). The triphosphate of these analogs are inhibitors of, and/or substrates for, the HSV DNA polymerase (ALLAUDEEN et al. 1981). Both BVdUrd and IVdUrd are extensively incorporated into HSV DNA (CHEN et al. 1981; LARSSON and OBERG 1981; ALLAUDEEN et al. 1982). Experimental herpes simplex keratitis in rabbits is effectively treated with BVdUrd (MAUGDAL et al. 1980) without associated drug toxicity; BVdUrd also has activity against intradermally inoculated HSV-1 in athymic nude mice (DECLERCQ et al. 1979a; DESCAMPS et al. 1979). Systemic administration of BVdUrd to mice was not associated with toxicity. Biologically active blood levels of BVdUrd persisted for 5 h after the drug was given orally in mice (DECLERCQ et al. 1979b). Retroviruses are not induced by BVdUrd in Balb 3T3 cells, a problem associated with a number of other antiviral agents (DECLERCQ et al. 1981). The use of BVdUrd in severe herpes zoster has been reported (DECLERCQ et al. 1980a).

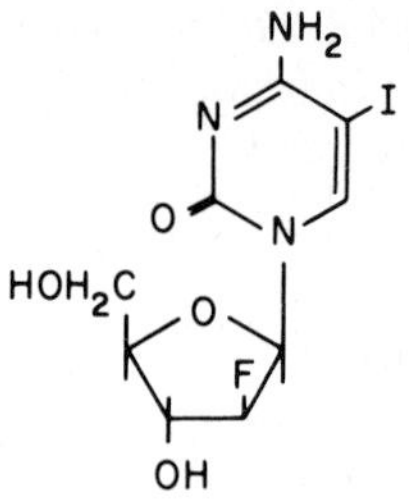

Fig. 4. Structure of 1-(2-deoxy-2-fluoro-β-D-arabinosyl)-5-iodocytosine

IV. 1-(2-Deoxy-2-fluoro-β-D-arabinosyl)-5-iodo-cytosine

Watanabe et al. (1979) synthesized an interesting series of 2′-fluoro derivatives of 2′-deoxyarabinofuranosyl-pyrimidine nucleosides, of which 1-(2-deoxy-2-fluoro-β-D-arabinosyl)-5-iodocytosine (FIAC) (Fig. 4) has excellent antiviral activity against HSV-1 and HSV-2, varicella-zoster virus, cytomegalovirus, and vaccinia virus in cell culture (Watanabe et al. 1979; Lopez et al. 1980). This compound is also effective against HSV-1 ecephalitis in mice (Lopez et al. 1980). It appeared to be effective against varicella-zoster virus or HSV infections in patients with underlying malignancies (C. Lopez, personal communication). A metabolic derivative of FIAC, 2′-fluoro-ara-T (FMAU), is as effective as acyclovir in reduction of mortality and prolongation of life (Fox et al. 1981; Schinazi et al., to be published). 2′-Fluoro-ara-T appears to be more potent and stable than FIAC. Chou et al. (1981) studied the pharmacologic and metabolic fate of FIAC in mice and rats and found FIAC to be deaminated at a rate comparable to 1-β-D-arabinofuranosylcytosine. In addition to 2′-fluoro-1-β-D-arabinofuranosyl-5-iodouracil (FIAU), the following metabolic products were formed: 2′-fluoro-ara-T and 2′-fluoro-ara-U. Both FIAC and FIAU are also potent cytotoxic agents.

V. 5-Iodo-5′-amino-2′,5′-dideoxyuridine

1. Synthesis

The toxicity of many antiviral agents results from their incorporation into DNA. In an effort to eliminate this problem, a series of nucleoside analogs were synthesized with 5′-modifications (Lin et al. 1976). It was hoped that a 5′-amino substituent such as that in 5-iodo-5′-amino-2′,5′-dideoxyuridine (AIdUrd) (Fig. 5) would prevent the phosphorylation of these compounds and thus their incorporation into DNA. Importantly, the work of Langen and his co-workers with 5′-halogenated nucleosides had previously indicated that biologically active nucleosides that are not phosphorylated could be developed (Langen and Kowollik 1968; Langen et al. 1969, 1972). More recently, Lin and Prusoff (1978 a) developed a new preparative synthesis of AIdUrd. The synthesis and development of AIdUrd have been reviewed (Prusoff et al. 1979 b).

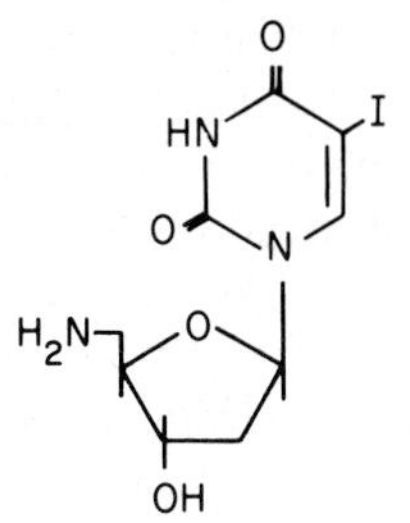

Fig. 5. Structure of 5-iodo-5′-amino-2′,5′-dideoxyuridine

2. Antiviral Activity

a) In Vitro

5-Iodo-5′-amino-2′,5′-dideoxyuridine is a highly selective inhibitor of HSV-1 replication in vitro (CHENG et al. 1975). Other herpesviruses including HSV-2 (PRUSOFF et al. 1977; DECLERCQ et al. 1980c), varicella-zoster virus (ILTIS et al. 1979), and Epstein-Barr virus (HENDERSON et al. 1979), are inhibited. Activity against the RNA leukemia viruses has also been reported (PRUSOFF et al. 1977).

Recently, an interesting approach to the chemotherapy of latent HSV infections was reported (HASCHKE et al. 1980). These investigators coupled AIdUrd to horseradish peroxidase by Schiff base formation. After corneal injection of this conjugate, retrograde transport by trigeminal ganglion neurons was demonstrated. Selective drug delivery may thus be achieved by this strategy, but its practical utility has not been established as yet.

b) In Vivo

The efficacy of AIdUrd administered as a solution or an ointment in the treatment of herpes simplex keratitis has been established (ALBERT et al. 1976; PULIAFITO et al. 1977). PARK et al. (1980a) have demonstrated the effectiveness of AIdUrd in the treatment of mice inoculated in the lip with HSV-2.

3. Effects on Normal Cells

5-Iodo-5′-amino-2′,5′-dideoxyuridine possesses very little toxicity for a large number of cell types (CHENG et al. 1975; PRUSOFF et al. 1977). At doses of 450 mg/kg given for 5 days, AIdUrd did not show toxicity in newborn or suckling mice (ALBERT et al. 1979). An analysis of the immunosuppressive properties of AIdUrd was done by KAN-MITCHELL et al. (1980). These investigators found the drug to have a very mild effect on both cell-mediated and humoral immunity. The degree of suppression was much less than that seen with IdUrd.

4. Mechanism of Action

The 5′-amino group of AIdUrd was introduced in an effort to prevent phosphorylation, and this is indeed the case in uninfected cells (CHEN et al. 1976a). This fact accounts for the low toxicity of AIdUrd. Interestingly, however, AIdUrd is phosphorylated to the 5′-diphosphate by the HSV-encoded multifunctional thymidine kinase (Chen and Prusoff 1979). It is this preferential activation involving the formation of a phosphoramidate bond that accounts for the antiviral selectivity of AIdUrd. The 5′-amino derivative of thymidine is also a selective inhibitor of herpesvirus replication (Lin et al. 1976; Lin and Prusoff 1978b) and it is preferentially phosphorylated by the virally specified thymidine kinase (Chen et al. 1980). The triphosphate of AIdUrd is present in HSV-1-infected cells, and is incorporated internally into the host cell and viral DNA of virus-infected cells only (Chen et al. 1976a). Chen et al. (1976b) have described the synthesis and chemical properties of 5-iodo-5′-amino-2′,5′-dideoxyuridine-5′-triphosphate (AIdUTP).

It is the incorporation of AIdUrd into the viral DNA which correlates most closely with the antiherpes activity of the drug (Fischer et al. 1980). Fragmentation and, in particular, single-stranded breakage, were evident in the viral DNA which contained the aminonucleoside. The role of such damage in the antiviral effects of AIdUrd is not clear, but it does not appear necessary for activity (Fischer et al. 1980). Other biochemical effects of AIdUrd in HSV-1-infected cells include a decreased rate of incorporation of thymidine into DNA and an expansion of the 2′-deoxyadenosine-5′-triphosphate, 2′-deoxyguanosine-5′-triphosphate, and 2′-deoxycytidine-5′-triphosphate pools (Y-C. Cheng and Prusoff, unpublished work). The incorporation of uridine into RNA or of amino acids into protein was not altered by AIdUrd. Otto et al. (1982) have recently investigated the effect of AIdUrd on the formation of HSV-proteins. Exposure of HSV-1-infected Vero cells to AIdUrd resulted in altered expression of HSV-1-induced β and γ proteins but had no effect on α proteins. In addition, virions in which AIdUrd was incorporated into the DNA were defective in their abilities to induce proteins upon subsequent infection of non-drug-treated host-cells.

VI. Phosphonoacetate and Phosphonoformate (Foscarnet)

1. Synthesis

The synthesis of phosphonoacetate (PAA) and phosphonoformate (PFA) was reported in 1924 by Nylén. The structures of these charged, highly water soluble compounds are shown in Fig. 6. The pharmacology and biochemistry of PAA have been extensively detailed by Boezi (1979), Newton (1979), and Overby et al. (1977). Hay et al. (1977) have also reviewed the subject. The pharmacology of PFA was recently surveyed by Helgstrand et al. (1979).

| | Phosphonoacetate | Phosphonoformate |

Fig. 6. Structures of phosphonoacetate and phosphonoformate (Foscarnet)

2. Antiviral Activity

a) In Vitro

The phosphonates are selective inhibitors of herpesviruses. Phosphonoacetate has been reported to inhibit replication of the following viruses: HSV-1 and HSV-2 (SHIPKOWITZ et al. 1973), equine abortion and varicella-zoster viruses (OVERBY et al. 1977), human cytomegalovirus (HUANG 1975), murine and simian cytomegalovirus (HUANG et al. 1976), Epstein-Barr virus (YAJIMA et al. 1976), herpesvirus saimiri (HAUNG et al. 1976), Marek's disease virus (LEE et al. 1976; NAZERIAN and LEE 1976), and frog virus 3 (ELLIOTT et al. 1980). Vaccinia virus is only moderately sensitive. Other DNA viruses, including SV40 and human adenovirus type 12, and RNA viruses are not inhibited by PAA (OVERBY et al. 1977).

Phosphonoformate inhibits the replication of HSV-1, HSV-2, pseudorabies virus, infectious bovine rhinotracheitis virus (HELGSTRAND et al. 1978; RENO et al. 1978), and Marek's disease virus (RENO et al. 1978).

b) In Vivo

Phosphonoacetate was first shown to be effective in treating herpes simplex keratitis in rabbits and herpes dermatitis in mice by SHIPKOWITZ et al. (1973). Efficacy has been confirmed (GERSTEIN et al. 1975; MEYER et al. 1976; KLEIN and FREIDMAN-KEIN 1975). Activity was also reported against HSV-induced skin infections in guinea pigs (ALENIUS and OBERG 1978; ALENIUS 1980), in genital herpes of mice (KERN et al. 1977) and of hamsters (RENIS 1977), and in mouse encephalitis (FITZ-WILLIAM and GRIFFITH 1976; KERN et al. 1978). Phosphonoacetate has effectiveness against cytomegalovirus infections in mice (OVERALL et al. 1976), delta herpesvirus in monkeys (FELSENFELD et al. 1978), and Shope fibroma and vaccinia virus infections in rabbits (FREIDMAN-KEIN et al. 1976).

The in vivo activity of PFA against cutaneous herpes infections in guinea pigs was recently reported (ALENIUS et al. 1978; HELGSTRAND et al. 1978). Phosphonoformate was also active in the treatment of HSV-2 genital infections in guinea pigs (ALENIUS and NORDLINDER 1979) and skin infections in hairless mice; however, the establishment of latent spinal or trigeminal ganglionic infections was not prevented (KLEIN et al. 1979 b). The effectiveness of PFA against experimental herpes simplex keratitis has now been demonstrated (ALENIUS et al. 1980).

3. Effects on Normal Cells

Phosphonoacetate is generally not toxic to uninfected cells at concentrations which produce an antiviral effect (OVERBY et al. 1974; HUANG 1975; LEE et al. 1976), and was found not to be mutagenic in in vitro tests (BECKER et al. 1977). However, treatment of cutaneous herpes infections has been associated with dermal toxicity (ALENIUS et al. 1978). Reversible punctate lesions of the cornea were associated with PAA treatment of herpes keratitis (GERSTEIN et al. 1975). Intravenous administration of PAA in high concentrations can produce muscle spasms and death in rabbits (MEYER et al. 1976). The drug is apparently not metabolized (BOPP et al. 1977).

Similarly, PFA is minimally toxic to uninfected cells in vitro. The cytotoxic effects seen at high concentrations are reversible (Stenberg and Larsson 1978). In contrast to PAA, PFA does not appear to produce local skin irritation (Alenius et al. 1978). Phosphonoformate was not toxic to rabbit eyes (Alenius et al. 1980), or when given subcutaneously to rats or dogs (Helgstrand et al. 1979). Although PFA was partially deposited in the bone, as is seen with PAA, no histological damage was apparent (Helgstrand et al. 1979).

4. Mechanism of Action

Phosphonoacetate exerts its selective antiherpes effects by preferentially inhibiting virally induced DNA polymerases. As such, PAA inhibition of viral DNA synthesis in HSV-infected cells (Overby et al. 1974) and in nuclei isolated from such cells (Bolden et al. 1975; Becker et al. 1977) has been demonstrated. The drug also inhibits viral DNA synthesis in cells infected with cytomegalovirus (Huang 1975; Huang et al. 1976), avian herpes virus (Lee et al. 1976), and Epstein-Barr virus (Summers and Klein 1976).

   Mao et al. (1975) first reported the inhibition of HSV-DNA polymerase by PAA. The key interaction is at the inorganic pyrophosphate binding site (Mao and Robishaw 1975; Leinbach et al. 1976; Eriksson et al. 1980). It appears that DNA polymerase α is sensitive to PAA inhibition but the other host cell polymerase (β or γ) are not (Bolden et al. 1975; Sabourin et al. 1978). Extensive characterization of PAA-resistant virus mutants has provided supporting data that the virally induced DNA polymerase is the target enzyme. Work from a number of laboratories involving different viruses indicates that mutants which are resistant to PAA induce an altered DNA polymerase activity. The enzyme is characterized by reduced sensitivity to PAA inhibition (Hay and Subak-Sharpe 1976; Honess and Watson 1977; Jofre et al. 1977; Purifoy and Powell 1977; Lee et al. 1978; Becker et al. 1977; Duff et al. 1978; Eriksson and Öberg 1979).

   Inhibition of viral DNA polymerases also appears to account for the selectivity of PFA (Reno et al. 1978; Helgstrand et al. 1978). DNA synthesis was preferentially inhibited by PFA in nuclei isolated from HSV-infected cells as compared to uninfected cells (Cheng et al. 1981 a).

References

Abel R Jr, Kaufman HE, Sugar J (1975) Effect of intravenous adenine arabinoside on herpes simplex keratouveitis in humans. In: Pavan-Langston D, Buchanan RA, Alford CA (eds) Adenine arabinoside: an antiviral agent. Raven, New York, pp 393–400

Abramson D (1979) The treatment of orbital rhabdomyosarcoma with irradiation and chemotherapy. Ophthalmology 86:1330–1335

Agarwal RP, Spector T, Parks RE Jr (1977) Tight binding inhibitors IV. Inhibition of adenosine deaminases by various inhibitors. Biochem Pharmacol 26:359–367

Albert DM, Lahav M, Bhatt PN, Reid TW, Ward RE, Cykiert RC, Lin T-S, Ward DC, Prusoff WH (1976) Successful therapy of herpes hominis keratitis in rabbits by 5-iodo-5′-amino-2′,5′-dideoxyuridine (AIU): a novel analog of thymidine. Invest Ophthalmol 15:470–478

Albert DM, Percy DH, Puliafito CA, Fritsch E, Lin T-S, Ward DC, Prusoff WH (1979) Postnatal treatment of mice with the antiviral nucleosides AIU or IdUrd. Adv Ophthalmol 38:89–98

Alenius S (1980) Inhibition of herpesvirus multiplication in guinea pig skin by antiviral compounds. Arch Virol 65:149–156

Alenius S, Nordlinger H (1979) Effect of trisodium phosphonoformate in genital infection of female guinea pigs with herpes simplex virus type 2. Arch Virol 60:197–206

Alenius S, Öberg B (1978) Comparison of the therapeutic effects of five antiviral agents on cutaneous herpesvirus infection in guinea pigs. Arch Virol 58:277–288

Alenius S. Dinter Z, Öberg B (1978) Therapeutic effect of trisodium phosphonoformate on cutaneous herpesvirus infection in guinea pigs. Antimicrob Agents Chemother 14:408–413

Alenius S, Laurent U, Öberg B (1980) Effect of trisodium phosphonoformate and idoxuridine on experimental herpes simplex keratitis in immunized and non-immunized rabbits. Acta Ophthalmol (Copenh) 58:167–173

Allaudeen HS, Kozarich JW, Bertino JR, DeClercq D (1981) On the mechanism of selective inhibition of herpesvirus replication by (E)-5-(2-bromovinyl)-2'-deoxyuridine. Proc Natl Acad Sci USA 78:2698–2702

Allaudeen HS, Chen MS, Lee JJ, DeClercq E, Prusoff WH (1982) Incorporation of E-5-(2-halovinyl)-2'-deoxyuridines into deoxyribonucleic acids of herpes simplex virus type-1 infected cells. J Biol Chem 257:303–306

Barrio JR, Bryant JD, Keyser GE (1980) A direct method for the preparation of 2-hydroxyethoxymethyl derivatives of guanine, adenine, and cytosine. J Med Chem 23:572–574

Bauer DJ, Collins P, Tucker ME, Macklin AW (1979) Treatment of experimental herpes simplex keratitis with acycloguanosine. Br J Ophthalmol 63:429–435

Becker Y, Hadar J (1980) Antivirals 1980 – an update. Prog Med Virol 26:1–44

Becker Y, Asher Y, Cohen A, Weinberg-Zahlering E, Schlomai (1977) Phosphonoacetic acid-resistant mutants of herpes simplex virus: effect of phosphonoacetic acid on virus replication and in vitro deoxyribonucleic acid synthesis in isolated nuclei. Antimicrob Agents Chemother 11:919–922

Bennett LL Jr, Shannon WM, Allan PW, Arnett G (1975) Studies on the biochemical basis for the antiviral activities of some nucleoside analogs. Ann NY Acad Sci 255:342–357

Berens K, Shugar D (1963) Ultraviolet absorption spectra and structure of halogenated uracils and their glycosides. Acta Biochim Pol 10:25–47

Biron KK, Elion GB (1980) In vitro susceptibility of varicella-zoster to acyclovir. Antimicrob Agents Chemother 18:443–447

Bishop JO, Madson EC (1975) Retinoblastoma: review of the current status. Surv Ophthalmol 19:342–366

Blyth WA, Harbour DA, Hill TJ (1980) Effect of acyclovir on recurrence of herpes simplex skin lesions in mice. J Gen Virol 48:417–419

Boezi JA (1979) The antiherpes action of phosphonoacetate. Pharmacol Ther 4:231–243

Bolden A, Aucker J, Weissbach A (1975) Synthesis of herpes simplex virus, vaccinia virus, and adenovirus DNA in isolated HeLa cell nuclei. J Virol 16:1584–1592

Bopp, BA, Estep LB, Anderson DJ (1977) Disposition of disodium phosphonoacetate-^{14}C in rat, rabbit, dog, and monkey. Fed Proc 36:939

Boston Interhospital Virus Study Group and the NIAID-Sponsored Cooperative Antiviral Clinical Study (1975) Failure of high dose 5-iodo-2'-deoxyuridine in the therapy of herpes simplex virus encephalitis. N Engl J Med 292:599–603

Bresnick E, Williams SS (1967) Effects of 5-trifluoromethyldeoxyuridine on deoxythymidine kinase. Biochem Pharmacol 16:503–507

Brink JJ, LePage GA (1964) Metabolic effects of 9-D-arabinosylpurines in ascites tumor cells. Cancer Res 24:312–318

Buettner W, Werchau H (1973) Incorporation of 5-iodo-2'-deoxyuridine (IUdR) into SV40 DNA. Virology 52:553–561

Calabresi P, Cardoso SS, Finch SC, Kligerman MS, Von Essen CF, Chu MY, Welch AD (1961) Initial clinical studies with 5-iodo-2'-deoxyuridine. Cancer Res 21:550–554

Cass CE (1979) 9-β-D-Arabinofuranosyladenine (ara-A). In: Hahn FE (ed) Antibiotics V-2, Springer, Berlin Heidelberg New York, pp 85–109

Cass CE, Ah-Yeung TH (1976) Enhancement of 9-β-D-arabinofuranosyladenine cytotoxicity to mouse leukemia L1210 *in vitro* by 2'-deoxycoformycin. Cancer Res 36:1486–1491

Centifanto YM, Kaufman HE (1979) 9-(2-Hydroxyethoxymethyl)guanine as an inhibitor of herpes simplex virus replication. Chemotherapy 25:279–281

Cha S (1975) Tight-binding inhibitors – I. Kinetic behavior. Biochem. Pharmacol 24:2187–2197

Chan T-S (1977) Induction of deoxycytidine deaminase activity in mammalian cell lines by infection with herpes simplex virus type 1. Proc Natl Acad Sci USA 74:1734–1738

Chang T-W, Syndman DR (1979) Antiviral agents: action and clinical use. Drugs 18:354–376

Chen MS, Prusoff WH (1978) Association of thymidylate kinase activity with pyrimidine deoxyribonucleoside kinase induced by herpes simplex virus. J Biol Chem 253:1325–1327

Chen MS, Prusoff WH (1979) Phosphorylation of 5-iodo-5'-amino-2',5'-dideoxyuridine by herpes simplex virus type 1 encoded thymidine kinase. J Biol Chem 254:10449–10452

Chen MS, Ward DC, Prusoff WH (1976 a) Specific herpes simplex virus-induced incorporation of 5-iodo-5'-amino-2',5'-dideoxyuridine into deoxyribonucleic acid. J Biol Chem 251:4833–4838

Chen MS, Ward DC, Prusoff WH (1976 b) 5-Iodo-5'amino-2',5'-dideoxyuridine-5'-*N'*-triphosphate synthesis, chemical properties, and effect on *Escherichia coli* thymidine kinase activity. J Biol Chem 251:4839–4842

Chen MS, Shiau GT, Prusoff WH (1980) 5'-Amino-5'-deoxythymidine: synthesis, specific phosphorylation by herpesvirus thymidine kinase, and stability to pH of the enzymically formed diphosphate derivative. Antimicrob Agents Chemother 18:433–436

Chen MS, Lee JJ, Allaudeen HS, DeClercq E, Prusoff WH (1981) Incorporation of E-5-(2-halovinyl)-2'-deoxyuridines into the deoxyribonucleic acid of herpes simplex virus type-1 infected Vero cells. Fed Proc 40:1826

Cheng Y-C (1976) Deoxythymidine kinase induced in HeLa TK-cells by herpes simplex virus type I and II. Substrate specificity and kinetic behavior. Biochim Biophys Acta 452:370–381

Cheng Y-C (1977) A rational approach to the development of antiviral chemotherapy. Alternate substrates of herpes simplex virus type 1 (HSV-1) and type 2 (HSV-2) thymidine kinase. Ann NY Acad Sci 284:594–598

Cheng Y-C, Goz B, Neenan JP, Ward DC, Prusoff WH (1975) Selective inhibition of herpes simplex virus by 5'-amino-2',5'-dideoxy-5-iodouridine. J Virol 15:1284–1285

Cheng Y-C, Domin BA, Sharma RA, Bobek M (1976) Antiviral action and cellular toxicity of four thymidine analogues: 5-ethyl-, 5-vinyl-, 5-propyl-, and 5-allyl-2'-deoxyuridine. Antimicrob Agents Chemother 10:119–122

Cheng Y-C, Grill S, Derse D, Chen J-Y, Caradonna SJ, Connor K (1981 a) Mode of action of phosphonoformate as an antiherpes simplex virus agent. Biochim Biophys Acta 652:90–98

Cheng Y-C, Dutschman G, DeClercq E, Jones AS, Rahim SG, Verhelst G, Walker RT (1981 b) Differential affinities of 5-(2-halogenovinyl-2'-deoxyuridines for deoxythymidine kinases of various origins. Mol Pharmacol 20:230–233

Ch'ien LT, Schabel FM Jr, Alford CA (1973) Arabinosyl nucleosides and nucleotides. In: Carter WA (ed) Selective inhibitors of viral functions. CRC Press, Cleveland, pp 227–256

Chou T-C, Feinberg A, Grant AJ, Vidal P, Reichman U, Watanabe KA, Fox JJ, Philips FS (1981) Pharmacological disposition and metabolic fate of 2'-fluoro-5-iodo-1-β-D-arabinofuranosylcytosine in mice and rats. Cancer Res 41:3336–3342

Clough DW, Parkhurst JR (1977) Experimental herpes simplex virus type 1 encephalitis: treatment with trifluoromethyl-2'-deoxyuridine. Antimicrob Agents Chemother 11:307–311

Coen DM, Schaffer PA (1980) Two distinct loci confer resistance to acycloguanosine in herpes simplex virus type 1. Proc Natl Acad Sci USA 77:2265–2269

Cohen GH (1972) Ribonucleotide reductase activity of synchronized KB cells infected with herpes simplex virus. J Virol 9:408–418

Cohen SS (1966) Introduction to the biochemistry of D-arabinosyl nucleosides. Prog Nucleic Acid Res Mol Biol 5:1–88

Cohen SS (1976) The lethality of aranucleotides. Med Biol 54:299–326

Colby BM, Shaw JE, Elion GB, Pagano JS (1980) Effect of acyclovir [9-(2-hydroxyethoxy-methyl)guanine] on Epstein-Barr virus DNA replication. J Virol 34:560–568

Collins P, Bauer DJ (1979) The activity in vitro of 9-(2-hydroxyethoxymethyl)guanine (acycloguanosine), a new antiviral agent. J Antimicrob Chemother 5:431–436

Collum LM, Benedict-Smith A, Hillary IB (1980) Randomized double-blind trial of acyclovir and idoxuridine in dendritic corneal ulceration. Br J Ophthalmol 64:766–769

Connor JD, Sweetman L, Carey S, Stuckey MA, Buchanan R (1975) Susceptibility in vitro of several large DNA viruses to the antiviral activity of adenine arabinoside: relation to human pharmacology. In: Pavang-Langston D, Buchanan RA, Alford CA Jr (eds) Adenine arabinoside: an antiviral agent. Raven, New York, pp 177–196

Coster DJ, McKinnon JR, McGill JI, Jones BR, Fraunfelder, FT (1976) Clinical evaluation of adenine arabinoside and trifluorothymidine in the treatment of corneal ulcers caused by herpes simplex virus. J Infect Dis S-133:A173–A177

Coster DJ, Wilkelmus JR, Michaud R, Jones BR (1980) A comparison of acyclovir and idoxuridine as treatment for ulcerative herpetic keratitis. Br J Ophthalmol 64:763–765

Crumpacker CS, Schnipper LE, Zaia JA, Lewis MJ (1979) Growth inhibition by Acycloguanosine of herpesviruses isolated from human infections. Antimicrob Agents Chemother 15:642–645

Crumpacker CS, Chartrand P, Subak-Sharpe JH, Wilkie NM (1980) Resistance of herpes simplex virus to acycloguanosine–genetic and physical analysis. Virology 105:171–184

Darby G, Larder BA, Bastow KF, Field HJ (1980) Sensitivity of viruses to phosphorylated 9-(2-hydroxyethoxymethyl)guanine revealed in TK-transformed cells. J Gen Virol 48:541–554

Darby G, Field HJ, Salisbury SA (1981) Altered substrate specificity of herpes simplex virus thymidine kinase confers acyclovir-resistance. Nature 289:81–83

Datta AK, Colby BM, Shaw JE, Pagano JS (1980) Acyclovir inhibition of Epstein-Barr virus replication. Proc Natl Acad Sci USA 77:5163–5166

Davis WB, Oakes JE, Taylor JA (1978) Effects of treatment with 5-ethyl-2′-desoxyuridine on herpes simplex virus encephalitis in normal and immunosuppressed mice. Antimicrob Agents Chemother 14:743–748

Davis WB, Oakes JE, Vacik JP, Rebert RR, Taylor JA (1979) 5-ethyl-2′-deoxyuridine as a systemic agent for treatment of herpes simplex virus encephalitis. Adv Ophthalmol 38:140–150

DeClercq E (1979) New trends in antiviral chemotherapy. Arch Int Physiol Biochim 81:353–395

DeClercq E, Shugar D (1975) Antiviral activity of 5-ethyl pyrimidine deoxyribonucleosides. Biochem Pharmacol 24:1073–1078

DeClercq E, Torrence PF (1978) Nucleoside analogs with selective antiviral activity. J Carbohydr Nucleosides Nucleotides 5:187–224

DeClercq E, Krajewska E, Descamps J, Torrence PF (1977) Antiherpes activity of deoxythymidine analogues: specific dependence on virus-induced deoxythymidine kinase. Mol Pharmacol 13:980–984

DeClercq E, Descamps J, Desomer P, Barr PJ, Jones AS, Walker RT (1979a) E-5-(2-Bromo-vinyl)-2′-deoxyuridine: a potent and selective antiherpes agent. Proc Natl Acad Sci USA 76:2947–2951

DeClercq E, Descamps J, Desomer P, Barr PJ, Jones AS, Walker RT (1979b) Pharmacokinetics of E-5-(2-bromo-vinyl)-2′-deoxyuridine in mice. Antimicrob Agents Chemother 16:234–236

DeClercq E, DeGreef H, Wildiers J, deJonge G, Drochmans A, Descamps J, deSomer P (1980a) Oral (E)-5-(2-bromovinyl)-2′-deoxyuridine in severe herpes zoster. Br Med J 281:1778

DeClercq E, Descamps J, Verhelst G, Jones AS, Walker RT (1980 b) Antiviral activity of 5-(2-halogenovinyl)-2'-deoxyuridines. In: Nelson JD, Grassi C (eds) Current chemotherapy and infectious disease. American Society for Microbiology. Washington DC, pp 1372–1374

DeClercq E, Descamps J, Verhelst G, Walker RT, Jones AS, Torrence PF, Shugar D (1980 c) Comparative efficiency of different antiherpes drug against different strains of herpes simplex virus. J Infect Dis 141:563–574

DeClercq E, Heremans H, Descamps J, Verhelst G, DeLey M, Billiau A (1981) Effects of E-5-(2-bromovinyl)-2'-deoxyuridine and other selective anti-herpes compounds on the induction of retrovirus particles in mouse Balb/3T3 cells. Mol Pharmacol 19:122–129

DeMiranda P, Whithley RJ, Blum MR, Keeney RE, Barton N, Cocchetto DM, Good S, Hemstreet GP, Kirk LE, Page DA, Elion GB (1979) Acyclovir kinetics after intravenous infusion. Clin Pharmacol Ther 26:718–728

Derse D, Cheng Y-C, Furman PA, St Clair HH, Elion GB (1981) Inhibition of purified human and herpes simplex virus-induced DNA polymerases by 9-(2-hydroxyethoxymethyl)guanine triphosphate. Effects on primer-template function. J Biol Chem 256:11447–11451

DeRudder J, Privat-Degarilhe M (1965/1966) Inhibitory effect of some nucleosides on the growth of various human viruses in tissue culture. Antimicrob Agents Chemother 578–584

Descamps J, DeClercq E (1981) Specific phosphorylation of E-5-(2-iodovinyl)-2'-deoxyuridine by herpes simplex virus-infected cells. J Biol Chem 256:5973–5976

Descamps J, CeClercq E, Barr PJ, Jones AS, Walker RT, Torrence PF, Shugar D (1979) Relative potencies of different anti-herpes agents in the topical treatment of cutaneous herpes simplex infection of athymic nude mice. Antimicrob Agents Chemother 16:680–682

Dexter DL, Oki T, Heidelberger C (1973) Fluorinated pyrimidines XLII. Effect of 5-trifluoromethyl-2'-deoxyuridine on transcription of vaccinia viral messenger ribonucleic acid. Mol Pharmacol 9:283–296

Doering A, Keller J, Cohen SS (1966) Some aspects of D-arabinosyl nucleosides on polymer synthesis in mouse fibroblasts. Cancer Res 26:2444–2450

Duff RG, Robishaw EE, Mao JC-H, Overby LR (1978) Characteristics of herpes simplex virus resistance to disodium phosphonoacetate. Intervirology 9:193–205

Elion GB, Furman PA, Fyfe JA, DeMiranda P, Beauchamp L, Schaeffer HJ (1977) Selectivity of action of an antiherpetic agent, 9-(2-hydroxyethoxymethyl)-guanine. Proc Natl Acad Sci USA 74:5716–5720

Elliott RM, Bateson A, Kelley DC (1980) Phosphonoacetic acid inhibition of frog virus 3 replication. J Virol 33:539–542

Elze K-L (1979) Ten years of clinical experiences with ethyldeoxyuridine. Adv Ophthalmol 38:134–139

Eriksson B, Öberg B (1979) Characteristics of herpesvirus mutants resistant to phosphonoformate and phosphonoacetate. Antimicrob Agents Chemother 15:758–762

Eriksson B, Larsson A, Helgstrand E, Johansson N-G, Oberg B (1980) Pyrophosphate analogues as inhibitors of herpes simplex virus type 1 DNA polymerase. Biochim Biophys Acta 607:53–64

Falcon MG, Jones BR (1979) Acycloguanosine: antiviral activity in the rabbit cornea. Br J Ophthalmol 63:422–424

Felsenfeld AD, Abee CR, Gerone PJ, Soike KF, Williams SR (1978) Phosphonoacetic acid in the treatment of simian varicella. Antimicrob Agents Chemother 14:331–335

Field HJ, Darby G (1980) Pathogenicity in mice of strains of herpes simplex virus which are resistant to acyclovir *in vitro* and *in vivo*. Antimicrob Agents Chemother 17:209–216

Field HJ, Wildy P (1978) The pathogenicity of thymidine kinase – deficient mutants of herpes simplex virus in mice. J Hyg Camb 81:267–277

Field HJ, Bell SE, Elion GB, Nash AA, Wildy P (1979) Effect of acycloguanosine treatment on acute and latent herpes simplex infections in mice. Antimicrob Agent Chemother 15:554–561

Fischer PH, Prusoff WH (1982) Pyrimidine nucleosides with selective antiviral activity. In: Came PE, Caliguiri LA (eds) Chemotherapy of viruses. Springer, Berlin Heidelberg New York, Handbook of experimental pharmacology, vol 61 pp 95–116

Fischer PH, Chen MS, Prusoff WH (1980) the incorporation of 5-iodo-5'-amino-2',5'-dideoxyuridine and 5-iodo-2'-deoxyuridine into herpes simplex virus DNA: a relationship to their antiviral activity and effects on DNA structure. Biochim Biophys Acta 606:236–245

Fitzwilliam JF, Griffith JF (1976) Experimental ecephalitis caused by herpes simplex virus: comparison of treatment with tilorone hydrochloride and phosphonacetic acid. J Infect Dis 133:A221–225

Foster CS, Pavan-Langston D (1977) Corneal wound healing and antiviral medication. Arch Ophthalmol 95:2062–2067

Fox JJ, Lopez C, Watanabe KA (1981) 2'-Fluoro-arabinosyl pyrimidine nucleosides: chemistry, antiviral, and potential anticancer activities. In: LaHeras FG, Vegas S (eds) Medicinal chemistry advances. Pergamon, Oxford, pp 27–40

Friedman-Kien AE, Fondak AA, Klein RJ (1976) Phosphonoacetic acid in the treatment of Shope fibroma and vaccinia virus skin infections in rabbits. J Invest Dermatol 66:99–102

Fujiwara Y, Heidelberger C (1970) Fluorinated pyrimidines XXXVIII. The incorporation of 5-trifluoromethyl-2'-deoxyuridine into the deoxyribonucleic acid of vaccinia virus. Mol Pharmacol 6:281–291

Fujiwara Y, Oki T, Heidelberger C (1970) Fluorinated pyrimidines XXXVII. Effects of 5-trifluoromethyl-2'-deoxyuridine on the synthesis of deoxyribonucleic acid of mammalian cells in culture. Mol Pharmacol 6:273–280

Furman PA, St Clair MH, Fyfe JA, Rideout JL, Keller PM, Elion GB (1979) Inhibition of herpes simplex virus-induced DNA polymerase activity and viral DNA replication by 9-(2-hydroxyethoxymethyl)guanine and its triphosphate. J Virol 32:72–77

Furman PA, McGuirt PV, Keller PM, Fyfe JA, Elion GB (1980) Inhibition of cell growth and DNA synthesis of cells biochemically transformed with herpes virus genetic information. Virology 102:420–430

Furth JJ, Cohen SS (1967) Inhibition of mammalian DNA polymerase by the 5'-triphosphate of 9-β-D-arabinofuranosyladenine. Cancer Res 27:1528–1533

Furth JJ, Cohn SS (1968) Inhibition of mammalian DNA polymerases by the 5'-triphosphate of 1-β-D-arabinofuranosylcytosine and the 5'-triphosphate of 9-β-D-arabinofuranosyladenine. Cancer Res 28:2061–2067

Fyfe JA, Keller PM, Furman PA, Miller RL, Elion GB (1978) Thymidine kinase from herpes simplex virus phosphorylates the new antiviral compound, 9-(2-hydroxyethoxymethyl)guanine. J Biol Chem 253:8721–8727

Gauri KK (1968) Subconjunctival application of 5-ethyl-2'-deoxyuridine in the chemotherapy of experimental keratitis in rabbits. Klin Monatsbl Augenheilkd 153:837–841

Gauri KK, Elze KL (1977) Concentration dependent effectiveness of 5-ethyl-2'-deoxyuridine in animal experiments and in the clinic. Klin Monatsbl Augenheilkd 171:459–463

Gauri KK, Malorny G (1967) Chemotherapy der Herpes-Infektion mit neuen 5-Akyl-uracildesoxyribosiden. Naunyn-Schmiedebergs Arch Exp Pathol Pharmakol 257:21–22

Gauri KK, Malorny G, Schiff W (1969) Immunobiological studies with the viro-statics 5-ethyl-2'-deoxyuridine and 1-allyl-3,5-diethyl-6-chlorouracil. Chemotherapy 14:129–132

Gerstein DD, Dawson CR, Oh JD (1975) Phosphonoacetic acid in the treatment of experimental herpes simplex keratitis. Antimicrob Agents Chemother 7:285–288

Goz B (1978) The effects of incorporation of 5-halogenated deoxyuridines into the DNA of eukaryotic cells. Pharmacol Rev 29:249–272

Goz B, Prusoff WH (1970) Pharmacology of viruses. Annu Rev Pharmacol 10:143–170

Haschke RH, Ordronneau JM, Bunt AH (1980) Preparation and retrograde axonal transport of an antiviral drug/horseradish peroxidase conjugate. J Neurochem 35:1431–1435

Hay J, Subak-Sharpe JH (1976) Mutants of herpes simplex virus type I and II that are resistant to phosphonoacetic acid induce altered DNA polymerase activities in infected cells. J Gen Virol 31:145–148

Hay J, Brown SM, Jamieson AT, Riyon FJ, Moss H, Dargan DA, Subak-Sharpe JH (1977) The effect of phosphanoacetic acid on herpes viruses. J Antimicrob Chemother 3 [Suppl A]: 63–70

Heidelberger C (1975a) On the molecular mechanism of the antiviral activity of trifluorothymidine. Ann NY Acad Sci 255:317–325

Heidelberger C (1975b) Fluorinated pyrimidines and their nucleosides. In: Sartorelli AC, Johns DG (eds) Antineoplastic and immunosuppressive agents, vol 2. Springer, Berlin Heidelberg New York, pp 193–231

Heidelberger C, Anderson SW (1964) Fluorinated pyrimidines XXI. The tumor-inhibitory activity of 5-trifluoromethyl-2'-deoxyuridine. Cancer Res 24:1979–1985

Heidelberger C, King DH (1979) Trifluorothymidine. Pharmacol Ther 6:427–442

Heidelberger C, Parsons DG, Remy DC (1964) Synthesis of 5-trifluoromethyluracil and 5-trifluoromethyl-2'-deoxyuridine. J Med Chem 7:1–5

Helgstrand E, Öberg B (1980) Enzymatic targets in virus chemotherapy. Antibiotics Chemother 27:27–69

Helgstrand E, Eriksson B, Johansson NG, Lannero B, Larsson A, Misiorny A, Noren JP, Sjoberg B, Stenberg K, Stening G, Stridh S, Öberg B, Alenius S, Philpson L (1978) Trisodium phosphonoformate, a new antiviral compound. Science 201:819–821

Helgstrand E, Öberg B, Alenius S (1979) Experimental studies on the antiherpetic agent phosphonoformic acid. Adv Ophthalmol 38:276–280

Henderson EE, Long WK, Ribecky K (1979) Effects of nucleoside analogs on Epstein-Barr virus-induced transformation of human umbilical cord leukocytes and Epstein-Barr virus expressions in transformed cells. Antimicrob Agents Chemother 15:101–110

Herrmann EC Jr (1961) Plaque inhibition test for detection of specific inhibitors of DNA containing viruses. Proc Soc Exp Biol Med 107:142–145

Herrmann EC Jr, Herrmann JA (1979) Diagnosis of viral disease and the advent of antiviral drugs. Pharmacol Ther 7:35–69

Hershfield MS (1979) Apparent suicide inactivation of human lymphoblast S-adenosyl-homocysteine hydrolase by 2'-deoxyadenosine and adenine arabinoside: a basis for direct toxic effects of analogs of adenosine. J Biol Chem 254:22–25

Hirsh MS, Swartz MN (1980) Antiviral agents (parts I and II). N Engl J Med 302:903, 949–953

Honess RW, Watson DH (1977) Herpes simplex virus resistance and sensitivity to phosphonoacetic acid. J Virol 21:584–600

Huang E-S (1975) Human cytomegalovirus. IV. Specific inhibition of virus induced DNA polymerase activity and viral DNA replication by phosphonoacetic acid. J Virol 16:1560–1565

Huang E-S, Huang C-H, Huong S-M, Selgrade M (1976) Preferential inhibition of herpes-group viruses by phosphonoacetic acid: effects on virus DNA synthesis and virus-induced DNA polymerase activity. Yale J Biol Med 49:93–98

Iltis JP, Lin T-S, Prusoff WH, Rapp F (1979) Effect of 5-iodo-5'-amino-2',5'-dideoxyuridine on varicella-zoster virus in vitro. Antimicrob Agents Chemother 16:92–97

Itoi M, Gefter JW, Kaneko N, Ishii Y, Ramer RM, Gassert S (1975) Teratogenicities of ophthalmic drugs I. Antiviral ophthalmic drugs. Arch Ophthalmol 93:46–51

Jamieson AT, Subak-Sharpe JH (1974) Biochemical studies on the herpes simplex virus-specified deoxypyrimidine kinase activity. J Gen Virol 24:481–492

Jamieson AT, Gentry GA, Subak-Sharpe JH (1974) Induction of both thymidine and deoxycytidine kinase activity by herpes viruses. J Gen Virol 24:465–480

Jofre JT, Schaffer PA, Parris DS (1977) Genetics of resistance to phosphonoacetic acid in strain KOS of herpes simplex type I. J Virol 23:833–836

Jones AS, Verhelst G, Walker RT (1979) The synthesis of the potent anti-herpes virus agent E-(5)-(2-bromovinyl)-2'-deoxyuridine and related compounds. Tetrahedron Lett 45:4415–4418

Jones BR, McGill JI, McKinnon JR, Holt-Wilson AD, Williams HP (1975) Preliminary experience with adenine arabinoside in comparison with idoxuridine and trifluorothymidine in the management of herpectic keratitis. In: Pavan-Langston D, Buchanan RA, Alford CA Jr (eds) Adenine arabinoside: a antiviral agent. Raven New York, pp 411–416

Juel-Jensen BE (1973) Herpes simplex and zoster. Med J 1:406–410

Juel-Jensen BE (1974) Virus diseases. Practitioner 213:508–518

Kan-Mitchell J, Prusoff WH (1979) Studies of the effects of 5-iodo-2′-deoxyuridine on the formation of adenovirus type 2 virions and the synthesis of virus induced polypeptides. Biochem Pharmacol 28:1819–1829

Kan-Mitchell J, Mitchell M, Lin T-S, Prusoff WH (1980) Comparative analysis of the immunosuppressive properties of two antiviral iodinated thymidine analogs, 5-iodo-2′-deoxyuridine and 5-iodo-5′-amino-2′,5′-dideoxyuridine. Cancer Res 40:3491–3494

Kaplan AS, Ben-Porat T (1966) Mode of antiviral action of 5-iodouracil deoxyriboside. J Mol Biol 19:302–332

Kaufman ER, Davidson RL (1979) Altered thymidylate kinase substrate specificity in mammalian cells selected for resistance to iododeoxyuridine. Exp Cell Res 123:355–363

Kaufman HE (1962) Clinical cure of herpes simplex keratitis by 5-iodo-2′-deoxyuridine. Proc Soc Exp Biol Med 109:251–252

Kaufman HE (1965) Problems in virus chemotherapy. Prog Med Virol 7:116–159

Kaufman HE (1977) Antiviral drugs. Int J Dermatol 16:464–475

Kaufman HE (1980) Antimetabolite therapy in herpes simplex. Ophthalmology 87:135–139

Kaufman HE, Heidelberger C (1964) Therapeutic antiviral action of 5-trifluoromethyl-2′-deoxyuridine in herpes simplex keratitis. Science 145:585–586

Kaufman HE, Maloney ED, Nesburn AB (1962a) Comparison of specific antiviral agents in herpes simplex keratitis. Invest Ophthalmol 1:686–692

Kaufman HE, Martola E, Dohlman C (1962b) Use of 5-iodo-2′-deoxyuridine (IDU) in treatment of herpes simplex keratitis. Arch Ophthalmol 68:235–239

Kaufman HE, Yarnell ED, Centifanto YM, Rheinstrom SD (1978) Effect of 9-(2-hydroxyethoxymethyl)guanine on herpesvirus-induced keratitis and iritis in rabbits. Antimicrob Agents Chemother 14:842–845

Keir HM, Gold E (1963) Deoxyribonucleic acid nucleotidyltransferase and deoxyribonuclease from cultured cells infected with herpes simplex virus. Biochim Biophys Acta 72:263–276

Kern ER, Richards JR, Overall JC, Glasgow LA (1977) Genital herpesvirus hominis infection in mice. II. Treatment with phosphonoacetic acid, adenine arabinoside, and adenine arabinoside 5′-monophosphate. J Infect Dis 135:557–567

Kern ER, Richards JR, Overall JC Jr, Glasgow LA (1978) Alteration of mortality and pathogenesis of three experimental *herpesvirus hominis* infections of mice with adenine arabinoside-5′-monophosphate, adenine arabinoside, and phosphonoacetic acid. Antimicrob Agents Chemother 13:53–60

Kit S (1979) Viral-associated and induced enzymes. Pharmacol Ther 4:501–585

Kit S, Dubbs DR (1963) Acquisition of thymidine kinase activity by herpes simplex-infected mouse fibroblast cells. Biochem Biophys Res Commun 11:55–59

Kit S, Dubbs DR, Pierkaraki JJ, Hsu TC (1963) Deletion of thymidine kinase activity from L cells resistant to bromodeoxyuridine. Exp Cell Res 31:297–312

Kitchin FD, Ellsworth RM (1980) Chemotherapy of ocular tumors. In: Srinivasan BD (ed) Ocular therapeutics. Masson, New York, pp 169–173

Klein RJ, Friedman-Kien AE (1975) Phosphonoacetic acid-resistant herpes simplex virus infection in hairless mice. Antimicrob Agents Chemother 7:289–293

Klein RJ, Friedman-Kien AE, DeStefano E (1979a) Latent herpes simplex virus infections in sensory ganglia of hairless mice prevented by acycloguanosine. Antimicrob Agents Chemother 15:723–729

Klein RJ, DeStefano E, Brady E, Friedman-Kien AE (1979b) Latent infections of sensory ganglia as influenced by phosphonoformate treatment of herpes simplex-virus-induced skin infections in hairless mice. Antimicrob Agents Chemother 16:266–270

Klein RJ, DeStefano E, Brady E, Friedman-Kien AE (1980) Experimental skin infection with acyclovir resistant mutant: response to antiviral treatment and protection against reinfection. Arch Virol 65:237–246

Kurtz SM (1975) Toxicology of adenine arabinoside. In: Pavan-Langston D, Buchanan RA, Alford CA (eds) Adenine arabinoside: an antiviral agent. Raven, New York, pp 145–157

Laibson PR, Arentsen JJ, Mazzanti WD, Eiferman RA (1977) Double-controlled comparison of IDU and trifluorothymidine in thirty-three patients with superficial herpetic keratitis. Trans Am Ophthalmol Soc 75:316–324

Langen P (1975) Antimetabolites of nucleic acid metabolism. Gordon and Breach, New York, pp 1–213

Langen P, Kowolik G (1968) 5'-Deoxy-5'-fluorothymidine, a biochemical analogue of thymidine-5'-monophosphate selectively inhibiting DNA synthesis. Eur J Biochem 6:344–351

Langen P, Kowollik G, Schutt M, Etzold G (1969) Thymidylate kinase as target enzyme for 5'-deoxythymidine and various 5'-deoxy-5'halogeno pyrimidine nucleosides. Acta Biol Med Ger 23:K19–K22

Langen P, Etzold G, Kowollik G (1972) Inhibition of DNA synthesis and thymidylate kinase by halogeno derivatives of 3',5'-dideoxythymidine. Acta Biol Med Ger 28:K5–K10

Langston RHS, Pavan-Langston D, Dohlman CH (1974) Antiviral medication and corneal wound healing. Arch Ophthalmol 92:509–513

Larsson A, Öberg B (1981) Selective inhibition of herpesvirus deoxyribonucleic acid synthesis by acycloguanosine, 2'-fluoro-5-iodo-aracytosine, and (E)-5-(2-bromovinyl)-2'-deoxyuridine. Antimicrob Agents Chemother 19:927–929

Lee LF, Nazerian K, Leinback SS, Reno JM, Boezi JA (1976) Effect of phosphonoacetate on Marek's disease virus replication. N Natl Cancer Inst 56:823–827

Lee LF, Nazerian K, Witter RL, Leinback SS, Boezi, JA (1978) A phosphonoacetate-resistant mutant of herpes virus of turkeys. J Natl Cancer Inst 60:1141–1145

Lee WW, Benitez A, Goodman L, Baker BR (1960) Potential anticancer agents. XL Synthesis of the β-anomer of 9-(D-arabinofuranosyl)adenine. J Am Chem Soc 82:2648–2649

Leinbach SS, Reno JM, Lee LF, Isbell AF, Boezi JA (1976) Mechanism of phosphonoacetate inhibition of herpesvirus-induced DNA polymerase. Biochemistry 15:426–430

LePage GA (1975) Purine arabinosides, xylosides and lyxosides. In: Sartorelli AC, Johns DG (eds) Antineoplastic and immunosuppressive agents, vol 2. Springer, Berlin Heidelberg New York, pp 426–433

Lin T-S, Prusoff WH (1978a) A novel synthesis and biological activity of several 5-halo-5'-amino analogues of deoxyribopyrimidine nucleosides. J Med Chem 21:106–109

Lin T-S, Prusoff WH (1978b) Synthesis and biological activity of several amino analogues of thymidine. J Med Chem 21:109–112

Lin TS, Neenan JP, Cheng Y-C, Prusoff WH, Ward DC (1976) Synthesis and antiviral activity of 5- and 5'-substituted thymidine analogs. J Med Chem 19:495–498

Lopez C, Watanabe KA, Fox JJ (1980) 2'-Fluoro-5-iodoaracytosine, a potent selective antiherpes agent. Antimicrob Agents Chemother 17:803–806

Maass G, Haas R (1966) Über die Bildung von virusspezifischen SV-40 Antigen in Gegenwart von 5-Iodo-2'-desoxyuridine. Arch Gesamte Virusforsch 18:253–256

Mao JC-H, Robishaw EE (1975) Mode of inhibition of herpes simplex virus DNA polymerase by phosphonoacetate. Biochemistry 14:5475–5479

Mao JC-H, Robishaw EE, Overby LR (1975) Inhibition of DNA polymerase from herpes simplex virus infected WI-38 cells by phosphonoacetic acid. J Virol 15:1281–1283

Martenet A-C (1975) The treatment of experimental deep herpes simplex keratitis with 5-ethyldeoxyuridine and iododeoxycytidine. Ophthalmol Res 7:170–180

Mathias AP, Fischer GA (1962) The metabolism of thymidine by murine leukemia lymphoblasts (L5178Y). Biochem Pharmacol 11:57–68

Maudgal PC, CeClercq E, Descamps J, Missotten L, Desomer P, Busson R, Vanderhaeghe H, Verhelst G, Walker RT, Jones AS (1980) (E)-5-(Bromovinyl)-2'-deoxyuridine in the treatment of experimental herpes simplex keratitis. Antimicrob Agents Chemother 17:8–12

McGill J, Holt-Wilson AP, McKinnon JR, Williams HP, Jones BR (1974) Some aspects of the clinical use of trifluorothymidine in the treatment of herpetic ulceration of the cornea. Trans Ophthalmol Soc UK 94:342–352

McGuffin RW, Shiota FM, Meyers JD (1980) Lack of toxicity of acyclovir to granulocyte progenitor cells in vitro. Antimicrob Agents Chemother 18:471–473

McKinnon JR, McGill JI, Jones BR (1975) A coded clinical evaulation of adenine arabinoside and trifluorothymidine in the treatment of ulcerative herpetic keratitis. In: Pavan-Langston D, Buchanan RA, Alford CA (eds) Adenine arabinoside: an antiviral agent. Raven, New York, pp 401–410

Meyer RF, Varnell ED, Kaufman HE (1976) Phosphonoacetic acid in the treatment of experimental ocular herpes simplex infection. Antimicrob Agents Chemother 9:308–311

Miller FA, Dixon GJ, Ehrlich J, Sloan BJ, McLean IW Jr (1969) Antiviral activity of 9-β-D-arabinofuranosyladenine. I. Cell culture studies. Antimicrob Agents Chemother 1:136–147

Miller WH, Miller RL (1980) Phosphorylation of acyclovir (acycloguanosine)-monophosphate by GMP kinase. J Biol Chem 255:7204–7207

Moore EC, Cohen SS (1967) Effects of arabino nucleotides on ribonucleotide reduction by an enzyme system from rat tumor. J Biol Chem 242:2116–2118

Müller WEG (1979) Mechanism of action and pharmacology: chemical agents. In: Galasso GJ (ed) Antiviral agents and virus diseases of man. Raven, New York, pp 77–149

Müller WEG (1980) Purines and their nucleosides. Antibiot Chemother 27:139–163

Müller WEG, Rohde HJ, Beyer R, Maidhof A, Lachmann M, Taschner H, Zahn RH (1975) Mode of action of 9β-D-arabinofuranosyladenine on the synthesis of DNA, RNA, and protein in vivo and in vitro. Cancer Res 35:2160–2168

Müller WEG Zahn RK, Beyer R, Falke D (1977a) 9-β-D-Arabinofuranosyladenine as a tool to study herpes simplex virus replication in vitro. Virology 76:787–796

Müller WEG, Zahn RK, Bittlingmaier K, Falke D (1977b) Inhibition of herpesvirus DNA synthesis by 9-β-D-Arabinofuranosyladenine in cellular and cell-free systems. Ann NY Acad Sci 284:34–38

Nazerian K, Lee LF (1976) Selective inhibition by phosphonoacetic acid of MDV DNA replication in a lymphoblastoid cell line. Virology 74–188–193

Newton AA (1979) Inhibition of the replication of herpes viruses by phosphonoacetate and related compounds. Adv Ophthalmol 38:267–275

Nishiyama Y, Rapp F (1979) Anticellular effects of 9-(2-hydroxyethoxymethyl)-guanine against herpes simplex virus-transformed cells. J Gen Virol 45:227–230

North TW, Cohen SS (1979) Aranucleosides and aranucleotides in viral chemotherapy. Pharmacol Ther 4:81–108

Nylén P (1924) Beitrag zur Kenntnis der organischen Phosphonerbindungen. Chem Ber 57B:1023–1035

O'Brien WJ, Edelhauser HF (1977) The corneal penetration of trifluorothymidine, adenine arabinoside and idoxuridine: a comparative study. Invest Ophthalmol Vis Sci 16:1093–1103

Oki T, Heidelberger C (1971) Fluorinated pyrimidine XXXIV. Effects of 5-trifluromethyl-2'-deoxyuridine on the replication of vaccinia viral messenger RNA and proteins. Mol Pharmacol 7:653–662

Ostrander M, Cheng Y-C (1980) Properties of herpes simplex virus type 1 and type 2 DNA polymerase. Biochim Biophys Acta 609:232–245

Otto MJ, Lee JJ, Prusoff WH (1982) Effects of nucleoside analogues on the expression of herpes simplex type 1 induced proteins. Antiviral Res 5:267–282

Overall JR Jr, Kern ER, Glasgow LA (1976) Effective antiviral chemotherapy in cytomegalovirus infection in mice. J Infect Dis 133:A237–A244

Overby, LR, Robishaw EE, Schleicher JB, Rueter A, Shipkowitz NL, Mao JC-H (1974) Inhibition of herpes simplex virus replication by phosphonoacetic acid. Antimicrob Agents Chemother 6:360–365

Overby LR, Duff RG, Mao JC-H (1977) Antiviral potential of phosphonoacetic acid. Ann NY Acad Sci 284:310–320

Oxford JS (1979) Inhibition of herpes virus by a new compound – acyclic guanosine. J Antimicrob Chemother 5:333–334

Park N-H, Pavan-Langston D, McLean SL (1979a) Acyclovir in oral and ganglionic herpes simplex infections. J Infect Dis 140:802–806

Park N-H, Pavan-Langston D, McLean SL, Albert DM (1979b) Therapy of experimental herpes simplex encephalitis with acyclovir in mice. Antimicrob Agents Chemother 15:775–779

Park N-H, Pavan-Langston D, Hettinger ME, McLean SL, Albert DM, Lin T-S, Prusoff WH (1980a) Topical therapeutic efficacy of 9-(2-hydroxyethoxymethyl)-guanine and 5-iodo-5′-amino-2′-5′-dideoxyuridine on oral infection with herpes simplex virus in mice. J Infect Dis 141:575–579

Park N-H, Pavan-Langston D, McLean SL, Lass JH (1980b) Acyclovir topical therapy of cutaneous herpes simplex virus infection in guinea pigs. Arch Dermatol 116:672–675

Parkhurst JR, Dannenberg PV, Heidelberger C (1976) Growth inhibition of cells in culture and of vaccinia virus infected HeLa cells by derivatives of trifluorothymidine. Chemotherapy 22:221–232

Pavan-Langston D (1979) Current trends in therapy of ocular herpes simplex: experimental and clinical studies. Adv Ophthalmol 38:82–88

Pavan-Langston D (1980) Ocular herpes simplex – current and future therapeutic trends. In: Srinivasan DB (ed) Ocular therapeutics. Masson, New York, pp 5–19

Pavan-Langston D, Buchanan RA (1976) Vidarabine therapy of simplex and IDU-complicated herpetic keratitis. Trans Am Acad Ophthalmol Otolaryngol 81:813–825

Pavan-Langston D, Dohlman CH (1972) A double blind clinical study of adenine arabinoside therapy of viral keratoconjunctivitis. Am J Ophthalmol 74:81–88

Pavan-Langston D, Foster CS (1977) Trifluorothymidine and iododeoxyuridine therapy of ocular herpes. Am J Ophthalmol 84:818–825

Pavan-Langston D, Buchanan RA, Alford CA Jr (1975) Adenine arabinoside: a antiviral agent. Raven, New York

Pavan-Langston D, Campbell R, Lass J (1978) Acyclic antimetabolite therapy of experimental herpes simplex keratitis. Am J Ophthalmol 86:618–623

Pavan-Langston D, Park N-H, Lass JH (1979) Herpetic ganglionic latency. Acyclovir and Vidarabine therapy. Arch Ophthalmol 97:1508–1510

Pelling JC, Drach JC, Shipman C Jr (1981) Internucleotide incorporation of arabinosyladenine into herpes simplex virus and mammalian cell DNA. Virology 109:323–325

Perkins ES, Wood RM, Sears ML, Prusoff WH, Welch AD (1962) Antiviral activities of several iodinated pyrimidine deoxyribonucleosides. Nature 194:985–986

Pietryzkowska I, Shugar D (1966) Replacement of thymine by 5-ethyluracil in bacteriophage DNA. Biochem Biophys Res Commun 25:567–572

Plunkett W, Cohen SS (1975) Two approaches that increase the activity of analogs of adenine nucleosides in animal cells. Cancer Res 35:1547–1554

Plunkett W, Lapi L, Oritz PJ, Cohen SS (1974) Penetration of mouse fibroblasts by the 5′-phosphate of 9-β-D-arabinofuranosyladenine and incorporation of the nucleotide into DNA. Proc Natl Acad Sci USA 71:73–77

Prusoff WH (1959) Synthesis and biological activities of iododeoxyuridine, an analog of the thymidine. Biochim Biophys Acta 32:295–296

Prusoff WH (1967) Recent advances in chemotherapy of viral diseases. Pharmacol Rev 19:209–250

Prusoff WH, Fischer PH (1979) Basis for the selective antiviral and antitumor activity of pyrimidine nucleoside analogs. In: Walker RT, DeClercq E, Eckstein F (eds) Nucleoside analogs. Plenum, New York, pp 281–318

Prusoff WH, Goz B (1973a) Potential mechanisms of action of antiviral agents. Fed Proc 32:1679–1687

Prusoff WH, Goz B (1973 b) Chemotherapy–molecular aspects. In: Kaplan AS (ed) The herpes viruses. Academic, New York, p 641

Prusoff WH, Goz B (1975) Halogenated pyrimidine deoxyribonucleosides. In: Sartorelli AC, Johns DG (eds) Antineoplastic and immunosuppressive agents. Springer, Berlin Heidelberg New York, pp 272–347

Prusoff WH, Ward DC (1976) Nucleosides with antiviral activity. Biochem Pharmacol 25:1233–1239

Prusoff WH, Bakhle YS, Sekely L (1965) Cellular and antiviral effects of halogenated deoxyribonucleosides. Ann NY Acad Sci 130:135–150

Prusoff WH, Ward DC, Lin T-S, Chen MS, Shiau GT, Chai C, Lentz E, Capizzi R, Idriss J, Ruddle NH, Black FL, Kumari HL, Albert D, Bhatt PN, Hsiung GD, Strickland S, Cheng YC (1977) Recent studies on the antiviral and biochemical properties of 5-halo-5′-amino-deoxyribonucleosides. Ann NY Acad Sci 284:335–341

Prusoff WH, Chen MS, Fischer PH, Lin T-S, Shiau GT (1979 a) 5-Iodo-2′-deoxyuridine. In: Hahn FE (ed) Antibiotics, vol 2. Springer, Berlin Heidelberg New York, pp 236–261

Prusoff WH, Chen MS, Fischer PH, Lin T-S, Schinazi RF, Walker J (1979 b) Antiviral iodinated pyrimidine deoxyribonucleosides: 5-iodo-2′-deoxyuridine; 5-iodo-2′-deoxycytidine; 5-iodo-5′-amino-2′,5′-dideoxyuridine. Pharmacol Ther 7:1–34

Puliafito CA, Robinson NL, Albert DH, Pavan-Langston D, Lin T-S, Ward DC, Prusoff WH (1977) Therapy of experimental herpes simplex keratitis in rabbits with 5-iodo-5′-amino-2′,5′-dideoxyuridine. Proc Soc Exp Biol Med 156:92–96

Purifoy DJM, Powell KL (1977) Herpes simplex virus DNA polymerase as the site of phosphonoacetate sensitivity: temperature-sensitive mutants. J Virol 24:470–477

Renis HE (1977) Chemotherapy of genital herpes simplex virus type 2 infections of female hamsters. Antimicrob Agents Chemother 11:701–707

Renis HE (1980) Pyrimidines and their nucleosides. Antibiot Chemother 27:164–207

Reno JM, Lee LF, Boezi JA (1978) Inhibition of herpesvirus replication and herpesvirus-induced deoxyribonucleic acid polymerase by phosphonoformate. Antimicrob Agents Chemother 13:188–192

Reyes P, Heidelberger C (1965) Fluorinated pyrimidines XXVI. Mammalian thymidylate synthetase, its mechanism of action and inhibition by fluorinated nucleotides. Mol Pharmacol 1:14–30

Roizman G, Aurelian L, Roane PR Jr (1963) The multiplication of herpes simplex virus I. The programming of viral DNA duplication in HEP-2 cells. Virology 21:482–498

Rosenbaum A, Parker RG, Falk P (1980) Retinoblastoma. In: Haskell CM (ed) Cancer treatment. Saunders, Philadelphia, pp 569–577

Sabourin CLK, Reno JM, Boezi JA (1978) Inhibition of eukaryotic DNA polymerases by phosphonoacetate and phosphonoformate. Arch Biochem Biophys 187:96–101

Schabel FM Jr (1968) The antiviral activity of 9-β-D-arabinofuranosyladenine. Chemotherapy 13:321–338

Schabel FM Jr, Montgomery JA (1972) Purines and pyrimidines. In: Bauer DJ (ed) Chemotherapy of virus diseases. Pergamon, Oxford, pp 231–363

Schaeffer JH, Gurwara S, Vince R, Bittner SJ (1971) Novel substrates of adenosine deaminase. J Med Chem 14:367–369

Schaeffer JH, Beauchamp L, de Miranda P, Elion GB, Bauer DJ, Collins P (1978) 9-(2-hydroxyethoxymethyl)guanine activity against viruses of the herpes group. Nature 272:583–585

Schinazi RF, Peters J, Nahmias AJ (to be published) The effect of FIAC and FMAU alone and in combination with ACV and ara-A in mice infected intracerebrally with herpes simplex virus type 2.

Schnipper LE, Crumpacker CS (1980) Resistance of herpes simplex virus to acycloguanosine: role of viral thymidine kinase and DNA polymerase loci. Proc Natl Acad Sci USA 77:2270–2273

Schwartz PM, Shipman C Jr, Drach JC (1976) Antiviral activity of arabinosyladenine and arabinosylhypoxanthine in herpes simplex virus-infected KB cells: selective inhibition of viral deoxyribonucleic acid synthesis in the presence of an adenosine deaminase inhibitor. Antimicrob Agents Chemother 10:64–74

Selby PJ, Powles RC, Jameson B, Kay HEM, Watson JG, Thornton R, Morgenstern G, Clink HM, McElwain TJ, Prentice HG, Corringham R, Ross MG, Hoffbrand HV, Bridgen D (1979) Parenteral acyclovir therapy for herpesvirus infections in man. Lancet II:1267–1270

Shannon WM (1975) Adenine arabinoside: antiviral activity *in vitro*. In: Pavan-Langston D, Buchanan RA, Alford CA (eds) Adenine arabinoside: an antiviral agent: Raven, New York, pp 1–43

Shiota H, Inou S, Yamane S (1979) Efficacy of acycloguanosine against herpetic ulcers in rabbit cornea. Br J Ophthalmol 63:425–428

Shipkowitz NL, Bower RR, Appell RN, Nordeen CW, Overby LR, Roderick WR, Schleicher JB, von Esch AM (1973) Suppression of herpes simplex virus infection by phosphonoacetic acid. Appl Microbiol 26:264–267

Shipman C Jr, Smith SH, Carlson RH, Drach JC (1976) Antiviral activity of arabinosyl-adenine and arabinosylhypoxanthine in herpes simplex virus-infected KB cells: selective inhibition of viral deoxyribonucleic acid synthesis in synchronized suspension cultures. Antimicrob Agents Chemother 9:120–127

Sidwell RW, Witkowski JT (1979) Antiviral agents. In: Wolf ME (ed) Burger's medicinal chemistry. Wiley, New York, pp 543–593

Silagi S, Balint RF, Gauri KK (1977) Comparative effects on growth and tumorigenicity of mouse melanoma cells by thymidine and its analogs, 5-ethyl- and 5-bromo-deoxyuridine. Cancer Res 37:3367–3373

Singh S, Willers I, Goedde HW, Gauri KK (1974) 5-Ethyl-2'-deoxyuridine: absence of effect on the chromosomes of human lymphocytes and fibroblasts in culture. Humangenetik 24:135–139

Sloan BJ, Miller FA, McLean IW (1973) Treatment of herpes simplex virus type 1 and 2 encephalitis in mice with 9-β-D-arabinofuranosyladenine (ara-A). Antimicrob Agents Chemother 3:74–80

Smith KO (1963) Some biologic aspects of herpesvirus-cell interactions in the presence of 5-iodo-2'-desoxyuridine (IDU). J Immunol 91:582–590

Smith KO, Dukes CD (1964) Effects of 5-iodo-2'-desoxyuridine (IDU) on herpes virus synthesis and survival in infected cells. J Immunol 92:550–554

Smith KO, Kennell WL, Poirier RH, Lynd FT (1980) In vitro and in vivo resistance of herpes simplex virus to 9-(2-hydroxytheoxymethyl)guanine (acycloguanosine). Antimicrob Agents Chemother 17:144–150

Smith RA, Sidwell RW, Robins RK (1980) Antiviral mechanism of action. Annu Rev Pharmacol Toxicol 20:259–284

St Clair MH, Furman PA, Lubbers CM, Elion GB (1980) Inhibition of cellular and virally induced deoxyribonucleic acid polymerases by the triphosphate of acyclovir. Antimicrob Agents Chemother 18:741–745

Steele RW, Marmer DJ, Kenney RE (1980) Comparative in vitro immunotoxicology of acyclovir and other antiviral agents. Infect Immun 28:957–962

Stenberg K, Larsson A (1978) Reversible effects on cellular metabolism and proliferation by trisodium phosphonoformate. Antimicrob Agents Chemother 14:727–730

Sugar J, Kaufmann HE (1973) Halogenated pyrimidines in antiviral therapy. In: Carter WA (ed) Selective inhibitors of viral funktions. CRC, Cleveland, pp 295–311

Sugar J, Varnell E, Centiafanto Y, Kaufman HE (1973) Trifluorothymidine treatment of herpetic iritis in rabbits and ocular penetration. Invest Ophthalmol 12:532–534

Summers WC, Klein G (1976) Inhibition of Epstein-Barr virus DNA synthesis and late gene expression by phosphonoacetic acid. J Virol 18:151–155

Swierkowski KM, Shugar D (1969) A nonmutagenic thymidine analog with antiviral activity. 5-Ethyldeoxyuridine. J Med Chem 12:533–534

Swierkowska KM, Jasinska JK, Steffen JA (1973) 5-Ethyl-2'-deoxyuridine: evidence for incorporation into DNA and evaluation of biological properties in lymphocte cultures grown under conditions of amethopterin-imposed thymidine deficiency. Biochem Pharmacol 22:85–93

Tone H, Heidelberger C (1973) Interaction of 5-trifluoromethyl-2'-deoxyuridine-5'-triphosphate with deoxyribonucleic acid polymerases. Mol Pharmacol 9:783–791

Travers JP, Patterson A (1978) A controlled trial of adenine arabinoside and trifluorothymidine in herpetic keratitis. J Int Med Res 6:102–104

Trousdale MD, Dunkel EC, Nesburn AB (1980) Effect of acyclovir on acute and latent herpes simplex virus infections in the rabbit. Invest Ophthalmol Vis Sci 19:1336–1341

Umeda M, Heidelberger C (1968) Fluorinated pyrimidines XXX. Comparative studies of fluorinated pyrimidines with various cell lines. Cancer Res 28:2529–2538

Umeda M, Heidelberger C (1969) Fluorinated pyrimidines XXXI. Mechanism of inhibition of vaccinia virus replication in HeLa cells by pyrimidine nucleosides. Proc Soc Exp Biol Med 130:24–29

Verbov J (1979) Local idoxuridine treatment of herpes simplex and zoster. J Antimicrob Chemother 5:126–128

Walter RD, Gauri KK (1975) 5-Ethyl-2′-deoxyuridine-5′-monophosphate inhibition of the thymidylate synthetase from Escherichia coli. Biochem Pharmacol 24:1025–1027

Waqar MA, Burgoyne LA, Atkinson MR (1971) Deoxyribonucleic acid synthesis in mammalian nuclei. Incorporation of deoxyribonucleotides and chain terminating nucleotide analogues. Biochem J 121:803–809

Watanabe KA, Reichman U, Hirota K, Lopez C, Fox JJ (1979) Nucleosides. 110. Synthesis and antiherpes virus activity of some 2′-fluoro-2′-deoxyarabinofuranosyl-pyrimidine nucleosides. J Med Chem 22:21–24

Webb JL (1963) Enzyme and metabolic inhibitors. Academic, New York, pp 104–105

Welch AD, Prusoff WH (1960) A synopsis of recent investigations of 5-iodo-2′-deoxyuridine. Cancer Chemother Rep 6:29–36

Wellings PC, Audry PN, Bors FH, Jones BR, Brown DC, Kaufman HE (1972) Clinical evaluation of trifluorothymidine in the treatment of herpes simplex corneal ulcers. Am J Ophthalmol 73:932–942

Whitley RJ, Ch'ien LT, Dolin R, Galasso GJ, Alford CA, and the collaborative study group (1976). Adenine arabinoside therapy of herpex zoster in the immunosuppressed. N Engl J Med 294:1193–1199

Whitley RJ, Soong SJ, Dolin R, Galasso GJ, Ch'ien LT, Alford CA (1977) Adenine arabinoside therapy of biopsy proved herpes simplex encephalitis. N Engl J Med 297:289–294

Whitley RJ, Nahmias AJ, Soong SJ, Galasso GJ, Fleming CL, Alford CA (1980a) Vidarabine therapy of neonatal herpes simplex virus infection. Pediatrics 66:495–501

Whitley RJ, Alford CA, Hess F, Buchanan R (1980b) Vidarabine: a preliminary review of its pharmacological properties and therapeutic use. Drugs 20:267–282

Wigand R, Klein W (1974) Properties of adenovirus substituted with iododeoxyuridine. Arch Gesamte Virusforschung 45:298–300

Yajima Y, Tanaka A, Nonoyama M (1976) Inhibition of productive replication of Epstein-Barr virus DNA by phosphonoacetic acid. Virology 71:352–354

York JL, LePage GA (1966) A proposed mechanism for the action of 9-β-D-arabinofuranosyladenine as an inhibitor of the growth of some ascites cells. Can J Biochem 44:19–26

CHAPTER 12

Immunosuppressive Drugs

I. GERY and R. B. NUSSENBLATT

A. Introduction

In addition to its pivotal beneficial function in defense against infection or malignancy, the immune system may participate in pathogenic processes which have been conventionally classified into the four types of hypersensitivity, i.e., immediate (type I), complement-mediated cytotoxic (II), immune-complex-mediated (III), and cell-mediated (IV). All four types of reaction may affect the eye, the antigens being either of foreign or of autologous origin. The immunopathogenic reactions threaten vision and therefore immunosuppressive drugs have been a welcome addition to the ophthalmologist's range of medications.

These immunopathogenic reactions are modulated or inhibited by a variety of pharmacologic agents, which may be divided into two main groups: (a) drugs which affect the early or inductive phases of the immune response, and (b) agents which are selectively directed against the later phases of the immunopathogenic reaction, namely, the inflammatory or allergic reactions. The present chapter deals mostly with the former group of agents, which are designated "immunosuppressive drugs" in the strict sense, whereas the anti-inflammatory and antiallergic drugs should be dealt with separately. It is noteworthy, however, that the different groups of drugs overlap to some extent. Many immunosuppressive agents may exert anti-inflammatory effects, mainly by reducing the numbers of leukocytes (BACH 1975; FAUCI et al. 1980). A family of drugs which affect most phases of the immunopathogenic processes, the steroids, is thoroughly discussed by POLANSKY and WEINREB (Chap. 10a).

The majority of immunosuppressive drugs affect the immune response by inhibiting the process of cellular proliferation, which is the main mechanism of clone expansion, whereby an antigenic stimulus triggers a small number of specifically committed lymphocytes to expand to a much larger clone of similarly committed lymphocytes. The group of drugs which inhibit lymphocyte proliferation consists mainly of alkylating agents and analogs of purines, pyrimidines, and folic acid, all of which have been used in the chemotherapy of cancer. These agents may affect nonlymphoid cells as well, and thus bring about adverse side effects. A great effort has been invested, therefore, in developing drugs with selective effects toward the immune system. This goal of selectivity has been partially achieved by drugs like cyclosporin A, or by specific antibodies against lymphocytes (see Sects. D and E).

The present chapter discusses the mode of action and specific effects on the immune system of the commonly used immunosuppressive drugs. Special attention

is focused on the effects of these drugs on ocular disorders of presumed immunologic origin.

Studies during the last two decades have revealed the tremendous complexity
of the immune system, particularly with regard to the variety of participating cell
types. Three major cell compartments comprise this system: macrophages and B
and T lymphocytes. In addition, each of the three cell compartments has been
shown to consist of subsets of cells which differ in their function and/or their
markers.

Macrophages (also designated "mononuclear phagocytes") serve in the immune reaction mainly as accessory cells, which (a) present the stimulating antigen
to reacting lymphocytes and (b) provide the latter cells with certain stimulating mediators (Moller 1978; Unanue 1981). In addition, macrophages play a major role
in the inflammatory processes, in particular of the chronic type, which are usually
triggered by lymphocyte-made mediators (see below).

The main function of B lymphocytes is antibody production. Antibodies play
the main role in three of the immunopathogenic reactions, i.e., the immediate type
(I), complement-mediated cytotoxicity (II), and immune-complex-mediated (III)
reactions. In addition, antibodies may attach to certain lymphoid cells to render
them specifically cytotoxic, a reaction which is designated "antibody-dependent
cell-mediated cytotoxity" (ADCC) (Perlmann and Cerottini 1979). On the other
hand, antibodies were shown to counteract in certain conditions the pathogenic effects of other immune responses, namely "blocking antibodies," which reduce the
allergic response, and "enhancing antibodies," which may inhibit the development
and/or effects of damaging cellular immune responses (Voisin 1980).

The highest level of cellular complexity is found in the T cell compartment. Subsets of T cells are engaged in multiple functions which include mainly (a) direct cytotoxicity, (b) release of mediators which bring about inflammation, and (c) activities regulatory of other compartments of the immune system. The former two
functions form the basis for the type IV or "cellular" hypersensitivity. The most
intriguing activity of T cells is their involvement in regulation of the immune response. Subsets of T lymphocytes were shown to help or suppress other lymphocytes of both the B and T cell compartments (Cantor and Gershon 1979), and
more recently a subset of T cells was found to cause "contrasuppression," i.e., inhibition of the suppressor cells (Gershon et al. 1981).

The various populations of the immune system differ in their metabolism and
are thus differently affected by various drugs. Most of the differences among lymphocyte populations in their susceptibility to drugs are quantitative, but high levels
of selectivity have been recently achieved with new drugs like cyclosporin A, which
affects only T cells at a wide range of concentrations (Sect. D). Selective effects
against certain lymphocyte populations have also been achieved by using specific
antisera (Sect. E). Selectivity in immunosuppression is desirable, since many immunopathogenic reactions are mediated by either B or T lymphocytes.

Macrophages are particularly susceptible to steroids. These agents affect the
macrophage involvement in both the immune response and the inflammatory reaction (Fauci et al. 1980) (see Chap. 10 a). B lymphocytes are relatively short-lived
and are therefore highly susceptible to agents which affect dividing cells, in particular the alkylating agents. The complexity of the T-lymphocyte population is ex-

pressed in the high variability in susceptibility of T-cell subsets to the effects of various drugs. Of special importance is the difference between the suppressor and inducer subpopulations; suppressor cells are highly affected by cyclophosphamide but are relatively resistant to cyclosporin A, while inducer T lymphocytes show the opposite pattern (see below). These differences between the various subsets of T lymphocytes should provide a useful approach to manipulating the immune system by selectively affecting one and not the other of these regulatory lymphocyte subsets.

Also of interest is the observation that secondary immune responses are more resistant to most immunosuppressive treatments than primary responses. The phenomenon is not well understood and more studies are needed for better dissection of the differences in biochemical processes between these two types of immune reaction.

Most immune responses are the outcome of interactions between cells of the aforementioned populations. These interactions are brought about by a large battery of cellular mediators which have been classified into two main groups, lymphocyte-made "lymphokines" and macrophage-derived "monokines." Little is known about the effect of drugs on the production or activities of these mediators, but studies in recent years have indicated that the effects of some drugs may be attributed at least in part to their activity on the production or effect of the mediators. Thus the immunosuppressive effect of cyclosporin A is partially related to its inhibition of the release of the lymphokine interleukin 2 (see Sect. D), while steroids were found to inhibit both the release of monokines by macrophages (OPPENHEIM and GERY 1982) and the effect of lymphokines on macrophages (FAUCI et al. 1980).

B. Alkylating Agents

The alkylating agents all have their origin in sulfur mustard, first synthesized in 1854. Though the vesicant properties of these agents were described in 1887, their profound effects on mankind became evident in July 1917, when sulfur mustard was used in chemical warfare. KRUMBHAAR and KRUMBHAAR (1919) first reported the leukopenia induced by the sulfur mustard in the survivors of these attacks, and on autopsy, aplasia of the lymphoid tissue was noted. Initial laboratory work using experimental animals confirmed the agent's profound effect on the lymphoid system. Nitrogen mustard was first administered to patients with lymphoma in the early 1940s, with beneficial results, and this sparked an interest in its use in human disease. The alkylating agents mainly used in immunosuppressive therapy today are cyclophosphamide and chlorambucil, both of which have a *bis*-(chlorethyl) amine end group (Fig. 1).

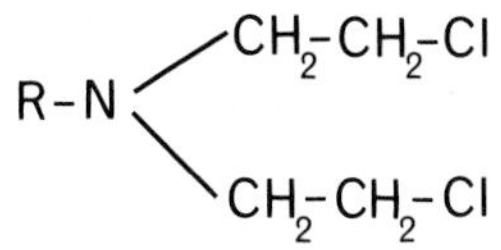

$$R-N \begin{cases} CH_2-CH_2-Cl \\ CH_2-CH_2-Cl \end{cases}$$

Fig. 1. Structure of *bis*-(chloroethyl) amine

I. Chemical Structure and Metabolism

Cyclophosphamide (Fig. 2) was developed by ARNOLD and BOURSEAUX (1958). In this modification of the original structure, the *bis*-chloroethyl amino group is attached to the phosphorus of oxazaphosphorine. This compound is stable, since the *bis*-(β-chlorethyl) segment of the molecule cannot be ionized until the cyclic group is cleaved at the phosphorous–nitrogen linkage by in vivo enzymatic processes. This factor was thought to have great potential importance, since various neoplastic tissues were found to have concentrations of phosphamidases and phosphatases (ARNOLD and BOURSEAUX 1958; ARNOLD et al. 1958). Therefore, it was postulated that the essentially inert cyclophosphamide would be selectively cleaved in the tissues where its effect was most desired. However, cyclophosphamide has been shown to be essentially metabolized by the liver-microsomal P-450 mixed-function oxidase system (BROCK and HOHORST 1963; COHEN and Jao 1970), with the initial oxidative process occurring in the cytosol of the cell. Cyclophosphamide is metabolized through several steps (CHABNER et al. 1977), ultimately yielding several compounds, not all of which have alkylating capacity. The metabolically inactive carboxyphosphamide, derived after oxidation of 4-ketocyclophosphamide and 4-hydroxycyclophosphamide (BAKKE et al. 1971; STRUCK et al. 1971), is important, since 50% of the ingested cyclophosphamide is excreted in the urine as this product (BAKKE et al. 1971; STRUCK et al. 1971). The observed effects of cyclophosphamide may be attributed to several of the metabolites of the parent compound. Phosphoramide mustard, a strong alkylating agent, may represent the most active of these metabolites (COLVIN et al. 1976; STRUCK et al. 1975). On the other hand, it has been shown (TAKAMIZAWA et al. 1973) that other metabolites, such as 4-hydroxycyclophosphamide, also have cytotoxic capabilities, and that these forms enter target cells more readily than does phosporamide mustard.

Chlorambucil, *p-β*-(di-2-chlorethyl) aminophenylbutyric acid (Fig. 3), was first synthesized at the Chester Beatty Research Institute in England (EVERETT et al. 1953). It is an aromatic derivative of mechlorethamine, and its structure makes it a relatively inert substance, thus permitting oral administration. The agent was shown to have a marked inhibitory effect on the Walker 256 tumor in rats (HAD-

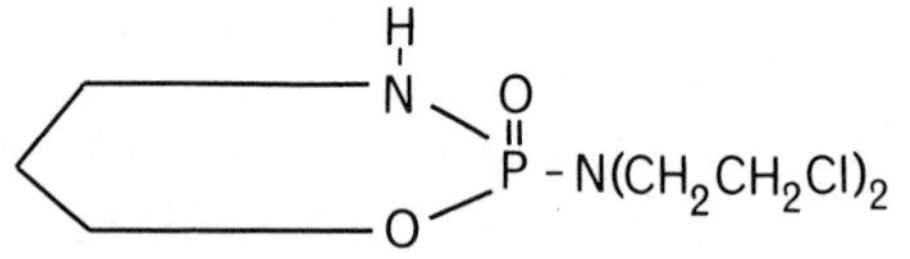

Fig. 2. Structure of cyclophosphamide

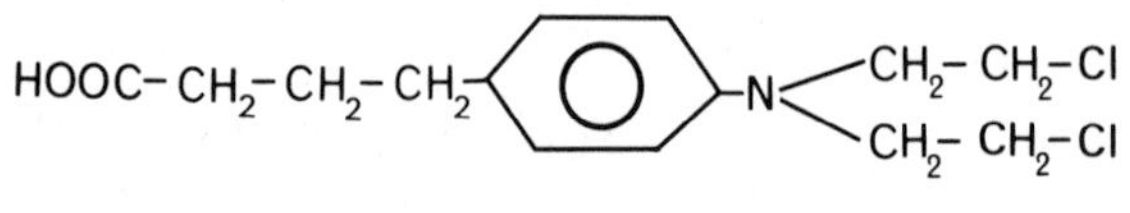

Fig. 3. Structure of chlorambucil

DOW 1954), and was introduced into the clinical sphere by GALTON et al. in 1955. An alkylating agent, its mechanisms of action are those outlined in the cyclophosphamide section. Animal studies (EVERETT et al. 1953) have shown that the effective alkylating agent phenyl acetic mustard is generated with the metabolism of chlorambucil. Human studies (McLEAN 1979) have also demonstrated the presence of this metabolite, a result of the β-oxidation of chlorambucil in patients treated for malignant disorders. A second, unidentified metabolite was also noted in these patients.

II. Mode of Action

Alkylating agents are electrophilic substances which alkylate nucleophilic substances. The agents used therapeutically all have a *bis*-(chloroethyl) amine end group (Fig. 1). These substances form carbonium ions which then can readily combine with nucleophilic compounds. The electrophilic ions will form covalent bonds with a variety of cell constituents. The alkylating agents appear to induce their cytotoxic effects by altering DNA. In particular, the 7-N guanine, a purine base and highly nucleophilic, appears to be the major site of action of these compounds (DORR and FRITZ 1980). Alkylation of this purine, as well as other positions in the DNA strands, could lead to several alterations. Perhaps the most common effect is the covalent cross-linking of DNA strands. The cross-linking efficacy of alkylating agents has been effectively demonstrated using such in vivo systems as bacterial DNA (KOHN et al. 1966). Another mode of action is a depurination of DNA, leading to a break in the sugar phosphate backbone of the structure. It is also possible that an altered base may remain in the DNA template, thus leading to the handing down of inaccurate information.

III. Effects on the Immune System

Both cyclophosphamide and chlorambucil are cytotoxic to cells of the lymphoid system. Most alkylating agents are cell-cycle-phase nonspecific, and therefore capable of affecting both rapidly proliferating and resting cells. Cyclophosphamide, however, appears to be unique in its ability to inhibit DNA synthesis, and therefore demonstrating a specificity for the S phase of the cell cycle (DORR and FRITZ 1980). Alkylating agents have been shown to have a profound effect on the immunocompetence of the organism being treated. In this regard, cyclophosphamide has been extensively evaluated both in man and in animals (STEINBERG et al. 1972; KAPLAN and CALABRESI 1973a, b; FAUCI et al. 1971), and its effects will be highlighted here. Cyclophosphamide has been found to be particularly useful in the treatment of nonneoplastic conditions (STEINBERG et al. 1972), such as Wegener's granulomatosis (FAUCI et al. 1971). Cyclophosphamide has been shown to have a dramatic effect on both primary and secondary humoral responses (SANTOS and OWENS 1966; MAIBACH and MAGUIRRE 1966). Studies in mice have revealed that cyclophosphamide caused a selective depletion of the thymus-dependent cortical regions of lymph nodes (MACKIEWICZ et al. 1978). Alterations in cell-mediated immunity, such as the delayed-type skin hypersensitivity reaction in both animals (WINKELSTEIN 1973; SCHWARTZ et al. 1978) and man (FAUCI et al. 1971), and the production of macrophage migration inhibitory factor and lymphocyte proliferation assays (WINKELSTEIN 1973; BALOW et al. 1975), have been seen with cyclophosphamide administration. HUNNINGHAKE and FAUCI (1976) reported that the dosage and mode of cyclophosphamide administration to experimental animals had a profound effect on the type of immune alteration elicited. Low daily doses of cyclophosphamide, as given to patients with autoimmune diseases, induced a moderate leukopenia and had essentially no effect on cytotoxic effector cells. With a marked increase in dosage, a concomitant profound neutropenia and decrease in mononuclear cell functioning was seen. This led to a severe alteration in host defenses.

The effect of cyclophosphamide on lymphocyte subpopulations remains unclear. The acute administration of the agent appears preferentially to affect B cells more than T cells (STOCKMAN et al. 1973). However, T cells in graft-versus-host disease appear to be sensitive to cyclophosphamide therapy (SCHWARTZ et al. 1976). Of special note is the finding that cyclophosphamide may eliminate suppressor T cells (SY et al. 1977; ROLLINGHOFF et al. 1977); consequently an increase in immune responses can be seen (MITSUOKA et al. 1976). It would seem that chronic therapy with cyclophosphamide depresses equally B- and T-cell populations (CLEMENTS et al. 1974; FAUCI et al. 1974).

C. Antimetabolic Drugs

I. Purine Analogs

The use of purine analogs was pioneered by HITCHINGS and his co-workers in 1942 (see ELION and HITCHINGS 1975). Since then, many compounds of this family have been synthesized and some of them have been found useful as immunosuppressive agents, while others are used as drugs for chemotherapy or antiviral activity (CRAB-

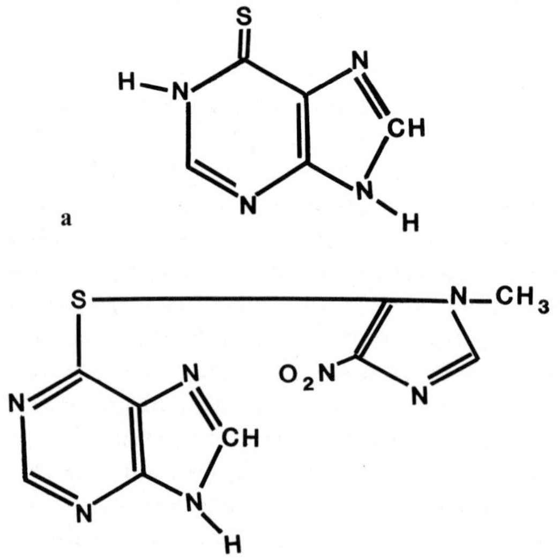

Fig. 4. Structures of **a** mercaptopurine and **b** azathioprine

TREE 1978) (see Chap. II). The major purine analogs in use as immunosuppressive agents are 6-mercaptopurine (6-MP) and azathioprine (AZA, Imuran); another compound, thioguanine, was found to be very active in experimental animals, but too toxic for human use. Azathioprine and 6-MP are analogs of hypoxanthine (Fig. 4), and both drugs were introduced and thoroughly investigated by Elion and her group (HITCHINGS and ELION 1963; ELION and HITCHINGS 1975). Azathioprine is assumed to be a prodrug, which reacts with sulfhydryl compounds (such as glutathione) to liberate 6-MP gradually.

1. Mode of Action

The mode of action of the thiopurines is not completely clear, but it seems these drugs act by multiple mechanisms, in particular by affecting the metabolism of nucleic acids.

6-Mercaptopurine affects the metabolism of RNA or DNA mainly after being converted (by hypoxanthine-guanine phosphoribosyltransferase) to a ribonucleotide form, 6-thioinosine-5′-phosphate (TIMP, thioisoinic acid). This nucleotide form is accumulated intracellularly and may affect the synthesis of nucleic acids. Possible mechanisms are reviewed in detail by BACH (1975), ELION and HITCHINGS (1975), and CRABTREE (1978). Inhibition of the normal metabolism of natural purine moieties and their incorporation into nucleic acids occurs. Other possible mechanisms by which TIMP may affect cells are apparently of marginal importance (see BACH 1975). These include: (a) "pseudofeedback" of the de novo synthesis of purines (McCOLLISTER et al. 1964), (b) direct incorporation of 6-MP into nucleic acids, and (c) interference with the synthesis or activation of coenzymes CoA and nicotinamide). Finally, it is noteworthy that the effects of purine analogs on lymphocytes may be related to some extent to the unique purine metabolism of lymphocytes, as shown by the extreme susceptibility of these cells to deficiency in adenosine deaminase (GIBLETT et al. 1972) (see Chap. 11).

2. Effects on the Immune System

The immunosuppressive effects of purine analogs have been investigated in numerous studies, which are reviewed in detail by SCHWARTZ (1965), MAKINODAN et al. (1970), BACH (1975), and SPREAFICO and ANACLERIO (1977).

Of practical importance are the studies in which 6-MP and AZA were compared. Azathioprine was found to be superior to 6-MP in inhibiting protein or antibody synthesis in vitro (FORBES and SMITH 1967; LEUNG and VOS 1968), and earlier reports suggested the superiority of AZA in vivo as well. Later studies (BERENBAUM 1971; SPREAFICO et al. 1973) could not confirm the superiority of AZA, but its use seems advantageous in view of its undisputedly better gastrointestinal absorption and lower toxicity (ELION and HITCHINGS 1975; SPREAFICO and ANACLERIO 1977).

The immunosuppressive effects of the thiopurines were demonstrated in numerous systems, both in vitro and in vivo. To mention a few, AZA or 6-MP inhibit lymphocyte cultures in their antibody production (e.g., DUTTON and PEARCE 1962), or mitotic responses to allogeneic antigens (BACH and BACH 1972). In vivo, thiopurines suppress antibody formation (e.g., BOREL et al. 1965), reactions of delayed hypersensitivity (BOREL and SCHWARTZ 1964), rejection of foreign grafts (CALNE

1960), and certain autoimmune diseases such as experimental allergic encephalo-myelitis (Hoyer et al. 1960).

The use of thiopurines in humans has been reported in a large number of pa-pers, which are thoroughly reviewed by Makinodan et al. (1970), Steinberg et al. (1972), Bach (1975), and Gerber and Steinberg (1976).

A noteworthy aspect of the immunosuppressive effects of purine analogs deals with the selectivity toward certain components of the immune system. Selectivity was found at three levels. Firstly, primary immune responses were found to be more susceptible than secondary responses (Spreafico and Anaclerio 1977). Se-condly, thiopurines are highly inhibitory of the inductive ("afferent") phases of the immune response, while having minimal effects on the later ("efferent") phases. Thus these drugs exert their maximal effect when administered early after the anti-genic stimulus but have minimal or no activity when given more than 48 h later (see Bach 1975; Spreafico and Anaclerio 1977). Further, AZA was found to be in-effective against cell-mediated cytotoxicity when presensitized lymphocytes were used (Spreafico and Anaclerio 1977). The third type of selectivity concerns the difference between T- and B-cell responses, the former being much more suscept-ible to thiopurines. This difference was particularly clear in culture: the antibody response to thymus-independent antigens was much more (300 times) resistant to AZA than the response to thymus-dependent antigens (Rollinghoff et al. 1973). Also, cell-mediated immune diseases such as experimental allergic encephalomyeli-tis (see above) are highly susceptible to thiopurines, while these drugs have minimal effects on the development of the autoimmune disease in New Zealand black mice, which is mainly antibody-mediated (Lemmel et al. 1971; Bach 1975).

II. Pyrimidine Analogs

The category comprised by pyrimidine analogs is quite diverse and consists of agents used for cancer chemotherapy, antiviral activity, and immunosuppression.

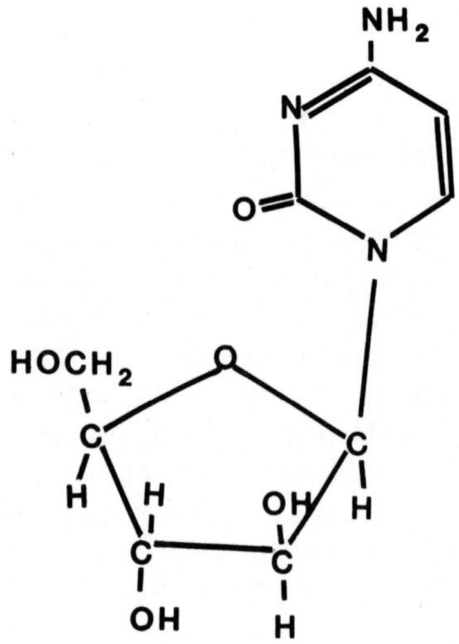

Fig. 5. Structure of cytarabine

Compounds with antiviral effect are thoroughly reviewed in Chap. 11. The major pyrimidine analog in use for immunosuppression is cytosine arabinoside (ara-C, cytarabine) (Fig. 5).

1. Mode of Action

It is generally assumed that ara-C exerts its metabolic effect after being converted enzymatically to the form of diphosphate or triphosphate nucleotide (ara-CDP or ara-CTP). The exact effect of the activated forms of ara-C is not completely defined, and at least two mechanisms have been suggested: (a) blocking of ribonucleoside diphosphate reductase, or (b) inhibition of DNA polymerases such as reverse transcriptase.

2. Effects on the Immune System

Little is known about the immunosuppressive activity of ara-C. A study by MITCHELL et al. (1969) demonstrated the immunosuppression which may develop during cancer chemotherapy with this drug, while HEPPNER and CALABRESI (1976) used ara-C to selectively suppress the humoral immune response while sparing the cellular immune capacity. On the other hand, ROLLINGHOFF et al. (1973) could not find a significant difference between the effect of ara-C on responses in culture of B or T lymphocytes.

III. Folic Acid Analogs

The folic acid analogs have been used extensively in cancer chemotherapy; agents of this group were the first to bring about remission of leukemia (FARBER et al. 1948). The major drug of this group, methotrexate (MTX, Fig. 6), has been used also as an immunosuppressive agent.

1. Mode of Action

The mechanism of action of folate analogs is primarily related to the capacity of these compounds to inhibit the enzyme dihydrofolate reductase. This enzyme converts dihydrofolate to tetrahydrofolate, which is the active metabolite of folate and transfers single carbon fragments to purine nucleotides such as thymidylate. These purines are needed for de novo synthesis of DNA and the folate analogs therefore inhibit this process.

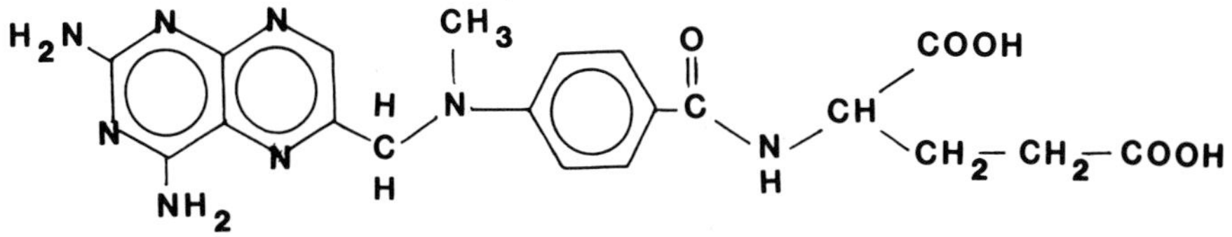

Fig. 6. Structure of methotrexate

An interesting feature of the folate analogs is the availability of compounds which may counteract their toxic activity and "rescue" normal cells. The rescue compounds include thymidine and/or leukovorin (citrovorum factor, N-formyl tetrahydrofolate).

2. Effects on the Immune System

Methotrexate was reported to be useful in selectively suppressing the humoral immune response without affecting the cellular immune compartment (HEPPNER and CALABRESI 1976). It is also of note that when given prior to the immunologic stimulus, MTX may actually stimulate the cellular immune response (LEVY and WHITEHOUSE 1974). In vitro, MTX was found to be unique among immunosuppressive drugs in that it was inhibitory even of lymphocytes activated 4 days earlier (BACH and BACH 1972). In man, MTX is used mainly for treatment of psoriasis (WEINSTEIN 1977). In addition, MTX has been used for various immune-related diseases, such as myasthenia gravis (see GERBER and STEINBERG 1976) or uveitis (see Sect. H), and has been found useful for prevention of graft-versus-host reaction in bone marrow recipients (RAMSAY et al. 1982).

D. Cyclosporin A

Cyclosporin A (CsA) is a peptide metabolite of the fungi *Trichoderma polysporum* Rifai and *Cylindrocarpon lucidom* Booth. The agent has been characterized as being a neutral cyclic endecapeptide with a molecular weight of 1202.6 (Fig. 7). Seven of the amino acids are N-methylated, giving CsA a highly nonpolar character (RÜEGGER et al. 1976; PETCHER et al. 1976).

Cyclosporin A has been demonstrated to have a narrow antifungal activity (DREYFUSS et al. 1976). However, its immunosuppressive characteristics have been

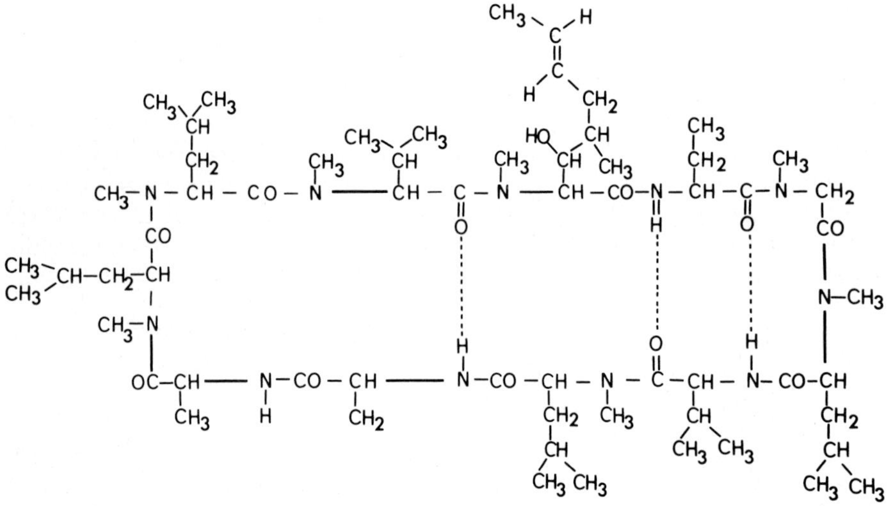

Fig. 7. Structure of cyclosporin A

the object of much study since BOREL et al. (1976) reported that CsA strongly depressed the appearance of plaque-forming cells, delayed skin graft rejection, and graft-versus-host disease in mice, and prevented rats from developing signs of the autoimmune neurological model, experimental allergic encephalomyelitis.

I. Mode of Action

Very little is known about the actual mechanism by which CsA affects cells. It is most intriguing that CsA's effects appear not to be mediated by cytotoxicity (BOREL et al. 1976; Wiesinger and BOREL 1979; BRENT 1980). Further, reports demonstrated early on that CsA's effect was limited to the T-cell portion of the immune system (BOREL et al. 1977; BURCKHARDT and GUGGENHEIM 1979). BOREL and co-workers (1977) demonstrated that CsA failed to inhibit production of antibodies to the T-cell-independent antigen lipopolysaccharide in nude mice (animals lacking T cells), and later reports (BRENT 1980) have supported this finding, thus making it the first immunosuppressive agent of its kind. However, CsA has been reported to have an exquisite effect on murine B cells responsive to a specific group of T-independent (TI-2) antigens (KUNKL and KLAUS 1980) and human B blast cells in vitro (PAAVONEN and HAYRY 1980).

Recent work would suggest that CsA's effect is by perturbating the delicate interleukin system needed for T-cell activation (Fig. 8). LARSSON (1980) compared CsA's effect on T cells with those induced by dexamethasone, and felt that the agents acted at distinctly different sites. At levels not capable of interfering with interleukin-2 (IL-2, T-cell growth factor) production, CsA appeared to inhibit re-

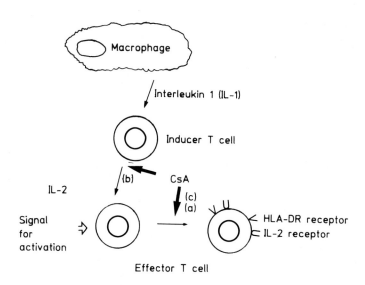

Fig. 8. Proposed mechanisms of action of cyclosporin A (*CsA*). CsA has been shown to block (*a*) the development of receptor for interleukin 2 (*IL-2*) (LARSSON 1980), (*b*) the production of IL-2 (BUNJES et al. 1981), and (*c*) the development of receptors for HLA DR antigens (PALACIOS and MÖLLER 1981)

ceptor formation to IL-2 on T cells, these receptors being mandatory for the acquisition of responsiveness to the factor. In contradistinction, dexamethasome appeared drastically to inhibit IL-2 production. Others (Bunjes et al. 1981; Hess et al. 1982) have demonstrated that CsA was also capable of interfering with IL-2 production, thereby breaking this communication chain in at least two positions. Further, Palacios and Möller (1981) have suggested that CsA may block the receptors for HLA-DR antigens on effector T cells. Bunjes et al. (1981) reported the apparent inhibition of IL-1 production by CsA, but this finding was not substantiated by further experimentation. Larsson's notion that CsA does not affect lymphocytes once they have developed receptors for IL-2 has been supported by data of Wiesinger and Borel 1979; Paavonen et al. 1981, and Hess et al. 1982. This is also in line with our finding (unpublished) that CsA at levels that inhibit thymocyte responses to concanavalin A (Con A) or to the combination of Con A and IL-1 or IL-2 had no effect on the direct mitogenic activity of these interleukins; only activated thymocytes react to the interleukins alone (Beller and Unanue 1979; Smith and Ruscetti 1981).

II. Effects on the Immune System

The effects of CsA have been extensively evaluated in vitro. It has been shown to suppress lymphocyte responses to stimulation by mitogens and alloantigens in primary and secondary mixed lymphocyte reactions, yet cytolytic effector lymphocytes did not seem to be effected (Hess and Tutschka 1980). A CsA-resistant murine cytotoxic splenic lymphocyte has been reported (Horsburgh et al. 1980). Several studies have suggested that CsA induction of a nonresponsive state may be mediated by a specific suppressor cell (Hess et al. 1981; Hutchinson et al. 1981; Wang et al. 1982), which may lead to a state of immune tolerance (Hess et al. 1981; Green et al. 1979). Further, CsA appears not to affect the generation or function of Con A induced suppressor cells (Leapman et al. 1980). Deeg et al. (1980), however, were unable to induce a state of immune tolerance in dogs. Cyclosporin A has been found most effective in suppressing various cell-mediated immune responses. Its effective inhibition of so-called T-cell-mediated autoimmune diseases was shown early on by Borel et al. (1976), and more recently CsA was reported to be effective in preventing the adoptive transfer of the T-cell-mediated experimental autoimmune encephalomyelitis (Bolton et al. 1982). Short-term CsA therapy was sufficient to prevent rejection of rabbit and kidney allografts for long periods (Green et al. 1979). Further, the use of CsA as the initial immunosuppressant agent in recipients of cadaveric kidneys, pancreases, and livers demonstrated a very high success rate with essentially no myelotoxicity (Calne et al. 1979, 1981). Allogeneic bone marrow transplantation has been successfully performed in CsA-treated rats (Tutschka et al. 1979) and in humans (Powles et al. 1980). It has been found effective in preventing graft-versus-host disease in rats (Tutschka et al. 1979), the most important cause of death after allogeneic bone marrow transplantation, and has been shown to modify the acute skin reaction in humans with this disease (Powles et al. 1978, 1980). Other transplant areas in which CsA has been found effective have been experimental lung transplantation (Veith et al. 1981) and liver transplantation (Starzl et al. 1981). Recent work has demonstrated CsA's effectiveness in heart-lung transplantation, with one patient demonstrating normal exercise tolerance 10 months after the procedure (REITZ et al. 1982).

E. Antilymphocyte Sera

Although the first preparation of antilymphocyte sera (ALS) was obtained by METCHNIKOFF in 1899, the observation that ALS may affect the immune response was made over five decades later (INDERBITZEN 1956). The possible application of ALS in prolongation of tissue grafts was indicated by WOODRUFF and ANDERSON (1963), and their observation has stimulated a great number of studies concerning this effect of ALS, in both experimental animals and man (see detailed reviews by TAUB 1970; TAUB and DEUTCH 1977; and BACH 1975).

I. Preparations

Immunosuppressive ALS are prepared by immunizing animals (mainly horses, rabbits, sheep, or goats) with lymphocytes from the species used later for treatment. Most ALS are prepared against thymocytes or enriched T cells; antisera against other lymphoid cells are less immunosuppressive. More recently, antisera against subsets of helper or suppressor T lymphocytes have become available (see CANTOR and BOYSE 1977; REINHERZ and SCHLOSSMAN 1980). Sera against subsets of lymphocytes were tested experimentally and found capable of modulating the immune system (PERRY et al. 1978, 1979). The ALS preparations consist of the whole serum, or of the IgG fraction (ALG), the latter being advantageous because of their lower adverse effects (see below). In addition, monoclonal antibodies have recently been prepared and proved capable of immunosuppression (COSIMI et al. 1981; SHERBURNE and CONDIE 1981) or of selective elimination of lymphocyte subpopulations (see MILLER et al. 1982).

II. Mode of Action

The mechanism of action of immunosuppressive ALS has not been completely clarified, and several hypothetical mechanisms have been considered, as discussed in detail by LEVEY and MEDAWAR (1966), TAUB (1970), and BACH (1975). Three of the hypothetical mechanisms are noteworthy: T-cell depletion, blindfolding (inactivation of the lymphocytes by coating with the antibodies), and sterile inactivation (loss of immune capacity by the lymphocytes following stimulation by the antibodies). The aforementioned mechanisms are not mutually exclusive and may all take place simultaneously. The most likely mechanism to play the major role in immunosuppression is the T-cell depletion, as supported by the following data:

1. Animals treated with ALS show a selective reduction in the number of circulating T cells and depletion of the thymus-dependent areas of spleen and lymph nodes (TAUB and LANCE 1968).
2. The immune responses most affected by ALS treatment are those carried out by T lymphocytes (see below).
3. The immunosuppressive state induced by ALS can readily be corrected by thymus cells (but not by bone marrow cells) (MARTIN and MILLER 1968).

The actual mechanism of T-cell depletion is mainly attributed to opsonization by the antibodies, which leads to lymphocyte elimination by the reticuloendothelial system (Bach 1975; Taub and Deutch 1977).

III. Effects on the Immune System

In accordance with the selective effects of ALS on the T-lymphocyte population, the immune responses mostly affected are those brought about by the T-cell populations. These responses include certain lymphocyte reactions in culture to stimuli like phytohemagglutinin or allogeneic antigens (e.g., Tursi et al. 1969; Schwartz et al. 1968) and a variety of cellular and humoral responses in vivo. Much attention has been focused on the capacity of ALS to inhibit the rejection of foreign grafts, as described in detail by Taub (1970), Taub and Deutch (1977), and Bach (1975). In addition, ALS inhibit a variety of cellular immune reactions in vivo, including delayed hypersensitivity (e.g., Inderbitzen 1956; Waksman et al. 1961), graft-versus-host reaction (e.g., Levey and Medawar 1966; Mandel and Asofsky 1968), or certain experimental autoimmune diseases such as encephalomyelitis (Waksman et al. 1961) or thyroiditis (Kalden et al. 1969).

The selectivity in the ALS effect on T lymphocytes is particularly clear when tested on humoral immune responses. Treatment with ALS significantly suppressed the antibody responses to all tested T-dependent antigens, such as sheep erythrocytes (e.g., Monaco et al. 1966), foreign serum albumin (Levey and Medawar 1966), or viruses (Strobel 1972). On the other hand, antibody responses to T-independent antigens were usually unaffected by ALS treatment (Kerbel and Eidinger 1971; Barth et al. 1973). Moreover, studies of Baker and his co-workers have shown that ALS treatment may actually increase the antibody response to type III pneumococcal polysaccharide (Baker et al. 1970). The latter finding has been interpreted to suggest that in these experiments ALS eliminated the suppressor T cells which regulate the response to this sugar (Baker 1975).

IV. Adverse Side Effects

Clinical use of ALS has been seriously hampered by the side effects provoked by this treatment. These effects are caused mainly by two mechanisms:
1. Preparations of ALS are often contaminated with antibodies against nonlymphoid cells, such as erythrocytes, platelets, or fibroblasts, which may damage these cells upon injection. Particularly pathogenic are antibodies which react with kidney components and may produce nephrotoxicity (Feltkamp-Vroom and Balner 1972).
2. The second pathogenic mechanism is mediated by the immune response of the host to the protein components of ALS, which may generate antigen–antibody complexes and can consequently cause serum sickness (see Bach 1975).

Various procedures have been introduced to reduce or prevent the development of the recipient's response to the ALS preparation. These include the use of the IgG fraction of the antiserum, which is much less immunogenic than the whole serum (Balner et al. 1970), and the suppression of the recipient's immune response by treatment with immunosuppressive drugs (Stockman et al. 1972), or its prevention by induction of immunotolerance toward the injected proteins (Balner et al. 1970; Fahey 1973).

F. Ionizing Irradiation

The immunosuppressive activity of ionizing radiation was recognized shortly after the introduction of this procedure for medical use (BENJAMIN and SLUKA 1908). Any extensive clinical use of irradiation for immunosuppression has been avoided, however, in view of its adverse effects. Recently, an irradiation procedure used for treatment of Hodgkin's disease patients has been applied as an immunosuppressive treatment. The procedure, termed "total lymphoid irradiation" (TLI), consists of a series of selective irradiation treatments of the lymphoid organs and has proved to be very effective in providing protection against rejection of various foreign grafts (see SLAVIN et al. 1980). Furthermore, in a series of recent studies TLI was found successful as a treatment for patients with severe rheumatoid arthritis (TRENTHAM et al. 1981; KOTZIN et al. 1981).

The mode of action of irradiation is not fully understood, and it seems that cells are affected by more than just one mechanism. However, the available data indicate that the immunosuppressive effects of irradiation are due mainly to gross damage to the genetic apparatus and to a consequent loss of the capacity of cells to divide. Accordingly, it is generally believed that cells in cycle show the highest levels of susceptibility to irradiation. Most B and T lymphocytes were found to be susceptible to irradiation effects, while macrophages show a remarkable level of radioresistance (see DUBOIS et al. 1981). It is also noteworthy that TLI affects helper T lymphocytes much more than suppressor T cells, an effect which may contribute to the total immunosuppression (KOTZIN et al. 1981).

G. Immunosuppressive Agents of Potential Future Use

Most immunosuppressive drugs in common use produce adverse side effects (see Sects. A and H). Much effort has therefore been focused on developing more selective drugs, to be effective on the immune system alone, or even just on the immuno-pathogenic response itself. These goals may be attainable by employing nature's processes of immunoregulation. Physiologically, immunosuppression is known to be produced by two classes of cell products, suppressor cell factors and anti-idiotypic antibodies. The activities of suppressor factors have been reviewed by numerous authors (see MÖLLER 1975; TADA and OKUMURA 1979). Experimentally, these factors have proved to be capable of suppressing specific immune responses (WHITAKER et al. 1981) and, as discussed by KRAKAUER and CLOUGH (1980), these agents may be used in man as well.

The concept of immunoregulation by anti-idiotypic antibodies has been championed by JERNE (1974), and has been experimentally confirmed in various systems (see URBAIN et al. 1981). Specific suppression or immunotolerance can be induced experimentally by antireceptor immunity of an autoanti-idiotypic nature (ANDERSSON et al. 1977), and conceivably could be applied for clinical use.

H. Immunosuppressive Agents in Ocular Conditions

Immunosuppressive drugs are used in the control of corneal graft rejection and in inflammations of the eye because immunopathogenic processes are believed to be involved.

I. Cyclophosphamide

Cyclophosphamide has been used not only in clinical ocular problems, but also in those found in the laboratory. Cyclophosphamide has been demonstrated to suppress both the ocular inflammation and the humoral response to an intravitreal administration of bovine γ-globulin (HALL et al. 1977). In primary herpes simplex infections of the cornea in rabbits, cyclophosphamide suppressed the secondary and presumed immune phase of the disease (OH 1978). In secondary herpes simplex uveitis in rabbits, cyclophosphamide had no significant effect on the severity of the disease, the increase in intraocular pressure seen in this model, or the host's immune responses (DENNIS and OH 1979). TICHO et al. (1974) have also used cyclophosphamide in order to study the immune-mediated aspects of lymphocytic choriomeningitis virus uveitis.

Cyclophosphamide has been reported as being effective in the treatment of peripheral uveitis (BUCKLEY and GILLS 1969), with a combination of cyclophosphamide and steroids being more effective. ONIKI et al. (1976) concluded that cyclophosphamide was more effective in treating Behçet's disease than corticosteroids and nonsteroidal anti-inflammatory agents. FOSTER (1980) found cyclophosphamide effective in treating patients with external ocular inflammatory disease due to Wegener's granulomatosis, Mooren's corneal ulcer, cicatricial pemphigoid, and rheumatoid arthritis. Cyclophosphamide has also been utilized in the management of advanced Graves' ophthalmopathy (BIGOS et al. 1979).

II. Chlorambucil

Chlorambucil was first described as useful in the treatment of Behçet's disease by MAMO and AZZAM (1970). Others (ABDALLA and BAHGAT 1973; DINNING and PERKINS 1975) have also reported the successful use of this drug in uveitis. A large series of cases in which chlorambucil was given for intractable idiopathic uveitis was reported by GODFREY et al. (1974). This form of therapy appeared to be useful in treating sympathetic ophthalmia, chronic cyclitis, and rheumatoid sclerouveitis, as well as Behçet's disease.

III. Azathioprine

Reports concerning the use of azathioprine are mixed. A relatively large study of 25 patients with Behçet's disease (AOKI and SUGIURA 1976) reported that more than half of the patients had no improvement or change in the course of their ocular disease. ROSSELET et al. (1968) felt that the extraocular manifestations of the disease did improve. However, patients with pars planitis (NEWELL et al. 1966) and one patient with sympathetic ophthalmia (MOORE 1968) have been reported to have been successfully treated with azathioprine.

More recently, ANDRASCH et al. (1978) utilized a combination of azathioprine and low-dose prednisone in treating patients with chronic uveitis. Adverse side effects were seen in some patients, and no therapeutic response was seen in others. FOSTER (1980) reported his experience with two cicatricial pemphigoid patients who received azathioprine, but side effects precluded continuation of this mode of therapy. This purine antimetabolite has also been recommended for use in difficult cases of corneal grafting (JAMES 1977).

IV. Methotrexate

Wong (1969) has reported his experience with 25 patients who were immunosuppressed for ocular inflammatory disease, most of whom received methotrexate. He found that a majority of patients demonstrated clinical improvement, including patients who had corneal grafting. However, side effects and refractoriness to methotrexate prevented continued administration in some cases. Foster (1980) found that methotrexate had a beneficial effect in patients with Mooren's corneal ulcer. Recent pharmacokinetic studies in patients receiving methotrexate revealed concentrations of the drug in tears equivalent to those in plasma at 24 and 48 h after treatment (Doroshow et al. 1981).

V. Cyclosporin A

Cyclosporin A is an unusual immunosuppressive agent which has already demonstrated its efficacy in ocular immunology. Several authors have demonstrated cyclosporin A's effective prolongation of corneal graft survival in rabbits, whether administered intramuscularly (Shepherd et al. 1980), by retrobulbar injection (Salisbury and Gebhardt 1981), or by topical administration (Hunter et al. 1981). In addition, cyclosporin A has been shown to be effective in preventing S-antigen-induced experimental autoimmune uveitis in rats (Nussenblatt et al. 1981, 1982). The drug was found to be effective in preventing the disease even when begun over a week after immunization. The striking findings in lower mammals have led to a pilot trial of cyclosporin A therapy in patients with bilateral posterior uveitis of a noninfectious etiology. The initial results appear very encouraging (Nussenblatt and Gery, unpublished results).

VI. Antilymphocyte Sera

Little experience has been accumulated concerning the use of ALS in ocular immunopathogenic conditions. They were found to be useful in partially protecting corneal grafts in rabbits (Polack et al. 1972), but had marginal effects in patients with complicated corneal transplants (Ring et al. 1978). Beneficial effects of ALS were reported in patients with sympathetic ophthalmia or chronic uveitis (Ring et al. 1978).

VII. Adverse Side Effects

All the drugs discussed in this section have proved beneficial in the treatment of human disease. As with almost any medication, harmful effects are known to occur, and some of the more common are listed in Table 1 (see Schein and Winokur 1975). Immunosuppressive agents do have a role in the treatment of sight-threatening disease. However, one must be made aware of possible long-term risk, including neoplasm and ocular complications (Cogan 1977; Griffin and Garnick 1981).

Table 1. Prominent side effects of immunosuppressive agents

Azathioprine	Methotrexate	Cyclophos-phamide	Chlorambucil	Cyclosporin A
Bone marrow suppression	Bone marrow suppression	Bone marrow suppression	Bone marrow suppression	Hepatotoxicity
Infection	Infection	Infection	Infection	Renal toxicity
Hepatotoxicity	Hepatotoxicity	Sterility	Hepatotoxicity	
Gastrointestinal upset	Alopecia	Alopecia	Sterility	
Skin eruptions	Oral ulcers	Hemorrhagic cystitis	Pulmonary fibrosis	
	Gastrointestinal upset		Skin eruptions	
	Skin eruptions			

Acknowledgments: We thank Joyce McIntyre and Gail Lozupone for their superb secretarial aassistance.

References

Abdalla MI, Bahgat NE (1973) Long-lasting remission of Behçet's disease after chlorambucil. Br J Ophthalmol 57:706–711

Anderson LC, Aguet M, Wight E, Andersson R, Binz H, Wigzell H (1977) Induction of specific unresponsiveness using purified MLC-activated T lymphoblasts as auto-immunogen. I. Demonstration of general validity as to species and histocompatibility barriers. J Exp Med 146:1124–1137

Andrasch RH, Pirofsky B, Burn RP (1978) Immunosuppressive therapy for severe chronic uveitis. Arch Ophthalmol 96:247–251

Aoki K, Sugiura S (1976) Immunosuppressive treatment of Behçet's disease. Mod Probl Ophthalmol 16:309–313

Arnold H, Bourseaux F (1958) Synthese und Abbau cytostatisch wirksamer cyclischer *N*-phosphamidester des *Bis*-(β-chlorathyl)-amins. Angew Chem (Engl) 70:539–544

Arnold H, Bourseaux F, Brock N (1958) Neuartige Krebs Chemotherapeutika aus der Gruppe der zyklischen N-lost-phosphamid-ester. Dtsch Med Wochenschr 83:458–462

Bach J-F (1975) The mode of action of immunosuppressive agents. North-Holland, Amsterdam

Bach MA, Bach J-F (1972) Activities of immunosuppressive agents in vitro II. Different timing of azathioprine and methotrexate in inhibition and stimulation of mixed lymphocyte reaction. Clin Exp Immunol 11:89–98

Baker PJ (1975) Homeostatic control of antibody responses: a model based on the recognition of cell-associated antibody by regulatory T cells. Transplant Rev 26:3–20

Baker PJ, Barth RF, Stashak PW, Amsbaugh DF (1970) Enhancement of the antibody response to type III pneumococcal polysaccharide in mice treated with antilymphocyte serum. J Immunol 104:1313–1315

Bakke JE, Feil VJ, Zaylskie RG (1971) Characterization of the major sheep urinary metabolites of cyclophosphamide, a defleecing chemical. J Agric Food Chem 19:788–790

Balner H, Yron I, Dersjant H, Zaalberg O, Betel I (1970) ALG treatment of rhesus monkeys. Attempts to reduce complications by the induction of tolerance. Transplantation 10:416–424

Balow JE, Hurley DL, Fauci AS (1975) Cyclophosphamide suppression of established cell-mediated immunity: quantitative vs qualitative changes in lymphocyte populations. J Clin Invest 56:65–70

Barth RF, Singla O, Ahlers P (1973) Effects of antilymphocyte serum on thymic independent immunity I. Lack of immunosuppressive action on the antibody response to *E. coli* lipopolysaccharide. Cell Immunol 7:380–388

Beller DI, Unanue ER (1979) Evidence that thymocytes require at least two distinct signals to proliferate. J Immunol 123:2890–2893

Benjamin E, Sluka E (1908) Antikörperbildung nach experimenteller Schädigung des haematopoietischen Systems durch Röntgenstrahlen. Wien Klin Wochenschr 21:311–312

Berenbaum MC (1971) Is azathioprine a better immunosuppressive than 6-mercaptopurine? Clin Exp Immunol 8:1–8

Bigos ST, Nisula BC, Daniels GH, Eastman RC, Johnston HH, Kohler PO (1979) Cyclophosphamide in the management of advanced Graves' ophthalmopathy. A preliminary report. Ann Intern Med 90:921–923

Bolton C, Allsopp G, Cuzner ML (1982) The effect of cyclosporin A on the adoptive transfer of experimental allergic encephalomyelitis in the Lewis rat. Clin Exp Immunol 47:127–132

Borel JF, Feurer C, Gubler HU, Stähelin H (1976) Biological effects of cyclosporin A: a new antilymphocytic agent. Agents Actions 6:468–475

Borel JF, Feurer C, Magnée C, Stähelin H (1977) Effects of the new anti-lymphocyte peptide cyclosporin A in animals. Immunology 32:1017–1025

Borel Y, Schwartz RS (1964) Inhibition of immediate and delayed hypersensitivity in rabbits by 6-mercaptopurine. J Immunol 92:754–761

Borel Y, Fauconnet M, Miescher PA (1965) Effect of 6-mercaptopurine (6-MP) on different classes of antibody. J Exp Med 122:263–275

Brent L (1980) Cyclosporin A: a discussion of its clinical and biological attributes – summary of a workshop. Transplant Proc 12:234–238

Brock N, Hohorst HJ (1963) Über die Aktivierung von Cyclophosphamid in vivo und in vitro. Arzneim Forsch 13:1021–1031

Bunjes D, Hardt C, Rollinghoff M, Wagner H (1981) Cyclosporin A mediates immunosuppression of primary cytotoxic T cell responses by impairing the release of interleukin 1 and interleukin 2. Eur J Immunol 11:657–661

Buckley CE, Gills JP (1969) Cyclophosphamide therapy of peripheral uveitis. Arch Intern Med 124:129–135

Burckhardt JJ, Guggenheim B (1979) Cyclosporin A: in vivo and in vitro suppression of rat T-lymphocyte function. Immunolgy 36:753–757

Calne RY (1960) The rejection of renal homografts inhibition in dogs by 6-mercaptopurine. Lancet I:417–418

Calne RY, Rolles K, White DJG, Thiru S, Evans DB, McMaster P, Dunn DC, Craddock GN, Henderson RG, Aziz S, Lewis P (1979) Cyclosporin A initially as the only immunosuppressant in 34 recipients of cadaveric organs: 32 kidneys, 2 pancreases, and 2 livers. Lancet II:1033–1036

Calne RY, Rolles K, White DJG, Thiru S, Evans DB, Henderson R, Hamilton DL, Boone N, McMaster P, Gibby O, Williams R (1981) Cyclosporin A in clinical organ grafting. Transplant Proc 13:349–358

Cantor H, Boyse EA (1977) Regulation of cellular and humoral immune responses by T-cell subclasses. Cold Spring Harbor Symp Quant Biol 41:23–32

Cantor H, Gershon RK (1979) Immunological circuits: cellular composition. Fed Proc 38:2058–2064

Chabner BA, Myers CE, Oliverio VT (1977) Clinical pharmacology of anticancer drugs. Semin Oncol 4:165–186

Clements PJ, Yu DTY, Levy J, Paulus HE, Barnett EV (1974) Effects of cyclophosphamide on B and T lymphocytes in rheumatoid arthritis. Arthritis Rheum 17:347–353

Cogan DG (1977) Immunosuppression and eye disease. Am J Ophthalmol 83:777–788

Cohen JL, Jao JY (1970) Enzymatic basis of cyclophosphamide activation by hepatic microsomes of the rat. J Pharmacol Exp Ther 174:206–210

Colvin M, Brundett RB, Kan MNN, Jardine I, Fenselau C (1976) Alkylating properties of phosphoramide mustard. Cancer Res 36:1121–1126

Cosimi AB, Burton RC, Kung PC, Colvin R, Goldstein G, Lifter J, Rhodes W, Russell PS (1981) Evaluation in primate renal allograft of monoclonal antibody to human T cell subclasses. Transplant Proc 13:499–503

Crabtree GW (1978) Mechanisms of action of pyrimidine and purine analogues. In: Brodsky I, Kahn SB, Conroy JR (eds) Cancer chemotherapy. Grune and Stratton, New York, pp 35–47

Deeg HJ, Storb R, Gerhard-Miller L, Shulman HM, Weiden PL, Thomas ED (1980) Cyclosporin A, a powerful immunosuppressant in vivo and in vitro in the dog, fails to induce tolerance. Transplantation 29:230–235

Dennis RF, Oh JO (1979) Aspirin, cyclophosphamide, and dexamethasone effects on experimental secondary herpes simplex uveitis. Arch Ophthalmol 97:2170–2174

Dinning WJ, Perkins ES (1975) Immunosuppressives in uveitis. A preliminary report of experience with chlorambucil. Br J Ophthalmol 59:397–403

Doroshow JH, Locker GY, Gaasterland DE, Hubbard SP, Young RC, Myers CE (1981) Ocular irritation from high-dose methotrexate therapy. Cancer 48:2158–2162

Dorr RT, Fritz WL (1980) Cancer chemotherapy handbook. Elsevier, New York

Dreyfuss M, Härri E, Hofmann H, Kobel H, Pache W, Ischerter H (1976) Cyclosporin A and C. New metabolites from *Trichoderma polysporum* (Link ex Pers.) Rifai. Eur J Appl Microbiol 3:125–133

Dubois JB, Serrou B, Rosenfeld C (eds) (1981) Immunopharmacologic effects of radiation therapy. Raven, New York

Dutton RW, Pearce JD (1962) A survey of the effect of metabolic antagonists on the synthesis of antibody in an in vitro system. Immunology 5:414–423

Elion GB, Hitchings GH (1975) Azathioprine. In: Sartorelli AC, Johns DG (eds) Antineoplastic and immunosuppressive agents, pt II. Springer, Berlin Heidelberg New York, pp 404–425 (Handbuch der Experimentellen Pharmakologie, vol 38)

Everett JL, Roberts JJ, Ross WCJ (1953) Aryl-2-halogenoalkylamines. Part XII. Some carboxylic derivaties of *NN*-di-2-chlorethylaniline. J Chem Soc 3:2386–2392

Fahey KJ (1973) Studies on goat anti CBA thymocyte globulin: the immunosuppressive activity of anti-lymphozyte globulin in mice tolerant to or sensitized to goat gammaglobulin. Aust J Exp Biol Med 51:501–511

Farber S, Diamond LK, Mercer RD, Sylvester RF, Wolff VA (1948) Temporary remissions in acute leukemia in children produced by folic antagonist 4-amethopteroylglutamic acid (aminopterin). N Engl J Med 238:787–793

Fauci AS, Wolff SM, Johnson JS (1971) Effect of cyclophosphamide upon the immune response in Wegener's granulomatosis. N Engl J Med 285:1493–1496

Fauci AS, Dale DC, Wolff SM (1974) Cyclophosphamide and lymphocyte subpopulations in Wegener's granulomatosis. Arthritis Rheum 17:355–361

Fauci AS, Haynes BF, Katz P (1980) Drug-induced T and B and monocyte dysfunction. In: Greico MH (ed) Infections complicating the abnormal host. York Medical, New York, pp 163–182

Feltkamp-Vroom T, Balner H (1972) Glomerular basement membrane –reactive antibodies in anti-lymphocyte sera: in vitro and in vivo characteristics. Eur J Immunol 2:166–173

Forbes IJ, Smith JL (1967) Effects of anti-inflammatory drugs on lymphocytes. Lancet II:334–335

Foster CS (1980) Immunosuppressive therapy for external ocular inflammatory disease. Ophthalmology 87:140–150

Galton DAG, Israels LG, Nabarro JDN, Till M (1955) Clinical trials of *p*-(di-2-chloroethylamino)-phenylbutyric acid (CB 1348) in malignant lymphoma. Br Med J 2:1172–1176

Gerber NL, Steinberg AD (1976) Clinical use of immunosuppressive drugs: part II. Drugs 11:90–112

Gershon RK, Eardley DD, Durum S, Green DR, Shen FW, Yamauchi K, Cantor H, Murphy DB (1981) Contrasuppression. A novel immunoregulatory activity. J Exp Med 153:1533–1546

Giblett ER, Anderson JE, Cohen F, Pollara B, Meuwissen HJ (1972) Adenosine-deaminase deficiency in two patients with severely impaired cellular immunity. Lancet II:1067–1069

Godfrey WA, Epstein MV, O'Connor GR, Kimura SJ, Hogan MJ, Nozik RA (1974) The use of chlorambucil in intractable idiopathic uveitis. Am J Ophthalmol 78:415–428

Green CJ, Allison AC, Precious S (1979) Induction of specific tolerance in rabbits by kidney allografting and short periods of cyclosporin-A treatment. Lancet II:123–125

Griffin JD, Garnick MB (1981) Eye toxicity of cancer chemotherapy: a review of the literature. Cancer 48:1539–1549

Haddow A (1954) Experimental and clinical aspects of the action of various carboxylic acid derivatives. In: Wolstenholme GEW, Cameron MP (eds) Leukemia research. Little, Brown, Boston, p 196

Hall JM, Ohno S, Pribnow JF (1977) The effect of cyclophosphamide on an ocular immune response. I. Primary response. Clin Exp Immunol 30:309–316

Heppner GH, Calabresi P (1976) Selective suppression of humoral immunity by antineoplastic drugs. Ann Rev Pharmacol Toxicol 16:367–379

Hess AD, Tutschka PJ (1980) Effect of cyclosporin A on human lymphocyte responses in vitro. I. CsA allows for the expression of alloantigen-activated suppressor cells while preferentially inhibiting the induction of cytolytic effector lymphocytes in MLR. J Immunol 124:2601–2608

Hess AD, Tutschka PJ, Santos GW (1981) Effect of cyclosporin A on human lymphocyte responses in vitro. II. Induction of specific alloantigen unresponsiveness mediated by a nylon wool adherent suppressor cell. J Immunol 126:961–968

Hess AD, Tutschka PJ, Santos GW (1982) Effect of cyclosporin A on human lymphocyte responses in vitro. III. CsA inhibits the production of T lymphocyte growth factors in secondary mixed lymphocyte responses but does not inhibit the response of primed lymphocytes to TCGF. J Immunol 128:355–359

Hitchings GH, Elion GB (1963) Chemical suppression of the immune response. Pharmacol Rev 15:365–405

Horsburgh T, Wood P, Brent L (1980) Suppression of in vitro lymphocyte reactivity by cyclosporin A: existence of a population of drug-resistant cytotoxic lymphocytes. Nature 286:609–611

Hoyer LW, Condie RM, Good RA (1960) Prevention of experimental allergic encephalomyelitis with 6-MP. Proc Soc Exp Biol Med 103:205–207

Hunninghake GW, Fauci AS (1976) Divergent effects of cyclophosphamide administration on mononuclear killer cells: quantitative depletion of cell numbers versus qualitative suppression of functional capabilities. J Immunol 117:337–342

Hunter PA, Wilhelmus KR, Rice NSC, Jones BR (1981) Cyclosporin A applied topically to the recipient eye inhibits corneal graft rejection. Clin Exp Immunol 45:173–177

Hutchinson IF, Shadur CA, Duarte JSA, Strom TB, Tilney NL (1981) Cyclosporin A spares selectively lymphocytes with donor-specific suppressor characteristics. Transplantation 32:210–216

Inderbitzen T (1956) The relationship of lymphocytes, delayed cutaneous allergic reactions and histamine. Int Arch Allergy 8:150–159

James GD (1977) Immunotherapy. Trans Ophthalmol Soc UK 97:468–473

Jerne NK (1974) Toward a network theory of the immune system. Ann Immunol (Paris) 125C:373

Kalden J, James K, Williamson WG, Irvine WJ (1969) The suppression of experimental thyroiditis in the rat by heterologous anti-lymphocyte globulin. Clin Exp Immunol 3:973–981

Kaplan SR, Calabresi P (1973a) Immunosuppressive agents, I. N Engl J Med 289:952–955

Kaplan SR, Calabresi P (1973b) Immunosuppressive agents, II. N Engl J Med 289:1234–1236

Kerbel RS, Eidinger D (1971) Variable effects of antilymphocyte serum on humoral antibody formation: role of thymus dependency of antigen. J Immunol 106:917–926

Kohn KW, Spears CL, Doty P (1966) Inter-strand crosslinking DNA by nitrogen mustard. J Mol Biol 19:266–288

Kotzin BL, Strober S, Engleman EG, Calin A, Hoppe RT, Kansas GS, Terrell CP, Kaplan HS (1981) Treatment of intractable rheumatoid arthritis with total lymphoiod irradiation. N Engl J Med 305:969–976

Krakauer RS, Clough JD (1980) Suppressor factors: potential for immunotherapy. Immunopharmacology 2:271–284

Krumbhaar EG, Krumbhaar HD (1919) The blood and bone marrow in yellow cross gas (mustard gas) poisoning: changes produced in the bone marrow of fatal cases. J Med Res 40:497–507

Kunkl A, Klaus GGB (1980) Selective effects of cyclosporin A on functional B cell subsets in the mouse. J Immunol 125:2526–2531

Larsson EV (1980) Cyclosporin A and dexamethasone suppress T cell responses by selectively acting at distinct sites of the triggering process. J Immunol 124:2828–2833

Leapman SB, Filo RS, Smith EJ, Smith PG (1980) In vitro effects of cyclosporin A on lymphocyte subpopulations. 1. Suppressor cell sparing by cyclosporin A. Transplantation 30:404–408

Lemmel E, Hurd ER, Ziff M (1971) Differential effects of 6-mercaptopurine and cyclophosphamide on autoimmune phenomena in NZB mice. Clin Exp Immunol 8:355–362

Leung FC, Vos SI (1968) Effects of immunosuppressive drugs on secondary antibody responses in vitro. Can J Microbiol 14:7–11

Levey RH, Medawar PB (1966) Nature and mode of action of antilymphocytic antiserum. Proc Natl Adad Sci USA 56:1130–1137

Levy L, Whitehouse MW (1974) Selective stimulation of a cellular immune response by methotrexate. Agents Actions 4:113–116

Mackiewicz U, Brelinska-Peczalska R, Konys J (1978) The influence of cyclophosphamide on lymph node and peripheral blood lymphocytes in mice. Arch Immunol Ther Exp (Warsz) 26:375–380

Maibach MI, Maguire HG Jr (1966) Studies on the inhibition of antibody formation in the guinea pig with cyclophosphamide, azathioprine, 5-fluorouracil, and urethane. Int Arch Allergy 29:209–212

Makinodan T, Santos GW, Quinn RP (1970) Immunosuppressive drugs. Pharmacol Rev 22:189–247

Mamo JG, Azzam SA (1970) Treatment of Behçet's disease with chlorambucil. Arch Ophthalmol 84:446–450

Mandel MA, Asofsky R (1968) The effects of heterologous antithymocyte sera in mice I. The use of a graft-versus-host assay as a measure of homograft reactivity. J Immunol 100:1319–1325

Martin WJ, Miller JFAP (1968) Cell to cell interaction in the immune response. IV Site of action of antilymphocyte globulin. J Exp Med 128:855–874

McCollister RJ, Gilbert WR, Ashton DM, Wyngaarden JB (1964) Pseudofeedback inhibition of purine synthesis by 6-MP ribonucleotide and other purine analogues. J Biol Chem 239:1560–1563

McLean A (1979) Pharmacokinetics and metabolism of chlorambucil in patients with malignant disease. Cancer Treat Rev [Suppl] 6:33–42

Miller RA, Maloney DG, Warnke R, Levy R (1982) Treatment of B-cell lymphoma with monoclonal anti-idiotype antibody. N Engl J Med 306:517–522

Mitchell MS, Wade ME, DeConti RC, Bertino JR, Calabresi P (1969) Immunosuppressive effects of cytosine arabinoside and methotrexate in man. Ann Intern Med 70:535–547

Mitsuoka A, Baba M, Morikawa S (1976) Enhancement of delayed hypersensitivity by depletion of suppressor cells with cyclophosphamide in mice. Nature 262:77–78

Möller G (ed) (1975) Suppressor T lymphocytes. Transplant Rev 26:1–205

Möller G (ed) (1978) Role of macrophages in the immune response. Immunol Rev 40:1–255

Monaco AP, Wood ML, Gray JG, Russell PS (1966) Studies on heterologous anti-lymphocyte serum in mice. II. Effect on the immune response. J Immunol 96:229–238

Moore CE (1968) Sympathetic ophthalmitis treated with azathioprine. Br J Ophthalmol 52:688–690

Newell FW, Krill AE, Thomson A (1966) The treatment of uveitis with 6-mercaptopurine. Am J Ophthalmol 61:1250–1255

Nussenblatt RB, Rodrigues MM, Wacker WB, Cevario SJ, Salinas-Carmona MC, Gery I (1981) Cyclosporin A. Inhibition of experimental autoimmune uveitis in Lewis rats. J Clin Invest 67:1228–1231

Nussenblatt RB, Rodrigues MM, Salinas-Carmona MC, Gery I, Cevario SJ, Wacker WB (1982) Modulation of experimental autoimmune uveitis with cyclosporin A. Arch Ophthalmol 100:1146–1149

Oh JO (1978) Effect of cyclophosphamide on primary herpes simplex uveitis in rabbits. Invest Ophthalmol 17:769–773

Oniki S, Kurakazu K, Kawata K (1976) Immunosuppressive treatment of Behçet's disease with cyclophosphamide. Jpn J Ophthalmol 20:32–40

Oppenheim JJ, Gery I (1982) Interleukin 1 is more than an interleukin. Immunol Today 3:113–119

Paavonen T, Häyry P (1980) Effect of cyclosporin A on T-dependent and T-independent immunoglobulin synthesis in vitro. Nature 287:542–544

Paavonen T, Järveläinen H, Kontiainen S, Häyry P (1981) Effect of cyclosporin A on in vitro proliferative activity and immunoglobulin synthesis of isolated human lymphoid cell subpopulations. Clin Exp Immunol 43:342–350

Palacios R, Möller G (1981) Cyclosporin A blocks receptors for HLA-DR antigens on T cells. Nature 290:792–794

Perlmann P, Cerottini JC (1979) Cytotoxic lymphocytes. In: Sela M (ed) The antigens, vol 5. Academic, New York, pp 173–181

Perry LL, Benacerraf B, McCluskey RT, Greene MI (1978) Enhanced syngeneic tumor destruction by in vivo inhibition of suppressor T cells using anti-I-J alloantiserum. Am J Pathol 92:491–506

Perry LL, Dorf ME, Benacerraf B, Greene MI (1979) Regulation of immune response to tumor antigen: interference with syngeneic tumor immunity by anti-IA alloantisera. Proc Natl Acad Sci USA 76:920–924

Petcher TJ, Weber HP, Rüegger A (1976) Crystal and molecular structure of an iodo-derivative of the cyclic endecapeptide cyclosporin A. Helv Chim Acta 59:1480–1489

Polack FM, Townsend WM, Waltman S (1972) Antilymphocyte serum and corneal graft rejection. Am J Ophthalmol 73:52–55

Powles RL, Barrett AJ, Clink H, Kay HEM, Sloane J, McElwain (1978) Cyclosporin A for the treatment of graft-versus-host disease in man. Lancet II:1327–1331

Powles RL, Clink HM, Spence D, Morgenstern G, Watson JG, Selby PJ, Woods M, Barrett A, Jameson B, Sloane J, Lawler SD, Kay HEM, Lawson D, McElwain TJ, Alexander P (1980) Cyclosporin A to prevent graft-versus-host disease in man after allogeneic bone-marrow transplantation. Lancet I:327–329

Ramsay NKC, Kersey JH, Robison LL, McGlave PB, Woods WG, Krivit W, Kim TH, Goldman AI, Nesbit ME (1982) A randomized study of the prevention of acute graft-versus-host disease. N Engl J Med 306:392–397

Reinherz EL, Schlossman SF (1980) The differentiation and function of human T lymphocytes. Cell 19:821–827

Reitz BA, Wallwork JL, Hunt SA, Pennock JL, Billingham ME, Oyer PE, Stinson EB, Shumway NE (1982) Heart-lung transplantation. N Engl J Med 306:557–564

Ring J, Dechant W, Seifert J, Lund O-E, Greite J-H, Stefani FH, Brendel W (1978) Immunosuppression with antilymphocyte globulin (ALG) in the treatment of ophthalmic disorders. Ophthalmic Res 10:82–97

Rollinghoff M, Schrader J, Wagner H (1973) Effect of azathioprine and cytosine arabinoside on humoral and cellular immunity in vitro. Clin Exp Immunol 15:261–269

Rollinghoff M, Starzinski-Powitz A, Pfizenmaier K, Wagner H (1977) Cyclophosphamide-sensitive T lymphocytes suppress the in vivo generation of antigen-specific cytotoxic T lymphocytes. J Exp Med 145:455–459

Rosselet E, Saudan Y, Zenklusen G (1968) Les effets de l'Azathioprine (Imuran) dans la maladie de Behçet. Premiers résultats thérapeutiques. Ophthalmologica 156:218–226

Rüegger A, Kuhn M, Lichti H, Loosli HR, Huguenin R, Quiquerez C, von Wartburg A (1976) Cyclosporin A, ein immunosuppressiv wirksamer Peptidmetabolit aus *Trichoderma polysporum* (Link ex Pers.) Rifai. Helv Chim Acta 59:1075–1092

Salisbury JD, Gebhardt BM (1981) Suppression of corneal allograft rejection by cyclosporin A. Arch Ophthalmol 99:1640–1643

Santos GW, Owens AH Jr (1966) 19S and 7S antibody production in the cyclophosphamide or methotrexate treated rat. Nature 209:622–624

Schein PS, Winokur SH (1975) Immunosuppressive and cytotoxic chemotherapy: long-term complications: Ann Intern Med 82:84–95

Schwartz A, Orbach-Arbouys S, Gershon RK (1976) Participation of cyclophosphamide-sensitive T cells in graft-vs-host reactions. J Immunol 117:871–875

Schwartz A, Askenase PW, Gershon RK (1978) Regulation of delayed-type hypersensitivity reactions by cyclophosphamide-sensitive T cells. J Immunol 121:1573–1577

Schwartz MR, Tyler RW, Everett NB (1968) Mixed lymphocyte reaction: an in vitro test for antilymphocytic serum activity. Science 160:1014–1017

Schwartz RS (1965) Immunosuppressive drugs. Prog Allergy 9:246–303

Shepherd WFI, Coster DJ, Chin Fook T, Rice NSC, Jones BR (1980) Effect of cyclosporin A on the survival of corneal grafts in rabbits. Br J Ophthalmol 64:148–153

Sherburne CG, Condie RM (1981) Immunosuppressive activity of monoclonal anti-thy-1.2: comparison of monoclonal IgM and IgG with xeno-anti-thymocyte preparations. Transplant Proc 13:504–508

Slavin S, Yatziv S, Zan-Bar I, Fuks Z, Kaplan HS, Strober S (1980) Nonspecific and specific immunosuppression by total lymphoid irradiation (TLI). In: Fougereau M, Dausset J (eds) Immunology 80, progress in immunology 4. Academic, London, pp 1160–1170

Smith KA, Ruscetti FW (1981) T-cell growth factor and the culture of cloned functional T cells. Adv Immunol 31:137–175

Spreafico F, Anaclerio A (1977) Immunosuppressive agents. In: Good RA, Day SB (eds) Comprehensive immunology, vol 3. Plenum, New York, pp 245–278

Spreafico F, Donelli MG, Bossi A, Vecchi A, Standen S, Garattini S (1973) Immunodepressant activity and 6-mercaptopurine levels after administration of 6-mercaptopurine and azathioprine. Transplantation 16:269–278

Starzl TE, Klintmalm GBG, Porter KA, Iwatsuki S, Schröter GPJ (1981) Liver transplantation with use of cyclosporin A and prednisone. N Engl J Med 305:266–269

Steinberg AD, Plotz PH, Wolff SM, Wong VG, Agus SG, Decker JL (1972) Cytotoxic drugs in treatment of nonmalignant diseases. Ann Intern Med 76:619–642

Stockman GD, Judd KP, Trentin JJ (1972) Cyclophosphamide-induced tolerance to equine-γ-globulin and equine antimouse thymocyte globulin in adult mice. II. Resulting prolongation of cardia allografts in ALG-treated animals. Transplantation 13:66–71

Stockman GD, Heim LR, South MA, Trentin JJ (1973) Differential effects of cyclophosphamide on the B- and T-cell compartments of adult mice. J Immunol 110:277–282

Strobel G (1972) The effect of thymectomy and anti-thymocyte serum on the immunological competence of adult mice. Eur J Immunol 2:475–476

Struck RF, Kirk MC, Mellett LB, El Dareer S, Hill DL (1971) Urinary metabolites of the antitumor agent cyclophosphamide. Mol Pharmacol 7:519–529

Struck RF, Kirk MC, Witt MH, Laster WR Jr (1975) Isolation and mass spectral identification of blood metabolites of cyclophosphamide; evidence for phosphoramide mustard as the biologically active metabolite. Biomed Mass Spectrom 2:46–52

Sy MS, Miller SD, Claman HN (1977) Immune suppression with supraoptimal doses of antigen in contact sensitivity. I. Demonstration of suppressor cells and their sensitivity to cyclophosphamide. J Immunol 119:240–244

Tada T, Okumura K (1979) The role of antigen-specific T cell factors in the immune response. Adv Immunol 28:1–87

Takamizawa A, Matsumoto S, Iwata T, Katagiri K, Tochino Y, Yamaguchi K (1973) Studies on cyclophosphamide metabolites and their related compounds. II. Preparation of an active species of cyclophosphamide and some related compounds. J Am Chem Soc 95:985–986

Taub RN (1970) Biological effects of heterologous antilymphocyte serum. Prog Allergy 14:208–258

Taub RN, Deutch V (1977) Antilymphocytic serum. Pharmacol Ther [A]2:89–111

Taub RN, Lance EM (1968) Histopathological effects in mice of heterologous antilymphocyte serum. J Exp Med 128:1281–1307

Ticho U, Silverstein AM, Cole GA (1974) Immunopathogenesis of LCM virus-induced uveitis. The role of T lymphocytes. Invest Ophthalmol 13:229–231

Trentham DE, Belli JA, Anderson RJ, Buckley JA, Goetzl EJ, David JR, Austen KF (1981) Clinical and immunologic effects of fractionated total lymphoid irradiation in refractory rheumatoid arthritis. N Engl J Med 305:976–982

Tursi A, Greaves MF, Torrigiani G, Playfair JHL, Roitt IM (1969) Response to phytohemagglutinin of lymphocytes from mice treated with anti-lymphocyte globulin. Immunology 17:801–811

Tutschka PJ, Beschorner WE, Allison AC, Burns WH, Santos GW (1979) Use of cyclosporin A in allogeneic bone marrow transplantation in the rat. Nature 280:148–151

Unanue ER (1981) The regulatory role of macrophages in antigenic stimulation. Part two: symbiotic relationship between lymphocytes and macrophages. Adv Immunol 31:1–136

Urbain J, Wuilmart C, Cazenave PA (1981) Idiotypic regulation in immune networks. Contemp Top Mol Immunol 8:113–148

Veith FJ, Norin AJ, Montefusco CM, Pinsker KL, Kamholz SL, Gliedman ML, Emeson E (1981) Cyclosporin A in experimental lung transplantation. Transplantation 32:474–481

Voisin GA (1980) Role of antibody classes in the regulatory facilitation reaction. Immunol Rev 49:3–59

Wang BS, Heacock EH, Chang-Hue Z, Tilney NL, Strom TB, Mannick JA (1982) Evidence for the presence of suppressor T lymphocytes in animals treated with cyclosporin A. J Immunol 128:1382–1385

Waksman BH, Arbouys S, Arnason GB (1961) The use of specific "lymphocyte" antisera to inhibit hypersensitive reactions of the "delayed" type. J Exp Med 114:997–1022

Weinstein GM (1977) Methotrexate. Ann Intern Med 86:199–204

Whitaker RB, Nepom JT, Sy M-S, Takaoki M, Gramm CF, Fox I, Germain RN, Nelles MJ, Greene MI, Benacerraf B (1981) Suppressor factor from a T cell hybrid inhibits delayed-type hypersensitivity responses to azobenzenearsonate. Proc Natl Acad Sci USA 78:6441–6445

Wiesinger D, Borel JF (1979) Studies on the mechanism of action of cyclosporin A. Immunobiol 156:454–463

Winkelstein A (1973) Mechanisms of immunosuppression: effects of cyclophosphamide on cellular immunity. Blood 41:273–284

Wong VG (1969) Immunosuppressive therapy of ocular inflammatory diseases. Arch Ophthalmol 81:628–637

Woodruff MFA, Anderson NF (1963) Effect of lymphocyte depletion by thoracic duct fistula and administration of antilymphocytic serum on the survival of skin homografts in rats. Nature 200:702

CHAPTER 13

Anticoagulants, Fibrinolytics, and Hemostatics

M. Pandolfi

A. Introduction: The Hemostatic Mechanism

Anticoagulants, fibrinolytics, and hemostatics are substances which interfere with
the mechanism of hemostasis. Hemostasis is the spontaneous cessation of bleeding
from a damaged vessel. The mechanism of hemostasis is summarized in Fig. 1. As
is apparent from the figure, three main processes are involved:
1. Adhesion and aggregation of platelets (primary hemostasis)
2. Blood coagulation
3. Fibrinolysis.
  As for primary hemostasis, opinions agree that baring of subendothelial collagen following vascular damage activates circulating platelets, which change in
shape, emit pseudopodia, and adhere to the vessel wall at the site of the damage.
A plasma factor (the von Willebrand factor: a macromolecule in complex with coagulation factor VIII) is necessary for the process of adhesion. Adherent platelets
release a host of substances active in hemostasis. In particular, they release
adenosine diphosphate (ADP), which causes platelets to adhere to one another
with the formation of a hemostatic plug hindering continuous blood escape. This
aggregation is enhanced by the presence of a substance (thromboxane, TXA_2)
which is produced in the cellular membrane of platelets.
  Besides stimulating platelets, collagen exposure activates one pathway (*the intrinsic pathway*) of the blood coagulation system (Fig. 2). It is believed that in the
intrinsic pathway a chain activation of the blood-clotting factors takes place as follows: factor XII (Hageman factor), factor XI (hemophilia C factor), factor IX (hemophilia B factor). The activated factor IX together with factor VIII (hemophilia
A factor) and platelet factor 3 (a phospholipidic membrane fragement released by
platelets during aggregation) from a complex activating factor X (Stuart–Prower
factor). Together with factor V (proaccelerin) and Ca^{++} the activated factor X
converts prothrombin into thrombin, a proteolytic enzyme which selectively attacks certain bond in the molecule of fibrinogen and splits off two pairs of peptides
(the A and B fibrinopeptides). The loss of these polypeptides activates the fibrinogen molecule, which acquires a strong tendency to polymerize, first end by end and
then side by side. The resulting molecule (fibrin) is no longer soluble and precipi-
tates. Fibrin formation is vital for an efficient hemostatic mechanism, since it rein-
forces the platelet plug, which otherwise would soon disgregate. At first the fibrin
network is held together only by weak hydrogen bonds, but later, under the action
of factor XIII (plasma transglutaminase, or fibrin-stabilizing factor, FSF), strong
covalent C–N bonds are formed which cross-link the molecules.

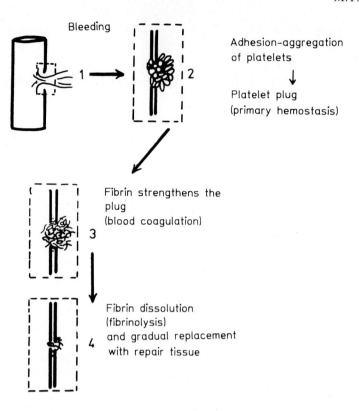

Bleeding

Adhesion-aggregation
of platelets

↓

Platelet plug
(primary hemostasis)

Fibrin strengthens the
plug
(blood coagulation)

Fibrin dissolution
(fibrinolysis)
and gradual replacement
with repair tissue

Fig. 1. Hemostatic process after trauma of a small vessel. Bleeding through the wound (*1*). Platelets adhere to the bared subendothelial collagen and aggregate, forming a hemostatic plug which arrests the hemorrhage (*2*). Following activation of the coagulation system, fibrin strengthening the plug is formed (*3*). The hemostatic plug is gradually dissolved by the fibrinolytic system and replaced by repair tissue (*4*)

Fibrin formation may also result from the activation of the *extrinsic pathway* of the blood coagulation system. A lipoprotein (tissue factor) liberated from damaged tissue interacts with factor VIII (proconvertin) and Ca^{++}, thereby activating factor X (Fig. 2). The subsequent events lead to the formation of fibrin and are identical to those of the intrinsic pathway.

Fibrin formation in the organism is usually followed by enzymatic fibrin breakdown (*fibrinolysis*). A very simplified scheme of the fibrinolytic system is shown in Fig. 2. Plasminogen, an inert plasma protein, is converted into plasmin, a endopeptidase with strong specificity for fibrin. Conversion of plasminogen into plasmin takes place by an activator-catalyzed cleavage of a carbamidic bond at the COOH end of the plasmin molecule, which exposes the catalytically active center. Activation of plasminogen is operated by a host of agents (plasminogen activators) released from the vascular endothelium (angiokinase), the kidney excretory system (urokinase), and various nonkeratinized epithelia. The numerous physiological

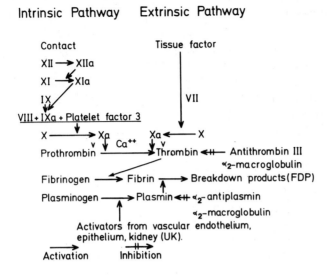

Fig. 2. Simplified mechanisms of blood coagulation and fibrinolysis. *UK,* urokinase; *FDP,* fibrin degradation products

plasminogen activators may be grouped into two main classes (PANDOLFI and LANTZ 1979). To one class belong the activator or activators produced by the endothelium and known in the literature as "tissue activator," but which should more properly be named "angiokinase"; to the other belong urokinase and the activator(s) produced in the epithelium of various mucous membranes. Angiokinase is supposed to act in blood, i.e., in an environment containing a powerful inhibitor of plasmin, the α_2-antiplasmin which immediately binds plasmin as soon as it is generated in the liquid phase. Fibrinolysis is possible because tissue activator shares with plasminogen the tendency to become bound to fibrin: consequently, plasmin formation takes place not in the liquid phase but in the fibrin meshwork, where plasmin is protected from the action of the inhibitor. The activators of the second class, urokinase and urokinase-like kinases, normally operate in fluids not containing inhibitors. The affinity of these to fibrin is far less than that of angiokinase.

The fibrinolytic mechanism is not only involved in hemostasis but has other functions, prevention of thrombosis and promotion of any dissolution of thrombi (thrombolysis).

Primary hemostasis and blood coagulation on the one hand and fibrinolysis on the other are in a continous dynamic equilibrium. A defect of primary hemostasis and/or blood coagulation causes a tendency to hemorrhages, while a defective fibrinolysis facilitates the occurrence of thrombosis. Conversely, stimulation of the fibrinolytic system impairs hemostasis, while hyperactive primary hemostasis/coagulation makes the organism prone to thrombosis.

B. Anticoagulants

Anticoagulant drugs antagonize one or more coagulation factors. The aim of anticoagulant treatment is to produce in the organism a controlled hemorrhagic diathesis; it is used in the prevention and treatment of thrombosis. Actually, anticoagulants have the ultimate effect of preventing formation of fibrin and they cannot be expected to have a direct thrombus-dissolving (thrombolytic) action. However, since they prevent thrombus growth by apposition of fibrin, they facilitate the task of the fibrinolytic system in dissolving the thrombus (physiological thrombolysis).

Anticoagulants are presently used in conditions such as venous thrombosis, pulmonary embolism, transient ischemic attacks (TIA), and heart disease with risk of embolism (e.g., where there is mitral stenosis or prosthetic heart valves), following thrombolytic therapy, and in various clinical situations often complicated by thrombosis (fractures, etc.). The value of anticoagulants in preventing recurrence of myocardial infarction is not yet established.

From the above list it can be concluded that the indications for anticoagulants are more often prophylactic than therapeutic. In ophthalmology the only conditions where anticoagulants are used are occlusion of the central retinal vein (VANNAS and RAITTA 1966) and amaurosis fugax associated with stenosis of the internal carotid. Sometimes the involvement of the ophthalmologist is indirect, e.g., when eye surgery is necessary in a patient under anticoagulant treatment.

I. Direct Anticoagulants (Heparin)

Heparin is a sulfated polysaccharide occurring in all tissues of the body, especially in the liver (hence the name) and lungs, but normally absent from the circulating blood. JAKOBSSON and LINDAHL (1979) failed to demonstrate heparin in normal blood using a method sensitive to concentrations as low as 2 ng/ml. The molecular weight of heparin is 20,000. Heparin has a strong negative charge and inhibits enzymes by binding them and blocking their active site. To have anticoagulant effect heparin needs the presence of a plasma glycoprotein called "antithrombin III" or "natural antithrombin" (AT III). This is a physiological anticoagulant which inhibits not only thrombin but also coagulation factors IX, X, XI, and XII in their active forms. This inhibition, normally quite slow, is strongly accelerated by the presence of heparin. Heparin binds AT III, and the molecular complex resulting is a much more powerful inhibitor than AT III alone. Hence the name of "heparin cofactor" proposed for AT III.

Heparin is generally given intravenously (not intramuscularly, since it can cause hematomas). Intermittent treatment (proposed doses: $15{,}000 + 10{,}000 + 10{,}000 + 12{,}500$ IU daily) is preferred to continuous infusion: 1,000 IU corresponds to 10 mg heparin.

The effect of heparin on coagulation can be monitored by a clotting test known as "kaolin cephalin time" or "activated partial thromboplastin time" (APTT). To attain a therapeutic level, heparin should be given in doses causing a prolongation of APTT by a factor of 2–4. In long-term anticoagulant treatment it is customary to begin simultaneously with both heparin to achieve an immediate effect and indirect anticoagulants. Heparin is withdrawn as soon as the indirect anticoagulants have depressed the vitamin K-dependent coagulation factors (see Sect. B.II) for therapeutic levels.

About 10 years ago, YIN et al. (1971) proposed a new hypothesis to explain the antithrombotic action of heparin. Such a hypothesis has clinical implications since it suggests that a therapeutic effect can be obtained with lower heparin doses. According to YIN et al., the main antithrombotic effect of heparin is not the result of a global inhibition of the clotting system but the result of inhibition of factor X. As is apparent from Fig. 2, factor X has a key role in the process of coagulation. Its activated form is especially sensitive to inhibition by heparin, a property explaining the antithrombotic effect of low-dose heparin tratment. According to KAKKAR (1975), an effective prophylaxis of postoperative thrombosis can be obtained with heparin dosages as low as 5,000 IU given subcutaneously 2 h before operation followed by the same dose every 12 h for 5 days. This subcutaneous treatment with single doses of only 5,000 IU hardly affects global blood clotting tests, such as APTT, but produces a significant inhibition of activated factor X (DENSON and BONNAR 1975). More clinical and laboratory research work is needed to give an answer to the problem of the optimal dosage of heparin.

If bleeding occurs during treatment, heparin should be withdrawn and protamine sulfate given: 10 mg protamine sulfate neutralizes 1,000 IU (10 mg) heparin in vitro. Protamine sulfate is usually injected in a 1% solution in doses not exceeding 50 mg of protamine every 2–4 h. It is estimated that heparin disappears within 4 h after intravenous injection of 5,000 IU and within 6–8 h after injection of 10,000–15,000 IU. Therefore, the optimal dosage of protamine sulfate has to be calculated from case to case.

II. Indirect Anticoagulants

Unlike heparin, which is active both in vivo and in vitro, indirect anticoagulants are active only in vivo. They are also called "oral anticoagulants." Indirect anticoagulants are coumarin derivatives (derivatives of 4-hydroxycoumarin, such as warfarin sodium) and indanedione derivatives (of indian-1:3-dione, such as diphenandione).

These substances act by interfering with the synthesis in the liver of the vitamin-K-dependent coagulation factors (factor II or prothrombin, factor VII, factor IX, and factor X). During treatment with indirect anticoagulants coagulation factors are still formed, but these factors are qualitatively defective and therefore no longer able to bind Ca^{++}. The formation of thrombin is inhibited as a consequence.

Compared to the short half-lives of the heparin drugs (1–3 h) the vitamin-K-dependent coagulation factors have a half-life time of from 6 (factor VII) to 80 h (prothrombin). Large loading doses to initiate therapy are recommended for this reason.

Indirect anticoagulants are given in deep venous thrombosis for 1–3 months and in pulmonary embolism for 6 months. Treatment for more than 6 months may be indicated in embolizing heart diseases, relapsing thrombosis, and TIA.

The method most commonly used to monitor treatment with anticoagulants is the one-stage prothrombin time of Quick. This method is sensitive to vitamin-K-dependent coagulation factors, but also to the level of factor V and fibrinogen.

Table 1. Drug interactions with the coumarin anticoagulants

Drug	Effect	Mechanism
Acetylsalicylic acid (ASA)	+	Competition with vitamin K_1 in the liver Displacement Antiaggregating effect on platelets
Anabolic steroids	+	Unknown
Barbiturates	−	Increased (liver) metabolism
Carbamazepine (Tegretol)	−	Increased metabolism
Chloramphenicol	+	Decreased metabolism
Clofibrate	+	Decreased metabolism
Disulfiram (Antabuse)	+	Decreased metabolism
Glutethimide (Doriden)	−	Increased metabolism
Griseofulvin	−	Decreased absorption Increased metabolism
Kinidin	+	Effect on receptors
Oxyphenbutazone	+	Displacement Decreased metabolism
Phenylbutazone	+	Displacement (from serum proteins) Decreased metabolism
Rifampicin	−	Increased metabolism

+, denotes increased; −, denotes decreased

Therefore the P- and P (prothrombin-proconvertin) test based on a system containing fibrinogen and factor V in excess seems preferable. Following this method the therapeutic level lies in the range of 10%–15% of control values. There is risk of hemorrhage when the P and P level is below 7%–8%. The most common complications involving bleeding are hemorrhages from the urinary tract, the gastrointestinal tract, and the mucous membranes. Sometimes anticoagulation reveals a hitherto silent malignancy of the urinary tract.

If the bleeding is only moderate, it is sufficient to withdraw the treatment for 2–3 days. If the bleeding is more severe, vitamin K_1 should be administered intravenously in doses of 10–20 mg. The bleeding generally ceases when the P and P rises above 20%.

Numerous drugs have been reported to interact with coumarin derivatives enhancing or decreasing their effect. They are listed in Table 1.

III. Contraindications: Precautions in Ophthalmology

Anticoagulants are contraindicated in any condition which directly or indirectly impairs hemostasis. Thus anticoagulants should not be given in congenital (hemophilia, von Willebrand's disease, etc.) or acquired hemorrhagic diathesis (secondary thrombocytopenia, prothrombin deficit due to liver disease, etc.). Other contraindications are gastroduodenal ulcer and arterial hypertension. Long-term treatment requires cooperation on the part of the patient and should not be prescribed in cases of poor mental health or alcoholism. Coumarin derivatives are contraindicated in pregnancy, since they are teratogenic and may produce hemorrhages in the fetus. Heparin, on the other hand, does not pass through the placental barrier.

Long term anticoagulation has been reported to be complicated by conjunctival and retinal hemorrhages (NEUMANN 1976; HAMBURGER 1970). Such cases are probably due to poor monitoring of the treatment leading to overdosage.

The ophthalmologist may be confronted with the problem of how to operate on a patient who is receiving anticoagulants. Such a situation may be difficult to solve, since interruption of anticoagulant treatment may result in a postoperative thrombosis, while its continuation in therapeutic doses strongly increases the risk of intra- or postoperative hemorrhages. Unfortunately, the ophthalmic literature offers almost no guidance as to how these situations should be coped with. As regards general surgery, opinions differ. Some authors claim that full anticoagulation can be continued (KLUFT et al. 1965), while others recommend a decreased dosage. According to NILSSON (1974), patients under dicumarol therapy should be operated upon only when the P and P level has reached 30%. Regarding ocular surgery, in the absence of specific reports the cautious approach seems preferable. According to my personal experience, it is possible to operate for cataract or glaucoma on patients receiving anticoagulants provided that the dosage is decreased enough to raise P and P level to 30%–40% on the day of operation. Full anticoagulant treatment can be reinstated 1 week after the operation.

C. Fibrinolytics

Fibrinolytics increase the fibrinolytic activity of the organism. Generally, they are given introvenously to increase the fibrinolytic activity of blood in order to dissolve an obstructing thrombus. In ophthalmology, fibrinolytics have been used intraocularly in cases of hemorrhage in the anterior chamber and in the vitreous body.

I. Commonly Used Fibrinolytic Agents

1. Streptokinase

Streptokinase is a protein with a molecular weight of about 50,000 which is produced by a strain of β-hemolytic streptococci. It activates plasminogen indirectly, reacting first in a stoichiometric way with a plasma protein – probably plasminogen itself – and forming a complex which catalytically converts plasminogen into plasmin.

2. Urokinase

Urokinase is a physiological activator of plasminogen and is produced by the kidney. Its molecular weight is about 55,000. It converts plasminogen into plasmin directly by cleavage of peptidic bonds of the molecule. Although urokinase shows esterase activity on certain synthetic substrates, it has a strict specificity for plasminogen and does not interact with other plasma proteins. It does not need the presence of fibrin to convert plasminogen into plasmin. Some confusion exists as regards its dosage, since the activity is currently expressed in two different units, Ploug units and IU (one IU is equivalent to about 0.7 Ploug unit). Being a commercial preparation made of human urokinase, this drug has the advantage of being nonantigenic. It is, however, very expensive.

3. Plasmin

To enhance blood fibrinolytic activity, preformed plasmin can be given. Plasmin induces fibrinolytic activity in blood directly, without needing to activate the patient's plasminogen. There are different plasmin preparations available, consisting of human or animal (porcine) plasminogen activated by streptokinase or trypsin. A drawback of some plasmin preparation is persisting contamination by the activating agent.

II. Therapeutic Thrombolysis: Effect on Hemostasis

Despite the differences between different thrombolytic agents, they have common clinical indications and contraindications and comparable modes of administration. According to NILSSON (1974), the indications of thrombolytic therapy are:
1. Acute arterial obstructions of the limbs (embolism and thrombosis)
2. Acute thrombosis of the veins of the limbs and pelvis
3. Acute pulmonary embolism
4. Occurrence of clots in artificial arteriovenous shunts for hemodialysis.

It is doubtful whether thrombolytic therapy is of any use in myocardial infarction, and many consider this therapy to be contraindicated in cerebrovascular occlusion because of the risk of hemorrhage.

Because plasmin has the effect of breaking down coagulation factors, thrombolytic therapy favors hemorrhages and has the same contraindications as anticoagulant therapy. However, in the case of thrombolytics the contraindications are more strict, since the risk of hemorrhage is higher.

The mechanisms of thrombolysis is still a matter of debate. According to the theory of the intrinsic thrombolysis (ALKJAERSIG et al. 1959), the interior of thrombi offers an unfavorable environment for the action of antiplasmins. Thus plasminogen activator diffuses into the thrombus and converts the plasminogen adsorbed to fibrin into plasmin, which, if uninhibited, digests the thrombus from inside. According to this theory, therapy with fibrinolytic activators is preferable to therapy with plasmin. Others (AMBRUS and MARKUS 1960) postulate that plasmin circulates in complex with antiplasmins: in the presence of fibrin the complex dissociates, since plasmin has a greater affinity for fibrin than for antiplasmin and plasmin can thus degrade fibrin. According to this theory, thrombolysis occurs on the surface of the thrombus; therapeutic thrombolysis can be achieved with activators and plasmin as well. These hypotheses are not mutually exclusive, and thrombolysis may occur according to both mechanisms simultaneously.

The recent discovery of the main physiological antiplasmin, the α_2-antiplasmin, has given us a better insight on the mechanism of therapeutic thrombolysis. It has been found that in order to produce thrombolysis by means of plasmin or activators without affinity to fibrin, such as urokinase or streptokinase, it is first necessary to bind all circulating antiplasmin. This situation occurs when about 70% of all plasminogen has been converted into plasmin – hence the necessity of giving large doses of fibrinolytic agents.

There is a drawback after effective fibrinolytic therapy from the infusion of large quantities of plasmin. Plasmin is an endopeptidase which attacks other clotting factors besides fibrin, including fibrinogen, factor VII, and factor VIII. During thrombolytic therapy there is always a decrease in the amounts of these factors, as well as a sharp fall in plasminogen if plasminogen activators are given. The result is an impairment of hemostasis with a tendency to bleeding.

Thrombolytic therapy is always brief (3 days or less) and requires hospitalization. For the doses see Table 2.

III. Fibrinolytics in Ophthalmology

1. Occlusion of the Central Retinal Vein

Although several authors (RABINOWICS et al. 1968; SEITZ 1964) tend not to attach importance to thrombosis in the pathogenesis of the occlusion of the retinal veins, cumulative evidence (PANDOLFI 1979) indicates that thrombosis plays an important role at least in converting a preexisting stenosis into occlusion – hence the indication of thrombolytic therapy.

A considerable number of reports on the use of thrombolytics in retinal vein occlusion are available. The agent most used is streptokinase (KHONER et al. 1976; KWAAN et al. 1977; and others); Urokinase (ALGAN et al. 1976; KWAAN et al. 1977; and others) and different plasmin preparations have been given (HOWDEN 1959; PANDOLFI and HEDNER, unpublished results; and others). All these authors claimed promising results except DEN OTTOLANDER and CRANDIJK (1968), who did not find streptokinase superior to heparin in a study of two small series of patients. According to KHONER et al. (1976) and also in my personal experience, treatment with con-

Table 2. Thrombolytic treatment of occlusion of retinal veins with streptokinase (Kabikinase Kabi), plasmin (Lysofibrin Novo), and urokinase (Abbot)

Indications
   Occlusion of the central retinal vein and its branches. Most authors do not treat occlusions older than 7–10 days; however, according to some other authors older occlusions (up to 120 days) may also benefit from the treatment

Contraindications
   Disorders of hemostasis, both congenital and acquired (thrombocytopenia, thrombocytopathia, coagulation defects), arterial hypertension, peptic ulcer, ulcerative colitis, postoperative states (during the first 10 days after surgery), previous cerebrovascular accidents, pregnancy

Dosage
   Streptokinase (Kabikinase Kabi)
      Continuous infusion (KHONER et al. 1976): loading dose of 600,000 IU i.v. followed by continuous infusion at the rate of 100,000 IU/h for 3–4 days
      Intermittent infusion (according to PANDOLFI and HEDNER, unpublished work): loading dose of 600,000 IU i.v. followed by three single doses of 250,000 IU i.v. after 24, 48, and 72 h
   Plasmin (Lysofibrin Novo) (PANDOLFI and HEDNER, unpublished work): loading dose of 2,000–3,000 NU (novo units) i.v. followed by single doses of 2,000–3,000 NU on the 1st, 2nd, and 3rd days
   Urokinase (Abbot) (KWAAN et al. 1977): loading dose of 6,000 CTA units/kg body wt. followed by one single dose of 6,000 CTA units/kg

tinuous infusion of streptokinase may be complicated by a massive vitreous hemorrhage.

Personally, I feel that thrombolytic treatment is worth trying in case of occlusion of retinal veins, especially if the patient is under 65, since in elderly subjects the arteriosclerotic component of the occlusion (which obviously cannot be influenced by thrombolytics) can be expected to be predominant. Indications, contraindications, and dosages of different thrombolytic agents for treatment of occlusion of retinal veins are summarized in Table 2. Continuous infusion of streptokinase is known to cause a prolonged depression of clotting factors which is probably responsible for the vitreous hemorrhages observed. Intermittent treatment with streptokinase and plasmin does not produce a persisting depression of clotting factors and therefore seems preferable.

2. Hemorrhages in the Anterior Chamber and Vitreous Body

Blood in the anterior chamber of the eye generally coagulates. As a rule the resulting clot is rapidly dissolved by the plasminogen activator deriving from the iris and the corneal endothelium (PANDOLFI 1978). The fluid "blood" commonly observed in hyphema is actually a dissolved clot, which in place of fibrinogen contains fibrin degradation products (FDP) and cannot coagulate any more.

Clot dissolution is the prerequisite for the eventual resorption of blood from the anterior chamber. Large amounts of clotted blood may exhaust the fibrinolytic capacity of the anterior chamber and fail to dissolve. In these cases, especially if intraocular pressure is increased, surgical removal of the clot from the anterior chamber is indicated. The clot extraction is facilitated by the previous irrigation of the anterior chamber with urokinase. After a few minutes of irrigation with urokinase (Leo) in a concentration of 2,500–5,000 Ploug units/ml the clot loosens, breaks down, and can be extracted through the irrigation opening (PIERSE and LE GRICE 1964; RAKUSIN 1972; and others). Apparently no side effects occur after the introduction of urokinase into the anterior chamber. The use of this fibrinolytic enzyme in the treatment of total hyphema is now accepted by many ophthalmologists. Commercially available urokinase can be purified further (HOLMBERG et al. 1976), a procedure which would permit the use of higher concentrations of urokinase.

Urokinase has also been injected in the vitreous cavity of the eye in order to accelerate the resorption of vitreous hemorrhages. The clinical results are encouraging also in consideration of the fact that the technique is far less traumatic than vitrectomy. According to CHAPMAN SMITH and CROCK (1977), urokinase should be used as a first line of attack in vitreous hemorrhages, vitrectomy being reserved for those patients who fail to respond. The clinical results are summarized in Table 3. The optimal dose of urokinase to be given intravitreally is debatable. Doses of 50,000 Ploug units/ml and more are clearly toxic in animals and should be avoided. The use of further purifications of commercially available preparations should be encouraged.

Intravitreal treatment with fibrinolytic activators poses a number of basic problems concerning its mechanism of action. Fibrinolysis can explain the beneficial effect of intravitreal urokinase when the agent is given in fresh hemorrhages.

Table 3. Clinical experience with the intravitreal injection of urokinase

Author(s)	No. of eyes	Concentration and amount injected	Remarks
FORRESTER and WILLIAMSON (1973)	5	10,000– 50,000 PU (0.5 ml)	Iritis Effect
DUGMORE and RAICHAND (1973)	3	50,000 PU (0.5 ml)	Effect
CLEARY et al. (1974)	15	8,000– 75,000 PU (0.2–0.6 ml)	Iritis No effect
HOLMES SELLORS et al. (1974)	5	100,000 PU (0.25 ml)	Iritis Doubtful effect
STENKULA and PANDOLFI (unpublished work)	3	25,000 PU (0.25 ml)	Effect
CHAPMAN SMITH and CROCK (1977)	34	25,000–300,000 PU (0.3 ml)	Iritis Effect

However, fibrin disappears from the vitreous after some weeks in experimental vitreous hemorrhages (FORRESTER et al. 1978) and is often absent in human vitreous obtained a vitrectomy (STENKULA and PANDOLFI, unpublished work). In the absence of fibrin the beneficial action of urokinase has to be explained in terms of other mechanisms, such as the proteolytic and macrophage-migration-promoting action of the plasmin formed (VASSALLI et al. 1976).

Presence of plasminogen in the vitreous body is another prerequisite for the occurrence of intravitreal fibrinolysis. Urokinase has only one known physiological substrate, i.e., plasminogen. Without plasminogen the action of urokinase in the vitreous amounts to nil. According to STENKULA and PANDOLFI, measurable amounts of plasminogen are present only in about 40% of the vitreous samples obtained at vitrectomy. In the same samples it was also found that fibrinolytic inhibitors (α_2-antiplasmin) were present in widely varying amounts.

In conclusion, in order for urokinase to stimulate fibrinolysis in the vitreous body the following conditions must prevail:
1. Fibrin must be present.
2. Plasminogen must be present.
3. Inhibitors must not exceed the amount of plasmin formed.

Available evidence speaks against the constant occurrence of such conditions in the vitreous body, and this may explain the varriable clinical results described in the literature. Further work is necessary to ascertain whether intraocular urokinase can be considered as a treatment of vitreous hemorrhages.

D. Hemostatics

Hemostatics are substances which facilitate the cessation of bleeding or prevent rebleeding. There is considerable confusion in this field, since many substances without any proven clinical effect are labeled hemostatics. Hemostatics can be di-

Table 4. Hemostatic agents used in surgery

Specific hemostatics (correct excessive surgical bleeding caused by disorders of hemostasis)

Disorder of hemostasis	Hemostatic
Congenital	Substitution therapy (e.g., factor VIII in hemophilia A, factor IX in hemophilia B, platelet concentrate in thrombocytopenia)
Acquired	Specific drugs (i.e., protamine sulfate in heparin treatment, vitamin K_1 in treatment with dicoumarolics, antifibrinolytics such as EACA or AMCA in general or local hyperfibrinolysis)

Nonspecific hemostatics (are claimed to reduce surgical bleeding by potentiating a normal hemostasis)

    Estrogens (Premarin, Styptanon)
    Ethamsylate (Dicynene)
    Calcium dobesilate (Doxium)
    Snake venom (Botropase, Reptilase)
    Vitamins C, K, and "P"
    Miscellaneous (Clauden, Tachostyptan, Sangostop)

---

vided in two groups. One group acts by correcting known disorders of local or general hemostasis. Among these substances are factor VIII and factor IX concentrates, vitamin K_1, and fibrinolytic inhibitors. Therapy with these substances, which is generally very effective, requires previous diagnosis of the hemostatic disorder. Obviously, no help can be expected from the infusion of factor VIII concentrate in hyperfibrinolysis or from injection of vitamin K_1 in any hemorrhagic disease which is not caused by a deficit of vitamin-K-dependent coagulation factors. The agents of this first group can be called "specific hemostatics" (Table 4).

The term "nonspecific hemostatics" should be reserved for the second group, which is made up of a host of substances claimed to "potentiate" a normal hemostasis. These substances are listed in Table 4. Their clinical effect is mostly unproven. Interestingly, the clinical use of no unspecific hemostatics is objectionable in view of their claimed mechanism of action. In principle, it is impossible to change a function of the normal organism without creating a pathological state. Thus potentiating hemostasis should induce in the organism a tendency to thrombosis. The fact that there are no reports of thromboembolic complications during treatment with nonspecific hemostatics casts an additional doubt on the efficacy of these drugs.

I. Specific

A few specific hemostatics are reviewed here with special reference to their use in ophthalmology. For a discussion of protamine sulfate see Sect. B.I. and for vitamin K see Sect. B.II.

1. Substitution Therapy

Congenital disorders of hemostasis caused by defective platelets or inactive coagulation factors are treated with infusion of healthy cells or factors. This therapy is especially indicated when patients with these conditions require surgery so as to avoid exaggerated surgical bleeding or postoperative rebleeding. As a rule, any operation on patients with a known tendency to bleeding should be carried out in close consultation with a coagulation laboratory.

Disorders of primary hemostasis should be treated by transfusion of platelet-rich plasma or platelet concentrates in amounts sufficient to correct the patient's bleeding time. The same applies for acquired disorders of hemostasis (uremia, myeloma, ingestion of aspirin, etc.).

The most common disorders of coagulation are von Willebrand's disease and hemophilia A. When operated upon, these patients should receive substitution therapy to raise the blood level of the missing factor before and after surgery. Such therapy may consist of transfusion of fresh plasma, plasma cryoprecipitate, or plasma fraction selectively rich in the missing factor, i.e., factor VIII in hemophilia A (Kabi fraction I-0) or factor IX in hemophilia B. For details on this treatment see NILSSON (1974). The plasma level of the missing factor should be raised to 30% –50% of normal on the operation day and first postoperative day. Lower levels (20%–30%) are sufficient for the following 6 days (OESTERLIND and NILSSON 1968). Antifibrinolytic drugs (tranexamic acid: see Sect. D.I.2) can also be given.

2. Antifibrinolytics

Of the antifibrinolytics only ε-aminocaproic acid (EACA) and *trans*-aminomethyl-cyclohexane carboxylic acid (tranexamic acid, AMCA) are reported because of their use in ophthalmology (Fig. 3). These two ω-aminocarboxylic acids inhibit fibrinolysis by blocking plasminogen's and plasmin's lysine-binding sites, which are largely responsible for the affinity plasminogen and plasmin have for fibrin. In the molecule of plasminogen and of plasmin there are at least six lysine-binding sites. The binding constant of EACA is higher than that of AMCA ($10^{-3}M$–$5 \times 10^{-3}M$ for EACA versus $10^{-6}M$–$10^{-5}M$ for AMCA). This difference is reflected in the different clinical dosage (0.1 g/Kg bodywt. three or four times daily for EACA, versus 0.1 g/10 kg bodywt. three or four times daily for AMCA). The necessity of a repeated daily administration derives from the rapid renal elimination of these drugs. Intravenously, EACA and AMCA are given in doses of 4 g and 0.5 g respectively three or four times daily.

As regards side effects, nausea, vomiting, and diarrhea have been reported following oral administration. Very rarely vertigo and lowering of blood pressure can occur. Although a decrease in the fibrinolytic activity of the organism is known

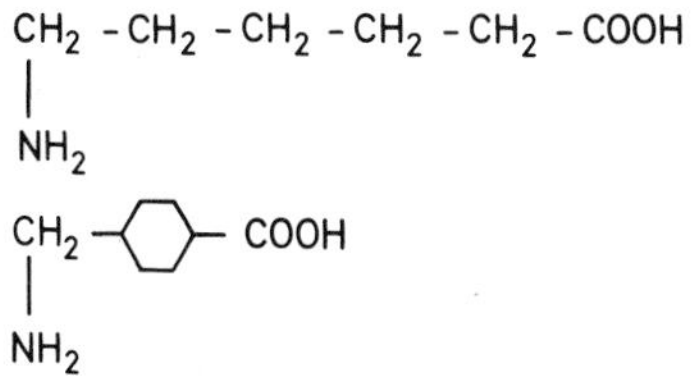

Fig. 3. Molecular structures of **a** ε-aminocaproic acid (EACA) and **b** tranexamic acid

Table 5. Suitable dosages of tranexamic acid (AMCA) in patients with varying degrees of renal insufficiency. (ANDERSSON et al. 1978)

Serum creatinine (μmol/l)	Dose of AMCA
120–150	10 mg/kg body wt. i.v. twice daily
250–500	10 mg/kg body wt. i.v. daily
> 500	10 mg/kg body wt. i.v. every 48 h

to favor the occurrence of thrombosis, thromboembolic complications during treatment with EACA and AMCA are rare. However, in special situations the risk of thrombosis may be significant. FODSTAD et al. (1978) and GELMERS (1980) have stressed the risk of thrombosis during antifibrinolitic treatment of subarachnoidal hemorrhages, a condition in which AMCA is given in doses twice as large as usual. Furthermore, in neurosurgery AMCA is suspected to cause cerebral ischemic complications. Although no thrombotic complications have been reported during the use of EACA or AMCA in ophthalmology, it seems advisable not to give these compounds in states predisposing to thrombosis (history of previous thrombosis, conditions causing hyperviscosity of blood, malignancies, etc.). Because EACA and AMCA are excreted by the kidney, caution is necessary in renal insufficiency to avoid accumulation of these substances in the blood. ANDERSSON et al. (1978) have elaborated suitable dosages of AMCA in various degrees of renal insufficiency (Table 5).

In ophthalmology, EACA and AMCA have been used to prevent secondary bleeding in traumatic hyphema or after surgery. It is known that secondary bleeding in the anterior chamber of the eye is generally severe and is often followed by increased intraocular pressure and loss of the eye. The rationale of the use of antifibrinolytics is reported in a review by PANDOLFI (1978). In blunt trauma the primary hemorrhage is generally caused by the rupture of a blood vessel located at the chamber angle. Because of the proximity of the iris, which is very rich in fibrinolytic activators, the platelet-fibrin plug sealing the vascular damage tends to dissolve prematurely, i.e., before the damaged vessel is definitely repaired by cellular proliferation. The prevailing prophylaxis of secondary bleeding is bed rest, with the intent of avoiding trauma and dislodgement of the weak hemostatic plug located at the chamber angle. Antifibrinolytics, on the other hand, act by locally delaying the dissolution of the fibrin plug. The advantage of the treatment with antifibrinolytics is to avoid hospitalization and prolonged immobility to the patient with considerable socioeconomical gains.

Favorable results have been reported with the use of EACA (CROUCH and FRENKEL 1976) and of AMCA (JERNDAL and FRISÉN 1976; BRAMSEN 1976, 1977, 1979; VARNEK et al. 1980). Summarizing these results, it was found that antifibrinolytic treatment significantly reduces the frequency of rebleeding and protects mobilized patients from secondary hemorrhages. A notable consequence of the treatment was a delay of resorption of clotted hyphemas, a direct proof of the antifibrinolytic effect of the drugs.

II. Nonspecific

Of the nonspecific hemostatic agents (Table 3), several have been used in ophthalmology, especially to reduce bleeding in surgery of the bulb. Their efficacy in ophthalmology – as in other specialities – is not proved, being generally claimed on the basis of uncontrolled studies. These substances have the disadvantage of offering a pseudocover against hemorrhagic complications: with an unjustified feeling of security the surgeon may not play attention to the hemostatic status of the patient and fail to give a specific hemostatic when necessary. On the other hand, some of these agents may be used according to personal beliefs and clinical experience, especially since they have no side effects, but only as a supplement to the specific hemostatic therapy.

References

Algan B, Leyder C, Marchal H, Geoffroy D, Marquis A (1976) Considerations sur l'étiologie des thromboses veneuses rétiniennes. Bull Soc Belge Ophtalmol 172:631–636

Alkjaersig N, Fletcher AP, Sherry S (1959) The mechanism of clot dissolution by plasmin. J Clin Invest 38:1086–1095

Ambrus CM, Markus G (1960) Plasmin-antiplasmin complex as a reservoir of fibrinolytic enzyme. Am J Physiol 199:491–494

Andersson L, Eriksson O, Hedlund PO, Kjellman H, Lindquist B (1978) Special considerations with regard to the dosage of tranexamic acid in patients with chronic renal diseases. Urol Res 6:83–88

Bramsen T (1976) Traumatic hyphaema treated with the antifibrinolytic drug tranexamic acid. I. Acta Ophthalmol 54:250–256

Bramsen T (1977) Traumatic hyphaema treated with the antifibrinolytic drug tranexamic acid. II. Acta Ophthalmol 55:616–620

Bramsen T (1979) Fibrinolysis and traumatic hyphaema. Acta Ophthalmol 57:447–454

Chapman Smith JS, Crock GW (1977) Urokinase in the treatment of vitreous haemorrhages. Br J Ophthalmol 61:500–505

Cleary AE, Davies EWG, Shilling JS, Hamilton AM (1974) Intravitreal urokinase in the treatment of vitreous haemorrhages. Trans Ophthalmol Soc UK 94:587–590

Crouch ER, Frenkel M (1976) Aminocaproic acid in the treatment of traumatic hyphema. Am J Ophthal 81:355–360

Den Ottolander GJH, Craandijk A (1968) Treatment of thrombosis of the central retinal vein with streptokinase. Thrombos Diathes Haemorrh 20:415–419

Denson KWE, Bonnar J (1975) Measurement of heparin in patients receiving subcutaneous heparin therapy. Br J Haemat 30:139–144

Dugmore WN, Raichand M (1973) Intravitreal urokinase in the treatment of vitreous haemorrhage. Am J Ophthalmol 75:779–781

Fodstad H, Liljequist B, Schannong M, Thulin CA (1978) Tranexamic acid in the preoperative management of ruptured intracranial anueurysm. Surg Neurol 10:9–15

Forrester J, Williamson J (1973) Resolution of intravitreal clots by urokinase. Lancet II:197–181

Forrester J, Lee WL, Williamson J (1978) The pathology of vitreous haemorrhages. Arch Ophthalmol 96:703–710

Gelmers HJ (1980) Prevention of recurrence of spontaneous subrachnoidal haemorrhage by tranexamic acid. Acta Neurochir 52:45–50

Hamburger FA (1970) Netzhautblutungen in beiden Augen nach Therapie mit Antikoagulantien. Wien Klin Wschr 82:549

Holmberg L, Bladh B, Aastedt B (1976) Purification of urokinase by affinity chromatography. Biochim Biophys Acta 445:215–222

Holmes Sellors PJ, Kanski JJ, Watson DM (1974) Intravitreal urokinase in the management of vitreous haemorrhages. Trans Ophthalmol Soc UK 94:591–596

Howden GD (1959) The successful treatment of a case of central retinal vein thrombosis with intravenous fibrinolysin. Can Med Assoc J 80:382–384

Jakobsson KG, Lindahl U (1979) Attempted determination of endogenous heparin in blood. Abstract 0195. Seventh international congress on thrombosis and haemostasis, London

Jerndal T, Frisén M (1976) Tranexamic acid (AMCA) and late hyphaema. A double blind study in cataract surgery. Acta Ophthalmol 54:417–429

Kakkar VV: Deep venous thrombosis; detection and prevention. Circulation 51:8–19

Khoner EM, Petit JE, Hamilton AM, Bulpit CJ, Dollery CT (1976) Streptokinase in central retinal vein occlusion: a controlled clinical trial. Br Med J I:550–553

Kluft O, Stortenbeck W, De Vries SI, Wieberdink J (1965) The postoperative dip in peroperative anticoagulation. Thrombos Diathes Haemorrh 13:218–234

Kwaan HC, Dobbie JG, Fetkenhour CL (1977) The use of anticoagulants and thrombolytic agents in occlusive retinal vascular diseases. In: Paoletti R, Sherry S (eds) Thrombosis and urokinase. Academic, New York, pp 191–198

Neumann L (1976) Les hémorragies conjonctivales, rétiniennes et vitréennes au cours des traitements anticoagulants de longue durée. Bull Soc Franc Ophtal 86:164–166

Nilsson IM (1974) Haemorrhagic and thrombotic disorders. Wiley, London

Oesterlind G, Nilsson IM (1968) Extraction of cataract in a patient with severe haemophilia. Acta Ophthalmol 42:176–181

Oehrstrom A (1972) Treatment of traumatic hyphaema with corticosteroids and mydriatics. Acta Ophthalmol 50:549–555

Pandolfi M (1978) Intraocular haemorrhages. A haemostatic therapeutic approach. Surv Ophthalmol 22:322–334

Pandolfi M (1979) Haemorrhages in ophthalmology. Thieme, Stuttgart

Pandolfi M, Lantz E (1979) Partial purification and characterization of keratokinase, the fibrinolytic activator of the cornea. Exp Eye Res 29:563–571

Pierse D, Le Grice H (1964) The use of urokinase in the anterior chamber of the eye. J Clin Path 17:362

Rabinowics IM, Litman S, Michaelson IC (1968) Branch venous thrombosis. A pathological report. Trans Ophthalmol Soc UK 88:191–210

Rakusin W (1972) Urokinase in the management of traumatic hyphaema. Br J Ophthalmol 55:826–832

Sears ML (1970) Surgical management of black ball hyphema. Trans Am Acad Ophth Otol 74:820–827

Seitz R (1964) The retinal vessels. Mosby, St. Louis, p 74

Vannas S, Raitta C (1966) Anticoagulant treatment of retinal venous occlusion. Am J Ophthalmol 62:874–884

Vassalli JD, Hamilton J, Reich E (1976) Macrophage plasminogen activator: modulation of enzyme production by anti-inflammatory steroids, mitotic inhibitors and cyclic nucleotides. Cell 8:271–281

Varnek L, Daalsgard C, Hansen A, Klie F (1980) The effect of tranexamic acid on secondary haemorrhage after traumatic hyphaema. Acta Ophthalmol 58:787

Yin ET, Wessler S, Stoll PJ (1971) Biological properties of the naturally occurring plasma inhibitors to the activated factor X. J Biol Chem 246:3703–3711

CHAPTER 14

Oxygen

R. W. FLOWER, M. O. HALL, and A. PATZ

A. Introduction

With the identification of oxygen overuse as the principal cause of the epidemic of retrolental fibroplasia, the retinopathy of prematurity, in the early 1950s, the effects of oxygen toxicity to the eye were established. In contrast to classic oxygen toxicity, usually associated with greater oxygen exposure, severe retinal damage resulting from inhalation of concentrations of oxygen of only 40%–50% at normal atmospheric pressure in the incubator occurred in retrolental fibroplasia. The unique susceptibility of the premature retinal vasculature to modest increases in blood oxygen was unparalleled in vascular or neural physiology.

Oxygen accounts for 20.946% of our normal gaseous environment at sea level. In the adult normal respiration in air produces arterial PO_2 levels from 80–100 torr. In utero the immature human retina receives a venous-like bloodflow ($PO_2 =$ 25 torr, $PCO_2 = 45$ torr) at a low arterial blood pressure (25–30 torr), but upon arterialization at birth, arterial blood oxygen tension rises ($PO_2 = 70$ torr, $PCO_2 = 35$ torr) along with blood pressure (35–40 torr). The premature infant with an essentially normal cardiopulmonary system, i.e., one without the idiopathic respiratory distress syndrome, has a significantly greater arterial PO_2 when breathing room air. For this reason, the gestational age at birth, as well as the oxygen concentration administered, are important in determining the ocular response of oxygen in the premature infant.

B. Oxygen and the Adult Eye

Prolonged continuous exposure to high oxygen concentrations (above 90%) at atmospheric pressure can produce severe toxic effects in the body as well as in the eye. The main route for oxygen to the eye is by circulating blood, although there is some transfer of atmospheric oxygen through the corneal epithelium. The importance of direct contact with atmospheric oxygen for integrity of the corneal epithelium is well established, a conclusion suggested initially by the corneal irritation and epithelial edema that occur in persons wearing tightly fitting hard contact lenses which are impermeable to oxygen. It is not clear, however, that atmospheric oxygen transfer is vital to maintenance of the corneal endothelium, a cell layer bathed by the aqueous having an oxygen tension of about 55 torr (FISCHER 1930). Although some studies have been aimed at the effects of reduced oxygen on the cornea, none have specifically concentrated on or reported the effects of increased oxygen, and to our knowledge there have been no reports that oxygen in itself has toxic effects on the cornea.

Chronic inhalation of elevated concentrations of oxygen has, on the other hand, been shown to produce changes in the adult retina. Localized detachments were produced in two of ten dogs maintained in 100% oxygen for 4 days at normal atmospheric pressure (BEEHLER et al. 1968), and in rabbits. Destruction of visual cells occurred after 2 days' exposure to 90% oxygen, and similar damage was noted after 5 days' exposure to 60% oxygen (NOELL 1955).

Under hyperbaric conditions, oxygen becomes more toxic; at 3 atm PO_2 levels of approximately 2,500 torr can be reached. In dogs so exposed for more than 4 h, a lesion typified by formation of globular bodies appeared in the retinal nerve fiber layer (MARGOLIS 1966). At the microscopic level, the lesion resembled the "cotton-wool or soft exudate" associated with several human retinopathies. The soft exudates in the retina were observed without apparent central nervous system damage.

Short-term exposure to oxygen also causes changes in the adult human eye. In 50 healthy human subjects breathing 100% oxygen at ambient pressure, a mean vessel caliber reduction of 12% in retinal arteries and 15% in retinal veins was observed (FRAZIER and HICKAM 1965; HICKAM et al. 1963); and in five human subjects, mean retinal circulation time was observed to rise to 6.1 s compared to 4.8 s while they were breathing air (HICKAM and FRAZIER 1965). As in the animal experiments, the observable effects of oxygen breathing are exaggerated at hyperbaric pressures. Breathing 100% oxygen at 2 atm resulted in a 42% reduction in retinal arterial caliber (DOLLERY et al. 1964); at 3.7 atm, breathing 100% oxygen reduced the retinal artery to less than one-half normal caliber, and mean circulation time increased to 6.3 s compared to 4.2 s during air breathing (FRAZIER et al. 1967). Also, the degree of narrowing of retinal vessels upon breathing high oxygen concentrations decreases in a linear fashion with increasing age (RAMALLO and DOLLERY 1968).

Oxyen administration has been employed as an emergency measure in treatment of central retinal artery occlusion. The rationale for this treatment is based on the dual blood supply to the retina. The inner retinal layers are supplied by the retinal vessels, and the outer layers by the choroidal circulation. Normally, approximately 50% of the oxygen in the retinal circulation is utilized by the retinal tissue. However, due to nearly ten times greater blood volume flow through the choroidal circulation, less than 5% of choroidal blood oxygen is utilized by the retina (BILL 1975). This relationship between the two ocular circulations suggests the possibility that when the retinal circulation is compromised, administration of a mixture of 95% oxygen and 5% carbon dioxide could significantly increase the oxygen capacity of circulating ocular blood, thereby increasing the effective gradient of oxygen diffusing from the choroidal circulation to the ischemic inner retinal layers. At the same time, the vasodilatory effects of carbon dioxide on the retinal vessels should overcome any oxygen-induced vasoconstriction. Such oxygen administration is done by mask or nasal catheter for approximately 10 min every hour. It may be used in conjunction with other measures, including Diamox (acetazolamide) and/ or paracentesis. There is little danger of inducing oxygen toxicity by this treatment because there is no reason to apply treatment for prolonged periods in retinal arterial occlusion. Since death of sensory retinal tissue occurs with in 1–2 h, prolonged treatment would be futile were retinal function not promptly restored.

Transient protection of the retina occurred in both experimental and clinical subjects with central retinal arterial occlusion (PATZ 1955). It was observed in the adult cat that following occlusion of the central retinal artery, oxygen tension of the vitreous dropped appreciably according to measurements made with a polarographic electrode introduced from the opposite pars plana. Following inhalation of oxygen, a measurable increase in PO_2 near the retinal surface was recorded, indicating that an increased range of diffusion of choroidal oxygen across the retina occurred. Experimental retinal arterial occlusion was also produced in the rat eye (PATZ 1955) by severing the optic nerve just posterior to the globe as originally performed by TURNBULL (1950). Control animals with experimental retinal arterial occlusion were placed in room air and compared with the treated group placed in an incubator at 80%–90% oxygen at ambient pressure. There was a definite reduction in the residual swelling and cell death in the inner layers of the retina in the oxygen-treated group, but the effect was short-lived. After several hours, the oxygen-treated animals showed no significant difference from the controls.

Paralleling the experimental studies, three patients with relatively fresh retinal arterial occlusions experienced improvement in their fields of vision and visual acuity during inhalation of oxygen by mask at ambient pressure. These studies were short-term. In patients with longer-standing occlusion no difference between the oxygen-treated and controls was noted (PATZ 1955).

The ophthalmologist rarely examines patients with complete blockage of blood flow during central retinal arterial occlusions; in most cases fluorescein angiography shows residual blood flow to the retina. The extent of this residual blood flow varies from patient to patient and, additionally, the state of a patient's choroidal circulation during central retinal arterial occlusion is not necessarily known – there could conceivably be simultaneous disruption to choroidal blood flow. Moreover, the interaction of the separate retinal and choroidal circulations in maintaining retinal tissue metabolism is not clearly understood. Considering the possible existence of residual retinal circulation during the acute stage of central retinal artery occlusion and the fact that the photoreceptors which initiate the sequence of events comprising the electroretinographic response are primarily dependent on the choroid, the status of the choroidal circulation is probably a critical factor in determining survival of overlying retinal tissue. It has been documented, in at least one case, that concomitant choroidal occlusion was responsible for irreversible retinal tissue damage (FLOWER et al. 1977). In any event, current clinical experience seems to support the opinion that breathing oxygen at atmospheric pressure alone is insufficient to meet the prolonged demands of the retina during central retinal arterial occlusion.

Under hyperbaric conditions the entire oxygen needs of the retina can be met by the choroidal circulation. In cats and rhesus monkeys a significantly attenuated choroidal circulation alone could supply the necessary retinal oxygen while 100% oxygen was breathed at 3.3 atm (FLOWER and PATZ 1971). It has also been theoretically calculated that with no choroidal attenuation, the entire oxygen needs of the retina can be met by breathing 100% oxygen at 2.36 atm (DOLLERY et al. 1969). The validity of such calculations, however, depends upon the accuracy of values assigned to the diffusion constant for oxygen in retina, the oxygen diffusion gradient present across the retinal tissue, and oxygen consumption by the sensory retina.

DOLLERY et al. (1969) assumed the value for oxygen diffusion constant to be that measured in muscle, 1.7×10^{-5} ml of oxygen per minute per square centimeter retina at 37 °C in a concentration gradient of 1 atm/cm² (KROGH 1929), and an assumed value for tissue oxygen uptake was utilized. Accurate numbers have been made available for these important factors. WEITER and ZUCKERMAN (1979) reported a retinal tissue oxygen diffusion coefficient of $2.91 \pm 0.23 \times 10^{-4}$ cm²/min and a total oxygen consumption of 2.57×10^{-3} ml/cm³ retina per minute. Nevertheless, practical limitations such as time preclude hyperbaric oxygenation as a routine method of treatment. Even if the oxygen needs of the retina were met during the acute stage of occlusion, insufficient supplies of other essential retinal nutrients might not be met, and the accumulation of toxic metabolites might ultimately be responsible for death of the retina.

In a related series of studies addressing the mechanism of photocoagulation to destroy neovascularization, WOLBARSHT and LANDERS (1980) suggested that the large oxygen capacity of the choroidal circulation may be masked from the retina by the photoreceptor layer. The photoreceptors contain approximately 90% of the mitochondria present in the retina and may account for more than 50% of total oxygen consumed by the sensory retina. The effectiveness of photocoagulation therapy of retinal neovascularization might result from destruction of photoreceptors because a consequent significant increase in the oxygen gradient from the choroid may cause constriction of the overlying new vessel growth.

C. Oxygen and the Immature Eye

I. Retrolental Fribroplasia

On the basis of retrospective studies conducted in Melbourne, CAMPBELL (1951) first suggested that overuse of oxygen was etiologically related to the development of retrolental fibroplasia (RLF). The first controlled trial implicating the role of oxygen in RLF was reported in 1952 (PATZ et al.), and the lesion was produced in experimental animals in 1953 (ASHTON et al. 1953; PATZ et al. 1953). The cooperative nursery study on oxygen involving 18 hospitals in the United States was reported in 1956 (KINSEY et al. 1956). The collaborative study gave final documentation of the etiology of oxygen in RLF.

Although the precise mechanism of oxygen injury to the premature retina is still not fully understood, the studies on kittens (ASHTON and COOK 1954) indicated that the incomplete vascularization of the retina was fundamental to the RLF experimental lesion; the fully vascularized retina showed no damage. The response of the immature retinal vasculature was directly proportional to the duration of oxygen administration and to the concentration of oxygen used, and inversely proportional to the degree of maturity of the retina. Experimental production of RLF in mice, kittens, and puppies (PATZ 1954) demonstrated the common susceptibility of the immature retina to oxygen.

From experimental observations, the response of the immature retina to oxygen can be divided into two distinct stages. In the primary stage prolonged oxygen breathing has a toxic effect on the immature retinal vasculature. The susceptible tissue, thought to be the capillary endothelium, causes obliteration of newly formed capillaries just posterior to the advancing border of mesenchyma. Normal vasculogenesis from the optic disc toward the retinal periphery is halted. The secondary stage occurs upon return to ambient air. Vasculogenesis, somewhat different from normal retinal vasculogenesis but nevertheless near normal, may resume. Posterior to the arteriovenous mesenchymal shunt, extraretinal intravitreal neovascularization may develop. Further progression beyond this stage, or regression and cicatrization, depend upon the degree of hemorrhage and subsequent traction on the new vessels by the posterior cortical vitreous.

During the secondary stage, the retinal neovascularization will leak fluorescein dye on angiography. Focal hemorrhages may also occur. We have demonstrated by fluorescein angiography in newborn kittens that the location and degree of vascular closure determine the locus of the secondary neovascularization. With prolonged high concentrations of oxygen (7 days at 80% concentration), the entire retinal vascular bed was frequently totally and permanently closed. Significant choroidal circulation remained, but velocity of the choroidal dye wave front was noticeably attenuated. Indeed, a form of experimental retinal arterial occlusion was produced. The retina never revascularized normally after returning to ambient air. Multiple fine twigs of vessels developed in the peripapillary area, but the remaining retina remained avascular. Thus neovascularization occurred and was confined to the peripapillary region.

Attempts have been made to determine safe guidelines for administration of oxygen to premature infants, the most notable being a five-hospital collaborative study started in 1969 (KINSEY et al. 1977). In this study arterial PO_2 levels were examined and did not correlate with the eye findings because of limited information available from intermittent sampling. The arterial oxygen tensions in the infants in this study were almost entirely within the range of 60–100 torr, and the authors conclude that it would have been misleading for them to make recommendations for premature infants in general.

Unfortunately, beyond linking occurrence of RLF with hyperoxia, progress toward elucidating the pathogenesis of RLF has been slow. To some extent this may be attributed to the obstacles to direct studies of human developmental retinal physiology. There is a paucity of human tissue available for histological examination. Consequently, much of the basic research on RLF has had to be done using experimental animal models. The full-term newborn kitten and puppy have been used most extensively. Because the full-term newborn of these two species has an incompletely vascularized retina comparable to that of a 6th–7th month human fetus, they are useful animal models for studying the pathogenesis of RLF and the mechanism of the oxygen effect on the immature retina.

Retinal vascular change in RLF has been said to proceed from an ischemic process secondary to retinal vascular closure, but results of preliminary studies using the beagle puppy eye suggest that the damage may actually be worse when vasoconstriction is inhibited (FLOWER et al. 1981). Data from the study suggest that retinal vasoconstriction may be a normal physiological mechanism to protect the immature retina from damaging effects of excessive oxygen; that is, retinal vasoconstriction may be a protective rather than a pathological process in response to hyperoxia. According to this view, vasoconstriction observed in the premature infant exposed to oxygen may be only an extreme manifestation of a normal physiological response by which retinal blood flow is modulated during in utero development of the retinal vasculature. It is conceivable that the susceptibility of an eye to oxygen-associated retinopathy at birth depends upon the extent to which the vasoconstrictive protective response is functional as well as upon the degree of retinal vascular "maturity" attained.

The fact that significantly more severe RLF was produced in oxygen-treated beagle puppies in which vasoconstriction was inhibited is compatible with the suggestion that retinal vascular damage may result from cytotoxic effects of oxygen on endothelial cells rather than being secondary to vasoconstriction and diminished blood flow (ASHTON and PEDDLER 1962). During oxygen breathing dilated retinal blood vessels would allow a larger than normal volume of blood to flow through immature retinal vessels; those vessel walls would then be in contact with oxygen radicals (probably derived from dissolved molecular oxygen) which are known to damage cell membranes. (The possibility that drugs which scavenge oxygen radicals may be of significant therapeutic value during oxygen administration is discussed below.)

II. Monitoring Oxygen Administration in the Nursery

Administration of oxygen to infants is indicated by clinical signs of respiratory distress. Of infants born before 37 weeks' gestation, approximately 10% might be expected to develop respiratory distress syndrome (RDS) and require some oxygen therapy during the first 2 weeks of life. Monitoring and regulating oxygen administration to these infants is difficult. It is more difficult because there are no definite upper limits for the safe range of arterial oxygen tension or for maximum duration of oxygen therapy.

Under any circumstances it is desirable to maintain a hemoglobin saturation greater than about 80% but not greater than that necessary to stabilize vital signs during oxygen administration. Because arterial oxygen tension can change very rapidly, even frequent sampling of arterial blood cannot assure against maintenance of levels that are too high or too low. For example, infants continuosly ventilated at constant inspired oxygen concentrations, ventilatory pressures, and respiratory frequencies have been observed to undergo a decrease in arterial PO_2 of as much as 80 torr and then abruptly return to their previous stable levels. Moreover, applying positive pressure to the airway of continuously ventilated infants with severe RDS can drastically change arterial PO_2; an infant ventilated on 30% O_2 without continuous positive airway pressure (CPAP) may have an arterial PO_2 of 100 torr, but on 40% O_2 with CPAP, his arterial PO_2 may quickly exceed 300 torr.

Under such circumstances it is not feasible to obtain serial arterial blood samples frequently and for long periods, either by arterial puncture or via umbilical catheter. Nor can cyanosis be used as an indicator for oxygen administration. Although the fetal hemoglobin dissociation curve is nearly linear between approximately 20% and 80% saturation, it is flat above 90% saturation. Therefore, once an infant on oxygen achieves a healthy color at a PO_2 of about 40 torr (approximately 80% saturation), no further change in color can occur to serve as a warning that an even higher PO_2 of as much as 400 torr has been achieved.

It is therefore unfortunate that there exists today no completely reliable method for continuous or even very frequent monitoring of arterial PO_2 level during prolonged periods of oxygen administration. Even if one did exist, the problem of what limits might safely be set on oxygen administration to avoid development of RLF has not yet been solved.

D. Oxygen Interaction with Other Drugs

I. Anti-Inflammatory Agents

The same preliminary study (FLOWER et al. 1981) suggests that aspirin administration, at a dosage producing plasma levels within the human therapeutic range, enhances the severity of oxygen-induced RLF in the puppy eye. Since the data in young puppies may not be directly applicable to human infants, specific clinical recommendations are not yet justified. However, these preliminary animal data, if confirmed independently by other investigators, should alert investigators using prostaglandin synthesis inhibitors to arrest labor or close the patent ductus to examine and possibly test this concept.

II. Antioxidants in Retrolental Fibroplasia

1. α-Tocopherol

The use of vitamin E (α-tocopherol) in the prevention of RLF was first advocated by OWENS and OWENS in the late 1940s. Although their initial controlled studies showed a protective effect, these observations were not repeatable as other investigators tested the prophylactic use of vitamin E (OWENS and OWENS 1949). Its use was discontinued in the early 1950s.

The rationale of therapy by OWENS and OWENS was based on the known deficiency of α-tocopherol in small premature infants, and the experimental findings in animals of a cerbral degeneration that developed in vitamin-E-deficient animals. At the time of the OWENS' nursery studies the role of oxygen in RLF was unknown, and the possible "antioxidant" protective effect of vitamin E was not considered. Some 20 years later, JOHNSON and co-workers initiated a nursery study utilizing α-tocopherol acetate by parenteral injection as a possible agent in the prevention, and also in the treatment, of early active RLF (JOHNSON et al. 1974; SCHAFFER and JOHNSON 1979). PHELPS and ROSENBAUM (1979), utilizing the experimental RLF model in kittens, demonstrated a protective effect of large doses of parenteral vitamin E. JOHNSON and her co-workers and PHELPS and co-workers are at present conducting controlled clinical trials in the nursery to test the prophylactic role of vitamin E administration.

Recently, PUKLIN et al. (1982) have reported on a controlled clinical trial involving 100 neonates who received intramuscular vitamin E injection. These infants received the vitamin during the acute phase of therapy for the RDS. Additional intramuscular doses were administered twice weekly to these infants as long as they remained in an oxygen-enriched environment and could not tolerate feedings and vitamin supplements by mouth. Control infants received intramuscular placebo injections and nutritional multivitamin supplements, including vitamin E. There was no difference noted in the incidence of RLF between the infants receiving vitamin E injections and their controls. The mean level of serum vitamin E in treated infants was significantly elevated over controls. For example, after 1 week the serum level in those infants receiving intramuscular vitamin E was approximately 3.9 mg/100 ml, in contrast to 0.8 mg/100 ml in the placebo group.

HITTNER et al. (1981) reported the results of a controlled clinical trial on the efficacy of 100 mg oral vitamin E per kilo administered daily from birth against RLF in infants who had the RDS. Control infants received 5 mg/kg. Plasma vitamin E levels in those infants on high doses of oral vitamin E averaged approximately 1.2 mg/100 ml, whereas the control group averaged approximately 0.6 mg/100 ml.

Using multivariate analysis, HITTNER's group reported that the severity of RLF was found to be significantly reduced in those infants who received large doses of vitamin E. HILLIS (1982) raised several questions on the statistical design of this study and questioned the data analysis reported. HILLIS cautioned that large doses of vitamin E, just as the high concentrations of oxygen administered in the 1950s, might have as yet unrecognized side effects. It would seem appropriate at this time to await the much larger controlled clinical trials that are being carried out by JOHNSON and co-workers and PHELPS and co-workers before drawing final conclusions on the efficacy of large doses of vitamin E on either the prevention of RLF or reduction in severity of this disease.

2. Superoxide Dismutase

Clinical interest in the occurrence of superoxide dismutase (SOD) in ocular tissues, and particularly in the retina, stems from the well-documented relationship between increased oxygen concentration and incidence of RLF in premature infants. The tolerance of a tissue to hyperoxia is directly related to an increased activity of SOD (FRIDOVICH 1975; CRAPO and TIERNEY 1974; CRAPO and McCORD 1976; CRAPO 1977). In general, gradual exposure to increased oxygen tension leads to tissue damage and death. Thus it was thought that SOD activity in the ocular tissues, particularly the retinas, of premature infants might be too low to deal with the increased oxygen levels to which they were exposed and could result in an increase in the level of damaging free radicals. In support of this suggestion is the recent demonstration (BOUGLE et al. 1980) that SOD levels are significantly lower in the retinas of newborn kittens exposed to ambient oxygen concentrations of 80% for 72 h, sufficient to produce irreversible retinal lesions. This study points out the need to use a suitable model for RLF and the need for exposure to oxygen for a sufficient length of time to observe gross retinal damage and effects on SOD levels (FRIED and MANDEL 1975).

Superoxide dismutases are enzymes which are found in all aerobic cells. They catalyze the dismutation of the superoxide anion radical, or simply superoxide, O_2^- (McCORD and FRIDOVICH 1968). The reaction catalyzed is:

$$O_2^- + O_2^- + 2H^+ \rightarrow H_2O_2 + O_2.$$

Cells evolved SOD in response to the transition from an anaerobic to an aerobic environment (FRIDOVICH 1974, 1978). Oxygen in the ground state is relatively unreactive. However, O_2^- is generated in a number of enzymatic and nonenzymatic reactions (FRIDOVICH 1975). The cytotoxic effects of O_2^- are numerous and include the generation of hydrogen peroxide (H_2O_2), inactivation of enzymes by oxidation of sulfhydryl ($-SH$) groups, formation of lipid peroxides, and the generation of the hydroxyl free radical (OH·) and of singlet oxygen $^1O_2^*$ (HALLIWELL 1978). Hydroxyl radicals are among the most reactive species known to organic chemistry, and will attack and damage almost every molecule found in living cells. Singlet oxygen, too, can oxidize many biomolecules. Thus, although superoxide is itself harmful to the cell, its real danger seems to lie in its ability to form OH· and singlet oxygen. The best protection for the cell lies in the rapid removal of the precursor (O_2^-) of these highly reactive substances. The dismutation reaction, which occurs spontaneously in the absence of SOD, is accelerated by a factor of 10^4 in the presence of this enzyme. Thus SOD appears to be the first line of defense against oxygen-free radicals, and the cell protects itself by keeping the steady-state level of O_2^- infinitesimally small ($\approx 10^{-10} M$) (FRIDOVICH 1975).

A major molecular species considered to be highly vulnerable to damage by free radicals are the polyunsaturated fatty acids (PUFAs) of cell membranes. The retinal phospholipids, and particularly those of the photoreceptor cell outer segment, contain a high level of these PUFAs, particularly docosahexaenoic acid (ANDERSON and MAUDE 1970), which appear to be extremely important in the maintenance of photoreceptor structure and function (WHEELER et al. 1975). It has been shown that exposure of frog retinas to light results in the accumulation of free radical oxidation products in the lipids of the photoreceptors (KAGAN et al. 1973). Additionally, the action spectrum of this process is similar to the absorption spectrum of rhodopsin, indicating that this photopigment might itself participate in the production of damaging free radicals. Thus intuitive reasoning would suggest that the retina, which is (a) highly vascularized, (b) contains high levels of PUFAs, (c) is enzymatically active, (d) has a high level of oxygen consumption, and (e) is known to be extremely susceptible to oxygen damage, would contain the enzyme SOD. The presence of SOD in the whole retina was first shown by FRIED and MANDEL (1975) and was later confirmed by other investigators (HALL and HALL 1975; CROUCH et al. 1978; BHUYAN and BHUYAN 1978). Of particular interest is the high concentration of this enzyme in the photoreceptor cell outer segment (HALL and HALL 1975), the part of the photoreceptor cell which contains the highest levels of PUFAs and, of course, rhodopsin. By keeping the levels of the superoxide anion (generated by the action of light and oxygen) extremely low in the outer segment, SOD would protect the functionally significant PUFAs and enzymes essential for the transduction process from damage by free radical oxidation. It has been suggested (RILEY and SLATER 1969; SLATER and RILEY 1970) that peroxidation of the membrane lipids in the developing retina, in the presence of a high oxygen concentration and light, may be sufficient to start the vasoobliterative phase of RLF.

As expected from its ubiquitous distribution, SOD is present in numerous other ocular tissues (CROUCH et al. 1978; BHUYAN and BHUYAN 1978). Although it is reported to be absent from bovine cornea (CROUCH et al. 1978), it is present in the corneal epithelium and endothelium of the rabbit (BHUYAN and BHUYAN 1978). This enzyme shows the highest specific activity in well-vascularized ocular tissues such as the iris, ciliary body, retina, and choroid, while its levels are lower in the avascular structures such as the cornea and lens. Since the toxic effect of ionizing radiation in animals is partly due to the formation of O_2^- (PETKAU 1978; MISRA and FRIDOVICH 1976), it is possible that the susceptibility of the lens to radiation cataracts is in part due to the low level of SOD in this tissue.

3. Other Antioxidants

Brief mention must also be made of other mechanisms which have been developed by cells to protect themselves against damage by O_2^-, $OH \cdot$, and singlet oxygen. These are the antioxidants glutathione and ascorbic acid (vitamin C). Glutathione exerts its protective effect by preferentially reacting with oxygen, as well as by reactivating enzymes damaged by high oxygen tension. Ascorbic acid reacts rapidly with both O_2^- and $OH \cdot$ (Allen and Hall 1973; Nishikimi 1975), while α-tocopherol (discussed earlier) is a powerful scavenger of singlet oxygen, as are other carotenoids. The retina is rich in all of these antioxidants, while the aqueous is rich in ascorbic acid, and the lens contains large concentrations of both ascorbic acid and glutathione. It thus appears that ocular tissues have evolved both enzymatic and chemical systems to protect them against oxygen toxicity.

E. Conclusions

The immature retina exhibits a striking susceptibility to toxic alteration by oxygen at ambient pressure. The combination of light and high oxygen concentrations may augment responsiveness of the retina to oxygen. Recent interest in the antioxidant vitamin E has prompted both clinical and experimental studies on the possible role of this agent in the prevention and therapy of retrolental fibroplasia. Clinical trials now under way should soon provide a clear answer to the potential therapeutic role of large doses of supplemental vitamin E for the premature infant.

References

Allen JF, Hall DO (1973) Superoxide reduction as mechanism of ascorbate-stimulated oxygen uptake by isolated chloroplasts. Biochem Biophys Res Commun 52:856–862

Anderson RE, Maude MB (1970) Phospholipids of bovine rod outer segments. Biochemistry 9:3624–3628

Ashton N, Cook C (1954) Direct observations of the effect of oxygen on developing vessels: preliminary report. Br J Ophthalmol 38::433–440

Ashton N, Peddler C (1962) Studies on developing retinal vessels: IX. Reaction of endothelial cells to oxygen. Br J Ophthalmol 46:257–276

Ashton N, Ward B, Serpell G (1953) Role of oxygen in the genesis of retrolental fibroplasia: a preliminary report. Br J Ophthalmol 37:513– 520

Beehler CC, Newton NL, Culver JF, Tredici TJ (1968) Retinal detachment in adult dogs resulting from oxygen toxicity. Arch Ophthalmol 79:759–762

Bhuyan KC, Bhuyan G (1978) Superoxide dismutase of the eye: relative functions of superoxide dismutase and catalase in protecting the ocular lens from oxidative damage. Biochem Biophys Acta 542:28–38

Bill A (1975) Ocular circulation. In: Moses RA (ed) Adler's physiology of the eye, 6th edn. Mosby, St. Louis, pp 210–231

Bougle D, Vert P, Reichert E, Hartemann D (1980) Retrolental fibroplasia and retinal superoxide in kittens. Lancet I:268

Campbell K (1951) Intensive oxygen therapy as a possible cause of retrolental fibroplasia: a clinical approach. Med J Aust 2:48–50

Crapo JD (1977) The role of the superoxide dismutases in pulmonary oxygen toxicity. In: Michelson AM, McCord JM, Fridovich I (eds) Superoxide and superoxide dismutases. Academic, New York, pp 231–238

Crapo JD, McCord JM (1976) O_2-induced changes in pulmonary superoxide dismutase assayed by antibody titrations. Am J. Physiol 231:1196–1203

Crapo JD, Tierney DG (1974) Superoxide dismutase and pulmonary oxygen toxicity. Am J Physiol 226:1401–1407

Crouch R, Priest DG, Duke EJ (1978) Superoxide dismutase activities of bovine ocular tissues. Exp Eye Res 27:503–509

Dollery CT, Hill DW, Mailer CM, Ramalho PS (1964) High oxygen pressure and the retinal blood vessels. Lancet II:291–294

Dollery CT, Bulpitt CJ, Kohner EM (1969) Oxygen supply to the retina from the retinal and choroidal circulation at normal and increased arterial oxygen tensions. Invest Ophthalmol 8:588–594

Fischer FP (1930) Über den Gasaustausch der Hornhaut mit der Luft. Arch Augenheilkd 102:146–164

Flower RW, Patz A (1971) The effect of hyperbaric oxygenation on retinal ischemia. Invest Ophthal 10:605–616

Flower RW, Speros P, Kenyon KR (1977) Electroretinographic changes and choroidal defects in a case of central retinal artery occlusion. Am J Ophthal 83:451–459

Flower RW, Blake DA, with Wajer SD, Egner PG, McLeod DS, Pitts SM (1981) Retrolental fibroplasia: evidence for a role of the prostaglandin cascade in the pathogenesis of oxygen-induced retinopathy in the newborn beagle. Pediatr Res 15:1293–1302

Frazier R, Hickam JB (1965) Effect of vasodilator drugs on retinal blood-flow in man. Arch Ophthalmol 73:640–642

Frazier R, Saltzman HA, Anderson B, Hickam JB, Sieker HO (1967) The effect of hyperbaric oxygenation on retinal circulation. Arch Ophthalmol 77:265–269

Fridovich I (1974) Superoxide and evolution. Horiz Biochem Biophys 1:1–37

Fridovich I (1975) Superoxide dismutases. Annu Rev Biochem 44:147–159

Fridovich I (1978) Superoxide radicals, superoxide dismutases and the aerobic lifestyle. Photochem Photobiol 28:733–741

Fried R, Mandel P (1975) Superoxide dismutase of mammalian nervous system. J Neurochem 24:533–438

Hall MO, Hall DO (1975) Superoxide dismutase in bovine and frog rod outer segments. Biochem Biophys Res Commun 67:1199–1204

Halliwell B (1978) Biochemical mechanisms accounting for the toxic action of oxygen on living organisms: the key role of superoxide dismutase. Cell Biol Int Rep 2:113–128

Hickam JB, Frazier R (1965) A photographic method for measuring the mean retinal circulation time using fluorescein. Invest Ophthalmol 4:876–884

Hickam JB, Frazier R, Ross JC (1963) A study of retinal venous blood oxygen saturation in human subjects by photographic means. Circulation 27:375–385

Hillis A (1982) Vitamin E in retrolental fibroplasia. Correspondence. N Engl J Med 306:866–867

Hittner HM, Godio LB, Rudolph AJ, et al. (1981) Retrolental fibroplasia: efficacy of vitamin E in a double-blind clinical study of preterm infants. N Engl J Med 305/23:1365–1371

Johnson L, Schaffer D, Boggs TR (1974) The premature infant, vitamin E deficiency and retrolental fibroplasia. Am J Clin Nutr 27:1158–1173

Kagan VE, Shvedova AA, Novikov KN, Koslov YP (1973) Light induced free radical oxidation of membrane lipids in photoreceptors of frog retina. Biochem Biophys Acta 330:76–79

Kinsey VE, Jacobus T, Hemphill FM (1956) Retrolental fibroplasia. Cooperative study of retrolental fibroplasia and the use of oxygen. Arch Ophthalmol 56:481–543

Kinsey VE, Arnold HJ, Kalina RE, Stern L, Stahlman M, Odell G, Driscoll JM Jr, Elliott JH, Payne JW, Patz A (1977) P_aO_2 levels and retrolental fibroplasia: a report of the cooperative study. Pediatrics 60:665–668

Krogh A (1929) The anatomy and physiology of the capillary. Yale University Press, New Haven

Margolis G (1966) Hyperbaric oxygenation: the eye as a limiting factor. Science 151::466–468

McCord JM, Fridovich I (1968) Reduction of cytochrome c by milk xanthine oxidase. J Biol Chem 243:5753–5760

Misra HP, Fridovich I (1976) Superoxide dismutase and the O_2 enhancement of radiation lethality. Arch Biochem Biophys 176:577–581

Nishikimi M (1975) Oxidation of ascorbic acid with O_2 generated by the xanthine-xanthine oxidase system. Biochem Biophys Res Commun 63:463–468

Noell WK (1955) Metabolic injuries of visual cells. Am J Ophthalmol 40:60–70

Owens WC, Owens EU (1949) Retrolental fibroplasia in premature infants. II. Studies on the prophylaxis of the disease: use of alpha-tocopherol acetate. Am J Ophthalmol 32:1631–1637

Patz A (1954) Clinical and experimental studies on the role of oxygen in retrolental fibroplasia. Trans Am Acad Ophthalmol Otolaryngol 58:45–50

Patz A (1955) Oxygen inhalation in retinal arterial occlusion: preliminary report. Am J Ophthalmol 40:789–795

Patz A, Hoeck LE, de La Cruz E (1952) Studies on the effect of high oxygen administration in retrolental fibroplasia: nursery observations. Am J Ophthalmol 35:1248–1253

Patz A, Eastham A, Higgenbotham DH, Kleh T (1953) Oxygen studies in retrolental fibroplasia: production of the microscopic changes of retrolental fibroplasia in experimental animals. Am J Ophthalmol 36:1511–1522

Petkau A (1978) Radiation protection by superoxide dismutase. Photochem Photobiol 28:765–774

Phelps DL, Rosenbaum AL (1979) Vitamin E in kitten oxygen-induced retinopathy. II. Blockage of vitreal neovascularization. Arch Ophthalmol 97:1522–1526

Puklin JE, Simon RM, Ehrenkranz RA (1982) Influence on retrolental fibroplasia of intramuscular vitamin E administration during respiratory distress syndrome. Ophthalmol 89:96–102

Ramalho PS, Dollery CT (1968) Hypertensive retinopathy: caliber changes in retinal blood vessels following blood-pressure reduction and inhalation of oxygen. Circulation 37:580–588

Riley PA, Slater TF (1969) Pathogenesis of retrolental fibroplasia. Lancet II:265

Schaffer DB, Johnson L (1979) A classification of retrolental fibroplasia to evaluate vitamin E therapy. Ophthalmology 86:1749–1760

Slater TF, Riley PA (1970) Free-radical damage in retrolental fibroplasia. Lancet II:467

Turnbull W (1950) Experimental retinal anemia in rats. Arch Ophthalmol 43:9–31

Weiter JJ, Zuckerman R (1979) Oxygen transport in the retina. Invest Ophthalmol Vis Sci [ARVO Suppl]:53

Wheeler TG, Benolken RM, Anderson RE (1975) Visual membranes: specificity of fatty acid precursors for the electrical response to illumination. Science 188:1312–1314

Wolbarsht ML, Landers MB III (1980) The rationale of photocoagulation therapy for proliferative diabetic retinopathy: a review and a model. Ophthalmic Surg 11:235–245

CHAPTER 15

The Aliphatic Alcohols

A. M. Potts

A. General

What may be called the "organic solvent properties" of the aliphatic alcohols manifest themselves in higher animals in narcosis and, eventually, death. These properties become more manifest with increasing length of the aliphatic chain (VON OETTINGEN 1943; MARDONES 1963). In this series ethanol has a special place. Its relatively high ratio of lethal to pharmacologic dose has led to its use and abuse throughout recorded history (cf. Gen. 9.20–21). Only with ethanol has reliable investigation been done on human subjects. Extensive studies of sublethal dose effects have been recorded. It has become clear that the organic solvent properties which ethanol shares with the other aliphatic alcohols and many other small organic molecules is the ability to act selectively on the central nervous system.

The physicochemical mechanism of this action still escapes us, but not from lack of attention to the problem. Pharmacologists concerned with the mechanism of anesthesia have done much experimentation with small organic molecules. Ethanol has frequently been included in the series of test substances. For relatively current work on anesthetics see the review of ROTH (1979). The review of KALANT (1971) deals with ethanol itself.

Some aspects are fairly well worked out. The postsynaptic membrane appears to be the only site where ethanol and anesthetics block neurotransmission at concentrations comparable to those that are attained after pharmacologic doses. It requires higher concentrations to block axonal conduction. Beyond this point all postulated mechanisms are speculative. There is no lack of speculation, but firm experimental evidence awaits the creative investigator.

Since so much of the central nervous system is dedicated to the eye and visual function, it is not astounding that there is a sizable catalog of effects of ethanol on the eye and vision. Since we are necessarily dealing with complex systems in the absence of a unifying theory, we must be content with a catalog only.

This work was supported in part by USPHS Research Grant Number EY 01591 from the National Eye Institute, National Institutes of Health, Bethesda, Maryland

B. Ocular Effects of Single Doses of Ethanol in Nonhabituated Individuals

I. Muscle Balance

The consensus is that at least for distance experimental doses of ethanol in humans cause esophoria (POWELL 1938; COLSON 1940; BRECHER et al. 1955). One of these workers (POWELL 1938) found exophoria for near vision, but this was not confirmed by the others. They agree with CHARNWOOD (1951) that there is no vertical phoria induced by ethanol.

In the experiments of BRECHER et al. (1955), blood alcohol levels were raised as high as 200 mg%. By the time these levels were reached, most of the subjects could not accomplish the fusion task no matter how much time was allowed. This explains and confirms the subjective diplopia reported by intoxicated individuals.

The experiments of COHEN and ALPERN (1969) were directed toward the more complex measurement of the accommodative convergence/accommodation ratio (AC/A). They found a uniform increase in tonic convergence agreeing with the esophoria reported by earlier workers above. They further found a decrease in AC/A ratio with increase in blood alcohol level. Since the conditions of the experiment fixed the ammount of accommodative stimulus, this means that accommodative convergence for any given accommodative stimulus must be less under the influence of alcohol than in the normal. This lower response to an accommodative stimulus is not the same physiological entity as the esophoria measured at a fixed distance by previous investigators, and is therefore not paradoxical.

II. Extraocular Muscles in Action

Still another task in which the extraocular muscles participate is the fixation of a moving target. If the motion of the target is rapid, the eye must make a rapid motion (saccade) to fix the target in its new position. If the target is moving slowly enough, it may be tracked by a smooth following movement. On the basis of measurement of velocity and acceleration patterns, there is reason to believe that saccadic and smooth following movements are mediated by different neural mechanisms.

A special situation in which both smooth following and saccadic movement play a role is optokinetic nystagmus. Unlike vestibular and other forms of neurogenic nystagmus (see Sect. B.III), optokinetic nystagmus is partially under voluntary control. In the most common testing situation, a striped drum is rotated relatively slowly before the eyes of the subject. The cooperative subject will fix a stripe on the drum and follow the stripe until it disappears around the edge of the drum (slow following); he will then rapidly refixate a new stripe (saccade) and follow it until it disappears. By measuring optokinetic responses to a series of stripe velocities, this system, whose final pathway is also the extraocular muscles, can be explored.

The literature contains studies of ocular motility influenced by ethanol under very specialized conditions, but all these studies are consonant with one another. DRISCHEL (1968) recorded the ability of the eye to follow a horizontally oscillating (projected) checkerboard target whose velocity changed sinusoidally. Over the frequency range 0.3–4 Hz the eyes of the subject could track easily at lower frequencies but were unable to track at the high-frequency end of the range. When amplitude versus frequency and phase angle versus frequency were plotted before and after administration of alcohol, it was found that amplitude decreased and phase-angle separation increased even at blood alcohol levels (BAL) of 30 mg%. At 90 mg% both effects were much more marked.

MIZOI et al. (1969) used optokinetic nystagmus elicited by a set of stripes whose speed accelerated $1°/s^2$ over 125 s, i.e., during the test time the rate of the stimulus increased from 0° to 125° per second. The slow phase of optokinetic nystagmus was measured electrically, and it was found that in the normal subject the total breakdown of ability to perform the task was preceded by a set of responses where the velocity of the slow phase fluctuated widely. The beginning of this phenomenon was taken as the point of measurement. The velocity of the eye in the slow phase at this point was reduced by 28% in 24 subjects who had BAL of 41–89 mg%.

Both smooth following movements (pendulum moving through 45° of visual angle) and maximum saccadic velocity were investigated by WILKINSON et al. (1974). With their doses, maximum BALs reached 80 mg% (average six subjects), and peak saccadic velocities were reduced by 20% in relation to controls. Errors on smooth following movements were scored for the pendulum task, which could be performed flawlessly before alcohol. Blood alcohol levels of 100 mg% made subjects commit large numbers of errors.

The task posed in the experiments of FRANCK and KUHLO (1970) was simply to look back and forth between targets placed 10° each side of primary position (straight ahead fixation position). This required a saccade of 20° of visual angle, which reached a maximum velocity in control trials of 460°–338° per second. At BALs of 60–120 mg% there was an average decrease in velocity of 24%.

An earlier report by MILES (1924) required a saccade of 40°. Both adductive and abductive saccades were slowed by a significant amount at a fixed time after a standard dose of alcohol in five subjects.

Still another parameter of saccadic movement was explored by LEVETT and HOEFT (1977). These researchers measured the latency between stimulus and response in a saccadic task. One might regard this as ocular reaction time. Once more, in six subjects whose BAL reached 108 mg% on average, there was a mean latency increase of 21%. The authors attribute this to effects on higher centers than the ocular motoneuromuscular system.

In each of the entities examined in this section (smooth following of sinusoidal motion, smooth following in the slow phase of optokinetic nystagmus, maximum saccadic velocity, and the latency of saccadic responses), efficiency of accomplishing the task was impaired by ethanol. The falloff in maximum saccadic velocity could be postulated to be located in the ocular motor nucleus-extraocular muscle system; but when one considers the earlier breakdown of optokinetic tracking (MIZOI et al. 1969), the breakdown of smooth tracking into fragmented saccades (WILKINSON et al. 1974), and the increase of latency of saccadic responses (LEVETT and HOEFT 1977), one is inevitably led to higher centers. The physical location of the necessary servomechanisms to coordinate eye movement is still unknown, but the need for them is real (see, e. g., BACH-Y-RITA et al. 1971), and the participation of cortical vision immediately moves them from brain stem to cortex. The effect of ethanol in lowest concentrations on other cortical functions makes this entirely believable.

III. Nystagmus

"Neurogenic" nystagmus, as differentiated from optokinetic nystagmus on the one hand and pendular nystagmus on the other, is a complex subject. Any competent treatment of the anatomy and physiology involved is well beyond the scope of this review. We must circumvent this complex area by simply defining neurogenic nystagmus as spontaneous rhythmic movement of the eyes, usually bilateral, usually synchronous, usually (but not invariably) horizontal, and exhibiting a fast and a slow component.

It has been known for more than 150 years that alcohol administration can cause this type of nystagmus. For a review of the early literature see Aschan et al. (1956a). The finding is real and it is inconstant. Howells (1956) found nystagmus in 4 of 12 subjects given alcohol (1–1.4 ml/kg). He did not measure BALs. Levett and Hoeft (1977) mention in passing (Fig. 3) the spontaneous nystagmus recorded in one of their six subjects at a BAL of 120 mg%.

Two patients have been reported by Bender and Gorman (1949) and one patient by Kroll (1969) who had spontaneous vertical nystagmus. They all had oscillopsia (the sensation of the world moving) as well. All three patients experienced relief of symptoms after receiving generous doses of alcohol. However, the two patients of Bender and Gorman were confirmed severe alcoholics with encephalopathy. The patient of Kroll disclaimed heavy drinking but required one-half to a whole pint of 80°–90° proof liquor to get relief from his nystagmus for a few hours. He had noticed this effect 4 months prior to his clinic visit. If his drinking was truly of only 4 months' duration, he could not be considered an alcoholic. One can go no further with this paradoxical effect at present.

Most curious of all is the well-authenticated entity, positional alcohol nystagmus. For an adequate exposition of this entity see the work of Aschan et al. (1956 a, b). An individual with medium BALs may show no nystagmus in primary position with eyes open. However, with eyes closed or with occlusive lenses, the act of turning from supine to lateral position induces horizontal nystagmus. Early after ingestion of alcohol the nystagmus has its fast component downward-turned (called "PAN I" by the Aschan group). Some 4 h after ingestion there is a period of inconstant response that lasts an hour or so; then the direction of the nystagmus reverses and the fast component is now upward (PAN II). PAN I appears within 30 min of ingestion at BALs of as little as 38 mg%. PAN II appears on the descending arm of the BAL curve and appears at an average BAL of 20 mg%. PAN II lasts after there is no detectable blood alcohol. Indeed, Hill et al. (1973) report than PAN II can last 15–16 h after the ingestion of 2.5 ml/kg of 100° proof liquor, which attained a maximum BAL of 90–100 mg% at 1 h. By their alcohol dehydrogenase determination, BAL was undetectable at 24 h. However, in some subjects they found some PAN I response at 24–32 h.

Clearly we have here one of the most sensitive physiological responses to alcohol intake. de Kleyn and Versteegh (1930) showed by ablation experiments that PAN in rabbits was dependent upon the presence of the labyrinths, not the saccules. This suggests that there is a vestibular stimulus via the median longitudinal fasciculus to the brain stem nuclei controlling the oculorotatory muscles whenever a head turn occurs. Under normal circumstances this stimulus, which must be a weak one, is counteracted by the stronger stabilizing forces of vision and of unidentified cortical centers. When vision is nullified by closing the eyes and when the unspecified cortical centers are inhibited by ethanol, the vestibular message can elicit a response. The idea that the alcohol effect can persist long after alcohol has disappeared from the body is truly impressive. It makes one wish to philosophize on the mechanism of this minihangover. One must take note of the opinion of MONEY and MYLES (1974), based on their findings with heavy water, that PAN is entirely due to density changes of the endolymph in relation to the cupula. They suggest that the cupula is more dense than the endolymph after the ingestion of heavy water and less dense after the ingestion of ethanol. This difference in density allows gravity to activate the labyrinth.

IV. Intraocular Muscles

1. The Iris

The relatively meager work on alcohol and pupil size is all based on low BALs. SKOGLUND'S (1943) four subjects received 15 ml 50% ethanol. Moderate dilation of the pupil measured from 16-mm frames was reported. However, BROWN et al. (1977), who raised BALs to 60 mg%, found no effect on pupillary size in their patients. In SKOGLUND'S studies, even though there was modest pupil dilation there was no effect of alcohol on the rate of response to light for that pupil size.

2. Accommodation

The experimental data available on the effect of alcohol on accommodation are confined to the time required to accommodate or relax accomodation by 2 diopters (LEVETT and KARRAS 1977). Objective measurement (presumably of the third Purkinje image) showed slowing of the time required; the higher the BAL, the greater the slowing.

V. Electrophysiological Measurements

By employing electrophysiological methods, we are making use of precision instruments, but the biological interpretation of results leaves something to be desired. The a wave of the electroretinogram (ERG) does precede the optic nerve discharge (OND), but it requires stimuli at least 3 log units more intense than the dark-adapted threshold to allow it to be recorded. What is triggering the optic nerve through those 3 log units? The b wave of the ERG peaks long after the OND has passed; thus the b wave can only be an after potential reflecting some aspects of the retinal response. The c wave of the ERG is intimately connected with the direct current potential across the eyeball. It is elicited only by stimuli of long duration 0,5–1 s).

An early and frequently quoted report is that of BERNHARD and SKOGLUND (1941). However, this work was done on the open eyecup of the frog, and 10%

ethanol gave the best effect. Such a concentration is two orders of magnitude higher than the 100 mg% BAL which produced the effects we have been discussing until now. This must necessarily be ignored. In a similar preparation, 200 mg% ethanol in the excised opened frog eyecup decreased lateral inhibition of the receptor field of individual ganglion cells to microelectrode recording. The latency of the response was increased (BÄCKSTRÖM 1977).

A single dose of 15 g ethanol per kilogram given by stomach tube caused rapid coma in cats and rabbits and eventual death, but at 2 h the b wave (200 µV at zero time) was abolished (PRAGLIN et al. 1955).

When the test object was the dark-adapted sheep and the stimulus 5 log units above b-wave threshold, BALs had to be raised to 140 mg% before a 15% decrease in a-wave and b-wave amplitude was observed. A BAL of 200 mg% caused a 22% decrease in a-wave and b-wave amplitude (BERNHARD et al. 1973).

VAN NORREN and PADMOS (1977) recorded the ERG in the monkey and paid particular attention to the first component – the cone contribution – of the b wave. The large effects of ethanol at 300 mg% (estimated) and of a number of inhalation anesthetics were to increase the latency of the cone component.

It is the consensus that alcohol increases the amplitude of the c wave of the ERG in sheep (KNAVE et al. 1974) and increases the amplitude of c wave oscillations with time in humans (SKOOG 1974), as well as the low-amplitude components of the off-effect (SKOOG et al. 1978). One must take cognizance of the report in one of the above papers (SKOOG 1974) of a moderate increase in b wave amplitude after alcohol in man with no change in a wave. However, the author is vague about correlating these effects with BALs. This finding agrees with that of IKEDA (1963) and partially with that of JACOBSON et al. (1969), who found an increase in amplitude of both a wave and b wave, and is contrary to the sheep data of BERNHARD et al. (1973) above.

The visually evoked response (VER) is recorded from the occipital scalp or from occipital-parietal scalp electrodes. Adequate stimuli are flashes of light, or checkerboard or bar patterns that reverse black for white and vice versa. Because each response is of the same order of magnitude as the ongoing electrical noise, it is usual to summate 100–200 responses synchronously with the stimulus, using a special-purpose or general-purpose computer. The summated response is easily read. If one considers the response to a full-field flash, perhaps 50% of the amplitude is due to the fovea centralis and the surrounding 1° of macula. Thus the VER with proper stimuli can be an adequate objective measure of visual acuity. Optic nerve disease causes increased latency of the occipital response. A great obstacle to widespread use of the VER for objective measurements is the wide variation between individuals in amplitude and configuration. If one wishes to compare a hypothetically injured eye to a fellow eye known to be normal, one is on safe ground. When both eyes are in question, the usefulness of the VER drops precipitously. However, in human experiments where each subject is his own control, as before and after alcohol administration, valid conclusions should be attainable.

The earliest report on alcohol and the VER after IKEDA (1963) used visual summation on a storage oscilloscope is that of MÜLLER and HAASE (1967). Blood alcohol levels were not measured but peak time of the major response was nearly doubled, so it is reasonable to believe that the finding is valid even with the inadequate instrumentation. Using summation of 100 responses of nine subjects to full-field flash on a PDP-9 computer, LEWIS et al. (1970) showed diminution in amplitude of the major components. This required 85 ml 95% ethanol, which produced blood levels of 70–100 mg%. This was confirmed by RHODES et al. (1975).

Only VAN LITH and VIJFVINKEL-BRUINENGA (1978) used alcoholics with initially subnormal VERs to a reversing-pattern stimulus as subjects. These individuals had further decrease in amplitude as well as increase in latency after 200 ml 35% ethanol.

It would seem that in normals the decrease in amplitude of the major components of the VER is a repeatable finding.

VI. Miscellaneous Measurements of Visual Function

One must deal here with the report of NEWMAN and FLETCHER (1941), who measured seven aspects of visual function in 50 subjects before and after alcohol administration. Blood alcohol levels ranged from 58 to 218 mg%. Neither investigator was an ophthalmologist. The tests and results follow:

1. Visual acuity (Keystone Telebinocular): 22% of subjects showed a drop of 20% or more in acuity after alcohol.
2. Depth perception (Keystone Telebinocular): 12% of subjects showed a 20% or more decrease in depth perception.
3. Distance judgment (Howard-Dohlman test): 18% showed 25-mm error in rod positioning after alcohol.
4. Lateral visual field (Brombach Perimeter). Used 20-mm white target. Only one subject showed 10° (?) narrowing of field.
5. Eye coordination (Keystone Telebinocular). "Used experience and judgment." Eighteen percent of subjects were judged to have major changes in this parameter.
6. Glare resistance (special apparatus from University of California, Berkeley): 12 of 50 subjects showed major changes.
7. Glare recovery (another special apparatus from University of California, Berkeley): 20% of subjects had major adverse changes.

The problem with this report is that there is no correlation between positive findings and BAL for the subject. Further, there is no tendency for a particular subject to have many changes and another subject to have few. Changes are scattered at random in relation to subject and in relation to BAL. For visual acuity decrease it was more than twice as likely for one eye to be affected as for both eyes. One is therefore likely to be dealing with some effect other than alcohol in this report. It is profitless to speculate at this distance on what the factor might be.

There is some confirming evidence on items 1 and 7. BRECHER et al. (1955) mention that 3 of 14 subjects showed decrease in visual acuity at higher alcohol levels. In their case this was 160–200 mg%.

The decreased visual acuity after alcohol in two subjects reported by MILES (1924) was small enough to be of questionable significance. At least it was in the same direction as the other reports.

Of the two more recent reports on glare recovery, one reports a glare recovery time shortened at BAL 21–142 mg% (TIBURTIUS et al. 1966). The second report describes glare recovery lengthened after ethanol dose that raised BAL to 60 mg% in 1 h (ADAMS et al. 1978). One can hardly draw conclusions on the data available.

In the same miscellaneous category is the light threshold increase of 30% in four subjects described by LANGE and SPECHT (JELLINEK and MCFARLAND 1940) and the 50% decrease in the threshold for intensity discrimination (same authors).

GOLDBERG (1943) described an alcohol effect on flicker fusion. At a constant frequency a brighter light was needed for fusion after alcohol. At constant brightness a lower frequency was needed.

VII. Intraocular Pressure

The only firmly established fact is that alcohol does lower the intraocular pressure. All authors are in agreement on that subject (PECZON and GRANT 1965; HOULE and GRANT 1967; RAMOS et al. 1969; OSTBAUM et al. 1973; LEYDHECKER et al. 1978; GIURLANI et al. 1978). It also appears that whereas BAL peaks 30–60 min after a single oral dose, the maximum intraocular-pressure-lowering effect is manifest 1–3 h after alcohol. Beyond this there is no agreement on mechanism of action or dose-dependence of action.

C. The Special Case of Disulfiram (Antabuse)

The principal pathway for the metabolism of ethanol is oxidation to acetaldehyde and thence to acetate. The first oxidation is catalyzed by alcohol dehydrogenase with NAD as cofactor. The second step is catalyzed by aldehyde oxidase and NAD is again the coenzyme involved. Inhibitors of aldehyde oxidase allow the accumulation of acetaldehyde in someone who has imbibed ethanol, and marked symptoms can result. Headache, flushing of the face, hyperventilation, increase in pulse rate, and fall in blood pressure are some of these. For a survey of the types of compounds that have this effect see MALING (1970). The substance that has been utilized in the therapy of alcoholism is tetraethylthiuram disulfide (disulfiram, Antabuse).

$$(C_2H_5)_2-N-\underset{\underset{S}{\|}}{C}-S-S-\underset{\underset{S}{\|}}{C}-N-(C_2H_5)_2$$

introduced by the JACOBSEN group (HALD et al. 1948; HALD and JACOBSEN 1948a; JACOBSEN 1952).

The ocular effect described following the use of alcohol by an individual who has taken disulfiram is scleral injection resulting in a bovine appearance (HALD and JACOBSEN 1948b).

D. Chronic Alcoholism and the Eye

In chronic alcoholism there are two major ways in which the eye is affected. The first of these is the complex constituting the ocular consequences of Wernicke's encephalopathy. The clinical findings include nuclear ocular palsies, internal ophthalmoplegias, ptosis, and nystagmus (DUKE-ELDER and SCOTT 1971). The histo-pathological findings are multiple hemorrhages with glial reaction, particularly in the gray matter surrounding the third ventricle (DE WARDENER and LENNOX 1947). Although the condition was originally ascribed to the direct toxicity of ethanol, it is now agreed that the proximal cause is thiamine deficiency (PHILLIPS et al. 1952; DREYFUS and VICTOR 1961). Such an indirect effect need not be considered further.

The second entity is alcohol (tobacco-alcohol) amblyopia. It is universally recognized that some chronic alcoholics present clinically with blurred or decreased central vision; that the chief additional finding is central or cecocentral scotoma in the visual field examination; and that beyond a certain point temporal pallor of the optic nerve head sets in, and the loss of central vision is irreversible. For multiple case histories see VICTOR et al. (1960). Histopathological examination shows loss of the papillomacular bundle, beginning with the perifoveal ganglion cells and traceable through optic nerve and chiasm to the lateral geniculate nucleus (VICTOR et al. 1960; VICTOR and DREYFUS 1965). Amblyopia in chronic alcoholics had been accepted as a phenomenon of alcohol toxicity until relatively recently (GALEZOWSKI 1978; DE SCHWEINITZ 1896; LEWIN and GUILLERY 1913). Only with the work of CARROLL (1944) has strong clinical evidence been produced which places tobacco-alcohol amblyopia in the category of nutritional deficiency diseases. For more recent publications see the review by POTTS (1973) and the paper of VICTOR et al. (1960). The weight of evidence is tipping strongly toward B_{12}-deficiency as the direct cause for the appearance of the symptom complex in alcoholics. The indirect cause is the deficient diet which alcoholics get. When most of their calories are supplied by alcohol, vitamin intake is insufficient. Thus this second eye disease seen in alcoholics is also not a direct pharmacologic effect of ethanol and need not be treated further.

E. Methanol

Methanol, the one-carbon member of the aliphatic alcohol series, has organic solvent properties as do the other members. One pharmacologic measure of this is systemic toxicity in mice. The LD_{50} is 11 g/kg in white mice. At this dosage level deep narcosis (another organic solvent property) is observable within a few minutes of injection. When 2 g ethanol per kilogram is added to methanol dosage, the LD_{50} for methanol is reduced to 5 g/kg. The more toxic and higher-molecular-weight ethanol lowers requirements for LD_{50} from 343 mmol/kg for methanol alone to 199 mmol total alcohols per kilogram when ethanol is added (GILGER et al. 1952).

When one considers methanol toxicity in humans and other primates, the picture is complicated by the fact that there are two additional and potentially lethal mechanisms at work. One of the two is systemic acidosis, which is a constant factor. Part of the acidosis is attributable to formate production, but calculation shows that even if 100% of a lethal dose of methanol were converted to formate, there would not be enough acid to reach the levels observed. There must be additional metabolic acidosis at work (VAN SLYKE and PALMER 1920; POTTS 1955).

The second additional factor is the effect on the central nervous system. This is seen in the effect on the retina, which is manifested in early retinal edema and early nerve head edema (ophthalmoscopy), and in late optic atrophy. A further effect on the central nervous system is necrosis of the caudate nucleus and putamen, described in humans by Orthner (1950) and in monkeys by Potts et al. (1955).

The existence of these facts makes the conditions for the investigation of methanol effects very different from those for ethanol. The organic solvent effect with methanol is much weaker than that for ethanol, so quite large doses are required to demonstrate it (recall the LD_{50} for mice of 11 g/kg). The additional effects mentioned above (metabolic acidosis and central nervous system damage) are obtainable with considerably lower doses of methanol. Since both effects are potentially fatal, there is in actuality little possibility of studying the effect of methanol in humans. In cases of accidental poisoning the saving of life is the first consideration. Thus there has been no opportunity to study subtle effects of methanol on the human eye such as those reported for ethanol. However, with the introduction of the monkey as a test animal (Gilger and Potts 1955), it became possible to study methanol toxicity in primates with the triple ramifications outlined above. All evidence presented so far suggests strongly that there is direct parallelism between methanol poisoning in the monkey and in man and that this parallelism does not exist between man and subprimates. The very confusing older literature on subprimates is reviewed in detail by Gilger and Potts (1955). For these reasons much of the unequivocal information on methanol poisoning in primates comes from experiments on monkeys, not from experience with humans, but there is enough observation of human disease to confirm that each of the clinical features observed in monkeys has been seen in man.

To go into somewhat greater detail, susceptibility to the organic solvent properties of methanol is shared by primates and nonprimates. If the dose is large enough the animal becomes semicomatose within 30–60 min after an oral dose and never recovers consciousness. Doses that cause this type of death are 11 g/kg parenterally for mice (LD_{50}); 4.75 g/kg orally for rats (LD_{70}); 9–10 g/kg orally für dogs; and 8 g/kg orally für monkeys (*Macaca rhesus*) (Gilger and Potts 1955).

Oral doses of less than half the above (3 g/kg) are fatal for monkeys because of systemic acidosis. The clinical findings in monkeys on 3 g/kg or more were characterized by early transient intoxication, followed by a latent period of almost 24 h during which symptoms were minimal. Then came the onset of dyspnea, asthenia, and collapse. These clinical findings were correlated with a sharp drop in CO_2-combining power of plasma and a rise in urinary output of organic acid. If the acidosis is untreated, death results (Gilger and Potts 1955). The finding of acidosis was confirmed in rhesus and pigtail monkeys by McMartin et al. (1975) and by Clay et al. (1975); only Cooper and Felig (1961) were incapable of reproducing these results.

It is possible to titrate the acid production in a monkey by administering base intravenously. With a little care, blood pH and CO_2 capacity can be maintained within normal limits (Potts 1955). Despite the lack of acidosis the central nervous system sustains damage which is manifested in at least two sites. Early damage is seen ophthalmoscopically as retinal edema and nerve-head edema (Potts 1955). The late manifestation of this same damage is optic atrophy (Potts et al. 1955). Relatively early cogwheel pupil contraction and dilated pupils unreactive to light are observed. Other central nervous system damage seems concentrated in the basal ganglia. It is manifested early in symptoms such as tremor, apraxia, and incoordination of limbs. Later anatomic findings are observable and appear as necrosis in the putamen and caudate nucleus.

The treatment of methanol poisoning is based on human and animal findings. RÖE (1950) and BENTON and CALHOUN (1953) used bicarbonate to combat the acidosis in methanol poisoning. WOOD and BULLER (1904), AGNER et al. (1949), and RÖE (1950) advocated the use of ethanol in methanol poisoning. In rhesus monkeys GILGER et al. (1956) and GILGER et al. (1959) demonstrated ethanol to be life-saving and to prevent central nervous system involvement. The laboratory support for these findings lies in the in vitro demonstration by ZATMAN (1946) and the in vivo demonstration by BARTLETT (1950) that ethanol inhibits the oxidation of methanol. An alternative method of prevention of oxidation of methanol is peritoneal dialysis or hemodialysis. Isolated reports (PFISTER et al. 1966; WENZL et al. 1968) and a review (WINCHESTER et al. 1977) report successful use of dialysis in human methanol poisoning.

It is clear on the basis of the above that methanol must be oxidized to exert its toxic effect. What is still quite unclear is the mechanism by which the toxic effects of methanol are mediated. From studies on in vitro inhibition of retinal metabolism (POTTS and JOHNSON 1952) and studies on the effect of disulfiram on methanol toxicity (GILGER et al. 1952), as well as studies on the electrophysiology of the eye (PRAGLIN et al. 1955), it was demonstrated that of the two oxidation products of methanol, formaldehyde and formate formaldehyde was clearly the more toxic. Free formaldehyde has not been isolated in the tissues of experimental animals, but this is not surprising because a highly active toxic agent might well react with tissue before being detectable chemically. However, the demonstration of formaldehyde in brain tissue by the Falck-Hillarp method has proved equivocal (A. M. POTTS unpublished work). This leads one to ask whether in the oxidation of methanol free formaldehyde ever exists, or whether this oxidation stage is always bound to normal carriers. Further, there have been claims that formate given to monkeys can produce optic nerve edema and dilated fixed pupils (MARTIN-AMAT et al. 1978). No reports of basal ganglion damage have appeared. MARTIN-AMAT et al. (1978) invoke the inhibition of cytochrome oxidase by formate at $10^{-2} M$ levels (NICHOLLS 1975) as a possible mechanism. MAKAR and TEPHLY (1977) can produce acidosis and increase in formate levels in the methanol-treated rat by rendering the animals folate-deficient.

To summarize, methanol has a unique toxic action in humans at a dosage level so low that the effects described above for ethanol never come into play. Methanol can cause blindness and death through several pathological modalities including metabolic acidosis, optic nerve atrophy, and basal ganglion necrosis. The biochemical mechanism for these manifestations is far from clear.

References

Adams AJ, Brown B, Haegerstrom-Portnoy G, Flom MC, Jones RT (1978) Marijuana, alcohol and combined drug effects on the time course of glare recovery. Psychopharmacology 56:81–86

Agner K, Höök O, von Porat B (1949) The treatment of methanol poisoning with ethanol. Q J Stud Alcohol 9:515–522

Aschan G, Bergstedt M, Goldberg L, Laurell L (1956a) Positional nystagmus in man during and after alcohol intoxication. Q J Stud Alcohol 17:381–405

Aschan G, Bergstedt M, Stahle J (1956b) Nystagmography; recording of nystagmus in clinical neuro-otological examinations. Acta Otolaryngol [Suppl] Stockh 129:1–103

Bach-y-Rita P, Collings CC, Hyde JE (1971) The control of eye movements. Academic, New York

Bäckström AC (1977) Effects of alcohol on ganglion cell receptive field properties sensitivity in the frog retina. In: Gross MM (ed) Alcohol intoxication and withdrawal – IIIb studies in alcohol dependence. Plenum, New York, pp 187–208

Bartlett GR (1950) Inhibition of methanol oxidation by ethanol in the rat. Am J Physiol 163:614–618

Bender MB, Gorman WF (1949) Vertical nystagmus on direct forward gaze with vertical oscillopsia. Am J Ophthalmol 32:967–972

Benton CD Jr, Calhoun EP (1953) The ocular effects of methyl alcohol poisoning. Am J Ophthalmol 36:1677–1685

Bernhard CG, Skoglund CR (1941) Selective suppression with ethyl alcohol of inhibition in the optic nerve and of the negative component P III of the electroretinogram. Acta Physiol Scand 2:10–21

Bernhard CG, Knave B, Persson HE (1973) Differential effects of ethyl alcohol on retinal functions. Acta Physiol Scand 88:373–381

Brecher GA, Hartman AP, Leonard DD (1955) Effect of alcohol on binocular vision. Am J Ophthalmol 39:44–52

Brown B, Adams AJ, Haegerstrom-Portnoy G, Jones RT, Flom MC (1977) Pupil size after use of marijuana and alcohol. Am J Ophthalmol 83:350–354

Carroll FD (1944) The etiology and treatment of tobacco-alcohol amblyopia. Am J Ophthalmol 27:713–725; 847–863

Charnwood L (1951) Influence of alcohol on fusion. Br J Ophthalmol 34:733–736

Clay KL, Murphy RC, Watkins WD (1975) Experimental methanol toxicity in the primate: analysis of metabolic acidosis. Toxicol Appl Pharmacol 34:49–61

Cohen MM, Alpern M (1969) Vergence and accomodation VI. The influence of ethanol on the AC/A ratio. Arch Ophthalmol 81:518–525

Colson ZW (1940) Effect of alcohol on vision. Experimental investigation. JAMA 115:1525–1527

Cooper JR, Felig P (1961) The biochemistry of methanol poisoning II. Metabolic acidosis in the monkey. Toxicol Appl Pharmacol 3:202–209

de Kleyn A, Versteegh C (1930) Experimentelle Untersuchungen über den sogenannten Lagenystagmus während akuter Alkoholvergiftung beim Kaninchen. Acta Otolaryngol (Stockh) 14:356–377

de Schweinitz GE (1896) The toxic amblyopias Lea, Philadelphia

de Wardener HE, Lennox B (1947) Cerebral beriberi (Wernicke's encephalopathy). Lancet I:11–17

Dreyfus PM, Victor M (1961) Effects of thiamine deficiency on the cenral nervous system. Am J Clin Nutr 9:414–425

Drischel H (1968) Frequency response of horizontal pursuit movements of the human eye and the influence of alcohol. In: Asratyan EA (ed) Brain reflexes. Elsevier, New York, pp 161–174

Duke-Elder S, Scott GI (1971) Wernicke's encephalopathy. In: Duke-Elder S (ed) A system of ophthalmology, vol 12. Kimpton, London, p 763 ff

Franck MC, Kuhlo W (1970) Die Wirkung des Alkohols auf die raschen Blickzielbewegungen (Saccaden) beim Menschen. Arch Psychiatr Nervenkr 213:238–245

Galezowski X (1878) Des amblyopies et des amauroses toxiques. Asselin, Paris

Gilger AP, Potts Am (1955) Studies on the visual toxicity of methanol V. The role of acidosis in experimental methanol poisoning. Am J Ophthalmol 39:63–86

Gilger AP, Potts AM, Johnson LV (1952) Studies on the visual toxicity of methanol II. The effect of parenterally administered substances on the systemic toxicity of methyl alcohol. AM J Ophthalmol 35:113–126

Gilger AP, Potts AM, Farkas IS (1956) Studies on the visual toxicity of methanol IX. The effect of ethanol on methanol poisoning in the rhesus monkey. Am J Ophthalmol 42:244–252

Gilger AP, Farkas IS, Potts AM (1959) Studies on the visual toxicity of methanol X. Further observations on the ethanol therapy of acute methanol. Am J Ophthalmol 48:153–161

Giurlani B, Obie LG, Petersen CG, Presley DD (1978) Alcohol and open angle glaucoma – influence on detection, IOP, BP/IOP ratios. J Am Optom Assoc 49:409–416

Goldberg L (1943) Quantitative studies on alcohol tolerance in man. Acta Physiol Scand 5 [Suppl]:1–128

Hald J, Jacobsen E (1948 a) The formation of acetaldeyhde in the organism after ingestion of Antabuse (tetraethylthiuramdisulphide) and alcohol. Acta Pharmacol Toxicol 4:305–310

Hald J, Jacobsen E (1948 b) A drug sensitizing the organism to ethyl alcohol. Lancet II:1001–1004

Hald J, Jacobsen E, Larsen V (1948) The sensitizing effect of tetraethylthiuramidisulphide (Antabuse) to ethyl alcohol. Acta Pharmacol Toxicol 4:258–296

Hill RJ, Collins WE, Schroeder DJ (1973) Influence of alcohol on positional nystagmus over 32-hour periods. Ann Oto Rhino Laryngol 82:103–110

Houle RE, Grant WM (1967) Alcohol, vasopressin, and intraocular pressure. Invest Ophthalmol 6:145–154

Howells DE (1956) Nystagmus as a physical sign in alcoholic intoxication. Br Med J 1:1405–1406

Ikeda H (1963) Effects of ethyl alcohol on the evoked potential of the human eye. Vision Res 3:155–169

Jacobsen E (1952) Deaths of alcoholic patients treated with disulfiram (tetraethyl-thiuramdisulfide) in Denmark. Q J Stud Alcohol 13:16–26

Jacobson JH, Hirose T, Stokes PE (1969) Changes in human ERG induced by intravenous alcohol. Ophthalmologica 158 [Suppl]:669–677

Jellinek EM, McFarland RA (1940) Analysis of psychological experiments on the effects of alcohol. Q J Stud Alcohol 1:272–371

Kalant H (1971) Absorption, diffusion, distribution, and elimination of ethanol effects on biological membranes. In: Kissin B, Begleiter H (eds) The biology of alcoholism, vol 1. Plenum, New York, pp 1–62

Knave B, Persson HE, Nilsson SEG (1974) A comparative study on the effects of barbiturate and ethyl alcohol on retinal functions with special reference to the c-wave of the electroretinogram and the standing potential of the sheep eye. Acta Ophthalmol 52:254–259

Kroll M (1969) Acquired idiopathic nystagmus and oscillopsia. Am J Ophthalmol 67:139–144

Levett J, Hoeft G (1977) Voluntary eye movements and alcohol. Aviat Space Environ Med 48:612–614

Levett J, Karras L (1977) Effects of alcohol on human accommodation. Aviat Space Environ Med 48:434–437

Lewin L, Guillery H (1913) Die Wirkungen von Arzneimitteln und Giften auf das Auge. Hirschwald, Berlin

Lewis EG, Dustman RE, Beck EC (1970) The effects of alcohol on visual and somatosensory evoked responses. EEG Clin Neurophysiol 28:202–205

Leydhecker W, Krieglstein GK, Uhlich E (1978) Experimentelle Untersuchungen zur Wirkungsweise alkoholischer Getränke auf den Augeninnendruck. Klin Monatsbl Augenheilkd 172:75–79

Makar A, Tephly TR (1977) Methanol poisoning VI. Role of folic acid in the production of methanol poisoning in the rat. J Toxicol Environ Health 2:1201–1209

Maling HM (1970) Toxicology of single doses of ethanol. In: Tremolieres J (ed) Alcohols and derivatives, vol 2. Pergamon, Oxford

Mardones J (1963) The alcohols. In: Root WS, Hoffmann FG (eds) Physiological pharmacolog, vol 1. Academic, New York

Martin-Amat G, McMartin KE, Hayreh SS, Hayreh MS, Tephly TR (1978) Methanol poisoning: ocular toxicity produced by formate. Toxicol Appl Pharmacol 45:201–208

McMartin KE, Makar AB, Martin-Amat G, Palese M, Tephly TR (1975) Methanol poisoning I. The role of formic acid in the development of metabolic acidosis in the monkey and the reversal by 4-methylpyrazole. Biochem Med 13:319–333

Miles WR (1924) Alcohol and human efficiency (Publication no. 333). Carnegie Institution of Washington, Washington

Mizoi Y, Hishida S, Maeba Y (1969) Diagnosis of alcohol intoxication by the optokinetic test. Q J Stud Alcohol 30:1–14

Money KE, Myles WS (1974) Heavy water nystagmus and effects of alcohol. Nature 247:404–405

Müller W, Haase E (1967) Das Verhalten der corticalen Antwort unter Alkoholeinwirkung. Albrecht von Graefes Arch Klin Exp Ophthalmol 173:108–113

Newman HW, Fletcher E (1941) The effect of alcohol on vision. Am J Med Sci 202:723–731

Nicholls P (1975) Formate as an inhibitor of cytochrome c oxidase. Biochem Biophys Res Commun 67:610–616

Orthner H (1950) Die Methylalkohol-Vergiftung. Springer, Berlin Göttingen Heidelberg

Ostbaum SA, Podos SM, Kolker AE (1973) Low-dose oral alcohol and intraocular pressure. Am J Ophthalmol 76:926–928

Peczon JD, Grant WM (1965) Glaucoma alcohol and intraocular pressure. Arch Ophthalmol 73:495–501

Pfister AK, McKenzie JV, Dinsmore HP, Edman CD (1966) Extracorporeal dialysis for methanol intoxication. JAMA 197:1041–1043

Phillips GB, Victor M, Admas RD, Davidson CS (1952) A study of the nutritional defect in Wernicke's syndrome. The effect of a purified diet, thiamine and other vitamins. J Clin Invest 31:859–871

Potts AM (1955) The visual toxicity of methanol VI. The clinical aspects of experimental methanol poisoning treated with base. Am J Ophthalmol 39:86–92

Potts AM (1973) Tobacco amblyopia. Surv Ophthalmol 17:313–339

Potts AM, Johnson LV (1952) Studies on the visual toxicity of methanol I. The effect of methanol and its degradation products on retinal metabolism. Am J Ophthalmol 35:107–113

Potts AM, Praglin J, Farkas IS, Orbison L, Chickering D (1955) Studies on the visual toxicity of methanol VIII. Additional observations on methanol poisoning. Am J Ophthalmol 40:76–82

Powell WH Jr (1938) Ocular manifestations of alcohol and a consideration of individual variations in 7 cases studied. J Aviat Med 9:97–103

Praglin J, Spurney R, Potts AM (1955) An experimental study of electroretinography I. The electroretinogram in experimental animals under the influence of methanol and its oxidation products. Am J Ophthalmol 39:52–62

Ramos L, Ramos AO, Giesbrecht AM (1969) Changes of intraocular pressure and of chloride, sodium and potassium concentrations in aqueous humor and serum of rabbits following ethanol. Ophthalmologica 159:430–435

Rhodes LE, Obitz FW, Creel D (1975) Effect of alcohol and task on hemispheric asymmetry of visually evoked potentials in man. Electroencephalogr Clin Neurophysiol 38:561–568

Röe O (1950) Methanol poisoning and treatment: its course, pathogenesis and treatment. Q J Stud Alcohol 11:107–112

Roth SH (1979) Physical mechanisms of anesthesia. Annu Rev Pharmacol Toxicol 19:159–178

Skoglund CR (1943) On the influence of alcohol on the pupillary light reflex in man. Acta Physiol Scand 6:94–96

Skoog K-O (1974) The c-wave of the human D. C. registered ERG III. Effects of ethyl alcohol on the c-wave. Acta Ophthalmol 52:913–923

Skoog K-O, Welinder E, Nilsson SEG (1978) The influence of ethyl alcohol on slow off-responses in the human D. C. registered electroretinogram. Vision Res 18:1041–1044

Tiburtius H, Wojahn H, Glass F (1966) Über Änderung der Readaptationszeit des menschlichen Auges nach fovealer Blendung unter Alkoholbelastung. Albrecht von Graefes
Arch Klin Exp Ophthalmol 169:318–327

van Lith G, Vijfvinkel-Bruinenga S (1978) Optic neuropathy due to alcohol abuse and
evoked cortical potentials. Doc Ophthalmol Proc Ser 15:221–225

van Norren D, Padmos P (1977) Influence of anesthetics, ethyl alcohol, and Freon on dark
adaptation of monkey cone ERG. Invest Ophthalmol 16:80–83

von Oettingen WF (1943) The aliphatic alcohols. US Public Health Bulletin 281. US Gov-
ernment Printing Office, Washington

van Slyke DD, Palmer WW (1920) Studies of acidosis XVI. The titration of organic acids
in urine. J Biol Chem 41:567–585

Victor M, Dreyfus PM (1965) Tobacco-alcohol amblyopia. Arch Ophthalmol 74:649–657

Victor M, Mancall EL, Dreyfus PM (1960) Deficiency amblyopia in the alcoholic patient.
Arch Ophthalmol 64:1–33

Wenzl JE, Mills SD, McCall JT (1968) Methanol poisoning in an infant. Am J Dis Child
116:445–447

Wilkinson IMS, Kime R, Purnell M (1974) Alcohol and human eye movement. Brain
97:785–792

Winchester JF, Gelfand MC, Knepshield JH, Schreiner GE (1977) Dialysis and hemoper-
fusion of poisons and drugs – update. Trans Am Soc Artif Int Organs 23:762–842

Wood CA, Buller F (1904) Poisoning by wood alcohol. JAMA 43:972–977, 1058–1062,
1117–1123

Zatman LJ (1946) The effect of ethanol on the metabolism of methanol in man. Biochem
J 40:1xvii–1xviii

CHAPTER 16

Photosensitizing Substances

A. M. POTTS

A. Direct Action of Ultraviolet Light on Skin

Sunburn must have been a basic fact of life since man evolved. Wavelengths between 280 and 315 nm are responsible, and the peak effect is found at 297 nm (COBLENTZ et al. 1932). However, some have said that scattering by superficial skin layers is responsible for the measured maximum, and that if the superficial layers are treated with clearing agents, the peak sensitivity shifts to 280 nm (LUCAS 1931). This is quite close to the absorption maximum of proteins in solution, chiefly mediated by the aromatic amino acids. This allows the Grotthuss–Draper Law (which states that only radiations which are absorbed by a reacting system are effective in producing chemical change) to be satisfied. Ultraviolet radiation in this wavelength band when absorbed by the skin can cause severe inflammatory signs and symptoms. Apparently all the mechanisms of inflammation can be activated, and all signs from mild erythema to the equivalent of a second-degree thermal burn can be generated by appropriate doses.

I. Mechanism of Ultraviolet Action

The exact steps which intervene between the absorption of a quantum of light by a protein molecule (the Stark–Einstein Law states that each molecule taking part in a chemical reaction induced by exposure to light absorbs 1 quantum of the radiation, causing the reaction) and the erythematous or inflammatory end result are by no means certain. Many assumptions are derived from the classic studies on the emission line spectrum of hydrogen done by the quantum chemists and physicists in the early years of this century. Those studies, at least, are on firm ground and the calculations derived from them are performable. The energetics of the absorption of a quantum of light by the hydrogen atom are well worked out. The energy of the quantum is transferred to the orbiting electron of hydrogen, causing it to enter a more energetic state (i.e., higher orbital). After an extremely brief period the excited electron can return to its ground state, losing its recently acquired energy in any of a number of ways. A common one is reemission of light, giving rise to one of the characteristic lines of the hydrogen spectrum.

If one goes on to special molecules such as the benzene molecule, precise calculations are impossible. However, it is known that in each benzene ring there are six electrons which are not bound to a single atom but are "delocalized." These so-

This work was supported in part by USPHS Research Grant number EY 01591 from the National Eye Institute, National Institute of Health, Bethesda, Maryland

called π electrons are less tightly bound than their less energetic relatives. They are considered to belong to the molecule as a whole and constitute the "π orbital" of the molecule. It is these electrons which participate in lowest-level energy transitions and become activated by incident photons.

One can extrapolate from benzene to the aromatic amino acids as components of proteins in the state in which they occur in tissues. The π electrons in phenylalanine, tyrosine, and tryptophane are the photon traps responsible for the reactivity of skin and cornea to ultraviolet wavelengths in the middle range, peaking at 280 nm.

When a molecule absorbs a quantum of light, it can reemit radiation at longer wavelengths as fluorescence or phosphorescence. However, there are radiationless transitions available to it as well. One of these is "internal conversion," whereby the energy of the photon is converted to vibrational energy of the molecule and is eventually dissipated to neighboring molecules as heat. Still another mode of energy disposition is rupture of the molecule into two stable molecules, or into free radicals, or the undergoing of molecular rearrangement.

It is reasonably certain that one or more of these mechanisms is the next step in the reaction chain of tissue to mid-band ultraviolet. Because of characteristic biological properties it has become useful for biomedical writers to consider the nonvacuum ultraviolet as composed of three bands. The band from 400 to 320 nm is long-wave ultraviolet and has cavalierly been labeled "UVA". The band from 320 to 270 nm is middle-wave ultraviolet, or UVB. The band from 270 to the vacuum limit at about 100 nm is short-wave ultraviolet and is designated "UVC". The C band is germicidal, the B band is erythemogenic, and the A band is primary in photoactivation. Electron spin resonance studies suggest that free radicals play a major role, but the exact chemical entries in this step are not known. It may be assumed, however, that whatever their identities, these substances turn on the whole panoply of the inflammatory mechanism, complete with histamine and prostaglandins. They further have the property of stimulating the melanin-forming mechanism causing increased pigmentation of skin in particular.

One final mechanism by means of which an absorbing molecule may dispose of its newly gained energy is to transmit the energy to a molecule of another species, in which second molecule a chemical reaction takes place. These reactions are sensitized reactions. The process is photoactivation and is the subject matter for the second portion of this chapter. For a more extensive treatment of these aspects of photobiology see Seliger and McElroy (1965), Shugar (1960), or Lerman (1980).

II. Direct Action of Light on the Eye

It is clear that as far as the skin of the eyelids is concerned, all the above considerations apply. If we ignore the very extensive subject of direct damage to the retina by visible and infrared wavelengths – that is beyond the scope of this discussion – the only other ocular structure affected directly by mid-range ultraviolet under real conditions is the cornea. Cogan and Kinsey (1946) used a large-aperture quartz monochromator and a 1000-W high-pressure mercury arc to measure the keratitis action spectrum in rabbits. The action spectrum gave a relatively narrow curve with a sharp peak at 288 nm – essentially identical under the conditions of the experiment with the 280-nm peak for skin. This, then, is the mechanism for snowblindness, arc-welding keratitis, and the miscellaneous other ultraviolet corneal burns encountered in industry. Curiously, the absorption maximum for corneal epithelium lies at 265 nm (KINSEY 1948). This maximum is attributed by KINSEY to nucleoprotein, which presumably does not mediate keratitis. Under ordinary circumstances the cornea appears to protect the interior structures from damage by mid-range ultraviolet. See KINSEY (1948) for a discussion of these relationships.

More recently PITTS and co-workers repeated the COGAN and KINSEY work using 5-kW xenon-mercury high-pressure arc and a single- or double-grating monochromator calibrated by an Edgerton, Germeshauser, and Grier radiometer. Under their conditions the threshold for corneal damage in the pigmented rabbit had its minimum at 270 nm and was attained with 0.005 J/cm^2 (PITTS 1978). Permanent lens damage threshold in the rabbit was obtained at 300 and 305 nm (rated 1+ on a scale of 4) with 0.5 J/cm^2 at the plane of the eye. Thus with enough power one can clearly get lens damage, but it requires 100 times the corneal damage threshold energy at the most sensitive wavelength to accomplish this.

B. Photosensitization

It is reported that as far back as the Ebers Papyrus (ca. 1550 B.C.) there are accounts that extracts of *Ammi majus,* a weed that grows along the Nile, can be used for the treatment of vitiligo (by exposure to sunlight after ingestion) (BENDETTO 1977). Further understanding had to wait until the mid-twentieth century, when

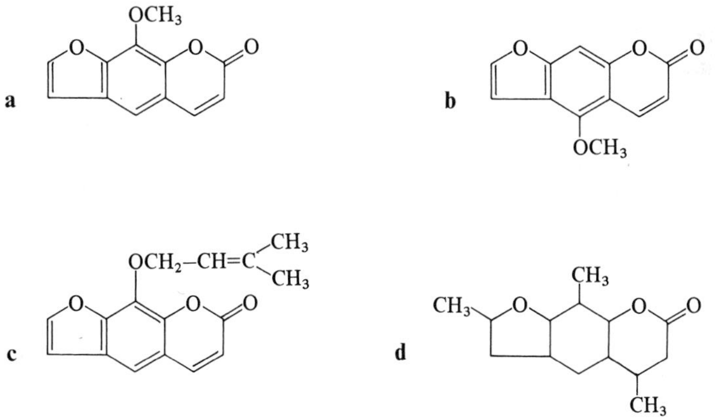

Fig. 1 a–d. Structures of the psoralens. **a** 8-methoxy furocoumarin (8-methoxypsoralen, methoxsalen, xanthotoxin, ammoidin, Oxsoralen); **b** 5-methoxy furocoumarin (5-methoxypsoralen, bergapten, majudin); **c** 8-isoamylenoxyfurocoumarin (imperatorin, ammidin); **d** 4,5′,8-trimethyl furocoumarin (4,5′,8-trimethylpsoralen, trioxsalen, Trisoralen) (synthetic)

three pure compounds were isolated from plant extracts (see Fig. 1). These had the same properties as *Ammi majus* extracts, i.e., causing exaggerated sunburn and thereby causing vitiligo spots to be pigmented. The same is true of a synthetic osypsoralen – trimethylpsoralen (TMP). Unlike the situation with sunburn, however, which requires medium-band ultraviolet, the wavelengths which activate the psoralens after ingestion or local application are in the long-wave ultraviolet (UVA) band. The treatment with psoralen and long-wave ultraviolet has been labeled "PUVA" by dermatologists. It was suggested by LERNER et al. (1953) that PUVA might be useful for psoriasis, and this was established as effective treatment by FITZPATRICK's group (PARRISH et al. 1974). More recently, PUVA has been found to be effective in the early stages – eczematous patch and plaque stages – of mycosis fungoides, although systemic progression continues nontheless. Other disease entities responsive to PUVA are palmoplantar pustulosis, atopic eczema, lichen planus, cutaneous mastocytosis, and alopecia areata (ANDERSON and VOORHEES 1980). Since so many entities are involved, including such a common trouble as psoriasis, we are dealing with a technique which promises to be of use to many patients. Thus we must ask quite seriously what ocular effects can occur.

I. Mechanism

It appears on the basis of available studies that in photosensitization the sensitizing molecule absorbs the quantum of light. This molecule has one or more of its electrons (most easily π electrons) raised to a higher orbital. The energy is then transferred to the susceptible tissue molecule. There is some evidence that psoralens are able to intercalate into the nucleic acid helix. However, it is by no means clear what the exact steps are in the process of photosensitization. What is known is that light contributes to the binding of psoralen to DNA, that the maximum quantum yield is at 365 nm, and that binding is by covalent bonds to pyrimidine bases only. Psoralen and long-wave ultraviolet cause both erythema and increase in pigmentation. However, erythema which peaks at 12–24 h in direct response to UVB does not peak until 36–72 h in response to PUVA. Indomethacin, an inhibitor of prostaglandin synthesis, reduces the reaction to UVB but has no effect on PUVA. For a review see ANDERSON and VOORHEES (1980).

Simply to distinguish the processes, we must take note of the "photodynamic action of light" phenomenon described first by RAAB (1900). He found that in the presence of acridine, ultraviolet light killed paramecia. It was later found that atmospheric oxygen was necessary for the effect. Oxygen is not necessary for the direct effect of UV, nor for the photosensitization phenomena of which PUVA is the most important in humans. Since the photodynamic effect has not been used in man and to only a limited extent in animals, it will not be pursued further here.

LERMAN et al. (1980) suggested on the basis of in vitro experiments that irradiation of solutions containing 8-methoxypsoralen (8-MOP) and tryptophane, or 8-MOP and α-, β-, or γ-crystallins at 360 nm, causes a photo adduct between 8-MOP and the aromatic amino acids of lens protein.

II. Ocular Effects

Since photosensitization by substances such as the psoralens is accomplished by UVA, we are dealing with wavelengths that pass the cornea, and in some instances the lens, with ease. The absorption of UVA at a given part of the eye is determined not by the content of aromatic amino acids but by the concentration of photosensitizing compound. In the case of the lens, yellow lens pigment can absorb UVA.

From the historical point of view the report of EGYED et al. (1975) is of more than passing interest. These workers force-fed ducklings with the seeds of *Ammi majus* and exposed them to sunlight 4–5 h per day for each of 5 days. These animals showed lesions on the beak and footwebs, a severe conjunctivitis, and transient corneal opacity in some birds. About 1 month after the external reaction all birds showed mydriasis and pigmentary retinopathy in the form of dense pigment clumps surrounded by seemingly normal retina. In a further publication EGYED and co-workers (BARISHAK et al. 1975) showed that atrophy of the muscle of the sphincter pupillae was responsible for the mydriasis observed a month after the start of the experiment. If this was the result of photosensitization it occurred despite the protection offered the iris sphincter by the iris pigment.

CLOUD et al. (1960) used 8-MOP in guinea pigs and exposed the animals to UVA from two Sylvania Blacklight Blue tubes for 24 h. Five of 11 white guinea pigs died within 10–14 days. In all white animals the ears and eyelids were severely burned. The conjunctiva showed chemosis. Of 22 eyes, 5 showed no corneal edema. The remaining eyes showed corneal edema ranging from slight to severe. In all eyes there was permanent mydriasis starting on the 5th–7th days. There were anterior cortical lens opacities in 21 of 22 eyes. Most of these opacities disappeared, but in 3 eyes lens opacities persisted until termination of the experiment. In black guinea pigs there was no lid or ear damage, conjunctival chemosis appeared in 2 of 8 eyes and was transient. Corneal edema was seen in 3 eyes and lasted 6 weeks in 1 eye only. The pupil did not dilate. Multiple white punctate opacities of the anterior lens cortex were found in 6 of 8 Lenses. In 3 of the 6, opacities persisted until termination of the experiment. No conclusions can be made about retinal changes because the retina in guinea pigs is difficult to observe.

In a chronic study CLOUD et al. (1961) used female Swiss albino mice. These animals were given 8-MOP daily and 1 h later they were exposed to UVA for 10 min. This was done 6 days a week for 5 months. The only significant difference between control and experimental groups at 5 months was the high incidence of anterior cortical cataract in the lower half of the lens. Later, damaged ears and a few dilated pupuls became evident.

As was mentioned above, the controlling factor here appears to be where the 8-MOP localizes in the eye. LERMAN and BORKMAN (1977) showed clearly that 8-MOP did localize in the lens, and the presence of cataract in the CLOUD group's acute and chronic animals is quite understandable.

Although the foregoing reports have described lesions of lids, cornea, iris, lens, and retina under experimental conditions, there is only one hypothesized report of damage to human eyes by PUVA. The protocol of treatment for psoriasis (and thousands of patients have been treated by now) has always required ultraviolet-absorbing goggles during treatment and UVA-absorbing spectacles for the day of treatment. The report of Cyrlin et al. (1980) deserves attention because it deals with a single patient whose stellate-shaped, zonularly distributed cataract is implied to be the result of PUVA treatment for vitiligo. Because this represents a single case of cataract among so many PUVA patients, one is forced to look carefully for an explanation of this finding. One possibility is that the cataract, which was present at the first eye examination, was nonprogressive, and reduced acuity to only 20/25− OD and 20/25+2 OS, was present before PUVA treatment and was unrelated to it. A second possibility is that because the patient wore no eye protection during 6 months of topical PUVA treatment, and because her eyewear during 2 years of systemic PUVA passed some UVA (see manufacturer's published curves for photoactivated sunglasses), we are dealing with an isolated case of PUVA cataract. Under any circumstances we will need a significant number of better documented cases before being convinced that PUVA therapy as now conducted represents a cataract hazard.

C. Photosensitizing Substances

I. Exogenous Photosensitizers

From the foregoing one should not get the notion that *Ammi majus* is the sole source of psoralens, or that furocoumarins are the only photosensitizing agents known. This is far from the truth.

Psoralens and related coumarins which potentiate sunburn are reported to occur in other Umbelliferae than *Ammi majus*. Parsnip, fennel, dill, parsley, carrots, masterwort, celery, *Angelica* species, and coriander have all been reported to have sunburn-potentiating properties excited by long-wave ultraviolet.

Similar properties are shared by members of the family Rutaceae. These include the common rue, bergamot and lime and other citrus species.

A miscellaneous group of other plants are reported to contain sunburn-potentiating substances. Among these are buttercup, mustard, bindweed, agrimony, yarrow, meadow grass, fig, and *Hypericum* species, e.g., St. John's wort. For a review see Fitzpatrick et al. (1963).

Numerous chemical substances, some of them with pharmacologic properties, can be activated by UVA to potentiate sunburn. Some of the numerous constituents of coal tar contribute to the therapeutic effect of locally applied coal tar followed by UVA. Likely candidates are the polycyclic hydrocarbons, which contain large numbers of π electrons.

Two reviews written from the dermatologic point of view are those of Sams (1960) and of Kirshbaum and Beerman (1964). These authors have documented lists of substances known to have caused photosensitization in the past. In addition, the latter review defines terminology which may have been confusing to nondermatologists. "Phototoxic" and "photoallergic" have been particularly troublesome. The simplification by Fowlks (1969) to "photosensitization" and its adaptation by Fitzpatrick et al. (1963) is welcome, but definitions of the earlier terms are useful.

One of the major categories of photosensitizing drugs is the sulfonamides and their congeners the sulfonylureas and the chlorothiazides. Sulfanilamide itself has been well documented as a photosensitizer, and numerous later-arriving sulfon-amides share its properties. Of the oral hypoglycemic agents, carbutamide, tolbut-amide, and chlorpropamide have been implicated. Of the chlorothiazide diuretics used against hypertension, chlorothiazide itself and hydrochlorothiazide have been reported as photosensitizers. With all the above compounds the action spectrum appears to lie in the UVB band (FITZPATRICK et al. 1963; Table III). Thus, al-though intensification of sunburn may be caused and eyelids may be involved, there is no unusual effect on the globe itself that would not be observed with an overdose of UVB.

A second major category of photosensitizers is the now sizeable group of phe-nothiazine drugs. Phenothiazine itself, although not now used in humans, is em-ployed as a vermifuge in veterinary medicine. WHITTEN and FILMER (1947) reported from New Zealand on a keratitis in young cattle caused by light and phenothiazine. Corneal opacity from the optic axis to the lateral canthus is the rule in this disease. Corneal ulceration and late vascularization may occur in severe cases. An almost identical report was published by DIRKSEN and TAMMEN (1964) from the Frisian coast and Schleswig-Holstein (West Germany). CLARE et al. (1947) suggest on the basis of known phenothiazine metabolites and the action spectrum of keratitis in sheep given phenothiazine that the actual photosensitizer is phenothiazine sulfox-ide. The phenothiazine tranquilizers and antihistamines, of which there are several dozen, are well-known photosensitizers whose action spectrum is in the long-wave ultraviolet band, with the exception of chlorpromazine. Photosensitization der-matitis has been recorded for chlorpromazine, promethazine, trimeprazine, and prochlorperazine. Chlorpromazine's action spectrum has been identified as being in the UVB range by EPSTEIN et al. (1957) and by SATANOVE and MCINTOSH (1967). Chlorpromazine is the only phenothiazine which is given to psychotic patients in doses which total one to several grams per day. At these levels there develops a typi-cal skin pigmentation seen only in the areas exposed to sunlight. The color is a dusky purple or, as described by BAN et al. (1965), *une coleur violacée metallique* (a metallic purple color). A color reproduction of this phenomenon appears in the article. The ocular effects in these patients were first described by GREINER and BERRY (1964). Tiny pigmented granules appear on the corneal endothelium and the anterior lens capsule. With time they enter the substance of the cornea and lens. It is my personal observation that the granules appear only on surfaces bathed by the aqueous humor. This suggests that they may be granules of uveal pigment re-leased after the chlorpromazine has adsorbed on them. No true cataracts that did not exist previously are observed in these patients. One may question whether light plays a role in this phenomenon, because the action spectrum for chlorpromazine and skin is in the UVB band and there is no observable corneal epithelial disease.

The ocular effects of thioridazine present a different set of facts. According to SATANOVE and MCINTOSH (1967), the action spectrum of thioridazine extends above the UVA band into the visible. These wavelengths can easily reach the retina and in particular the retinal pigmented epithelium, which is one of the locations where phenothiazines concentrate. When thioridazine is administered in doses higher than 800 mg/day, a pigmentary retinopathy develops with severe loss of vi-sion. On cessation of dosage some vision is recovered, but if this does not happen promptly much permanent damage results. It is the suggestion of SATANOVE and

McIntosh (1967) that thioridazine retinopathy is a photosensitivity reaction. Arguing against this is the finding that many phenothiazines whose action spectrum is in the long-wave ultraviolet band bind to melanin as avidly as does thioridazine, or more so (e.g., prochlorperazine; Potts 1964), yet these compounds do not cause pigmentary retinopathy. A more direct answer will come from experiments now under way in the University of Louisville laboratory on photosensitivity behavior of retinal pigmented epithelium in tissue culture, where all conditions are amenable to precise control.

Still another group of photosensitizing drugs is the tetracyclines. All these substances have one aromatic ring able to resonate with the conjugated double bonds of the three remaining alicyclic rings. Indeed, the pale yellow color of these substances indicates that they absorb at the short-wavelength end of the visible spectrum. Photodermatitis has been observed with tetracycline, chlortetracycline, demethylchlortetracycline, and oxytetracycline (see Kirshbaum and Beerman 1964). There appear to be no reports of severe damage to the globe due to this mechanism.

A miscellaneous assortment of other exogenous substances cause photodermatitis. Griseofulvin, the antimycotic 4-chloro-2-hydroxybenzoic acid-N-n-butylamide, Tridione (trimethadione), Dilantin (diphenylhydantoin), Benadryl (diphenhydramine), tetrachlorsalicylanalide, and 9-aminoacridine have all been reported to cause photodermatitis. There appear to be no other ocular effects apart from the expected lid skin involvement. One report by Bernstein et al. (1970) describes corneal and lens opacities in dogs after feeding 2,6-dichloro-4-nitroaniline (a fungicide) and keeping the animals in sunlight. The severity of the response was a function of dose, and at 24 mg/kg/day abnormalities were seen. At lower doses they did not appear and at higher doses they appeared sooner. The authors postulate a parallelism in cataractogenesis between this compound and dinitrophenol, suggesting that both give rise to benzoquinone, the fungicide via paraquinoneimine. They do not make it clear what role sunlight has in this oxidation.

II. Endogenous Photosensitizers

The details of porphyrin metabolism are complex, and the inborn errors of metabolism which result in abnormally high levels of free porphyrin in blood and urine are rare. An excellent treatment of the subject may be found in Meyer and Schmid (1978). One aspect of interest is the growing conviction that George III of England and subsequent Hanoverian monarchs until Victoria (whose line was not involved) suffered, particularly mentally, from the effects of variegate porphyria (Ware 1968). More importantly for the purposes of this chapter, elevated blood levels of porphyrins cause photosensitization. The action spectrum is in the visible range, peaking near 400 nm. The presence of oxygen is essential for the skin effect and protection is given by β-carotene, which quenches excited oxygen molecules. The forms of porphyria in which photic skin effects are prominent are:

1. Heriditary coproporphyria, characterized by unremitting excretion of coproporphyrin in urine and feces secondary to a defect in coproporphyrinogen oxidase in liver.
2. Variegate porphyria, characterized by increased excretion of fecal protoporphyrin and (to a lesser extent) coproporphyrin secondary to a decrease in liver protoporphyrinogen oxidase.

3. Porphyria cutanea tarda, characterized by urinary excretion of large amounts of uroporphyrin secondary to a deficiency of uroporphyrinogen decarboxylase.

Since the second of these diseases has been intensively studied in the Dutch population of South Africa, where the records of over 1400 affected individuals with a common ancestry are on file, and since the third disease has its highest incidence in the Bantu population of South Africa, the report of BARNES and BOSHOFF (1952) on 38 whites and 46 blacks from South Africa with eye involvement secondary to porphyria takes on special significance (Table 1). The authors at that time did not have complete appreciation of the differences in disease entities, but they did report a roughly equivalent incidence of clinical findings separately for whites and blacks. There were disturbances in every part of the eye and adnexa. Cornea and sclera appeared to be more frequently affected in blacks (Table 2).

Perhaps the white patients exhibit the effects of variegate porphyria and the black patients show effects of porphyria cutanea tarda.

In addition, the authors mention that the iris participates in adherent leukoma. One white woman had a partly disintegrated cataract in a badly damaged globe. However, primary disease of iris, ciliary body, or lens does not appear to be characteristic of these entities. Since generalized cerebral involvement is characteristic of variegate porphyria, one might wonder how many of the fundus findings were connected with increased intracranial pressure secondary to brain swelling. However, the authors describe only two cases where the discs were "slightly blurred and hyperemic" (Table 3).

Table 1. Findings in conjunctiva and eyelids (BARNES and BOSHOFF 1952)

Condition	Whites	Blacks	Total
External scarring of lids	5	4	9
Internal scarring of lids	1	2	3
Ectropion	1	2	3
Blepharochalasis	8	3	11
Symblepharon	3	1	4
Hyaloid thickening of conjunctiva	2	4	6
Pemphigoid occlusion of fornix	0	1	1
Acute bulbar conjunctivitis	2	0	2

Table 2. Findings in cornea and sclera (BARNES and BOSHOFF 1952)

Conditions	Whites	Blacks	Total
Scleromalacia perforans	1	1	2
Scleromalacia "semiperforans"	1	4	5
Extension on to cornea	0	3	3
Limbal phlyctenulosis later developed farther	0	2	2
Adherent leukoma	1	4	5
Keratitic scars	1	4	5

Table 3. Findings on funduscopic examination (Barnes and Boshoff 1952)

Condition	Whites	Blacks	Total
Cotton wool patches	1	2	3
Cotton wool patches and hemorrhage	1	0	1
Flat striate edema	3	1	4
Discrete annular choroiditis	5	5	10
En plaque choroiditis	5	1	6
En plaque choroiditis with edema and hemorrhage	1	0	1
Lanceolate and striate scars	8	5	13
Granular diffuse lesions	2	8	10
Macular pigment shift	4	6	12
Globular pigment scars	6	3	9
Depigmented patches	1	4	5
Hemorrhages present	1	2	3

Just as the diseases we have discussed are due to inherited genetic disorders which affect individual liver enzymes, it is possible to get specific liver damage and porphyria from exogenous substances. The hypnotic drugs Sulfonal (sulfonmethane) and Trional (sulfonethylmethane) were noted for causing acquired porphyria. They were eventually withdrawn from use for this reason. Studies of acquired porphyria have not pinpointed a metabolic defect, and indeed there may be more than a single enzyme affected in toxic disease. Jaffe (1950) described a single case of what he thinks was a case of toxic porphyria in a 22-year-old woman. No medical details were given that would allow closer categorization. Jaffe described in this patient bilateral ptosis, bilateral incomplete oculomotor palsy, pupils dilated and unreactive to light and near, bilateral blurred discs, and numerous hemorrhages near the disc – preretinal, nerve fiber, and choroidal. The patient became comatose on the 6th hospital day, then began to recover rapidly, and by the 10th day was virtually recovered. It should be marked that almost all these findings could go with increased intracranial pressure and central nervous system involvement.

Experimental porphyria was reproduced in pigmented rabbits by Freeman and Troll (1967). These authors gave daily intraperitoneal injections of hematoporphyrin at 37 mg/kg and exposed the experimental group to a 100-W incandescent blub for 4 h/day, 6 days a week. There was a bulb on each side of the cage ca. 15 cm from the animal's eye. The chief finding was extensive retinal degeneration in all layers, with adherence of the vestigial retina to the choroid at numerous places. This is another strong proof that the pathological effects of photosensitization are dependent on the depth of penetration of the light, which in turn depends on the balance between action spectrum of the photosensitizing substance and absorption of cornea and lens. Retinal damage is only a factor when the action spectrum is in the visible. The second determining factor is the diffusion behavior of the photosensitizing substance. The porphyrins seem to remain in vascular tissues. Thus skin, conjunctiva, sclera, and retina are highly involved in porphyria, and avascular structures such as cornea and lens are affected secondarily or not at all.

D. Conclusions

The subject of photosensitivity and the eye is a significant one that requires much additional study. Our continued intimate contact with more and more varied chemical compounds is a necessity. Thus we must learn how best to cope with photosensitizers – to use them to our advantage, as in PUVA treatment for psoriasis, and to avoid damage from them, as in hereditary and acquired porphyria. Extension of our knowledge of quantum biochemistry can only enhance these efforts.

References

Anderson TF, Voorhees JJ (1980) Psoralen photochemotherapy of cutaneous disorders. Ann Rev Pharmacol Toxicol 20:235–257

Ban TA, Lehmann HE, Gallai Z, Warnes H, Lee H (1965) Rapport entre la photosensibilité et la pigmentation pathologique de la peau avec des doses elevées de chlorpromazine. Union Med Can 94:305–307

Barishak YR, Beemer AM, Egyed MN, Shlosberg A, Eilat A (1975) Histology of the iris in geese and ducks photosensitized by ingestion of *Ammi majus* seeds. Acta Ophthalmol 53:585–590

Barnes HD, Boshoff PH (1952) Ocular lesions in patients with porphyria. Arch Ophthalmol 48:567–580

Bendetto AV (1977) The psoralens: an historical perspective. Cutis 20:469–471

Bernstein HN, Curtis J, Earl FL, Kuwabara T (1970) Phototoxic corneal and lens opacities. Arch Ophthalmol 83:336–348

Clare NT, Whitten LK, Filmer DB (1947) A photosensitized keratitis in young cattle following the use of phenothiazine as an anthelmintic III. Identification of the photosensitizing agent. Aust Vet J 23:344–348

Cloud TM, Hakim R, Griffin AC (1960) Photosensitization of the eye with methoxsalen I. Acute effects. Arch Ophthalmol 64:346–351

Cloud TM, Hakim R, Griffin AC (1961) Photosensitization of the eye with methoxsalen II. Chronic effects. Arch Ophthalmol 66:105–110

Coblentz WW, Stair R, Hogue JM (1932) The spectral erythemic reaction of the untanned human skin to ultraviolet light radiation. Bur Stand J Res 8:541–547

Cogan DG, Kinsey VE (1946) Action spectrum of keratitis produced by ultraviolet radiation. Arch Ophthalmol 35:670–677

Cyrlin MN, Pedvis-Leftick A, Sugar J (1980) Cataract formation in association with ultraviolet photosensitivity. Ann Ophthalmol 12:786–790

Dirksen G, Tammen C (1964) Keratitis bei Jungrindern infolge Photosensibilität nach Dauermedikation. Dtsch Tierärztl Wochenschr 71:545–548

Egyed MN, Singer L, Eilat A, Shlosberg A (1975) Eye lesions in ducklings fed *Ammi majus* seeds. Zentralbl Veterinaermed 22:764–768

Epstein JH, Brunsting LA, Petersen MC, Schwarz BE (1957) A study of photosensitivity occurring with chlorpromazine therapy. J Invest Dermatol 28:329–338

Fitzpatrick TB, Pathak MA, Magnus IA, Curwen WL (1963) Abnormal reactions of man to light. Annu Rev Med 14:195–214

Fowlks WL (1959) The mechanism of the photodynamic effect. J Invest Dermatol 32:233–247

Freeman RG, Troll D (1967) Hematoporphyrin photosensitization of rabbit eye to visible light. Arch Ophthalmol 78:766–768

Greiner AC, Berry K (1964) Skin pigmentation and corneal and lens opacities with prolonged chlorpromazine therapy. Can Med Assoc J 90:663–665

Jaffe NS (1950) Acute porphyria associated with retinal hemorrhages and bilateral oculomotor palsy. Am J Ophthalmol 33:470–472

Kinsey VE (1948) Spectral transmission of the eye to ultraviolet radiations. Arch Ophthalmol 39:508–513

Kirshbaum BA, Beerman H (1964) Photosensitization due to drugs. Am J Med Sci 248:445–468

Lerman S (1980) Radiant energy and the eye. Macmillan, New York

Lerman S, Borkman RF (1977) A method for detecting 8-methoxypsoralen in the ocular lens. Science 197:1287–1288

Lerman S, Megaw J, Willis I (1980) The photoreactions of 8-methoxypsoralen with tryptophan and lens proteins. Photochem Photobiol 31:235–242

Lerner AB, Denton CR, Fitzpatrick TB (1953) Clinical and experimental studies with 8-methoxypsoralen in vitiligo. J Invest Dermatol 20:299–314

Lucas NS (1931) The permeability of human epidermis to ultraviolet irradiation. Biochem J 25:57–70

Meyer UA, Schmid R (1978) The porphyrias. In: Stanbury JB, Wyngaarden JB, Fredrickson DS (eds) The metabolic basis of inherited disease, 4th edn. McGraw-Hill, New York, chap 50

Parrish JA, Fitzpatrick TB, Tannenbaum L, Pathak MA (1974) Photochemotherapy of psoriasis with oral methoxysalen and long wave ultraviolet light. N Engl J Med 291:1207–1222

Pitts DG (1978) The ocular effects of ultraviolet radiation. Am J Optom Physiol Opt 55:19–35

Potts AM (1964) The reaction of uveal pigment in vitro with polycyclic compounds. Invest Ophthalmol 3:405–416

Raab O (1900) Über die Wirkung fluoreszierender Stoffe auf Infusorien. Z Biol (Munich) 39:524–546

Sams WM (1960) Photosensitizing therapeutic agents. JAMA 174:2043–2048

Satanove A, McIntosh JS (1967) Phototoxic reactions induced by high doses of chlorpromazine and thioridazine. JAMA 200:209–212

Seliger HH, McElroy WD (1965) Light: physical and biological action, chap 2. Academic, New York

Shugar D (1960) Photochemistry of the nucleic acids and their constituents. In: Chargaff E, Davidson JN (eds) The nucleic acids, vol 3. Academic, New York, chap 30

Ware M (ed) (1968) Porphyria – a royal malady. British Medical Association, London

Whitten LK, Filmer DB (1947) A photosensitized keratitis in young cattle following the use of phenothiazine as an anthelmintic I. A clinical description with a note on its widespread occurrence in New Zealand. Aust Vet J 23:336–340

CHAPTER 17

Trace Elements in the Eye

T. R. JONES and T. W. REID

A. Introduction

More than 96% by weight of the human body consists of hydrogen, oxygen, carbon, and nitrogen. Other elements, including calcium, chlorine, magnesium, phosphorus, potassium, sodium, and sulfur, are constituents of some macromolecules and important components in both intracellular and extracellular fluids. Their concentrations are such that they can be quantified easily and are expressed often as grams per kilogram or grams per day (MERTZ 1981). Found in very much lower concentrations, however, are another group of elements which are also important to homeostasis and, in some cases, survival. These are designated "trace elements" because the concentrations found in the body by early investigators were at or near the sensitivity of the assays they used (UNDERWOOD 1977). The classification of these elements on a purely chemical basis correlated poorly with biological characteristics (i.e., concentration, localization, function, and essentiality). MERTZ (1981) simply divides them into two categories: those essential in some or all mammals to either organismal survival or optimal performance, and those elements for which proof of essentiality does not exist. Those elements now considered proved to be essential are arsenic, chromium, cobalt, copper, iodine, iron, manganese, molybdenum, nickel, selenium, silicon, vanadium, and zinc. There is also some evidence suggesting that tin and fluorine are necessary for proper growth regulation (MERTZ 1981) (Fig. 1).

These elements, found in such low concentrations, are able to exact their physiological effects by coupling, in a variety of ways, to biomolecules. Iodine, for example, is a required component of thyroxine and triiodothyronine. Copper is part of several metalloenzymes including cytochrome c oxidase, tyrosinase, and dopamine β-hydroxylase (O'DELL 1976), and iron, of course, is required for the synthesis of hemoglobin, myoglobin, and the cytochrome proteins (PRASAD 1978).

Although the optimal systemic levels and ingestion rates for every trace element are not yet clear, a relationship between essential nutrient level and optimal health and function has been discussed (UNDERWOOD 1977; MERTZ 1981). When percentage optimal function is charted against nutrient intake, a bell-like curve is generated. The extremes of the curve represent deficiency-induced death and toxicity-induced death, while the central plateau represents optimal function. Obviously, the breadth of the plateau and the slope of the trailing sides vary with each element. What this formulation suggests, however, is that each element has a safe and optimal concentration range within which homeostatic mechanisms function properly, and that when this concentration is exceeded, toxicity and death may result. In-

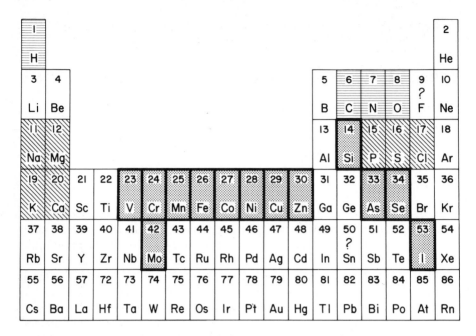

Fig. 1. Those elements which constitute the bulk of animal tissue are designated in this periodic table by *horizontal hatching*. Elements found in lower concentrations but which are important as components of biomolecules and as electrolytes are noted with *diagonal hatching*. The essential trace elements, several of which are required for normal ocular function, are *heavily outlined*

sufficient levels of required elements, on the other hand, would lead to deficiency states and perhaps death (MERTZ 1981). One also expects that different organs and tissues will have different sensitivities to trace element deficiency and overload. The importance of iodine to thyroid function and the relationship between iron and anemia are perhaps the best-known examples of this.

Intake levels of trace elements can be viewed in a variety of ways. "Recommended" levels are usually those levels needed to meet the highest level required by any given individual in a population. Minimum required levels, on the other hand, often are considerably lower. Recommended iron intake is 10–18 mg/day (MERTZ 1981), while estimated iron loss per day is only 1–1.5 mg (HARPER 1976). Table 1 lists both average daily intake (not recommended or minimum levels) and average body burden (SCHROEDER 1965; FOOD AND NUTRITION BOARD 1974; UNDERWOOD 1977; MERTZ 1981).

Trace element deficiency states cannot be remedied with similar elements; in fact, other elements often exacerbate them. A molybdenum-deficient animal fed tungsten, a metal similar to molybdenum and from the same family on the periodic table, will not show a recovery from the molybdenum deficiency. It will, rather, have its molybdenum deficiency actually aggravated (HIGGINS et al. 1956). Rainbow trout suffering from zinc-deficiency-induced cataracts were successfully protected from cataracts by treatment with ethylenediamine tetraacetic acid, a metal-

Table 1. Approximate daily intake and human body burden of selected essential trace elements. (SCHROEDER 1965; FOOD AND NUTRITION BOARD 1974; UNDERWOOD 1977; MERTZ 1981)

Elements	Daily intake (mg/day)	Body burden (mg/70 kg)
Iron	10–18	4,100
Zinc	12–15	2,300
Copper	2–3.2	100
Selenium	0.05–0.2	25
Vanadium	2	20
Chromium	0.05–0.2	< 6
Manganese	5	20
Cobalt	0.075	3
Nickel	0.45	< 10
Molybdenum	0.35	5

Table 2. Concentrations of iron, zinc, copper, and selenium in parts of the bovine eye. Values are mg/100 g in wet tissue. (TAUBER and KRAUSE 1943; OKSALA 1954; TAUSSKY et al. 1966)

	Iron	Zinc	Copper	Selenium
Cornea	0.26–0.5	0.02–0.2	0.05–0.18	0.0025
Stroma	0.20	0.12	0.13	
Epithelium	0.62	0.38	0.46	
Lens	0.032–0.6	0.003–0.75	0.04–0.17	0.014
Optic nerve	0.34	0.24	0.35	
Retina	0.38–1.1	0.04–0.3	0.08–0.26	0.014
Sclera	0.36–0.8	0.02–0.27	0.04–0.22	0.005
Uvea	7.1	0.5	0.08	
Choroid	1.8	0.22	0.34	
Iris	0.34	0.4	0.32	0.076
Vitreous humor	0.012–0.2	0.03	0.03–0.1	

ion-chelating agent, which apparently reduced levels of other metal ions which were interfering with zinc metabolism (KETOLA 1979).

Several investigators have measured the concentrations of a variety of elements in parts of the eye (Table 2) (TAUBER and KRAUSE 1943; OKSALA 1954; SWANSON et al. 1968; ECKERT 1979; STARZYCKA et al. 1979; UJIIE 1979a), but these studies, while giving absolute amounts present of a given element, do not describe the state in which the element exists. It may be in the prosthetic group of a metalloenzyme, bound by a carrier protein, pigment-bound, metallothionein-bound, or free. Pathological conditions which do not primarily involve an element's concentration can indirectly affect it through changes in the macromolecules which interact with it. For several elements, these macromolecule–element relationships have been deciphered; a discussion of their relationship to ocular physiology, pharmacology, and disease constitutes the majority of the material in this review.

Those readers also interested in the systemic distribution, general physiology, and pharmacology of trace elements are referred to the following reviews: Underwood (1977), Mertz (1977), Prasad (1978), Chesters (1979), Prasad (1979), Mertz (1981), and Yolton (1981).

B. Iron

In aqueous solution, iron exists in two stable oxidation states: ferrous (Fe^{2+}), and ferric (Fe^{3+}). It is the interconversion of these two states that forms the basis for all reactions of iron in living organisms. These reactions are as diverse as the synthesis of DNA, the binding of oxygen to hemoglobin, the bioenergetic pathways, and the activation of molecular oxygen. Because Fe^{2+} can be oxidized readily to Fe^{3+} by molecular oxygen, and because of the insolubility of Fe^{3+} under physiological conditions (solubility of about $10^{-17}M$), organisms have been compelled to evolve specific iron-sequestering molecules to maintain the element in a soluble form available for transport and for the biosynthesis of essential iron proteins and enzymes (Aisen and Listowsky 1980). Most iron is bound to hemoglobin (60% –70%), but the transport and storage proteins of iron metabolism are transferrin and ferritin. They have high enough binding constants to avoid the formation of significant amounts of free iron, but the release rate is fast enough to make the metal available on demand to the cell.

An average human diet contains approximately 15 mg iron per day; about 1 mg is absorbed daily. This is enough to compensate for small losses from the body, principally through bile secretion, sloughing of epithelial cells, and menses. The human body appears to have no mechanism for the excretion of excessive amounts of iron. The iron content of the body is regulated solely by the rate of uptake. The mechanism of control of iron absorption is still uncertain, but once in the body, Fe^{3+} is bound to transferrin, an 80,000-dalton protein which contains two iron-binding sites (Aisen and Listowsky 1980). The principle function of transferrin is the transport of iron throughout the body. Transferrin may also serve as an iron buffer; it is possible that the inflow of iron through the intestinal mucosa is regulated by the state of saturation of transferrin in the blood. Iron is stored in ferritin, a 450,000-dalton protein where iron exists as polynuclear aggregates of variable size and composition. Over 2,500 iron atoms may be accommodated easily by each ferritin molecule (Fischbach and Anderegg 1965).

Transferrin may be of importance to the eye, since it was shown recently that this compound, at a concentration of $4 \times 10^{-8}M$, caused a dramatic increase in rate of growth of retinoblastoma-derived cultured cells growing in serum-free culture. Transferrin is also required for selenium to have its stimulatory effect on the same cells (T. W. Reid and D. L. Antonetti, unpublished data). Thus the effects of two critical metal ions on ocular cell growth appear to be regulated by this metal transport protein.

Iron concentrations throughout the eye vary greatly. Tauber and Krause (1943) found that, in the bovine eye, iron levels were highest in the choroid at approximately 2 mg/100 g wet tissue. The aqueous and vitreous humors were lowest at 0.012–0.016 mg/100 g wet tissue; the remainder of the eye tissues varied within a range of 0.03–0.6 mg/100 g wet tissue. Oksala (1954), also studying wet tissue, found values that agreed well with those of TAUBER and KRAUSE (1943) (Table 2). In each tissue, it was not determined in which form the iron exists (i.e., free iron, protein-bound, pigment-bound, cytochrome prosthetic group, or metalloenzyme component). During melanin synthesis, quinone intermediates generate free radicals (RILEY 1970). These free radicals may bind and hold substantial numbers of metal ions, including iron; this could explain why the pigmented tissues of the eye appear to act as "metal sinks" (BRUENGER et al. 1967; POTTS and AU 1976).

In some normal subjects and in a few pathological conditions, iron deposits often appear as lines traversing the superficial cornea (GASS 1964). The Hudson-Stähli line is seen in normal, often elderly patients; it runs horizontally across the lower one-third of the cornea. In 59 of 62 apparently normal corneas, GASS (1964) found detectable levels of iron in the epithelium near the junction of the inferior and middle one-third of the cornea. Other iron lines, probably abberrations of the Hudson-Stähli line, can be noted in two pathological conditions. The corneas of patients with pterygium, a hyperplastic lesion in which the conjunctiva encroaches upon the cornea (SCHEIE and ALBERT 1977), can display a horizontal iron line which bifurcates near the point where the pterygium touches the cornea. This iron line is known as Stocker's line (GASS 1964). In keratoconus, the cornea gradually thins at its apex and becomes conical. An iron line, present in 50% of the cases, encircles the cone and is called Fleischer's line (GASS 1964). In an electron microscopic study of Fleischer's line, IWAMOTO and DEVOE (1976) found an accumulation of 6-nm particles in widened intracellular spraces and cytoplasmic vacuoles of the corneal epithelium. The morphology of these granules was consistent with the iron core of the ferritin molecule. Because these iron lines are apparently benign and because the conditions with which they are commonly associated are not treated with iron-chelating agents, their sensitivity to such agents is unknown. URRETS-ZAVALIA and KATZ (1971) reported a case of corneal dystrophy where a diffuse opacity in the anterior third of the stroma was formed of minute, slightly refringent dots. The dots contained nucleic acids and hemosiderin. The authors regarded this as a nonsystemic, eye-localized case of hemochromatosis. In three cases of primary hemochromatosis, ROTH and FOOS (1972) reported iron granules only in the stroma and epithelium of the ciliary body, and in the sclera. No diabetic oculopathy was seen. In other cases of verified hemochromatosis, DAVIES et al. (1972) found that 29% of the patients examined had pigmentation of the conjunctiva and/or lid margin. Biopsies revealed the presence of iron in the pigmented conjunctivae studied. Three eyes were inspected at autopsy and free ferric iron was found in both the cornea and in the nonpigmented epithelium of the ciliary body.

An iron-chelating agent, deferoxamine, has been used to treat ocular siderosis induced by the presence of a ferruginous foreign body (siderosis bulbi). Deferoxamine has very high affinity for ferric iron ($K = 10^{31}$), and readily competes for iron with ferritin and hemosiderin but removes only small amounts from transferrin. The iron in hemoglobin and the cytochrome proteins is inaccessible to deferoxamine (KLAASSEN 1980). WISE (1966) used deferoxamine to treat experimental ocular siderosis, and found that subconjunctival administration prevented siderosis but was ineffective in the treatment of advanced, well-established siderosis. VALVO (1967), on the other hand, used a 10% solution topically applied to treat successfully a long-standing case of ocular siderosis in man. Deferoxamine by itself is not very efficient in iron removal. However, when ascorbate is administered along with deferoxamine, a more effective negative iron balance is reached (Propper et al. 1976). High concentrations of ascorbate in the aqueous humor may explain why topical deferoxamine is effective in the eye. The extremely high binding affinity of deferoxamine for iron is not the only factor important to its success as a drug. The drug must gain entry to the appropriate parts of the eye and then, once having bound iron, must be amenable to mobilization and excretion. Untoward ocular effects caused by deferoxamine are rare (Grant 1974; Fraunfelder 1976). Although several studies of patients receiving the drug for long periods of time have revealed no ocular pathology (Grant 1974), one report of cataracts appearing in three patients has been published (Ciba 1969).

Experiments in which systemic siderosis was induced in dogs (Cibis et al. 1957) demonstrated that high daily doses of iron given for up to 300 days produced ocular lesions as long as 5 years later. Stainable iron had long since disappeared from the eyes, but long-term changes such as retinal degeneration, optic nerve atrophy and gliosis, and a reduction in the pigmented epithelium were noted. Syversen (1979) reported a similar case in man. An anemic patient received a total body dose of 100 g iron over a 20-year period and exhibited reduced visual acuity, a narrowing of visual fields, and tapetoretinal degeneration. No systemic siderosis or hemochromatosis was demonstrated.

Intravitreal homologous hemoglobin and $FeSO_4$ injections both induced DNA synthesis in the rabbit eye. A biphasic response was noted with many ^3H-thymidine-labeled cells moving toward the vitreous from the retinal outer layers in the first phase. These cells appeared to be hematogenous in origin. In the second phase, cells appeared to be moving back through the retina and toward the choroid. By days 2–4, retinal necrosis and disorganization were apparent. Some labeling of Müller cells was also noted (Burke and Smith 1981). The authors suggest that this proliferative response may aggravate the progression of some nonvascular proliferative retinopathies.

A recent report by Eaton et al. (1982) demonstrated that bacterial infection is prevented by haptoglobin, a hemoglobin-binding plasma protein. The apparent mode of action of haptoglobin involves the denial to the bacteria of a critical iron source by preventing the liberation of iron from hemoglobin. Haptoglobin may, in the future, prove to be an effective natural antibacterial agent useful in treating a variety of ocular infections.

C. Zinc

The whole-body zinc level in a normal 70-kg man is estimated at 1.4–2.3 g, about half that of iron, with 20% found in the skin (Underwood 1977).

Although all areas of the eye tested contain detectable levels of zinc, the concentrations vary by an order of magnitude. The cornea, relatively poor in zinc, has approximately 5 mg/100 g dry weight, while the retina and uvea contain some of the highest levels of zinc in the body, 50 mg/100 g dry weight (Vallee 1959; Galin et al. 1962; O'Rourke et al. 1972; Ujiie 1979 a). Zinc levels measured in wet bovine eye tissue also show very high levels of zinc in both the pigmented eye tissues and the lens (Table 2) (Tauber and Krause 1943; Oksala 1954). As with iron, free radicals in the melanin-containing portions of the eye may act as a metal sink and bind large amounts of zinc. Systemic zinc levels are of direct importance to the eye because of the part played by zinc in vitamin A (retinol) metabolism. Zinc is required for the mobilization into the serum of liver vitamin A. Insufficient zinc levels lead to a depression in the rate of synthesis of retinol-binding plasma protein. This in turn reduces the amount of retinol mobilized from the liver and the amount available to the retina (SMITH et al. 1973). Although the concentrations of ocular zinc have been documented, the forms in which it exists have not been described thoroughly. Its high levels in the uveal and retinal tissues are explained, to some degree, by zinc metalloenzymes operating there. In the retina, the zinc metalloenzyme alcohol dehydrogenase catalyzes the conversion of retinol to retinal, a required precursor of rhodopsin. Low systemic zinc levels translate into an alcohol dehydrogenase deficiency and insufficient retinal (HUBER and GERSHOFF 1975). This results in poor dark adaptation (SCHEIE und ALBERT 1977).

Carbonic anhydrase, another zinc metalloenzyme, is found in the ciliary body, a part of the uveal tract. This enzyme has been implicated in the formation of aqueous humor. Inhibitors of carbonic anhydrase can reduce the formation of aqueous humor by 50%–60% (BECKER 1959), but the mechanism by which this reduction is effected is unclear. It is possible that, by slowing the rate of movement of bicarbonate into the aqueous humor of the posterior chamber, the rate of entry of water or the rate of aqueous flow may be reduced (ZIMMERMANN et al. 1976). The action of acetazolamide (Diamox), a carbonic anhydrase inhibitor, is reversible. This effect probably results from the drug's interaction with the zinc complexed at the active site of the enzyme. Ocular or, more specifically, ciliary body zinc levels are not reduced, however (GALIN et al. 1962). Ethambutol, on the other hand, is an antitubercular agent known to chelate zinc (FIGUEROA et al. 1971). An untoward effect of this drug in humans is retrobulbar neuritis (GRANT 1974). It is conceivable that the basis of this side effect lies in the requirement of zinc for the integrity of neuronal microtubules and rapid axonal transport (EDSTROM and MATTSSON 1975). When given to cats and dogs, this drug disrupts the tapetum lucidum, the green, refractile layer behind the retina of many nocturnal animals; this layer contains the highest zinc levels measured in animal tissue. A major component of this layer is zinc cysteinate monohydrate (KOHLER 1981); ethambutol significantly reduces the zinc levels normally found there. Ethambutol studies in rabbits (UJIIE 1979b) showed that while the drug had little effect on zinc levels in extraocular tissues, the cornea, sclera, iris, and optic nerve selectively exhibited significantly depressed zinc concentrations. D-Penicillamine was also evaluated and it induced a decrease in zinc levels in the cornea, iris, choroid, and optic nerve. Diphenylthiocarbazone (Dithizone) is another agent capable of chelating zinc. BUDINGER (1961) tested the ocular effects of diphenylthiocarbazone on dogs and discovered that the drug caused edema and inflammation in the tapetum lucidum. The retina overlying the tapetum appeared normal but later detached. AGUIRRE and RUBIN (1979) corroborated this but found that areas of retina not overlying the tapetum became necrotic. BUDINGER (1961) also studied monkeys and found that doses of diphenylthiocarbazone higher than those given to the dogs caused no detectable ocular changes. Monkeys, like humans, lack a tapetum lucidum. When given to rabbits, however, diphenylthiocarbazone caused nerve-fiber swelling and extensive retinal disorganization within 48 h. These effects were unlike those seen in the dog and the authors suggested that they were not due to the chelation of zinc but to another, undescribed phenomenon (SORSBY and HARDING 1962). LEURE-DU-PREE (1981) was able to induce unique cytoplasmic inclusions in the retinal pigmented epithelium of rats with both diphenylthiocarbazone and 1,10-phenanthroline. These inclusion bodies were osmophilic, were not membrane-bound, and had scalloped edges. The number of inclusion bodies was dose dependent. The origin of the bodies is not known but the author suggests that they are induced by the loss of zinc from the retinal pigmented epithelium, which interferes with zinc-dependent normal functions such as zinc metalloenzyme activity. This view is partially supported by evidence that zinc dietary deficiency can also produce these lesions and that 1,5-phenanthroline, an analog of 1,10-phenanthroline which does not chelate zinc, does not induce the lesions (LEURE-DUPREE and McCLAIN 1982).

Bovine rod outer segments contain a metalloenzyme, superoxide dismutase, which appears to be identical with Cu-Zn-containing superoxide dismutase of erythrocytes. The enzyme activity in the rod outer segments is 200–400 times greater than in the rest of the retina. The enzyme may be important in inhibiting free radical oxidation of polyunsaturated fatty acids. Premature infants exposed to high concentrations of O_2 may develop retrolental fibroplasia, a condition exhibiting gray-white, opaque membranes about the retina. This could be the result of levels of superoxide dismutase insufficient to prevent cytotoxic superoxide radicals from causing lipid peroxidation (HALL 1975). A selenoenzyme, glutathione peroxidase (see Sect. E), is another enzyme important in the protection of the lens and retina from oxidative damage. Studies in the rat have demonstrated that this enzyme is highly sensitive to inhibition by zinc. The K_i for zinc with regard to the enzyme is only $3.7 \times 10^{-6} M$. If the human enzyme is as sensitive to zinc, there is sufficient zinc in the plasma, $1.5 \times 10^{-5} M$ (SPLITTGERBER and TAPPEL 1979), to inhibit glutathione peroxidase. Failure to see this inhibition may be due to the relationship between zinc and albumin. CHARLWOOD (1979) reported that, once zinc has entered the blood from the gastrointestinal tract through a mechanism involving transferrin, the zinc is selectively bound by albumin. Once bound, it may be unable to enter the aqueous humor as free zinc. GERHARD et al. (1980) reported aqueous humor zinc levels to be 0.036 mg/100 g ($5.5 \times 10^{-6} M$). This is sufficient to neutralize 80% of the lenticular glutathione peroxidase if the human enzyme is as sensitive as the rat enzyme. The failure of the lenticular glutathione peroxidase to be inhibited suggests that the zinc in the aqueous humor is bound in some manner, making it unavailable to inhibit the glutathione peroxidase.

D. Copper

Total human body copper levels have been estimated to be 100 mg. Normal blood contains approximately 0.5–1.5 µg/ml (UNDERWOOD 1977).

Remarkably high levels of copper are found in the pigmented tissues of the bovine eye; the iris and ciliary body contain 2–5 mg copper/100 g dry tissue (BOWNESS et al. 1952). The copper is associated with melanin and is largely protein-bound (BOWNESS and MORTON 1953). Although the exact relationship between ocular melanin and copper is unclear, tyrosinase, an enzyme instrumental in melanin synthesis, is a copper-carrying metalloenzyme (O'DELL 1976) and may be responsible in part for these high levels of melanin-associated copper. Melanin content in nonocular pigmented substances such as hair and wool is very sensitive to organismal copper status and also suggests a close relationship between copper and melanin (UNDERWOOD 1977). Nonpigmented bovine eye tissues also contain measurable amounts of copper, although in substantially lower concentrations (TAUBER and KRAUSE 1943; BOWNESS et al. 1952; SWANSON and TRUESDALE 1971; STARZYCKA et al. 1979).

The major pathological condition involving both the eye and copper metabolism is Wilson's disease. Patients with this inherited disorder have insufficient levels of circulating ceruloplasmin, a copper-carrying protein; this results in increased free serum copper, increased urinary excretion of copper, postnecrotic cirrhosis, and focal lesions within the central nervous system (SASS-KORTSAK and BEARN 1978). The pathognomonic sign in Wilson's disease is, however, the Kayser-Fleischer ring found at the limbus of the cornea. The Kayser-Fleischer ring lies on the inner surface of the cornea in the posterior one-third of Descemet's membrane. The width and intensity is greatest at the superior and inferior aspects of the cornea. The basis for this distribution is unknown, but it has been suggested that the vertical flow of aqueous humor which rises along the outer surface of the iris and descends along the inner aspect of the cornea leads to preferential deposition of copper in the better-irrigated regions (SASS-KORTSAK and BEARN 1978). The brown to black granules that form the ring can range from 5 to 180 nm in diameter. The larger granules appear to be conglomerates of smaller granules. Rubeanic stains have revealed the presence of copper in these granules but the form it takes is unknown (JOHNSON 1973).

Control of copper levels in Wilson's disease is now possible through the use of heavy metal chelators. The drug of choice is D-penicillamine (D-β,β-dimethylcysteine). It is an effective chelator of copper, mercury, zinc, and lead, and facilitates urinary excretion of the metal. Under penicillamine therapy, systemic copper levels drop and the Kayser-Fleischer ring partially or totally resolves (SUSSMAN and SCHEINBERG 1969; DINGLE and HAVENER 1978; KLAASSEN 1980). BELKIN et al. (1976) used noninvasive X-ray excitation spectrometry to measure the copper levels in the corneas of seven Wilson's disease patients. Their findings correlated reasonably well with the status of the Kayser-Fleischer ring and well with drug therapy status. Because it is quantitative and more sensitive, this method gives a more accurate estimate of corneal copper levels than does the observation of changes in the Kayser-Fleischer ring.

Cases of suspected penicillamine toxicity have been recorded. Anecdotal reports of chronic follicular conjunctivitis and retinal pigment changes (DINGLE and HAVENER 1978), recurrent asymptomatic superficial retinal hemorrhage (BIGGER 1968), and optic neuritis possibly secondary to a pyridoxine (vitamin B_6) deficiency (TU et al. 1963; GOLDSTEIN et al. 1966) have been published. The dextro form of penicillamine is less toxic than the levo form which is, along with dextro-levo form combinations, responsible for most reported cases of toxicity (KLAASSEN 1980). UJIIE (1979 b) showed that while D-penicillamine did not affect ocular copper levels in normal rabbits, another agent capable of metal-ion chelation did.

Ethambutol induced significant copper level decreases in the cornea and ciliary body without significant changes in the copper status of extraocular tissues.

Two other heavy-metal chelators, triethylene tetramine dihydrochloride and 2,3-dimercaptopropanol (BAL, dimercaprol), have been used as alternatives to penicillamine when penicillamine proved ineffective or toxic. Triethylene tetramine dihydrochloride is, however, effective in a lower percentage of cases (Walshe 1969; Dixon et al. 1972), while 2,3-dimercaptopropanol can induce abscesses at the site of injection, nausea, vomiting, and fever (Sass-Kortsak and Bearn 1978).

Menkes' kinky hair disease is a sex-linked recessive genetic disorder characterized by abnormally low levels of serum copper, copper oxidase, and ceruloplasmin. Wray et al. (1976) studied the ocular lesions in this disease and found a progressive degeneration of retinal ganglion cells, loss of nerve fibers, and optic atrophy. The pigmented epithelium was also abnormal. Its melanin granules were small and irregularly distributed. The authors felt that this could be due to a disruption of normal tyrosinase activity. Tyrosinase is a copper metalloenzyme.

E. Selenium

There are few data on selenium levels in whole human tissues, but generally levels seem to range from 0.01 to 0.03 mg/100 g wet tissue. Tissue concentrations are unusually sensitive to changes in dietary selenium levels (Underwood 1977).

Taussky et al. (1966) quantified the levels of selenium in the bovine eye and found the greatest concentrations in the iris at approximately 0.07 mg/100 g wet tissue. The aqueous humor, vitreous humor, sclera, and cornea all contained trace levels in the range of 0.00016–0.005 mg/100 g wet tissue. Levels in lens and retina were approximately one order of magnitude greater. Swanson and Truesdale (1971) found that lenticular selenium levels normally increased 40-fold during life, but that in cataractous lenses the selenium concentrations were only one-sixth of the levels found in normal lenses of the same age.

Ocular selenium, like ocular zinc, has its most important known function as the metallic component of a metalloenzyme found in the retinal pigmented epithelium (Stone et al. 1979). In 1973, Rotruck et al. showed that gluthathione peroxidase, a selenium metalloenzyme, was important in the protection of hemoglobin from oxidation.

$$2\,G\text{–}SH + H_2O_2 \rightarrow G\text{–}S\text{–}S\text{–}G + 2\,H_2O$$

Hemolyzed erythrocytes from selenium-deficient rats were incubated with ascorbate or H_2O_2 and glutathione. Oxidative damage to the hemoglobin occurred in the absence of glutathione peroxidase due to a failure to degrade the H_2O_2. Most pathological lesions seen in selenium-deficient animals result from peroxidation of unsaturated lipids in cell membranes. Glutathione peroxidase helps to prevent this lipid peroxidation (Flohe et al. 1973). Farnsworth et al. (1979) showed that rats deficient in α-tocopherol (vitamin E) and selenium demonstrated a marked decrease in total polyunsaturated fatty acids in the retinal pigmented epithelium. Both α-tocopherol and glutathione peroxidase are thought to be important in preventing the accumulation of oxidants near the retinal rod outer segments, thereby preventing the oxidation of membrane polyunsaturated fatty acids. These rod outer segments are particularly sensitive in vitro to peroxidation, and both α-tocopherol (FARNSWORTH and DRATZ 1976) and selenium (FLOHE et al. 1973) are capable of offering protection. Their actions appear to be synergistic (FLOHE et al. 1973).

KATZ et al. (1978) showed that when rats were fed a high polyunsaturated fatty acid diet deficient in selenium, α-tocopherol, sulfur-containing amino acids, and chromium, yellow autofluorescent pigment appeared in the retinal pigmented epithelium. This lipofuscin or ceroid pigment is generally thought to be the product of membrane autooxidation. All four of the previously mentioned components in which the diet was deficient appear to function as antioxidants. Dietary supplemention with these components substantially reduced the pigment levels. An apparently identical autofluorescent pigment is also seen in human eyes. Aged, normal eyes and eyes from patients with some forms of retinitis pigmentosa can contain it. In rats deficient in α-tocopherol and selenium, STONE and DRATZ (1980) noted the induction of glutathione-S-transferase. This was apparently in response to the lowered levels of other antioxidants. This prevented significant levels of lipofuscin from accumulating in the central nervous system, liver, testes, and retinal pigmented epithelium. The retina, on the other hand, did not show increased levels of glutathione-S-transferase and did contain elevated levels of lipofuscin.

A glutathione peroxidase similar to the retinal enzyme just described is also found in the lens. Lenticular glutathione peroxidase is also a selenoenzyme with a 4:1 molar ratio of selenium to enzyme (BERGAD et al. 1982). LAWRENCE et al. (1974) showed an 85% reduction in lenticular glutathione peroxidase in rats selenium-deficient in the long term, while SPRINKLER et al. (1971) demonstrated cataracts in second-generation selenium-deficient rats. RATHBUN and HANSON (1979), working with bovine eyes, and GIBLIN et al. (1982), studying rabbits, have described lenticular enzyme systems which revolve around the action of glutathione peroxidase. These enzyme systems scavenge for electrophiles and hydroperoxides, thereby protecting the lens from potentially cataractogenic damage.

OSTADALOVA et al. (1978) and SHEARER et al. (1980) induced cataracts in neonatal rats by selenium salt injections at doses between 0.25 mg/kg and 2.4 mg/kg. In both cases, the cataracts were nuclear in nature. OSTADALOVA et al. (1978) noted that some were permanent while others appeared and disappeared intermittently. SHEARER et al. (1980) thought calcifications might be present and noted that the nuclear lens fibers were abnormally enlarged. With increasing doses of selenite, vacuolization in the equatorial region of lens increased.

The ability to induce cataracts in rats by either significant increases or decreases in systemic selenium levels represents an example of the bell-like curve of trace element dependency discussed in Sect. A. Both deficiency and toxicity states induce lesions; only by maintaining selenium levels within certain physiological limits can normal ocular function be assured.

According to BURK (1976), no specific treatment exists for selenium toxicity. The only treatment involves the removal of the selenium from the immediate environment. Penicillamine, 2,3 dimercaptopropanol, and bromobenzene were all either impractical or ineffective.

F. Vanadium

Vanadium deficiency is found to cause impaired growth, reproduction, and lipid metabolism in mammals (SCHWARZ and MILNE 1971; NIELSEN and SANDSTEAD 1974), and is found in most mammalian tissues in concentrations of 0.1–1 μM. Data from rats and chicks do indicate essentiality, but exact levels are unknown. Required levels in man are not known, but humans can consume 75 mg/day for several weeks without noticeable affects (SOMMERVILLE and DAVIES 1962), and ordinarily consume an estimated 1–4 mg vanadium per day (SCHROEDER et al. 1963 a). However, BECKER (1980) found that very little systemically administered ^{48}V-labeled vanadate entered the rabbit eye.

Through a fortuitous set of circumstances, vanadate, a vanadium salt, was discovered to inhibit sodium-potassium-dependent adenosine triphosphatase (Na–K–ATPase) (CHARNEY et al. 1975; CANTLEY et al. 1977). It has since been shown to inhibit other enzymes, including alkaline phosphatase (LOPEZ et al. 1976), phosphofructokinase (CHOATE and MANSOUR 1978), and adenylate kinase (DEMASTER and MITCHELL 1973). Vanadate appears to block the action of Na–K–ATPase by acting on an intermediate phosphoenzyme. It reversibly binds to a high-affinity ATP site on the enzyme and by doing so also blocks the binding of ATP at another, lower-affinity site (CANTLEY et al. 1977). Because of its action on Na–K–ATPase, vanadate is of interest in ophthalmology; Na–K–ATPase has been implicated in aqueous humor formation. Treatment of the ciliary epithelium with either vanadate ($3 \times 10^{-3}M$) or ouabain ($10^{-6}M$) (also capable of blocking ciliary epithelium Na–K–ATPase) markedly reduces the accumulation of Na–K–ATPase reaction products seen by histochemical localization (BECKER 1980), and vanadate also reduces the uptake by the ciliary epithelium of ^{86}Rb, an element which can compete with potassium. Another interesting facet of the relationship between vanadate and Na–K–ATPase is the effect upon them of ascorbate. Ascorbate can reduce vanadate so that it no longer inhibits Na–K–ATPase, and can reverse the inhibition of ^{86}Rb uptake induced by vanadate (BECKER 1980). V^{+5} is also reduced to V^{+4} by gluthathione (MACARA et al. 1980). It was shown that V^{+4} can form a complex with ATP. The stability constant for this complex is similar to the stability constants for magnesium ATP and manganese ATP at the same pH. Although high V^{+5} concentrations may exist transiently in the body following addition to tissues, within a few hours almost all vanadium is present in V^{+4} complexes with proteins and small molecules such as ATP. As shown by CANTLEY and AISEN (1979), V^{+4} is a much less potent inhibitor of the Na–K–ATPase than V^{+5}, but its effect on other cytoplasmic proteins is unknown. Thus the interplay between ascorbate and gluthathione and V^{+5} at pharmacologic doses may be important to our understanding of the regulatory mechanism of aqueous humor production.

Vanadate has been shown to activate adenylate cyclase in rat fat cells (SCHWABE et al. 1979) and to affect the cAMP–protein kinase system in rat liver (CATALÁN et al. 1980). However, no change in aqueous humor cAMP concentration in rabbit eyes in vivo (BECKER 1980) was noted after vanadate treatment. Vanadate has been shown to lower intraocular pressure (BECKER 1980; KRUPIN et al. 1980) and to inhibit the membrane Na–K–ATPase of the ciliary epithelium in rabbits. This combined effect is consistent with results seen with compounds, such as timolol (10^{-2}

M) and propranolol $3 \times 10^{-4} M$), which also block the Na–K–ATPase. Previously, it was felt that these compounds exhibited their effect by acting as β-adrenergic blocking agents. Recently, however, A. UNGRICHT and D. GREGORY (personal communication) showed that the concentration of timolol necessary to cause changes in intraocular pressure is over two orders of magnitude greater than its binding constant for the adrenergic receptors of the ciliary epithelium, which would suggest the existence of another receptor. At the same time, this concentration is three orders of magnitude less than that required to show 50% inhibition of the Na–K–ATPase. This tends to rule out a role for Na–K–ATPase in timolol action and points to some other mechanism for aqueous humor dynamics. These data may bear on the conflict presented by adrenergic agonists and antagonists having the same effect on aqueous secretion (GREGORY et al. 1981).

The usefulness of vanadate as a therapeutic agent for controlling aqueous humor production is questionable. Vanadate inhibits the active transport of chloride and sodium in the cornea (CANDIA and PODOS 1981), and an agent with an action similar to vanadate, i.e., Na–K–ATPase inhibition, has been implicated in cataractogenesis in Nakano mice (FUKUI et al. 1978).

G. Chromium

SCHWARTZ and MERTZ established in 1959 that rats deficient in chromium grew poorly and had a reduced life expectancy. This was due to an impaired glucose tolerance. This same effect of chromium deficiency was later shown in mice (SCHROEDER et al. 1963 b) and squirrel monkeys (DAVIDSON and BLACKWELL 1968). More recently, glucose intolerance, insulin resistance, and central and peripheral nervous system disorders were described in two separate cases where patients were sustained entirely on intravenous fluids. All symptoms were relieved by parenteral chromium but not insulin (JEEJEEBHOY et al. 1977; FREUND et al. 1979).

Chromium appears to exert its effects through naturally occurring chromium–peptide complexes called "glucose tolerance factors" (GTF). The chromium in the GTF is thought to react with insulin and in some way potentiate its effect (EVANS et al. 1973; ROGINSKI 1974). Consistent with this is the observation that normal serum levels of chromium, 0.03 mM, decrease sharply when glucose is injected (PEKAREK et al. 1974). Also, in genetically diabetic mice in which hyperglycemia and hyperinsulinemia coexist, crude GTF supplementation to the diet (but not inorganic chromium) was effective in reducing the elevated blood glucose levels to normal. It is theorized that these diabetic mice cannot convert inorganic chromium to GTF (TUMAN and DOISY 1977; TUMAN et al. 1978).

Although the chemical structure of GTF remains unclear, several characteristics are currently known (MERTZ 1975; TUMAN and DOISY 1977). The richest source of GTF is brewer's yeast, but it is also found in the liver and kidney of mammals (MERTZ 1969; MERTZ et al. 1974). Studies with crude GTF show that it is capable of binding to insulin (ANDERSON and BRANTNER 1977). More recent work with GTF has suggested that it may be more than one factor and that chromium binds to more than one peptide, although the active fraction appears to result from chromium binding tightly to a peptide similar to glutathione in conjugation with nicotinic acid (ANDERSON and BRANTNER 1977; ANDERSON et al. 1978). In mammals, however, much larger complexes have been found to occur (Yamamoto et al. 1981).

In human studies, there is evidence to suggest that chromium supplementation may improve glucose tolerance (Levine et al. 1968). However, 250 μg of chromium has no effect on the glucose removal rate of normal newborns (Saner et al. 1980), and 1 mg/day for 6 days was found to have no effect in adults (Wise 1978). Recently, though, Offenbacher and Pi-Sunyer (1980) demonstrated that chromium-rich yeast caused significant improvement in glucose tolerance and blood lipids in non-insulin-dependent diabetic subjects, while chromium-poor yeast did not. This would appear to be due to the effect of GTF rather than that of free chromium. These data are consistent with the finding of a decrease in total urine chromium concentration with age (Canfield and Doisy 1976). In this study, healthy subjects had the highest concentration of volatile chromium (thought to be GTF) in their urine, while elderly and diabetic subjects had lower concentrations. In addition, the decrease in urinary chromium was greater in the volatile form than in the nonvolatile form, which would appear to indicate a loss of GTF.

In the eye, the role of chromium is not documented. However, Reid and Antonetti (unpublished data) have shown that GTF preparations from yeast, but not free chromium, will stimulate the growth of human retinoblastoma-derived cultured cells growing in a totally serum-free environment. Thus GTF may play a role in cell growth in the eye.

H. Conclusion

Although much is unknown about ocular trace elements, several have been shown to be critical to ocular function. Most are important because they are components of biomolecules which play important roles in the normal physiology of the eye. Selenium, an integral part of glutathione peroxidase, is necessary for the protection of both the lens and the retina from oxidative damage. Zinc, as a component of superoxide dismutase, serves a similar function. Vanadium, on the other hand, may at pharmacologic concentrations exert an effect on aqueous humor dynamics as an inorganic metal salt, not as a metal ion in complex with a biomolecule.

The bell-like curve of trace element dependency may appear intuitively obvious, but it is nonetheless very important in at least two areas of therapy. Any drug which can chelate metal ions, whether or not that is its major function, must be used judiciously to avoid inducing trace element deficiencies. This should be stressed, because some chelating agents, including penicillamine, are capable of binding a variety of metal ions. The advent of total parenteral nutrition regiments has created another source of iatrogenic trace element imbalance. As with the case of cataracts induced by both selenium deficiency and selenium toxicity, supplementation of total parenteral nutrition regimens with trace elements can lead to either deficiency or toxicity states. A change in the concentration of one trace element can affect the function of systems dependent on another trace element; the ability of zinc to inhibit the selenoenzyme glutathione peroxidase is an excellent example of this. These relationships require that each element be carefully titrated to avoid disrupting both systemic and ocular homeostasis.

Acknowledgments. The authors thank MARY V. BANNON for the rapid and accurate preparation of the manuscript, Dr. MIGUEL COCA-PRADOS for his invaluable assistance in translating portions of the literature, and Dr. DOUGLAS S. GREGORY for his illuminating comments on the manuscript.

References

Aguirre G, Rubin L (1979) Disease of the retinal pigment epithelium in animals. In: Zinn KM; Marmor MF (eds) The retinal pigment epithelium. Harvard University Press, Cambridge, p 334

Aisen P, Listowsky I (1980) Iron transport and storage proteins. Ann Rev Biochem 49:357 393

Anderson RA, Brantner JH (1977) Binding of chromium by porcine insulin. Fed Proc 36:1123

Anderson RA, Polansky MM, Roginski ED, Mertz W (1978) Factors affecting the retention and extraction of yeast chromium. J Agric Food Chem 26:858–861

Becker B (1959) Carbonic anhydrase and the formation of the aqueous humor. Am J Ophthalmol 47:342–361

Becker B (1980) Vanadate and aqueous humor dynamics. Invest Ophthalmol Vis Sci 19:1156–1165

Belkin M, Chajek T, Zeimer R, Friedman G, Melamed E (1976) Non-invasive quantitation of corneal copper in hepatolenticular degeneration (Wilson's disease). Lancet I:391–392

Bergad PL, Rathbun WB, Linder W (1982) Glutathione peroxidase from bovine lens: a selenoenzyme. Exp Eye Res 34:131–134

Bigger JF (1968) Retinal hemorrhages during penicillamine therapy of cystinuria. Am J Ophthalmol 66:954–955

Bowness JM, Morton RA (1953) The association of zinc and other metals with melanin and a melanin-protein complex. Biochem J 53:620–626

Bowness JM, Morton RA, Shakir MN, Stubbs AL (1952) Distribution of copper and zinc in mammalian eyes. Occurrence of metals in melanin fractions from eye tissues. Biochem J 51:521–530

Bruenger FW, Stover BJ, Atherton DR (1976) The incorporation of various metal ions in vivo- and in vitro-produced melanin. Radiat Res 32:1–12

Budinger JM (1961) Diphenylthiocarbazone blindness in dogs. Arch Pathol 71:304–310

Burk RF (1976) Selenium in man. In: Prasad AS (ed) Trace elements in human health and disease, vol 2. Academic, New York, p 105

Burke JM, Smith JM (1981) Retinal proliferation in response to vitreous hemoglobin or iron. Invest Ophthalmol Vis Sci 20:582–592

Candia OA, Podos SM (1981) Inhibition of active transport of chloride and sodium by vanadate in the cornea. Invest Ophthal Vis Sci 20:733–739

Canfield WK, Doisy RJ (1976) Chromium and diabetes in the aged. In: Hsu JM, Davis RL, Neithamer RW (eds) The biochemical role of trace elements in aging. Eckerd College, St. Petersburg, p 119

Cantley LC, Aisen P (1979) The fate of cytoplasmic vanadium. J Biol Chem 254:1781–1784

Cantley LC, Josephson L, Warner R, Yanagisawa M, Lechene C, Guidotti G (1977) Vanadate is a potent (Na, K)-ATPase inhibitor found in ATP derived from muscle. J Biol Chem 252:7421–7423

Catalán RE, Martínez AM, Aragonés MD (1980) Effects of vanadate on the cyclic AMP-protein kinase system in rat liver. Biochem Biophys Res Com 96:672–677

Charlwood PA (1979) The relative affinity of transferrin and albumin for zinc. Biochim Biophys Acta 581:260–265

Charney AN, Silva P, Epstein FN (1975) An in vitro inhibitor of Na–K–ATPase present in an adenosine triphosphate preparation. J Appl Physiol 39:156–158

Chester JK (1979) Biochemical functions of zinc in animals. World Rev Nutr Diet 32:135–164

Choate GL, Mansour TE (1978) Inhibition of sheep heart phosphofructokinase by ortho vanadate. Fed Proc 37:1433

Ciba Pharmaceutical Company (1969) Deferoxamine mesylate (Desferal mesylate). Clin Pharmacol Ther 10:595–596

Cibis PA, Brown EB, Hong S-M (1957) Ocular effects of systemic siderosis. Am J Ophthalmol 44:158–172

Davidson IWF, Blackwell WL (1968) Changes in carbohydrate metabolism of squirrel monkeys with chromium dietary supplementation. Proc Soc Exp Biol Med 127:66–70

Davies G, Dymock I, Harry J, Williams R (1972) Deposition of melanin and iron in ocular structures in haemochromatosis. Br J Ophthalmol 56:338–342

DeMaster EG, Mitchell RA (1973) A comparison of arsenate and vanadate as inhibitors or uncouplers of mitochondrial and glycolytic energy metabolism. Biochemistry 12:3616–3621

Dingle J, Havener WH (1978) Ophthalmoscopic changes in a patient with Wilson's disease during long-term penicillamine therapy. Ann Ophthalmol 10:1227–1230

Dixon HBF, Gibbs K, Walshe JM (1972) Preparation of triethylenetetramine dihydrochloride for the treatment of Wilson's disease. Lancet I:853

Eaton JW, Brandt P, Mahoney JR, Lee JT (1982) Haptoglobin: a natural bacteriostat. Science 215:691–693

Eckert CD (1979) A comparative study of the concentrations of Ca, Fe, Zn, Cu, and Mn in ocular tissues. Fed Proc 38:872

Edstrom A, Mattsson H (1975) Small amounts of zinc stimulate rapid axonal transport in vitro. Brain Res 86:162–167

Evans GW, Roginski EE, Mertz W (1973) Interaction of the glucose tolerance factor (GTF) with insulin. Biochem Biophys Res Commun 50:718–722

Farnsworth CC, Dratz EA (1976) Oxidative damage of retinal rod outer segment membranes and the role of vitamin E. Biochim Biophys Acta 443:556–570

Farnsworth CC, Stone WL, Dratz EA (1979) Effects of vitamin E and selenium deficiency of the fatty acid composition of rat retinal tissues. Biochim Biophys Acta 552:281–293

Figueroa R, Weiss H, Smith JC, Hackley BM, McBean LD, Swassing CR, Halsted JA (1971) Effect of ethambutol on the ocular zinc concentration in dogs. Am Rev Respir Dis 104:592–594

Fischbach FA, Anderegg JW (1965) An X-ray scattering study of ferritin and apoferritin. J Mol Biol 14:458–473

Flohe L, Günzler WA, Schock HH (1973) Glutathione peroxidase: a selenoenzyme. FEBS Lett 32:132–134

Food and Nutrition Board (1974) Recommended daily allowances, 8th edn National 1 Academy of Sciences, Washington, DC

Fraunfelder FT (1976) Drug-induced ocular side effects and drug interactions. Lea and Febiger, Philadelphia

Freund H, Atamian S, Fischer JE (1979) Chromium deficiency during total parenteral nutrition. JAMA 241:496–499

Fukui HN, Merola LO, Kinoshita JN (1978) A possible cataractogenic factor in Nakano mouse lens. Exp Eye Res 26:477–485

Galin MA, Nano HD, Hall T (1962) Ocular zinc concentration. Invest Ophthalmol 1:142–148

Gass JDM (1964) The iron lines of the superficial cornea. Arch Ophthalmol 71:348–358

Gerhard JP, Calmé P, Kraeminger E (1980) À propos du zinc de l'humeur aqueuse. Klin Monatsbl Augenheilkd 176:652–654

Giblin FJ, McCready JP, Reddy VN (1982) The role of glutathione metabolism in the detoxification of H_2O_2 in rabbit lens. Invest Ophthalmol Vis Sci 22:333–335

Goldstein NP, Hollenhorst RW, Randall RV, Gross JB (1966) Possible relationship of optic neuritis, Wilson's disease and DL-penicillamine therapy. JAMA 196:734–735

Grant WM (1974) Toxicology of the eye, 2nd edn Thomas, Springfield

Gregory DS, Bausher LP, Bromberg BB, Sears ML (1981) The beta-adrenergic receptor and adenyl cyclase of rabbit ciliary processes. In: Sears ML (ed) New directions in ophthalmic research. Yale University Press, New Haven, p 127

Hall MO (1975) Superoxide dismutase of bovine and frog rod outer segments. Biochem Biophys Res Commun 67:1199–1204

Harper AE (1976) Basis of recommended dietary allowances for trace elements. In: Prasad AS (ed) Trace elements in human health and disease, vol 2. Academic, New York, p 371

Higgins ES, Richert DA, Westerfeld WW (1956) Molybdenum deficiency and tungstate inhibition studies. J Nutr 59:539–559

Huber AM, Gershoff SN (1975) Effects of zinc deficiency on the oxidation of retinol and ethanol in rats. J Nutr 105:1486–1490

Iwamoto T, DeVoe AG (1976) Electron microscopical study of the Fleischer ring. Arch Ophthalmol 94:1579–1584

Jeejeebhoy KN, Chu RC, Marliss EB, Greenberg GR, Bruce-Robertson A (1977) Chromium deficiency, glucose intolerance and neuropathy reversed by chromium supplementation, in a patient receiving long-term total parenteral nutrition. Am J Clin Nutr 30:531–538

Johnson BL (1973) Ultrastructure of the Kayser-Fleischer ring. Am J Ophthalmol 76:455–461

Katz ML, Stone WL, Dratz EA (1978) Fluorescent pigment accumulation in retinal pigment epithelium of antioxidant-deficient rats. Invest Ophthalmol Vis Sci 17:1049–1058

Ketola HG (1979) Influence of dietary zinc on cataracts in rainbow trout (*Salmo gairdneri*). J Nutr 109:965–969

Klaassen CD (1980) Heavy metals and heavy-metal antagonists. In: Gilman AG, Goodman LS, Gilman A (eds) The pharmacological basis of therapeutics, 6th edn MacMillan, New York, p 1615

Kohler T (1981) Histochemical and cytochemical demonstration of zinc cysteinate in the tapetum lucidum of the cat. Histochemistry 70:173–178

Krupin T, Becker B, Podos SM (1980) Topical vanadate lowers intraocular pressure in rabbits. Invest Ophthalmol Vis Sci 19:1360–1363

Lawrence RA, Sunde RA, Schwartz GL, Hoekstra WG (1974) Glutathione peroxidase activity in rat lens and other tissues in relation to dietary selenium intake. Exp Eye Res 18:563–569

Leure-duPree AE (1981) Electron-opaque inclusions in the rat retinal pigment epithelium after treatment with chelators of zinc. Invest Ophthalmol Vis Sci 21:1–9

Leure-duPree AE, McClain CJ (1982) The effect of severe zinc deficiency on the morphology of rat retinal pigment epithelium. Invest Ophthalmol Vis Sci 23:425–434

Levine RA, Streeten DPH, Doisy RJ (1968) Effects of oral chromium supplementation on the glucose tolerance of elderly human subjects. Metabolism 17:114–125

Lopez V, Stevens T, Lindquist RN (1976) Vanadium ion inhibition of alkaline phosphatase-catalyzed phosphate ester hydrolysis. Arch Biochem Biophys 175:31–38

Macara IG, Justin K, Cantley LC (1980) Glutathione reduces cytoplasmic vanadate mechanism and physiological implications. Biochim Biophys Acta 629:95–106

Mertz W (1969) Chromium occurrence and function in biological systems. Physiol Rev 49:163–239

Mertz W (1975) Effects and metabolism of glucose tolerance factor. Nutr Rev 33:129–135

Mertz W (1977) Human requirements: Basic and optimal. NY Acad Sci 199:191–201

Mertz W (1981) The essential trace elements. Science 213:1332–1338

Mertz W, Toepfer EW, Roginski EE, Polansky MM (1974) Present knowledge of the role of chromium. Fed Proc 33:2275–2280

Nielsen FH, Sandstead HH (1974) Are nickel, vanadium, silicon, fluorine, and tin essential for man? A review. Am J Clin Nutr 27:515–520

O'Dell BL (1976) Biochemistry and physiology of copper in vertebrates. In: Prasad AS (ed) Trace elements in human health and disease, vol 1. Academic, New York, p 391

Offenbacher EG, Pi-Sunyer FX (1980) Beneficial effect of chromium-rich yeast on glucose tolerance and blood lipids in elderly subjects. Diabetes 29:919–925

Oksala A (1954) On the occurrence of some trace metals in the eye. Acta Ophthalmol 32:235–244

O'Rourke J, Durrani J, Benson C (1972) Uveoretinal uptake of [69m]Zn. Ophthalmol Res 3:289–297

Ostadalova I, Babicky B, Obenberger J (1978) Cataract induced by administration of a single dose of sodium selenite to suckling rats. Experientia 34:222–223

Pekarek RS, Hauer EC, Rayfield EJ, Wannemacher RW, Beisel WR (1974) Relationship between serum chromium and glucose utilization in normal and infected subjects. Fed Proc 33:660

Potts AM, Au PC (1976) The affinity of melanin for inorganic ions. Exp Eye Res 22:487–491

Prasad AS (1978) Trace elements and iron in human metabolism. Plenum, New York

Prasad AS (1979) Clinical, biochemical and pharmacological role of zinc. Annu Rev Pharmacol Toxicol 19:393–426

Propper RD, Shurin SB, Nathan DG (1976) Reassessment of the use of desferrioxamine B in iron overload. N Engl J Med 294:1421–1423

Rathbun WB, Hanson SK (1979) Glutathione metabolic pathway as a scavenging system in the lens. Ophthalmol Res 11:172–176

Riley PA (1970) Mechanism of pigment-cell toxicity produced by hydroxyanisole. J Pathol 101:163–169

Roginsky EE (1974) Effects of nicotinic acid-chromium complexes on glucose oxidation by rat epididymal fat tissue. Fed Proc 33:659

Roth AM, Foos RY (1972) Ocular pathologic changes in primary hemochromatosis. Arch Ophthalmol 87:507–514

Rotruck JT, Pope AL, Ganther HE, Swanson AB, Hafeman DG, Hoekstra WG (1973) Selenium: biochemical role as a component of glutathione peroxidase. Science 179:588–590

Saner G, Türkan Y, Gürson CT (1980) Effect of chromium on insulin secretion and glucose removal rate in the newborn. Am J Clin Nutr 33:232–235

Sass-Kortsak A, Bearn AG (1978) Hereditary disorders of copper metabolism. In: Stanbury JB, Wyngaarden JB, Fredrickson DS (eds) The metabolic basis of inherited disease, 4th edn McGraw-Hill, New York, p 1098

Scheie HG, Albert DM (1977) Textbook of ophthalmology, 9th edn Saunders, Philadelphia

Schroeder HA (1965) The biological trace elements. J Chronic Dis 18:217–228

Schroeder HA, Balassa JJ, Tipton IH (1963a) Abnormal trace metals in man – vanadium. J Chronic Dis 16:1047–1071

Schroeder HA, Vinton WH, Balassa JJ (1963b) Effect of chromium, cadmium and other trace metals on the growth and survival of mice. J Nutr 80:39–47

Schwabe U, Puchstein C, Hannemann H, Söchtig E (1979) Activation of adenylate cyclase by vanadate. Nature 277:143–145

Schwarz K, Metz W (1959) Chromium III and the glucose tolerance factor. Arch Biochem Biophys 85:292–295

Schwarz K, Milne DB (1971) Growth effects of vanadium in the rat. Science 174:426–428

Shearer TR, McCormack DW, DeSart DJ, Britton JL, Lopez MT (1980) Histological evaluation of selenium induced cataracts. Exp Eye Res 31:327–333

Smith JC, McDaniel EG, Fan FF, Halsted JA (1973) Zinc: a trace element essential in vitamin A metabolism. Science 181:954–955

Somerville J, Davies B (1962) Effect of vanadium on serum cholesterol. Am Heart J 64:54–56

Sorsby A, Harding R (1962) Experimental degeneration of the retina – VIII. Vision Res 2:149–155

Splittgerber AG, Tappel AL (1979) Inhibition of glutathione peroxidase by cadmium and other metal ions. Arch Biochem Biophys 197:534–542

Sprinkler L, Harr J, Newberne P, Whanger D, Weswig P (1971) Selenium deficiency lesions in rats fed vitamin E supplemented rations. Nutr Rep Int 4:335–340

Starzycka M, Kowalski A, Kedziora M (1979) Some inorganic constituents of the subretinal fluid. Ophthalmologica 179:220–224

Stone WL, Dratz EA (1980) Increased glutathione-S-transferase activity in antioxidant-deficient rats. Biochim Biophys Acta 631:503–506

Stone WL, Katz ML, Lurie M, Marmon MF, Dratz EA (1979) Effects of dietary vitamin E and selenium on light damage to the rat eye. Photochem Photobiol 29:725–730

Sussman, W, Scheinberg IH (1969) Disappearance of Kayser-Fleischer rings. Arch Ophthalmol 82:738–741

Swanson AA, Truesdale AW (1971) Elemental analysis in normal and cataractous human lens tissue. Biochem Biophys Res Commun 45:1488–1496

Swanson AA, Jeter J, Tucker P (1968) Inorganic cations in the crystalline lens from young and aged rats. J Gerontol 23:502–505

Syversen K (1979) Intramuscular iron therapy and tapetoretinal degeneration. Acta Ophthalmol 57:358–361

Tauber FW, Krause AC (1943) The role of iron, copper, zinc, and manganese in the metabolism of the ocular tissues, with special reference to the lens. Am J Ophthalmol 26:260–266

Taussky HH, Washington A, Zubillaga E, Mihorat AT (1966) Distribution of selenium in the tissues of the eye. Nature 210:949–950

Tu J-B, Blackwell RQ, Lee P-F (1963) DL-Penicillamine as a cause of optic axial neuritis. JAMA 185:83–86

Tuman RW, Doisy RJ (1977) Metabolic effects of the glucose tolerance factor (GTF) in normal and genetically diabetic mice. Diabetes 26:820–826

Tuman RW, Bilbo JT, Doisy RJ (1978) Comparison and effects of natural and synthetic glucose tolerance factor in normal and genetically diabetic mice. Diabetes 27:49–56

Ujiie M (1979a) Studies on metabolism of trace metals, especially of zinc, in biological fluids and tissues (1). Nippon Ganka Gakkai Zasshi 83:105–113

Ujiie M (1979b) Studies on metabolism of trace metals, especially of zinc, in biological fluids and tissues (2). Nippon Ganka Gakkai Zasshi 83:114–121

Underwood EJ (1977) Trace elements in human and animal nutrition, 4th edn. Adacemic, New York

Urrets-Zavalia A, Katz C (1971) Corneal hemochromatosis. Am J Ophthalmol 72:88–96

Vallee BL (1959) Biochemistry, physiology and pathology of zinc. Physiol Rev 39:443–490

Valvo A (1967) Desferrioxamine B in ophthalmology. Am J Ophthalmol 63:98–103

Walshe JM (1969) Management of penicillamine nephropathy in Wilson's disease: a new chelating agent. Lancet II:1401–1402

Wise A (1978) Chromium supplementation and diabetes. JAMA 240:2045–2046

Wise JB (1966) Treatment of experimental siderosis bulbi, vitreous hemorrhage, and corneal blood staining with deferoxamine. Arch Ophthalmol 75:698–707

Wray SH, Kuwabara T, Sanderson P (1976) Menkes' kinky hair disease: a light and electron microscopic study of the eye. Invest Ophthalmol 15:128–138

Yamamoto A, Wada O, Ono T (1981) A low-molecular-weight chromium-binding substance in mammals. Toxicol Appl Pharmacol 59:515–523

Yolton D (1981) Nutritional effects of zinc on ocular and systemic physiology. J Am Optom Assoc 52:409–414

Zimmerman TJ, Garg LC, Vogh BP, Maren TH (1976) The effect of acetazolamide on the movements of anions into the posterior chamber of the dog eye. J Pharmacol Exp Ther 196:510–516

CHAPTER 18

Clinical Trials

D. SEIGEL

A. A Strategy of Research

Clinical trials of pharmacologic agents in ophthalmology consist of randomized allocation of eyes or patients to alternative treatments in order to evaluate the efficacy and toxicity of each. At their best, they give careful attention to ethical factors, masking, appropriate sample size, well-defined questions and procedures, quality control, follow-up, data monitoring, and statistical analysis, though none of these is unique to clinical trials.

The clinical trial is only one of the several ways in which information on the role of a drug in therapy is accumulated. Several well-defined stages (DOLLERY and BENNETT 1975; WHO SCIENTIFIC GROUP 1968) are generally required to bring a drug into widespread use, each with its own design characteristics. As the drug moves from the laboratory to use in man, the number of subjects under investigation will be small, and the principal goal is to determine whether the drug has marked toxicity. Normal volunteers may be used and tissues and organs that might be affected are screened for toxicity. If no significant unanticipated toxicity emerges, the dose–response relationship can be explored in patients. The goal is to obtain the minimal effective dose. Once the appropriate dose has been defined, a clinical trial with sufficient controls and patients to evaluate the drug's efficacy and toxicity is then needed to permit an informed judgment on whether the drug should be marketed.

Our interest in learning more about drugs continues after marketing. Premarketing studies rarely permit evaluation of long-term effects of drugs, or of less common side effects. Even agents that are as familiar to the clinician as salicylic acid continue to reveal new aspects of their physiological response. Guidelines for such continued study vary. They may require additional clinical trials, or other research designs familiar to the epidemiologist (MACMAHON and PUGH 1970).

The role of the randomized clinical trial within this research strategy is still unfolding. Credit for popularizing the clinical trial is usually given to Bradford Hill, a British physician who participated in a study (MEDICAL RESEARCH COUNCIL 1948) which demonstrated the efficacy of streptomycin in tuberculosis therapy, and wrote a textbook on medical statistics that remains one of the foremost primers (HILL 1971). Advocates of the method regard it as most likely to provide a valid evaluation of the merits of alternative treatments. KUPFER (1979) writes:

... there are isolated instances in medicine where the results of certain therapies were so dramatic in their immediate benefit that extensive clinical testing was not necessary. However, one can be confronted with chronic diseases characterized by remissions and exacerbations in which, even after many years of experience with a treatment modality, the efficacy of the therapy still remains uncertain.

He goes on to show how clinical trials have yielded results that markedly altered views previously held on portacaval shunt for cirrhosis of the liver with varices, tolbutamide therapy in diabetic patients, and tamoxifen use in the treatment of breast carcinoma.

The successful conduct of clinical trials requires the collaboration of personnel trained in a variety of disciplines. These include statistics and computer sciences. Because the technical aspects of the subject are complex, and would be difficult to describe in a single chapter, the objective here will be limited to indicating what the current thinking is on some of the major issues. They will be discussed in the order in which they actually occur: planning and conducting the trial, and analysis of the data.

B. Planning the Trial

There is much to be said for spending ample time "sharpening pencils" prior to beginning a clinical trial. Several months are likely to be required to state the research questions carefully, demonstrate that the study will answer them, and write a detailed protocol.

I. Defining the Research Goals

Inexperienced investigators tend to underestimate the importance of carefully stating all the research questions that a study is intended to address. Such questions are likely to fall into one of three general types.
1. Which drug has greater efficacy and which has more side effects? (Main effects)
2. Do the differences appear to be the same in all types of patients, or do they vary in individual subgroups? (Interactions)
3. Aside from treatment, what factors appear to govern the progress of the disease? (Natural history)

An understanding of these three questions will facilitate the planning of a study. For instance, does a new β-blocker decrease intraocular pressure, and what complications accompany its use? Does its effectiveness vary with racial group, age, or duration of disease? Do patients with hypertension progress more rapidly to loss of visual function?

Some general principles that might be kept in mind when discussing the role of these questions in any clinical trial are:
1. A study will do well if it answers main effect questions alone.
2. Though the pursuit of interactions may be attractive, they require increased sample sizes and are found to be present less often than is generally supposed.
3. Natural history questions can be pursued outside of randomized clinical trials, frequently by research designs that are considerably less costly.

Planners of a trial are greatly tempted to add on as many incidental data as they can think of, in what may be called the "Wouldn't it be interesting...?" syndrome. When trials involve several clinics and long follow-up, some may view them like Noah's Ark, the last boat out, and add items to the protocol as though seeking two of every beast in the kingdom. Modern trials are not constructed as was Noah's Ark, however, and when over loaded may float with the safe water line submerged.

Every laboratory measurement, every clinical observation, and every item on the questionnaire will have some cost. This cost may be in data processing, entry, verification, storage, and recall. It may appear in patient fatigue, leading to decreased participation. The increased examination protocol may be accompanied by a lower quality of data acquisition throughout, since time and personnel may no longer be generously dedicated to essential items. Finally, financial costs are likely to be increased.

II. Sample Size

If there is any role with which the statistician is identified, it is determination of the sample size. He does this by assisting the investigator in specifying at least two essential pieces of information: (a) the principal end point(s) of the study, and (b) the degree of difference in rates that is clinically significant (and must therefore be detected by the study). The manual of procedures (Diabetic Retinopathy Vitrectomy Study, Manual of operations, unpublished, 1970) for the National Eye Institute study of early versus late vitrectomy states: "To demonstrate a 25% change in the success rate of 0.41, a combined sample size of 826 eyes is required." "Success" rate refers to the principal end point, attaining 20/200 or better visual acuity; 25% change in the number achieving this end point was perceived as clinically important.

Some simple rules govern sample size computations:
1. "Small" samples suffice only in those remarkable instances when treatment effects turn out to be overwhelming.
2. No sample size is ever truly large enough. There are always groups of patients of special interest that one wishes to look at separately. Further, there are often secondary "end points," some of which may require larger sample sizes than do the main end points.
3. Two factors generally argue for minimal sample sizes. The first is limited resources (of patients, of investigators, of money); the second is the need to arrive at decisions governing patient care as early as possible.
4. Studies of uncommon complications tend to require very large sample sizes. In studies of the safety of intraocular lens implants in cataract surgery, for example, evaluating visual function requires fewer patients than estimating the rate of postoperative corneal decompensation.

A recent nomogram (FEIGL 1978) is one of several published sources to assist the investigator (and statistician) in specifying reasonable sample sizes.

III. The Ethical Basis

When is it appropriate to initiate a clinical trial? When there is considerable doubt as to which of the available treatments is better, with the weight of evidence favoring each roughly in balance and each having a reasonable chance of turning out to be a sizeable "winner."

But what is meant by "better?" Does it refer to effectiveness of the treatments? What about complications? If these are implied, which measures of effectiveness, which complications? How does one combine the assessment of effectiveness and complications? Should we divide the two, as in the risk/benefit ratio? Though the assessment of potential risks and benefits of alternative treatments is not likely to lend itself to a formal analysis, we are obliged nevertheless to satisfy ourselves that informed opinion does not strongly favor one treatment more than the others, and that there is ample opportunity for each treatment to emerge from the trial clearly preferred. In order to do so, the planners of a trial need to review the major goals of treatment and the major complications, and satisfy themselves that an "overall" balance exists. Such a review will include anecdotal information, previous clinical experience, animal research, and theoretical arguments that draw upon outside information.

C. Conducting the Trial

I. Bias

We tend to be less aware of our own susceptibility to introduce bias into our research then we are of others. GEORGE CORNER and WILLARD ALLEN collaborated to discover progesterone, but prior to publishing their results, CORNER found himself frustrated at being unable to replicate their experimental results independently. CORNER (1963) explains:

> ...our rabbits ranged from 600 to 1,200 g. When we went to the cages to inject them, WILLARD ALLEN's idea of what constitutes a nice rabbit led him to choose the larger ones, while I must have had a subconscious preference for the infants. My extracts had been as good as his all the while, but my rabbits were insensitive. It is staggering to think how often the success or failure of research may hang upon such an unimaginable contingency.

In 1794, BENJAMIN RUSH expressed "sublime joy" in describing his success in treating yellow fever by bloodletting. "Of the one hundred patients whom I have visited, or prescribed for, this day, I have lost none" (RUSH 1794). The study was uncontrolled and Rush's sublime joy established bloodletting as a standard therapy for a half century.

Randomization and masking (blinding) help to constrain our natural inclinations to make sure that the therapies we investigate turn out to be safe and effective. Randomization (allocation of patients to treatments by a chance device, such as coin tossing) has as its principal goal the creation of treatment groups that are similar. COCHRAN and COX (1957) describe randomization as "one of the few characteristics of modern experimental design that appears to be really modern. One can find experiments made 100 to 150 years ago that embody the principles that are now regarded as sound, with the conspicuous exception of randomization." Rather than tossed coins, investigators commonly use random numbers, either from published tables or as generated by computers. Shortcuts such as alternating days for subject assignment are less foolproof than randomization in restraining the investigator's bias.

Assignment of a treatment to the "worse" eye is likely to lead to confusing results. That eye may be worse because of temporary random variation. If so, changes in function before and after treatment may be greater in the worse eye for reasons unrelated to the treatment. Moreover, determining which is the worse eye may not be straightforward, and the investigator may then have the freedom to make his assignment by criteria that remain unknown.

Wherever possible the treatment to which the patient is assigned should be coded, or unavailable. Such masking of the patient and the investigator ensures that data collection is free of bias. Masking takes over where randomization ends. It may require omission of the treatment on forms, evaluation of patient progress by someone other than the therapist, or other precautions. Where a placebo is possible, it is preferable to no treatment. The chances of success of such placebos will be proportional to the effort expended to make them similar in appearance, taste, and smell to the drug being evaluated. The investigator who believes these several measures to eliminate bias unnecessary should consider them nevertheless, since journal reviewers and his professional peers may have higher levels of scientific skepticism than he does.

II. Data Monitoring

In many trials, data may be available for analysis while patients are still being randomized to treatment. Review of such data may reveal strong trends favoring one or more treatment to others. The weight of opinion of those reviewing the data may shift, causing cracks to appear in the ethical foundation supporting the trial. Modern practice of clinical trials requires that for each one "data and safety monitoring committees" be established, whose responsibility it is to review the accumulating data and recommend changes in protocol that are indicated. Such changes may mean eliminating a treatment, or even stopping the trial. The committee may have to investigate high complication rates in an individual clinic. Their analyses typically anticipate those that will be employed at completion of the study. Their primary responsibility is to ensure that the trial does not continue longer than it needs to. Though complicated statistical procedures have been devised to adapt to this continued monitoring of the data, none are really satisfactory, and at best one hopes for wise decisions from a committee of experts. Knowledge of the subject matter, the details of the trial, and statistics needs to be represented. Where possible, those who are involved in treating study patients or evaluating their progress should not be members of the monitoring committee. Otherwise they may find themselves in an awkward position when discussing the trial with new patients. The committee should meet sufficiently frequently for large shifts in the data not to go unnoticed. Members need to guard against the twin dangers of continuing the trial after the research questions have been answered, and stopping the trial prematurely on the basis of weak early trends.

Even in trials where randomized allocation of treatment has been terminated, data monitoring is desirable. Preferable treatments need to be detected and reported as early as possible.

III. Follow-up

The general principles relating to follow-up of patients are among the simplest and yet most poorly appreciated. If a sizable proportion of patients who should have had 3 years' follow-up did not return for examinations in the 3rd year, then the study results for 3 years after treatment will simply not be convincing. The same can be said for any other duration of follow-up. The study will be capable, then, of reporting results of treatment only for a period of time for which losses to follow-up are kept low.

If the percentage lost to follow-up is high, then critics will properly inquire whether results for such patients are fairly represented by those for whom examination data remain available. Are patients lost because of poor visual outcome and dissatisfaction with the study? Are they lost because their condition is improved, and tiring clinic visits seem unnecessary? Has their health deteriorated, including their eye condition?

The best way to avoid problems with losses to follow-up, it has been suggested, is not to have any. But that is rarely achieved. Some measures can be taken to minimize the problem:

1. Only include patients who appear stable and committed to participation in the trial. Patients who are uncertain may help to meet recruiting quotas but will be costly to the quality of the study.
2. Obtain personal information that will help to locate a patient who has moved. Social Security numbers and names and addresses of close relatives not living with the patient are examples.
3. Some patients may need help in getting to the clinic.
4. Consideration should be given to conducting examinations in the patient's home when no other choice is available.
5. If a patient has moved, a lesser amount of information may be helpful, either self-reported or obtained by another physician.
6. Newsletters might be sent to patients periodically to keep interest high. These could include reports on the progress of the study, or general information on health care.
7. Where possible, the reasons why patients are no longer participating in a study should be obtained and tabulated. Have they moved, become very ill, sought medical care elsewhere, or refused to return to the clinic? Tabulating such reasons may assist in evaluating the impact of the losses to follow-up.
8. Compare characteristics of patients who remain in the study with those who do not. Though such comparisons do not demonstrate that these two groups have similar outcomes after patients are lost, they may provide a measure of reassurance.

One commonly suggested means of dealing with the problem of losses to follow-up is to replace these patients with an equal number of cooperative patients. Though this suggestion helps to restore satisfactory sample sizes to the study, it does not provide a solution to the problem of bias resulting from loss-to-follow-up patients being markedly different from those who remain.

D. Analysis of the Results

I. Adherence

Some patients may not receive the treatment to which they are randomized. The investigator may feel that the medical condition in a patient has changed, so that the treatment is no longer indicated, or the patient may refuse. Where the treatment is repetitive, as with glaucoma medication, the patient may miss treatments, or stop completely. If such deviations from the assigned therapy occur, two principles govern at the time of analysis:

1. All patients should be analyzed within the treatment groups to which they are assigned. [As WALTER STARK points out, in studies of intraocular lens implants in cataract surgery, it is important to retain "aborted" cases, in which implants are planned but not actually inserted, in the implant series (STARK et al. 1977).]
2. Patients who do not adhere to their treatments should be included in the analysis along with those who do. The analysis should not be restricted to those who completely undergo the treatment.

These two principles sometimes appear to defy common sense. They imply that if a patient is randomized to treatment A, but by mistake receives treatment B, he should be retained in group A in analyses. They also imply that in comparing regimens for achieving control in diabetics to assess their impact on prognosis, all patients should be retained in the analysis, regardless of their cooperation or of their blood sugar levels. The reasoning behind these two principles is that the benefits of randomization will no longer be realized if some members of the randomized group are retained while others are set aside. The concern is that those patient groups which remain to be analyzed will not necessarily be comparable. Furthermore, a similar proportion of adhering patients in each group is not a reason to set aside these principles, since the reasons for nonadherence in each treatment group may be very dissimilar.

As a result, randomized trials evaluate "strategies" of treatment. When adherence is near 100%, there is no important difference between the strategy of treatment and the actual treatment employed. When adherence is markedly less than 100%, then the trial will disappoint those who insist on a comparison of efficacy in those who use the treatment as prescribed. Such investigators need to take special care that adherence will be high. Ways in which this can be accomplished are:

1. Be careful to screen potential patients to ensure that they are likely to cooperate with the protocol.
2. Develop procedures to evaluate patient adherence. (In studies in which aspirin therapy is prescribed, three different methods have been used to evaluate adherence: questions asked at follow-up visits, pill counts of bottles returned at visits, and analysis of urine specimens.)
3. If adherence appears to be falling off, the importance of staying on treatment should be reinforced. Incidentally, where the study is masked, the monitoring of adherence should be done without affecting the masking.

The temptation to compare results for treatment groups including only those patients who adhere to their treatment if often yielded to, in spite of the warnings by strict constructionists of the Clinical Trials Constitution. Descriptions and interpretations of such analysis ought to be done with great caution, given considerably less emphasis, and invested with less authority than primary analyses.

II. Eyes Come in Twos

The fact that patients have two eyes presents special opportunities in clinical trials in ophthalmology, but analytic methods need to be appropriate. The opportunities are those of matched studies in which one eye receives one treatment, the other the alternate. The DIABETIC RETINOPATHY STUDY (1976) randomized one eye of eligible patients to photocoagulation therapy; the other was untreated. Analyses of such paired treatment allocations are different from those in unpaired studies. The details of such analytic methods are described in elementary statistical texts (Snedecor and Cochran 1967).

Care is also required in analyzing data when the same treatment is allocated to the two eyes, as when a drug is administered orally. Most characteristics of eyes are correlated within individuals. If intraocular pressure is elevated in one eye, it is likely to be elevated in the other. Lens changes in one eye tend to be associated with lens changes in the other. Measurements in two eyes from the same individual cannot be regarded as independent pieces of information. Analyses that regard the data from 2 n eyes from n persons as though they were independent will have biased significance tests and standard errors. The results will appear to have more precision than they actually do. Some ways of analyzing such data that yield unbiased results are:

1. Conduct all analyses on one eye only, that eye being selected in a uniform way (right eye, left eye, the eye with the higher value, an eye selected at random, etc.).
2. Take the average value of the two eyes (or the sum).
3. Categorize the patient as having a score of 0, 1, or 2 (for neither, one, or both eyes affected).

The device in each of these approaches is to convert the two pieces of information from each patient into a single number and proceed with the analysis of such numbers.

III. Variable Duration of Follow-up

It is very common in clinical trials, at close of study, for patients to vary in the duration of their follow-up experience. Patients recruited initially will have the longest follow-up, those recruited most recently the shortest. Within a study, the range of duration of follow-up may be from several months to several years. Efficient analysis of data from patients with varying duration of follow up may require use of some technique such as life table analysis (Cutler and Ederer 1958). Even without such procedures, some elementary rules can be helpful:

1. Do not combine results for all patients, ignoring their duration of follow up. "Follow-up ranged from 6 months to 2 years; 40% of patients lost two lines of visual acuity" is a very imprecise statement. It leaves one unsure of the status of patients at 6 months, 2 years, or at any other time, for that matter.
2. Do present results specific for important durations of follow up. For example, provide the reader with average intraocular pressure at entry to study, at 6 months follow-up, 1 year, 18 months, etc. For each of these periods tabulate the number with that duration of follow-up and the results.
3. For complications, report the rate in the first time interval among those with follow up-through the first interval, rates in the second interval among those with such follow-up, etc.
4. Some events will only happen once to an eye or patient. Death is an example, but it is not commonly a primary variable in eye research. Reaching some level of visual acuity may be of interest, or experiencing some very serious complication, such as phthisis. In such cases life table analysis will be considerable help,

and will require the skills of someone trained in medical statistics. If life table analysis is not used, then the preceding rules are still appropriate.

IV. Tests of Significance and Data Analysis

There are many misconceptions about the process by which clinical trial data are analyzed and interpreted. Some think that there are computer programs (that "computerize" the data) by which the analysis can be conducted, without involvement of a sensitive human being. Some express surprise when trials do not settle issues once and for all. They assume there is a unique and unavoidable set of inferences following a clinical trial.

The results of a trial may not be easily summarized. There may be more than one treatment group. Complications of treatment may appear in some clinics but not in others. Efficacy may be variable in different types of patients. The amount of credence given to the many findings in a clinical trial depends on the investigator's experience with the subject matter, his skills in analysis of data, and to a surprising extent, his personality. We need to be wary of that part of ourselves that likes to root among the data, only too surely to come up with a bag full of truffles. We need to remember that out of every 100 contrasts, 5 will be significant (at the 0.05 level), even when there is no "real" difference. Analytic methodologies have been suggested that attempt to ensure the validity of tests of significance in the presence of multiple contrasts. At best, however, the statistical methods will constitute a set of slender aids for the process of evaluating the data.

A few simple guidelines may protect against many of the pitfalls of data analysis.

1. Persons with diverse professional skills need to work together in looking at the data and attempting to summarize them. Of primary importance among these are a statistician and a clinical specialist. The statistician needs to have a background in medical applications.

2. Results that are complex should be viewed with skepticism. If a drug is on the average ineffective, but shows favorable results for a subgroup of patients (e.g., women between 40 and 49 years of age), there may be a temptation to create a complex hypothesis on the drug's mechanism of action (e.g., an interaction with hormonal changes around menopause). Every data set will have some such results created by chance alone. The investigator is not obliged to offer an elegant hypothesis for each.

3. If an unexpected result does appear that demands interpretation, criteria for credibility should be tightened. Lower levels for significance tests should be used. Ask whether there is consistency in the data. For example, if favorable results appear in women of 40–49, are there similar though less striking results in adjoining age cells? How about men in the same age group?

4. If the data set is to be explored for unexpected finds, explore half the data and confirm tentative conclusions using the second half. If they do not appear in the second half, treat the results as chance variation.

E. A Greater Awareness

This chapter began by pointing out the recency of randomized trials in clinical research. Practitioners may find themselves challenged on the need for this method by those accustomed to more traditional approaches. A continuing dialogue on these questions may broaden all of our perceptions as to how randomized clinical trials should be used in the future.

Some argue that randomized clinical trials are dull and unimaginative. This point of view expresses personal preferences, to which the adage applies *de gustibus non disputandum est* (there is no arguing about tastes). Personal preferences aside, the research questions can be as exciting as any experiment allows, with the possibility of obtaining results that govern large segments of medical practice. As with any clinical experiment, moreover, the results can provide impetus to activities elsewhere in the research community. For example, knowledge of whether aspirin is effective in slowing the progress of diabetic retinopathy can have a profound impact on general research into the role of platelets in vascular disease.

Some critics say that randomized clinical trials are very expensive. If they are expensive, it is not because of randomization, which constitutes a minor technical element. The cost is for good clinical research, including careful observation, successful follow-up, unbiased data collection, adequate protection of the patient (and of the trial), and competent data management and analysis. If we believe that research can influence medical care, then we must insure that the influence is a good one. From this point of view, the cost of randomized clinical trials needs to be compared with that of poor research and poor medical care.

Finally, many find randomized trials difficult to do. It is important to recognize that this is a real problem for many investigators and patients at this time. Physicians are unaccustomed to acknowledging to patients that they are uncertain as to which treatment is preferable. Patients may have prejudices against being subjects or research studies. They may have preferences for one treatment over another. They may be disappointed in a physician who does not appear to be omniscient. For these reasons we need to extend the public and professional understanding of how randomized clinical trials can promote good medical care.

In writing of the difficulty of conducting clinical trials, and of the need for extending responsibility for them, past Director of the National Institutes of Health, DONALD FREDERICKSON (1968) wrote:

> The total burden cannot be borne by a few portions of the population. We also have an obligation to educate all of society to a keener sophistication in the matter of determining how one must determine the usefulness of measures pertinent to health care. The decision making groups of society need full understanding of the need for scientific techniques in lightening the burdens imposed by mystique or indifference. . . .
>
> Field trials are indispensable. They will continue to be an ordeal. They lack glamour, they strain our resources and patience, and they protract the moment of truth to excruciating limits. Still, they are among the most challenging tests of our skills. . . . If, in major medical dilemmas, the alternative is to pay the cost of perpetual uncertainty, have we really any choice?

References

Cochran WG, Cox GM (1957) Experimental designs, 2nd edn. Wiley, New York

Corner G (1963) The hormones in human reproduction. Antheneum, New York

Cutler SJ, Ederer F (1958) Maximum utilization of the life table method of analyzing survival. J Chronic Dis 8:699–712

Diabetic Retinopathy Study Research Group (1976) Preliminary report on effects of photocoagulation therapy. Am J Ophthalmol 81:383–396

Dollery CT, Bennett PN (1975) Clinical trials. Br J Clin Pharmacol 2:479–480 (editorial)

Feigl P (1978) A graphical aid for determining sample size when comparing two independent proportions. Biometrics 34:111–122

Frederickson DS (1968) The field trial: some thoughts on the indispensable ordeal. Bull NY Acad Med 44:983–985

Hill B (1971) Principles of medical statistics, 9th edn. Oxford University Press, New York

Kupfer C (1979) The role of clinical drug trial methodology with respect to studies of new drugs. Clinical trials of timolol. Surv Ophthalmol 23:399–401

MacMahon B, Pugh TF (1970) Epidemiology. Principles and methods. Little, Brown, Boston

Medical Research Council (1948) Streptomycin in tuberculosis trials committee. Br Med J 2:769

Rush B (1794) An account of the bilious remitting yellow fever as it appeared in the city of Philadelphia in 1793. Dobson, Philadelphia

Snedecor GW, Cochran WG (1967) Statistical methods, 6th edn. Iowa State University Press, Ames

Stark WJ, Hirst LW, Snip RC, Maumenee AW (1977) A two-year trial of intraocular lenses at the Wilmer Institute. Am J Ophthalmol 84:769–774

WHO Scientific Group (1968) Principles for the clinical evaluation of drugs. WHO Tech Rep Ser 403

Diagnostic Agents in Ophthalmology: Sodium Fluorescein and Other Dyes

L.M. JAMPOL and J. CUNHA-VAZ

A. Sodium Fluorescein

I. Introduction

Sodium fluorescein ($C_{20}H_{10}O_5Na_2$, resorcinolphthalein sodium, uranin, uranine yellow) is the disodium salt of fluorescein, a weakly acidic dye of the xanthene series (Fig. 1). It is an orange-red, odorless powder that is hygroscopic, freely soluble in water, and sparingly soluble in alcohol. Its molecular weight is 376 and its radius is 5.5 Å. Fluorescein is synthesized by heating resorcinol with phthalic anhydride.

Several properties of fluorescein contribute to its widespread use in ophthalmology. It is virtually nontoxic, shows only weak reversible tissue binding, and demonstrates the property of fluorescence. A fluorescent molecule absorbs light energy at a given wavelength. This results in excitation of electrons from the ground state to an excited state. Within a very short period of time (about 10^{-9} s), the electrons return from the excitation state to the ground state and emit energy at a longer wavelength of light than that previously absorbed. The wavelengths at which fluorescein absorbs and emits light will vary, depending upon the pH of the solution, the thickness and concentration of the solution, the solvent, the presence of protein binding, the presence of hemoglobin, and other factors. Circulating fluorescein in the blood absorbs maximally at about 465–490 nm and has a peak emission at 520–530 nm. In the ocular fluids, the absorption peak is 480 nm and the emission peak is 520 nm. Fluorescein is a very efficient fluorescent molecule with a high quantum yield. Because of this, it can be detected at very low concentrations.

Several additional properties of fluorescein mut be understood in order to appreciate its clinical uses. In general, the more intense the exciting light source, the greater will be the amount of fluorescence. Up to a point, increasing the concentration of fluorescein will result in increased fluorescence. At high concentrations, however, dimerization and polymerization occur and result in decreased fluorescence, with a shift in the emission spectrum to longer wavelengths. Quenching, a nonradiative dissipation of the absorbed energy, also occurs in concentrated solutions. Self-absorption of emitted light reduces fluorescence and the emission spectrum shifts toward longer wavelengths. For these reasons, highly concentrated so-

This work was supported in part by grant PHS HL 15168 from the National Heart, Lung, and Blood Institute, and grants EY 02214 and EY 03106, and core grant EY 1792 from the National Eye Institute, Bethesda, Maryland

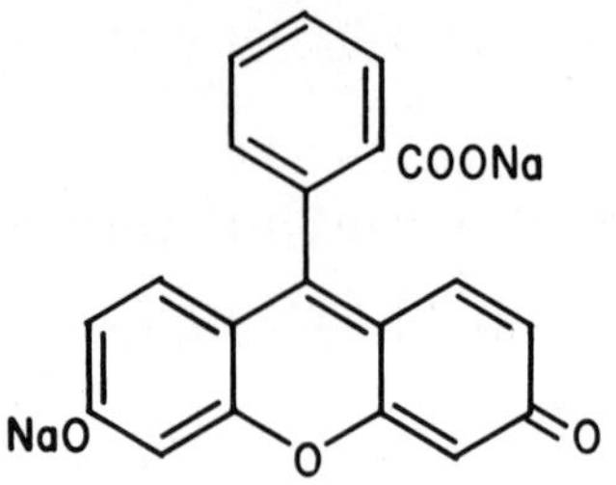

Fig. 1. Molecular structure of sodium fluorescein

lutions appear yellow-orange. Diluted solutions appear greener. Other factors besides high concentration may also cause quenching. For example, the intensity of fluorescence decreases when fluorescein is bound to protein (despite the fact that the bond to protein is weak). In the presence of protein binding, the emission spectrum of fluorescein shifts to longer wavelengths (Delori et al. 1978). Fluorescein also binds to erythrocytes; in addition, hemoglobin will cause quenching of fluorescence (Delori et al. 1978). Thus the blood of anemic patients will fluoresce more efficiently, allowing high-quality fluorescein angiograms (see below). The fluorescence of a solution of sodium fluorescein decreases markedly as the pH decreases from 8 to 5. However, at physiological levels of pH (e.g., aqueous humor 7.3, tears 7.4) this factor is unimportant.

Fluorescein was first synthesized by Adolf von Baeyer in 1871. It was subsequently used by Pflüger in detection of epithelial defects of the cornea in 1882 (Passamore and King 1955; Norn 1974). Ehrlich, in 1882, used fluorescein to study the formation of aqueous humor. Following systemic injection, he noted that fluorescein entered the anterior chamber (Maurice 1967):

The following uses of sodium fluorescein in ophthalmology will be described:
Detection of corneal and conjunctival epithelial defects
Applanation tonometry
Contact lens fitting
Assessment of the patency of the lacrimal system, the thickness of the tear film, and the rate of tear turnover
The Seidel test
Measurement of the rate of aqueous humor formation
Intravenous administration of fluorescein with measurements of the arm-to-retina circulation time and retinal transit times
Fundus and iris fluorescein angiography
Aqueous and vitreous fluorophotometry
Assessment of the blood–ocular barriers using fluorescein and fluorescein-labeled dextrans as histological markers.

II. Defects of the Corneal and Conjunctival Epithelia

The intact corneal and conjunctival epithelia have a high lipid content and resist the penetration of water-soluble sodium fluorescein. Disruption of junctions between epithelial cells results in staining of the extracellular fluid between these cells

(NORN 1974). An example of this is the punctate keratitis seen as a sign of micro-cystic edema of the cornea. Breaks in the corneal or conjunctival epithelium allow fluorescein to pass into the underlying stroma. Because the anterior portions of the stroma "stain" intensely, the epithelial defects are readily visible.

To assess the corneal and conjunctival epithelia, a drop of 0.5%–2% sodium fluorescein can be placed on the eye, or a strip of fluorescein-impregnated filter paper can be used to instill fluorescein into the cul-de-sac. Intense green staining of epithelial defects can be observed with a handlight, but the cobalt blue filter of the slit-lamp biomicroscope enhances visualization. With a cobalt blue light, normal epithelium and tears appear dark, while epithelial defects are seen as bright yellow-green. The cobalt blue light penetrates deeply into the highly concentrated fluorescein in the tear film, and the fluorescent light emitted is self-absorbed – hence the dark color of the normal tear film noted initially. The less concentrated but more fluorescent fluorescein in the corneal stroma is easily seen. Normally, the fluorescein in the cul-de-sac disappears completely within 15–30 min. Any epithelial defect remains stained for a longer period of time.

Fluorescein can also be used in the operating room to stain temporarily Ziegler or other knife tracts through the cornea into the anterior chamber so that they can be identified later in the operative procedure. Methylene blue can also be used for this purpose and is somewhat longer-lasting.

III. Use for Applanation Tonometry

In applanation tonometry (with the Goldmann and Perkins tonometers), sodium fluorescein allows visualization of the tear film throughout the applanator. If no fluorescein is instilled into the cul-de-sac, applanation can be done using the normal tear menisci; however, gross underestimation of the intraocular pressure occurs (ROPER 1980). With the proper concentration of fluorescein in the tear film, an accurate measurement of intraocular pressure is possible with the Goldmann (and other) applanators. A commonly used solution contains 0.25% sodium fluorescein in combination with 0.4% benoxinate hydrochloride (a topical anesthetic) and 1% chlorbutanol (to prevent contamination with bacteria or fungi). When instilled into the cul-de-sac, this results in an anesthetic cornea with the proper pH and appropriate concentration of sodium fluorescein in the tear film for applanation (ROPER 1980; HAVENER 1978). The solution is also bacteriostatic and can actually sterilize itself if pathogenic organisms are introduced. The benoxinate anesthetic does not quench fluorescence, as some other topical anesthetic agents do.

IV. Fitting of Contact Lenses

Sodium fluorescein is frequently utilized for assessing contact lens fit (OBRIG 1947). After contact lens wear, epithelial defects or epithelial edema can be detected by placing sodium fluorescein in the eye after the lens is removed. In addition, fluorescein can be used to visualize the tear film in assessing the fit of the hard contact lens. Because the thickness of the tear film affects the amount of fluorescence seen, areas of lens–cornea contact are dark and can be identified. In these areas, there is thinning of the fluorescein layer with decreased fluorescence.

In assessing the fit of a hard contact lens, the lens is inserted in the patient's eye and allowed to adjust for 20–30 min. A drop of 1% sodium fluorescein is then added to the tear film and the patient is examined with a cobalt blue light. On a spherical cornea, the fluorescein pattern shows a thin uniform tear film under the central portion of the lens and then thickening under the peripheral portions of the lens. Abnormal patterns may indicate corneal astigmatism, corneal irregularity, or a need for modification of the lens. Fluorescein may also be seen to flow beneath the lens periphery with each blink, which provides evidence of oxygenated tear pumping to the cornea.

Sodium fluorescein cannot be used in the eye at the same time as hydrophilic soft contact lenses, because it enters pores in the lens and results in staining of the lens. Fluorexon (REFOJO et al. 1972), a fluorescein derivative with a larger molecular size than sodium fluorescein (molecular weight 710 vs 376), can be used in these eyes to evaluate lens fit or to identify epithelial defects. It does not stain soft contact lenses. Fluorexon has also been used (POLSE 1979) to establish that oxygenation of the cornea occurs by diffusion through a soft lens and not by tear pumping, as in hard lenses.

V. Assessment of the Lacrimal System

The normal and abnormal tear film in the eye and the functioning of the lacrimal system can be assessed using sodium fluorescein. MAURICE (1967) measured the normal thickness of the precorneal tear film using fluorescein as a marker. Comparing the amount of fluorescence of solutions of known concentrations and varying thickness with measurements made in patients, the thickness of the corneal tear film (6.5 μm) was calculated. The rate at which fluorescein disappears from the tear film can be used as a measure of tear turnover, dependent on the rate of formation of new tears and the drainage into the nose (MISHIMA et al. 1966). Introduction of a known amount of fluorescein and measurement of its decreasing concentration allow calculation of the normal tear volume (6.2 μl) and average tear flow (1.2 μl/min). A similar method can determine the effect of various drug vehicles on ocular contact time (BARENDSEN et al. 1979). Radioisotopes have also been utilized for this calculation (HARDBERGER et al. 1975).

Patients with markedly decreased tears may demonstrate corneal and conjunctival staining with sodium fluorescein. Rose bengal, however, is a more sensitive detector in this situation (see Sect. B).

Sodium fluorescein is quite important in the assessment of lacrimal drainage using the primary and secondary dye tests (see PUTTERMAN 1980). The primary dye test is performed in a patient with complaints of tearing or in whom lack of proper lacrimal drainage is suspected. Several drops of fluorescein are placed in the eye. After several minutes, the patient's eye is observed to see if the fluorescein dye is retained. Normally, only a small amount of fluorescein is left at the tear interface of the lower eyelid margin and cornea. If lacrimal excretion is abnormal, a marked retention of dye is noted in this eye. A cotton-tipped applicator can be passed into the nose under the inferior meatus at the opening of the nasolacrimal duct. Dye on the applicator tip indicates that there is no obstruction of the excretory system, whereas absence of dye may imply obstruction. The patient can also be asked to blow his nose and the presence of fluorescein-stained solution on the tissue is an indication that sodium fluorescein has drained into the nose and the lacrimal system is patent and functioning.

If the primary dye test is abnormal, and there is retention of dye in the cul-de-sac, a secondary dye test is done. Following the primary test, a syringe with normal saline is passed by way of the inferior canaliculus into the lacrimal sac, and several milliliters of fluid are irrigated into the sac. The patient holds his head forward with tissue paper beneath the nostrils. If fluorescein-stained saline comes out of the nostrils, this indicates that there is a partial obstruction of the nasolacrimal system between the sac and nose; the dye is able to pass into the sac, but not into the nose without irrigation. If saline that is not stained with fluorescein comes out of the nose, this indicates that the obstruction must be between the puncta and the lacrimal sac, because no dye entered the lacrimal sac. If no saline comes out of the nose, then there is complete obstruction of the nasolacrimal system at some point.

VI. The Seidel Test – Documentation of Appearance of Aqueous Humor in the Cul-de-sac

SEIDEL in 1920 suggested using a 2% solution of sodium fluorescein to demonstrate the flow of aqueous humor through the conjunctiva in patients who have had filtering procedures (ROMANCHUK 1979). The Seidel test has attained wide usage in ophthalmology for the detection of conjunctival, corneal, or scleral wound leaks after intraocular surgery or ocular perforation. It is an aid in demonstrating passage of aqueous humor from the anterior chamber into the tearfilm or the cul-de-sac.

The standard Seidel test utilizes 2% sodium fluorescein drops. It has been suggested, however, that a 10% solution enhances the visualization and allows a longer time for observation (ROMANCHUK 1979). A drop of the sodium fluorescein is placed in the cul-de-sac. The patient is then examined with a cobalt blue light at a slit lamp. The highly concentrated fluorescein solution in the cul-de-sac and over the cornea appears dark yellow-orange. If aqueous humor is leaking through a wound in the cornea or sclera, a dilution of the highly concentrated film of sodium fluorescein occurs. This results in increased fluorescence and a shift of the wavelength of fluorescence of the sodium fluorescein toward shorter wavelengths (green). Thus a rivulet of highly fluorescent green solution is seen passing externally down over the cornea or sclera from the site of leakage. Slight pressure on the globe may be necessary to see the leakage. HAVENER (1978) attributes the green fluorescent color of the rivulet to the more alkaline pH of aqueous humor compared with tears, but this explanation appears to be incorrect, as there is little difference in pH between the two. Dilution of the fluorescein seems to be more important. Passage of aqueous humor can also be documented through full-thickness conjunctiva in patients with thin filtering blebs, or along a suture tract or fistula.

In the operating room, if an apparent wound leak is present and cannot be localized, fluorescein-stained balanced salt solution can be injected into the anterior chamber through a separate (Ziegler) tract or an incision. The eye can then be visualized with the operating microscope (ideally with a cobalt blue filter). Leakage of fluorescing aqueous humor through the defect helps to locate the site of leakage. Cyolodialysis clefts can sometimes be ascertained in this way via sclerotomies.

VII. Measurement of the Rate of Aqueous Humor Formation

Many investigators have utilized sodium fluorescein to calculate the rate of aqueous humor formation in the human and animal eye. Goldmann (1950) delivered fluorescein into the aqueous humor by intravenous injection. He estimated the concentration of fluorescein by color-matching the aqueous with projected fluorescein standards and then following over time the fluorescein concentration in the aqueous, plasma, and plasma ultrafiltrate. These data were then fitted to theoretical curves to measure aqueous flow rate and blood–aqueous permeability coefficients.

The accuracy of this type of experiment was increased substantially by the development of an objective fluorophotometer that could measure aqueous fluorescein concentrations in vivo. Langham and Wybar (1954) were the first to use an objective photodetection system that included a photomultiplier tube. Maurice (1963) developed a much more practical system with a moderately intense light source, an appropriate excitation and barrier filter combination to decrease background nonfluorescent light, and a sensitive objective photodetection system. Subsequent modifications in the fluorophotometer have been described by Waltman and Kaufman (1970) and Brubaker and Coakes (1978).

Jones and Maurice (1966) also calculated aqueous formation rates, but they utilized the corneal route to deliver fluorescein into the anterior chamber. Iontophoresis was used to deposit fluorescein in the corneal stroma and aqueous. Either of two different methods was then employed to calculate the rate of aqueous formation. The first method measured the fluorescein concentration in the anterior chamber with time, from which the turnover of aqueous humor was calculated. The second method measured the ratio of total fluorescence of the eye to that of the aqueous humor, leading to a direct evaluation of aqueous flow rate.

Nagataki (1975), Coakes and Brubaker (1979), and others (Bloom et al. 1976) have applied similar methods to measure the rate of aqueous humor formation. Calculations can also be made of corneal endothelial permeability to fluorescein. It should be noted that these methods are not as accurate in inflamed eyes, because breakdown of the blood–aqueous barrier with increased leakage of protein and fluorescein into the aqueous nullifies many of the assumptions of this methodology. Nagataki and Mishima (1976) have used anterior chamber fluorophotometry to study the entrance of fluorescein into the aqueous in patients with glaucomatocyclitic crisis.

VIII. Measurement of Arm–Retina Circulation Times and Retinal Transit Times

Several commercial brands of sodium fluorescein for intravenous injections are presently on the market. These contain 5%, 10%, or 25% sodium fluorescein solutions, with a pH of approximately 8–9. The usual dosage in an adult is 500 mg (e.g., 5 ml 10% sodium fluorescein). After the intravenous injection of sodium fluorescein, the passage of fluorescein to the eye can be recorded. The time interval from its rapid injection into a vein in the arm (usually the antecubital fossa) until its visualization in the fundus (often with use of the fundus camera and appropriate filters) is the arm-to-retina circulation time. Normal values are approximately 9–12 s. In patients with congestive heart failure, elevated central venous pressure, carotid or ophthalmic artery disease, or elevated intraocular pressure, this time interval may be considerably lengthened. Patients with increased cardiac output may have decreased circulation times. Investigators have also used the passage of sodium fluorescein through the retinal circulation to measure retinal transit times and retinal blood flow (BEN-SIRA and RIVA 1973; CUNHA-VAZ and LIMA 1978). In these methods, passage of the bolus of sodium fluorescein through a retinal arteriole is recorded on videotape, by photograph, or with light-sensitive fiberoptic probes. The time from the passage of the fluorescein wave through the arteriole to its passage in the adjacent venule is a measure of the retinal transit time in that portion of the retina. Abnormal transit times may result from systemic factors (e.g., anemia-decreased transit time), or local factors (e.g., vein occlusion-increased transit time). Measurement of the passage of fluorescein by two different points in the same arteriole allows an estimation of retinal blood flow in the arteriole (CUNHA-VAZ and LIMA 1978; VILSER et al. 1979).

IX. Fundus and Iris Fluorescein Angiography

Following the intravenous injection of fluorescein, the dye spreads rapidly throughout the intravascular space of the body. As noted, the absorption peak for sodium fluorescein in blood is approximately 465–490 nm. Peak emission is between 520 and 530 nm. This fluorescent property of the blood column can be used to study the retinal and choroidal circulations with a technique called "fluorescein angiography" (see SCHATZ et al. 1978).

MCLEAN and MAUMENEE (1960) used fluorescein injections to visualize the blood vessels in choroidal hemangiomas. FLOCKS et al. (1959) employed trypan blue and fluorescein in the cat to measure retinal circulation times. Shortly afterward, NOVOTNY and ALVIS (1961) first described the modern technique of fluorescein angiography.

After the intravenous injection of fluorescein (usually 500 mg), the fundus is visualized through a fundus camera. If only late views of the fundus are required, the fluorescein can be given orally (KELLEY et al. 1980). An appropriate filter is placed over the illuminating light to produce excitation near the peak of the absorption spectrum of sodium fluorescein. Photographs of the fundus are then taken with high-sensitivity black and white film through a barrier filter that allows passage of light at wavelengths near the peak fluorescent emission of the fluorescein. The barrier filter must exclude reflected nonfluorescent excitation light energy. The passage of sodium fluorescein through the retinal and choroidal circulations is sequentially photographically recorded.

Shortly after intravenous injection, the intravascular concentration of fluorescein begins to fall as the fluorescein gains access to the extravascular space. This reduction in concentration continues as fluorescein is actively transported into the urine by the renal tubules. The capillaries of the body are freely permeable to sodium fluorescein, with the exception of those of the brain, retina, and (to a lesser degree) the iris. This property of relative impermeability to sodium fluorescein allows accurate assessment of the retinal circulation. The intravascular fluorescein binds weakly to serum proteins, which somewhat changes its fluorescent properties (see Sec. A.I). However, approximately 20%–30% of the sodium fluorescein remains free (NAGATAKI 1975; CUNHA-VAZ and MAURICE 1969; BRU-BAKER et al. 1982), and the bond to plasma protein is reversible (IANACONE et al. 1980). After intravenous injection, the patient's skin and mucous membranes develop a yellow coloration that lasts for several hours. The urine also becomes a yellow-orange color for up to 36 h following injection. In patients with impaired renal function, the fluorescein may remain in the body for even longer periods of time. The majority of the fluorescein is eliminated by the kidney (in the urine) and a smaller amount by the liver (in bile).

Normal retinal vessels will not allow sodium fluorescein to exit in significant amounts from the intravascular space. The vascular pattern of the retina can thus be seen as the retinal arterioles, the capillary bed, and then the venules fill. An avascular zone, approximately 500 µm in size, is visualized in the foveal area. Interestingly, the blood vessel will appear wider with fluorescein angiography than with ophthalmoscopy or fundus photography. This is because fluorescein fills the entire lumen, whereas red blood cells are absent from a peripheral rim of plasma in the vessel.

The choroidal circulation can also be seen with fluorescein angiography. Normally, a choroidal "flush" occurs just prior to the appearance of fluorescein in the retinal arterioles. The choriocapillaris is permeable to sodium fluorescein, so fluorescein leaks into the choroidal stroma. However, because of tight junctions between the retinal pigmented epithelial cells and retinal vessel impermeability, minimal amounts of sodium fluorescein penetrate to the retina under normal circumstances.

Many pathological processes can result in abnormal patterns of fluorescence. Neovascular tissue rapidly leaks sodium fluorescein into the vitreous cavity (retinal neovascularization) or into the subretinal space and deeper layers of the retina (subretinal neovascularization). Damaged retinal vessels and tumor vessels also leak fluorescein. Areas of retinal or choroidal vascular nonperfusion can be visualized. Abnormalities in the retinal pigmented epithelium may also be detected. Disruption of the retinal pigmented epithelium may cause leakage of fluorescein from the choroid into or under the retina. A good example of this is central serous retinopathy. If the amount of pigment in the retinal pigmented epithelium is decreased, increased choroidal fluorescence is visualized through this area. This hyperfluorescence without leakage, called a "window defect," may be noted in areas of retinal pigmented epithelial pigmentary loss or thinning. Areas of hypofluorescence in the angiograms may be caused by decreased perfusion or blockage by pigment, blood, or other materials.

Some structures in the fundus may demonstrate autofluorescence; that is, they have fluorescent characteristics and can absorb the exciting light and fluoresce without fluorescein. An example of this is drusen of the optic nerve head. Pseudofluorescence may also occur during fluorescein angiography. If the barrier and excitation filters are not close to ideal, a white or otherwise highly reflective structure in the fundus may reflect enough of the excitation light for some light to exit through the barrier filter. Thus there is apparent fluorescence of a structure that is not fluorescing. In addition, light on its way into the eye may cause fluorescence of fluorescein that has leaked into the aqueous or vitreous; if enough of this light reflects from a fundus lesion, this will also appear fluorescent, although the lesion itself is not truly fluorescent.

Sodium fluorescein is nontoxic and adverse reactions to fluorescein angiography are rare (LEVACY and JUSTICE 1976). It should probably not be used in pregnant women until its teratogenic potential has been clarified, however. About 10% –20% of patients undergoing fluorescein angiography will feel nausea and a smaller number will have vomiting. In addition, occasionally, urticaria can be seen. If the fluorescein extravasates, induration and rarely skin necrosis may occur (SCHATZ 1978). Other more serious side effects, including bronchospasm, anaphylaxis, myocardial infarction, shock, pulmonary edema, and cardiorespiratory arrest, have been reported rarely (WESLEY et al. 1979). Because of these side effects, it is necessary to take precautions for handling emergencies if they do occur. An apparatus for institution of an airway and respiratory support should be present in the area. Intravenous cannulas should also be at hand along with drugs for a cardiorespiratory resuscitation, including epinephrine (0.1%), hydrocortisone, and antihistamines. Trained personnel should be available to institute these supportive measures in the event of complications.

Fluorescein angiography can also be used to visualize normal and abnormal vessels in the anterior segment (KOTTOW 1978). The iris vessels are relatively impermeable to fluorescein, although they appear to be leakier than the cerebral and retinal vesseles (RAPOPORT 1976). In patients with lightly pigmented (blue, gray, light green) irides, the normal pattern of iris vascular filling can be visualized with fluorescein angiography. In patients with more darkly pigmented irides, the normal vascular pattern is not visible. Abnormal leakage from iris vessels and areas of nonperfusion of the iris can be detected using this technique (JAMPOL et al. 1974). Neovascularization of the iris (rubeosis iridis) can occur in association with many conditions, including diabetes mellitus, central retinal vein occlusion, uveitis, and ocular tumors. Leakage from normal iris vessels is not apparent on angiography, although some elderly patients may have a slight peripupillary leakage. In patients with neovascularization of the iris, marked leakage may be seen. Corneal neovascularization can also be documented using fluorescein angiography. The same filter combinations specified for fundus fluorescein angiography can be used for iris or corneal fluorescein angiography.

X. Assessment of the Blood–Ocular Barriers

Examples of restricted permeability of substances between the blood and the eye are numerous. The term "blood–ocular barrier" (CUNHA-VAZ 1979; SEARS 1981), akin to the blood–brain barrier (RAPOPORT 1976), has been used to describe these restricted permeabilities. Two main factors are responsible for the presence of a blood–ocular barrier: (a) the existence of many active physiological transport systems from the blood into the eye and in the opposite direction, and (b) the presence of tight junctions between the cells that control the access passages between the blood and the eye. The presence of the blood–ocular barrier serves largely to exclude certain substances from the eye and to prevent fluctuations in the concentrations of other substances.

The blood–ocular barrier can be divided into two main parts. The first system, which regulates exchanges between the blood and the aqueous humor, is frequently called the "blood–aqueous barrier." It has two components, the epithelial barrier located in the nonpigmented layer of the ciliary body, and the vascular endothelial barrier that restricts molecular movements across the walls of the iridial blood vessels.

A second barrier system limits movement of substances from the blood into the eye in the region of the retina. It is responsible for homeostasis of the neural retina. This barrier also has two components, the tight junctions of the retinal vascular endothelium (the inner blood–retinal barrier), and the tight junctions between the retinal pigmented epithelial cells (the outer blood–retinal barrier). Assessment of the blood–ocular barriers can be performed using fluorophotometry.

1. Aqueous Fluorophotometry

In the quiet, uninflamed eye, sodium fluorescein gradually gains access to the anterior chamber. Diffusion of fluorescein through the ciliary processes and/or the iris results in the slow appearance of fluorescein into the anterior chamber. This appearance can be documented with a fluorophotometer. With disruption of the blood–aqueous barrier, fluorescein will appear in the anterior chamber more rapidly and reach a higher concentration. This may be associated with the leakage of other substance into the aqueous, including protein. Leakage of fluorescein can occur into the posterior chamber from the ciliary processes, or into the anterior chamber from the iris. Aqueous fluorophotometry has been used to assess the blood–aqueous barrier in experimental situations (e.g., breakdown of the barrier from topical nitrogen mustard in the rabbit eye, JAMPOL and NOTH 1979), or in clinical situations (e.g., increased leakage following cataract surgery with intraocular lens insertion [KRAFF et al. 1980; SANDERS et al. 1982]). Aqueous fluorophotometry allows quantitation of the breakdown of the barrier and facilitates evaluation of therapeutic modalities to reestablish the blood–aqueous barrier.

2. Vitreous Fluorophotometry

In a study of the blood–retinal barrier using fluorescein as a tracer, CUNHA-VAZ and MAURICE (1967) found that the passage of fluorescein from the blood to the retina and vitreous is highly restricted, and the movement of fluorescein is mainly unidirectional: from the inside of the eye to the blood. This movement is associated with an active transport system for organic anions, apparently located in the ciliary body and the retina. Using a fluorophotometer similar to that described by WALTMAN and KAUFMAN (1970), CUNHA-VAZ et al. (1975) noted abnormal leakage of fluorescein into the vitreous in patients with diabetes mellitus, even those without ophthalmoscopically detectable retinopathy. Leakage was more marked in patients with long-standing diabetes and in those whose control of the diabetes was poor.

Vitreous fluorophotometry is presently used to detect abnormalities of the blood–retinal barrier. Possible problems and errors associated with this methodology have been studied in detail (ZEIMER et al. 1982). Apparent abnormalities in the blood–retinal barrier have been demonstrated in patients with diabetes mellitus (CUNHA-VAZ et al. 1975, 1979) or hypertension (JAMPOL et al. 1981), retinitis pigmentosa (FISHMAN et al. 1981), and optic neuritis (BRAUDE et al. 1981), and in carriers of X-linked retinitis pigmentosa (GIESER et al. 1980). Vitreous fluorophotometry is usually performed 1 h after an intravenous injection of 14 mg sodium fluorescein per kilogram, or as a kinetic study in which the vitreous levels are observed at hourly intervals after oral or intravenous fluorescein administration. Using both of these methods, information can be obtained regarding the permeability of the blood-retinal barrier and the direction and rate of movement of fluorescein in the vitreous. It should be noted, of course, that an apparent increase in the concentration of fluorescein in the vitreous as measured by fluorophotometry can be caused by factors other than an increase in blood–retinal barrier permeability (PALESTINE and BRUBAKER 1981).

3. Histopathology

Using fluorescein angiography, the normal retinal and iris vessels are minimally permeable to sodium fluorescein. The retinal pigmented epithelium will also not allow sodium fluorescein to pass from the area of the choriocapillaris into the retina. Although careful histopathological studies reveal some leakage of fluorescein into normal retina and ciliary epithelium (GRIMES et al. 1982), sodium fluorescein has been utilized as a marker to assess the integrity of the blood–ocular barriers in experimental situations. An intravenous injection of sodium fluorescein is given to the experimental animal. The animal is killed, and the eye is rapidly enucleated and frozen in isopentane that has been cooled to $-110\ °C$ by immersion in liquid nitrogen. Subsequently, the eye is freeze-dried for several weeks, embedded in paraffin, and sectioned. This method traps the sodium fluorescein in the regions it had access to during life (GRAYSON and LATIES 1971; MIZUNO et al. 1973, 1974; MCMAHON et al. 1975). Using fluorescent microscopy with appropriate filters, these areas can then be visualized. In the normal situation, sodium fluorescein is visualized primarily in the vascular lumina of the retina and the iris. Leakage does occur in the choroid. Only slight leakage into the retina is seen. With abnormal retinal vascular leakage or breakdown of the outer blood–retinal barrier in the region of the retinal pigmented epithelium, gross leakage of sodium fluorescein into the retina and vitreous can be demonstrated. This may occur in a variety of abnormal situations, including experimental diabetes and experimental hypertension (LATIES et al. 1979). Sodium fluorescein is a much smaller tracer than other frequently utilized histopathological markers, such as horseradish peroxidase, and thus the data obtained are complementary to horseradish peroxidase studies.

Carboxyfluorescein is a fluorescein derivative with the same fluorescence characteristics as sodium fluorescein but much lower lipid solubility at physiological pH. Because of its polarity and decreased lipid solubility, carboxyfluorescein will normally not enter the retina, ciliary epithelium, or iris epithelial cells (while careful studies do reveal some penetration of sodium fluorescein). It has been suggested that carboxyfluorescein can allow a better definition of the blood–ocular barriers than sodium fluorescein (GRIMES et al. 1982). Another alternative is to bind fluorescein to dextrans to assess the size of defects in the blood–ocular barriers.

Fluorescein isothiocyanate is conjugated to dextrans which vary in molecular weight from 3,000 to 150,000; these compounds can then be used experimentally in animals for iris fluorescein angiography (Burns-Bellhorn et al. 1978), fundus angiography (Bellhorn et al. 1977; Rabkin et al. 1977), and aqueous and vitreous fluorophotometry. Following intravenous injections of these fluorescein-labeled dextrans, passage of the dextrans into the anterior chamber can be assessed using anterior segment angiography or aqueous fluorophotometry. Fundus angiography and vitreous fluorophotometry can also be performed. In addition, histopathological studies can be made utilizing the technique described above for localization of the fluorescein-labeled dextrans in the eye. Fluorescence microscopy is employed to visualize the fluorescein. Fluorescein isothiocyanate dextran can be used in the experimental animal to trace the pathway of aqueous outflow in vivo and in postmortem material (Cole and Monro 1976).

Fluorescein isothiocyanate can also be conjugated with specific antibodies for histopathological localization of the antigen with which these antibodies react (immunofluorescence). The tissue sections are again viewed with a fluorescence microscope. With increasing interest in ocular immunology, these techniques are being applied to the eye more frequently (Jampol et al. 1975).

B. Rose Bengal

Rose bengal, a derivative of fluorescein, was synthetized in 1882 by Gnehm (Norn 1974). It stains devitalized epithelial cells bright red. It is used to stain infected cells surrounding herpetic epithelial defects or to detect exposure keratitis or a dry eye with a tear deficiency (keratoconjunctivitis sicca). When 1% rose bengal is placed in the cul-de-sac, normal corneal and conjunctival epithelia do not stain; devitalized cells do. Van Bijsterveld (1969) has developed a scoring system for the dry eye based upon staining of the medial conjunctiva, the lateral conjunctiva, and the cornea. In each area, staining is scored from 0 to +3. The total score for the eye is thus 0 to +9. Rose bengal staining is a more sensitive indicator than fluorescein staining in the detection of keratoconjunctivitis sicca.

C. Indocyanine Green

Fluorescein angiography provides excellent visualization of the retinal blood vessels, but visualization of the choroidal circulation is much inferior because of blockage by melanin and lipofuscin pigments in the pigmented epithelium and macular xanthophyll and leakage of fluorescein out of choroidal capillaries. Indocyanine green (ICG, Cardio-Green) is a cyanine dye with a molecular weight of 775. It has been used extensively by cardiovascular physiologists to quantify blood flow. Because it is highly bound to serum albumin (98%), it remains within the choroidal blood vessels. This feature enhances visualization of the choroidal vasculature (Brown and Strong 1973; Flower and Hochheimer 1973). Angiograms using intravenous ICG can be made using fluorescence of the ICG dye or absorption of infrared light by the ICG dye. Both types of angiography employ infrared light, which is more readily transmitted through the retinal pigmented epithelium and macular xanthophyll than the visible light used in fluorescein angiography. Indocyanine green has an absorption peak of 790 nm and fluoresces near 830 nm. Angiograms are done with high-speed infrared film. The fluorescence angiograms (with an excitation filter range of 750–800 nm and a barrier filter peak transmission at 835 nm) show both large and small choroidal vessels. The absorption angiograms (using only a band pass filter with a peak of 800–810 nm) demonstrate only large choroidal vessels.

Indocyanine green is removed from the blood by the liver and is excreted in bile. Because it contains iodine it should be used with caution in patients known to be iodine-sensitive. To date, this technique has not gained widespread acceptance in ophthalmology.

D. Other Dyes for Retinal and Choroidal Angiography

The search for new dyes for use in fundus angiography continues (HOCHHEIMER and D'ANNA 1978). Sodium fluorescein is an almost ideal dye for retinal visualization, but other substances may improve choroidal visualization. In the future, the ophthalmologist may well have a variety of dyes of varying molecular sizes and properties from which to choose.

E. Other Dyes for Vital Staining of the Conjunctiva and Cornea (NORN 1974)

Alcian blue, a complex cyclic compound that contains copper, is used to dye wool. As a 1% solution, it can stain mucus threads in the fornix bluish green. It does not stain epithelial cells. It should not be used in the presence of epithelial defects, as it may permanently tatoo the corneal stroma.

Tetrazolium is a colorless dye that is converted by degenerating but not dead cells to the red substance formazan. Its corneal and conjunctival epithelial staining pattern is similar to that of rose bengal when used as a 1% solution. Other vital stains less commonly used in the external eye include trypan blue (1% solution stains dead cells and mucus), lissamine green (1% solution stains degenerating and dead cells and mucus), and bromothymol blue (0.2% solution stains degenerating and dead cells and mucus). Trypan blue has also been used alone and in combination with alizarin red S to assess corneal endothelial cell viability (SPENCE and PEYMAN 1976).

Methylene blue in a 0.5% solution can be used to mark the sclera temporarily during an operative procedure. It will also stain a suture tract or a knife tract through the cornea. It is also used to stain the inside of the lacrimal sac to facilitate identification during lacrimal sac surgery.

Acknowledgments. Joel Sugar, Ronald Krefman, Allen Putterman, Donald Sanders, and Gerald Fishman reviewed the manuscript. Maxine Gere edited the manuscript and Susan Schneeweiss provided secretarial assistance.

References

Barendsen H, Oosterhuis JA, van Haeringen NJ (1979) Concentration of fluorescein in tear film after instillation as eye-drops I. Isotonic eye-drops. Ophthalmic Res 11:73–82

Bellhorn MB, Bellhorn RW, Poll DS (1977) Permeability of fluorescein-labelled dextrans in fundus fluorescein angiography of rats and birds. Exp Eye Res 24:595–605

Ben-Sira I, Riva CE (1973) Fluorophotometric recordings of fluorescein dilution curves in human retinal vessels. Invest Ophthalmol 12:310–312

Bloom JN, Levine RZ, Thomas G, Kimura R (1976) Fluorophotometry and the rate of aqueous flow in man. Arch Ophthalmol 94:435–443

Braude LS, Cunha-Vaz JG, Goldberg MF, Frenkel M, Hughes JR (1981) Diagnosing acute retrobulbar neuritis by vitreous fluorophotometry. Am J Ophthalmol 91:764–773

Brown N, Strong R (1973) Infrared fundus angiography. Br J Ophthalmol 57:797–802

Brubaker RF, Coakes RL (1978) Use of a xenon flash tube as the excitation source in a new slit-lamp fluorophotometer. Am J Ophthalmol 86:474–484

Brubaker RF, Penniston JT, Grotte DA, Nagataki S (1982) Measurement of fluorescein binding in human plasma using fluorescence polarization. Arch Ophthalmol 100:625–630

Burns-Bellhorn MS, Bellhorn RW, Benjamin JV (1978) Anterior segment permeability to fluorescein-labeled dextrans in the rat. Invest Ophthalmol Vis Sci 17:857–862

Coakes RL, Brubaker RF (1979) Method of measuring aqueous humor flow and corneal endothelial permeability using a fluorophotometry nomogram. Invest Ophthalmol Vis Sci 18:288–302

Cole DF, Monro PAG (1976) The use of fluorescein-labelled dextrans in investigation of aqueous humour outflow in the rabbit. Exp Eye Res 23:571–585

Cunha-Vaz JG (1979) The blood-ocular barriers. Surv Ophthalmol 23:279–296

Cunha-Vaz JG, Lima JJP (1978) Studies on retinal blood flow I. Estimation of human retinal blood flow by slit-lamp fluorophotometry. Arch Ophthalmol 96:893–897

Cunha-Vaz JG, Maurice DM (1967) The active transport of fluorescein by the retinal vessels and retina. J Physiol (Lond) 191:467–486

Cunha-Vaz J, Maurice D (1969) Fluorescein dynamics in the eye. Doc Ophthalmol 26:61–72

Cunha-Vaz JG, Abreu JR, Campos AJ, Figo G (1975) Early breakdown of the blood-retinal barrier in diabetes. Br J Ophthalmol 59:649–656

Cunha-Vaz JG, Goldberg MF, Vygantas C, Noth J (1979) Early detection of retinal involvement in diabetes by vitreous fluorophotometry. Ophthalmology 86:264–275

Delori FC, Castany MA, Webb RH (1978) Fluorescence characteristics of sodium fluorescein in plasma and whole blood. Exp Eye Res 27:417–425

Fishman G, Cunha-Vaz J, Salzano T (1981) Vitreous fluorophotometry in patients with retinitis pigmentosa. Arch Ophthalmol 99:1202–1207

Flocks M, Miller J, Chao P (1959) Retinal circulation time with the aid of fundus cinematography. Am J Ophthalmol 48:3–6

Flower RW, Hochheimer BF (1973) A clinical technique and apparatus for simultaneous angiography of the separate retinal and choroidal circulations. Invest Ophthalmol 12:248–261

Gieser DK, Fishman G, Cunha-Vaz JG (1980) X-linked recessive retinitis pigmentosa and vitreous fluorophotometry. A study of female heterozygotes. Arch Ophthalmol 98:307–310

Goldmann H (1950) Über Fluorescein in der menschlichen Vorderkammer. Ophthalmologica 119:65–95

Grayson MC, Laties Am (1971) Ocular localization of sodium fluorescein. Arch Ophthalmol 85:600–609

Grimes PA, Stone RA, Laties AM, Li W (1982) Carboxyfluorescein. Arch Ophthalmol 100:635–639

Hardberger R, Hanna C, Boyd CM (1975) Effects of drug vehicles on ocular contact time. Arch Ophthalmol 93:42–45

Havener WH (1978) Ocular pharmacology. Mosby, St. Louis, pp 413–424

Hochheimer BF, D'Anna SA (1978) Angiography with new dyes. Exp Eye Res 27:1–16

Ianacone DC, Feldberg NT, Federman JL (1980) Titrated fluorescein binding to normal human plasma proteins. Arch Ophthalmol 98:1643–1645

Jampol LM, Noth J (1979) Further studies of the ipsilateral and contralateral responses to topical nitrogen mustard. Exp Eye Res 28:591–600

Jampol LM, Rosser MJ, Sears ML (1974) Unusual aspects of progressive essential iris atrophy. Am J Ophthalmol 77:353–357

Jampol LM, Lahav M, Albert DM, Craft J (1975) Ocular clinical findings and basement membrane changes in Goodpasture's syndrome. Am J Ophthalmol 79:452–463

Jampol LM, White S, Cunha-Vaz J (1981) Vitreous fluorophotometry in patients with hypertension. Invest Ophthalmol Vis Sci [Suppl] 20:11

Jones RF, Maurice DM (1966) New methods of measuring the rate of aqueous flow in man with fluorescein. Exp Eye Res 5:208–220

Kelley JS, Kincaid M, Hoover RE, McBeth C (1980) Retinal fluorograms using oral fluorescein. Ophthalmology 87:805–811

Kottow MH (1978) Anterior segment fluorescein angiography. Williams and Wilkins, Baltimore

Kraff MC, Sanders DR, Peyman GA, Lieberman HL, Tarabishy S (1980) Slit lamp fluorophotometry in intraocular lens patients. Ophthalmology 87:877–880

Langham M, Wybar KC (1954) Fluorophotometric apparatus for the objective determination of fluorescence in the anterior chamber of the living eye. Br J Ophthalmol 38:52–57

Laties AM, Rapoport SI, McGlinn A (1979) Hypertensive breakdown of cerebral but not of retinal blood vessels in rhesus monkey. Arch Ophthalmol 97:1511–1514

Levacy RA, Justice J Jr (1976) Adverse reactions to intravenous fluorescein. Int Ophthalmol Clin 16:53–61

Maurice DM (1963) A new objective fluorophotometer. Exp Eye Res 2:33–38

Maurice DM (1967) The use of fluorescein in ophthalmological research. Invest Ophthalmol 6:464–477

McLean AL, Maumenee AE (1960) Hemangioma of the choroid. Am J Ophthalmol 50:3–11

McMahon RT, Tso MOM, McLean IW (1975) Histologic localization of sodium fluorescein in human ocular tissues. Am J Ophthalmol 80:1058–1065

Mishima S, Gasset A, Klyce Jr SD, Baum JL (1966) Determination of tear volume and flow. Invest Ophthalmol 5:264–276

Mizuno K, Ohtsuki K, Sasaki K (1973) Histochemical interpretation of fluorescein angiogram. Jpn J Ophthalmol 17:202–209

Mizuno K, Sasaki K, Ohtsuki K (1974) Histochemical identification of fluorescein in ocular tissue. In: Shimizu K (ed) Fluorescein angiography. Proceedings of ISFA, Tokyo, 1971. Igaku-shoin, Tokyo

Nagataki S (1975) Aqueous humor dynamics of human eyes as studied using fluorescein. Jpn J Ophthalmol 19:235–249

Nagataki S, Mishima S (1976) Aqueous humor dynamics in glaucomatocyclitic crisis. Invest Ophthalmol 15:365–370

Norn MS (1974) External eye: methods of examination. Scriptor, Copenhagen, pp 51–72

Novotny HR, Alvis DL (1961) A method of photographing fluorescence in circulating blood in the human retina. Circulation 24:82–86

Obrig TE (1947) Contact lenses. Chilton, Philadelphia

Palestine AG, Brubaker RF (1981) Pharmacokinetics of fluorescein in the vitreous. Inv Ophthalmol Vis Sci 21:542–549

Passamore JW, King JH Jr (1955) Vital staining of conjunctiva and cornea. Arch Ophthalmol 53:568–574

Polse KA (1979) Tear flow under hydrogel lenses. Invest Ophthalmol 18:409–413

Putterman AM (1980) Basic oculoplastic surgery. In: Peyman GA, Sanders DR, Goldberg MF (eds) Principles and practice of ophthalmology. Saunders, Philadelphia, pp 2276–2277

Rabkin MD, Bellhorn MB, Bellhorn RW (1977) Selected molecular weight dextrans for in vivo permeability studies of rat retinal vascular disease. Exp Eye Res 24:607–612

Rapoport SI (1976) Blood-brain barrier in physiology and medicine. Raven, New York, p 218

Refojo MF, Miller D, Fiore AS (1972) A new fluorescent stain for soft hydrophilic lens fitting. Arch Ophthalmol 87:275–277

Romanchuk KG (1979) Seidel's test using 10% fluorescein. Can J Ophthalmol 14:253–256

Roper DL (1980) Applanation tonometry with and without fluorescein. Am J Ophthalmol 90:668–671

Sanders DR, Kraff MC, Lieberman HL, Peyman GA, Tarabishy S (1982) Breakdown and reestablishment of blood-aqueous barrier with implant surgery. Arch Ophthalmol 100:588–590

Schatz H (1978) Sloughing of skin following fluorescein extravasation. Ann Ophthalmol 10:625

Schatz H, Burton TC, Yannuzzi LA, Rabb MF (1978) Interpretation of fundus fluorescein angiography. Mosby, St. Louis

Sears ML (1981) The aqueous. In: Moses RA (ed) Adler's physiology of the eye. Mosby, St. Louis, pp 204–226

Spence DJ, Peyman GA (1976) A new technique for the vital staining of the corneal endothelium. Invest Ophthalmol 15:1000–1002

van Bijsterveld OP (1969) Diagnostic tests in the sicca syndrome. Arch Ophthalmol 82:10–14

Vilser W, Brandt HP, Konigsdorffer E, Wittwer B, Jutte A, Dietze U, Deufrains A (1979) Messungen zur Ermittlung des Blutvolumendurchflusses in großen retinalen Gefäßen des Menschen. Albrecht von Graefes Arch Ophthalmol 212:41–47

Waltman SR, Kaufman HE (1970) A new objective slit-lamp fluorophotometer. Invest Ophthalmol 9:247–249

Wesley RE, Blount WC, Arterberry JF (1979) Acute myocardial infarction after fluorescein angiography. Am J Ophthalmol 87:834–835

Zeimer RC, Cunha-Vaz JG, Johnson ME (1982) Studies on the technique of vitreous fluorophotometry. Invest Ophthalmol Vis Sci 22:668–674

CHAPTER 19b

Diagnostic Agents in Ophthalmology: Drugs and the Pupil

M. ROSENBERG and L. M. JAMPOL

A. Introduction

The pupil size at any moment is determined by the relative actions of the dilator and sphincter muscles of the iris, which act independently but simultaneously. Pupillary reactivity, whether dilation or constriction, is determined by the pattern and amount of autonomic innervation to the muscles of the iris. The dilator muscle of the iris is innervated by neurons from the sympathetic (adrenergic) autonomic nervous system, while the sphincter muscle is innervated by neurons of the parasympathetic (cholinergic) autonomic nervous system.

Abnormalities of pupillary size and reactivity are most often due to anatomic or pharmacologic disturbances of autonomic innervation (ISHIKAWA et al. 1977; THOMPSON and PILLEY 1976). Less often, abnormalities are the result of anatomic lesions of the iris or its muscles. This chapter describes pharmacologic agents that aid in the diagnosis of pupillary abnormalities caused by disorders of autonomic innervation.

B. The Sympathetic Nervous System

The sympathetic innervation of the dilator muscle of the iris (and other ocular structures) originates in the hypothalamus, and can be divided into three neurons termed "central" (First), "preganglionic" (second), and "postganglionic" (third). The central neuron passes from the hypothalamus through the tegmentum of the brain stem to the spinal cord, and reaches the intermediolateral column of gray (the ciliospinal center of Budge) at the levels of C_7 to T_2. There it synapses with the preganglionic neuron, which passes from the intermediolateral column via the ventral spinal roots and the white rami to the paravertebral sympathetic chain. The nerve fiber then passes to the superior cervical ganglion, where it synapses with the postganglionic neuron. This neuron extends from the superior cervical ganglion along the walls of first the common and then the internal carotic artery to the Gasserian (trigeminal) ganglion. Fibers that subserve sweating on the ipsilateral side of the face diverge from these pupillary fibers and follow the external carotid artery rather than the internal carotid artery. The pupillomotor fibers enter the orbit with the nasociliary branch of the trigeminal nerve and pass within the ciliary nerves to reach the dilator muscle of the iris.

This work was supported in a part by core grant EY 1792 from the National Eye Institute, Bethesda, Maryland

A defect in the sympathetic innervation of the ocular structures results in Horner's syndrome. This syndrome is characterized by pupillary miosis, ptosis, a narrowed palpebral fissure, and apparent endophthalmos. Facial sweating on the ipsilateral side may be diminished (see above). Less consistent abnormalities include hyperemia of the conjunctiva and increased amplitude of accommodation. All these signs result from partial or total loss of sympathetic innervation. The miosis is due to decreased iris dilator function. The ptosis and elevation of the inferior lid are caused by paresis of the retractor muscles of the lids. Hyperemia of the conjunctiva may be caused by the loss of sympathetic tone to the conjunctival vessels. The increased amplitude of accommodation is thought to be a result of loss of inhibitory adrenergic innervation to the ciliary body.

Horner's syndrome may be caused by lesions that affect the central, preganglionic, or postganglionic neurons. Localization of Horner's syndrome is often important as an aid in determining the etiology of the sympathetic paresis. Testing to localize the lesion has included the use of epinephrine, cocaine, and hydroxyamphetamine (GRIMSON and THOMPSON 1975). The pharmacologic basis for the use of these agents will now be reviewed.

I. Epinephrine

Norepinephrine is the catecholamine neurotransmitter of the sympathetic innervation of the iris. Following stimulation of the postganglionic neuron, norepinephrine is released and diffuses across the synapse to the dilator muscle of the iris. There, an α-receptor mediates dilation of the iris. The action of norepinephrine is terminated largely by reuptake of norepinephrine by the presynaptic neuron. With destruction of the postganglionic neuron (but not the central or preganglionic neurons), supersensitivity to norepinephrine may develop (CANNON 1939). Much lower concentrations of norepinephrine will result in dilation of the iris. Epinephrine is a closely related catecholamine that has significant α and β effects. While it is not a true neurotransmitter, it is synthesized by the adrenal medulla. In topical concentrations of 0.5%–2%, epinephrine is used to treat glaucoma, and usually does not cause dilation of the iris. Epinephrine solutions are lipophobic and penetrate the cornea poorly, and following the application of 0.1% epinephrine, the iris will not dilate. Patients with denervation hypersensitivity due to destruction of the postganglionic neuron may show dilation of the iris with 0.1% epinephrine solution (Table 1). This test, however, has not proved reliable, as positive results are rarely seen. Marked individual variations in sensitivity to topical epinephrine oc-

Table 1. Pupillary dilation after weak (0.1%) epinephrine

Larger (normal) pupil	No dilation
Smaller (Horner's) pupil	
Location of defect	
Central neuron	No dilation
Preganglionic neuron	No dilation
Postganglionic neuron	Dilation in some cases

cur. Phenylephrine in a 1% solution has been similarly disappointing. It should also be noted that corneal abnormalities may result in increased penetration of epinephrine into the anterior chamber, which causes dilation of the pupil following application of a dilute solution of epinephrine to an eye without postganglionic Horner's syndrome. Topically applied cocaine can disrupt the corneal epithelium; the epinephrine test should therefore never be performed after the cocaine test.

II. Cocaine

Cocaine is a naturally occurring alkaloid obtained from the leaves of *Erythroxylon coca* and other species of trees indigenous to Peru and Bolivia (GILMAN et al. 1980). It is an ester of benzoic acid and a nitrogen-containing base. Cocaine has no intrinsic sympathomimetic effect, but it blocks neuronal reuptake of norepinephrine. Cocaine's primary use in ophthalmology has been as a topical anesthetic agent. It has also been used, however, to detect the presence of Horner's syndrome. Because cocaine prevents reuptake of normally released norepinephrine at the synapse of the postganglionic neuron with the dilator muscle, norepinephrine accumulates at the synapse following the application of cocaine and causes pupillary dilation in normal eyes. In patients with lesions of the sympathetic pathway, the release of norepinephrine is absent or minimal due to the interruption conduction of impulses to this area. Thus if no norepinephrine is released, none accumulates and no pupillary dilation occurs. Absent or decreased pupillary dilation in response to cocaine is thus evidence of sympathetic paresis.

The cocaine test is most likely to be positive (show no dilation) in patients with lesions of the preganglionic or postganglionic neurons (Table 2). However, patients with lesions of the central nervous system may also have a positive cocaine test result. Because it has no localizing value, cocaine is of use only in diagnosing Horner's syndrome. To perform the cocaine test, a drop of 4% or 5% solution is instilled into each eye simultaneously. A second drop is instilled 10 min later. The pupil size is then checked at 10-min intervals. Dilation is maximal at 45–60 min in normally pigmented eyes. Lightly pigmented irides respond sooner, while heavily pigmented irides, particularly in black patients, respond less readily. The absence of pupil dilation in the miotic eye with dilation of the normal pupil confirms the presence of Horner's syndrome.

III. Hydroxyamphetamine

The most useful test for localizing the lesion in Horner's syndrome is the Paredrine (hydroxyamphetamine) test (THOMPSON and MENSHER 1971). Hydroxyamphet-

Table 2. Pupillary dilation after cocaine (4% or 5%)

Larger (normal) pupil	Dilation
Smaller (Horner's) pupil	
Location of defect	
Central neuron	Some dilation, often less than opposite eye
Preganglionic neuron	No dilation
Postganglionic neuron	No dilation

Table 3. Pupillary dilation after hydroxyamphetamine (1%)

Larger (normal) pupil	Dilation
Smaller (Horner's) pupil	
Location of defect	
Central neuron	Dilation
Preganglionic neuron	Dilation
Postganglionic neuron	No dilation

amine hydrobromide is an indirect-acting sympathomimetic. Hydroxyamphetamine works primarily by displacing norepinephrine from sympathetic nerve terminals. A 1% solution applied to the cornea is an effective mydriatic in the normal eye. In patients with postganglionic neuron Horner's syndrome, there is no norepinephrine to release, and thus dilation does not occur in response to hydroxyamphetamine instillation (Table 3). In fact, because of dilation of the contralateral (normal) eye, the pupil on the side with Horner's syndrome actually contracts because more light enters into the other eye. This test should not be performed within 2 days of the cocaine test because cocaine can block uptake of hydroxyamphetamine. In patients with central or preganglionic neuronal lesions, the response to hydroxyamphetamine is normal. A solution of 5% tyramine has a similar action to that of hydroxyamphetamine and has also been used for localizing postganglionic lesions.

C. The Parasympathetic Nervous System

The sphincter of the iris is innervated by the parasympathetic nervous system. This innervation begins in the Edinger-Wesphal nucleus, located in the periaqueductal gray region inferior to the sylvian aqueduct at the level of the superior colliculus. The parasympathetic innervation runs with the third (oculomotor) cranial nerve. It enters the orbit with the third nerve via the superior orbital fissure. It then passes with the inferior branch of the third nerve and synapses in the ciliary ganglion. The postganglionic fibers pass from the ciliary ganglion in the ciliary nerves to the anterior segment, where they innervate the iris sphincter and the ciliary muscle.

Interruption of the parasympathetic pathways to the iris results in pupillary mydriasis. A tonic (Adie's) pupil results from interruption of the postganglionic parasympathetic neurons with subsequent aberrant regeneration (THOMPSON 1977). Characteristics of a tonic pupil include mydriasis in average room light, absent or very poor reaction to light, tonic (slow) segmental pupillary constriction to light and/or near stimulation, and tonic segmental redilation. Accommodative paresis is present initially. Examination with a slit lamp shows vermiform movements of the sphincter with light or near stimulation. With time, the tonic pupil gradually becomes smaller and accommodation recovers, although it may remain tonic.

Tonic pupil is unilateral in 80% of cases and bilateral in 20%. It is found most often in young females. The association of a tonic pupil in many patients with diminished deep tendon reflexes, especially at the ankle, is called "Adie's syndrome." The etiology of this syndrome is uncertain.

Table 4. Pupillary constriction after 0.1% pilocarpine or 2.5% methacholine

Smaller (normal) pupil	No constriction
Larger pupil	
Location of parasympathetic defect	
Preganglionic neuron	No constriction
Postganglionic neuron	Constriction

Interruption of the preganglionic parasympathetic neuron, as seen with more common oculomotor nerve palsies, results in mydriasis but usually not a tonic pupil (Table 4). Agents used in testing for the tonic pupil include 2.5% methacholine (ADLER and SCHEIE 1940) and dilute pilocarpine.

Mecholyl (methacholine bromide) is a parasympathomimetic compound with properties similar to those of acetylcholine but more resistant to cholinesterase. Topical solutions of less than 10% methacholine do not cause miosis in the normal eye. Patients with postganglionic parasympathetic denervation may develop denervation hypersensitivity (CANNON 1939). This is the basis for the methacholine test for a tonic pupil. The application of a drop of 2.5% methacholine will often cause miosis (and accommodation) in an eye with postganglionic parasympathetic denervation (Table 4).

Methacholine solutions are no longer commercially available. As a result, dilute solutions of pilocarpine have been utilized. Pilocarpine is a cholinomimetic alkaloid that is derived from the *Pilocarpus* genus of South American shrubs (GILMAN et al. 1980). It is widely used clinically in the treatment of glaucoma. In the normal eye, solutions of 0.2% pilocarpine may produce miosis; however, in concentrations of approximately 0.0625%–0.125%, there is usually no constriction. In eyes with postganglionic parasympathetic denervation, 0.0625%–0.1%, or 0.125% pilocarpine will usually cause pupillary constriction (Table 4) (COHEN and ZAKOV 1975; PILLEY and THOMPSON 1975; YOUNGE and BUSKI 1976).

Hypersensitivity to 2.5% methacholine or dilute pilocarpine is seen in other conditions beside tonic pupil. It has been noted in patients with familial dysautonomia (SMITH et al. 1965), amyloidosis, and diabetes mellitus.

D. Distinction Between Pharmacologic Blockade and Oculomotor Nerve Palsy

Acute pupillary mydriasis and areflexia may result from an anatomic interruption of the parasympathetic innervation of the eye by a lesion such as an aneurysm, or alternatively from a pharmacologic blockade of the neuroeffectors (e.g., atropinization of the pupil). Pilocarpine in a 0.5% or 1% solution has been used to distinguish between pharmacologic and denervation mydriasis (THOMPSON et al. 1971). These solutions will cause pupillary constriction in patients with parasympathetic paresis but will not cause significant constriction in patients with pharmacologic blockade. In order for this test to work, the sphincter of the iris must be intact. This test helps the ophthalmologist to distinguish between inadvertent or intentional pharmacologic mydriasis and parasympathetic denervation.

E. Diagnosis of Accommodative Esotropia

Echothiophate iodide (phospholine iodide), demecarium bromide (Humorsol), and diisopropyl fluorophosphate are cholinesterase inhibitors. The administration of these drugs results in a buildup of acetylcholine at the various parasympathetic neuroeffector sites, including the iris sphincter and the ciliary muscle. These drugs may be utilized topically in patients who have esotropia to distinguish accommodative esotropia with or without hyperopia from nonaccommodative esotropia (MILLER 1960; ABRAHAMSON and ABRAHAMSON 1964). Improvement of the esotropia after administration of these drugs implies a significant accommodative component to the esotropia and, in many cases, a high accommodative convergence/accommodation (AC/A) ratio. After administration of these drugs, a decrease in the AC/A ratio is seen (SLOAN et al. 1960).

Acknowledgements. Maxine Gere edited and Cindy Gustman typed the manuscript.

References

Abrahamson IA Jr, Abrahamson IA Sr (1964) Preliminary report on 0.06-percent phospholine (echothiophate) iodide in the management of esotropia. Am J Ophthalmol 57:290–298

Adler FH, Scheie HG (1940) The site of the disturbance in tonic pupils. Trans Am Ophthalmol Soc 38:183–192

Cannon WB (1939) A law of denervation. Am J Med Sci 198:737–750

Cohen DN, Zakov ZN (1975) The diagnosis of Adie's pupil using 0.0625% pilocarpine solution. Am J Ophthalmol 79:883–885

Gilman AG, Goodman LS, Gilman A (eds) (1980) The pharmacologic basis of therapeutics, 6th ed. Macmillan, New York

Grimson BS, Thompson HS (1975) Drug testing in Horner's syndrome. In: Glaser JS, Smith JL (eds) Neuroophthalmology, vol 8. Mosby, St. Louis, pp 265–270

Ishikawa S, Oono S, Hikita H (1977) Drugs affecting iris muscle. In: Dikstein S (ed) Drugs and ocular tissues. Karger, Basel, pp 288–374

Miller JE (1960) A comparison of miotics in accommodative esotropia. Am J Ophthalmol 49:1350–1355

Pilley SFJ, Thompson HS (1975) Cholinergic supersensitivity in Adie's syndrome: pilocarpine vs mecholyl. Am J Ophthalmol 80:955

Sloan LL, Sears ML, Jablonski MD (1960) Convergence-accommodation relationships. Arch Ophthalmol 63:283–306

Smith AA, Dancis J, Breinin G (1965) Ocular responses to autonomic drugs in familial dysautonomia. Invest Ophthalmol 4:358–361

Thompson HS (1977) Adie's syndrome: some new observations. Trans Am Ophthalmol Soc 75:587–626

Thompson HS, Mensher JH (1971) Adrenergic mydriasis in Horner's syndrome: hydroxyamphetamine test for diagnosis of postganglionic defects. Am J Ophthalmol 72:472–480

Thompson HS, Pilley SFJ (1976) Unequal pupils: a flow chart for sorting out the anisocorias. Surv Ophthalmol 21:45–48

Thompson HS, Newsome DA, Loewenfeld IE (1971) The fixed dilated pupil: sudden iridoplegia or mydriatic drops? A simple diagnostic test. Arch Ophthalmol 86:21–27

Younge B, Buski ZJ (1976) Tonic pupil: a simple screening test. Can J Ophthalmol 11:295–299

Subject Index

Abel, J.J.   15
Accommodation   163, 171–173
Aceclidine   150–153
Acetaminophen (π-hydroxyacetanilide)   124, 142
Acetazolamide
  acidosis   293
  aqueous humor dynamics   290
  as carbonic anhydrase inhibitor   279–281
  Diamox and oxygen administration   268
  IOP   294
  miscellaneous uses   298, 299
  ouabain   293
  properties and effects   281–283, 287, 300, 673
Acetylation   130, 131
Acetylcholine (ACh)   54, 149, 150, 152, 156, 229
  corneal role of   157, 158
  lenticular role of   159
Acetylcholinesterase (AChE)   149, 150, 152, 156, 159, 168
Acetylsalicylic acid   542, 543
Acridine, ultraviolet light and   658
ACTH   461, 489, 503
Activated partial thromboplastin time (APTT)   614
Acyclovir   553, 561
  antiherpes action of   561–564
Acyl-CoA: amino N-acyltransferase   131, 132
Adenine dinucleotide   119
Adenohypophysis   343
Adenosine diphosphate   611
Adenosine diphospho-ribosyltransferase   220
Adenylate cyclase
  adrenergic action   210–214, 218, 258
  prostaglandins   320
  vanadate   678
Adenylate cyclase receptor complex, see Intraocular pressure
Adenylate kinase   678
Adie's syndrome   174, 175, 718

Adrenal glands   459, 460
Adrenaline   202, 208
Adrenergic agonists   193–195, 201, 202, 226
  β-agonists and IOP   261
  glaucoma treatment   207, 208
  mydriatic response to   205
α-Adrenergic antagonists   270–272
β-Adrenergic antagonists   258, 259, 261
  aqueous humor dynamics   257, 258, 268
  as antiglaucomatous drugs   207, 208
  intraocular pressure   249, 254–257
  mechanisms of action on IOP   262–264, 269
  ocular penetration and distribution   264, 265, 269, 270
  prostaglandins   323
  structures and properties   250, 251
  studies of   252–255
Adrenergic nervous system   38, 193–197, 226, 249, 715, 716
Adrenocortical function and vitamin A   367
Adrenocorticotropic hormone   231
Aesculapius   3
Agranulocytosis   436
Ah (aromatic hydrocarbon) locus   136, 142
Albumin   470, 674
Albuterol   261
Alcian blue   711
Alcohol dehydrogenase   646
Aldehyde oxidase   646
Aliphatic alcohol
  alcoholism and the eye   642, 646, 647
  disulfiram   646
  saccadic movement   640, 641
  see also Nystagmus
Alizarin red S   711
Alkaline phosphatase   678
Alkylating agents   587
  chemical structure and metabolism   588, 589
  effects on immune system   589, 590
  mode of action   589
Alprenolol   212, 213, 261

Amacrine cells   168, 231, 232, 338, 343, 349
Amaurosis fugax   328, 548
Amblyopia   647
Amikacin   385, 426, 427
Amine oxidase   118, 119
Amines, sympathomimetic   204
4-Aminoantipyrine   130
p-Aminobenzoic acid   130
ε-Aminocaproic acid   623, 624
β-Aminoethylimidazole, *see* Histamine
Aminofluorene   130
Aminoglycosides   385, 423
Aminopeptidase   135
p-Aminosalicylic acid   130
Ammi majus   657–660
Amoxicillin   418
Amphicillin   93, 94, 418
Amphotericin B   442, 443
Amyloidosis   719
Angiography, fluorescein   79, 705–707
    fundus   710, 711
Angiokinase   612, 613
Angiotensin II   194
Anilines   34, 130
Anionic dye   37
Anisocoria   174
Antabuse, *see* Disulfiram
Anthranilic acid derivatives   548
Anti-inflammatory agents   459, 539
    see also Steroids *and individual agents*
Antibiotics
    adverse drug interactions   406–409
    antagonism   404, 405
    described   358–390
    dosage determination of   390–393
    limiting factors in dosage   391–393
    routes of administration   393–398
    subconjunctival injections   401, 402
    synergism   405, 406
    topically applied drops   398–401
    used in combination   402, 403
    see also Endophthalmitis *and individual*
        agents
Anticoagulants   611, 614–617
    contraindications   616, 617
    direct   614, 615
    indirect   615, 616
Antidiuretic hormone   344–346, 349
Antidromic vasodilation   331
Antifibrinolytic drugs   623–625
Antilymphocyte sera   597–599, 601
Antimetabolic drugs   590
Antiplasmin   618
α$_2$-Antiplasmin   613
Antiviral agents
    9-β-D-arabinofuranosyladenine   557–
        559

    described   553, 554
    5-ethyl-2′-deoxyuridine   564, 565
    idoxuridine   554–557
    other new agents under development
        565–568
    phosphonoacetate   568–570
    5-trifluoromethyl-2′-deoxyuridine   559–
        561
    see also Herpes viral infections
Aphakic cystoid macular edema   328, 329
Aqueous flow
    adrenergic effects   215, 216, 218, 219,
        225, 226
    antibiotics   391
    carbonic anhydrase inhibitors   289–293
    concept of   201, 207–210
    effects of adenylate cyclase receptor
        complex   215, 220, 221
    prostaglandins   322
    substance P   341
    see also Aqueous humor dynamics
Aqueous humor
    described   37
    drug concentration   31
    fluorescein use   703, 704
    pharmacokinetic studies   23
    trace elements in   670, 674, 676
Aqueous humor dynamics
    β-adrenergic agonist   193 ff
    β-adrenergic antagonists   249 ff, 268
    carbonic anhydrase inhibition   288–293
    changes in aqueous concentration   88,
        89
    cholinergic effects   149 ff, 161, 162, 167,
        168
    exchange with cornea   88, 89
    formation of   84–86, 167
    Na-K-ATPase   678
    prostaglandins   321, 322
    pseudofacility   167, 168, 208, 209, 289,
        322
    substance P   341
Ara-C (cytosine arabinoside)   593
Arachidonic acid   230, 312, 314, 513, 540
Areflexia   719
Argon-laser irradiation   327
Aristotle   3
Aromatic amino acids   658
Aromatic carboxyl group   131, 132
Aryl hydrocarbon hydroxylase   138–140
Arylsulfotransferase   129, 130
Ascorbic acid   636
Aspergillus   415
Aspirin   312, *see also* Acetylsalicylic acid
Atenolol   254, 256, 298
ATPases   222, 224
Atropine   40, 54, 61, 176

Atropine esterase   40
Autacoids   143, 163, 311, 349
    described   311–314
    see also Histamine; Prostaglandins;
        Substance P; and individual agents
Autofluorescence   706
Autoradiography   165, 316, 375, 521
Avitaminosis C   331
Azathioprine   591, 600
Azlocillin   421

Bacillus subtilis   414
Bacitracin   431
Bacon, Francis   7
Barriers, ocular
    blood-aqueous   78, 79
    blood-vitreous   79, 80
    cornea   31, 34
    described   20–22
    endothelium   31
    systemic dosage   25
    tears   27
    zonula occludens   38
    see also Blood-aqueous barrier
Barth, Joseph   10
Bartisch, Georg   3, 8
Basophils   511
Bathorhodopsin   378, 379
Bayley, Walter   9
Beer, George Joseph   10
Befunolol   59
Behçet's disease   328, 489, 600
Belladonna   11, 12
Benemid, see Probenecid
Benoxinate   57, 58
Benzodiazepines   231
Benzylpenicillin   95, 100
Bessey-Lowry procedure   371
Blepharitis   5
Blinking patterns   25, 65
Blood-aqueous barrier   78, 79, 167
    aspirin   542
    cholinergic processes   162, 163, 167, 168
    disruption of   91, 98, 315–317, 321, 325,
        336, 340, 346, 539
    permeability of to antibiotics   390
    prostaglandins   317, 320
    substance P   340, 341
Blood flow   23, 26, 99, 205
    adrenergic stimulation   205–207
    aqueous humor dynamics   84–86, 222–
        224
    blood-vitreous barrier   79, 80
    changes in aqueous concentration   88,
        89
    chemical factors in drug penetration
        80–82

drug distribution in eye   82–84
    kinetics of intracameral penetration
        89–91
    loss of drug to blood   52
    penetration into cornea and lens   93–95
    posterior chamber concentration   86, 87
    prostaglandins   316, 317
    structures related to drug entry from
        blood   78, 79
    substance P   340, 341
    uveal blood supply   140
    vitreous kinetics   91–93
Blood-vitreous barrier   79, 80, 100, 101
Botulinum toxin   149, 169
Bradykinin   334, 336, 341, 349, 539
Brisseau, Michel   10
Brombach Perimeter   645
Bromcresol green   316
Bromobenzene   677
Bromothymol blue   711
Bromovinyldeoxyuridine   553
Bruch's membrane   204
Bupranolol   298
Butadrine   254
Butoxamine   256
Butyrophenones   231

^{14}C-Sucrose   73
Caffeine   230
Calabar bean   12, 154
cAMP (cyclic adenosine monophosphate)
    adrenergic processes   202, 203, 214, 217,
        220, 232
    prostaglandins   320
    steroid effects   518–521
    vanadate   678
Candida   415
Candidiasis   443
Capsaicin   325, 338
Carbachol   54, 149, 154, 156
    as muscarinic agent   150–153
Carbamates   154–156
Carbamylation   156
Carbenicillin   70, 82, 100, 101, 418, 419
Carbomycin   429, 430
Carbonic anhydrase   673
    history of   279–281
Carbonic anhydrase inhibitors   209, 279
    acidosis and alkalosis   293
    aqueous humor dynamics   228–293
    clinical uses   297–299
    compounds used in glaucoma
        treatment   281–288, 297, 298
    hypercapnia   294
    hypercarbia   293
    IOP, effects on   289, 290

Carbonic anhydrase inhibitors
ocular effect and enzyme inhibition 293–297
permeability of cornea 33
toxic effects 300–303
urolithiasis 299, 300
Carinamide 420
Carr-Price colorimetric reaction 371–373
Cataractogenesis 175, 176
Cataracts
anticoagulation 617
carbonic anhydrase inhibitors 297, 298
psoralens 660
removal of and drug kinetics 96
zinc deficiency 668
Cataracts, posterior subcapsular 500–502
Cataracts, steroid 484, see also Steroids
Catechol O-methyltransferase 40, 132, 133, 199
Catecholamines 38, 193, 197, 198, 210, 230
Cefamandole 84
Cefazaflur 423
Cefazolin 71
Cefoperazone 422
Ceforanide 423
Cefotaxime 422
Cefsulodin 422
Ceftazidime 422
Ceftizoxime 422
Cell junctions 22, 79, 97, 98, 163
desmosomal 222
gap junctions 39, 222
see also Zonulae occludentes
Cellular retinoic acid binding protein 372, 375, 376
Celsus 4, 6, 9
Cephaloridine 422
Cephalosporins 420–423, see also individual agents
Cephalothin 422
Cephamycin 422
Ceruloplasmin 675
cGMP 158, 228, 232
Chelators, heavy-metal 676
Chlorambucil 587–589, 600
Chloramphenicol 31, 84
penetration of into lens 95
probenecid 82
structure and use 434, 435
toxicity and side effects 435–438
Chloroquine 138
Chlorothiazides 660, 661
Chlorpromazine 661
Chlortetracycline 435
Cholecystokinin 348, 349
Cholera toxin 215, 216, 219, 220, 222
Cholinergics 149
anticholinesterases 154–156

aqueous humor composition/blood-aqueous barrier 162, 163, 167, 168
aqueous humor formation and drainage 161, 162
cataractogenesis 175–178
classification of drugs 149
direct-acting agonists 150–154
lacrimation 156, 157
neurotransmission 149, 150
oculorotary and respiratory skeletal muscles 169, 170
prostaglandins 324
sensitivity in ocular smooth muscles 170–175
structures of 151
tissue sensitivity 178, 180
trabecular outflow 163–165
see also Carbamates; Muscarinic agents; Nicotinic agents; and individual structures
Cholinergic nervous system 38, 718, 719
Cholinesterases 125, 154, 719
Cholinolytics 157
Cholinomimetics 157, 164, 165, 167, 174, 179, 226, 256
Choriocapillaris 22, 78, 206, 706
Chorionic gonadotropin 215
Choroid 78, 628, 629, 635, 706
Christison, Robert 12, 13
Chromium 679, 680
Chronic echothiophate treatment 256
α-Chymotrypsin 207, 254, 298
Ciliary body 23, 28, 38, 39
β-adrenergic receptors in 259
described 38
hydroxylase activity of 140
pharmacokinetic studies on 23
porphyria 663
prostaglandins in 320
superoxide dismutase in 635
trace elements in 671, 673, 674, 678
transport mechanisms in 81
Ciliary muscle 164, 165
and cholinergic subsensitivity 178, 180
Ciliary processes 25, 37, 38
adenylate cyclase receptor complex in 211, 212, 220–222, 227
Cimetidine 331
Cinchona bark 9
Circadian rhythm 202
Clindamycin 57, 429
Clinical trials
analysis of results 692–695
data monitoring and follow-up 691, 692, 694
development of 687, 688
planning and goals 688–690
randomization and masking 690, 691

Clobetasone butyrate   488
Clonidine   194, 206
Clostridium perfringens   414
Clotrimazole   443
Cloxacillin   82, 93, 94, 100
Cocaine   717
Colchinine   205
Colistin   385, 432, 433
Collyria   4, 5
Compartments, ocular   19, 21, 22
    anterior chamber, hemorrhages in   620, 621
    anterior chamber kinetics   88
    area under tear curve   64
    biological responses to drugs   53, 54
    blink reflex   28
    compartmentation   41, 43
    cycloplegic response   57
    dose-response relationship in pupil   54, 55
    dynamics of substance exchange   84–86
    endothelial permeability   62, 63
    endothelial transfer coefficient   59, 61, 62
    epithelial permeability values   64–66
    identification of compartments   41
    IOP response   58, 59
    kinetics of intracameral penetration   89–91
    kinetics of pupil responses   55–57
    limbal exchange   52
    mass entering the cornea   63, 64
    pharmacokinetics of surface anesthetics in cornea   57–58
    posterior chamber kinetics   86–88
    posterior reservoir   52, 53
    tear patterns   28, 49–52
    three-compartment situation   95
    two-compartment model   43–48
Compound E, *see* Cortisone
Conjunctiva
    antibiotics in   391
    anticoagulation   617
    conjunctival epithelium as barrier   36
    conjunctival epithelium as reservoir for lipid-soluble drugs   36
    described   36
    dyes for staining   711
    fluorescein   700, 701
    histamine   331
    indomethacin   543
    permeability of   36
    porphyria   663, 664
    prophylactic antibiotics   415
    subconjunctival injection   24
    trace elements in   671
    transconjunctival penetration   24
Conjunctivitis   486, 491, 659, 675

Contact lenses   701, 702
Copernicus   7
Copper   667, 674–676
Cordus, Valerius   8
Cornea
    adrenergic action in   202, 203, 266
    cholinergic processes and   157, 158
    corneal epithelia and fluorescein   700, 701
    described   31
    drug penetration in   63, 64, 93–95
    dyes for staining   711
    endothelium   31, 93, 99
    oxygen effects   627
    permeability of   25, 31, 34
    porphyria   663, 664
    psoralens   659
    steroid metabolism in   475
    stroma, corneal   32
    superoxide dismutase in   635
    topical drug application   66, 67
    trace elements in   671–673, 676, 679
    ultraviolet light   656
Corneal dystrophy   671
Corneal graft   599–601
Corpus Hippocraticum   4
Corticosteroids, *see* Steroids
Corticosteroid-binding globulin   470
Corticosterone   460
Cortin   460
Cortisol, *see* Hydrocortisone
Cortisone   461
Coumarin derivatives   615–617
Crede, Karl   14
Cushing's syndrome   493, 503
Cyclic AMP, *see* cAMP
Cyclic GMP, *see* cGMP
Cyclic nucleotides   222, 229, 232
    guanyl nucleotide binding protein   215
Cyclitis   600
Cyclocryotherapy   542
Cyclooxygenase pathway   312, 315, 323, 540
Cyclophosphamide   554, 587–590, 600
Cycloplegia   161, 175
Cycloplegic drugs   57
Cyclosporin A   587, 594–597, 601
Cytochemical localization studies   259
Cytochrome P-450 system   117, 119, 120, 125
    conjugation reactions   127, 128
    dehalogenation   126
    in eye   138
    inducible forms of   135
    oxidative reactions   121–126
    reductive reactions   126, 127
Cytosol   32
Cystoid macular edema   200, 545

9-β-D-Arabinofuranosyladenine 557–559
Decamethonium 149
Deferoxamine 671, 672
Dehalogenation 126
Dehydroretinol 369
Demecarium 154, 159
Demecarium bromide 720
Demeclocycline 439
1-(2-Deoxy-2-fluoro-beta-D-arabinosyl)-5-
    iodo-cytosine 566
Deoxycorticosterone 460
Deoxycytidine deaminase 554
Deoxyribonuclease 554
Desaturase system 121
Descartes, Reneé 7
Descemet's membrane 675
De Universa Medicina 4
Dexamethasone 94, 463, 464, 482
    cyclosporin A 595
    glucocorticoid receptors 517
    penetration of 93
    potency of 466
    systemic application 100
    topical therapy 476
Dexamethasone alcohol 478
Dexamethasone phosphate 99, 478
Diabetes mellitus 227, 232, 504
Diamox, see Acetazolamide
Dibenamine 270
Dibutyryl cyclic adenosine monophosphate
    (DBcAMP) 202
Dichloroisoproterenol (DCI) 207, 251
Dichlorphenamide 281, 288, 301
Diethoxyphosphinylthiocholine iodide
    (echothiophate iodide) 156
Diethylcarbamazine 444–446
Dihydrofolate reductase 593
Dihydrostreptomycin 423
Diisopropyl fluorophosphate 720
Diisopropylphosphorofluoridate 156
2,3-Dimercaptopropanol 676, 677
Dimethylaminopropylisothiourea 331
D-β, β-Dimethylcysteine (D-penicillamine)
    673, 675
Dimethyloxazolidinedione 293
Dioscorides 3–6, 9
Diphenylthiocarbazone (Dilhizone) 673,
    674
Dipivalyl epinephrine 41, 200
Diplopia 169, 640
Dismutation reaction 635
Disodium cromoglycate (Cromolyn) 486
Disulfiram 646
DNA polymerases 553, 554, 570
Donders, Frans 11, 12
Dopamine 193, 194, 229, 332
Doxycycline 93, 100

Drops, eye 23, 34
    anti-inflammatory 478
    hypertonic 35
    hypotonic 35
    osmotic effects of 35
    size of drop 28, 29
    viscosity of 28, 30
Drug administration
    aqueous humor concentration 68–70
    concentration of drug 24, 34, 35, 44–48
    continuous delivery 30, 479
    distribution of drug in eye 82–84
    depot dynamics 68
    drug binding 153
    drug metabolism 141, 142
    human application of data 77
    injection, intravitreal 72
    injection, subconjunctival 67
    local injection 24, 25
    ocular responses 53–59
    ointments 30
    penetration, chemical factors in 80–82
    pulsed delivery system 30, 50
    regurgitation 24, 67, 68, 70
    retrobulbar injection 71
    side effects 29
    sustained delivery system 30, 51
    systemic administration 25, 77
    tear patterns 49, 50
    topical administration 23, 24, 26
Dry eyes 99
D-Tubocurarine 149
Dyes 699, see also Fluorescein;
    Fluorophotometry; and individual agents
Dysautonomia 719

E-5-(2-bromovinyl)-2'-deoxyridine 565
Ebers Papyrus 2, 657
Echothiophate 171, 173, 178, 180
    cataractogenesis 176
    in lens 159
Echothiophate iodide 720
Econazole 444
Edema, epithelial 99
Edwin Smith Papyrus 2
Ehrlich, Paul 15
5,8,11,14,17-Eicosapentaenoic acid 312
5,8,11,14-Eicosatetraenoic acid, see
    Arachidonic acid
8,11,14-Eicosatrienoic acid (dihomo-γ-
    linolenic acid) 312, 314
Electron spin resonance studies 656
π-Electrons 656, 658, 660
Electrooculogram 268
Electroretinography 54, 298, 548, 629,
    643–645

Endophthalmitis   24
  causes of   413–415
  incidence of   412, 413
  treatment of   404–412, 415, 416
Endothelium, capillary   630
Endothelium, corneal
  active transport by   62
  oxygen   627
  pharmacokinetics   66
Enkephalins   342
Enzymatic hydrolysis   40
Enzymes, drug-metabolizing   117, 118
Enzymes, induction of   117, 118, 135–138
Epinephrine   54, 193, 716
  adrenergic action   196, 208
  as metabolite   40, 41
  mydriasis and   24
Epithelialitis   486
Epithelium   34, 63–65
Epithelium, corneal
  as barrier to pilocarpine   67
  oxygen transfer and   627
  pharmacokinetics   63–66
Epithelium, retinal pigmented   676
Eosinophils   511
Erasistratus   4
Erythema   655, 658
Erythromycin   427, 428
Escherichia coli   414, 418
Eserine, see Physostigmine
Esophoria   640
Esotropia   175, 720
Esthesiometer, Cochet-Bonnet   57
Ethambutol   673
Ethanol   345, 640–642, 644, 647
Ethers
  alkyl thio   125
  alkylaryl   124
7-Ethoxycoumarin   124
Ethoxzolamide   281, 288, 294, 300
5-Ethyl-2'-deoxyuridine (aedurid)   553,
  564, 565
Ethylenediamine tetraacetic acid   668, 669
Ethylmorphine N-demethylation   121
Evans' blue   80
Exophoria   640
Extrinsic pathway   612
Eyelids   656, 659, 661, 663

Falck-Hillarp method   649
Fanconi's syndrome   439
Ferritin   670, 671
Fibrin   611, 612
Fibrin degradation products   620
Fibrin-stabilizing factor   611
Fibrinogen   615
Fibrinolysis   612, 613

Fibrinolytics   611, 617
  in ophthalmology   619–621
  plasmin   618
  streptokinase   617
  therapeutic thrombolysis   618, 619
  urokinase   617
Fibrinopeptides, A and B   611
Fibroblast   37
Flavine mononucleotide   121
Fleisher's line   671
Fluocinolone acetonide   463, 464
Fluorescein   22, 25, 30, 32, 70, 704, 705
  aqueous humor dynamics and   86
  described   699, 700
  in pharmacokinetic studies   67
  metabolism of   41
  removal rate of   75
Fluorescein angiography   316, 329, 545,
  629, 631
Fluorescein isothiocyanate   710
Fluorescein photometry, see
  Fluorophotometry
Fluorescence microscopy   372
9α-Fluorocortisol   463
5-Fluorocytosine   443
Fluorexon   702
Fluorometholone   465, 476, 494, 495
Fluorometholone alcohol   478
Fluorometholone crystals   31
Fluorophotometry   208, 209
  aqueous fluorophotometry   708, 710
  concentration of fluorescein in
    conjunctival sac   27
  fluorescein in corneal stroma   31, 70
  pseudofacility and uveoscleral flow   209,
    215
  use of thodamine B   95
  vitreous fluorophotometry   708–710
Flurbiprofen   323, 324
Folic acid analogs   593, 594
Formazan   711
Forskolin   215, 219, 220, 222, 228
Fraser, Thomas   12, 13, 15
Fuchs' heterochromic iridocyclitis   485
Fuchs' syndrome   512
Fundus angiography   710, 711
Fusarium   415

Galen   4, 6, 9
Gas liquid chromatography   265
Gastrin   348, 349
Gel electrophoresis   516
Gentamicin   36, 84
  injection of   69–79, 101
  kinetics of   75–77
  structure and use   424

Gentamicin
   systemic administration of   100
   topical application of   99
Gibson, Benjamin   14
Glaucoma
   adrenergic action   267
   anticoagulation   617
   cholinergic drugs   169
   steroid   498
   treatment of with adrenergic
      compounds   193
   see also Carbonic anhydrase inhibitors
Glaucoma, angle-closure   272, 297
Glaucoma, open-angle   298, 492, 498
Glaucoma, steroid   491
   biochemical studies   499, 500
   dose-response relationships   493–496
   IOP response to steroids   492, 493
   triamcinolone acetonide   481, 484
Glaucomatocyclitis crisis   328
Glucagon   348
Glucocorticoid receptors   514, 517–523
   target cell   515–517
Glucocorticoid receptor assay   470
Glucosamine   130
Glucose-6-phosphate dehydrogenase
   deficiency   392
Glucose tolerance factors   679, 680
Glucuronidation   128, 129
Glucuronide   41, 86
Glucuronosyltransferase   128
Glutamine   130
Glutamine synthetase   521
γ-Glutamyl dopa   143
γ-Glutamyltranspeptidase   135
Glutathione   133–135, 314, 636
Glutathione peroxidase   674, 676
Glutathione S-transferase   133–135, 140,
   677
Glycoprotein hormones   343
Glycosaminoglycan   32, 499
Glycosylation reactions   368
Gonadotropin hormones   215
Graefe, Albrecht von   10–12
Graefe, Alfred Carl   14
Graefe, Carl Friedrich von   10
Grassus, Benvenutus   6
Graves' ophthalmopathy   600
Griseofulvin   441–443
Grotthuss-Draper Law   655
Guanethidine   197
Guanosine triphosphatase (GTP) activity
   215, 216, 219, 222
Guanyl cyclase   228, 229
Guanyl nucleotide binding protein   215,
   220
Guillemeau, Jacques   8, 9

Haab, Otto   15
Haemophilus influenza   414
Hageman factor   611
Haloperidol   231
Hamster cheek pouch chamber technique
   329
Haptoglobin   672
Harderian glands   347, 348
[3]H-dihydroalprenolol   259, 261
Hemangioma, choroidal   705
Hemicholinium   149
Hemochromatosis   671, 672
Hemoglobin saturation   632
Hemophilia   611, 616, 623
Hemosiderin   671
Hemostatics   611, 621, 622
   antifibrinolytics   623–625
   hemophilia factors A, B, and C   611, 623
   nonspecific   625
   specific   622–625
Hemostasis
   mechanism of   611–613
   see also Anticoagulants; Fibrinolytics;
      Hemostatics
Heparin   614, 615, 617
Heracleides of Tarentum   4
Hermetic Books of Thoth   3
Herodotus   3
Herophilus of Chalcedon   4
Herpes virus infections   553, 554, 559, 560
   acyclovir   561–564
   herpes simplex   486, 487, 553, 556, 600
   herpes zoster   486, 558, 565
Hexamethonium   149
High-pressure arc   656, 657
High-pressure liquid chromatography
   371, 373
Hill, Bradford   687
Himly, Karl   6
Hippocrates   3
Hippurate synthesis   131
Hirschberg, Julius   15
Histamine   97, 98, 132, 311
   described   329, 330
   histamine metabolism   133
   inflammation   539
   IOP   331
   ocular occurrence and effects of   330,
      331
   ocular response to injury   331, 332
Histamine N-methyltransferase   132
Histamine receptors   329
Histidine   154, 329
Histopathology   709, 710
Homatropine   57
Horner's syndrome   195, 716–718
Horseradish peroxidase   317, 709

Howard-Dohlman test   645
³H-quinuclidenylbenzilate   170
Hudson-Stahli line   671
Huygens, Constantijn   7
Hyaloid membrane   72, 91
Hyaluronic acid   75
Hyaluronidase   499
Hydrocarbons, aromatic   133, 135, 136,
  140
Hydrocortisone   68, 462, 463, 466, 476
Hydrocortisone solution   23
Hydroguinone   314
Hydroperoxidase   312
Hydroperoxides   312
Hydrophilic drugs   32
Hydroxyamphetamine test   717, 718
6-Hydroxydopamine   197, 230
9-(2-Hydroxyethoxymethyl)guanine, see
  Acycloguanosine
5-Hydroxyindolacetic acid   332
Hydroxyindole-O-methyltransferase
  activity   333
Hydroxylases   136
Hydroxylation   119, 121–123
Hydroxyl radicals   635
5-Hydroxytryptamine   332–334, 539
Hyoscyamine   6, 11
Hyperemia   214, 323, 324
Hyperfibrinolysis   622
Hyperopia   720
Hyperoxia   631
Hypertension, ocular   267
Hyphema   620
Hypochromia   230, 231
Hypokalemia   301, 442
Hypothalamic peptides   343
Hypothalamic-pituitary-adrenal (HPA)
  axis   482, 483, 505
Hypothalamic-pituitary axis   493

I-hydroxybenzylpindolol   210–212, 214
¹²⁵I-hydroxybenzylpindolol   259
I-serum albumin   73
Imidazoles   443, 444
Immune system   585
  alkylating agents   589, 590
  ALS   598
  ara-C   593
  cyclosporin A   596, 597
  methotrexate   594
  pathogenic processes   585–587
  purine analogs   591, 592
Immunofluorescence   315
Immunosuppressive drugs   585, 599, 601,
  602
  agents in ocular conditions   599–602

agents of potential future use   599
antilymphocyte sera   597–599
B lymphocytes   586, 587
cyclosporin A   594–597
folic acid analogs and methotrexate
  593, 594
lymphokines   587
macrophages   586, 587
monokines   587
purine analogs   590–592
pyrimidine analogs   592, 593
T lymphocytes   586, 587
see also Alkylating agents
Indanedione derivatives   615
Indocyanine green   710, 711
Indomethacin
  ACME   328
  blocking of prostaglandin transport
    system   313, 314, 316, 324
  flurbiprofen compared   546–548
  inhibition of IOP rise   543, 544
  inhibition of prostaglandin synthesis
    541, 543, 544
  side effects   545
  systemic dosage   81
  topical administration   328, 329, 528
  ultraviolet light   658
Indoxole   543
Interleukins   595, 596
Intraocular pressure (IOP)   162, 169
  adenylate cyclase receptor complex   212,
    215, 220–222, 227
  β-adrenergic antagonists   207, 249–251,
    254–257, 262–264, 267, 268
  alcohol, effects of   646
  aniridia, effects of   164
  ChE inhibitors   178
  epinephrine and   199
  episcleral venous pressure   201
  inflow and carbonic anhydrase
    inhibitors   209, 210
  pharmacologic effects of adrenergic
    compounds   209
  pilocarpine and   165, 168
  resistance to outflow   201
  response to drugs   58, 59
  response to steroids   490, 491
  secretory ciliary epithelia, role of   207
  substance P   341
  vasopressin extracts, effects of on   345
  see also Aqueous flow; Aqueous humor
    dynamics; cAMP; Glaucoma, steroid;
    Pseudofacility; Uveoscleral flow
Intrinsic pathway   611
Iodine   667, 668
5-iodo-5′-amino-2′,5′-dideoxyuridine
  566–568

5-iodo-2deoxyuridine (idoxuridine)   554–
   557
Iodopyracet   68, 74, 75
Ionic procion   39
Ionizing irradiation   599
Iontophoresis   24, 35, 36, 45, 49, 70, 86,
   317
Iridial smooth muscles   339, 340
Iridocyclitis   461, 480
Iris
   adrenergic action   203–205, 266
   alcohol, effects on   643
   cholinergic subsensitivity   170, 173, 178
   described   37
   pharmacokinetic studies   23, 66
   prostaglandins and iris sphincter tone
      324
   psoralens   659
   superoxide dismutase   635
   trace elements in   673, 674
Iritis   480
Iron   667, 668, 670–672
Isomerization   133, 134
Isoniazid   130, 392
Isoprene   368
Isoprenoids   368
Isoproterenol   54, 196, 197, 208, 211, 225,
   324
Isozymes   129, 130, 133
IU   617

Julliard, Étienne   14

Kainic acid   344
Kallidin   334
Kanamycin (Kantrex)   426
Kaolin cephalin time, see Activated partial
   thromboplastin time
Kayser-Fleischer ring   675
Kepler, Johannes   7
Keratitis   463, 478, 486, 487, 657
Keratoconjunctivitis   486
Keratoconus   671
Keratocytes   32
Keratomalcia   367, 370
Keratopathy, bullous   99
Keratoplasty   327
Keratouveitis   487
Keto steroids   475
Keystone Telebinocular   645
Kinanase II   337, 349
Knapp, Hermann   14
Koller, Karl   14

Labetalol   271, 272
Lacrimal system   201, 202, 267, 702, 703
   see also Tears
β-Lactamases   420, 421

Laqueur, Ludwig   12
Lens
   adrenergic action   202, 203
   cholinergic processes   158, 159
   described   39
   penetration of drugs into   95
   pharmacokinetic studies   23
   porphyria   663
   psoralens   659
   superoxide dismutase   635
   trace elements in   672, 676
Leukocytes   298, 327, 506–512
Leukomata   5
Leukopenia   587, 590
Leukotrienes   312, 313, 316, 323, 514, 541,
   542, 545
Leukovorin   594
Levamisole   444
Lidocaine   57, 58
Lincomycin   70, 99, 428, 429
Lipid solubility   31, 33, 34, 48, 65, 81, 95
Lipofuscin   677
Lipoxygenase pathway   312, 315, 323, 540
Liquid chromatography   338
Liquid scintillation   265
Lissamine green   711
Lundsgard, K.K.   14
Luteinizing-hormone-releasing hormone
   344
Lymphocytes
   B   586, 590, 599
   T   586, 587, 590, 597–599
Lymphokine   507, 587
Lymphoma   587

Mackenzie, William   11
Macrophages   585, 586, 589
   monocyte-macrophage system   510
   see also Immunosuppressive drugs
Macula occludens   38
Maitre-Jan, Antoine   10
Mandrake Root   6
Manometric measurements   208, 225
Mattioli   8
Mebendazole   444
Mecolyl   719
Mediflow lens   401
Medrysone   465, 476, 494, 495
Meibomian gland secretion   27
Melanin, intraocular   80, 140, 230, 674,
   675
Melanocyte-stimulating hormones   230,
   231, 346, 347
Melanogenesis, iris stromal   231
Melanoma   26
Menkes' kinky hair disease   676
6-Mercaptopurine   591

Mercapturate 135, 140
Metalloenzymes 667, 669
Methacholine 149–153, 719
Methanol 647–649
β-Methasone 254, 256
Methazolamide 281, 285–287, 293, 300, 301
Methicillin 82
Methotrexate, *see* Immune system; Immunosuppressive drugs
8-Methoxypsoralen 658, 659
Methylation 132, 133, 216, 219
3-Methylcholanthrene 117
α-Methyldopa 195
Methylene blue 701, 711
α-Methylnorepinephrine 195
Methylprednisolone 466
6α-Methylprednisolone 463, 464
Methyltransferases 132, 133
Metroprolol 254, 256
Meyer, Hans 15
Mezocillin 421
Miconazole 443
Mineralocorticoid potency 466
Minocycline 439
Miosis
    adrenergic action 272
    drug response 55
    pharmacokinetics and 53
    thymoxamine 205
    vasopressin extracts 345
Mitochondrial enzymes 131
Mitochondrial hydroxylation system 119
Monoamine oxidase 40, 198
Monochromator 656, 657
Monokine 587
Mononuclear phagocytes, *see* Macrophages
Monooxygenase activities 117, 135, 136
Mooren's ulcer 485, 600, 601
Moxalactam 422
Mucin 27
Mucopolysaccharide metabolism 208
Mucopolysaccharide synthesis 367
Murine B cells 595
Muscarinic agents 150, 153, 194
    carbachol 154
    muscarinic receptors 149, 150, 153, 158, 161, 171
Myasthenia gravis 169, 227
Mydriasis 718, 719
    adrenergic action 195, 199, 272
    drug response 55
    pharmacokinetics 53
    psoralens 659
    steroids 502
    vasopressin extracts 345
Myrrh 5

N-Acetylimidoquinone 124
N-Acetyltransferase 130–132, 135
N-Acyloxylarylamines 131
N-Alkyl *p*-aminobenzoate ester 34
N-Dealkylation 123
N-Hydroxylation
Na-K-ATPase 223, 678, 679
NADH·cytochrome b$_5$ reductase 121
NADPH·cytochrome P-450 reductase 118, 120, 121
Naphthylamine 33
Naphthylazopenicillin 80
Neisseria meningitidis 414
Neomycin 425, 426
Neostigmine 154
Neovascularization 630, 631, 707
Netilmicin 427
Neuritis, optic 709
    steroid therapy 489
Neurohypophysis 344
Neuropeptides, *see* Autacoids
Neurospora sitophila 415
Neurotensin 342, 343
Neutrophil kinetics 511
Nicotine 149
Nicotinic agents 153, 154
    nicotinic receptors 149, 153, 154, 158, 169
NIH shift 122
Nitrogen mustard 587, *see also* Alkylating agents
Nitrosamines 228
Norepinephrine 193, 716, 717
    adrenergic action 196, 207
    L- and D-norepinephrine
    prostaglandins 323, 324
Nouveau Traité des Maladies des Yeux 5
Novobiocin (Albamycin, Cathomycin) 430
Nyctalopia 2
Nystagmus 4, 642, 643, 647
    neurogenic 642
    optokinetic 640, 641
    pendular 642
Nystatin 442, 443

O$_2$ 634–636
O-Dealkylation 124
O-Methylating system 199
Occlusion, central retinal arterial 228, 629
Oculorotary muscles 169, 170
Ocusert 30, 61
15-*OH*-Dehydrogenase 312
Oleandomycin 429
Onchocerciasis 444–446
Ophthalmia 5, 6, 600

Ophthalmic therapeutics, history of
  Age of Enlightenment   10–13
  cataract classified   11
  cataract treatment   9
  Dark Ages   6
  diseases treated   2–6, 11–15
  drugs and treatments discovered   11–15
  Egypt's contribution   1–3
  glaucoma   10, 12
  Greece's contributions   3, 4
  modern era   15, 16
  mysticism   1–3
  nineteenth century   14, 15
  physostigmine   11–14
  plants and minerals used   5–6, 11, 12, 14
  Renaissance   7–10
  Rome's contribution   4–6
Ophthalmoplegia   647
Ophthalmoscopy   11, 12, 647
Ophthalmoxipis   4
Opium   5
Organophosphorous compounds   156
Oscillopsia   642
Oxypsoralen   658
Ouabain   81, 678
Oxprenolol   254, 256, 261
Oxygen   627–630
  anti-inflammatory agents   633
  consumption   630
  ocular response to   628
  PO_2 629, 631, 632
  superoxide dismutase   634–636
  vitamin E   633, 634, 636
  see also Retrolental fibroplasia
Oxygen, singlet   635, 636
Oxyphenbutazone   543, 545, 546
Oxytetracycline   435
Oxytocin   346

$\alpha^{32}P$-Adenosine triphosphatase   215
P- and P (prothrombin-proconvertin) test
  616
P-Chlorophenylalanine   334
Palpebral aperture   27
Palsy, ocular   646
Pancreozymin, see Cholecystokinin
Panretinal scatter photocoagulation   175
Paracelsus   7, 8
Paracentesis   100, 327, 628
Paramecia   658
Parasympathetic nervous system, see
  Cholinergic nervous system
Paré, Ambrose   9
Paredine test, see Hydroxyamphetamine
  test
Pargyline   198
Pasteurella septica   414
Penethamate   41

Penicillamine   676, 677
Penicillin   36, 76, 77, 81, 93, 99
Penicillin derivatives   417, 418
Pentobarbital   340
Peptic ulcer disease   504
Peptide hormones   344–346
Peptidyldipeptidase   337
Perikarya   333
Perilimbal suction cup technique   322
Pharmacokinetics
  abbreviations of symbols used   19
  adrenergic nervous system   200, 201
  aqueous humor   37
  basic concepts   20–22, 25, 26
  binding of drugs to proteins   80
  compartment theory   52, 53
  drug chemistry   33, 34
  dose-response curve   218
  experimental limits of   95–98
  K_I and K_d 212, 214
  least effective dose   58, 59, 200, 201
  methotrexate   601
  steroids   467, 471, 472
  studies   101, 102
  tissue distribution   84
  see also Barriers, ocular; Compartments,
    ocular; Drug administration
Phenacetin (p-ethoxyacetanilide)   124
1,5- and 1,10-Phenanthroline   674
Phenothiazine drugs   661
Phenoxybenzamine   211, 270, 324
Phentolamine   270, 324
Phenylacetone   124
Phenylalanine   130
Phenylbutazolidine   543, 545
Phenylephrine   194, 196, 230, 717
Phenyltrimethylammonium   149
Phorbol myristate acetate   231
Phosphatidate phosphohydrolase   266
Phosphodiesterase   216, 219, 232
Phosphofructokinase   678
Phospholipase A_2 312
Phosphonoacetate   568–570
Phosphonoformate (foscarnet)   568–570
Phosphorylases   223
Phosphorylation   156, 223
Photocoagulation   630
Photodermatitis   662
Photofluorometry, see Fluorophotometry
Photogrammetric methods   289
Photophobia   4, 461
Photoreceptors   141, 231, 232, 629, 635
Photosensitizing substances   665, 660–665
  mechanism of   658
  ocular effects   659, 660
  photosensitization   657–660
  see also Porphyria; Psoralens; Ultraviolet
    light

Physostigmine   154, 159
Picosecond absorption spectroscopy   379
Pigment, ocular   57, 675
  adrenergic action   199, 229–232
  pigmented tissues and trace elements
    671, 672
Pilocarpine   719
  as cholinergic agonist   163–165, 178
  as muscarinic agent   150–153
  cataractogenesis   176
  kinetics of   61, 70–75
  in lens   159
  metabolism of   40
  penetration of   35, 65
  pseudofacility   168
  tear flow rate   54
Pimaricin   444
Pindolol   251, 254
Pirprofen   543
Pivalic acid diester   200, 227
Plasma dialysate   27
Plasma kinins   334–336
Plasma transglutaminase   611
Plasmin   612, 618
Plaminogen   612, 619, 621
Platelet factor 3   611
Pliny the Elder   5, 6
Ploug units   617
Pneumococcus   414
PO$_2$ 627–629, 631, 632
Polycyclic hydrocarbons   660
Polymyxins   431, 432
Polyphloretin phosphate   316, 317
Porphyria   662, 663
Porphyrin   662, 664
Porphyropsins   369
Practolol   254, 261
Prazosin   194, 195, 270
Prednisolone   463, 466, 476, 482
Prednisolone acetate   65, 68
Prednisolone phosphate   99
Prednisone   463, 482
Proaccelerin   611
Probenecid   82, 316, 420
Procaine   34, 35, 170
Prodrug   40, 41
Proparacaine   58
Propionic acid derivatives   546–548
Propranolol   207, 254, 256, 261, 324, 679
Prostacyclin   312, 323
Prostacyclin synthetase   312
Prostaglandins
  adrenergic action   194, 228, 229
  aspirin   543
  blood-ocular barrier   315, 316
  described   312–314
  endoperoxides   312, 314
  glucocorticoids and synthesis of   313

  in eye   314, 315
  indomethacin   543, 544
  naturally occurring   318, 319
  ocular blood flow   316, 317
  ocular response to injury   325–329
  steroids   499, 513
  transport system of   315, 316
Protamine sulfate   615
Proteus   414, 420
Prothrombin   615
Pseudofacility, see Aqueous humor
  dynamics
Pseudofluorescence   706
Pseudomonas   418, 420
  P. aeruginosa   414, 422
Psoralen   657–660
Psoriasis   658
Ptosis   169, 323, 502, 647
Pupil   54, 55
  adrenergic action in   266
  dose-response relationship   54, 55
  kinetics of pupil response   55, 57
  pupillary movement and cholinergic
    processes   159, 161
  tonic pupil   718, 719
Purine analogs   590–592
Pyrazolon derivatives   545, 546
Pyridoxamine   130
Pyrimethamine   439–441
Pyrimidine analogs   592, 593
Pythagoras   3

Radioimmunoassay   328, 370
Radiolabeled microsphere technique   206
Radioligand-binding analysis   194, 195
Radioligand techniques   195, 202
Radiometer   657
Raman spectroscopy   379
Regurgitation, see Drug administration
Renin-angiotensin system   336, 337
Resinger, Franz   11
Respiratory distress syndrome   632, 633
Reticulum, endoplasmic   117, see also
  Tissues
Retina
  adrenergic action   230–232
  anticoagulation   617
  cholinergic processes   168
  fibrinolytics   619, 620
  hemorrhage, retinal   675
  light, direct action of   656
  methanol   647
  oxygen   629, 630
  porphyria   664
  retinal circulation and oxygen   628, 629
  retinal phospholipids   635
  substance P in   339
  superoxide dismutase   635

Retina
  trace elements   672, 676
  transport mechanisms   81
  vasoconstriction   631
Retinal (retinene)   368, 373
Retinitis pigmentosa   709
Retinochoroiditis   486
Retinohypothalmic pathway   333
Retinoic acid   368, 374, 380
Retinoids
  described   368–373
  glycoprotein biosynthesis   379
  hormone-like action   380
  metabolism   373–375
  uptake   375, 376
  visual process   377–379
Retinol   367, 368
Retinomotor pigment migration   231
Retinopathy   138, 659, 662
  diabetic retinopathy   175, 328
Retinyl-*P*   379
Retinyl-*P*-mannose   379, 380
Retrobulbar neuritis   673
Retrolental fibroplasia (RLF)   627, 630,
  632, 674
  antioxidants   633–636
  vitamin E   633
Rhazes   6
Rhodamine B   39
Rhodopsin   367, 377, 378
Rhodopsin moiety   368
Ribonucleotide diphosphate reductase
  554
Rifampin   385, 392
Ristocetin (Spontin)   430
Rivière, Lazare   9
RNA replicases   554
RNA transcriptases   554
Robertson, Douglas Argyll   12
Rose bengal   710, 711
Roux, Ernst   15
Rubeanic stains   675
Rush, Benjamin   690

S-Adenosyl-L-methionine   132, 133
S-Dealkylation   125
Saccadic movement   640, 641
Saint Yves, Charles de   5, 10
Sala, Angelus   14
Salbutamol   197, 261
Salicylates   36, 542, 543
Sarcoid   512
Schlemm's canal   98, 161, 163–165
Schmidt, J.A.   10
Sclera   36, 37, 663, 664
  trace elements in   671, 673, 676
Sclerotomics   704
Sclerouveitis   489, 600

Scopolamine   61
Scotoma   647
Seidel test   703, 704
Selenium   676, 677, 680
Serotonin, *see* 5-Hydroxytryptamine
Serum retinol-binding protein (RBP)   371
Siderosis   671, 672
Sisomicin   427
Slit lamp biomicroscope   701
Snowblindness   657
Sodium azide   229
Sodium nitroprusside   228
Somatostatin   343
Sotalol   254
Soterenol   197
Spectinomycin   427
Spectrofluorometric techniques   264
Spiramycin   430
Staphylococcus aureus   414
Staphylococcus epidermidis   414
Stark-Einstein Law   655
Stereoisomerism   197, 198, 371
Steroids
  absorption and distribution   470–473
  adrenergic action   228
  antibiotics   416
  clinical problems   485, 486
  complications   490
  cyclophosphamide   600
  dilution of   84
  glucocorticoid effects   466–468
  historical development   459–465
  hormone effects in tissues   523, 524
  immunologic processes   514
  immunopathogenic processes   585
  injection   67, 484
  leucocyte kinetics and function   506–512
  metabolism   40, 473–475
  ocular allergy   486
  ocular changes induced by   502, 503
  ophthalmic therapeutics, steroids used
    461–465
  penetration   65, 66
  periocular injection   480–482
  permeability of cornea   34
  potency of   466–470
  selectivity in use   524
  steroid-withdrawal syndrome   504
  sulfoconjugation   129
  systemic complications   503–505
  systemic therapy   482–484
  temporal aspects of steroid therapy
    496–499
  topical therapy   475–480
  vascular and inflammatory effects   512–
    514
  see also Glaucoma, steroid; Intraocular
    pressure

Stevens-Johnson syndrome   393
Stocker's line   671
Strabismus   4, 169
Streptococcus   414
Streptokinase   617, 619, 620
Streptomycin   75–77, 423
Stroma   37
Stuart-Prower factor   611
Substance P   337–341, 349, 540
Succinylcholine   169, 170
Sulfacetamide   75–77
Sulfadiazine   441
Sulfamethoxazole   84
Sulfanilamide   279, 661
Sulfation   129, 130
Sulfonamides   289, 290, 433, 434, 660, 661
Sulfonethylmethane   664
Sulfonmethane   664
Sulfonylureas   660
Sulfotransferase   129, 130
Sulfur mustard   587
Superoxide, *see* O$_2$
Superoxide dismutase   634, 635, 674
Suprachoroid   23, 37, 78
Suprarenal capsules, *see* Adrenal glands
Sympathectomy   340
Sympathetic autonomic nervous system, *see*
    Adrenergic nervous system

Tachyphylaxis   228, 322
Tadkirat   6, 9
Tapetoretinal degeneration   672
Tapetum lucidum   673
Tears
    area under tear curve   64
    cholinergic stimulation   156, 157
    drug kinetics   27
    drug penetration   26, 29
    histamine content   330
    lacrimation system, assessment of and
        fluorescein   702, 703
    precorneal tear film   27, 28
    tear patterns   49–52
    see also Cholinergics; Tissues
Technetium loss   28
Tenon's capsule   24
Terrien's marginal corneal disease   485
Tetracaine   170
Tetracycline   93–95
    as photosensitizing drug   662
    fluorescence   438
    side effects of   439
    structure and use   437, 438
    systemic administration   100
Tetraethylthiuram disulfide, *see* Disulfiram
Tetrahydrotriamcinolone   40, 465
Tetrahydrotriamcinolone acetonide   494,
    495

Tetrazolium   711
Tetrodoxin   325
Thioguanine   591
Thioltransferase   133
Thiolysis   134
Thiopurines   592
Thioridazine   661, 662
Thodamine B   95
Thrombocytopenia   436
Thrombolysis   613, 614
    therapeutic thrombolysis   618, 619
    see also Fibrinolytics
Thrombophlebitis   442
Thrombosis   613, 614
    indirect anticoagulants   615
    occlusion of retinal veins   619, 620
Thromboxane   312, 323, 328, 611
Thymidine   594
Thymoxamine   231, 270
Thyroidectomy   331
Thyrotropin   331
Thyrotropin-releasing hormone   343, 344
Thyroxin   331
Ticarcillin   419, 420
Timolol   678
    as β-adrenergic antagonist   195, 226,
        254, 256
    and carbonic anhydrase inhibitors   209,
        298
    IOP   201, 207, 221, 258, 261
Tissues
    blood vessels   25, 26, 38, 77, 78, 205, 206
    ciliary body   200, 206
    ciliary channels   221, 222
    ciliary epithelium   24, 25, 31, 215, 219,
        222
    ciliary processes   38, 200, 212, 221
    conjunctival epithelium   29
    corneal endothelium   31, 32
    corneal epithelium   31
    corneal stroma   23, 31, 32, 33, 66
    glucocorticoid receptors in   521–523
    iris   200, 203–205, 214
    iris epithelium   38, 85
    lens   72, 85, 203
    lids   27, 30, 169
    optic nerve   26
    orbit   25
    retina   25, 77, 231, 232
    retinal pigment epithelium   25, 230–232
    sclera   23, 27, 36, 37, 77
    sensitivity of tissues to cholinergic
        drugs · 171
    subconjunctiva   24, 208
    tear film   26–28, 30, 34
    tissue binding   390
    uvea   77, 86, 102, 206

Tissues
  see also Aqueous humor; Blood flow;
    Conjunctiva; Cornea; Tears; Vitreous
    body, and other individual structures
Tobramycin   69, 70, 424, 425
α-Tocopherol   676, 677, see also Vitamin E
Tonicity, of tears   35
Tonography   167, 208, 280, 289
Tonometry, applanation   701
TPI effect   205
Trabecular meshwork   161, 162
  outflow and cholinergic drug effects
    163–165, 178
  steroids   499, 500
  trabecular compression   298
Trace elements   667–670, 680, see also
  individual elements
Trachoma   2, 4
Trans-aminomethylcyclohexane carboxylic
  acid (tranexamic acid)   623, 624
Transferrin   670
Transport systems   20, 22, 162, 163
  entry routes into anterior chamber   70,
    71
  exit routes from vitreous chamber   72–
    75
  in ciliary body and retina   81
  in vitreous body   71
  see also Indomethacin; Retina
Tranylcypromine   198, 315
Triamcinolone   466
Triamcinolone acetonide   463, 464
Triethylene tetramine dihydrochloride
  676
Trifluormethazolamide   294
5-Trifluoromethyl-2′-deoxyuridine   559–
  564
Trimethoprim-sulfamethoxazole   434
Trimethylpsoralen   658
Trisulfapyrimidines   441
Trypan blue   711
Tuberculosis, ocular   462
D-Tubocurarine   149
Tumors, ocular   230, 553, 554
Tyndall effect   167
Tyrosinase   230, 676
Tyrosine aminotransferase   518

UDP-glucuronosyltransferase   139, 140
Ultraviolet light
  long-wave ultraviolet (UVA)   656, 659–
    661
  mechanism of   655, 656
  middle-wave (UVB)   656, 658, 661
  short-wave (UVC)   656
Urokinase   612, 613, 617, 619–621
Urolithiasis   299, 300
Urticaria   707

Uveal tract
  adrenergic action   206, 226
  indomethacin   543
  trace elements in   672
  see also Uveoscleral flow
Uveitis   542
  cholinergic drugs   169
  cyclophosphamide   600
  cyclosporin A   601
  methotrexate   594
  prostaglandins   327, 328
  steroid therapy   480, 488, 489
  sarcoid   488
Uveoscleral flow   165, 209, 215
  antibiotics   391
  cholinergic drug effects   165
  concept of   209

Vanadate   678, 679
Vanadium   678, 680
Vancomycin   430, 431
Vasculogenesis   631
Vasoactive intestinal polypeptide   347, 348
Vesalius, Andreas   7
Vinblastine   205
Vincristine   554
Vitamin A   367, 368, 673, see also Retinoid
Vitamin E   633, 634, 636
Vitamin K   616
Vitamin-K-dependent coagulation factors
  615, 622
Vitiligo   657, 660
Vitrectomy   416, 417, 621
Vitreous body   91–93, 620, 670, 678
  see also Blood flow; Fluorophotometry;
    Transport systems
Volutella   415
von Willebrand factor   611
von Willebrand's disease   616, 623

Ware, James   14
Warfarin sodium   615
Wegener's granulomatosis   589
Williams, Henry Willard   14
Wilson's disease   675

Xanthelasma   3
Xenobiotics   117, 136
Xerophthalmia   367, 444

Yersinia pestus   414
Yohimbine   194, 195

Zinc   672–674, 680
Zonulae occludentes   38, 39, 78, 79, 162,
  222
Zoxazolamine   136

Handbook of Experimental Pharmacology

Continuation of "Handbuch der experimentellen Pharmakologie"

Editorial Board
G.V.R.Born, A.Farah,
H.Herken, A.D.Welch

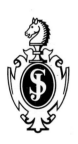

Springer-Verlag
Berlin
Heidelberg
New York
Tokyo

Volume 22: Part 1
Die Gestagene I

Part 2
Die Gestagene II

Volume 23
Neurohypophysial Hormones and Similar Polypeptides

Volume 24
Diuretica

Volume 25
Bradykinin, Kallidin and Kallikrein

Volume 26
Vergleichende Pharmakologie von Überträgersubstanzen in tiersystematischer Darstellung

Volume 27
Anticoagulantien

Volume 28: Part 1
Concepts in Biochemical Pharmacology I

Part 3
Concepts in Biochemical Pharmacology III

Volume 29
Oral wirksame Antidiabetika

Volume 30
Modern Inhalation Anesthetics

Volume 32: Part 2
Insulin II

Volume 34
Secretin, Cholecystokinin, Pancreozymin and Gastrin

Volume 35: Part 1
Androgene I

Part 2
Androgens II and Antiandrogens/Androgene II und Antiandrogene

Volume 36
Uranium – Plutonium – Transplutonic Elements

Volume 37
Angiotensin

Volume 38: Part 1
Antineoplastic and Immunosuppressive Agents I

Part 2
Antineoplastic and Immunosuppressive Agents II

Volume 39
Antihypertensive Agents

Volume 40
Organic Nitrates

Volume 41
Hypolipidemic Agents

Volume 42
Neuromuscular Junction

Volume 43
Anabolic-Androgenic Steroids

Volume 44
Heme and Hemoproteins

Volume 45: Part 1
Drug Addiction I

Part 2
Drug Addiction II

Volume 46
Fibrinolytics and Antifibrinolytics

Handbook of Experimental Pharmacology

Continuation of "Handbuch der experimentellen Pharmakologie"

Editorial Board
G.V.R.Born, A.Farah,
H.Herken, A.D.Welch

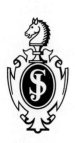

Springer-Verlag
Berlin
Heidelberg
New York
Tokyo

Volume 47
Kinetics of Drug Action

Volume 48
Arthropod Venoms

Volume 49
Ergot Alkaloids and Related Compounds

Volume 50: Part 1
Inflammation

Part 2
Anti-Inflammatory Drugs

Volume 51
Uric Acid

Volume 52
Snake Venoms

Volume 53
Pharmacology of Gang-lionic Transmission

Volume 54: Part 1
Adrenergic Activators and Inhibitors I

Part 2
Adrenergic Activators and Inhibitors II

Volume 55
Psychotropic Agents

Part 1
Antipsychotics and Antidepressants I

Part 2
Anxiolytis, Gerontopsycho-pharmacological Agents and Psychomotor Stimulants

Part 3
Alcohol and Psychotomime-tics, Psychotropic Effects of Central Acting Drugs

Volume 56, Part 1 + 2
Cardiac Glycosides

Volume 57
Tissue Growth Factors

Volume 58
Cyclic Nucleotides
Part 1: Biochemistry
Part 2: Physiology and Pharmacology

Volume 59
Mediators and Drugs in Gastrointestinal Motility
Part 1: Morphological Basis and Neurophysiological Control
Part 2: Endogenis and Exogenous Agents

Volume 60
Pyretics and Antipyretics

Volume 61
Chemotherapy of Viral Infections

Volume 62
Aminoglycosides

Volume 64
Inhibition of Folate Metabolism in Chemotherapy

Volume 65
Teratogenesis and Reproductive Toxicology

Volume 66
Part 1: Glucagon I
Part 2: Glucagon II

Volume 67
Part 1
Antibiotics Containing the Beta-Lactam Structure I

Part 2
Antibiotics Containing the Beta-Lactam Structure II